Dietary Supplements

Dietary Supplements

FOURTH EDITION

Pamela Mason

BSc, MSc, PhD, MRPharmS
Nutrition and Pharmaceutical Writer and Consultant Usk,
Monmouthshire, UK

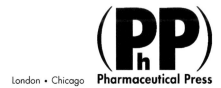

London • Chicago   **Pharmaceutical Press**

Published by the Pharmaceutical Press

1 Lambeth High Street, London SE1 7JN, UK

© Royal Pharmaceutical Society of Great Britain 2012

(**PhP**) is a trade mark of Pharmaceutical Press

Pharmaceutical Press is the publishing division of the
Royal Pharmaceutical Society

First edition published by Blackwell Science Ltd 1995
Reprinted 1998
Second edition 2001
Third edition 2007
Fourth edition 2012

Typeset by Thomson Digital, Noida, India
Printed in Great Britain by T J International, Padstow

ISBN 978 0 85369 883 8

A catalogue record for this book is available from the British Library

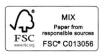

Contents

Preface

SINCE THE THIRD EDITON of this book was published four years ago, the global market for food supplements has continued to grow and diversify. Vitamins and minerals – in multiple-ingredient products and as single ingredients – remain very popular. Indeed, multivitamins and minerals have the largest share of the market in most countries. However, since the last edition, interest in other supplements, such as antioxidants, carotenoids, flavonoids, glucosamine, isoflavones, omega-3 fatty acids and probiotics has continued to grow. Technological advances are increasingly making it possible to include such ingredients in both dietary supplements and foods; hence the blurring of boundaries between 'supplements', 'functional foods' and the 'nutraceutical' ingredients that go into them. As the range of components identified in foods, and knowledge of their potential benefits in health, continues to grow, it is likely that many more such substances will be included in food supplements in the future.

The amount of information about food supplements has grown exponentially during the past few years, most of it appearing on the Internet and fully accessible to the public, added to which is the huge variety of food supplements on the shelves of pharmacies, health food shops, supermarkets and on the Internet. Finding an evidence-based path through the maze of information and products continues to be an enormous challenge for the health professional, and it is very confusing for the potential buyer who wants to know 'what really works'.

Few health professionals, including pharmacists, nurses, doctors or dieticians, have an in-depth knowledge of dietary supplements, yet the public expects them to be able to answer questions on these products. Although there is an abundance of spurious information, there is, alongside this, a growing evidence base for dietary supplements. A large number of peer-reviewed, high-quality trials, systematic reviews and meta-analyses have been published since the third edition of this book, offering health professionals a better evidence base from which to offer information to the public.

There are still, of course, many uncertainties, and the inevitable 'more research needed' will continue to apply to many dietary supplements for some time to come. However, this should not prevent health professionals from giving evidence-based information where it exists and being honest enough to say 'research has not yet provided the answers' where appropriate.

So, what has changed in the fourth edition of *Dietary Supplements*? The answer to this lies mainly in the depth of information provided in the monographs, which has arisen entirely because of the growth in the research base. Trial evidence has been summarised in tabular form for supplements, such as calcium, fish oils, folic acid, isoflavones and probiotics where the evidence base has grown significantly. Twenty one new monographs have also been added making a total of 103 monographs for this new edition.

The European Union Food Supplements Directive has been force since 2006. Since the third edition of this book, the European Food Safety Authority (EFSA) has given opinions on health claims submitted by EU member states. As opinions, these are not yet enshrined in European Commission (EC) law and at the time of going to press, these opinions of EFSA had yet to be considered by the EC. What the outcomes of these considerations will be is not yet known, but the labelling and marketing of supplements produced in the EU member states is likely to change in the future.

The easy-to-use encyclopaedic format for *Dietary Supplements* continues to be retained and it is my intention that this book is primarily a reference source, which I hope will continue to be useful to many colleagues around the world.

Pamela Mason
2011

About the author

PAMELA MASON is a pharmaceutical and nutrition writer and consultant based in Usk, Monmouthshire. She qualified as a pharmacist at Manchester University and worked as a community pharmacist for several years before studying at King's College London, where she completed an MSc and PhD in nutrition. Most recently, she has completed an MSc in food policy at City University London. Her interest in food supplements began as a result of her studies in nutrition and her experience in community pharmacy, where she was often asked questions about these products. She is the author of three other books, several open learning programmes and over 300 articles. She has taught nutrition to pharmacists at both undergraduate and postgraduate level and gives conference presentations about supplements both in the UK and abroad.

Introduction

There is now considerable interest in dietary supplements, and significant numbers of people are using them. In the UK, sales of vitamin and mineral supplements in 2009 were approximately £324.2 million in 'bricks and mortar' shops (excluding health food shops), £2.2 million more than 2008, representing an increase of 0.7%.[1] An increasing number of people buy vitamins and supplements via mail order or the Internet. According to a 2009 US report[2] total sales of dietary supplements in the UK in 2006 were approximately £506m compared with £497m in 2005; presumably this includes sales from all outlets. The largest market shares were held by multivitamins and fish oils, followed by single vitamins, glucosamine, evening primrose and starflower oils and minerals (see Table 1)

According to a 2009 report from Keynote, the value of the market for vitamins, minerals and supplements (VMS) in Great Britain fell by 8.5% in the year ending April 2009. Sales of VMS products have tended to rise when the economy is growing and fall during recessions, revealing their partly discretionary nature. Between 2001 and 2007, virtually all of the market's growth was in supplements: in 2006/2007, vitamins accounted for 31% of the market and minerals/supplements for 69%. However, this situation has now changed: by 2008/2009, vitamins had increased their share to 35%.[3]

What are dietary supplements?

Definition

Various definitions for dietary supplements exist worldwide. In the UK, the definition developed by the Proprietary Association of Great Britain (PAGB), British Herbal Manufacturers' Association (BHMA) and the Health Food Manufacturers' Association (HFMA) is that they are:

> foods in unit dosage form, e.g. tablets, capsules and elixirs, taken to supplement the diet. Most are products containing nutrients normally present in foods which are used by the body to develop cells, bone, muscle etc, to replace co-enzymes depleted by infection and illness, and generally to maintain good health.

In addition to vitamins and minerals, this definition also covers ingredients such as garlic, fish oils, evening primrose oil and ginseng, which can be taken to supplement dietary intake or for their suggested health benefits.

For the purposes of the European Union (EU) Directive on food supplements the term 'food supplements' means:

> foodstuffs the purpose of which is to supplement the normal diet and which are concentrated sources of nutrients or other substances with a nutritional or physiological effect, alone or in combination, marketed in dose form, namely forms such as capsules, pastilles, tablets, pills and other similar forms, sachets of powder, ampoules of liquids, drop dispensing bottles, and other similar forms of liquids and powders designed to be taken in measured small unit quantities.

Table 1 Annual UK Dietary Supplement Sales (£m)[2]

Supplement	Sales 2005	Sales 2006
Multivitamins	104	105
Other supplements	101	104
Fish oils	102	103
Single vitamins	54	51
Glucosamine	43	49
Evening primrose and starflower oils	35	34
Minerals	29	29
Garlic	12	13
Ginkgo	9	10
St John's wort	7	7
Ginseng	1	1
Total	497	506

In the USA, the Dietary Supplement Health Education Act (DSHEA) 1994 defines a dietary supplement as:

> *a product (other than tobacco) that is intended to supplement the diet which bears or contains one or more of the following dietary ingredients: a vitamin, a mineral, a herb or other botanical, an amino acid, a dietary substance for use by man to supplement the diet by increasing the total daily intake, or a concentrate, metabolite, constituent, extract or combinations of these ingredients. It is intended for ingestion in pill, capsule, tablet or liquid form, is not represented for use as a conventional food or as the sole item of a meal or diet and is labelled as a dietary supplement.*

This definition, like that in the UK, also expands the meaning of dietary supplements beyond essential nutrients, to include such substances as ginseng, garlic, psyllium, other plant ingredients, enzymes, fish oils and mixtures of these. The EU definition does not currently include substances apart from vitamins and minerals, but other substances may be included in the future.

One of the key points in these definitions is that dietary supplements are products consumed in unit quantities in addition to normal food intake. This differentiates supplements from other foods, such as fortified foods and functional foods, to which nutrients are added. However, a major difference in the US definition is the explicit inclusion of 'herbs or other botanicals' in the list of dietary ingredients. In the UK, herbal products are currently marketed under a variety of arrangements – either as fully licensed medicines, under the Traditional Herbal Medicines Product (THMP) Directive, 'medicines exempt from licensing' under section 12 of the 1968 Medicines Act, or as cosmetics or foods, so they do not fall entirely in the food supplements category.

Enteral feeds (e.g. Complan and Ensure) and slimming aids are also classified as dietary supplements by nutritionists and dietitians, but for the purposes of this book, these products will not be treated as dietary supplements and will be ignored.

Classification

Dietary supplements fall into several categories in relation to ingredients. These are:

1 Vitamins and minerals
   - Multivitamins and minerals. These normally contain around 100% of the Recommended Daily Allowance (RDA) for vitamins, with varying amounts of minerals and trace elements.
   - Single vitamins and minerals. These may contain very large amounts, and when levels exceed ten times the RDA, they are often termed 'megadoses'.
   - Combinations of vitamins and minerals. These may be marketed for specific population groups, e.g. athletes, children, pregnant women, slimmers, teenagers, vegetarians, etc.
   - Combinations of vitamins and minerals with other substances, such as evening primrose oil and ginseng.
2 'Unofficial' vitamins and minerals, for which a requirement and a deficiency disorder in humans has not, so far, been recognised, e.g. boron, choline, inositol, silicon.
3 Natural oils containing fatty acids for which there is some evidence of beneficial effects, e.g. evening primrose oil and fish oils.
4 Natural substances containing 'herbal' ingredients with recognised pharmacological actions but whose composition and effects have not been fully defined, e.g. echinacea, garlic, ginkgo biloba and ginseng.
5 Natural substances whose composition and effects are not well defined but which are marketed for their 'health giving properties', e.g. *Chlorella*, royal jelly and spirulina.
6 Enzymes with known physiological effects, but of doubtful efficacy when taken by mouth, e.g. superoxide dismutase.
7 Amino acids or amino acid derivatives, e.g. *N*-acetyl cysteine, *S*-adenosyl methionine.

Who takes supplements?

Several surveys in the UK and Ireland have addressed the question of who takes food supplements. Overall, surveys show that supplements are more popular among women than men and use increases with age and higher socio-economic class. In the largest British dietary survey, the National Diet and Nutrition Survey (NDNS) of adults aged 19–64 years, 40% of the surveyed population were taking supplements.[4] Use of supplements increased with age to 55% of women in the 50–64 age group. Cod liver oil and other fish oil based supplements and multi-vitamins and multi-minerals were the most commonly used types of supplements in this age group.

A 2008 report from the Scientific Advisory Committee on Nutrition (SACN) summarised findings on supplement usage from NDNS reports in other age groups.[5] A fifth of children aged $1^1/_2 – 4^1/_2$ years and a fifth of 4–18 year olds were taking non-prescribed supplements, mainly vitamins A, C and D and multivitamins. Among people overt the age of 65 years, 31% of free-living individuals (28% of men and 34% of women) were taking supplements, most commonly cod-liver oil based. In the institution group the proportion that reported taking supplements was much lower – 5% of men and 9% of women. The proportion of older people reported, by 4 day dietary record, to be taking vitamin D supplements (including prescribed supplements) was also lower in the institutional group (3%) than in those living independently in the community (16%).

A questionnaire survey of 21,923 adults (70.5% response) in the metropolitan boroughs of Bolton and Wigan in the north west of England found that 35.5% of the surveyed population was taking supplements. Use of vitamin, mineral and/or antioxidant supplements was associated with eating more fruits and vegetables and taking fish oil supplements was associated with eating oil-rich fish.[6] In this survey, supplement users were more likely to be women, white, home-owners, non-smokers and physically active. A history of CVD or risk factors for CVD reduced the likelihood of taking vitamins, minerals and/or antioxidants or fish oil supplements. Those reporting musculoskeletal disorders such as arthritis were more likely to take fish oil supplements.

A 1997 survey evaluating the factors associated with vitamin use in children (4–12 years) in 56 areas of England and Scotland found that greater likelihood of supplement use occurred among younger children, those whose mothers reached further education, whose fathers were in non-manual occupations or who lived in the Midlands or South, as were children from smaller families or whose parents were non-smokers. Children of Afro-Caribbean, Asian or other origin were more likely to take a supplement compared to white English and Scottish groups.[7]

In the most recent Irish food survey (covering both the North and the South), which included 1379 (662 male and 717 female) randomly selected Irish adults aged 18–64 years, 28% reported using food supplements.[8] A total of 83.5% of the respondents who reported currently using supplements consumed them at least once during the subsequent week. Twice as many women used supplements as men and this ratio did not change with age. People in the 36–50 and 51–64 year age categories had a slightly higher rate of supplement use than the 18–35 year olds. Almost 27% of the total number of supplements used by respondents were single-vitamin preparations, 16.3% were multivitamins and 10.3% were fish oil/cod liver oil preparations. Non-nutritional supplements, e.g. garlic, ginseng and aloe vera juice, were also widely used and accounted for 20% of the 184 supplements recorded.

Attitudes to use of supplements

Individuals take supplements for may different reasons, which are often complex, combining social, psychological, knowledge and economic factors and may include lack of time to eat a healthy diet, desire to improve overall health and fitness, prolong vitality and delay the onset of age associated problems or because supplements have been recommended by a complementary medical practitioner, a health professional, a friend or relative. The increased use of vitamin supplements (and herbal remedies) in the UK over the past 30 years or so has been attributed to several factors, including positive discussion in the media and health programmes, growing use of the Internet, training of more nutritional therapists as a result of the greater availability of courses, increases in affluence and improvements in living standards, as well as a desire to minimise exposure to prescription medication.[9]

A survey of 442 women (data available for 411 women) over 60 years of age in Hull found that 269 (65.4%) were currently taking food supplements.[10] There was no difference in terms of age, smoking, consumption of fruit and vegetables, life-style and attitude towards conventional medicine between current or past users of supplements and never-users. The majority of users thought that food supplements help maintain good health. Overall long-term (5 years) adherence was achieved in 244 cases of supplement uses (36%). Among users, 150 (43%) thought that supplements were very effective, and 171 (49.5%) women had noticed an improvement of various symptoms. Although the majority of users ($n = 176$, 51%) believed that supplements might have adverse effects, over 66% would not associate side-effects with the food supplement. Information regarding supplements was obtained primarily from the media, particularly magazine and newspaper articles (27%), with health professionals rarely being consulted (16%).

Dietary supplement use was also explored in a cohort of 400 women selected from the UK Womens' Cohort Study (UKWCS) database. The aim was to use the Theory of Planned Behaviour (TPB) as a basis for eliciting beliefs about dietary supplements among supplement users and non-users.[11,12] Supplement users displayed stronger intentions to use supplements, more positive attitudes, perceiving more normative pressure to use supplements and reporting greater perceived behavioural control over the use of supplements. Users were significantly more likely to believe that use of supplements protected against various health conditions.

The most striking differences in beliefs between users and non-users were that users believed supplements would help to 'keep me healthy' and 'stop me getting ill' followed by supplements would 'not do me any harm' and 'be the best I can do for myself'. These results suggest that for supplement users, taking dietary supplements was an 'act of faith' in that there was a strong belief that they would help them to be healthy, would not do any harm and provide an opportunity to do something positive. Other factors making respondents more likely to use supplements were 'having a hectic lifestyle', 'being diet conscious', 'problems eating a balanced diet', 'poor food quality' and 'being in control'. Factors judged likely to inhibit supplement use included 'dietary supplements are expensive', 'exaggerated claims' and 'difficulty seeing any benefit from taking supplements.' In terms of illnesses, supplement users felt that taking dietary supplements made them less likely to develop colds/flu and arthritis/rheumatism.

Approaches to supplement use

There are two main approaches to the use of supplements. They can be used to:

- treat or prevent nutritional deficiency; and to
- reduce the risk of non-deficiency disease and promote optimal health.

When vitamins were first discovered during the early years of the 20th century, their only indication was for the prevention and treatment of deficiency disease such as scurvy, beri-beri, pellagra, etc. This led to the development of dietary standards such as RDAs and, more recently, to the Dietary Reference Values (DRVs).[13] These values were based on amounts of nutrients required to prevent deficiency, and even though subject to various limitations, they are still the best measure of dietary adequacy.

After the Second World War, it was thought that nutritional deficiencies had largely disappeared and scientific interest in vitamins and minerals waned. However, with the increase in various chronic diseases such as cardiovascular disease and cancer, vitamins became an area of growing interest again, and it was suggested that supplements might help to reduce the risk of such disease. During these early years of the 21st century, there is growing concern among the public to improve quality of life and supplements are increasingly used to promote so-called optimum health.

Findings from dietary surveys

Despite the idea that nutritional deficiency had disappeared, recent UK national diet and nutrition surveys have shown that there is no room for complacency. Although average dietary intakes may appear adequate, some groups of the surveyed populations are clearly at risk of marginal deficiencies. The most recent National Diet and Nutrition Survey (NDNS) involving British adults aged 19–64 years[4] found that mean intakes of all nutrients in men are $\geq 100\%$ of the RNI. For women, mean intakes of iron, magnesium and copper were below the RNI. However, mean intakes fail to show the proportion of people that do not achieve the RNI. For women, mean magnesium intake was 85% of the RNI, but 74% in this survey failed to achieve the RNI. Mean intakes also fail to show that intakes in some age groups are particularly poor. Iron intake in women overall was 82% of the RNI while in 19–24-year-old women it was 60% of the RNI. Overall, 91% of women failed to achieve the RNI for iron while 41% of women aged 19 to 34 had intakes of iron below the LRNI. For magnesium and copper, intake overall in women is 85% and 86% of the RNI, respectively, but for women aged 19–24 years it was 76% of the RNI for both minerals. Indeed, men and women aged 19–24 had significantly poorer intakes of all vitamins and minerals than those aged 50–64, with mineral and trace element intakes in the women aged 19–24 years a particular cause for concern.

Similar to the NDNS in adults, national surveys in children and teenagers have shown that some groups fail to achieve recommended intakes. The NDNS in pre-school children[14] showed that 8% of the surveyed youngsters aged $1\frac{1}{2}$ to $4\frac{1}{2}$ were anaemic, a further 12% were mildly iron-deficient and 15% had a poor intake of zinc. Vitamin A deficiency was present in 8%, vitamin B_2 deficiency in 23% and vitamin C deficiency in 3%.

A similar nutritional survey of older children[15] again showed average nutrient intakes were largely fine, but anaemia was present in 1.5% of boys and 5% of girls, with respective totals of 13% and 27% having low serum ferritin – an indication of iron deficiency. In addition, zinc was found to be low in the diets of 10% of boys and 20% of girls. Also of concern were calcium intakes, which were below the Lower Reference Nutrient Intake (LRNI) in 6% of boys and 12% of girls. For magnesium, the respective figures were 12% and 27% and for vitamin A, 10% and 11%. Furthermore, some of the surveyed youngsters also appeared to have poor status for vitamin B_{12}, vitamin C, vitamin D, folate, riboflavin and thiamine.

The National Diet and Nutrition Survey of people aged 65 years and over[16] showed that there were nutritional problems in some individuals. Up to 38% of the survey population was deficient in vitamin D, up to 38% were deficient in vitamin C, up to 18% in folate, up to 15% in vitamin B_{12} and up to 30% in iron. Of the free-living individuals, 11% of men and 9% of women were anaemic.

More recent data from the NDNS were published in 2010.[17] This survey is the first of a new rolling programme covering people of all ages and involved a sample of 500 adults and 500 children using a 4-day diet diary (rather than a 7-day diet record). This showed that intake of vitamins and minerals in the UK has not improved, though because the methodology is different from that used in the 2001 survey in adults and earlier surveys in children and teenagers, the data cannot be directly compared.

As in previous NDNS surveys among the UK population, intakes of minerals are particularly worrying. Mean intakes fell below the Reference Nutrient Intake (RNI) for a number of minerals, in particular iron, magnesium, potassium and selenium. This was particularly the case for boys and girls aged 11 to 18 years. For girls in this age group, the mean iron intake was 58% of the RNI, the same proportion as in the previous survey of this age group. Mean intakes of magnesium and potassium also fell bellow the RNI for both boys and girls aged 11–18 years, as did zinc, calcium and iodine for girls. Substantial proportions of older girls had mineral intakes below the LRNI (a level at which deficiency is likely); 46% of girls aged 11–18 years had intakes of iron and magnesium below the LRNI; the equivalent figure for potassium was 30% and for zinc 15%. Among boys of this age group, 26% failed to achieve the LRNI for magnesium. Intakes of calcium were of particular concern in 11–18 year old girls, an age at which calcium is particularly important for bone development. More than one in ten girls in this age group failed to achieve the LRNI for calcium. Among younger children, 7% of those aged 4–10 years had intakes of zinc below the LRNI while 6% of toddlers had intakes of iron below the LRNI. Significant numbers of adults also had low intakes. One fifth of adult women failed to achieve the LRNI for iron, while one in ten men and one in ten women failed to achieve the LRNI for magnesium. Intakes of selenium, which have not been reported in the NDNS before, fell below the RNI in both older children and adults. Adult women overall achieved 72% of the RNI while adult men achieved 74% of the RNI. Around half of adult women and older girls and a fifth of men and older boys had intakes below the LRNI.

Intakes of vitamins have not improved since the last dietary surveys with the exception of vitamin C and vitamin A. Intakes of thiamine, riboflavin, niacin, folic acid and vitamin D have remained approximately the same or fallen slightly in adult men and women since the 2000/01 NDNS.

The Low Income Diet and Nutrition Survey (LIDNS)[18] found patterns of vitamin and intake in this population group to be broadly similar to that of the general population. For those where mean intakes fell below the RNI in specific age groups, this was usually the case for the same groups in both surveys. For example, women aged 19–64 years in both surveys had mean daily intakes of total iron, magnesium, potassium and copper below the RNI. However, low income women had lower mean intakes of these minerals, especially for iron (68% of RNI in LIDNS, compared with 82% of RNI in NDNS).

Evidence suggests that other population sub-groups such as prisoners,[19] hospital patients,[20] and patients in mental care establishments[21,22] have poor vitamin status. Dietary surveys of pregnant women in the UK have also found that intakes of micronutrients can be lower than reference values.[23–26] Pregnant women at most risk of low nutrient intake are adolescents[27] and those from ethnic minority groups.[28]

Although good diet is the most appropriate route to achieving improved nutrition in these population groups, there is no evidence to suggest that risk of deficiency is a thing of the past.

Populations are at risk of deficiency

Various groups of the population could be at risk of nutrient deficiency and could benefit from supplementation. These include:

- People in a particular demographic category, e.g. infants and children, adolescents, women during pregnancy and lactation and throughout the reproductive period, the elderly and ethnic minorities.
- People whose nutritional status may be compromised by lifestyle (enforced or voluntary), e.g. smokers, alcoholics, drug addicts, slimmers, strict vegetarians (i.e. vegans), food faddists, individuals on low incomes and athletes.
- People whose nutritional status may be compromised by surgery and/or disease, e.g. malabsorption syndromes, hepato-biliary disorders, severe burns and wounds, and inborn errors of metabolism.
- People whose nutritional status may be compromised by long-term drug administration (e.g. anticonvulsants may increase the requirement for vitamin D).

Increasingly, people are taking supplements for reasons other than prevention of deficiency and at amounts higher than the RDA. Moreover, evidence is increasing that, at least for some nutrients (e.g. folic acid, vitamin D), there may be benefits in achieving higher intakes than the RDA.

However, while there is agreement about the beneficial effects of nutrients in the prevention of deficiency disease and the amounts required to achieve such effects, there is controversy about amounts required for reduction in risk of chronic disease and so-called 'optimum health'. Some would argue that higher amounts are required and that basing requirements for nutrients only on the prevention of deficiency disease is inadequate. But what other end points should be used is open to debate: longevity, increased resistance to cancer and coronary heart disease, improved athletic performance, etc. Higher levels of intake cannot always easily be obtained from diet alone, and supplementation is required. However, excessive intake of some nutrients can lead to toxicity, and it is with this in mind that several committees worldwide have established safe upper limits for supplement intake.

Legal status

The UK

In the UK, the majority of dietary supplements are classified legally as foods, and sold under UK food law. There are just a few exceptions (e.g. Abidec, Pregaday, Maxepa and some generic vitamin and mineral preparations) which are licensed medicines. Unlike medicines, most supplements do not, therefore, require marketing authorisations, they do not have to go through such rigorous clinical trials, and are therefore much cheaper to put on the market than medicines.

Dietary supplements are not controlled by quite the same strict conditions of dosage, labelling, purity criteria and levels of ingredients as medicines. The retail supply of those vitamins that have marketing authorisations (i.e. licensed medicines) are subject to limitations which depend on their strength and maximum daily dose, as shown in Table 2.

Dietary supplements containing levels of vitamins in excess of those in prescription-only medicines are available to the public. However, in recognition of the fact that consumers are increasingly using high-dose products, the

Table 2 Limitations on the sale or supply of licensed medicines containing certain vitamins

Vitamin	Legal status
Vitamin A	Up to 2250 µg (7500 units) GSL Over 2250 µg (7500 units) POM
Vitamin D	Up to 10 µg (400 units) GSL Over 10 µg (400 units) P
Cyanocobalamin	Up to 10 µg GSL Over 10 µg P
Folic acid	Up to 200 µg GSL 200–500 µg P Over 500 µg POM

GSL = subject to control under the Medicines (General Sales List) Order, 1977.
POM = subject to control under the Medicines (Prescriptions Only) Order, 1977.
P = Pharmacy only products.

Food Standards Agency (FSA) Expert Group on Vitamins and Minerals (EVM) has published safe levels of intake for vitamins and minerals[29] (see Appendix 3).

Claims that can be made for supplements are regulated by UK food law, and increasingly at European level. Advertising of dietary supplements is regulated by various advertising codes for both the broadcast media (TV and radio advertising standards codes) and the non-broadcast media. These codes are policed by the Advertising Standards Authority (ASA), an independent body set up by the advertising industry.

Europe

Across the countries of the European Union (EU), the diversity of regulation for food supplements has been wide, with several approaches to regulating vitamin and mineral supplements such that one product of the same strength (e.g. vitamin C 1000 mg) can be a food in one country but a medicine in another.

However, the regulatory environment in Europe has changed in recent years. The European Commission (EC) has adopted Directive 2002/46/EC, which lays down specific rules for vitamins and minerals used as ingredients for food supplements. All food supplements containing vitamins or minerals as well as other ingredients should conform to the specific rules for vitamins and minerals laid down in the Directive. The Directive was implemented in the UK in August 2005.

The Directive includes a 'positive list' of vitamins and minerals permitted in food supplements (Annex 1), and a second list identifying the chemical substances that can be used in their manufacture (Annex 2). Only vitamins and minerals in the forms listed may be used in the manufacture of food supplements. Specific rules concerning nutrients, other than vitamins and minerals, or other substances with a nutritional or physiological effect used as ingredients of food supplements (e.g. fatty acids, amino acids, fibre, and herbal ingredients) will be laid down at a later stage.

The Directive will also establish maximum permitted levels of vitamins and minerals for food supplements. These will take into account upper safe levels of vitamins and minerals established by scientific risk assessment based on generally accepted scientific data, intake of vitamins and minerals from other dietary sources and the varying degrees of sensitivity of different consumer groups. Figures for upper levels of vitamins and minerals unlikely to have adverse effects have been published by official groups such as the EU Scientific Committee on Food (SCF),[30] the UK Expert Vitamin and Mineral Group[29] and the US National Academy of Sciences[31] (see Appendix 3).

The Directive also pays attention to advertising, presentation, purity criteria and labelling of content and dosage. Labels on dietary supplements express their nutrient content in terms of RDAs. EU RDAs are based on the requirements of men and are said to apply to average adults. They take no account of differences in nutritional requirements according to age, sex and other factors, and are therefore simple approximations used for labels only.

Labelling should not imply that a varied and adequate diet cannot provide sufficient quantities of nutrients. In addition, 'medicinal' claims relating to the prevention, treatment or cure of disease in the labelling, advertising or promotion of food supplements are prohibited.

Health claims are regulated by the Health and Nutrition Claims Regulation, which was adopted in 2006. Under this Regulation, there are several categories of health claims:

- Article 13(1): 'general function' claims refer to the role of a nutrient or substance in growth, development and body functions; psychological and behavioural functions; slimming and weight control, satiety or reduction of available energy from the diet. These claims do not include those related to child development or health or disease risk reduction. Proposed claims were gathered by each member state and across the EU more than 44,000 claims were submitted to the EC. The EC consolidated the list and a final list of 4637 claims was submitted to the European Food Safety Authority (EFSA) for consideration. As of April 2011, EFSA had published 263 opinions providing scientific advice on more than 2150 'general function' health claims. A significant number of submitted health claims have been rejected on the basis of insufficient evidence and/or insufficient characterisation of the food supplement. EFSA's opinions can be found at http://www.efsa.europa.eu/cs/ Satellite. The EC will consider the EFSA opinions and decide which health claims will be permitted under EC law.
- Article 13(5): 'new function' claims are those based on newly developed scientific evidence and/or for which protection of proprietary data is requested. For these health claims authorisation is required on a case-by-case basis, following the submission of a scientific dossier to EFSA for assessment.
- Article 14: claims referring to reduction of disease risk or to children's development or health.

The USA

In the USA, the Food and Drug Administration (FDA) regulates dietary supplements according to the Dietary Supplement Health and Education Act (DSHEA) 1994. Under this law, supplements are regulated in a similar manner to food products, while prohibiting their regulation as medicines or food additives. This Act includes a framework for safety, guidelines for third-party literature provided at the point of sale, guidance on good manufacturing practice (GMP) and labelling standards. Under DSHEA, manufacturers are responsible for marketing safe and properly labelled products, but the FDA bears the burden of proving that a product is unsafe or improperly labelled. However, the FDA has insufficient resources for doing this, and there is concern that not all supplements are marketed according to best standards of practice.

DSHEA regulates the labelling of supplements and the claims that can be made. This includes permissible statements describing the link between a nutrient and a deficiency or between a nutrient and its effect on the body's structure or function, or its effect on well-being. Examples include 'promotes relaxation' or 'builds strong bones'. But to make these claims, the supplement label must also carry the disclaimer: 'This statement has not been validated by the Food and Drug Administration. This product is not intended to diagnose, treat, cure or prevent any disease.'

Under the US Nutrition Labelling and Education Act of 1990, a number of specific health claims are also permitted. These describe the link between a specific nutrient and the reduction in risk of a particular disease or condition and they are based on significant scientific agreement. Claims applicable to dietary supplements include those in relation to calcium and osteoporosis, folic acid and neural tube defects, soluble fibre (from oat bran and psyllium seed) and coronary heart disease and soya and coronary heart disease.

Patient/client counselling

The following questions may be used by health professionals before making any recommendations about supplement use:

1 Who is the supplement for? The individual buying the product may not be the consumer; requirements for vitamins and minerals vary according to age and sex.
2 Why do you think you need a supplement? The individual may have misconceptions about the need for and benefits of supplements that should be addressed.
3 What are your symptoms (if any) and how long have you had them? The individual could have a serious underlying disorder that should be referred for appropriate diagnosis and treatment.
4 What do you eat? A simple dietary assessment should be undertaken to give some

indication as to whether vitamin and mineral deficiency is likely.

5 Is your diet restricted in any way? Slimming, vegetarianism or religious conviction could increase the risk of nutritional deficiency.

6 Do you take any prescription or over-the-counter medicines? This information can be used to assess possible drug–nutrient interactions.

7 Do you take other supplements? If so, which ones? This information can be used to assess potential overdosage of supplements which could be toxic.

8 Do you suffer from any chronic illness, e.g. diabetes, epilepsy, Crohn's disease? Nutrient requirements in patients with chronic disease may be greater than in healthy individuals.

9 Are you pregnant or breast-feeding? Nutrient requirements may be increased.

10 Do you take part in sports or other regular physical activity?

11 Do you smoke? Requirements for some vitamins (e.g. vitamin C) may be increased.

12 How much alcohol do you drink? Excessive alcohol consumption may lead to deficiency of the B vitamins.

Guidelines for supplement use

The following guidelines may be useful in making recommendations:

- Compare labels with dietary standards (usually RDAs).
- In the absence of an indication for a specific nutrient, a balanced multivitamin/mineral product is normally preferable to one that contains one or two specific nutrients.
- Use a product that provides approximately 100% of the RDA for as wide a range of vitamins and minerals as possible.
- Avoid preparations containing unrecognised nutrients or nutrients in minute amounts; this increases the cost, but not the value.
- Avoid preparations that claim to be natural, organic or high potency; this increases the cost and, in the case of high-potency products, the risk of toxicity.
- Distinguish between credible claims and unsubstantiated claims.
- If there is uncertainty about product quality, check with the companies concerned. Ask about quality assurance. For example, is the final product analysed to guarantee the contents in the bottle match the label declarations? Are tests for disintegration, dissolution or other tests for bioavailability conducted?

Role of the health professional

When asked about supplements, health professionals should emphasise the importance of consuming a diet based on healthy eating guidelines. This is a diet rich in starchy, fibrous carbohydrates, including fruit and vegetables, and low in fat, sugar and salt. Dietary supplements do not convert a poor diet into a good one.

Health professionals should be aware of dietary standards and good food sources for nutrients. They should be able to assess an individual's risk of nutrient deficiency and need for further referral, by asking questions to detect cultural, physical, environmental and social conditions which may predispose to inadequate intakes.

There is a need to be aware of the potential for adverse effects with supplements. Thus, when a client or patient presents with any symptoms, questions should be asked about the use of dietary supplements. Individuals will not always volunteer this information without prompting because they believe that supplements are 'natural' and therefore safe.

Pharmacists have a particular responsibility, simply because they sell these products. When supplying any supplement with perceived health benefits, pharmacists must be careful to avoid giving their professional authority to a product that may lack any health or therapeutic benefit and has risks associated with its use. In accordance with the Code of Ethics of the Royal Pharmaceutical Society of Great Britain, this may involve not stocking or selling the product. Pharmacists must not give the impression that any dietary supplement is efficacious when there is no evidence for such efficacy.

However, providing a product is not harmful for a particular individual, the freedom to use it should be respected. What is important is that consumers are able to make informed and intelligent choices about the products they buy.

References

1 PAGB. Symphony IRI Group 2009 UK OTC Market Summary. 2010. http://www.pagb.co.uk/information/PDFs/2009marketfigures.pdf (accessed 3 August 2010).

2 Themedica. The UK Dietary Supplements Industry Overview. 2009. http://www.themedica.com/articles/2009/03/the-uk-dietary-supplement-indu.html (accessed 3 August 2010).

3 Keynote. Vitamins, Minerals & Supplements Market Assessment. Summary only. 2009. http://www.keynote.co.uk/market-intelligence/view/product/2276/vitamins-minerals-%26-supplements (accessed 3 August 2010).

4 Henderson L, Irving K, Gregory J, et al. The National Diet and Nutrition Survey: adults aged 19 to 64 years. Vol. 3: Vitamin and Mineral Intake and Urinary Analysis. London: The Stationery Office, 2003.

5 Scientific Advisory Committee on Nutrition (SACN). The Nutritional Wellbeing of the British Population. 2008. http://www.sacn.gov.uk/pdfs/nutritional_health_of_the_population_final_oct_08.pdf (accessed 3 August 2010).

6 Harrison RA, Holt D, Pattison DJ, et al. Are those in need taking dietary supplements? A survey of 21 923 adults Br J Nutr 2004; 91(4): 617–623.

7 Bristow A, Qureshi S, Rona RJ, et al. The use of nutritional supplements by 4–12 year olds in England and Scotland. Eur J Clin Nutr 1997; 51 (6): 366–369.

8 Kiely M, Flynn A, Harrington KE, et al. The efficacy and safety of nutritional supplement use in a representative sample of adults in the North/South Ireland Food Consumption Survey. Public Health Nutr 2001; 4(5A): 1089–1097.

9 Ritchie MR. Use of herbal supplements and nutritional supplements in the UK: what do we know about their pattern of usage? Proc Nutr Soc 2007; 66(4): 479–482.

10 Albertazzi P, Steel SA, Clifford E, et al. Attitudes towards and use of dietary supplementation in a sample of postmenopausal women. Climacteric 2002; 5(4): 374–382.

11 Conner M, Kirk SF, Cade JE, et al. Why do women use dietary supplements? The use of the theory of planned behaviour to explore beliefs about their use Soc Sci Med 2001; 52(4): 621–633.

12 Conner M, Kirk SF, Cade JE, et al. Environmental influences: factors influencing a woman's decision to use dietary supplements. J Nutr 2003; 133(6): 1978S–1982S.

13 Department of Health. Dietary Reference Values for Food Energy and Nutrients for the United Kingdom. Report on Health and Social Subjects No 41. London: HMSO, 1991.

14 Gregory J, Collins D, Davies P, et al. National Diet and Nutrition Survey: children aged $1^1/_2$ to $4^1/_2$ years. Vol. 1: Report of the Diet and Nutrition Survey. London: HMSO, 1995.

15 Gregory J, Lowe S, Bates C, et al. National Diet and Nutrition Survey: Young People aged 4 to 18 years. Vol. 1: Report of the Diet and Nutrition Survey. London: The Stationery Office, 2000.

16 Finch S, Doyle W, Lowe C, et al. National Diet and Nutrition Survey: People aged 65 years and over. Vol. 1: Report of the Diet and Nutrition Survey. London: The Stationery Office, 1998.

17 Bates B, Lennox A, Swan G. National Diet and Nutrition Survey. Headline Results from Year 1 of the Rolling Programme (2008/2009). A Survey Carried out on Behalf of the Food Standards Agency and the Department of Health. London: The Stationery Office, 2010, http://www.food.gov.uk/multimedia/pdfs/publication/ndnsreport0809.pdf and http://www.food.gov.uk/multimedia/pdfs/publication/ndnstables0809.pdf (accessed 16 May 2011).

18 Nelson M, Lowes K, Hwang V. The contribution of school meals to food consumption and nutrient intakes of young people aged 4–18 years in England. Public Health Nutr 2007; 10(7): 652–662.

19 Gesch CB, Hammond SM, Hampson SE, et al. Influence of supplementary vitamins, minerals and essential fatty acids on the antisocial behaviour of young adult prisoners: randomised, placebo-controlled trial. Br J Psychiatry 2002; 181(1): 22–28.

20 Gan R, Eintracht S, Hoffer LJ. Vitamin C deficiency in a university teaching hospital. J Am Coll Nutr 2008; 27(3): 428–433.

21 Hancock MR, Hullin RP, Aylard PR, et al. Nutritional state of elderly women on admission to mental hospital. Br J Psychiatry 1985; 147(4): 404–407.

22 Tiangga E, Gowda A, Dent JA. Vitamin D deficiency in psychiatric in-patients and treatment with daily supplements of calcium and ergocalciferol. Psychiatr Bull 2008; 32(10): 390–393.

23 Black AE, Wiles SJ, Paul AA. The nutrient intakes of pregnant and lactating mothers of good socio-economic status in Cambridge UK: some implications for recommended daily allowances of minor nutrients. Br J Nutr 1986; 56(1): 59–72.

24 Rogers I, Emmett P. Diet during pregnancy in a population of pregnant women in South West England. ALSPAC Study Team. Avon Longitudinal Study of Pregnancy and Childhood. Eur J Clin Nutr 1998; 52(4): 246–250.

25 Emmett P, Rogers I, Symes C. Food and nutrient intakes of a population sample of 3-year-old children in the south west of England in 1996. Public Health Nutr 2002; 5(1): 55–64.

26 Mouratidou T, Ford F, Prountzou F, et al. Dietary assessment of a population of pregnant women in Sheffield, UK. Br J Nutr 2006; 96(5): 929–935.

27 Baker PN, Wheeler SJ, Sanders TA, et al. A prospective study of micronutrient status in adolescent pregnancy. Am J Clin Nutr 2009; 89(4): 1114–1124.

28 Rees G, Brooke Z, Doyle W, et al. The nutritional status of women in the first trimester of pregnancy attending an inner-city antenatal department in the UK. J R Soc Promot Health 2005; 125(5): 232–238.

29 Expert Group on Vitamins and Minerals. Safe Upper Levels for Vitamins and Minerals. 2003. http://

www.food.gov.uk/multimedia/pdfs/vitmin2003.pdf
(accessed 7 May 2011).

30 Scientific Committee on Food. *Tolerable upper
intake levels for vitamins and minerals. Scientific
Panel on Dietetic Products, Nutrition and Allergies.*
2006. http://www.efsa.europa.eu/en/ndatopics/docs/
ndatolerableuil.pdf (accessed 7 May 2011).

31 National Academy of Sciences Institute of
Medicine, Food and Nutrition Board. *Dietary
Reference Intakes: UL for Vitamins and Elements.*
2010 (updated). http://iom.edu/Activities/Nutrition/
SummaryDRIs/~/media/Files/Activity%20Files/
Nutrition/DRIs/ULs%20for%20Vitamins%20and
%20Elements.pdf (accessed 7 May 2011).

How to use this book

This book covers 108 commonly available dietary supplements, including vitamins, minerals, trace elements and other substances, such as garlic, ginseng and fish oils. For ease of reference, they are arranged in alphabetical order and give information, where appropriate, under the following standard headings.

Description

States the type of substance, e.g. a vitamin, mineral, fatty acid, amino acid, enzyme, plant extract.

Nomenclature

Lists names and alternative names in current usage.

Units

Includes alternative units and conversion factors.

Constituents

Lists active ingredients in supplements that are not pure vitamins or minerals (e.g. evening primrose oil contains gamma-linolenic acid).

Human requirements

Lists for different ages and sex (where established):

- UK Dietary Reference Values and safe upper levels;
- US Recommended Dietary Allowances (RDAs) and Tolerable Upper Intake Levels (ULs);

- World Health Organization (WHO) Reference Nutrient Intakes;
- European Union Recommended Dietary Allowances (RDAs).

Definitions

The UK
Dietary reference values (DRVs) were established in 1991[1] to replace recommended daily amounts (RDAs).

- EAR: Estimated Average Requirement. An assessment of the average requirement for energy or protein for a vitamin or mineral. About half the population will need more than the EAR, and half less.
- LRNI: Lower Reference Nutrient Intake. The amount of protein, vitamin or mineral considered to be sufficient for the few people in a group who have low needs. Most people will need more than the LRNI and if people consistently consume less they may be at risk of deficiency of that nutrient.
- RNI: Reference Nutrient Intake. The amount of protein, vitamin or mineral sufficient for almost every individual. This level of intake is much higher than many people need.
- Safe Intake. A term used to indicate intake or range of intakes of a nutrient for which there is not enough information to estimate RNI, EAR or LRNI. It is considered to be adequate for almost everyone's needs but not large enough to cause undesirable effects.
- DRV: Dietary Reference Value. A term used to cover LRNI, EAR, RNI and safe intake.

The USA
The US Institute of Medicine and the Food and Nutrition Board have established a set of reference values to replace the previous RDAs.[2–5] The

Dietary Reference Intakes encompass EARs, RDAs, AI (adequate intakes) and Tolerable Upper Intake Levels (UIs). RDAs and AIs are set at levels that should decrease the risk of developing a nutritional deficiency disease.

- RDA: Recommended Dietary Allowance. The average amount of energy or a nutrient recommended to cover the needs of groups of healthy people.
- Safe Intake and Adequate Daily Dietary Intakes. These are given for some vitamins and minerals where there is less information on which to base allowances, and figures are provided in the form of ranges.
- Tolerable Upper Intake Levels.[6] Defined by the Food and Nutrition Board of the US National Academy of Sciences as the highest total level of a nutrient (diet plus supplements) which could be consumed safely on a daily basis and is unlikely to cause adverse health effects to almost all individuals in the general population. As intakes rise above the UL, the risk of adverse effects increases. The UL describes long-term intakes, so an isolated dose above the UL need not necessarily cause adverse effects. The UL defines safety limits and is not a recommended intake for most people most of the time.

Europe
RDA: Recommended Dietary Allowance. Provides sufficient for most individuals. The EU RDA is used on dietary supplement labels.

The following points should be noted in relation to dietary standards:

- Dietary standards are intended to assess the diets of populations, not of individuals. Thus, both the RDA and the UK Reference Nutrient Intake (RNI) are set at two standard deviations above the average population requirement and are intended to cover the needs of 95% of the population. So, if an individual is typically consuming the RDA or the RNI for a particular nutrient, it can be assumed that his or her diet provides adequate amounts (or more than adequate amounts) of that nutrient to prevent deficiency. If intake is regularly below the RNI, it cannot necessarily be assumed that the diet is inadequate, because the person may have a lower requirement for that nutrient. However, if an individual is consistently consuming less than the Lower Reference Nutrient Intake (LRNI) for a nutrient, it can be assumed that the diet is deficient in that nutrient. Nevertheless, individuals differ in the amounts of nutrients they need and the quantities they absorb and utilise, and although the dietary standards are the best figures currently available, they were never intended to assess the adequacy of individual diets.
- Dietary standards are estimates which are assessed from a variety of epidemiological, biochemical and nutritional data, including:
  - the intake of a nutrient required to prevent or cure clinical signs of deficiency;
  - the intake of a nutrient required to maintain balance (i.e. intake – output = zero);
  - the intake of a nutrient required to maintain a given blood level, tissue concentration or degree of enzyme saturation; and
  - the intake of a nutrient in the diet of a healthy population.
- Dietary standards apply only to healthy people and not to those with disease, whose nutrient needs may be very different. Requirements may be increased in patients with disorders of the gastrointestinal tract (GI), liver and kidney, and in those with inborn errors of metabolism, cancer, severe infections, wounds, burns and following surgery. Drug administration may also alter nutrient requirements.

Dietary intake

States amounts of nutrients provided by the average adult diet in the UK.[7,8]

Action

Describes the role of the substance in maintaining physiological function and identifies pharmacological actions where appropriate.

Dietary sources

Lists significant food sources based on average portion sizes. In addition, a food may be described as an *excellent* or *good* source of a nutrient. This does not describe any food as 'excellent' or 'good' overall. It defines only the amount of the nutrient (per portion or serving) in relation to the Reference Nutrient Intake (RNI) of the nutrient for the average adult male.

Thus, an excellent source provides 30% or more of the RNI; a good source provides 15–30% of the RNI.

Where no RNI has been set for a particular nutrient, *excellent* and *good* are numerically defined.

Metabolism

Discusses absorption, transport, distribution and excretion.

Bioavailability

Includes the effects of cooking, processing, storage methods and substances in food which may alter bioavailability.

Deficiency

Lists signs and symptoms of deficiency.

Uses

Discusses potential indications for use with the level of evidence. Evidence for use of supplements is obtained from several types of studies:

- Epidemiological studies. These are population-based studies and early evidence for the potential value of a nutrient usually comes from epidemiological research. For example, the idea that antioxidant supplements could reduce the risk of cancer came from studies in populations in which high intake of fruit and vegetables was associated with a low risk of cancer.
- *In vitro* (laboratory) studies and animal studies. Data from these studies can be used to support evidence, but is not enough on its own. Although both types of study allow for good control of variables such as nutrients and more aggressive intervention, each suffers from uncertainties of extrapolating any observed effects to human.
- Observational studies. These may be prospective and retrospective and include, in decreasing order of persuasiveness, cohort studies, case–control studies and uncontrolled studies. In prospective studies, subjects are recruited and observed prior to the occurrence of the outcome. In retrospective studies, investigators review the records

of subjects and interview subjects after the outcome has occurred. Retrospective studies are more vulnerable to recall bias and measurement error but less likely to suffer from the subject selection bias that can occur in prospective studies. In all observational studies, the investigator has no control of the intervention.
- Intervention studies. The investigator controls whether subjects receive an intervention or not. The randomised controlled trial (RCT) is the gold standard. Intervention trials with supplements differ from those for drugs. Unlike studies with drugs, those with foods and nutrients may have additional confounders secondary to the intervention itself. For example, results from intervention studies with antioxidant supplements (e.g. vitamins A, C and E) in the prevention of cancer are inconsistent, even though epidemiological studies have consistently shown that diets high in these nutrients are associated with reduced cancer risk. This could be because such diets contain a range of other substances apart from those in the tested supplements and the antioxidants are merely acting as markers for a type of diet that is protective. Moreover, chronic disease, such as cancer and coronary heart disease, develops over many years and to investigate the effect of a supplement on disease risk, therefore, requires a prolonged study period (e.g. 20–30 years) as well as a huge number of subjects, and this makes such studies difficult and expensive to conduct. However, without such trials, evidence for efficacy of many supplements will remain sparse.
- Systematic reviews and meta-analyses. These may include RCTs only or they may also include observational studies. Decisions on the part of reviewers to include or leave out certain types of studies can lead to differing conclusions from the analysis.

Precautions/contraindications

Lists diseases and conditions in which the substance should be avoided or used with caution.

Pregnancy and breastfeeding

Comments on safety or potential toxicity during pregnancy and lactation.

Adverse effects

Describes the risks that may accompany excessive intake, and signs and symptoms of toxicity.

Interactions

Lists drugs and other nutrients that may interact with the supplement. This includes drugs that affect vitamin and mineral status and supplements that influence drug metabolism.

Dose

Gives usual recommended dosage (if established).

References

1 Department of Health. *Dietary Reference Values for Food Energy and Nutrients for the United Kingdom*. Report on Health and Social Subjects No 41. London: HMSO, 1991.

2 Institute of Medicine Food and Nutrition Board. *Dietary Reference Intakes for Calcium, Phosphorus, Magnesium, Vitamin D and Fluoride*. Washington DC: National Academies Press, 1999.

3 Institute of Medicine Food and Nutrition Board. *Dietary Reference Intakes for Thiamin, Riboflavin, Niacin, Vitamin B_6, Folate, Vitamin B_{12}, Pantothenic Acid, Biotin and Choline*. Washington DC: National Academies Press, 2000.

4 Institute of Medicine Food and Nutrition Board. *Dietary Reference Intakes for Vitamin C, Vitamin E, Selenium and Carotenoids*. Washington DC: National Academies Press, 2000.

5 Institute of Medicine Food and Nutrition Board. *Dietary Reference Intakes for Vitamin A, Vitamin K, Arsenic, Boron, Chromium, Copper, Iodine, Iron, Manganese, Molybdenum, Nickel, Silicon, Vanadium and Zinc*. Washington DC: National Academies Press, 2002.

6 National Academy of Sciences Institute of Medicine Food and Nutrition Board. *Dietary Reference Intakes: UL for Vitamins and Elements*. Washington DC: National Academies Press, 2010 (updated) http://iom.edu/Activities/Nutrition/SummaryDRIs/~/media/Files/Activity%20Files/Nutrition/DRIs/ULs%20for%20Vitamins%20and%20Elements.pdf (accessed 7 May 2011).

7 Henderson L, Irving K, Gregory J, *et al*. *The National Diet and Nutrition Survey: Adults aged 19 to 64 years*, Vol. 3: *Vitamin and Mineral Intake and Urinary Analysis*. London: The Stationery Office, 2003.

8 Bates B, Lennox A, Swan G. *National Diet and Nutrition Survey. Headline Results from Year 1 of the Rolling Programme (2008/2009). A Survey Carried Out on Behalf of the Food Standards Agency and the Department of Health*. London: The Stationery Office, 2010, http://www.food.gov.uk/multimedia/pdfs/publication/ndnsreport0809.pdf and http://www.food.gov.uk/multimedia/pdfs/publication/ndnstables0809.pdf (accessed 16 May 2011).

Abbreviations

ACE	angiotensin-converting enzyme	EAR	Estimated Average Requirement
ADP	adenosine 5′-diphosphate	HDL	high-density lipoprotein
ARMD	age-related macular degeneration	HIV	human immunodeficiency virus
ATP	adenosine triphosphate	HRT	hormone replacement therapy
BCAAs	branched-chain amino acids	IBS	irritable bowel syndrome
BMD	bone mineral density	LDL	low-density lipoprotein
CHD	coronary heart disease	NSAID	non-steroidal anti-inflammatory drug
CHF	congestive heart failure	PMS	premenstrual syndrome
CNS	central nervous system	PUFAs	polyunsaturated fatty acids
COPD	chronic obstructive pulmonary disease	RCT	randomised controlled trial
		RDA	Recommended Daily Allowance
CVD	cardiovascular disease	RNA	ribonucleic acid
DNA	deoxyribonucleic acid	RNI	Reference Nutrient Intake
DRI	Dietary Reference Intake	SLE	systemic lupus erythematosus
DRV	Dietary Reference Value	VLDL	very-low-density lipoprotein

Acai

Description

Acai, as a dietary supplement, is derived from the acai fruit, which is the fruit of *Euterpe oleracea*, a multi-stemmed palm of the Arecaceae family. Eight species are native to Central and South America and grow mainly in swamps and floodplains. The fruit is green when young and ripens to a dark purple colour.

Acai fruit contains a variety of anthocyanins, proanthocyanidins and other flavonoids.[1–4] The most abundant are cyanidin-3-glucoside, cyanidin-3-rutinoside, ferulic acid, epicatechin, *p*-hydroxybenzoic acid and pelargonidin-3-glucoside. Others include cyanidin-3-sambubioside, peonidin-3-glucoside and peonidin-3-rutinoside, gallic acid and several derivatives, catechin and ellagic acid.

Action

Anthocyanins are antioxidants. Increased plasma antioxidant capacity has been demonstrated following consumption of acai in a trial involving 12 human beings.[5] A specific freeze-dried acai fruit pulp and skin powder (OptiAcai, K2A LLC) has potent *in vitro* antioxidant activity against superoxide and peroxyl radical that is higher than that of other fruits. But it has only mild antioxidant activity against peroxynitrite and hydroxyl radical. This extract also appears to inhibit cyclooxygenase (COX) 1 and 2 *in vitro*.[6] *In vitro* studies have demonstrated the antiproliferative potential of acai in a human colon cancer cell model[7] and a vasodilator effect in the rat.[8]

Possible uses

Acai is marketed as a supplement on the basis of its antioxidant content. People use it for osteoarthritis, hypercholesterolaemia, erectile dysfunction, weight loss and obesity, detoxification and for improving general health. It has been claimed to reverse diabetes and to improve men's virility. There are no clinical trials in humans to support these uses and claims.

In mice, acai seed extract has been shown to reduce glucose intolerance and symptoms of metabolic syndrome.[9] Supplementation of rats with acai pulp has been shown to reduce biomarkers of oxidative stress and improve lipid profile.[10]

Precautions/contraindications

Insufficient reliable information.

Conclusion
Acai fruit contains a variety of anthocyanins with antioxidant potential. It is marketed as a dietary supplement, but no clinical trials in humans are available to support any of the claims made for this preparation.

Pregnancy and breastfeeding

Insufficient data.

Adverse effects

Insufficient data.

Interactions

Insufficient data.

Dose

No dose established.

References

1 Schauss AG, Wu X, Prior RL, *et al*. Phytochemical and nutrient composition of the freeze-dried Amazonian palm berry. *Euterpe oleraceae* Mart. (acai). *J Agric Food Chem* 2006; 54: 8598–8603.

2 DelPozo-Insfran D, Brenes CH, Talcott ST. Phytochemical composition and pigment stability of Acai (*Euterpe oleracea* Mart.). *J Agric Food Chem* 2004; 52: 1539–1545.

3 Pacheco-Palencia LA, Mertens-Talcott S, Talcott ST. Chemical composition, antioxidant properties, and thermal stability of a phytochemical enriched oil from Acai (*Euterpe oleracea* Mart.). *J Agric Food Chem* 2008; 56: 4631–4636.

4 Rodrigues RB, Lichtenthaler R, Zimmermann BF, *et al.* Total oxidant scavenging capacity of *Euterpe oleracea* Mart. (acai) seeds and identification of their polyphenolic compounds. *J Agric Food Chem* 2006; 54: 4162–4167.

5 Mertens-Talcott SU, Rios J, Jilma-Stohlawetz P, *et al.* Pharmacokinetics of anthocyanins and anti-oxidant effects after the consumption of anthocyanin-rich acai juice and pulp (*Euterpe oleracea* Mart.) in human healthy volunteers. *J Agric Food Chem* 2008; 56: 7796–7802.

6 Schauss AG, Wu X, Prior RL, *et al.* Antioxidant capacity and other bioactivities of the freeze-dried Amazonian palm berry, *Euterpe oleraceae* Mart. (acai). *J Agric Food Chem* 2006; 54: 8604–8610.

7 Pacheco-Palencia LA, Talcott ST, Safe S, Mertens-Talcott S. Absorption and biological activity of phytochemical-rich extracts from acai (*Euterpe oleracea* Mart.) pulp and oil in vitro. *J Agric Food Chem* 2008; 56: 3593–3600.

8 Rocha AP, Carvalho LC, Sousa MA, *et al.* Endothelium-dependent vasodilator effect of *Euterpe oleracea* Mart. (acai) extracts in mesenteric vascular bed of the rat. *Vascul Pharmacol* 2007; 46: 97–104.

9 DeOliveira PR, da Costa CA, de Bem GF, *et al.* Effects of an extract obtained from fruits of *Euterpe oleracea* Mart. in the components of metabolic syndrome induced in C57BL/6J mice fed a high-fat diet. *J Cardiovasc Pharmacol* 2010; 56(6): 619–626.

10 DeSouza MO, Silva M, Silva ME, Oliveira Rde P, Pedrosa ML. Diet supplementation with acai (*Euterpe oleracea* Mart.) pulp improves biomarkers of oxidative stress and the serum lipid profile in rats. *Nutrition* 2009; 26: 804–810.

Aloe vera

Description

Aloe vera is the mucilaginous substance obtained from the central parenchymatous tissues of the large blade-like leaves of *Aloe vera*. It should not be confused with aloes, which is obtained by evaporating water from the bitter yellow juice that is drained from the leaf.

Constituents

Aloe vera contains polysaccharides, tannins, sterols, saponins, vitamins, minerals, cholesterol, gamma-linolenic acid and arachidonic acid.[1] Unlike aloes, aloe vera does not contain anthraquinone compounds and does not therefore exert a laxative action.

Action

Used externally, aloe vera acts as a moisturiser and reduces inflammation. Internally, it may act as an anti-inflammatory, hypoglycaemic and hyperlipidaemic agent. It also has anti-platelet activity.

Possible uses

Topical

Topical aloe vera has been investigated for its effects on wound healing and psoriasis, while oral aloe vera has been investigated in patients with diabetes mellitus and hyperlipidaemia.

A review in 1987 concluded that topical application of aloe vera gel reduces acute inflammation, promotes wound healing, reduces pain and exerts an antipruritic effect.[2] A further review in 1999[1] stated that research had continued to confirm these benefits.

A double-blind, placebo-controlled study of 60 people with psoriasis of mean duration 8.5 years found that applying aloe vera to skin lesions three times a day for 8 months led to significant improvement in 83% of aloe vera patients but in only 6% of those who used placebo.[3] A further randomised, comparative, double-blind, 8-week study in 80 patients with psoriasis compared topical aloe vera with 0.1% triamcinolone acetonide cream. After 8 weeks of treatment, the severity of psoriasis measured according to the Psoriasis Area Severity Index had decreased significantly compared with that in the steroid group. However, both treatments had similar efficacy in improving the quality of life of patients with mild to moderate psoriasis.[4]

In rabbits, aloe vera cream was found to be better than placebo and as effective as oral pentoxifylline in improving tissue survival after frostbite.[5] Aloe vera has also been shown to reduce inflammation[6] and enhance wound healing[7] in rats with burns. In a study of 27 patients, aloe vera gel healed burns faster than Vaseline gauze.[8] A systematic review of four studies with a total of 371 patients, using duration of wound healing as an outcome measure, found that the weighted mean difference in healing time of the aloe vera group was 8.79 days shorter than those in the control group ($P = 0.006$). Because of the differences in products and outcome measures, no specific conclusion could be reached; however, cumulative evidence tends to support the view that aloe vera might be an effective intervention for healing of first or second degree burns.[9] Further, well-designed trials with sufficient details of the contents of aloe vera products should be carried out to determine the effectiveness of aloe vera.

However, a recent Cochrane review identified a single trial of aloe vera supplementation that suggested delayed wound healing with aloe vera, but the reviewers concluded that the results of the trial were not easily interpretable.[10]

Systemic

Oral aloe vera has been investigated for a number of applications including reduction of blood glucose and inflammatory bowel disease.

A systematic review of 10 studies[11] showed that oral aloe vera might be useful as an adjunct for lowering blood glucose concentrations in diabetes and for reducing blood lipid levels in hyperlipidaemia. A recent study in mice showed that oral aloe vera gel could slow the progression of type 2 diabetes mellitus, reducing blood glucose, insulin resistance and plasma triglyceride concentrations.[12] A further trial in rats with induced diabetes found that oral aloe vera restored levels of HDL, LDL and VLDL cholesterol to normal.[13] These two animal trials provide a rationale for the use of aloe vera in diabetes, but controlled clinical trials in humans are required.

There is some evidence that the anti-inflammatory actions of aloe vera might have therapeutic potential in inflammatory bowel disease. An *in vitro* study found that aloe vera gel had a dose-dependent inhibitory effect on the production of reactive oxygen metabolites and eicosanoids in human colorectal mucosa.[14]

Aloe vera has also been suggested to be beneficial in irritable bowel syndrome. A randomized controlled trial in 58 patients with irritable bowel syndrome (of whom 49 completed 1 month's treatment) found that 11 of 31 (35%) patients taking aloe vera and 6 of 27 (22%) patients taking placebo responded at 1 month, but the difference was statistically insignificant ($P = 0.763$). Patients with diarrhoea as their predominant symptoms showed a trend towards a response to treatment at 1 month and the authors recommended that aloe vera should be further investigated in this group of patients.[15]

An RCT in 44 patients with ulcerative colitis found that aloe vera gel 100 ml four times weekly produced a clinical response more often than placebo, reducing histological disease activity. The researchers recommended that further evaluation of aloe vera in inflammatory bowel disease is needed.[16]

Although topical aloe vera gel is known to have moisturising properties, few studies have evaluated the effects of aloe vera on the skin when taken orally. In a small study among 30 healthy women over the age of 45 years, aloe vera in two daily doses (1200 and 3600 mg) significantly improved wrinkles and skin elasticity, with an increase in collagen production. No dose–reponse relationship was found with the two doses.[17]

More recently, aloe vera oral gel has been shown to have immunomodulatory activity. Oral administration of aloe vera gel significantly reduced the growth of *Candida albicans* in the spleen and kidney following intravenous injection of *C. albicans* in normal mice.[18]

Conclusion

A huge number of *in vitro* and animal studies have examined aloe vera over the past 30 years. However, there have been few studies in humans, and these have been poorly controlled.

Topical aloe vera may be helpful in psoriasis, but whether it is useful for wound healing is unclear. There is some – albeit limited – evidence that oral aloe vera may be useful for lowering blood glucose in diabetes, reducing blood lipids in hyperlipidaemia and it may have therapeutic potential in inflammatory bowel disease.

Precautions/contraindications

None established, although the potential hypoglycaemic effect means that it should be used with caution in patients with diabetes mellitus. Preliminary research in rats has suggested that aloe vera has a hypoglycaemic effect.[19]

Pregnancy and breast-feeding

No problems have been reported, but there have not been sufficient studies to guarantee the safety of aloe vera in pregnancy and breast-feeding.

Adverse effects

None reported apart from occasional allergic reactions. However, there are no long-term studies investigating the safety of aloe vera. Research in mice showed that oral aloe vera had no subacute toxic effects over 4 weeks but reduced male kidney weights.[20] This finding requires further investigation.

Interactions

Aloe vera has antiplatelet activity and could theoretically interact with drugs with antiplatelet effects. A case study in one individual found a potential interaction between aloe vera and sevoflurane, in which the woman lost 5 L of blood during surgery.[21]

Dose

Aloe vera is available in the form of creams, gels, tablets, capsules and juice. The International Aloe Science Council operates a voluntary approval scheme that gives an official seal ('IASC – certified') on products containing certified raw ingredients processed according to standard guidelines.

Used internally, there is no established dose. Product manufacturers suggest $1/2$ to $1/4$ cup of juice or 1 to 2 capsules three times a day. The juice in the product should ideally contain at least 98% aloe vera and no aloin.

Used externally, aloe vera should be applied liberally as needed. The product should contain at least 20% aloe vera.

Upper safety levels

A 1-month study in mice found that the lowest observed adverse effect level (LOAEL) of an active aloe product was 120 mg/kg body weight in male ICR mice, and the daily upper level was 0.4 mg/kg body weight [(120 mg/kg)/(100 for safety factor) × (3 for modifying factor)], or 24 mg for a 60-kg adult human (24 mg × 200 = 4.8 g aloe gel daily), assuming that consumers utilise active aloe for a month.[20]

References

1 Reynolds T, Dweck AC. Aloe vera leaf gel: a review update. *J Ethnopharmacol* 1999; 68(13): 3–37.
2 Heggers JP, Kucukcelebi A, Listengarten D, *et al.* Beneficial effect of aloe on wound healing in an excisional wound model. *J Altern Complement Med* 1996; 2(2): 271–277.
3 Syed TA, Ahmad SA, Holt AH, *et al.* Management of psoriasis with aloe vera extract in a hydrophilic cream: a placebo-controlled, double-blind study. *Trop Med Int Health* 1996; 1(4): 505–509.
4 Choonhakarn C, Busaracome P, Sripanidkulchai B, *et al.* A prospective, randomized clinical trial comparing topical aloe vera with 0.1% triamcinolone acetonide in mild to moderate plaque psoriasis. *J Eur Acad Dermatol Venereol* 2009; 24(2): 168–172.
5 Miller MB, Koltai PJ. Treatment of experimental frostbite with pentoxifylline and aloe vera cream. *Arch Otolaryngol Head Neck Surg* 1995; 121(6): 678–680.
6 Duansak D, Somboonwong J, Patumraj S. Effects of Aloe vera on leukocyte adhesion and TNF-alpha and IL-6 levels in burn wounded rats. *Clin Hemorheol Microcirc* 2003; 29(34): 239–246.

7 Somboonwong J, Thanamittramanee S, Jariyapongskul A, *et al.* Therapeutic effects of Aloe vera on cutaneous microcirculation and wound healing in second degree burn model in rats. *J Med Assoc Thai* 2000; 83(4): 417–425.

8 Visuthikosol V, Chowchuen B, Sukwanarat Y, *et al.* Effect of aloe vera gel to healing of burn wound a clinical and histologic study. *J Med Assoc Thai* 1995; 78(8): 403–409.

9 Maenthaisong R, Chaiyakunapruk N, Niruntraporn S, *et al.* The efficacy of aloe vera used for burn wound healing: a systematic review. *Burns* 2007; 33(6): 713–718.

10 Vermeulen H, Ubbink D, Goossens A, *et al.* Dressings and topical agents for surgical wounds healing by secondary intention. *Cochrane Database Syst Rev* 2004; 2(2): CD003554.

11 Vogler BK, Ernst E. Aloe vera: a systematic review of its clinical effectiveness. *Br J Gen Pract* 1999; 49 (447): 823–828.

12 Kim K, Kim H, Kwon J, *et al.* Hypoglycemic and hypolipidemic effects of processed Aloe vera gel in a mouse model of non-insulin-dependent diabetes mellitus. *Phytomedicine* 2009; 16(9): 856–863.

13 Rajasekaran S, Ravi K, Sivagnanam K, *et al.* Beneficial effects of aloe vera leaf gel extract on lipid profile status in rats with streptozotocin diabetes. *Clin Exp Pharmacol Physiol* 2006; 33(3): 232–237.

14 Langmead L, Makins RJ, Rampton DS. Anti-inflammatory effects of aloe vera gel in human colorectal mucosa in vitro. *Aliment Pharmacol Ther* 2004; 19(5): 521–527.

15 Davis K, Philpott S, Kumar D, *et al.* Randomised double-blind placebo-controlled trial of aloe vera for irritable bowel syndrome. *Int J Clin Pract* 2006; 60(9): 1080–1086.

16 Langmead L, Feakins RM, Goldthorpe S, *et al.* Randomized, double-blind, placebo-controlled trial of oral aloe vera gel for active ulcerative colitis. *Aliment Pharmacol Ther* 2004; 19(7): 739–477.

17 Cho S, Lee S, Lee MJ, *et al.* Dietary aloe vera supplementation improves facial wrinkles and elasticity and it increases the type I procollagen gene expression in human skin in vivo. *Ann Dermatol* 2009; 21(1): 6–11.

18 Im SA, Lee YR, Lee YH, *et al.* In vivo evidence of the immunomodulatory activity of orally administered Aloe vera gel. *Arch Pharm Res* 2010; 33(3): 451–456.

19 Rajasekaran S, Sivagnanam K, Ravi K, *et al.* Hypoglycemic effect of Aloe vera gel on streptozotocin-induced diabetes in experimental rats. *J Med Food* 2004; 7(1): 61–66.

20 Kwack SJ, Kim KB, Lee BM. Estimation of tolerable upper intake level (UL) of active aloe. *J Toxicol Environ Health A* 2009; 72(2122): 1455–1462.

21 Lee A, Chui PT, Aun CS, *et al.* Possible interaction between sevoflurane and Aloe vera. *Ann Pharmacother* 2004; 38(10): 1651–1654.

Alpha-lipoic acid

Description

Alpha-lipoic acid is a naturally-occurring sulphur-containing cofactor. It is synthesised in humans.

Nomenclature

Alternative names include alpha-lipoate, thioctic acid, lipoic acid, 2-dithiolane-3-pentatonic acid, and 1,2-dithiolane-3-valeric acid.

Action

Alpha-lipoic acid functions as a potent antioxidant and as a cofactor for various enzymes (e.g. pyruvate dehydrogenase and alpha-ketoglutarate dehydrogenase) in energy-producing metabolic reactions of the Krebs cycle.

In addition, it appears to improve recycling of other antioxidant compounds, including vitamins C and E,[1] coenzyme Q[2] and glutathione.[3] It may also protect against arsenic,[4] cadmium,[5] lead[6] and mercury[7] poisoning.

Dietary sources

Alpha-lipoic acid is present in foods such as spinach, meat (especially liver) and brewer's yeast, but it is difficult to obtain amounts used in clinical studies (i.e. possibly therapeutic amounts) from food.

Metabolism

Alpha-lipoic acid is both fat-soluble and water-soluble, and this facilitates its diffusion into lipophilic and hydrophilic environments. It is metabolised to dihydrolipoic acid (DHLA), which also demonstrates antioxidant properties.

Possible uses

As a dietary supplement, alpha-lipoic acid is claimed to improve glucose metabolism and insulin sensitivity in diabetes, and to reduce replication of the human immunodeficiency virus (HIV). It has been investigated for possible use in patients with diabetes mellitus, glaucoma, HIV, hypertension and Alzheimer's disease.

Diabetes mellitus

Alpha-lipoic acid has long been of interest as a potential therapeutic agent in diabetes, including both the microvascular and neuropathic pathologies. This stems from alpha-lipoic acid's metabolic role and also because diabetes results in chronic oxidative stress. Alpha-lipoic acid appears to increase muscle cell glucose uptake and increase insulin sensitivity in individuals with type 2 diabetes mellitus. *In vitro*, alpha-lipoic acid has been found to stimulate glucose uptake by muscle cells in a manner similar to insulin.[8]

In an uncontrolled study, patients with type 2 diabetes given 1000 mg lipoic acid intravenously experienced a 50% improvement in insulin-stimulated glucose uptake.[9] In a further uncontrolled pilot study,[10] 20 patients with type 2 diabetes were given 500 mg lipoic acid intravenously for 10 days. Glucose uptake increased by an average of 30%, but there were no changes in either fasting blood glucose or insulin levels. A controlled parallel design trial involving 30 patients with type 2 diabetes mellitus showed that intravenous alpha-lipoic acid improved endothelium-dependent vasodilatation.[11] Whether this translates into vascular risk reduction remains to be established.

In a study involving 10 lean and 10 obese patients with type 2 diabetes,[12] oral alpha-lipoic acid 600 mg twice daily improved glucose effectiveness and prevented hyperglycaemia-induced increases in serum lactate and pyruvate. In the lean diabetic patients, but not the obese patients, alpha-lipoic acid resulted in improved insulin sensitivity and lower fasting glucose.

In a placebo-controlled, multicentre pilot study,[13] 74 patients with type 2 diabetes were randomised to receive alpha-lipoic acid 600 mg once, twice or three times a day, or placebo. When compared with placebo, significantly more patients had an increase in insulin-stimulated glucose disposal. As there was no dose effect, all three treatment groups were combined into one active group and compared with placebo. The increase in insulin-stimulated glucose disposal was then statistically significant, suggesting that oral administration of alpha-lipoic acid can improve insulin sensitivity in patients with type 2 diabetes.

A further trial (not placebo-controlled) in 12 patients with type 2 diabetes showed that alpha-lipoic acid 600 mg twice a day for 4 weeks increased peripheral insulin sensitivity.[14]

Data from preliminary trials indicate that alpha-lipoic acid may reduce plasma levels of asymmetric dimethylarginine (a risk factor for cardiovascular disease) in patients with type 2 diabetes.[15,16]

Diabetic neuropathy

Alpha-lipoic acid has been used extensively in Germany for the treatment of diabetic neuropathy. An *in vitro* study showed that lipoic acid reduced lipid peroxidation of nerve tissue.[17] A study in rats with diabetes induced by streptozotocin showed that alpha-lipoic acid reversed the reduction in glucose uptake that occurs in diabetes, and that this change was associated with an improvement in peripheral nerve function.[18]

In a randomised, double-blind, placebo-controlled multicentre trial, 73 patients with non-insulin-dependent diabetes mellitus were assigned to receive oral alpha-lipoic acid 800 mg daily or placebo for 4 months. Of the total, 17 patients dropped out of the study, but the results suggested that alpha-lipoic acid might slightly improve cardiac autonomic neuropathy (assessed by measures of heart rate variability) in non-insulin-dependent diabetic patients.[19]

In a randomised, placebo-controlled study involving 24 patients with type 2 diabetes,[20] oral treatment with 600 mg alpha-lipoic acid three times a day for 3 weeks appeared to reduce the chief symptoms of diabetic neuropathy. A further placebo-controlled, randomised, double-blind trial showed that oral alpha-lipoic acid 600 mg once or twice a day appeared to have a beneficial effect on nerve conduction in patients with both type 1 and type 2 diabetes.[21]

A review[22] of the evidence of the effect of alpha-lipoic acid in the treatment of diabetic neuropathy concluded that short-term treatment with oral or intravenous alpha-lipoic acid appears to reduce the chief symptoms of diabetic neuropathy, but this needs to be confirmed by larger studies.

A meta-analysis of four trials of alpha-lipoic acid involving 1258 patients found a benefit of 16–25% (compared with placebo) in signs and symptoms of neuropathy (e.g. ankle reflexes, pain, burning, numbness, pin-prick and touch-pressure sensation) after 3 weeks of treatment. This is supported by three more recent trials, which have also shown favourable results with alpha-lipoic acid in diabetic neuropathy.[23] Three non-blinded trials (one in Korea and two in Bulgaria) tested alpha-lipoic acid in a dose of 600 mg daily. In the Korean study, total symptom score was significantly reduced at 8 weeks, as were individual symptom scores for pain, burning sensation, paraesthesia and numbness.[24] In one of the Bulgarian trials, there was a significant improvement in several aspects of autonomic function, including postural blood pressure change and overall cardiovascular autonomic neuropathy score.[25] In the second Bulgarian study, alpha-lipoic acid was found to be effective in peripheral and autonomic diabetic neuropathy and also diabetic mononeuropathy of the cranial nerves, leading to full recovery of the patients.[26] A recent Australian trial found that oral treatment with alpha-lipoic acid for 5 weeks improved neuropathic symptoms in patients with diabetic neuropathy.[27] An oral dose of 600 mg once daily appears to provide the optimum risk-to-benefit ratio.

Glaucoma

In a study involving 75 patients with open-angle glaucoma,[28] alpha-lipoic acid was administered in a dose of either 75 mg daily for 2 months or 150 mg daily for 1 month. Improvements in biochemical parameters and visual function were found, particularly in the group receiving 150 mg lipoic acid.

Human immunodeficiency virus

Alpha-lipoic acid blocks activation of NF-κB, which is required for HIV virus transcription, and has also been noted to improve antioxidant status, T-helper lymphocytes, and the T-helper/suppressor cell ratio in HIV-infected T-cells.[29] However, it is not known whether supplementation would improve survival in individuals who are HIV positive.

Burning mouth syndrome

A systematic review from the Cochrane Collaboration stated that alpha-lipoic acid may help in the management of burning mouth syndrome.[30] Because all of the data on alpha-lipoic acid came from a single group, it has been stressed that its effectiveness should be reproduced in other populations. An 8-week double-blind, randomised, placebo-controlled study in 54 men and 12 women (of whom 52 completed the study) evaluated the efficacy of alpha-lipoic acid (400 mg) and alpha-lipoic acid (400 mg) plus vitamins in the treatment of burning mouth syndrome.[31] Symptoms were evaluated by using a Visual Analogue Scale (VAS) and the McGill Pain Questionnaire (MPQ) at 0, 2, 4, 8 and 16 weeks. All three groups had significant reductions in the VAS score and in the mixed affective/evaluative subscale of the MPQ; the responders' rate (at least 50% improvement in the VAS score) was about 30%. No significant differences were observed among the groups either in the response rate or in the mean latency of the therapeutic effect. This study failed to support a role for alpha-lipoic acid in the treatment of burning mouth syndrome, and the fairly high placebo effect was similar to data obtained from patients affected by atypical facial pain. Two further RCTs in 38 patients[32] and 60 patients[33] with burning mouth syndrome found that alpha-lipoic acid was no more effective than placebo.

Miscellaneous

Results of preliminary studies suggest that alpha-lipoic acid may lower blood pressure,[34] and improve T-cell functions *in vitro* in patients with advanced stage cancer.[35] Alpha-lipoic acid has also been investigated for a potential role in dementia, but there is only very limited evidence available.[36–38] Alpha-lipoic acid has been investigated for an effect in conditions such as cancer cachexia, liver disease, ischaemia reperfusion injury, photoageing of the skin and cataract.

Data from one preliminary trial suggest that alpha-lipoic acid could ameliorate the adverse metabolic effects (including weight gain) associated with atypical antipsychotic drugs.[39] Preliminary data also suggest that alpha-lipoic acid 600 mg daily may confer pain relief in patients with peripheral arterial disease.[27] However, there are no convincing data as yet from human RCT in these areas.

> ### Conclusion
> There is evidence that alpha-lipoic acid might have a role in patients with diabetes mellitus in improving glucose utilisation, insulin sensitivity and diabetic neuropathy. Very limited evidence also exists that alpha-lipoic acid may be helpful in glaucoma, dementia, hypertension, peripheral arterial disease, adverse metabolic effects of atypical antipsychotic drugs and slowing the replication of HIV and cancer cells, but evidence of benefit in all these conditions, including diabetes, is too limited to make recommendations for supplementation.

Precautions/contraindications

Alpha-lipoic acid should be used with caution in patients predisposed to hypoglycaemia, including patients taking antidiabetic agents.

Pregnancy and breast-feeding

No problems have been reported, but there have not been sufficient studies to guarantee the safety of alpha-lipoic acid in pregnancy and breast-feeding.

Adverse effects

None reported, apart from occasional skin rashes. Studies investigating the effect of alpha-lipoic acid have suggested that it is a safe supplement at reasonable doses. However, there are no long-term studies assessing the safety of alpha-lipoic acid.

Interactions

Drugs

Oral hypoglycaemics and insulin: theoretically, alpha-lipoic acid could enhance the effects of these drugs.

Dose

Alpha-lipoic acid is available in the form of tablets and capsules.

The dose is not established. Studies have used 300–1800 mg daily. Dietary supplements provide 50–300 mg daily.

References

1 Scholich H, Murphy ME, Sies H. Antioxidant activity of dihydrolipoate against microsomal lipid peroxidation and its dependence on alpha-tocopherol. *Biochim Biophys Acta* 1989; 1001(3): 256–261.

2 Kagan V, Serbinova E, Packer L. Antioxidant effects of ubiquinones in microsomes and mitochondria are mediated by tocopherol recycling. *Biochem Biophys Res Commun* 1990; 169(3): 851–857.

3 Busse E, Zimmer G, Schopohl B, *et al.* Influence of alpha-lipoic acid on intracellular glutathione in vitro and in vivo. *Arzneimittelforschung* 1992; 42 (6): 829–831.

4 Grunert RR. The effect of DL-alpha-lipoic acid on heavy-metal intoxication in mice and dogs. *Arch Biochem Biophys* 1960; 86: 190–194.

5 Muller L, Menzel H. Studies on the efficacy of lipoate and dihydrolipoate in the alteration of cadmium2$^+$ toxicity in isolated hepatocytes. *Biochim Biophys Acta* 1990; 1052(3): 386–391.

6 Gurer H, Ozgunes H, Oztezcan S, *et al.* Antioxidant role of alpha-lipoic acid in lead toxicity. *Free Radic Biol Med* 1999; 27(12): 75–81.

7 Keith RL, Setiarahardjo I, Fernando Q, *et al.* Utilization of renal slices to evaluate the efficacy of chelating agents for removing mercury from the kidney. *Toxicology* 1997; 116(13): 67–75.

8 Estrada DE, Ewart HS, Tsakiridis T, *et al.* Stimulation of glucose uptake by the natural coenzyme alpha-lipoic acid/thioctic acid: participation of elements of the insulin signaling pathway. *Diabetes* 1996; 45(12): 1798–1804.

9 Jacob S, Henriksen EJ, Schiemann AL, *et al.* Enhancement of glucose disposal in patients with type 2 diabetes by alpha-lipoic acid. *Arzneimittelforschung* 1995; 45(8): 872–874.

10 Jacob S, Henriksen EJ, Tritschler HJ, *et al.* Improvement of insulin-stimulated glucose-disposal in type 2 diabetes after repeated parenteral administration of thioctic acid. *Exp Clin Endocrinol Diabetes* 1996; 104(3): 284–288.

11 Heinisch BB, Francesconi M, Mittermayer F, *et al.* Alpha-lipoic acid improves vascular endothelial function in patients with type 2 diabetes: a placebo-controlled randomized trial. *Eur J Clin Invest* 2009; 40(2): 148–154.

12 Konrad T, Vicini P, Kusterer K, *et al.* Alpha-lipoic acid treatment decreases serum lactate and pyruvate concentrations and improves glucose

effectiveness in lean and obese patients with type 2 diabetes. *Diabetes Care* 1999; 22(2): 280–287.

13 Jacob S, Ruus P, Hermann R, *et al*. Oral administration of RAC-alpha-lipoic acid modulates insulin sensitivity in patients with type-2 diabetes mellitus: a placebo-controlled pilot trial. *Free Radic Biol Med* 1999; 27(34): 309–314.

14 Kamenova P. Improvementof insulin sensitivity in patients with type 2 diabetes mellitus after oral administration of alpha-lipoic acid. *Hormones (Athens)* 2006; 5(4): 251–258.

15 Chang JW, Lee EK, Kim TH, *et al*. Effects of alpha-lipoic acid on the plasma levels of asymmetric dimethylarginine in diabetic end-stage renal disease patients on hemodialysis: a pilot study. *Am J Nephrol* 2007; 27(1): 70–74.

16 Mittermayer F, Pleiner J, Francesconi M, *et al*. Treatment with alpha-lipoic acid reduces asymmetric dimethylarginine in patients with type 2 diabetes mellitus. *Transl Res* 2010; 155(1): 6–9.

17 Nickander KK, McPhee BR, Low PA, *et al*. Alpha-lipoic acid: antioxidant potency against lipid peroxidation of neural tissues in vitro and implications for diabetic neuropathy. *Free Radic Biol Med* 1996; 21(5): 631–639.

18 Kishi Y, Schmelzer JD, Yao JK, *et al*. Alpha-lipoic acid: effect on glucose uptake, sorbitol pathway, and energy metabolism in experimental diabetic neuropathy. *Diabetes* 1999; 48(10): 2045–2051.

19 Ziegler D, Schatz H, Conrad F, *et al*. Effects of treatment withthe antioxidant alpha-lipoic acid on cardiac autonomic neuropathy in NIDDM patients. A 4-month randomized controlled multicenter trial (DEKAN Study). Deutsche Kardiale Autonome Neuropathie. *Diabetes Care* 1997; 20(3): 369–373.

20 Ruhnau KJ, Meissner HP, Finn JR, *et al*. Effects of 3-week oral treatment with the antioxidant thioctic acid (alpha-lipoic acid) in symptomatic diabetic polyneuropathy. *Diabet Med* 1999; 16(12): 1040–1043.

21 Reljanovic M, Reichel G, Rett K, *et al*. Treatment of diabetic polyneuropathy with the antioxidant thioctic acid (alpha-lipoic acid): a two year multicenter randomized double-blind placebo-controlled trial (ALADIN II). Alpha Lipoic Acid in Diabetic Neuropathy. *Free Radic Res* 1999; 31(3): 171–179.

22 Ziegler D, Reljanovic M, Mehnert H, *et al*. Alpha-lipoic acid in the treatment of diabetic polyneuropathy in Germany: current evidence from clinical trials. *Exp Clin Endocrinol Diabetes* 1999; 107(7): 421–430.

23 Ziegler D, Nowak H, Kempler P, *et al*. Treatment of symptomatic diabetic polyneuropathy with the antioxidant alpha-lipoic acid: a meta-analysis. *Diabet Med* 2004; 21(2): 114–121.

24 Hahm JR, Kim BJ, Kim KW. Clinical experience with thioctacid (thioctic acid) in the treatment of distal symmetric polyneuropathy in Korean diabetic patients. *J Diabetes Complications* 2004; 18 (2): 79–85.

25 Tankova T, Koev D, Dakovska L. Alpha-lipoic acid in the treatment of autonomic diabetic neuropathy (controlled, randomized, open-label study). *Rom J Intern Med* 2004; 42(2): 457–464.

26 Tankova T, Cherninkova S, Koev D. Treatment for diabetic mononeuropathy with alpha-lipoic acid. *Int J Clin Pract* 2005; 59(6): 645–650.

27 Vincent HK, Bourguignon CM, Vincent KR, *et al*. Effects of alpha-lipoic acid supplementation in peripheral arterial disease: a pilot study. *J Altern Complement Med* 2007; 13(5): 577–584.

28 Filina AA, Davydova NG, Endrikhovskii SN, *et al*. Lipoic acid as a means of metabolic therapy of open-angle glaucoma. *Vestn Oftalmol* 1995; 111(4): 6–8.

29 Baur A, Harrer T, Peukert M, *et al*. Alpha-lipoic acid is an effective inhibitor of human immunodeficiency virus (HIV-1) replication. *Klin Wochenschr* 1991; 69(15): 722–724.

30 Zakrzewska JM, Forssell H, Glenny AM. Interventions for the treatment of burning mouth syndrome. *Cochrane Database Syst Rev* 2005; 25 (1): CD002779.

31 Carbone M, Pentenero M, Carrozzo M, *et al*. Lack of efficacy of alpha-lipoic acid in burning mouth syndrome: a double-blind, randomized, placebo-controlled study. *Eur J Pain* 2009; 13(5): 492–496.

32 Cavalcanti DR, daSilveira FR. Alpha lipoic acid in burning mouth syndrome–a randomized double-blind placebo-controlled trial. *J Oral Pathol Med* 2009; 38(3): 254–261.

33 Lopez-Jornet P, Camacho-Alonso F, Leon-Espinosa S. Efficacy of alpha lipoic acid in burning mouth syndrome: a randomized, placebo-treatment study. *J Oral Rehabil* 2009; 36(1): 52–57.

34 Vasdev S, Ford CA, Parai S, *et al*. Dietary alpha-lipoic acid supplementation lowers blood pressure in spontaneously hypertensive rats. *J Hypertens* 2000; 18(5): 567–573.

35 Mantovani G, Maccio A, Melis G, *et al*. Restoration of functional defects in peripheral blood mononuclear cells isolated from cancer patients by thiol antioxidants alpha-lipoic acid and N-acetyl cysteine. *Int J Cancer* 2000; 86(6): 842–847.

36 Savitha S, Sivarajan K, Haripriya D, *et al*. Efficacy of levo carnitine and alpha lipoic acid in ameliorating the decline in mitochondrial enzymes during aging. *Clin Nutr* 2005; 24(5): 794–800.

37 Sauer J, Tabet N, Howard R. Alpha lipoic acid for dementia. *Cochrane Database Syst Rev* 2004; 1(1): CD004244.

38 Hager K, Kenklies M, McAfoose J, *et al*. Alpha-lipoic acid as a new treatment option for Alzheimer's disease–a 48 months follow-up analysis. *J Neural Transm Suppl* 2007; 72(72): 189–193.

39 Kim E, Park DW, Choi SH, *et al*. A preliminary investigation of alpha-lipoic acid treatment of antipsychotic drug-induced weight gain in patients with schizophrenia. *J Clin Psychopharmacol* 2008; 28 (2): 138–146.

Androstenedione

Description

Androstenedione is a naturally occurring adrenal androgen that is a precursor of testosterone and oestrone in men and women. It is secreted by the testes, ovaries and adrenal glands. Production peaks during the third decade and declines after the age of 30.

Action

Androstenedione is used by men as a hormone replacement and as an enhancer for athletic performance. The effects of androstenedione on testosterone levels and muscle have been studied in men of various ages with normal testosterone levels.

An 8-week trial in 30 men aged 19–29 years found that androstenedione supplementation did not increase serum testosterone concentrations or enhance skeletal muscle adaptations to resistance training.[1] A study in 42 men aged 20–40 years found that androstenedione, when given in a dose of 300 mg/day, increased serum testosterone and oestradiol concentrations, but there was marked variability in individual responses for all measured sex steroids.[2] A further study in 55 men aged 30–56 years found that administration of 100 mg androstenedione, three times per day, did not increase serum total testosterone concentrations but did elicit increases in androstenedione, free testosterone and oestradiol, and decreased serum high-density lipoprotein cholesterol concentrations.[3] In a 5-day study of six healthy young men, oral androstenedione (100 mg/day) did not increase plasma testosterone concentrations and had no anabolic effect on muscle protein metabolism.[4]

In a study of 30 healthy postmenopausal women, acute administration of both 50 mg and 100 mg androstenedione increased both serum testosterone and oestrone levels, but not oestradiol levels. The authors concluded that if these hormonal effects were sustained during long-term administration, regular use of this supplement by postmenopausal women could cause both beneficial and adverse effects.[5]

Possible uses

Androstenedione has been employed in an attempt to enhance athletic performance and as hormone replacement for men. Advertisements for androstenedione have linked this substance with improved body mass and increased muscle mass, so supplements have been used by bodybuilders and other athletes hoping to increase muscle bulk quickly. When administered to achieve higher than physiological levels in the body, androstenedione can increase muscle size, enhance mood and change lipid profiles.

Precautions/contraindications

Avoid use of this substance.

Androstenedione is banned by several organisations, including the International Olympic Committee. Currently, it is available in the UK as an over-the-counter dietary supplement, but it is considered to be unsafe for sports use. In early 2008, the government classified androstenedione as a Class C drug and warned people about using it to enhance their physical performance and appearance leading up to the 2012 Olympic games.[6]

Pregnancy and breast-feeding

Avoid in pregnancy and breast-feeding.

Adverse effects

Common adverse effects of androstenedione include acne, hepatic dysfunction, hirsutism, gynaecomastia, adolescent stunted growth, psychiatric problems (e.g. moodiness, anxiety) and cancer (e.g. tumour of the liver and leukaemia).

Interactions

Androstenedione may exacerbate the effects of exogenously administered oestrogens.

Dose

Avoid use.

Conclusion

Androstenedione has been used in an attempt to enhance athletic performance, build muscle mass and as hormone replacement in men. It is considered to be unsafe and should be avoided. Several organisations ban this substance for use in sports.

References

1 King DS, Sharp RL, Vukovich MD, *et al.* Effect of oral androstenedione on serum testosterone and adaptations to resistance training in young men: a randomized controlled trial. *JAMA* 1999; 281: 2020–2028.

2 Leder BZ, Longcope C, Catlin DH, *et al.* Oral androstenedione administration and serum testosterone concentrations in young men. *JAMA* 2000; 283: 779–782.

3 Brown GA, Vukovich MD, Martini ER, *et al.* Endocrine responses to chronic androstenedione intake in 30- to 56-year-old men. *J Clin Endocrinol Metab* 2000; 85: 4074–4080.

4 Rasmussen BB, Volpi E, Gore DC, Wolfe RR. Androstenedione does not stimulate muscle protein anabolism in young healthy men. *J Clin Endocrinol Metab* 2000; 85: 55–59.

5 Leder BZ, Leblanc KM, Longcope C, *et al.* Effects of oral androstenedione administration on serum testosterone and estradiol levels in postmenopausal women. *J Clin Endocrinol Metab* 2002; 87: 5449–5454.

6 Home Office. *Home Office Circular 21/2009. A Change to the Misuse of Drugs Act 1971: Control of GBL, 1,4-BD, BZP and related piperazine compounds, a further group of anabolic steroids and 2 non-steroidal agents, synthetic cannabinoid receptor agonists and oripavine.* London: The Stationery Office; 2009, http://www.homeoffice.gov.uk/ (accessed 9 May 2010).

Antioxidants

Description

Various antioxidant systems have evolved to offer protection against free radicals and prevent damage to vital biological structures such as lipid membranes, proteins and DNA. Antioxidant capacity is a concept used to describe the overall ability of tissues to inhibit processes mediated by free radicals.[1] It is dependent on the concentrations of individual antioxidants and the activity of protective enzymes. The most common and important antioxidant defences are shown in Table 1.

The antioxidant vitamins can be divided into those that are water-soluble and exist in aqueous solution – primarily vitamin C – and those that are fat-soluble and exist in membranes or lipoproteins – primarily vitamin E. Lipid membranes are particularly vulnerable to oxidative breakdown by free radicals. Vitamin E protects cell membranes from destruction by undergoing preferential oxidation and destruction. Carotenoids, such as beta-carotene, which are found in most dark green, red or yellow fruits and vegetables and some quinones, such as ubiquinone (coenzyme Q) also appear to have antioxidant properties. Flavonoids and other phenols and polyphenols found in foods such as green tea, red wine, olive oil, grapes and many other fruits are also antioxidants. All these substances can act as free radical scavengers and can react directly with free radicals.

Some trace elements act as essential components of antioxidant enzymes – copper, magnesium or zinc for superoxide dismutase and selenium for glutathione peroxidase.

Table 1   Antioxidant defences

- **Intracellular antioxidants**
  Enzymes
    catalase
    glutathione peroxidase
    superoxide dismutase
- **Extracellular antioxidants**
  Vitamin C
  Sulphydryl groups
- **Membrane antioxidants**
  Carotenoids
  Ubiquinone
  Vitamin E
- **Substances essential for synthesis of antioxidant enzymes**
  Copper
  Manganese
  Selenium
  Zinc

Supplements that are marketed as having antioxidant activity include:

- vitamin A (usually as beta-carotene), vitamins C and E (ACE vitamins, often with selenium)
- alpha-lipoic acid (see Alpha-lipoic acid)
- carnitine (see Carnitine)
- carotenoids (see Carotenoids)
- coenzyme Q (see Coenzyme Q)
- green tea (see Green tea extract)
- zinc (see Zinc).

Action

Antioxidants are believed to protect against certain diseases by preventing the deleterious effects of processes mediated by free radicals in cell membranes and by reducing the susceptibility of tissues to oxidative stress.

Free radicals

Each orbital surrounding the nucleus of an atom is occupied by a pair of electrons. If an orbital in the outer shell of a molecule loses an electron, the molecule becomes a free radical. As a result of the unpaired electron, the molecule becomes unstable and, therefore, highly reactive. The free radical may then react with any other nearby molecule, also converting that molecule to a free radical which can then initiate another reaction. Some free radicals are capable of severely damaging cells.

Theoretically, a single free radical can ultimately cause an endless number of reactions. This chain reaction is terminated either by the free radical's reaction with another free radical, resulting in the formation of a covalently bound molecule, or by the free radical's reaction with an antioxidant, an antioxidant enzyme, or both. Fortunately, many enzyme systems have evolved to provide protection from free radical production.

Because antioxidant defences are not completely efficient, increased free radical formation in the body is likely to increase damage. The term 'oxidative stress' is often used to refer to this effect. If mild oxidative stress occurs, tissues often respond by increasing their antioxidant defences. However, severe oxidative stress can cause cell injury and cell death.

There is evidence that free-radical damage is involved in the development of many diseases, such as atherosclerosis, cancer, Parkinson's disease and other neurodegenerative disorders, inflammatory bowel disease and lung disease. However, free radical production is essential for health and the 'antioxidant theory' appears to be more complex than was first thought. It is likely that a balance of antioxidant and pro-oxidant activity is beneficial.

Possible uses

Epidemiological evidence suggests that low plasma levels of antioxidant nutrients and low dietary intakes are related to an increased risk of diseases such as coronary heart disease (CHD) and cancer. There is also increasing evidence that these diseases can be prevented or delayed to some extent by dietary changes, in particular by increased consumption of fruits and vegetables. Several substances in fruit and vegetables (e.g. beta-carotene, vitamin C and vitamin E) may act to diminish oxidative damage *in vivo* and, because endogenous antioxidant defences are not completely effective, dietary antioxidants may be important in diminishing the cumulative effects of oxidative damage in the human body.

A question of particular interest is whether supplementation of adequately nourished subjects with antioxidant nutrients will reduce the incidence of such diseases. Intervention trials of antioxidants and meta-analyses reported so far have shown little evidence for the value of supplements. Some have shown harmful effects. A recent meta-analysis of 68 randomised controlled trials including 232 606 participants found that low-bias risk trials were significantly associated with increased mortality (relative risk (RR), 0.998; 95% confidence interval (CI), 0.997 to 0.9995). In low-bias risk trials, beta-carotene, vitamin A and vitamin E, singly or combined, significantly increased mortality. However, vitamin C and selenium had no significant effect on mortality.[2] Any possible benefits are more likely to be seen in those with poor diets rather than in well-nourished populations.[3]

Cardiovascular disease

Epidemiological studies

Experimental studies suggest an inverse association between CHD mortality and vitamins C, E and beta-carotene, and argue strongly in favour of a protective role of antioxidants in the development of atherosclerosis.

In a cross-cultural study of middle-aged men representing 16 European populations,[1] differences in mortality from ischaemic heart disease were primarily attributable to plasma levels of vitamin E. Twelve of the 16 populations had similar blood cholesterol levels and blood pressure but differed greatly in tocopherol levels and heart disease death rates. For vitamin E, mean plasma levels lower than 25 μmol/L were associated with a high risk of CHD, whereas plasma levels above this value were associated with a higher risk of the disease. In the case of vitamin C, mean plasma levels less than 22fs.7 μmol/L were found in those regions that had a moderate to high risk of CHD, whereas plasma levels in excess of this level tended to be found in those areas at low risk.

In a large case-control study in Scotland,[4] 6000 men aged 35–54 were studied for a possible association between antioxidant status and risk of angina pectoris. Highly significant correlations between low plasma concentrations of beta-carotene, vitamin C, vitamin E and risk of angina were found.

The Health Professionals' Study,[5] a large prospective investigation that looked at 39 910 US male health professionals aged 40–75, showed that men who took more than 100 IU of vitamin E daily for over 2 years had a 37% reduction in risk of heart disease. The Nurses' Health Study,[6] in which 87 245 female nurses aged 34–59 took part, showed that women who took more than 200 IU of vitamin E daily for more than 2 years had a 41% reduction in risk of CHD.

Intervention trials

The first intervention trial published was a study of 333 male physicians aged between 40 and 84 with angina pectoris and/or coronary revascularisation, which showed that 50 mg of beta-carotene on alternate days resulted in a 44% reduction in major coronary events.[7]

However, another study[8] tested aspirin, vitamin E and beta-carotene in the prevention of cardiovascular disease (CVD) and cancer in 39 76 women aged 45 and older. Among those randomly assigned to receive 50 mg beta-carotene or a placebo every other day, there were no statistically significant differences in incidence of CVD, cancer or overall death rate after a median of 2 years of treatment and 2 years of follow-up.

In a study of 1862 smoking men aged 50 to 59 (participants in the Finnish Alpha-Tocopherol, Beta-Carotene Cancer Prevention (ATBC) Study)[9] who were followed for a median of 5.3 years, dietary supplements of alpha-tocopherol (50 mg a day), beta-carotene (20 mg a day), both, or a placebo were given. There were significantly more deaths from CHD among those who took beta-carotene supplements, and a non-significant trend towards more deaths in the vitamin E group. This same study also found that neither alpha-tocopherol nor beta-carotene had a preventive effect for large abdominal aortic aneurysm.[10] During the 6-year post-trial follow-up in the ATBC study, beta-carotene increased the post-trial risk of first-ever non-fatal myocardial infarction, suggesting that these supplements should not be used in the prevention of CVD among male smokers.[11]

Another large trial involving 20 536 UK adults aged 40–80 with coronary disease, other occlusive arterial disease or diabetes, randomly allocated participants to receive antioxidant vitamin supplementation (600 mg vitamin E, 250 mg vitamin C and 20 mg beta-carotene daily) or matching placebo over 5 years. There were no significant differences in all-cause mortality, or in deaths due to vascular or non-vascular causes. Nor were there any significant differences in the number of participants having non-fatal myocardial infarction or coronary death, non-fatal or fatal stroke, or coronary or non-coronary revascularisation. For the first occurrence of these major vascular events, there were no material differences overall and no significant differences in cancer incidence and hospitalisation for any other non-vascular disease.[12]

A double-blind clinical trial[13] found that taking high doses of vitamin C (500 mg twice a day) and E (700 IU twice a day) and beta-carotene (30 000 units twice a day) did not reduce the risk of arteries re-clogging after balloon coronary angioplasty. The patients took probucol, probucol plus three antioxidants, the antioxidants alone or placebo. All patients also received aspirin. After 6 months the rates of repeated angioplasty were 11% in the probucol group, 16.2% in the combined treatment group, 24.4% in the multivitamin group and 26.6% in the placebo group.

A trial in postmenopausal women with coronary disease found that supplementation with vitamin E 400 IU twice daily and vitamin C 500 mg twice daily did not retard atherosclerosis and provided no cardiovascular benefit.[14] Results from the SU.VI.MAX trial also suggested that a combination of antioxidants (120 mg vitamin C, 30 mg vitamin E, 6 mg beta-carotene, 100 μg selenium, 20 mg zinc) over an average of 7.2 years had no beneficial effects on carotid atherosclerosis and arterial stiffness[15] or risk of hypertension[16] in healthy patients. A further trial in 520 smoking and non-smoking men and postmenopausal women (all of whom had serum cholesterol > 5 mmol/L) found that supplementation with combination vitamin E and slow-release vitamin C slows down atherosclerotic progression.[17]

The Women's Antioxidant Cardiovascular Study evaluated the effects of vitamin C (500 mg daily), vitamin E (600 IU every other day) and beta-carotene (50 mg every other day) on the combined outcome of myocardial infarction, stroke, coronary revascularisation, or CVD death among 8171 female health professionals (≥ 40 years) with a history of CVD or three or more CVD risk factors. They were followed up for a mean duration of 9.4 years. A total of 1450 women experienced one or more CVD outcomes. There was no overall effect of any of the antioxidants on the primary combined end point or on the individual secondary outcomes of myocardial infarction, stroke, coronary revascularisation or CVD death.[18]

More recent trials have shown some beneficial effect of antioxidant supplements on certain aspects of CVD. A Polish trial involving 800 patients with acute myocardial infarction found that supplementation with vitamin C 1200 mg daily and vitamin E 600 mg daily over 30 days had a positive influence on primary end points (i.e. in-hospital cardiac mortality, non-fatal new myocardial infarction) and concluded that a larger study is warranted to generate further evidence for this particular regimen.[19]

An RCT involving 100 patients with asymptomatic or mildly symptomatic moderate aortic stenosis found that supplementation with vitamin E (400 IU) and vitamin C (1000 mg) daily had modest anti-inflammatory effect, although the clinical relevance requires further clarification.[20] A 15-day clinical trial in patients with early-stage untreated type 2 diabetes mellitus or impaired glucose tolerance found that supplementation with N-acetylcysteine 600 mg daily, vitamin E 300 mg daily and vitamin C 250 mg daily reversed unfavourable oxidative changes occurring after a moderate fat meal and may therefore have decreased oxidative stress.[21] A further trial involving 48 acute ischaemic stroke patients (evaluated within 12 h of symptom onset) found that compared with placebo, alpha-tocopherol 800 IU daily and vitamin C 500 mg daily over 14 days increased antioxidant capacity, reduced lipid peroxidation products and may have an anti-inflammatory effect.[22]

There is some evidence that folate status could have an influence on the response to antioxidant supplementation in patients at cardiovascular risk. One study found that folate deficiency may amplify the effect of other risk factors such as elevated homocysteine or variant methylene tetrahydrofolate reductase (MTHFR genotype), as well as influencing the ability of antioxidant supplementation to protect against genetic damage.[23] A reduction in systolic blood pressure has been observed in young healthy men supplemented with both folic acid (10 mg daily) and antioxidants (vitamin C 100 mg, vitamin E 800 mg).[24] However, in a further study involving patients in the immediate aftermath of stroke, supplementation with antioxidant vitamins (vitamin E 800 IU and vitamin C 500 mg daily), or B group vitamins (5 mg folic acid, 5 mg vitamin B_2, 50 mg vitamin B_6, 0.4 mg vitamin B_{12}), both vitamins together or no supplements found that supplementation with antioxidant vitamins with or without B-group vitamins enhances antioxidant capacity, mitigates oxidative damage and may have an anti-inflammatory effect immediately post-infarct in stroke.[25]

The effect of antioxidant supplementation in CVD has been evaluated in systematic reviews and meta-analyses. One systematic review assessed whether antioxidants in food or supplements can offer primary prevention against myocardial infarction or stroke.[26] Eight RCTs were included, six of which tested supplements of beta-carotene, four tested alpha-tocopherol and two ascorbic acid. None of the RCTs showed any benefit of antioxidant supplementation on CVD. In one study there was a significantly increased risk for fatal or non-fatal intracerebral and subarachnoid haemorrhage in participants taking alpha-tocopherol. The reviewers concluded that from these RCTs (which had limitations) antioxidants as food supplements had no beneficial effects in the primary prevention of myocardial infarction and stroke and cannot be recommended for such purposes.

A meta-analysis that looked at the effect of antioxidant vitamins on long-term cardiovascular outcomes included 12 RCTs, of which seven examined vitamin E and eight beta-carotene.[27] Over all the studies there was no statistically significant difference between vitamin E and control for all-cause mortality, cardiovascular mortality or cerebrovascular accident. Beta-carotene was associated with a slight statistically significant increase in all-cause mortality and cardiovascular death compared with control. The authors concluded that the routine use of vitamin E cannot be recommended and that the use of supplements containing beta-carotene should be actively discouraged.

The US Agency for Healthcare Research and Quality (AHRQ) commissioned an extensive report on the efficacy and safety of antioxidant supplements (vitamins C, E and coenzyme Q_{10}) for the prevention and treatment of CVD.[28] From a review and analysis of the 144 clinical

trials the authors identified, the following conclusions were reached. Firstly, the evidence does not suggest a benefit of supplements containing vitamin E or vitamin C (either alone or in combination) on either CVD or all-cause mortality, but there was no suggestion of harm. Secondly, there was no consistent support for a beneficial effect on fatal or non-fatal myocardial infarction or upon plasma lipid levels. Evidence on coenzyme Q_{10} was judged to be insufficient to reach conclusions on its effects in CVD.

A pooled analysis of nine cohort studies evaluated the relationship between the intake of antioxidant vitamins and CHD risk. Dietary intake of antioxidants was only weakly related to CHD risk. However, subjects with a higher supplemental vitamin C intake had a lower CHD incidence, while supplemental vitamin E intake was not significantly associated with CHD risk.[29]

In 2004, the American Heart Association Council on Nutrition, Physical Activity and Metabolism concluded that antioxidant supplements have little or no proven value for preventing or treating CVD.[30]

A 2008 Cochrane review of 46 trials including 68 111 participants found overall that antioxidant supplements had no significant effect on mortality, with no evidence to support an influence on primary or secondary mortality. When trials were assessed separately, vitamin A, beta-carotene and vitamin E were associated with increased mortality, but there was no significant detrimental effect of vitamin C or selenium.[31]

Cancer

Epidemiological studies
There is now good evidence linking high intake of fruit and vegetables with lower incidence of certain cancers, and it is presumed that the protective nutrients are some or all of the antioxidant nutrients.

In a study of 25 802 volunteers in Washington County, Maryland,[32] prediagnostic blood samples from 436 cancer cases at nine cancer sites were compared with 765 matched control cases. Serum beta-carotene levels showed a strong protective association with lung cancer, suggestive protective associations with melanoma and bladder cancer, and a suggestive but non-protective association with lung cancer.

Serum vitamin E levels showed a protective association with lung cancer, but none of the other cancer sites studied showed impressive associations. Low levels of serum lycopene (a carotenoid occurring in ripe fruits) were strongly associated with pancreatic cancer and less strongly associated with cancer of the bladder and rectum.

The Basel study from Switzerland[33] demonstrated that patients who had died from all cancers, including cancer of the bronchus and stomach, had statistically lower mean carotene levels compared with a matched group of healthy survivors.

In a Finnish study,[34] individuals with low serum levels of vitamin E had about a 1.5-fold risk of cancer compared with those with a higher serum level of vitamin E. The strength of the association between serum vitamin E level and cancer risk varied for different cancer sites and was strongest for some gastrointestinal cancers and for the combined group of cancers unrelated to smoking.

In a US prospective study, which evaluated the intakes of vitamins C, E and A and carotenoids and risk of oral premalignant lesions in men, high intakes of beta-carotene and vitamin E were associated with increased risk, while vitamin C from dietary sources, but not supplements, was associated with reduced risk.[35]

In an Italian case–control study, a significant inverse association was found for vitamin E and vitamin C intake in relation to the risk of renal cell cancer. No significant trend was observed for other antioxidants (e.g. lycopene, lutein/zeaxanthin).[36]

Intervention trials

An intervention trial in Linxian, China,[37] provided some of the earliest clinical data on the effects of specific vitamin–mineral supplementation on cancer incidence and disease-specific mortality. Linxian County has one of the world's highest rates of oesophageal and gastric cancers. Combined daily doses of 15 mg beta-carotene, 30 mg vitamin E and 50 µg selenium taken over 5 years were associated with a 13% reduction in deaths from cancer, and an overall reduction in mortality of 9%. These results, although impressive, might have been achieved because the population studied had low intakes and were deficient in the nutrients investigated.

A similar study is required in a well-nourished population.

Not all studies have shown positive results. The ATBC Study in Finland[38] found no reduction in the incidence of lung cancer among male smokers after 5 to 8 years of dietary supplementation with vitamin E or beta-carotene; incidence of lung cancer increased by 18% and overall death rate by 8% in the group receiving beta-carotene. However, these results should be considered in the context of the population studied – the subjects had smoked an average of 20 cigarettes a day for 36 years. Most studies with antioxidants suggest that their protective properties are associated with the early stages of cancer and it is likely that this intervention took place too late in the carcinogenic process. In addition, the study could have employed too low a dose (50 mg vitamin E and/or 20 mg beta-carotene were used) or was of too short a duration. The excess risks of beta-carotene on lung cancer were no longer evident 4–6 years after the intervention had ended.[39] More recent data from this study suggest no association between dietary vitamin C or E, alpha- or gamma-tocopherol, alpha- or beta-carotene, lycopene or lutein and risk for colorectal cancer.[40] No overall preventive effect of long-term supplementation with alpha-tocopherol or beta-carotene on gastric cancer was found.[41]

Another trial,[42] which tested a combination of beta-carotene and vitamin A, was terminated after 4 years because it appeared that those taking the supplements and who also smoked had a 28% higher incidence of lung cancer and a 17% higher death rate.

In the Nurses' Health Study,[43] large intakes of vitamin C or E did not protect women from breast cancer. In contrast, there was a significant inverse association of vitamin A intake with risk of this disease. The authors concluded, however, that vitamin A supplements are unlikely to influence the risk of breast cancer among women whose dietary intake of this vitamin is already adequate.

In the Polyp Prevention Study,[44] there was no evidence that supplements of either beta-carotene or vitamins C and E reduced the incidence of colorectal adenomas. Compared with placebo, alpha-tocopherol supplementation increased the occurrence of second primary cancers in head and neck patients.[45]

A further study found that low-dose antioxidant supplementation (over 7.5 years) lowered total cancer incidence and all-cause mortality in men, but not in women. The authors suggested that the effectiveness of supplementation in men may have been because of their lower baseline status of certain antioxidants, especially beta-carotene.[46] In a further study, supplemental beta-carotene intake at a dose of at least 2000 µg daily was associated with a decreased risk of prostate cancer in men with low dietary beta-carotene intake. Among current and recent smokers, increasing dose (>400 IU daily) and duration (>10 years) of supplemental vitamin E use was also associated with reduced prostate cancer risk.[47] A meta-analysis of nine RCTs found no evidence of benefit for beta-carotene, vitamins C and E on risk of prostate cancer.[48]

AHRQ commissioned a report to investigate the effectiveness of vitamin E, vitamin C and coenzyme Q_{10} in the prevention and treatment of cancer.[49] They found no evidence to support the beneficial effects of vitamin E and/or vitamin C in the prevention of new tumours, the development of colonic polyps or in the treatment of patients with advanced cancer.[49] A systematic review and meta-analysis found no evidence that antioxidant supplements (beta-carotene, vitamin A, C and E) can prevent gastrointestinal cancers, but rather that they seemed to increase overall mortality. There was evidence from four of the included trials that selenium has a beneficial effect on the incidence of gastrointestinal cancer. However, good clinical trials are needed to confirm this benefit.[50] A further meta-analysis in 2009 of both primary and secondary prevention trials also found no preventive effect of antioxidant supplements on cancer.[51]

More recent trials have continued to show a similar picture. Supplementation with antioxidants (vitamin C, E and beta-carotene) was not effective in the regression and progression of pre-cancerous gastric lesions in a high-risk population in Venezuela.[52] In a RCT investigating the effect of high-dose antioxidants (vitamin E 400 IU daily and beta-carotene 30 mg daily) on head and neck cancer patients, both all-cause mortality and cause-specific mortality were higher in the supplemented group than in the placebo group. Moreover, supplementation with beta-carotene was discontinued during the trial.[53] A 2008 systematic review of 20 RCTs found no evidence that the studied antioxidant supplements prevented gastrointestinal cancers.[31]

A trial conducted within the framework of the French Supplementation in Vitamins and Mineral Antioxidants (SU.VI.MAX) study found that an antioxidant supplement (vitamin C 120 mg, vitamin E 30 mg, beta-carotene 6 mg, selenium 100 µg and zinc 20 mg) over a median follow-up period of 7.5 years was associated with a higher incidence of skin cancer in women. In men, incidence of skin cancer did not differ between the antioxidant and placebo groups. The incidence of melanoma was also higher in the antioxidant group for women. The incidence of non-melanoma skin cancer did not differ between the antioxidant and placebo groups for men or women. The authors concluded that their findings suggest that antioxidant supplementation affects the incidence of skin cancer differently in men and women.[54]

Cataract

Antioxidants are also being investigated for a possible protective effect in cataract. Low vitamin C intakes have been associated with increased risk of cataract.[55] Increased levels of supplementary vitamins C and E correlated with a 50% reduction in the risk of cataracts,[56] while the Nurses' Health Study[57] found that dietary carotenoids, although not necessarily beta-carotene, and long-term vitamin C supplementation may reduce the risk of cataracts.

The Age-Related Eye Disease Study (AREDS), an 11-centre trial, evaluated the effect of a high-dose antioxidant supplement (vitamin C 500 mg, vitamin E 400 IU, beta-carotene 15 mg) on the development and progression of age-related lens opacities and visual acuity loss. Of 4757 participants enrolled, 4629 who were aged from 55 to 80 had at least one natural lens present and were followed up for an average of 6.3 years. No statistically significant effect of the antioxidant formulation was seen on the development or progression of age-related lens opacities or visual acuity loss.[58]

A further trial – the Roche European American Cataract Trial (REACT) – randomised 445 patients with age-related cataract (in English and American outpatient settings) to a mixture of oral antioxidant micronutrients (beta-carotene 18 mg daily, vitamin C 750 mg daily and vitamin E 600 mg daily) or placebo and followed them for 2–4 years. After 2 years of treatment, there was a small positive treatment effect in the US group and after 3 years a positive effect was apparent in both the US and UK groups. The positive effect in the US group was even more positive after 3 years, but the benefit in the UK group did not reach statistical significance.[59]

Age-related macular degeneration

Research is being conducted to determine whether taking supplements or consuming foods rich in antioxidants can protect against age-related macular degeneration (ARMD), a disease in which the central portion of the retina deteriorates so that only peripheral vision remains. A study following 3654 individuals aged 49 or older found no statistically significant association between ARMD and dietary intake of either carotene, zinc or vitamins A or C, either from diet, supplements or both.[60] An earlier study involving 156 subjects with ARMD showed that neither serum alpha-tocopherol nor beta-carotene was significantly associated with age-related maculopathy.[61]

In 29 000 smoking males aged 50 to 69 randomly assigned to alpha-tocopherol (50 mg a day), beta-carotene (20 mg a day), placebo or both, no beneficial effect of supplementation on the occurrence of ARMD was found.[62] However, in a study involving 21 120 male physicians,[63] those who used vitamin E supplements or multivitamins had a possible but non-significant reduced risk of ARMD, but the authors concluded that large reductions in the risk of ARMD were unlikely.

A Cochrane review[64] (which included one study) concluded in 2000 that there was no evidence to date that people without ARMD should take antioxidant vitamin and mineral supplements to prevent or delay the onset of the disease.

The AREDS (see Cataract above) also evaluated the effect of antioxidants with the addition of zinc (80 mg daily) and copper (2 mg daily) on ARMD. All patients had best eye visual acuity of 20/32 or better in at least one eye. They had category 2, 3 or 4 disease, meaning that they had small to intermediate drusen. The main outcome was progression to advanced macular degeneration. Antioxidants combined with zinc were associated with lower rates of development of advanced ARMD and loss of visual acuity. Both zinc and antioxidants plus zinc significantly reduced the odds of developing advanced ARMD in the higher-risk group. In conclusion this trial showed that the combination of antioxidants plus zinc was worthwhile in people with extant macular degeneration to prevent or slow further development to the advanced form.[65] This study did not show this supplement had benefits at other stages of ARMD.

A recent Dutch cohort study involving 4170 participants aged 55 or older in a suburb of Rotterdam found that dietary intake of both vitamin E and zinc was inversely associated with incident ARMD. An above median intake of beta-carotene, vitamin C, vitamin E and zinc was associated with a 35% reduced risk of ARMD.[66]

In a RCT of 22 071 US male physicians, beta-carotene 50 mg every other day for 12 years had no beneficial or harmful effect on the incidence of ARMD.[67]

Two systematic reviews concluded that evidence for the effectiveness of antioxidant vitamin and mineral supplementation in halting progression of ARMD comes mainly from the AREDS. They also concluded that the generalisability of these findings to other populations is unknown and further large trials are required.[68,69]

Pre-eclampsia

Antioxidants have also been evaluated for possible prevention of pre-eclampsia, with mixed results.[70–72] A Cochrane review of seven (mostly poor quality) trials found that antioxidant supplementation seems to reduce the risk of pre-eclampsia, with a reduction in risk of having a small-for-dates baby associated with antioxidants, although there is an increase in the risk of pre-term birth. Several large trials are ongoing and the results of these are needed before antioxidants can be recommended for clinical practice.[73] A more recent trial found that antioxidant supplementation (vitamins A 1000 units, B_6 2.2 mg, B_{12} 2.2 µg, C 200 mg, E 400 IU; folic acid 400 µg, N-acetylcysteine 200 mg, copper 2 mg, zinc 15 mg, manganese

0.5 mg, iron 30 mg, calcium 800 mg, selenium 100 μg) early in pregnancy (8–12 weeks) in women with low antioxidant status was associated with better maternal and neonatal outcome than supplementation with iron and folic acid alone.[74] Evidence from a Cochrane review of 10 trials does not support routine antioxidant supplementation during pregnancy to reduce the risk of pre-eclampsia and other serious complications of pregnancy.[75]

Physical exercise

Intense physical exercise has been associated with an increase in free radical production and an increase in oxidative stress. Antioxidant supplements have been evaluated for an effect on exercise stress. Supplementation has been associated with a decrease in oxidative stress markers in basketball players,[76] an increase in antioxidant enzymes in athletes,[77] enhancement in neutrophil oxidative burst in trained runners,[78] prevention of decreases in serum iron in endurance athletes,[79] prevention of exercise-induced lipid peroxidation in ultra-marathon runners,[80] but not prevention of muscle damage in response to an ultra-marathon run.[81]

Fertility

Infertility and the conditions that contribute to it are associated with a pro-oxidant state. Antioxidants are used to protect fertility in veterinary practice. Several human trials of variable quality suggest, but do not yet prove, that antioxidant supplements may have a role in treatment of infertility, particularly in men. Two meta-analyses have combined studies on oxidative stress and male infertility. One combined three studies[82] comparing reactive oxygen species (ROS) with *in vitro* fertilisation (IVF) rate, and found that ROS levels inversely correlated with the IVF rate. The other meta-analysis considered 22 observational studies[83] of oxidation status in variocoele-linked infertility and found that both ROS level and total antioxidant capacity were lower in the variocoele patients than in the controls. A recent trial that gave antioxidants (astaxanthin) to 30 men who were part of a couple diagnosed with infertility of at least 12 months' duration (where the female partner has no demonstrable contributing infertility cause) found that pregnancy rates were higher in couples with the antioxidant-taking male.[84] Further larger RCTs are needed where the outcome measure is the number of healthy pregnancies.

Cognitive function

Studies are also examining the relationship between antioxidants and Alzheimer's disease. A recent prospective cohort study showed no association between supplemental use of vitamin E and C, alone or in combination, with Alzheimer's disease or overall dementia.[85] However, data from 3376 elderly patients in a US cohort study found that those who used supplements of vitamins C and E and non-steroidal anti-inflammatory drugs (NSAIDs) experienced less cognitive decline than those not taking supplements, a benefit that was observed entirely in participants with a specific gene (APOEε4 allele).[86] In addition, an intervention trial in 16 adults with type 2 diabetes mellitus involving consumption of vitamin C (1000 mg) and vitamin E (800 IU) reduced meal-induced memory impairment, with significant improvement in naming of words and colours.[87] In the US Womens' Antioxidant Cardiovascular Study (with secondary prevention of CVD as the main outcome measure), vitamin E (402 mg every other day), beta-carotene (50 mg every other day), and vitamin C (500 mg daily) did not slow cognitive decline in those with CVD risk factors or pre-existing CVD. However, there was a possible benefit of vitamin C and beta-carotene emerging late in the trial, which suggested the need for further study.[88]

Miscellaneous

Antioxidant supplements have been investigated for a wide range of other conditions. Research interests include asthma, lung function, mountain sickness and critical illness in hospital. Recent trials have found that antioxidant supplements may improve quality of life and reduce pain in patients suffering from chronic pancreatitis,[89] and may also improve certain parameters related to skin structure (roughness and scaling),[90] Higher maternal intakes of antioxidants in pregnancy have been associated with reduced risk for wheezing illness in early childhood.[91] Low intakes of vitamins A and C have been associated with increased risk of asthma.[92] A single trial found no evidence of benefit of an antioxidant supplement in mountain sickness.[93]

Adverse effects

Antioxidants are considered to be largely safe in low doses. However, routine use of combinations of antioxidants exceeding the Recommended Daily Allowance (RDA) should not be recommended for long-term use. In high doses, antioxidants may act as pro-oxidants, although there is no consensus on how much of a real clinical problem this could be. One study has found that antioxidants (vitamins E and C, beta-carotene and selenium) could block the favourable effects of statins combined with niacin (a drug combination used in the USA). This interaction could have implications for the management of CVD.[94] A Cochrane review involving trials where supplements were largely given in high doses concluded that vitamin A, beta-carotene and vitamin E were associated with increased mortality.[31]

> **Conclusion**
> Biochemical evidence suggests that oxidative stress caused by accumulation of free radicals is involved in the pathogenesis of several diseases. Appropriate levels of antioxidant nutrients might therefore be expected to delay or prevent these diseases. Several epidemiological studies have found lower serum levels of antioxidant nutrients in patients with CVD, cancer and cataract, but there is no good evidence that supplements of antioxidant nutrients prevent CVD or cancer. Evidence suggests that some may cause harm and increase mortality. However further intervention trials with different combination of antioxidants in different doses could produce different outcomes. Before conducting such trials further study of antioxidant substances at a mechanistic level would be valuable. An antioxidant combination has been found to delay progression of ARMD.

Interactions

Chemotherapy

A systematic review of 19 RCTs evaluating various antioxidants (glutathione, melatonin, vitamin A, an antioxidant mixture, vitamin C, *N*-acetylcysteine, vitamin E and ellagic acid) concluded that antioxidant supplementation during chemotherapy resulted in either increased survival times or increased tumour responses, or both, as well as fewer toxicities than controls. However, many of the trials lacked statistical power and the authors concluded that further well-designed trials of antioxidant supplementation in patients on chemotherapy are warranted.[95]

References

1 Gey KF, Puska P, Jordan P, *et al.* Inverse correlation between plasma vitamin E and mortality from ischaemic heart disease in cross-cultural epidemiology. *Am J Clin Nutr* 1991; 53: 326S–334S.

2 Bjelakovic G, Nikolova D, Gluud LL, *et al.* Mortality in randomized trials of antioxidant supplements for primary and secondary prevention: systematic review and meta-analysis. *JAMA* 2007; 297(8): 842–857.

3 Czernichow S, Vergnaud AC, Galan P, *et al.* Effects of long-term antioxidant supplementation and association of serum antioxidant concentrations with risk of metabolic syndrome in adults. *Am J Clin Nutr* 2009; 90(2): 329–335.

4 Riemersma RA, Wood DA, MacIntyre CCA, *et al.* Risk of angina pectoris and plasma concentrations of vitamins A, C and E and carotene. *Lancet* 1991; 337: 1–5.

5 Rimm EB, Stampfer MJ, Ascherio A, *et al.* Vitamin E consumption and the risk of coronary heart disease in men. *N Engl J Med* 1993; 328: 1450–1456.

6 Stampfer MJ, Hennekens CH, Manson JE, *et al.* Vitamin E consumption and the risk of coronary heart disease in women. *N Engl J Med* 1993; 328: 1444–1449.

7 Gaziano JM, Manson JE, Ridker PM, *et al.* Beta carotene therapy for chronic stable angina. *Circulation* 1990; 82(Suppl III): 201 (Abstr. 0796).

8 Rapola JM, Virtamo J, Ripatti S, *et al.* Randomised trial of alpha-tocopherol and beta-carotene supplements on incidence of major coronary events in men with previous myocardial infarction. *Lancet* 1997; 349: 1715–1720.

9 Hennekens CH, Buring JE, Manson JE, *et al.* Lack of effect of long term supplementation with beta-carotene on the incidence of malignant neoplasms and cardiovascular disease. *N Engl J Med* 1996; 334: 1145–1149.

10 Tornwall ME, Virtamo J, Haukka JK, *et al.* Alpha-tocopherol (vitamin E) and beta-carotene supplementation does not affect the risk for large abdominal aortic aneurysm in a controlled trial. *Atherosclerosis* 2001; 157: 167–173.

11 Tornwall ME, Virtamo J, Korhonen PA, *et al.* Effect of alpha-tocopherol and beta-carotene supplementation on coronary heart disease during the

6-year post-trial follow-up in the ATBC study. *Eur Heart J* 2004; 25: 1171–1178.

12 Heart Protection Study Collaborative Group. MRC/BHF Heart Protection Study of antioxidant vitamin supplementation in 20,536 high-risk individuals: a randomised placebo-controlled trial. *Lancet* 2002; 360: 23–33.

13 Tardif JC. Probucol and multivitamins in the prevention of restenosis after coronary angioplasty. *N Engl J Med* 1997; 337: 365–372.

14 Waters DD, Alderman EL, Hsia J, *et al.* Effects of hormone replacement therapy and antioxidant vitamin supplements on coronary atherosclerosis in postmenopasal women. *JAMA* 2002; 288: 2432–2440.

15 Zureik M, Galan P, Bertrais S, *et al.* Effects of long-term daily low-dose supplementation with antioxidant vitamins and minerals on structure and function of large arteries. *Arterioscler Thromb Vasc Biol* 2004; 24: 1485–1491.

16 Czernichow S, Bertrais S, Blacher J, *et al.* Effect of supplementation with antioxidants upon long-term risk of hypertension in the SU.VI.MAX study: association with plasma antioxidant levels. *J Hypertens* 2005; 23: 2013–2018.

17 Salonen RM, Nyyssonen K, Kaikkonene J, *et al.* Six-year effect of combined vitamin C and E supplementation on atherosclerotic progression: the Antioxidant Supplementation in Atherosclerotic Prevention (ASAP) Study. *Circulation* 2003; 107: 947–953.

18 Cook NR, Albert CM, Gaziano JM, *et al.* A randomized factorial trial of vitamins C and E and beta carotene in the secondary prevention of cardiovascular events in women: results from the Women's Antioxidant Cardiovascular Study. *Arch Intern Med* 2007; 167(15): 1610–1618.

19 Jaxa-Chamiec T, Bednarz B, Drozdowska D, *et al.* Antioxidant effects of combined vitamins C and E in acute myocardial infarction. The randomized, double-blind, placebo controlled, multicenter pilot Myocardial Infarction and VITamins (MIVIT) trial. *Kardiol Pol* 2005; 62: 344–350.

20 Tahir M, Foley B, Pate G, *et al.* Impact of vitamin E and C supplementation on serum adhesion molecules in chronic degenerative aortic stenosis: a randomized controlled trial. *Am Heart J* 2005; 150: 302–306.

21 Signorelli NS, Torrisi B, Pulvirenti D, *et al.* Effects of antioxidant supplementation on postprandial oxidative stress and endothelial dysfunction: a single-blind, 15-day clinical trial in patients with untreated type 2 diabetes, subjects with impaired glucose tolerance, and healthy controls. *Clin Ther* 2005; 27: 1764–1773.

22 Ullegaddi R, Powers HJ, Gariballa SE. Antioxidant supplementation enhances antioxidant capacity and mitigates oxidative damage following acute ischemic stroke. *Eur J Clin Nutr* 2005; 59: 1367–1373.

23 Smolkova B, Dusinska M, Raslova K, *et al.* Folate levels determine effect of antioxidant supplementation on micronuclei in subjects with cardiovascular risk. *Mutagenesis* 2004; 19: 469–476.

24 Schutte AE, Huisman HW, Oosthuizen W, *et al.* Cardiovascular effects of oral supplementation of vitamin C, E and folic acid in young healthy males. *Int J Vitam Nutr Res* 2004; 74: 285–293.

25 Ullegaddi R, Powers HJ, Gariballa SE. Antioxidant supplementation with or without B-group vitamins after acute ischaemic stroke: a randomised controlled trial. *J Parenter Enteral Nutr* 2006: 108–114.

26 Asplund K. Antioxidant vitamins in the prevention of cardiovascular disease: a systematic review. *J Intern Med* 2002(251): 372–392.

27 Vivekananthan DP, Penn MS, Sapp SK, *et al.* Use of antioxidant vitamins for the prevention of cardiovascular disease: meta-analysis of randomized trials. *Lancet* 2003; 361: 2017–2023.

28 Agency for Healthcare Research and Quality. *Effect of supplemental antioxidants vitamin C, vitamin E and co-enzyme Q10 for the prevention and treatment of cardiovascular disease.* [Evidence report/ Technology Assessment 83, AHRQ Publication Number 03-E042] Rockville, MD: Agency for Healthcare Research and Quality, 2003, http://www.ahrq.gov/clinic/epcsums/antioxsum.htm. (accessed 9 May, 2011).

29 Knekt P, Ritz J, Pereira MA, *et al.* Antioxidant vitamins and coronary heart disease risk: a pooled analysis of 9 cohorts. *Am J Clin Nutr* 2004; 80: 1508–1520.

30 Kris-Etherton PM, Lichtenstein AH, Howard BV, *et al.* Antioxidant vitamin supplements and cardiovascular disease. *Circulation* 2004; 110: 637–641.

31 Bjelakovic G, Nikolova D, Simonetti RG, *et al.* Systematic review: primary and secondary prevention of gastrointestinal cancers with antioxidant supplements. *Aliment Pharmacol Ther* 2008; 28 (6): 689–703.

32 Comstock GW, Helzlsouer KJ, Bush T. Prediagnostic serum levels of carotenoids and vitamin E as related to subsequent cancer in Washington County, Maryland. *Am J Clin Nutr* 1991; 53: 260S–264S.

33 Stahelin HB, Gey KF, Eichholzer M, *et al.* β-Carotene and cancer prevention: the Basel study. *Am J Clin Nutr* 1991; 53: 265S–269S.

34 Knekt P, Aromaa A, Maatela J, *et al.* Vitamin E and cancer prevention. *Am J Clin Nutr* 1991; 53: 283S–286S.

35 Maserejian NN, Giovannucci E, Rosner B, Joshipura K. Prospective study of vitamins C, E, and A and carotenoids and risk of oral premalignant lesions in men. *Int J Cancer* 2007; 120(5): 970–977.

36 Bosetti C, Scotti L, Maso LD, *et al.* Micronutrients and the risk of renal cell cancer: a case-control study from Italy. *Int J Cancer* 2007; 120(4): 892–896.

37 Blot WJ, Li JY, Taylor PR. Nutrition intervention trials in Linxian, China: supplementation with specific vitamin/mineral combinations, cancer

incidence, and disease-specific mortality in the general population. *J Natl Cancer Inst* 1993; 85: 1483–1492.

38 The Alpha Tocopherol Beta-Carotene Cancer Prevention Study Group. The effect of vitamin E and beta carotene on the incidence of lung cancer in male smokers. *N Engl J Med* 1994; 330: 1029–1035.

39 Virtamo J, Pietinen P, Huttunen JK, *et al.* Incidence of cancer and mortality following alpha-tocopherol and beta-carotene supplementation: a postintervention follow-up. *JAMA* 2003; 290: 476–485.

40 Malila N, Virtamo J, Virtanen M, *et al.* Dietary and serum alpha-tocopherol, beta-carotene and retinol, and risk for colorectal cancer in male smokers. *Eur J Clin Nutr* 2002; 56: 615–621.

41 Malila N, Taylor PR, Virtanen MJ, *et al.* Effects of alpha-tocopherol and beta-carotene supplementation on gastric cancer incidence in male smokers (ATBC Study Finland). *Cancer Causes Control* 2002; 13: 617–623.

42 Omenn GS, Goodman GE, Thornquist MD, *et al.* Effects of a combination of betacarotene and vitamin A on lung cancer and cardiovascular disease. *N Engl J Med* 1996; 334: 1150–1155.

43 Hunter DJ, Manson JE, Colditz GA, *et al.* A prospective study of vitamins C, E and A and the risk of breast cancer. *N Engl J Med* 1993; 329: 234–240.

44 Greenberg ER, Baron JA, Tosteson TD, *et al.* A clinical trial of antioxidant vitamins to prevent colorectal adenoma. *N Engl J Med* 1994; 331: 141–147.

45 Bairati I, Meyer F, Gelinas M, *et al.* A randomized trial of antioxidant vitamins to prevent second primary cancers in head and neck cancer patients. *J Natl Cancer Inst* 2003; 97: 468–470.

46 Hercberg S, Galan P, Preziosi P, *et al.* The SU.VI.MAX study: a randomized, placebo-controlled trial of the health effects of antioxidant vitamins and minerals. *Arch Intern Med* 2004; 164: 2335–2342.

47 Kirsch VA, Hayes RB, Mayne ST, *et al.* Supplemental vitamin E, beta-carotene, and vitamin C intakes and prostate cancer risk. *J Natl Cancer Inst* 2006; 98: 245–254.

48 Jiang L, Yang KH, Tian JH, *et al.* Efficacy of antioxidant vitamins and selenium supplement in prostate cancer prevention: a meta-analysis of randomized controlled trials. *Nutr Cancer* 2010; 62(6): 719–727.

49 Agency for Healthcare Research and Quality. *Effect of the supplemental use of antioxidants vitamin C, vitamin E, and the coenzyme Q10 for the prevention and treatment of cancer.* [Evidence report/Technology Assessment 75, Publication Number 04-E002] Rockville, MD: Agency for Healthcare Research and Quality, 2003, http://www.ahrq.gov/clinic/epcsums/aoxcansum.htm (accessed 9 May 2011).

50 Bjelakovic G, Nikolova D, Simonetti RG, *et al.* Antioxidant supplements for prevention of gastrointestinal cancers: a systematic review and meta-analysis. *Lancet* 2004; 364: 1219–1228.

51 Myung SK, Kim Y, Ju W, *et al.* Effects of antioxidant supplements on cancer prevention: meta-analysis of randomized controlled trials. *Ann Oncol* 2009; 21(1): 166–179.

52 Plummer M, Vivas J, Lopez G, *et al.* Chemoprevention of precancerous gastric lesions with antioxidant vitamin supplementation: a randomized trial in a high-risk population. *J. Natl. Cancer Inst* 2007; 99(2): 137–146.

53 Bairati I, Meyer F, Jobin E, *et al.* Antioxidant vitamins supplementation and mortality: a randomized trial in head and neck cancer patients. *Int J Cancer* 2006; 119(9): 2221–2224.

54 Hercberg S, Ezzedine K, Guinot C, *et al.* Antioxidant supplementation increases the risk of skin cancers in women but not in men. *J Nutr* 2007; 137(9): 2098–2105.

55 Jacques PF, Chylack LT. Epidemiologic evidence of a role for the antioxidant vitamins and carotenoids in cancer prevention. *Am J Clin Nutr* 1991; 53: 352S–355S.

56 Robertson J McD, Donner AP, Trevithick JR. A possible role for vitamins C and E in cataract prevention. *Am J Clin Nutr* 1991; 53: 346S–351S.

57 Hankinson SE, Stampfer MJ, Seddon JM, *et al.* Nutrient intake and cataract extraction in women: a prospective study. *Br Med J* 1992; 305: 335–339.

58 Age-Related Eye Disease Study Research Group. A randomized, placebo-controlled, clinical trial of high-dose supplementation with vitamins C and E and beta-carotene for age-related cataract and vision loss: AREDS Report No. 9. *Arch Ophthalmol* 2001; 119: 1439–1452.

59 Chylack LT, Jr Brown NP, Bron A, *et al.* The Roche American Cataract Trial (REACT): a randomised clinical trial to investigate the efficacy of an oral antioxidant micronutrient mixture to slow progression of age-related cataract. *Ophthalmic Epidemiol* 2002; 9: 49–80.

60 Smith W, Mitchell P, Webb K, *et al.* Dietary antioxidants and age-related maculopathy: The Blue Mountains Study. *Ophthalmology* 1999; 106: 761–767.

61 Smith W, Mitchell P, Rochester C., *et al.* Serum betacarotene, alpha tocopherol and age-related maculopathy: the Blue Mountain study. *Am J Ophthalmol* 1997; 124: 839–840.

62 Teikari JM, Laatikainen L, Virtamo J, *et al.* Six-year supplementation with alpha-tocopherol and beta-carotene and age-related maculopathy. *Acta Ophthalmol Scand* 1998; 76: 224–229.

63 Christen WG, Ajani UA, Glynn RG, *et al.* Prospective cohort study of antioxidant vitamin supplement use and the risk of age-related maculopathy. *Am J Epidemiol* 1999; 149: 476–484.

64 Evans JR, Henshaw K. Antioxidant vitamin and mineral supplementation for preventing age related macular degeneration. *Cochrane Database Syst Rev* 2008; (1): CD000253.

65 Age-Related Eye Disease StudyResearch Group. A randomized, placebo-controlled, clinicaltrial of high-dose supplementation with vitamins C and E, beta-carotene and zinc for age-related cataract andvision loss: AREDS Report No. 8. *Arch Ophthalmol* 2001; 119: 1417–1436.

66 van Leeuwen R, Boekhoorn S, Vingerling JR, *et al.* Dietary intake of antioxidants and risk of age-related macular degeneration. *JAMA* 2005; 294: 3101–3107.

67 Christen WG, Manson JE, Glynn RJ, *et al.* Beta carotene supplementation and age-related maculopathy in a randomized trial of US physicians. *Arch Ophthalmol* 2007; 125(3): 333–339.

68 Evans JR. Antioxidant vitamin and mineral supplements for slowing the progression of age-related macular degeneration. *Cochrane Database Syst Rev* 2006; (2): CD000254.

69 Evans J. Antioxidant supplements to prevent or slow down the progression of AMD: a systematic review and meta-analysis. *Eye (Lond)* 2008; 22(6): 751–760.

70 Beazley D, Ahokas R, Livingston J, *et al.* Vitamin C and E supplementation in women at high risk for preeclampsia: a double-blind, placebo-controlled trial. *Am J Obstet Gynecol* 2005; 192: 520–521.

71 Rumbold AR, Crowther CA, Haslam RR, *et al.* Vitamins C and E and the risks of preeclampsia and perinatal complications. *N Engl J Med* 2006; 354: 1796–1806.

72 Poston L, Briley AL, Seed PT, *et al.* Vitamin C and vitamin E in pregnant women at risk for preeclampsia (VIP) trial: randomised placebo-controlled trial. *Lancet* 2006; 367: 1145–1154.

73 Rumbold A, Duley L, Crowther C, *et al.* Antioxidants for preventing preeclampsia. *Cochrane Database Syst Rev* 2005; (4): CD004227.

74 Rumiris D, Purwosunu Y, Wibowo N, *et al.* Lower rate of preeclampsia after antioxidant supplementation in pregnant women with low antioxidant status. *Hypertens Pregnancy* 2006; 25(3): 241–253.

75 Rumbold A, Duley L, Crowther CA, *et al.* Antioxidants for preventing pre-eclampsia. *Cochrane Database Syst Rev* 2008; 23(1): CD004227.

76 Schroder H, Navarro E, Mora J, *et al.* Effects of alpha-tocopherol, beta-carotene and ascorbic acid on oxidative, hormonal and enzymatic exercise stress markers in habitual training activity of professional basketball players. *Eur J Clin Nutr* 2001; 40: 178–184.

77 Tauler P, Aguilo A, Fuentespina E, *et al.* Diet supplementation with vitamin E, vitamin C and beta-carotene cocktail enhances basal neutrophil antioxidant enzymes in athletes. *Pflugers Arch* 2002; 443: 791–797.

78 Robson PJ, Bouic PJ, Myburgh KH. Antioxidant supplementation enhances neutrophil oxidative burst in trained runners following prolonged exercise. *Int J Sport Nutr Exerc Metab* 2003; 13: 369–381.

79 Aguilo A, Tauler P, Fuentespina E, *et al.* Antioxidant diet supplementation influences blood iron status in endurance athletes. *Int J Sport Nutr Exerc Metab* 2004; 14: 147–160.

80 Mastaloudis A, Morrow JD, Hopkins DW, *et al.* Antioxidant supplementation prevents exercise-induced lipid peroxidation, but not inflammation, in ultramarathon runners. *Free Radic Biol Med* 2004; 36: 1329–1341.

81 Mastaloudis A, Traver MG, Carstensen K, *et al.* Antioxidants did not prevent muscle damage in response to an ultramarathon run. *Med Sci Sports Exerc* 2006; 38: 72–80.

82 Agarwal A, Allamaneni SS, Nallella KP, *et al.* Correlation of reactive oxygen species levels with the fertilization rate after in vitro fertilization: a qualified meta-analysis. *Fertil Steril* 2005; 84(1): 228–231.

83 Agarwal A, Prabakaran S, Allamaneni SS. Relationship between oxidative stress, varicocele and infertility: a meta-analysis. *Reprod Biomed Online* 2006; 12(5): 630–633.

84 Comhaire FH, El Garem Y, Mahmoud A, *et al.* Combined conventional/antioxidant 'Astaxanthin' treatment for male infertility: a double blind, randomized trial. *Asian J Androl* 2005; 7(3): 257–262.

85 Gray SL, Anderson ML, Crane PK, *et al.* Antioxidant vitamin supplement use and risk of dementia or Alzheimer's disease in older adults. *J Am Geriatr Soc* 2008; 56(2): 291–295.

86 Fotuhi M, Zandi PP, Hayden KM, *et al.* Better cognitive performance in elderly taking antioxidant vitamins E and C supplements in combination with nonsteroidal anti-inflammatory drugs: the Cache County Study. *Alzheimers Dement* 2008; 4(3): 223–227.

87 Chui MH, Greenwood CE. Antioxidant vitamins reduce acute meal-induced memory deficits in adults with type 2 diabetes. *Nutr Res* 2008; 28(7): 423–429.

88 Kang JH, Cook NR, Manson JE, *et al.* Vitamin E, vitamin C, beta carotene, and cognitive function among women with or at risk of cardiovascular disease: The Women's Antioxidant and Cardiovascular Study. *Circulation* 2009; 119(21): 2772–2780.

89 Kirk GR, White JS, McKie L, *et al.* Combined antioxidant therapy reduces pain and improves quality of life in chronic pancreatitis. *J Gastrointest Surg* 2006; 10(4): 499–503.

90 Heinrich U, Tronnier H, Stahl W, *et al.* Antioxidant supplements improve parameters related to skin structure in humans. *Skin Pharmacol Physiol* 2006; 19(4): 224–231.

91 Litonjua AA, Rifas-Shiman SL, Ly NP, *et al.* Maternal antioxidant intake in pregnancy and wheezing illnesses in children at 2 y of age. *Am J Clin Nutr* 2006; 84(4): 903–911.

92 Allen S, Britton JR, Leonardi-Bee JA. Association between antioxidant vitamins and asthma outcome

measures: systematic review and meta-analysis. *Thorax* 2009; 64(7): 610–619.

93 Baillie JK, Thompson AA, Irving JB, *et al*. Oral antioxidant supplementation does not prevent acute mountain sickness: double blind, randomized placebo-controlled trial. *Q J Med* 2009; 102(5): 341–348.

94 Cheung MC, Zhao XQ, Chait A. Antioxidant supplements block the response of HDL to simvastatin-niacin therapy in patients with coronary artery disease and low HDL. *Arterioscler Thromb Vasc Biol* 2001; 21: 1320–1326.

95 Block KI, Koch AC, Mead MN, *et al*. Impact of antioxidant supplementation on chemotherapeutic efficacy: a systematic review of the evidence from randomized controlled trials. *Cancer Treat Rev* 2007; 33(5): 407–418.

Arginine

Description

Arginine is a non-essential amino acid.

Action

Arginine has several functions.[1,2] It:
- is involved in the synthesis of urea in the liver
- is a substrate for nitric oxide synthetase and therefore a precursor to nitric oxide (NO); NO causes vasodilatation in endothelial cells
- regulates pH in blood and in the extracellular environment
- has antihypertensive and antioxidant properties
- influences blood viscosity and the coagulation/fibrinolysis system
- influences risk of atherosclerosis
- influences endothelial function
- it becomes essential (indispensable) during growth and catabolic states because it is thought to promote secretion of anabolic hormones (human growth hormone and insulin).

Dietary sources

Arginine is found naturally in foods, such as red meat, poultry, fish and dairy products.

Bioavailability

Arginine is well utilised in humans with low absolute and relative urinary excretion and rapid return to basal blood values.[3] There are no pharmacokinetic studies on the long-term administration of arginine in healthy human subjects. Data from animal studies suggest that humans should be able to tolerate supplemental doses of 6–15 g arginine daily in addition to the dietary intake which averages 4–6 g daily.[4]

Possible uses

Because arginine is a substrate for NO synthesis, supplements have been evaluated for a role in cardiovascular disease. L-Arginine has also been evaluated for potential benefit in erectile dysfunction, as an ergogenic aid during physical training, in glucose metabolism, immune function, wound healing and cancer management.

Cardiovascular disease

Preliminary studies have shown that oral L-arginine supplementation can improve endothelial function and blood flow and reduce cell adhesion. A RCT in 27 young hypercholesterolaemic subjects found that L-arginine 7 g three times daily for 4 weeks significantly improved endothelium-dependent dilatation.[5] A further trial in hypercholesterolaemic patients demonstrated that L-arginine 8.4 g daily restores NO activity and inhibits platelet aggregation.[6] However, another RCT in 47 subjects with hypercholesterolaemia given 3.3 g L-arginine twice daily for 2 weeks (in the form of HeartBar) found no favourable effects on either endothelial or platelet function.[7]

A trial in 10 men with angiographically proven atherosclerosis also found that L-arginine 7 g three times daily improved endothelium-dependent dilatation and reduced endothelial cell adhesion.[8] Adhesiveness of mononuclear cells in hypercholesterolaemia was shown in a further study to be reversed by administration of L-arginine 8.4 g daily for 2 weeks.[9] In a placebo-controlled trial involving 35 patients, oral administration of 6 g daily of L-arginine acutely improved endothelium-dependent, flow-mediated dilatation of the brachial artery in patients with essential hypertension.[10] Other trials have found that L-arginine increases exercise capacity in patients with angina[11] and improves functional status in heart failure.[12] The administration of L-arginine (700 mg four times daily) modified or prevented the development of nitrate tolerance during continuous glyceryl trinitrate therapy.[13]

In patients with coronary artery disease, oral supplementation of L-arginine (6 g daily) did not affect exercise-induced changes in QT interval duration, QT dispersion or the magnitude of ST segment depression. However, it significantly increased exercise tolerance, most likely due to improved peripheral vasomotion.[14]

A trial in 10 healthy postmenopausal women showed no effect of L-arginine 9 g daily on either nitric oxide production or vascular dilatation.[15]

Arginine supplementation has also been evaluated in patients with peripheral arterial disease (PAD). In one trial, 39 patients with intermittent claudication were randomly assigned to receive 2×8 g L-arginine daily, or 2×40 µg prostaglandin E_1 (PGE_1) daily, or no haemodynamically active treatment for 3 weeks. Arginine improved pain-free walking distance, absolute walking distance and endothelium-dependent vasodilatation in the femoral artery. These effects were associated with improvements in the clinical symptoms of intermittent claudication in these patients.[16] A further trial also found that L-arginine supplementation increased pain-free walking distance and absolute walking distance in patients with PAD.[17]

However, a more recent pilot study (for a larger trial) found no difference in symptom of intermittent claudication between groups given 0, 3, 6 or 9 g L-arginine daily for 12 weeks. However, a trend was observed for a greater increase in walking distance in the group treated with 3 g L-arginine daily, and there was a trend for an improvement in walking speed in patients treated with L-arginine.[18] A long-term trial of 3 g arginine daily for 6 months in 133 patients

with PAD found no increase in NO synthesis or vascular reactivity and concluded that L-arginine is not useful in patients with intermittent claudication and PAD.[19]

Erectile dysfunction

On the basis that L-arginine is a precursor of NO and impaired penile endothelial L-arginine NO activity appears to play a role in erectile dysfunction,[20] arginine supplementation has been investigated for a role in this condition. Similar mechanisms have been established for alterations in L-arginine–NO pathways for both erectile dysfunction and atherosclerosis, supporting the concept that there is a reduction in NO bioavailability contributing to vascular changes in both conditions.[21] Studies have also shown correlations between the presence of erectile dysfunction and clinical or subclinical ischaemic heart disease.[22]

Human clinical trials of L-arginine for erectile dysfunction have yielded mixed results. In one small, uncontrolled trial of men with erectile dysfunction who were administered 2.8 g arginine daily for 2 weeks, 40% of men in the treatment group reported improvement, compared to none in the placebo group.[23] In a larger, double-blind trial, 50 men with confirmed erectile dysfunction were administered 5 g L-arginine daily or matching placebo for six weeks. Of the men taking L-arginine, 31% reported a significant subjective improvement in sexual function, although objective variables assessed remained unchanged. All patients reporting subjective improvements had had initially low urinary NO excretion, which had doubled by the end of the study.[24] L-Arginine may therefore be more effective in erectile dysfunction patients with alterations in endothelial L-arginine–NO activity and a reduction in NO availability. A further randomised, placebo-controlled, crossover study evaluating 1.5 g L-arginine daily (a lower dose than other studies) for 17 days found no benefit in erectile dysfunction.[25]

In a further study of 40 men aged 25–45 years given a combination of L-arginine and pycnogenol (oligomeric proanthocyanidins; OPCs) from pine bark in a 3-month trial, during the first month patients received 1.7 g L-arginine daily; during the second month 40 mg pycnogenol twice daily was added and during the third month the dose of pycnogenol was increased to 40 mg three times daily. After the first month 5% of patients experienced a normal erection. The following month, with the addition of 80 mg pycnogenol, 80% of men reported normal erection, and after the third month of treatment this increased to 92.5%. These men also experienced a decrease in time until erection developed in response to stimulation, as well as extended duration of erection.[26]

In a more recent study of randomised, double-blind, placebo-controlled, crossover design, 50 patients with mild to moderate erectile dysfunction were treated for 1 month with placebo or a combination of L-arginine aspartate and pycnogenol (Prelox). Patients reported sexual function from diaries. Testosterone levels and endothelial NO synthetase were monitored along with routine clinical chemistry. Intake of this product for 1 month restored erectile function to normal. Intercourse frequency doubled while endothelial NO synthetase in spermatozoa and testosterone levels in blood increased significantly. Cholesterol levels and blood pressure were lowered. No unwanted effects were reported. The authors concluded that Prelox is a promising alternative to treat mild to moderate erectile dysfunction.[27] Pycnogenols have been associated with increased NO synthesis[28] and pycnogenol and L-arginine may act synergistically to increase the synthesis of NO.

Physical training

Amino acids, including arginine, are commonly ingested as ergogenic acids in the belief that they enhance protein synthesis, strength and stimulate growth hormone (GH) release. In one RCT, arginine (1 g daily) and ornithine (1 g daily) in conjunction with a high-intensity strength training programme, increased total strength and lean body mass and aided in recovery from chronic stress by quelling tissue breakdown as evidenced by lower urinary hydroxyproline levels.[29]

Arginine supplementation does not appear to influence GH. In one study, seven male bodybuilders were supplemented on four occasions after an 8 h fast with either a placebo, a 2.4 g arginine/lysine supplement, a 1.85 g ornithine/tyrosine supplement, or a 20 g Bovril drink. The main finding was that serum GH concentrations were not altered consistently in these healthy young men.[30] In a further study, ingestion of 1500 mg arginine and 1500 mg lysine immediately before resistance exercise did not alter exercise-induced changes in GH in young men. However, when the same amino acid mixture was ingested under basal conditions, the acute secretion of GH is increased.[31] In a study involving 20 young and eight older volunteers, oral arginine (5 g daily) did not stimulate GH secretion and may impair GH release during resistive exercise.[32]

Glucose metabolism

In a study involving 33 patients with diabetes, oral L-arginine treatment (8.3 g daily) for 21 days resulted in an additive effect compared with a diet and exercise training programme alone on glucose metabolism and insulin sensitivity. Furthermore, it improved endothelial function, oxidative stress and adipokine release in obese type 2 diabetic patients with insulin resistance.[33]

In a study involving 12 lean, type 2 diabetic patients, L-arginine treatment (3 g three times daily) significantly improved but did not completely normalise peripheral and hepatic insulin sensitivity.[34]

A 10 g oral dose of L-arginine was found to have no effect on blood glucose disposal in human subjects after oral carbohydrate ingestion, either when rested or after different modes of exercise known to differentially affect glucose disposal.[35]

Immune function

Preliminary *in vitro* studies have suggested that arginine may improve immune response. However, arginine (8.5 g or 17 g daily for 4 weeks) did not enhance lymphocyte proliferation or interleukin 2 production in nursing home residents with pressure ulcers.[36] In a randomised, double-blind, placebo-controlled study in 55 HIV-infected outpatients, arginine supplementation (7.4 g daily) had no effect on immunological parameters (CD4 and CD8 lymphocyte counts, tumour necrosis factor soluble receptors, viraemia) or body weight.[37]

Wound healing

Arginine supplementation (in doses of 17 g daily or 24.8 g daily) has been shown to significantly enhance the amount of collagen deposited in a wound, suggesting that arginine may be of clinical benefit in improving wound healing and immune response.[38] In a double-blind, placebo-controlled trial, 30 healthy men and women received supplements containing 17 g of arginine each day. Arginine supplementation for 2 weeks significantly enhanced wound catheter hydroxyproline accumulation (a measure of collagen deposition) and total protein content. Arginine did not influence the DNA content or the rate of epithelialisation of the skin defect. Peripheral blood lymphocyte responses to mitogenic and allogenic stimulation were greater in the arginine supplemented group. Serum insulin-like growth factor-1 levels were significantly elevated in the arginine group. The authors concluded that arginine supplementation may improve wound healing and immune responses in the elderly.[39]

Cancer

High doses of arginine prior to chemotherapy have been shown to improve some immune parameters in those with breast and colon cancer. A small study involving 10 patients with breast cancer found that 30 g L-arginine administered before chemotherapy delayed the onset and severity of immunosuppression compared to placebo and also stimulated natural killer and lymphokine-activated killer cell activity.[40] A larger trial in which 96 breast cancer patients were randomised to receive 3 g L-arginine or placebo for 3 days before each of six chemotherapy treatments during 21 days found no difference in response between the groups. However, in patients with tumours less than 6 cm in initial diameter, histopathological responses were significantly improved with L-arginine.[41] In a study involving 18 patients with colorectal cancer, L-arginine 30 g daily significantly altered the spectrum of tumour infiltrating lymphocytes.[42]

> ## Conclusion
> There is preliminary evidence that L-arginine improves endothelial function and blood flow in people with hypercholesterolaemia and atherosclerosis, but not all trials have shown benefit in people with coronary heart disease. Evidence also exists that L-arginine

> supplementation can improve symptoms and ability to walk in patients with peripheral arterial disease but, again, not all trials show benefit.
> Evidence of benefit for L-arginine in erectile dysfunction is mixed but promising. Evidence that L-arginine is of benefit in sporting activities, glucose metabolism and immune function is very limited.

Precautions/contraindications

Caution should be taken in patients with herpes simplex virus since arginine is required for the replication of the virus. Theoretically, arginine supplementation may exacerbate outbreaks of herpes. Caution is also required in patients on medication for hypertension, angina and other cardiovascular disease. Arginine should not be taken in any medical condition without medical supervision.

Pregnancy and breast-feeding

No problems reported. L-Arginine 12 g daily for 2 days has been used with apparent safety in women with gestational length of 28 to 36 weeks.[43] There are no longer term data in pregnancy, so arginine is best avoided.

Adverse effects

Arginine is well tolerated but supplements may increase sodium and water loss. Arginine may or may not affect lysine levels. Supplementation may deplete glycine levels. Gastrointestinal side-effects have been reported.

Interactions

None reported. However, high intakes of any amino acid may interfere with the metabolism of other amino acids.

Dose

Not established. Doses used in studies have varied between 3 and 20 g daily depending on the condition (usually 3–6 g daily in cardiovascular conditions). Products (i.e. tablets, capsules, drinks, powders) containing various doses (0.5–3 g) are available.

References

1 Tousoulis D, Antoniades C, Tentolouris C, *et al.* L-Arginine in cardiovascular disease: dream or reality? *Vasc Med* 2002; 7: 203–211.

2 Tousoulis D, Boger RH, Antoniades C, *et al.* Mechanisms of disease: L-arginine in coronary atherosclerosis–a clinical perspective. *Nat Clin Pract Cardiovasc Med* 2007; 4: 274–283.

3 Cynober L. Pharmacokinetics of arginine and related amino acids. *J Nutr* 2007; 137(Suppl2): 1646S–1649S.

4 Wu G, Bazer FW, Cudd TA, *et al.* Pharmacokinetics and safety of arginine supplementation in animals. *J Nutr* 2007; 137(Suppl2): 1673S–1680S.

5 Clarkson P, Adams MR, Powe AJ, *et al.* Oral L-arginine improves endothelium-dependent dilation in hypercholesterolemic young adults. *J Clin Invest* 1996; 97: 1989–1994.

6 Wolf A, Zalpour C, Theilmeier G, *et al.* Dietary L-arginine supplementation normalizes platelet aggregation in hypercholesterolemic humans. *J Am Coll Cardiol* 1997; 29: 479–485.

7 Abdelhamed AI, Reis SE, Sane DC, *et al.* No effect of an L-arginine-enriched medical food (HeartBars) on endothelial function and platelet aggregation in subjects with hypercholesterolemia. *Am Heart J* 2003; 145: E15.

8 Adams MR, McCredie R, Jessup W, *et al.* Oral L-arginine improves endothelium-dependent dilatation and reduces monocyte adhesion to endothelial cells in young men with coronary artery disease. *Atherosclerosis* 1997; 129: 261–269.

9 Theilmeier G, Chan JR, Zalpour C, *et al.* Adhesiveness of mononuclear cells in hypercholesterolemic humans is normalized by dietary L-arginine. *Arterioscler Thromb Vasc Biol* 1997; 17: 3557–3564.

10 Lekakis JP, Papathanassiou S, Papaioannou TG *et al.* Oral L-arginine improves endothelial dysfunction in patients with essential hypertension. *Int J Cardiol* 2002; 86: 317–323.

11 Ceremuzynski L, Chamiec T, Herbaczynska-Cedro K. Effect of supplemental oral L-arginine on exercise capacity in patients with stable angina pectoris. *Am J Cardiol* 1997; 80: 331–333.

12 Rector TS, Bank AJ, Mullen KA, *et al.* Randomized, double-blind, placebo-controlled study of supplemental oral L-arginine in patients with heart failure. *Circulation* 1996; 93: 2135–2141.

13 Parker JO, Parker JD, Caldwell RW, *et al.* The effect of supplemental L-arginine on tolerance development during continuous transdermal nitroglycerin therapy. *J Am Coll Cardiol* 2002; 39: 1199–1203.

14 Bednarz B, Wolk R, Chamiec T, *et al.* Effects of oral L-arginine supplementation on exercise-induced QT dispersion and exercise tolerance in stable angina pectoris. *Int J Cardiol* 2000; 75: 205–210.

15 Blum A, Hathaway L, Mincemoyer R, *et al.* Effects of oral L-arginine on endothelium-dependent vasodilation and markers of inflammation in healthy postmenopausal women. *J Am Coll Cardiol* 2000; 35: 271–276.

16 Boger RH, Bode-Boger SM, Thiele W, *et al.* Restoring vascular nitric oxide formation by L-arginine improves the symptoms of intermittent claudication in patients with peripheral arterial occlusive disease. *J Am Coll Cardiol* 1998; 32: 1336–1344.

17 Maxwell AJ, Anderson BE, Cooke JP. Nutritional therapy for peripheral arterial disease: a double-blind, placebo-controlled, randomized trial of HeartBar. *Vasc Med* 2000; 5: 11–19.

18 Oka RK, Szuba A, Giacomini JC, Cooke JP. A pilot study of L-arginine supplementation on functional capacity in peripheral arterial disease. *Vasc Med* 2005; 10: 265–274.

19 Wilson AM, Harada R, Nair N, *et al.* L-Arginine supplementation in peripheral arterial disease: no benefit and possible harm. *Circulation* 2007; 116: 188–195.

20 Gonzalez-Cadavid NF, Rajfer J. Therapeutic stimulation of penile nitric oxide synthase (NOS) and related pathways. *Drugs Today (Barc)* 2000; 36: 163–174.

21 Sullivan ME, Thompson CS, Dashwood MR, *et al.* Nitric oxide and penile erection: is erectile dysfunction another manifestation of vascular disease? *Cardiovasc Res* 1999; 43: 658–665.

22 Greenstein A, Chen J, Miller H, *et al.* Does severity of ischemic coronary disease correlate with erectile function? *Int J Impot Res* 1997; 9: 123–126.

23 Zorgniotti AW, Lizza EF. Effect of large doses of the nitric oxide precursor, L-arginine, on erectile dysfunction. *Int J Impot Res* 1994; 6: 33–35 discussion 36.

24 Chen J, Wollman Y, Chernichovsky T, *et al.* Effect of oral administration of high-dose nitric oxide donor L-arginine in men with organic erectile dysfunction: results of a double-blind, randomized, placebo-controlled study. *BJU Int* 1999; 83: 269–273.

25 Klotz T, Mathers MJ, Braun M, *et al.* Effectiveness of oral L-arginine in first-line treatment of erectile dysfunction in a controlled crossover study. *Urol Int* 1999; 63: 220–223.

26 Stanislavov R, Nikolova V. Treatment of erectile dysfunction with pycnogenol and L-arginine. *J Sex Marital Ther* 2003; 29: 207–213.

27 Stanislavov R, Nikolova V, Rohdewald P. Improvement of erectile function with Prelox: a randomized, double-blind, placebo-controlled, crossover trial. *Int J Impot Res* 2008; 20: 173–180.

28 Fitzpatrick DF, Bing B, Rohdewald P. Endothelium-dependent vascular effects of pycnogenol. *J Cardiovasc Pharmacol* 1998; 32: 509–515.

29 Elam RP, Hardin DH, Sutton RA, Hagen L. Effects of arginine and ornithine on strength, lean body mass and urinary hydroxyproline in adult males. *J Sports Med Phys Fitness* 1989; 29: 52–56.

30 Lambert MI, Hefer JA, Millar RP, Macfarlane PW. Failure of commercial oral amino acid supplements to increase serum growth hormone concentrations

in male body-builders. *Int J Sport Nutr* 1993; 3: 298–305.

31 Suminski RR, Robertson RJ, Goss FL, *et al.* Acute effect of amino acid ingestion and resistance exercise on plasma growth hormone concentration in young men. *Int J Sport Nutr* 1997; 7: 48–60.

32 Marcell TJ, Taaffe DR, Hawkins SA, *et al.* Oral arginine does not stimulate basal or augment exercise-induced GH secretion in either young or old adults. *J Gerontol A Biol Sci Med Sci* 1999; 54: M395–M399.

33 Lucotti P, Setola E, Monti LD, *et al.* Beneficial effects of a long-term oral L-arginine treatment added to a hypocaloric diet and exercise training program in obese, insulin-resistant type 2 diabetic patients. *Am J Physiol Endocrinol Metab* 2006; 291: E906–E912.

34 Piatti PM, Monti LD, Valsecchi G, *et al.* Long-term oral L-arginine administration improves peripheral and hepatic insulin sensitivity in type 2 diabetic patients. *Diabetes Care* 2001; 24: 875–880.

35 Robinson TM, Sewell DA, Greenhaff PL. L-Arginine ingestion after rest and exercise: effects on glucose disposal. *Med Sci Sports Exerc* 2003; 35: 1309–1315.

36 Langkamp-Henken B, Herrlinger-Garcia KA, Stechmiller JK, *et al.* Arginine supplementation is well tolerated but does not enhance mitogen-induced lymphocyte proliferation in elderly nursing home residents with pressure ulcers. *J Parenter Enteral Nutr* 2000; 24: 280–287.

37 Pichard C, Sudre P, Karsegard V, *et al.* A randomized double-blind controlled study of 6 months of oral nutritional supplementation with arginine and omega-3 fatty acids in HIV-infected patients. Swiss HIV Cohort Study. *Aids* 1998; 12: 53–63.

38 Barbul A, Lazarou SA, Efron DT, *et al.* Arginine enhances wound healing and lymphocyte immune responses in humans. *Surgery* 1990; 108: 331–336; discussion, 336–337.

39 Kirk SJ, Hurson M, Regan MC, *et al.* Arginine stimulates wound healing and immune function in elderly human beings. *Surgery* 1993; 114: 155–159; discussion 160.

40 Brittenden J, Heys SD, Ross J, *et al.* Natural cytotoxicity in breast cancer patients receiving neoadjuvant chemotherapy: effects of L-arginine supplementation. *Eur J Surg Oncol* 1994; 20: 467–472.

41 Heys SD, Ogston K, Miller I, *et al.* Potentiation of the response to chemotherapy in patients with breast cancer by dietary supplementation with L-arginine: results of a randomised controlled trial. *Int J Oncol* 1998; 12: 221–225.

42 Heys SD, Segar A, Payne S, *et al.* Dietary supplementation with L-arginine: modulation of tumour-infiltrating lymphocytes in patients with colorectal cancer. *Br J Surg* 1997; 84: 238–241.

43 Staff AC, Berge L, Haugen G, *et al.* Dietary supplementation with L-arginine or placebo in women with pre-eclampsia. *Acta Obstet Gynecol Scand* 2004; 83: 103–107.

Bee pollen

Description

Bee pollen consists of flower pollen and nectar from male seed flowers. It is collected by the worker honey bee, mixed with secretions from the bee such as saliva, which contains digestive enzymes, and is then carried back to the beehive on the hind legs of the bee. The pollen is harvested at the entrance to the beehive as bees travel through the wire mesh brushing their legs against a collecting vessel. Commercial quantities of pollen can also be collected directly from the flowers.

Constituents

Bee pollen consists of protein, carbohydrates, minerals, and essential fatty acids such as alpha-linolenic acid and linoleic acids. It also contains small amounts of B vitamins, vitamin C, flavonoids and various amino acids, hormones, enzymes and coenzymes. In nutritional terms the amounts of vitamins and minerals are too small to be significant.

Action

Bee pollen may have antioxidant and anti-inflammatory activity.

Possible uses

Bee pollen has been claimed to be useful for improving prostatitis and benign prostatic hypertrophy, although all the studies conducted so far have been uncontrolled and none published in English. Bee pollen has also been claimed to be beneficial in reducing the risk of atherosclerosis, hypertension and varicose veins, but there are no clinical studies to support these claims.

Two double-blind, placebo-controlled trials in humans have investigated the effects of bee pollen in cross-country runners,[1] and in elderly patients with memory deterioration.[2] However, there were no improvements in running speed or memory function in these two studies.

Precautions/contraindications

Bee pollen is contraindicated in people with a known history of atopy or allergy to pollen or plant products because of the risk of hypersensitivity.[3,4]

Pregnancy and breast-feeding

No problems have been reported, but there have not been sufficient studies to guarantee the safety of bee pollen in pregnancy and breast-feeding.

Adverse effects

Bee pollen may cause allergic reactions, including nausea, vomiting and anaphylaxis. One 19-year-old man with asthma had a fatal reaction to bee pollen.[5] Anecdotally, bee pollen has been shown to promote hyperglycaemia in diabetes.

Interactions

In one case study, consumption of bee pollen led to increased international normalised ratios in a patient taking warfarin.[6]

Dose

Bee pollen is available in the form of capsules and powder.

The dose is not established. Product manufacturers tend to recommend doses of 500–1500 mg daily from capsules or $^1/_2$ to 1 teaspoon of the powder.

References

1 Steben R, Boudreaux P. The effects of pollen and protein extracts on selected blood factors and performance of athletes. *J Sports Med Phys Fitness* 1978; 18: 221–226.

2 Iversen T, Fiirgaard KM, Schriver P, *et al.* The effect of NaO Li Su on memory functions and blood chemistry in elderly people. *J Ethnopharmacol* 1997; 56 (2): 109–116.

3 Pitsios C, Chliva C, Mikos N, *et al.* Bee pollen sensitivity in airborne pollen allergic individuals. *Ann Allergy Asthma Immunol* 2006; 97(5): 703–706.

4 Martin-Munoz MF, Bartolome B, Caminoa M, *et al.* Bee pollen: a dangerous food for allergic children. Identification of responsible allergens. *Allergol Immunopathol (Madr)* 2010; 38(5): 263–265.

5 Prichard M, Turner KJ. Acute hypersensitivity to ingested processed pollen. *Aust N Z J Med* 1985; 15 (3): 346–347.

6 Hurren KM, Lewis CL. Probable interaction between warfarin and bee pollen. *Am J Health Syst Pharm* 2010; 67(23): 2034–2037.

Beta-alanine

Description

Beta-alanine is the rate-limiting precursor of carnosine, a dipeptide with a high concentration in mammalian skeletal muscle.

Action

Beta-alanine leads to muscle carnosine loading, which results in improved performance in high-intensity exercise in both untrained and trained individuals.[1–5] Carnosine is not involved in the classic adenosine triphosphate (ATP)-generating metabolic pathways, suggesting that it has a role in the homeostasis of contracting muscle cells. Carnosine may also attenuate acidosis by acting as a pH buffer, and chronic beta-alanine supplementation can attenuate the fall in blood pH during high-intensity exercise.[6] However, improved contractile performance may also be obtained by an influence of carnosine on improved excitation–contraction coupling and as a defence against reactive oxygen species.[2] High carnosine concentrations are found in individuals with a high proportion of fast-twitch fibres, because these fibres are enriched with the dipeptide. Sprint-trained athletes also display markedly high muscular carnosine, but the acute effect of several weeks of training on muscle carnosine is limited.[2] Beta-alanine availability appears to be more significant than physical training in affecting muscle carnosine synthesis.[7]

Beta-alanine is derived from the diet in omnivorous individuals. Muscle carnosine content is, therefore, probably lower in vegetarians. It is also lower in women and declines with age.[2]

Possible uses

Orally, beta-alanine is used for improving athletic performance and exercise capacity, building lean muscle mass and improving physical functioning in the elderly. Preliminary evidence suggests that beta-alanine might improve some measures of physical performance, especially during high-intensity exercise and strength training.

A 28-day study in 50 untrained healthy men evaluated the effect of beta-alanine and/or creatine monohydrate supplementation on time to fatigue following a cycling test. The results suggested that beta-alanine supplementation may delay the onset of neuromuscular fatigue.[8] In a similar study in young women, beta-alanine supplementation improved cycling performance and time to exhaustion.[9] In a study in experienced resistance-trained men, beta-alanine significantly improved muscular endurance during resistance training, but these effects were not associated with the expected changes in testosterone.[10] However, in a further study in which subjects were given beta-alanine or placebo in addition to simultaneously participating in 10 weeks of resistance training, there was no significant effect of beta-alanine on any exercise parameters measured (whole body strength, isokinetic force production, muscular endurance, body composition).[11]

Beta-alanine has also been shown to improve muscle endurance in older people, a factor that could help to prevent falls.[12]

Precautions/contraindications

None reported.

Pregnancy and breast-feeding

Insufficient data.

Adverse effects

Orally, beta-alanine in healthy volunteers can cause dose-dependent flushing and paraesthesiae, starting on the scalp within 20 minutes of the dose and spreading to most of the body, and lasting for about an hour. This was described as severe with a dose of 40 mg/kg, tolerable with 20 mg/kg, and very mild with 10 mg/kg.[4]

Interactions

None reported.

Dose

Typical doses in studies vary between 3200 mg and 6400 mg daily.

Conclusion

Beta-alanine is rapidly developing as a popular ergogenic nutritional supplement for athletes worldwide, and the currently available scientific literature suggests that its use is evidence based. However, many aspects of the supplement, such as the potential side-effects and the mechanism of action, require additional and thorough investigation by the sports science community.

References

1 Baguet A, Reyngoudt H, Pottier A, *et al.* Carnosine loading and washout in human skeletal muscles. *J Appl Physiol* 2009; 106: 837–842.

2 Derave W, Everaert I, Beeckman S, Baguet A. Muscle carnosine metabolism and β-alanine supplementation in relation to exercise and training. *Sports Med* 2010; 40: 247–263.

3 Derave W, Ozdemir MS, Harris RC, *et al.* Beta-alanine supplementation augments muscle carnosine content and attenuates fatigue during repeated isokinetic contraction bouts in trained sprinters. *J Appl Physiol* 2007; 103: 1736–1743.

4 Harris RC, Tallon MJ, Dunnett M, *et al.* The absorption of orally supplied beta-alanine and its effect on muscle carnosine synthesis in human vastus lateralis. *Amino Acids* 2006; 30: 279–289.

5 Hill CA, Harris RC, Kim HJ, *et al.* Influence of beta-alanine supplementation on skeletal muscle carnosine concentrations and high intensity cycling capacity. *Amino Acids* 2007; 32: 225–233.

6 Baguet A, Koppo K, Pottier A, Derave W. Beta-alanine supplementation reduces acidosis but not oxygen uptake response during high-intensity cycling exercise. *Eur J Appl Physiol* 2009; 108: 495–503.

7 Kendrick IP, Kim HJ, Harris RC, *et al.* The effect of 4 weeks beta-alanine supplementation and isokinetic training on carnosine concentrations in type I and II human skeletal muscle fibres. *Eur J Appl Physiol* 2009; 106: 131–138.

8 Stout JR, Cramer JT, Mielke M, *et al.* Effects of twenty-eight days of beta-alanine and creatine monohydrate supplementation on the physical working capacity at neuromuscular fatigue threshold. *J Strength Cond Res* 2006; 20: 928–931.

9 Stout JR, Cramer JT, Zoeller RF, *et al.* Effects of beta-alanine supplementation on the onset of neuromuscular fatigue and ventilatory threshold in women. *Amino Acids* 2007; 32: 381–386.

10 Hoffman J, Ratamess NA, Ross R, *et al.* Beta-alanine and the hormonal response to exercise. *Int J Sports Med* 2008; 29: 952–958.

11 Kendrick IP, Harris RC, Kim HJ, *et al.* The effects of 10 weeks of resistance training combined with beta-alanine supplementation on whole body strength, force production, muscular endurance and body composition. *Amino Acids* 2008; 34: 547–554.

12 Stout JR, Graves BS, Smith AE, *et al.* The effect of beta-alanine supplementation on neuromuscular fatigue in elderly (55–92 years): a double-blind randomized study. *J Int Soc Sports Nutr* 2008; 5: 21.

Beta-glucan

Description

Beta-glucan is a polysaccharide derived from oat and barley fibre, the cell wall of baker's yeast, and many medicinal mushrooms, such as maitake. Oats and barley contain a mixture of beta-1,3-glucan and beta-1,4-glucan. Yeast and mushrooms contain a mixture of beta-1,3-glucan and beta-1,6-glucan. As a dietary supplement, beta-glucan is available in liquid form, capsules and tablets.

Action

Beta-glucans appear to have antibacterial, antiviral and anti-cancer[1–5] activity and may enhance the anti-tumour activity of monoclonal antibodies.[6,7] Some types of beta-glucan also appear to have cholesterol-lowering capacity.[8]

Possible uses

Oral beta-glucan has been most intensively studied for its influence on plasma cholesterol levels. In a study in 62 healthy men and women, a low dosage of beta-glucan (3 g/day) did not significantly reduce total cholesterol or low-density lipoprotein (LDL) cholesterol.[9] A crossover trial in 18 men with mild hyperlipidaemia involving administration of 8.1–11.9 g beta-glucan daily for 4 weeks found the effect on plasma cholesterol was highly variable between subjects, and there was no evidence of a clinically significant improvement in cardiovascular disease risk across this group.[10] A 5-week parallel design trial in healthy people found that beta-glucan incorporated into fruit juice significantly lowered total and LDL cholesterol.[11]

In a further trial involving 75 men with hypercholesterolaemia, 6 g/day of concentrated oat beta-glucan for 6 weeks significantly reduced total and LDL cholesterol; the LDL cholesterol reduction was greater than the change in the control group.[8] A trial in 38 overweight men with mild hypercholesterolaemia found that 6 g/day of beta-glucan from oats improved lipid profile, reducing total and LDL cholesterol, blood glucose and body weight.[12] Barley beta-glucan has been found to improve the lipid profile in some studies;[13,14] in another study it had a more limited effect dependent on the molecular weight of the beta-glucan.[15] However, a study in rats concluded that the molecular weight of beta-glucan had no influence on the lowering of cholesterol.[16] Nevertheless, an extruded breakfast cereal containing 3 g/day of oat beta-glucan with a high molecular weight (2 210 000 g/mol) or a medium molecular weight (530 000 g/mol) lowered LDL cholesterol similarly by $\approx$0.2 mmol/L (5%), but efficacy was reduced by 50% when molecular weight was reduced to 210 000 g/mol.[17] A trial in 53 people with type 2 diabetes showed that a dose of 3.5 g/day of beta-glucan for 8 weeks did not change the lipid profile and HbA1c in this group.[18]

A systematic review of eight trials showed that the use of barley significantly lowered total cholesterol, LDL cholesterol and triglycerides but did not appear to significantly alter high-density lipoprotein (HDL) cholesterol.[19] A meta-analysis of 112 randomised controlled trials found that overall barley and beta-glucan isolated from barley lowered total and LDL cholesterol concentrations by 0.30 mmol/l (95% CI, −0.39 to −0.21, $P < 0.00001$) and 0.27 mmol/l (95% CI, −0.34 to −0.20, $P < 0.00001$), respectively, compared with control. The pattern of cholesterol-lowering action of barley in this analysis could not be viewed as a dose-dependent response. There were no significant subgroup differences by type of intervention and food matrix.[20]

Conclusion

Beta-glucan from oat and barley fibre has been studied for an effect on cholesterol lowering. Trials to date suggest that doses of 6–15 g daily can improve lipid profile, reducing total and LDL cholesterol.

Precautions/contraindications

Insufficient reliable information.

Pregnancy and breast-feeding

Insufficient data.

Adverse effects

None reported in animal studies.[21,22]

Interactions

None reported.

Dose

Trials of beta-glucan that have been linked with cholesterol lowering have used 6–15 g beta-glucan daily.

References

1 Kobayashi H, Yoshida R, Kanada Y, *et al*. Suppressing effects of daily oral supplementation of beta-glucan extracted from *Agaricus blazei Murill* on spontaneous and peritoneal disseminated metastasis in mouse model. *J Cancer Res Clin Oncol* 2005; 131: 527–538.

2 Zhang M, Chiu LC, Cheung PC, Ooi VE. Growth-inhibitory effects of a beta-glucan from the myce-lium of *Poria cocos* on human breast carcinoma MCF-7 cells: cell-cycle arrest and apoptosis induc-tion. *Oncol Rep* 2006; 15: 637–643.

3 Li B, Cai Y, Qi C, *et al*. Orally administered partic-ulate beta-glucan modulates tumor-capturing den-dritic cells and improves antitumor T-cell responses in cancer. *Clin Cancer Res* 2010; 16: 5153–5164.

4 Volman JJ, Mensink RP, Ramakers JD, *et al*. Dietary (1→3), (1→4)-beta-D-glucans from oat activate nuclear factor-kappaB in intestinal leukocytes and enterocytes from mice. *Nutr Res* 2010; 30: 40–48.

5 Murphy EA, Davis JM, Brown AS, *et al*. Benefits of oat beta-glucan on respiratory infection following exercise stress: role of lung macrophages. *Am J Physiol Regul Integr Comp Physiol* 2008; 294: R1593–R1599.

6 Cheung NK, Modak S, Vickers A, Knuckles B. Orally administered beta-glucans enhance anti-tumor effects of monoclonal antibodies. *Cancer Immunol Immunother* 2002; 51: 557–564.

7 Hong F, Yan J, Baran JT, *et al*. Mechanism by which orally administered beta-1,3-glucans enhance the tumoricidal activity of antitumor monoclonal antibodies in murine tumor models. *J Immunol* 2004; 173: 797–806.

8 Queenan KM, Stewart ML, Smith KN, *et al*. Concentrated oat beta-glucan, a fermentable fiber, lowers serum cholesterol in hypercholesterolemic adults in a randomized controlled trial. *Nutr J* 2007; 6: 6.

9 Lovegrove JA, Clohessy A, Milon H, Williams CM. Modest doses of beta-glucan do not reduce concen-trations of potentially atherogenic lipoproteins. *Am J Clin Nutr* 2000; 72: 49–55.

10 Keogh GF, Cooper GJ, Mulvey TB, *et al*. Randomized controlled crossover study of the effect of a highly beta-glucan-enriched barley on cardio-vascular disease risk factors in mildly hypercholes-terolemic men. *Am J Clin Nutr* 2003; 78: 711–718.

11 Naumann E, vanRees AB, Onning G, *et al*. Beta-glucan incorporated into a fruit drink effectively lowers serum LDL-cholesterol concentrations. *Am J Clin Nutr* 2006; 83: 601–605.

12 Reyna-Villasmil N, Bermudez-Pirela V, Mengual-Moreno E, *et al*. Oat-derived beta-glucan signifi-cantly improves HDLC and diminishes LDLC and non-HDL cholesterol in overweight individuals with mild hypercholesterolemia. *Am J Ther* 2007; 14: 203–212.

13 Keenan JM, Goulson M, Shamliyan T, *et al*. The effects of concentrated barley beta-glucan on blood lipids in a population of hypercholesterolaemic men and women. *Br J Nutr* 2007; 97: 1162–1168.

14 Shimizu C, Kihara M, Aoe S, *et al*. Effect of high beta-glucan barley on serum cholesterol concentra-tions and visceral fat area in Japanese men: a ran-domized, double-blinded, placebo-controlled trial. *Plant Foods Hum Nutr* 2008; 63: 21–25.

15 Smith KN, Queenan KM, Thomas W, Fulcher RG, Slavin JL. Physiological effects of concen-trated barley beta-glucan in mildly hypercho-lesterolemic adults. *J Am Coll Nutr* 2008; 27: 434–440.

16 Immerstrand T, Andersson KE, Wange C, *et al*. Effects of oat bran, processed to different molecular weights of beta-glucan, on plasma lipids and caecal formation of SCFA in mice. *Br J Nutr* 2010; 104: 364–373.

17 Wolever TM, Tosh SM, Gibbs AL, *et al*. Physicochemical properties of oat beta-glucan influence its ability to reduce serum LDL choles-terol in humans: a randomized clinical trial. *Am J Clin Nutr* 2010; 92: 723–732.

18 Cugnet-Anceau C, Nazare JA, Biorklund M, *et al*. A controlled study of consumption of beta-glucan-enriched soups for 2 months by type 2 diabetic free-living subjects. *Br J Nutr* 2009; 103: 422–428.

19 Talati R, Baker WL, Pabilonia MS, White CM, Coleman CI. The effects of barley-derived soluble fiber on serum lipids. *Ann Fam Med* 2009; 7: 157–163.

20 Abumweis SS, Jew S, Ames NP. Beta-glucan from barley and its lipid-lowering capacity: a meta-analysis of randomized, controlled trials. *Eur J Clin Nutr* 2010; 64: 1472–1480.

21 Delaney B, Carlson T, Frazer S, *et al*. Evaluation of the toxicity of concentrated barley beta-glucan in a 28-day feeding study in Wistar rats. *Food Chem Toxicol* 2003; 41: 477–487.

22 Jonker D, Hasselwander O, Tervila-Wilo A, Tenning PP. 28-day oral toxicity study in rats with high purity barley beta-glucan (Glucagel). *Food Chem Toxicol* 2009; 48: 422–428.

Betaine

Description

Betaine is a cofactor in various methylation reactions.

Action

Betaine works with choline, vitamin B_{12}, and also *S*-adenosyl methionine (SAMe), a derivative of the amino acid methionine, from which homocysteine is synthesised. It reduces homocysteine levels by remethylating homocysteine to produce methionine.

Possible uses

As a supplement, betaine is available in the form of the hydrochloride and as such contains 23% hydrochloric acid. It has been used as a digestive aid to treat people with achlorhydria and to reduce high levels of homocysteine. Whether it can reduce near normal levels of homocysteine is open to question.

Homocysteine reduction

Betaine has been reported to play a role in reducing plasma homocysteine levels, which may reduce the risk of heart disease. A study in 15 healthy men and women aged 18–35 years showed that betaine 6 g daily for 3 weeks reduced plasma homocysteine concentration after 2 weeks by 0.9 μmol/L and after 3 weeks by 0.6 μmol/L.[1] However, the extent of the decrease was much smaller than that in patients with homocystinuria[2] and appears to be smaller than that established by interventions with folic acid.[3] A RCT in 42 obese subjects[4] found that betaine supplementation (6 g daily for 12 weeks) decreased plasma homocysteine concentration by 8.76 ± 1.63 μmol/L/L at the start of the study and 7.93 ± 1.52 μmol/L at the end of the study. More recent research has shown that doses of 3 to 6 g daily (but not 1 g daily) are needed to reduced plasma homocysteine.[5] However, there is insufficient evidence to recommend betaine supplements for the prevention of coronary heart disease. A recent placebo-controlled trial in 63 healthy young people found that betaine 4 g daily had no influence on plasma lipid profile.[6] A further trial in 39 people aged 50–70 years showed that betaine supplementation 6 g daily had no influence on flow mediated dilatation.[7]

Sports performance

Betaine supplementation has been evaluated for sports performance. A placebo-controlled trial in 24 college men found that 2 weeks of betaine supplementation appeared to improve muscle endurance (in a squat exercise, but not a bench press exercise), and increase the quality of exercises performed.[8] A further trial found that betaine supplementation for 14 days improved performance in various squat and jump tests.[9]

Precautions/contraindications

Betaine should be avoided in patients with peptic ulcer.

Pregnancy and breast-feeding

No problems have been reported, but there have not been sufficient studies to guarantee the safety of betaine in pregnancy and breast-feeding.

Adverse effects

Betaine may cause gastrointestinal irritation.

Interactions

None reported.

Dose

Betaine is available in the form of tablets and capsules.

The dose is not established. Dietary supplements provide 250–500 mg in each dose. Doses of up to 6 g daily have been used in studies. An oral dose of 500 mg daily has been found to raise plasma betaine concentration.[10]

References

1 Brouwer IA, Verhoef P, Urgert R. Betaine supplementation and plasma homocysteine in healthy volunteers. *Arch Intern Med* 2000; 160(16): 2546–2547.
2 Wilcken DE, Dudman NP, Tyrrell PA. Homocystinuria due to cystathionine beta-synthase deficiency: the effects of betaine treatment in pyridoxine-responsive patients. *Metabolism* 1985; 34 (12): 1115–1121.
3 Homocysteine Lowering Trialists' Collaboration. Lowering blood homocysteine with folic acid based supplements: meta-analysis of randomised trials. *BMJ* 1998; 316: 894–898.
4 Schwab U, Torronen A, Toppinen L, *et al.* Betaine supplementation decreases plasma homocysteine concentrations but does not affect body weight, body composition, or resting energy expenditure in human subjects. *Am J Clin Nutr* 2002; 76(5): 961–967.
5 Schwab U, Torronen A, Meririnne E, *et al.* Orally administered betaine has an acute and dose-dependent effect on serum betaine and plasma homocysteine concentrations in healthy humans. *J Nutr* 2006; 136(1): 34–38.
6 Schwab U, Alfthan G, Aro A, *et al.* Long-term effect of betaine on risk factors associated with the metabolic syndrome in healthy subjects. *Eur J Clin Nutr* 2010; 65: 70–76.
7 Olthof MR, Bots ML, Katan MB, *et al.* Effect of folic acid and betaine supplementation on flow-mediated dilation: a randomized, controlled study in healthy volunteers. *PLoS Clin Trials* 2006; 1(2): e10.
8 Hoffman JR, Ratamess NA, Kang J, *et al.* Effect of betaine supplementation on power performance and fatigue. *J Int Soc Sports Nutr* 2009; 6(7): 7.
9 Lee EC, Maresh CM, Kraemer WJ, *et al.* Ergogenic effects of betaine supplementation on strength and power performance. *J Int Soc Sports Nutr* 2010; 7 (27): 27.
10 Atkinson W, Elmslie J, Lever M, *et al.* Dietary and supplementary betaine: acute effects on plasma betaine and homocysteine concentrations under standard and postmethionine load conditions in healthy male subjects. *Am J Clin Nutr* 2008; 87 (3): 577–585.

Biotin

Description

Biotin is a water-soluble vitamin and a member of the vitamin B complex.

Nomenclature

Biotin was formerly known as vitamin H or coenzyme R.

Human requirements

See Table 1 for Dietary Reference Values for biotin.

Dietary intake

In the UK, the average dietary intake in adult women is 28 µg daily and in adult men is 39 µg daily. Biotin is also produced by colonic bacteria, but the effect of this on biotin requirements is not known.

Action

Biotin functions as an integral part of the enzymes that transport carboxyl units and fix carbon dioxide. Biotin enzymes are important

Table 1 Dietary Reference Values for biotin (µg/day)

	EU RDA = 150 µg			
Age	UK safe intake	UK EVM	USA AI	FAO/WHO RNI
Males and females				
0–6 months			5	5
7–12 months			6	6
1–3 years			8	8
4–6 years			–	12
4–8 years			12	–
7–9 years			–	20
9–13 years			20	–
10–18 years			–	25
14–18 years			25	–
19–50 years			30	45
51+ years			30	45
11–50+ years	10–20	970	–	–
Pregnancy			30	30
Lactation			35	35

AI = Adequate Intake.
EVM = likely safe daily intake from supplements alone.
RNI = Reference Nutrient Intake.
TUL = Tolerable Upper Intake Level (not determined for biotin).

in carbohydrate and lipid metabolism, and are involved in gluconeogenesis, fatty acid synthesis, propionate metabolism and the catabolism of amino acids.

Dietary sources

Biotin is ubiquitous in the diet. The richest sources of biotin are liver, kidney, eggs, soya beans and peanuts. Meat, wholegrain cereals, wholemeal bread, milk and cheese are also good sources. Green vegetables contain very little biotin.

Metabolism

Absorption

Biotin is absorbed rapidly from the gastrointestinal tract by facilitated transport (at low concentrations) and by passive diffusion (at high concentrations). Absorption is greater in the jejunum than the ileum and minimal in the colon.

Distribution

Biotin is bound to plasma proteins.

Elimination

Excess biotin is excreted largely unchanged in the urine. It also appears in breast milk.

Deficiency

Biotin deficiency is a risk only in those patients on prolonged parenteral nutrition (who will automatically be given multivitamin supplements). Deficiency has been induced by the ingestion of large amounts of raw egg white, which contain the biotin-binding protein, avidin, to a diet low in biotin.[1] Marginal biotin deficiency may also occur in pregnancy.[2]

Symptoms of biotin deficiency include anorexia, nausea, vomiting, dry scaly dermatitis, glossitis, loss of taste, somnolence, panic and an increase in serum cholesterol and bile pigments.

Possible uses

Biotin has been claimed to be of value in the treatment of brittle finger nails, acne, seborrhoeic dermatitis, hair fragility and alopecia, but such claims need further confirmation by controlled clinical trials.

A trial of biotin (2.5 mg four times daily) in women with brittle nails found a 25% increase in nail thickness, as assessed by electron microscopy.[3]

Biotin deficiency has been associated with sudden infant death syndrome (SIDS). In one study, the median biotin levels in the livers of infants who died from SIDS were significantly lower than those of infants who died from explicable causes.[4] However, evidence that biotin deficiency is an important contributory factor in SIDS is circumstantial and there is no unequivocal proof. There is no requirement for biotin supplements in newborn or young infants. Supplements should *not* be sold to parents for this purpose.

Precautions/contraindications

No problems have been reported.

Pregnancy and breast-feeding

No problems have been reported.

Adverse effects

None reported.

Interactions

Drugs

Anticonvulsants (carbamazepine, phenobarbitone, phenytoin and primidone): requirements for biotin may be increased.

Dose

Biotin is available in the form of tablets and capsules. However, it is available mainly in multivitamin preparations.

The dose is not established. Dietary supplements provide 100–300 µg daily.

Upper safety levels

The UK Expert Group on Vitamins and Minerals (EVM) has identified a likely safe total daily intake of biotin from supplements alone of 970 µg.

References

1 Baugh CM, Malone JW, Butterworth Jr, CE. Human biotin deficiency. A case history of biotin deficiency induced by raw egg consumption in a cirrhotic patient. *Am J Clin Nutr* 1968; 21: 173–182.
2 Mock DM, Quirk JG, Mock NI. Marginal biotin deficiency during normal pregnancy. *Am J Clin Nutr* 2002; 75: 295–299.
3 Colombo VE, Gerber F, Bronhofer M, *et al.* Treatment of brittle fingernails and onychoschizia with biotin: scanning electron microscopy. *J Am Acad Dermatol* 1990; 23: 1127–1132.
4 Heard GS, Hood RL, Johnson AR. Hepatic biotin and sudden infant death syndrome. *Med J Aust* 1983; 2: 305–306.

Boron

Description

Boron is an ultratrace mineral.

Human requirements

Boron is essential in plants and some animals, and evidence of essentiality is accumulating in humans; however, requirements have not so far been defined. The Food Standards Agency Expert Vitamins and Minerals (EVM) group set a safe upper level from supplements alone of 5.9 mg daily.

Dietary intake

Most UK diets appear to provide about 2 mg daily.

Action

Boron appears to be important in calcium metabolism, and can affect the composition, structure and strength of bone. It may also influence the metabolism of copper, magnesium, phosphorus, potassium and vitamin D. In addition, boron affects the activity of certain enzymes. It also affects brain function; boron deprivation appears to depress mental alertness.

Dietary sources

Foods of plant origin, especially non-citrus fruits, leafy vegetables and nuts, are rich sources of boron, but there is little in meat, fish and poultry. Beer, wine and cider contain significant amounts.

Metabolism

Absorption

Dietary boron is rapidly absorbed. The mechanism of absorption from the gastrointestinal tract has not been elucidated.

Distribution

Boron is distributed throughout the body tissues; the highest concentrations are found in the bone, teeth, fingernails, spleen and thyroid.

Elimination

Boron is excreted mainly in the urine.

Deficiency

No precise signs and symptoms of boron deficiency have been defined.

Possible uses

Boron has been claimed to prevent osteoporosis and to both prevent and relieve the symptoms of osteoarthritis, as well as to improve memory.

Bone

In a study of 12 post-menopausal women,[1] boron supplementation (3 mg daily) reduced urinary excretions of calcium and magnesium, and elevated serum concentrations of oestradiol and ionised calcium.

A further study[2] has provided evidence that boron can both enhance and mimic some effects of oestrogen ingestion in post-menopausal women. In women receiving oestrogen therapy, an increase in boron intake increased serum oestradiol concentrations to higher levels than when boron intake was low. However, there is no evidence that boron supplements can relieve the symptoms of the menopause. The effects seen in this study did not occur in men or in women not receiving oestrogen therapy. However, another study[3] in men found that supplementation with boron (10 mg a day) significantly increased oestradiol concentrations, and there was also a trend for plasma testosterone to increase. These findings support the contention that, if oestrogen is beneficial to calcium metabolism, then boron might also be beneficial.

However, another study[4] in post-menopausal women showed that 3 mg boron daily had no effect on bone mineral absorption and excretion, plasma sex steroid levels and urinary excretion of pyridinium crosslink markers of bone turnover. Moreover, in this study a low-boron diet appeared to induce hyperabsorption of calcium because positive calcium balances were found in combination with elevated urinary calcium excretion. The authors concluded that this phenomenon may have inhibited or obscured any effect of boron supplementation.

Arthritis

Boron has been claimed to relieve the symptoms of arthritis, but evidence is very weak. Epidemiological studies suggest that incidence of arthritis is higher in areas of the world where boron intake is low, and subjects with arthritis have been found to have lower bone boron concentrations.[5] One double-blind controlled (but not randomised) trial in 20 patients with osteoarthritis found that boron (6 mg daily) improved symptoms in five out of 10 subjects in the treated group, and one out of 10 subjects in the placebo group. However, statistical analysis was not performed because of the small number of subjects.[6]

Brain function

Three placebo-controlled, double-blind randomised trials in 28 healthy adults showed that low dietary boron (0.25 mg/2000 kcal) was associated with poorer performance of a variety of cognitive and psychomotor tasks and also depression of mental alertness than higher intake (3.25 mg/2000 kcal).[7]

Conclusion

There is preliminary evidence that boron has beneficial effects on calcium metabolism in post-menopausal women by preventing calcium loss and bone demineralisation, but no evidence that it can prevent or be of benefit in treating osteoarthritis. There is some evidence that diets low in boron impair cognitive function.

Precautions/contraindications

No problems have been reported.

Pregnancy and breast-feeding

No problems have been reported, but there have not been sufficient studies to guarantee the safety of boron in pregnancy and breast-feeding. However, supplements are probably best avoided because of possible changes in oestrogen metabolism.

Adverse effects

Boron is relatively non-toxic when administered orally at doses contained in food supplements. High oral doses (> 100 mg daily) are associated with disturbances in appetite and digestion, nausea, vomiting, diarrhoea, dermatitis and lethargy.

Toxicity has occurred, especially in children, from the application of boron-containing dusting powders and lotions (in the form of borax or boric acid) to areas of broken skin and mucous membranes. Such preparations are no longer recommended.

Interactions

Nutrients

Riboflavin: large doses of boron may increase excretion of riboflavin.

Magnesium: boron supplementation may reduce urinary magnesium excretion and increase serum magnesium concentrations.

Dose

Boron is available in the form of tablets and capsules.

The dose is not established. Dietary supplements provide, on average, 3 mg per daily dose.

Upper safety levels

The UK Expert Group on Vitamins and Minerals (EVM) has identified a safe total intake of boron for adults from supplements alone of 5.9 mg daily.

The US Tolerable Upper Intake Level (UL) for boron, the highest total amount from diet and supplements unlikely to pose no risk for most people, is 20 mg daily for adults; 17 mg daily for youngsters aged 14–18; 11 mg daily for youngsters aged 9–13; 6 mg daily for children aged 4–8; and 3 mg daily for children aged 1–3.

References

1   Nielsen FH, Hunt CD, Mullen LM, Hunt JR. Effect of dietary boron on mineral, estrogen and testosterone metabolism in postmenopausal women. *FASEB J* 1987; 1: 394–397.
2   Nielsen FH, Mullen LM, Gallagher SK. Effect of boron depletion and repletion on blood indicators of calcium status in humans fed a magnesium-low diet. *J Trace Elem Exp Med* 1990; 3: 45–54.
3   Naghii MR, Samman S. The effect of boron supplementation on its urinary excretion and selected cardiovascular risk factors in healthy male subjects. *Biol Trace Elem Res* 1997; 56: 273–286.
4   Beattie JH, Peace HS. The influence of a low-boron diet and boron supplementation on bone, major mineral and sex steroid metabolism in postmenopausal women. *Br J Nutr* 1993; 69: 871–884.
5   Newnham RE. Essentiality of boron for healthy bones and joints. *Environ Health Perspect* 1994; 102(Suppl. 7): 83–85.
6   Travers RL, Rennie GC, Newnham RE. Boron and arthritis: the results of a double-blind, pilot study. *J Nutr Med* 1990; 1: 127–132.
7   Penland JG. Dietary boron, brain function, and cognitive performance. *Environ Health Perspect* 1994; 102(Suppl. 7): 65–72.

Branched-chain amino acids

Description

Branched-chain amino acids (BCAAs) are a group of essential amino acids. They are all found in the muscle, accounting for one-third of all amino acids in muscle protein.

Constituents

L-Leucine, L-isoleucine, L-valine.

Action

As with all amino acids, the primary function of BCAAs is as precursors for the synthesis of proteins. In addition, they may be broken down if necessary to serve as an energy source. They may be used directly by skeletal muscle, as opposed to other amino acids, which require prior gluconeogenesis in the liver to produce a useful energy source. Muscle tissue appears to demonstrate an increased need for these amino acids during times of intense physical exercise, and there is some evidence that serum BCAA levels fall during exercise.

In addition, because BCAAs are not readily degraded by the liver, they circulate in the blood and compete with the amino acid tryptophan for uptake into the brain. Tryptophan is a precursor of serotonin (5-hydroxytryptamine), which may produce symptoms of fatigue. It appears that exercise increases the ratio of free tryptophan: BCAA, thus raising serotonin levels in the brain. Some researchers think that supplementation with BCAAs will reduce this ratio and raise serum levels of BCAAs, so improving mental and physical performance.

Possible uses

Exercise performance
Researchers have been interested in the potential role of BCAAs in exercise and whether they can improve performance.

A placebo-controlled (not blinded) study involving 193 experienced runners given 16 g BCAAs or placebo showed that running performance was improved in the slow runners but not the fast runners with BCAAs. A second part of the study showed that 7.5 g BCAAs improved mental performance during exercise compared with placebo, but the study has been criticised for lack of dietary control and poor choice of performance measures.[1]

Another placebo-controlled, but in this case double-blind, study in 16 subjects, participating in a 21-day trek at a mean altitude of 3255 m found that supplementation with BCAAs (11.52 g) improved indices of muscle loss and concluded that BCAAs could prevent muscle loss during chronic hypoxia of high altitude.[2]

In a double-blind, placebo-controlled study, 10 endurance-trained male athletes were studied during cycle exercise while ingesting in random order drinks containing sucrose, sucrose plus tryptophan, sucrose plus BCAAs (6 g) or sucrose plus BCAAs (18 g). There were no differences between the treatment groups in time to exhaustion, suggesting that BCAAs did not improve exercise performance. However, BCAAs reduced brain tryptophan uptake and

significantly increased plasma ammonia levels compared to the control group.[3]

In a double-blind, placebo-controlled, randomised, crossover study, nine well-trained male cyclists performed three laboratory trials consisting of 100 km cycling after ingesting either glucose, glucose plus BCAA, or placebo. Neither the glucose nor the BCAAs enhanced performance in these cyclists.[4]

In a further study of seven well-trained male cyclists, perceived exhaustion was 7% lower and ratings of mental fatigue were 15% lower than when they were given placebo, but there was no difference in physical performance. However, the ratio of tryptophan:BCAA, which increased during exercise, remained unchanged or decreased when BCAAs were ingested.[5]

In a double-blind, placebo-controlled trial, six women and seven women participated in a cycle trial in the heat. Cycle time to exhaustion increased with BCAAs, indicating that BCAA supplementation prolongs moderate exercise performance in the heat.[6]

In a further double-blind, placebo-controlled trial, eight subjects performed three exercise trials and were given carbohydrate drinks, carbohydrate plus BCAAs (7 g) or placebo 1 h before and then during exercise. Subjects ran longer with both carbohydrate and carbohydrate plus BCAAs, but there were no differences between the carbohydrate and carbohydrate and BCAA groups, indicating that BCAAs are of no added benefit in exercise.[7]

Other studies have suggested that BCAAs could prevent or decrease the net rate of protein degradation seen in heavy exercise[8,9] while others have not.[10] One study indicated that BCAAs might have a sparing effect on muscle glycogen degradation during exercise[11] while other studies have suggested that BCAA supplementation may reduce the muscle damage associated with endurance exercise[12–15] and muscle soreness.[16] There is also some evidence that BCAAs can alter mood and cognitive performance during exercise[17] and may improve the immune response, reducing the incidence of infections.[18,19]

Miscellaneous
BCAAs can activate glutamate dehydrogenase, an enzyme deficient in amyotrophic lateral sclerosis. In one double-blind, randomised, placebo-controlled trial of BCAA, supplements

helped maintenance of muscle strength and continued ability to walk in such patients.[20] However, a larger study was ended early when BCAAs not only failed to cause benefit, but also led to excess mortality.[21] BCAAs have also been investigated for potential value in anorexia and cachexia. A review concluded that they could exert significant anti-anorectic and anti-cachectic effects and that their supplementation may represent a viable intervention for patients suffering from chronic disease such as cancer, chronic renal failure and liver cirrhosis[22] and for patients at risk of muscle wasting due to age, immobility or bed rest.[23] Increase intake of BCAAs has also been associated with a reduced prevalence of obesity in adults.[24]

> **Conclusion**
> Evidence from well-controlled trials shows no benefit of BCAAs in exercise performance. Benefit has been shown mainly in poorly controlled trials.

Precautions/contraindications

No problems have been reported, but BCAAs should probably not be used in hepatic and renal impairment without medical supervision. However, BCAAs are used occasionally in patients with these conditions but in a medical setting.

Pregnancy and breast-feeding

No problems have been reported, but there have not been sufficient studies to guarantee the safety of BCAAs in pregnancy and breast-feeding.

Adverse effects

None reported, but there are no long-term studies assessing the safety of BCAAs. Large doses of BCAAs ($> 20\,g$) may increase plasma ammonia levels and may impair water absorption, causing gastrointestinal discomfort.

Interactions

None reported. BCAAs compete with aromatic amino acids (e.g. phenylalanine, tyrosine, tryptophan) for transport into the brain.

Dose

BCAAs are available in tablet and powder form.

The dose is not established. Dietary supplements provide 7–$20\,g$ per dose.

References

1 Blomstrand E, Hassmen P, Ekblom B, *et al.* Administration of branched-chain amino acids during sustained exercise – effects on performance and plasma concentrations of some amino acids. *Eur J Appl Physiol Occup Physiol* 1991; 63: 83–88.

2 Schena F, Guerrini F, Tregnaghi P, Kayser B. Branched-chain amino acid supplementation during trekking at high altitude. The effects on loss of body mass, body composition and muscle power. *Eur J Appl Physiol Occup Physiol* 1992; 65: 394–398.

3 VanHall G, Raaymakers J, Saris W, *et al.* Ingestion of branched chain amino acids and tryptophan during sustained exercise in man: failure to affect performance. *J Physiol* 1995; 486: 789–794.

4 Madsen K, MacLean DA, Kiens B, *et al.* Effects of glucose, glucose plus branched chain amino acids or placebo on bike performance over 100 km. *J Appl Physiol* 1996; 81: 2644–2650.

5 Blomstrand E, Hassmen P, Ek S, *et al.* Influence of ingesting a solution of branched chain amino acids on perceived exertion during exercise. *Acta Physiol Scand* 1997; 159: 41–49.

6 Mittleman KD, Ricci MR, Bailey SP. Branched-chain amino acids prolong exercise during heat stress in men and women. *Med Sci Sports Exerc* 1998; 30: 83–91.

7 Davis JM, Welsh RS, DeVolve KL, Alderson NA. Effects of branched-chain amino acids and carbohydrate on fatigue during intermittent, high intensity running. *Int J Sports Med* 1999; 20: 309–314.

8 Blomstrand E, Newsholme EA. Effect of branched-chain amino acid supplementation on the exercise induced change in aromatic amino acid concentration in human muscle. *Acta Physiol Scand* 1992; 146: 293–298.

9 MacLean DA, Graham TE, Saltin B. Branched-chain amino acids augment ammonia metabolism while attenuating protein breakdown during exercise. *Am J Physiol* 1994; 267: E1010–E1022.

10 Blomstrand E, Andersson S, Hassmen P, *et al.* Effect of branched-chain amino acid and carbohydrate supplementation on the exercise-induced change in plasma and muscle concentration of amino acids in human subjects. *Acta Physiol Scand* 1995; 153: 87–96.

11 Blomstrand E, Ek S, Newsholme EA. Influence of ingesting a solution of branched-chain amino acids on plasma and muscle concentrations of amino acids during prolonged submaximal exercise. *Nutrition* 1996; 12: 485–490.

12 Coombes JS, McNaughton LR. Effects of branched-chain amino acid supplementation on serum creatine kinase and lactate dehydrogenase after prolonged exercise. *J Sports Med Phys Fitness* 2000; 40(3): 240–246.

13 Greer BK, Woodard JL, White JP, *et al*. Branched-chain amino acid supplementation and indicators of muscle damage after endurance exercise. *Int J Sport Nutr Exerc Metab* 2007; 17(6): 595–607.

14 Koba T, Hamada K, Sakurai M, *et al*. Branched-chain amino acids supplementation attenuates the accumulation of blood lactate dehydrogenase during distance running. *J Sports Med Phys Fitness* 2007; 47(3): 316–322.

15 Shimomura Y, Inaguma A, Watanabe S, *et al*. Branched-chain amino acid supplementation before squat exercise and delayed-onset muscle soreness. *Int J Sport Nutr Exerc Metab* 2010; 20(3): 236–244.

16 Jackman SR, Witard OC, Jeukendrup AE, *et al*. Branched-chain amino acid ingestion can ameliorate soreness from eccentric exercise. *Med Sci Sports Exerc* 2010; 42(5): 962–970.

17 Hassmen P, Blomstrand E, Ekblom B, Newsholme EA. Branched chain amino acid supplementation during 30-km competitive run: mood and cognitive performance. *Nutrition* 1994; 10: 405–410.

18 Bassit RA, Sawada LA, Bacurau RF, *et al*. The effect of BCAA supplementation upon the immune response of triathletes. *Med Sci Sports Exerc* 2000; 32(7): 1214–1219.

19 Bassit RA, Sawada LA, Bacurau RF, *et al*. Branched-chain amino acid supplementation and the immune response of long-distance athletes. *Nutrition* 2002; 18(5): 376–379.

20 Plaitakis A, Smith J, Mandeli J, Yahr MD. Pilot trial of branched-chain amino acids in amyotrophic lateral sclerosis. *Lancet* 1988; 1: 1015–1018.

21 The Italian ALS Study Group. Branched-chain amino acids and amyotrophic lateral sclerosis: a treatment failure? *Neurology* 1993; 43: 2466–2470.

22 Charlton M. Branched-chain amino acid enriched supplements as therapy for liver disease. *J Nutr* 2006; 136(Suppl1): 295S–298S.

23 Laviano A, Muscaritoli M, Cascino A, *et al*. Branched-chain amino acids: the best compromise to achieve anabolism? *Curr Opin Clin Nutr Metab Care* 2005; 8: 408–414.

24 Qin LQ, Xun P, Bujnowski D, *et al*. Higher branched-chain amino acid intake is associated with a lower prevalence of being overweight or obese in middle-aged East Asian and Western adults. *J Nutr* 2011; 141(2): 249–254.

Brewer's yeast

Description

Brewer's yeast is *Saccharomyces cerevisiae*.

Constituents

The average nutrient composition of dried brewer's yeast is shown in Table 1.

Possible uses

Brewer's yeast is a useful source of B vitamins and several minerals (see Table 1).

Brewer's yeast has been used to treat diarrhoea caused by *Clostridium difficile*.[1] A review concluded that it appears successful in many cases, but it is unclear whether it acts as a probiotic or as a source of B vitamins.[2]

A specific yeast-based supplement has also been evaluated for the common cold and allergic rhinitis. In a 12-week, randomised, double-blind, placebo-controlled clinical trial, 116 participants who had received influenza vaccination received daily supplementation with 500 mg EpiCor or placebo for 12 weeks. Participants receiving the yeast-based product had significantly fewer symptoms and significantly shorter duration of symptoms compared with subjects taking a placebo.[3] A concurrent trial in 116 subjects with no history of influenza vaccination found that subjects receiving the intervention experienced a statistically significant reduction in the incidence $(P = 0.01)$, a

Table 1 Average nutrient composition of dried brewer's yeast

Nutrient	Per teaspoon 8 g	RNI, approx. (%)[1]
Vitamin A	Trace	–
Thiamine (mg)	1.2	133
Riboflavin (mg)	0.4	33
Niacin (mg)	2.0	14
Vitamin B_6 (mg)	0.2	16
Folic acid (µg)	320	160
Pantothenic acid (mg)	0.9	–
Biotin (µg)	16	–
Vitamin C	Trace	–
Calcium (mg)	6	0.9
Magnesium (mg)	18	6
Potassium (mg)	160	4.5
Phosphorus (mg)	103	19
Iron (mg)	1.6	13
Zinc (mg)	0.6	7
Copper (mg)	0.4	33
Chromium (µg)		
Selenium (µg)		

[1]Reference Nutrient Intake for men aged 19–50 years.
Note: Brewer's yeast tablets contain approximately 300 mg brewer's yeast per tablet; extra B vitamins are often added.

non-significant reduction in duration ($P = 0.10$), with no impact on the severity ($P = 0.90$) of colds or flu-like symptoms, but a more favorable safety profile compared with subjects receiving placebo.[4]

A further 12-week RCT in 96 subjects found that the same supplement significantly reduced the mean severity of specific allergic rhinitis symptoms, including a significant reduction in nasal congestion ($P = 0.04$) and rhinorrhoea ($P = 0.005$), and a non-significant reduction in ocular discharge symptoms. A significantly reduced total number of days with nasal congestion (12.5 fewer days; $P = 0.04$) favoured EpiCor compared with placebo, as did the nasal congestion section of the quality of life questionnaire ($P = 0.04$). Subjects receiving the intervention also experienced significantly ($P = 0.03$)

higher salivary IgA levels. Adverse events were similar to placebo.[5]

Because brewer's yeast contains chromium it has been claimed to help in the control of blood glucose levels. It is also claimed to prevent hypercholesterolaemia. However, there is insufficient evidence for these claims.

Conclusion

Brewer's yeast has a suggested value in controlling blood glucose levels, preventing hypercholesterolaemia and controlling diarrhoea caused by *Clostridium difficile*. Little evidence is available to support its efficacy in all but the last of these conditions. A specific yeast supplements has been associated with reduced incidence and duration of the common cold and with reduction in symptoms in allergic rhinitis.

Precautions/contraindications

Brewer's yeast should be avoided by patients taking monoamine oxidase inhibitors (see Interactions). It is also best avoided by patients with gout; this is because of high concentrations of nucleic acids, which may lead to purine formation.

Pregnancy and breast-feeding

No problems have been reported.

Adverse effects

None reported except flatulence.

Interactions

Drugs
Monoamine oxidase inhibitors: may provoke hypertensive crisis.

Dose

Brewer's yeast is available in the form of tablets and powder.

The dose is not established.

References

1 Schellenberg D, Bonington A, Champion CM, *et al.* Treatment of *Clostridium difficile* diarrhoea with brewer's yeast. *Lancet* 1994; 343: 171.

2 Sargent G, Wickens H. Brewers' yeast in *C. difficile* infection: probiotic or B group vitamins. *Pharm J* 2004; 273: 230–231.

3 Moyad MA, Robinson LE, Zawada ETJr, *et al.* Effects of a modified yeast supplement on cold/flu symptoms. *Urol Nurs* 2008; 28(1): 50–55.

4 Moyad MA, Robinson LE, Zawada ET, *et al.* Immunogenic yeast-based fermentate for cold/flu-like symptoms in nonvaccinated individuals. *J Altern Complement Med* 2010; 16(2): 213–218.

5 Moyad MA, Robinson LE, Kittelsrud JM, *et al.* Immunogenic yeast-based fermentation product reduces allergic rhinitis-induced nasal congestion: a randomized, double-blind, placebo-controlled trial. *Adv Ther* 2009; 26(8): 795–804.

Bromelain

Description

Bromelain is the name for the protease enzymes extracted from the stem and fruit of fresh pineapple. The commercial supplement is usually obtained only from the stem of the pineapple, which contains a higher concentration of the enzymes than the fruit.

Constituents

Bromelains are sulphydryl proteolytic enzymes, including several proteases. In addition, bromelain also contains small amounts of non-proteolytic enzymes (including acid phosphatase, peroxidase and cellulase), polypeptide protease inhibitors and organically bound calcium.

Action

Bromelain is an anti-inflammatory agent and is thought to act through direct or indirect effects on inflammatory mediators, such as bradykinin. It inhibits the enzyme thromboxane synthetase, which converts prostaglandin H_2 into pro-inflammatory prostaglandins and thromboxanes. Bromelain also stimulates the breakdown of fibrin, which stimulates pro-inflammatory prostaglandins responsible for fluid retention and clot formation. It also appears to promote the conversion of plasminogen to plasmin, causing an increase in fibrinolysis. Bromelain also appears to have effects on the immune system, activating natural killer cells and increasing production of tumour necrosis factor-alpha, interferon-gamma, interleukin-1, interleukin-2, interleukin-6 and granulocyte–macrophage colony-stimulating factor *in vitro*.[1]

Possible uses

Various claims are made for the value of bromelain supplementation, but much of the research underpinning these claims was carried out in the 1960s and 1970s, and there are very few well-controlled human studies.

Bromelain has been associated with improvement in symptoms of sinusitis, acceleration of wound healing, potentiation of antibiotic action, healing of gastric ulcers, treatment of inflammation and soft tissue injuries, reduction in severity of angina, reduction in sputum production in patients with chronic bronchitis and pneumonia and decrease in symptoms of thrombophlebitis.[2]

Sinusitis

Two double-blind, placebo-controlled studies showed that bromelain 160 mg (400 000 units) could reduce some symptoms of sinusitis.[3,4] However, headache was not improved in either study. In a more recent study in children with acute sinusitis, treatment with bromelain shortened the duration of symptoms and speeded recovery compared with usual care.[5]

Musculoskeletal injuries

In animals, bromelain promotes healing after acute injury.[6] Human studies suggest similar benefits. In a double-blind, placebo-controlled trial,[7] 146 boxers with bruises to the face and haematomas to the eyes, lips, ears, arms and chest received either 160 mg bromelain daily or placebo for 14 days. At day 4, 78% of the bromelain-treated group was completely cured of bruises compared with 15% of the placebo group. However, this result was not tested for statistical significance. In injuries to the musculoskeletal system resulting in strains and torn ligaments, bromelain produced a reduction in swelling, pain at rest and during movement, and tenderness.[8] Bromelain, in combination with other enzymes, has been found to to reduce soreness and soft tissue injury associated with unaccustomed exercise.[9,10] However, in a trial comparing ibuprofen and bromelain for muscle soreness as result of exercise, there was no difference between treatments.[11]

Arthritis

There is preliminary clinical evidence that the anti-inflammatory and analgesic properties of bromelain help to reduce symptoms of osteo- and rheumatoid arthritis. In an open-label trial involving 77 subjects suffering from mild knee pain, ingestion of bromelain (200 and 400 mg) resulted in improvements in total symptoms, stiffness and physical function in a dose-dependent manner. The authors concluded that double-blind, placebo-controlled studies are now warranted to confirm these results.[12] A combination of bromelain, trypsin and rutin was compared with diclofenac in 103 patients with osteoarthritis of the knee. After 6 weeks, both treatments resulted in significant and similar reductions in pain and inflammation.[13] In another 6-week trial, diclofenac or a combination of bromelain, trypsin and rutin in patients with osteoarthritis of the hip reduced pain and joint stiffness equally well.[14] In another study, bromelain given to individuals with knee osteoarthritis for 12 weeks resulted in no improvement compared with the placebo group.[15]

Surgical procedures

Bromelain has been reported in at least two studies[16,17] to reduce the degree and duration of swelling and oral pain with oral surgery. However, one study was not controlled and the other had no statistical analysis.

Antibacterial action

Bromelain could be useful as an anti-diarrhoeal agent. In an *in vitro* study,[18] bromelain was shown to prevent intestinal fluid secretion mediated by *Escherichia coli* and *Vibrio cholerae*, and in other studies[19,20] to protect piglets from diarrhoea. *In vitro* evidence also suggest potential effects against *Candida albicans*.[21] Pitryasis lichenoides chronica is an infectious skin disease of unknown aetiology and bromelain reportedly caused complete resolution of this condition.[22]

Cardiovascular disease

Bromelain has been reported to reduce the severity of angina,[23] and several *in vitro* studies have demonstrated that bromelain reduces platelet aggregation,[24,25] is an effective fibrinolytic agent, and inhibits thrombus formation.[25] Animal studies suggest that bromelain limits myocardial injury in ischaemia reperfusion experiments, aiding functional recovery of the heart.[26,27] In humans, a decrease in the incidence of coronary infarct after administration of bromelain plus potassium and magnesium orotate has been reported.[28]

Ulcerative colitis

Animal studies have shown that bromelain can reduce the incidence and severity of colonic inflammation and colitis.[29,30] A letter from two US consultants[31] stated that two patients with ulcerative colitis not responding to medical therapy achieved complete clinical and endoscopic remission after initiation of therapy with bromelain.

Cystitis

One double-blind study in humans revealed that bromelain was effective in treating non-infectious cystitis.[32]

Cancer

Several animal and human studies suggest that bromelain might have some anticancer activity.[33–35] Bromelain, in doses over 1000 mg daily, has been combined with chemotherapeutic agents such as fluoruracil and vincristine, resulting in tumour regression.[33,34]

> **Conclusion**
>
> Many claims have been made for bromelain, based largely on studies conducted in the 1960s and 1970s. Many of the published trials are uncontrolled human studies or animal or *in vitro* studies, and well-controlled clinical trials are required to establish the role of bromelain as a potential supplement.

Precautions/contraindications

No problems have been reported, but based on the potential pharmacological activity of bromelain, i.e. that it may inhibit platelet aggregation, bromelain should be used with caution in patients with a history of bleeding or haemostatic disorders.

Pregnancy and breast-feeding

No problems have been reported, but there have been insufficient studies to guarantee the safety of bromelain in pregnancy and breast-feeding.

Adverse effects

None reported, but there are no long-term studies assessing the safety of bromelain.

Interactions

Drugs

Bromelain has been documented to increase blood and urine levels of some antibiotics in humans.[36–38]

Theoretically, bleeding tendency may be increased with anticoagulants, aspirin and antiplatelet drugs.

Dose

Bromelain is available in the form of tablets, capsules and powders. A variety of designations have been used to indicate the activity of bromelain. These include rorer units (ru), gelatine-dissolving units (gdu) and milk-clotting units (mcu). One gram of bromelain standardised to 2000 mcu would be approximately equal to 1 g with 1200 gdu of activity or 8 g with 100 000 ru of activity.[1]

The dose is not established. Dietary supplements provide 125–500 mg in a dose.

References

1 Anon. Bromelain monograph. *Altern Med Rev* 2010; 15(4): 361–368.
2 Anon. Bromelain. *Altern Med Rev* 1998; 3: 302–308.
3 Seltzer AP. Adjunctive use of bromelains in sinusitis: a controlled study. *Eye Ear Nose Throat Mon* 1967; 46(10): 1281–1288.
4 Ryan RE. A double-blind clinical evaluation of bromelains in the treatment of acute sinusitis. *Headache* 1967; 7(1): 13–17.
5 Braun JM, Schneider B, Beuth HJ. Therapeutic use, efficiency and safety of the proteolytic pineapple enzyme Bromelain-POS in children with acute sinusitis in Germany. *In Vivo* 2005; 19(2): 417–421.
6 Aiyegbusi AI, Duru FI, Anunobi CC, *et al.* Bromelain in the early phase of healing in acute crush Achilles tendon injury. *Phytother Res* 2010; 25(1): 49–52.
7 Blonstein J. Control of swelling in boxing injuries. *Practitioner* 1960; 185: 78.
8 Masson M. Bromelain in blunt injuries of the locomotor system. A study of observed applications in general practice. *Fortschr Med* 1995; 113(19): 303–306.
9 Miller PC, Bailey SP, Barnes ME, *et al.* The effects of protease supplementation on skeletal muscle function and DOMS following downhill running. *J Sports Sci* 2004; 22(4): 365–372.
10 Buford TW, Cooke MB, Redd LL, *et al.* Protease supplementation improves muscle function after eccentric exercise. *Med Sci Sports Exerc* 2009; 2: 2.
11 Stone MB, Merrick MA, Ingersoll CD, *et al.* Preliminary comparison of bromelain and ibuprofen for delayed onset muscle soreness management. *Clin J Sport Med* 2002; 12(6): 373–378.
12 Walker AF, Bundy R, Hicks SM, *et al.* Bromelain reduces mild acute knee pain and improves well-being in a dose-dependent fashion in an open study of otherwise healthy adults. *Phytomedicine* 2002; 9 (8): 681–686.
13 Akhtar NM, Naseer R, Farooqi AZ, *et al.* Oral enzyme combination versus diclofenac in the treatment of osteoarthritis of the knee–a double-blind prospective randomized study. *Clin Rheumatol* 2004; 23(5): 410–415.
14 Klein G, Kullich W, Schnitker J, *et al.* Efficacy and tolerance of an oral enzyme combination in painful osteoarthritis of the hip. A double-blind, randomised study comparing oral enzymes with non-steroidal anti-inflammatory drugs. *Clin Exp Rheumatol* 2006; 24(1): 25–30.
15 Brien S, Lewith G, Walker AF, *et al.* Bromelain as an adjunctive treatment for moderate-to-severe osteoarthritis of the knee: a randomized placebo-controlled pilot study. *Q J Med* 2006; 99(12): 841–850.

16 Tassman G, Zafran JN, Zayon GM. Evaluation of a plant proteolytic enzyme for the control of inflammation and pain. *J Dent Med* 1964; 19: 73–77.

17 Tassman GC, Zafran JN, Zayon GM. A double-blind crossover study of a plant proteolytic enzyme in oral surgery. *J Dent Med* 1965; 20: 51–54.

18 Mynott TL, Guandalini S, Raimondi F, *et al.* Bromelain prevents secretion caused by *Vibrio cholerae* and *Escherichia coli* enterotoxins in rabbit ileum in vitro. *Gastroenterology* 1997; 113(1): 175–184.

19 Mynott TL, Luke RK, Chandler DS. Oral administration of protease inhibits enterotoxigenic *Escherichia coli* receptor activity in piglet small intestine. *Gut* 1996; 38(1): 28–32.

20 Chandler D, Mynott TL. Bromelain protects piglets from diarrhoea caused by oral challenge with K88-positive enterotoxigenic *Escherichia coli*. *Gut* 1998; 43: 196–202.

21 Brakebusch M, Wintergerst U, Petropoulou T, *et al.* Bromelain is an accelerator of phagocytosis, respiratory burst and killing of *Candida albicans* by human granulocytes and monocytes. *Eur J Med Res* 2001; 6(5): 193–200.

22 Massimiliano R, Pietro R, Paolo S, *et al.* Role of bromelain in the treatment of patients with pityriasis lichenoides chronica. *J Dermatolog Treat* 2007; 18(4): 219–222.

23 Nieper H. Effect of bromelain on coronary heart disease and angina pectoris. *Acta Med Empir* 1978; 5: 274–278.

24 Heinicke RM, van der Wal L, Yokoyama M. Effect of bromelain (Ananase) on human platelet aggregation. *Experientia* 1972; 28(7): 844–845.

25 Metzig C, Grabowska E, Eckert K, *et al.* Bromelain proteases reduce human platelet aggregation in vitro, adhesion to bovine endothelial cells and thrombus formation in rat vessels in vivo. *In Vivo* 1999; 13(1): 7–12.

26 Neumayer C, Fugl A, Nanobashvili J, *et al.* Combined enzymatic and antioxidative treatment reduces ischemia-reperfusion injury in rabbit skeletal muscle. *J Surg Res* 2006; 133(2): 150–158.

27 Bahde R, Palmes D, Minin E, *et al.* Bromelain ameliorates hepatic microcirculation after warm ischemia. *J Surg Res* 2007; 139(1): 88–96.

28 Nieper HA. Decrease in the incidence of coronary heart infarct by Mg- and K-orotate and bromelain. *Acta Med Empir* 1977; 12: 614–618.

29 Hale LP, Greer PK, Trinh CT, *et al.* Treatment with oral bromelain decreases colonic inflammation in the IL-10-deficient murine model of inflammatory bowel disease. *Clin Immunol* 2005; 116(2): 135–142.

30 Onken JE, Greer PK, Calingaert B, *et al.* Bromelain treatment decreases secretion of pro-inflammatory cytokines and chemokines by colon biopsies in vitro. *Clin Immunol* 2008; 126(3): 345–352.

31 Kane S, Goldberg MJ. Use of bromelain for mild ulcerative colitis. *Ann Intern Med* 2000; 132(8): 680.

32 Lotti T, Mirone V, Imbimbo C, *et al.* Controlled clinical studies of nimesulide in the treatment of urogenital inflammation. *Drugs* 1993; 46(Suppl1): 144–146.

33 Baez R, Lopes MT, Salas CE, *et al.* In vivo antitumoral activity of stem pineapple (*Ananas comosus*) bromelain. *Planta Med* 2007; 73(13): 1377–183.

34 Gerard G. Anticancer treatment and bromelains. *Agressologie* 1972; 13(4): 261–274.

35 Taussig SJ, Szekercze J, Batkin S. Inhibition of tumour growth in vitro by bromelain, an extract of the pineapple plant (*Ananas comosus*). *Planta Med* 1985; 51(6): 538–539.

36 Tinozzi S, Venegoni A. Effect of bromelain on serum and tissue levels of amoxicillin. *Drugs Exp Clin Res* 1978; 4: 21–23.

37 Luerti M, Vignali M. Influence of bromelain on serum and tissue levels of amoxicillin. *Drugs Exp Clin Res* 1978; 4: 45–48.

38 Renzini G, Varengo M. Absorption of tetracycline in presence of bromelain after oral administration. *Arzneimittelforschung* 1972; 22: 410–412.

Calcium

Description

Calcium is an essential mineral.

Human requirements

Dietary Reference Values for calcium are shown in Table 1.

Dietary intake

In the UK, the average diet provides: for men, 1007 mg daily; women, 774 mg daily.

Action

Calcium has a structural role in bones and teeth. Some 99% of calcium is found in the skeleton. Bone mineral density (BMD) increases during the first three decades of life, reaching its peak at about the age of 30. After this age, BMD declines, and the decline increases more rapidly in women after the menopause. However, BMD also declines in older men. Calcium is also essential for cellular structure, blood clotting, muscle contraction, nerve transmission, enzyme activation and hormone function.

Dietary sources

Dietary sources of calcium are shown in Table 2.

Metabolism

Absorption
Calcium is absorbed in the duodenum, jejunum and ileum by an active saturable process that involves vitamin D. At high intakes, some calcium is absorbed by passive diffusion (independent of vitamin D). It can also be absorbed from the colon.

Distribution
More than 99% of the body's calcium is stored in the bones and teeth. The physiologically active form of calcium is the ionised form (in the blood). Blood calcium levels are controlled homeostatically by parathyroid hormone, calcitonin and vitamin D and a range of other hormones.

Elimination
Excretion of calcium occurs in the urine, although a large amount is reabsorbed in the kidney tubules, the amount excreted varying with the quantity of calcium absorbed and the degree of bone loss. Elimination of unabsorbed and endogenously secreted calcium occurs in the faeces. Calcium is also lost in the sweat and is excreted in breast milk.

Bioavailability

Bioavailability is dependent to some extent on vitamin D status. Absorption is reduced by phytates (present in bran and high-fibre cereals), but high-fibre diets at currently recommended levels of intake do not significantly affect calcium absorption in the long term. Absorption is reduced by oxalic acid (present in cauliflower, spinach and rhubarb). High sodium intake may reduce calcium retention.

The efficiency of absorption is increased during periods of high physiological requirement (e.g. in childhood, adolescence, pregnancy and breast-feeding) and impaired in the elderly.

Deficiency

Simple calcium deficiency is not a recognised clinical disorder. However, low dietary intake during adolescence and young adulthood may reduce peak bone mass and bone mineral content and increase the risk of osteoporosis in later life.

However, requirements may be increased and/or and supplements may be necessary in:

- children, adolescents, pre- and postmenopausal women;

Table 1 Dietary Reference Values for calcium (mg/day)

							EU RDA = 800 mg
Age	UK			EVM	USA		WHO RNI
	LRNI	EAR	RNI		AI	TUL	
0–6 months	240	400	525		210	–	300[1]
7–12 months	240	400	525		270	–	400
1–3 years	200	275	350		500	2500	500
4–6 years	275	350	450		–	–	600
4–8 years	–	–	–		800	2500	–
7–10 years	325	425	550		800	–	700[2]
9–18 years	–	–	–		1300	2500	–
Males							
11–14 years	450	750	1000		–	–	1300[3]
15–18 years	450	750	1000		–	–	1300
19–24 years	400	525	700	1500	–	2500	1000
25–50 years	400	525	700	1500	1000	2500	1000
50+ years	400	525	700	1500	1200	2500	1000[4]
Females							
11–14 years	480	625	800		–	–	1300[3]
15–18 years	480	625	800		–	–	1300
19–50 years	400	525	700	1500	1000	2500	1000
50+ years	400	525	700	1500	1200	2500	1300
Pregnancy	*	*	*		1000[5]	2500	1200[6]
Lactation			+550		1000[5]	2500	1000

* No increment.
[1] 400 mg for cows' milk feed;   [2] 7–9 years;   [3] 10–14 years;   [4] 1300 mg for men > 65 years;   [5] ≤ 18 years, 1300 mg;   [6] third trimester.
AI = Adequate Intake.
EAR = Estimated Average Reference value.
EVM = Likely safe daily intake from supplements alone.
LRNI = Lowest Reference Nutrient Intake.
RNI = Recommended Nutrient Intake.
TUL = Tolerable Upper Intake Level from diet and supplements.
Note: The National Osteoporosis Society has produced separate guidelines for recommended daily calcium intake as follows:
7–12 years, 800 mg; 13–19 years, 1000 mg; men 20–45 years, 1000 mg; men > 45 years, 1500 mg; women 20–45 years,
1000 mg; women > 45 years, 1500 mg; women > 45 years (using HRT), 1000 mg; pregnant and breast-feeding women, 1200 mg;
pregnant and breast-feeding teenagers, 1500 mg.

- pregnant and breast-feeding women;
- vegans and others who avoid milk and milk products; and
- those with lactose intolerance (because of avoidance of milk and milk products).

Possible uses

The role of calcium has been investigated in a number of conditions, including osteoporosis, hypertension, colon cancer, obesity, menstrual symptoms and pre-eclampsia.

Osteoporosis, fracture and bone health
Calcium supplements may have a role in the prevention of osteoporosis and fracture. Most of the available evidence has been obtained from studies looking at three different population groups (i.e. children and adolescents, pre- and postmenopausal women) (see Table 3).

Table 2 Dietary sources of calcium

Food portion	Calcium content (mg)
Cereal products	
Bread, brown, 2 slices	70
white, 2 slices	70
wholemeal, 2 slices	35
1 chapati	20
Milk and dairy products	
¹/₂ pint (280 ml) **milk, whole, semi-skimmed or skimmed**	350
¹/₂ pint (280 ml) soya milk	50
1 pot *yoghurt, plain* (150 g)	300
fruit (150 g)	*250*
Cheese, Brie (50 g)	270
Camembert (50 g)	*175*
Cheddar (50 g)	360
Cheddar, reduced fat (50 g)	420
Cottage cheese (100 g)	73
Cream cheese (30 g)	35
Edam (50 g)	350
Feta (50 g)	*180*
Fromage frais (100 g)	85
White cheese (50 g)	280
1 egg, size 2 (60 g)	35
Fish	
Pilchards, canned (105 g)	*105*
Prawns (80 g)	*120*
Salmon, canned (115 g)	100
Sardines, canned (70 g)	350
Shrimps (80 g)	100
Whitebait (100 g)	860
Vegetables	
Broccoli (100 g)	40
Spinach (100 g)	*150*
Spring greens (100 g)	75
1 small can baked beans (200 g)	106
Dahl, chickpea (150 g)	100
Lentils, kidney beans or chick peas (105 g)	40–70
(105 g)	40–70
Soya beans, cooked (100 g)	85
Tofu (60 g)	*300*
Fruit	
1 large orange	70
Nuts	
20 almonds	50
1 tablespoon *sesame seeds* (20 g)	*140*
Tahini paste on 1 slice bread (10 g)	70
Milk chocolate (100 g)	*240*

[8] Excellent sources (**bold**); good source (*italics*).

Children and adolescents

Adequate intake of calcium is important throughout life, but seems to be particularly important during skeletal growth and development of peak bone mass.[29,30] There are also data to show that high intake of milk and dairy produce increases bone mineralisation and bone growth in adolescence – effects that may not be due entirely to the high calcium content of milk.[31,32] In addition to other minerals, such as magnesium, phosphorus and zinc (which are themselves important for bone health), milk also provides energy and protein, both of which may stimulate bone growth through their influence on insulin growth factor 1.

Several controlled intervention studies[3,4,8,12] using calcium supplements in children and adolescents have shown that calcium intakes above the current British Reference Nutrient Intake are effective in increasing bone mineral accretion, particularly in those youngsters with habitually low calcium intakes. However, another study has demonstrated that calcium supplementation (500 mg daily) has only a modest effect on BMD in girls aged 12–14 years, and this effect was independent of habitual calcium intake.[14]

Whether any benefits are sustained if calcium intake is reduced is not clear. However, a follow-up study of a trial in which 1000 mg calcium was given to adolescent girls for 1 year has shown that increased bone mineral accretion may be sustained for a period of 3.5 years after supplementation has been discontinued.[16] A further RCT has demonstrated that calcium supplementation given from childhood to young adulthood significantly improved bone accretion during the pubertal growth spurt with a diminishing effect thereafter.[17]

A Cochrane review[33] (also published in the *British Medical Journal*[18]) including 19 trials, has assessed the effectiveness of calcium supplementation for improving BMD in children. There was no effect of calcium supplementation on femoral neck or lumbar spine BMD. There was a small effect on total body bone mineral content and upper limb BMD, but only the effect in the upper limb persisted after supplementation stopped. This effect is unlikely to result in a clinically significant reduction in fracture risk and the review concluded that the results do not support the use of calcium supplementation in healthy children as a public health intervention.

Table 3 Clinical trials and systematic reviews evaluating the effect of calcium on bone

Reference	Duration and type of trial	Dose of calcium	Study group	Outcome measures	Observed effects
Dawson-Hughes et al. (1990)[1]	2-year double-blind, placebo-controlled, randomised trial (US)	500 mg/day calcium	301 healthy postmenopausal women, half of whom had a daily calcium intake <400 mg and half an intake of 400–650 mg	Bone loss from the spine, femoral neck, and radius	In the group with intake of <400 mg, increasing calcium intake to 800 mg daily significantly reduced bone loss
Chapuy et al. (1992)[2]	18 month randomised controlled trial (US)	1200 mg calcium + 800 IU vitamin D_3	3270 elderly women	Frequency of hip fractures and other non-vertebral fractures	Risk of hip fractures and other non-vertebral fractures reduced
Johnston et al. (1992)[3]	3-year, double-blind, placebo-controlled trial (US)	1000 mg/day calcium citrate malate	70 pairs of identical twins (mean age 10±2 years)	BMD in hip and spine	Calcium supplementation increased the rate of increase in BMD
Lloyd et al. (1993)[4]	18 month placebo-controlled study (US)	500 mg/day calcium citrate malate	94 girls (mean age 11.9±0.5 years)	BMD and BMC of the lumbar spine and total body	Significant increase in total body and spine BMD
Reid et al. (1993)[5]	2 year RCT (US)	Calcium 1000 mg/day	122 normal women at least 3 years after they had reached menopause who had a mean dietary calcium intake of 750 mg/day	BMD of total body, lumbar spine, proximal femur	Calcium supplementation significantly slowed axial and appendicular bone loss
Chevalley et al. (1994)[6]	18-month RCT (Switzerland)	800 mg/day calcium	93 elderly vitamin D-replete people, (63 with recent hip fracture)	BMD and incidence of vertebral fracture	Calcium prevented femoral BMD decrease and lowered vertebral fracture rate in the elderly
Rico et al. (1994)[7]	1 year longitudinal study	1 g/day elemental calcium or placebo daily	72 women (mean age 39±4 years)	Total body and regional BMC	Correlation between cumulative calcium dose at the end of treatment and gain in total body BMC

Study	Design	Intervention	Participants	Outcome	Results
Lee et al. (1995)[8]	18-month randomised, double-blind, controlled trial (US)	800 mg/day calcium total, from diet and 300 mg supplement	84 7-year-old Hong Kong Chinese children	Bone mass	Positive effect on bone mass of the spine and radius but no effects on femoral-neck and height increase
Reid et al. (1995)[9]	2-year double-blind RCT (New Zealand)	1 g/day calcium	86 postmenopausal women	BMD total body and regional sites	A sustained reduction in the rate of loss of total body BMD with calcium
Dawson-Hughes et al. (1997)[10]	3-year RCT (US)	500 mg of calcium + 700 IU vitamin D_3	176 men and 213 women living at home (≥ 65 years)	BMD, biochemical measures of bone metabolism, the incidence of non-vertebral fractures	Calcium + vitamin D moderately reduced bone loss at the femoral neck, spine, and total body over the 3-year study period and reduced the incidence of non-vertebral fractures
Chapuy et al. (2002)[11]	A 2-year, multicentre, randomised, double-masked, placebo-controlled trial (Decalyos II, France)	Calcium (1200 mg), vitamin D (800 IU) alone or combined, or placebo	583 ambulatory institutionalised women (mean age 85.2 years)	Bone loss, risk of hip fracture	Calcium + vitamin D reduced both hip bone loss and the risk of hip fracture
Rozen et al. (2003)[12]	A 12 month double-blind, placebo-controlled study (Israel)	Calcium 1000 mg	100 girls with a with habitual calcium intakes < 800 mg/day (mean age 14 ± 0.5 years)	Bone mass accretion	Calcium enhanced bone mineral acquisition, especially in girls > 2 years past the onset of menarche
Di Daniele et al. (2004)[13]	A 30-month randomised placebo-controlled, double-blind trial (Italy)	Calcium 1200 mg + vitamin D 800 IU	120 women (> 45 years)	BMD and BMC	Calcium enhanced BMD
Molgaard et al. (2004)[14]	A 1 year a randomised, double-blind, placebo-controlled trial (Denmark)	Calcium 500 mg/day	113 girls (12–14 years)	BMD and BMC	Calcium supplementation enhanced BMD
Shea et al. (2004)[15]	Meta-analysis	Various	15 trials (1806 participants)	BMD and fractures in postmenopausal women	A small positive effect of calcium on BMD; a trend toward reduction in vertebral fractures, but it is unclear if calcium reduces the incidence of non-vertebral fractures

(Continued)

Table 3 *(continued)*

Reference	Duration and type of trial	Dose of calcium	Study group	Outcome measures	Observed effects
Dodiuk-Gad et al. (2005)[16]	Follow-up study 3.5 years after 1 year RCT[12] (Israel)	1000 mg calcium during previous supplementation study	96 adolescent girls	Bone mineral accretion 3.5 years after RCT	Bone mineral accretion was sustained in the previously calcium-supplemented group
Matkovic et al. (2005)[17]	4 year RCT (optional extension to 7 years) (US)	640 mg calcium	354 adolescent girls with mean dietary calcium of 830 mg daily	Distal and proximal radius BMD, total-body BMD, metacarpal cortical indexes	Calcium supplementation significantly influenced bone accretion
Winzenberg et al. (2006)[18]	Meta-analysis	Various	19 studies involving 2859 children	BMD	Small effect of calcium supplementation on BMD in the upper limb
Jackson et al. (2006)[19]	7 year RCT (US)	1000 mg calcium + vitamin D 800 IU	36 282 postmenopausal women (50–79 years)	Hip fracture	Calcium resulted in a small but significant improvement in hip BMD, but did not significantly reduce hip fracture
Prince et al. (2006)[20]	5-year, double-blind, placebo-controlled study (Australia)	Calcium carbonate 600 mg twice daily	1460 women (>70 years)	Osteoporotic fractures, vertebral deformity, adverse events	Calcium ineffective in preventing fracture through poor compliance; effective in people who are compliant
Zhu et al. (2007)[21]	5-year randomised controlled double-blind trial (Australia)	Calcium 1200 mg/day with placebo, with 1000 IU/day vitamin D₂; or double placebo (control).	120 community-dwelling women (70–80 years)	Hip BMD	Hip BMD was preserved with calcium + vitamin D and calcium alone but not with placebo; benefits seen mainly in those with low 25-hydroxyvitamin D
Bischoff-Ferrari et al. (2007)[22]	Meta-analysis	Various	12 cohort studies, 5 clinical studies	Hip fracture risk	No reduction in hip fracture risk with calcium supplementation

Study	Design	Intervention	Participants	Outcome	Results
Lambert et al. (2008)[23]	18 month RCT (UK)	Calcium 792 mg/day	96 girls with low calcium intakes (mean: 636 mg/day) (mean age 12 years)	Change in total-body, lumbar spine, and total hip BMC during supplementation and 2 years after supplement withdrawal	BMC and BMD increased with calcium but after 42 months gains in BMD and BMC were not evident
Lappe et al. (2008)[24]	2-year RCT (US)	2000 mg/day calcium + 800 IU/day vitamin D	5201 female Navy recruit volunteers	Incidence of stress fracture	21% lower incidence of stress fracture in supplemented group
Bischoff-Ferrari et al. (2008)[25]	4-year RCT (US)	1200 mg calcium daily	930 health participants (mean age 61 years)	Risk of fracture	Calcium reduced risk of all fractures
Reid et al. (2008)[26]	2-year double-blind RCT (New Zealand)	Calcium 600 or 1200 mg/day	323 healthy men (mean age 57 years)	BMD	Calcium 1200 mg/day but not 600 mg/day improved BMD
Nordin et al. (2009)[27]	Meta-analysis	Various	24 trials in postmenopausal women	Bone loss	Calcium supplementation of about 1000 mg daily had a significant preventive effect on bone loss in postmenopausal women for at least 4 years
Yin et al. (2010)[28]	24 month RCT (China)	Calcium 63, 354, 660, or 966 mg/day	257 healthy Chinese adolescents (12–15 years)	Bone mineral accretion	Calcium supplementation more than 230 mg/day for 2 years can improve bone mineral accretion in Chinese male adolescents

BMC, bone mineral content; BMD, bone mineral density.

Pre-menopausal women

In pre-menopausal women, results from studies examining the relationship between dietary calcium intake and bone mass and also those from calcium supplementation studies are contradictory. Some show a positive effect of calcium[7,34] on BMD, but others do not.[35–37]

Postmenopausal women

After the menopause, bone loss occurs at an increasing rate, and while calcium may help to slow the loss, it does not prevent it. Moreover, the influence of calcium at this stage of life seems to vary with the length of time that has passed since the menopause. Most studies fail to show a relationship between calcium intake, from either food or supplements, and bone loss during the 5 years immediately following the menopause. The rapid loss of oestrogen causes a very high rate of bone resorption, which increases serum calcium concentrations and inhibits intestinal absorption of calcium.[38]

In one study,[1] women who had undergone the menopause within the last 5 years had rapid bone loss that was not affected by a calcium supplement of 500 mg a day. However, one RCT in women over 45 showed that calcium and vitamin D supplementation during a 30-month period showed a positive effect on BMD in both peri- and postmenopausal subjects.[13]

In women who were more than 6 years after the menopause (and had a calcium intake of < 400 mg a day), the same supplement significantly reduced bone loss. Another study in women 10 years after the menopause[5] showed that a calcium supplement of 1000 mg a day had a benefit on both total and site-specific bone mass even though their habitual calcium intake was satisfactory, and that this effect of supplementation could last for 4 years and result in fewer fractures.[9]

Using fracture rather than bone loss as the end point, some recent studies have demonstrated a benefit of calcium given with vitamin D in older people. A French study (Decalyos I),[2] showed considerable reduction in fracture rates in a large group of elderly people (mean age 84 ± 6 years) who were living in a nursing home and given 1200 mg calcium with 800 units of vitamin D. Protection became apparent after 6–12 months, and after 3 years the probability of hip fractures was reduced by 29%.

In a further study,[6] also in elderly people, similar results were obtained from calcium supplementation alone, but the subjects were vitamin D replete. Researchers in the USA[10] looked at the effects of 500 mg calcium plus 700 units vitamin D for 3 years in 176 men and 213 women aged 65 or older who were living at home. The supplemented group had a reduced incidence of non-vertebral fracture and lower bone loss in the femoral neck and the total body than the non-supplemented group.

A further study conducted by the French group (Decalyos II) has confirmed the results of Decalyos I and found that calcium (1200 mg) plus vitamin D (800 units) reduces both hip bone loss and the risk of hip fracture in elderly institutionalised women.[11] Analysis of the Decalyos data showed that this supplementation strategy is cost saving.[39] A meta-analysis has confirmed that calcium supplementation slows bone loss in postmenopausal women, with a trend towards a reduction in vertebral fractures.[15]

A trial involving 36 282 postmenopausal women aged 50–79 randomised participants to receive 1000 mg elemental calcium with 400 units vitamin D_3 daily or placebo. There was a small but significant 1% improvement in hip BMD for those taking calcium combined with vitamin D compared with those taking placebo. There was also a 12% reduction in hip fracture, but this was non-significant. However, women who consistently took the full supplement dose experienced a 29% decrease in hip fracture. Women older than 60 had a significant 21% reduction in hip fracture. The supplements had no significant effect on spine or total fractures and were associated with an increased risk of kidney stones.[19]

A 5-year, double-blind, placebo-controlled study involving 1460 women over the age of 70 found that 1200 mg calcium daily was effective in preventing fracture in those who are compliant, but as a public health intervention in the ambulatory elderly population would be ineffective because of poor long-term compliance.[20]

A recent meta-analysis which included 29 trials, involving 63 897 subjects, 58 785 of whom were women, concluded that calcium, or calcium in combination with vitamin D supplementation, is effective in the preventive treatment of osteoporosis in people aged 50 years or older.[40] Supplementation was associated with a reduced rate of bone loss of 0.54% (95%

confidence interval (CI), 0.35 to 0.73; $P < 0.0001$) at the hip and 1.19% (0.76–1.61; $P < 0.001$) in the spine. Treatment was also associated with a 12% risk reduction in fractures of all types (relative risk, 0.88; 95% CI, 0.83 to 0.95; $P = 0.0004$). The fracture risk reduction was significantly greater (24%) in trials in which compliance rate was high ($P < 0.0001$). In addition, the treatment effect was better with calcium doses of 1200 mg or more than with doses <1200 mg and with vitamin D doses of 800 units or more than with doses <800 units.

A systematic review of 32 controlled trials found that calcium supplementation of about 1000 mg daily had a significant preventive effect on bone loss in postmenopausal women, which lasted for 4 years. Doses of less than 700 mg daily were not effective.[27]

Corticosteroid-induced osteoporosis

Steroids cause bone loss and it has been suggested that patients on steroids should receive preventive treatment (e.g. calcium, vitamin D, bisphosphonates, oestrogens). A Cochrane meta-analysis of five trials involving 274 patients found a clinically and statistically significant prevention of bone loss at the lumbar spine and forearm with vitamin D and calcium in corticosteroid treated patients. The authors recommended that because of low toxicity and low cost, all patients being started on corticosteroids should receive prophylactic therapy with calcium and vitamin D.[41]

Hypertension

Epidemiological studies[42,43] support an inverse relationship between the amount of calcium in the diet and blood pressure. However, based on multivariate analyses, the absolute contribution of calcium is very small. Some clinical intervention studies have reported reduction in blood pressure in normotensive and hypertensive subjects[44–46] or no effect.[47] A meta-analysis of 33 RCTs concluded that calcium (800–2000 mg daily) may lead to a small reduction in systolic blood pressure.[48] Another meta-analysis of 22 randomised clinical trials showed that calcium supplements (500–1000 mg daily) produced a significant decrease in systolic but not diastolic blood pressure, but the authors concluded that the effect was too small to support the use of calcium supplementation in hypertension.[49] Calcium may be most effective in patients with hypertension who are Afro-Caribbean[50] or who are responsive to manipulation of dietary sodium.[51]

A Cochrane review of 13 RCTs found that calcium supplementation was associated with a statistically significant reduction in systolic blood pressure (mean difference –2.5 mmHg; 95% CI, –4.5 to –0.6) but not diastolic blood pressure (mean difference –0.8 mmHg; 95% CI, 2.1 to 0.4). The review concluded that evidence in favour of causal association between calcium supplementation and blood pressure reduction is weak and that longer duration, better quality studies are needed.[52]

Cardiovascular events

Individuals with vascular or valvular calcification are at increased risk for coronary events and the risk of such events was evaluated in a RCT of 36 282 postmenopausal women (50–79 years) given calcium carbonate 500 mg with vitamin D 200 units twice daily or placebo. During 7 years of follow-up, calcium/vitamin D supplementation neither increased nor decreased coronary or cerebrovascular risk in this group of women.[53]

Some more recent studies have shown increased risk of cardiovascular events with calcium supplementation[54] while others have not.[55–57] A meta-analysis of 15 studies found that calcium without coadministered vitamin D increased the risk of myocardial infarction.[58] When this meta-analysis was extended, calcium with or without vitamin D was found to increase the risk of cardiovascular events, particularly myocardial infarction.[59] This paper included a post-hoc analysis of the Women's Health Initiative Study, which evaluated the effect of calcium (1200 mg) and vitamin D (800 IU) on cardiovascular events. No influence of calcium and vitamin D was found in the original study but in this later analysis, women who were taking calcium supplements at the time of randomisation did not have increased risk of cardiovascular events, while those not taking calcium supplements at the time of randomisation did have an increased risk. This suggests that a rapid change in calcium intake could have been the factor increasing risk, although separation of the two groups of women for the post hoc analysis could have influenced the results in that appropriate randomisation was not assured (as was the case in the original study).[59]

Cancer

Calcium supplementation may reduce the occurrence of colorectal cancer, but study results are inconsistent. High calcium intake (1200–1400 mg daily) has been linked with reduced colon cancer risk in epidemiological studies, and high dietary and supplemental calcium have been associated with reduced recurrence of adenomatous polyps,[60–62] and reduced colorectal cancer risk.[63] Other studies have shown no significant effects of calcium supplementation on colorectal cell proliferation in subjects at high risk for colorectal cancer.[64,65] There is also evidence that vitamin D acts with calcium in reducing risk of colorectal adenomal recurrence.[66] A pooled analysis of 10 cohort studies found that higher consumption of calcium is associated with lower risk of colorectal cancer.[67]

Evidence from the Calcium Polyp Prevention Study, which involved patients with recent colorectal adenoma, showed that calcium (1200 mg daily) may have a more pronounced antineoplastic effect on advanced colorectal lesions than on other types of polyp.[68] Follow-up to this study, which tracked adenoma occurrence for an average of 7 years after the end of randomised treatment, found that the protective effect of calcium supplementation on risk of colorectal adenoma recurrence extended to 5 years.[69] In the Polyp Prevention Trial, calcium and vitamin D intake was inversely associated with recurrence of adenomatous polyps in the large bowel.[70] A recent Cochrane review concluded that evidence from two RCTs suggests that calcium supplementation might contribute to a moderate degree to the prevention of colorectal adenomatous polyps, but that this does not constitute sufficient evidence to recommend the general use of calcium supplements to prevent colorectal cancer.[71] A systematic review and meta-analysis of three trials also suggested that calcium supplementation prevents recurrent colorectal adenomas.[72] Two further observational studies found that total calcium intake (from food and supplements) was inversely associated with colorectal cancer in women[73] and also in both men and women,[74] so supporting the hypothesis for a protective role of calcium. A recent meta-analysis of six studies found that that supplemental calcium was effective for the prevention of adenoma recurrence in populations with a history of adenomas, but no similar effect was apparent in populations at higher or lower risk.[75]

Calcium has been associated with increased risk of prostate cancer. In the Physicians' Health Study, men consuming > 600 mg calcium a day from dairy products had a 32% higher risk of prostate cancer compared with men consuming < 150 mg daily.[76] However, in a recent RCT involving 672 men, calcium 1200 mg daily was not associated with increased prostate cancer risk.[77] A meta-analysis of 12 studies found that high intake of dairy products and calcium may be associated with an increased risk of prostate cancer, although the effect appeared to be small.[78]

Animal studies suggest potential anticarcinogenic effects of calcium on breast cancer development. However, epidemiological data in women have been conflicting. In the Women's Health Study, involving 10 578 pre-menopausal women and 20 909 postmenopausal women, higher intakes of calcium (and vitamin D) were associated with lower risk of breast cancer in pre-menopausal women, but not in postmenopausal women.[79]

Menstrual symptoms

Calcium supplementation (1200 mg daily for three menstrual cycles) was effective in reducing premenstrual but not menstrual pain in a prospective, randomised, double-blind, placebo-controlled trial.[80] In another trial, calcium (1336 mg daily), when given with manganese, reduced menstrual pain and undesirable behavioural symptoms.[81] A further trial showed that calcium (1000 mg daily) reduced both premenstrual and menstrual symptom scores, and there was a significant effect of calcium on menstrual pain.[82]

Pre-eclampsia

Use of calcium supplements during pregnancy may reduce the risk of pre-eclampsia. An analysis of clinical trials that examined the effects of calcium intake on pre-eclampsia and pregnancy outcomes in 2500 women found that those who consumed 1500–2000 mg of calcium a day were 70% less likely to suffer from hypertension in pregnancy.[83] However, a large study involving 4589 healthy first-time mothers found that calcium supplementation

(2000 mg daily) had no effect on the incidence of hypertension, protein excretion or complications of childbirth.[84]

A Cochrane systematic review of pregnancy-induced hypertension[85] (and later published in the *British Journal of Obstetrics and Gynaecology*[86]) identified nine placebo-controlled RCTs. Calcium significantly reduced the relative risk of hypertension, especially in women at high risk of hypertension and with low dietary calcium.[85]

Obesity

Dietary calcium plays a pivotal role in the regulation of energy metabolism. High-calcium diets reduce adipose tissue accretion and weight gain during periods of overconsumption and increase fat breakdown to preserve thermogenesis during energy restriction, thereby accelerating weight loss.[87] A review analysing data from six observational studies and three controlled trials has shown that high calcium intakes are associated with lower weight gain at mid-life.[88] An RCT looking at the effect of calcium supplementation (1000 mg daily) in 100 women found no significant differences between body weight or fat mass changes between the placebo and calcium-supplemented groups. However, there was a trend to increased loss of body weight in the calcium group, which the authors suggested to be consistent with a small effect.[89] A more recent RCT involving 36 282 postmenopausal women (aged 50–79 years) found that calcium (1000 mg daily) and vitamin D (400 units) had a small effect on the prevention of weight gain, which was observed primarily in women who reported inadequate calcium intakes.[90]

> ### Conclusion
> There is evidence that calcium supplementation can improve BMD in adolescents. Calcium may also help to reduce the decline in BMD in postmenopausal women, particularly when given in conjunction with vitamin D. However, there is less evidence that calcium supplementation attenuates the reduction in BMD around the time of the menopause. Calcium supplementation may lower blood pressure, but the effect is too small to recommend its use in hypertension. Evidence linking calcium to colon cancer and prostate cancer is conflicting. There is preliminary evidence that calcium supplementation may help symptoms of premenstrual syndrome, particularly pain, and may also reduce the risk of pre-eclampsia. Evidence of the value of calcium supplements in obesity is limited.

Precautions/contraindications

Calcium supplements should be avoided in conditions associated with hypercalcaemia and hypercalcuria, and in renal impairment (chronic). They should be used with caution and with medical supervision in hypertension because blood pressure control may be altered.

Traditionally, a low-calcium diet was advised in patients with or at risk of kidney stones. Recent studies have suggested that the risk of kidney stones is not increased by calcium.[91–94] In two studies, however, supplemental calcium was positively associated with risk.[19,95] A recent review on developments in stone prevention[96] states: 'Calcium should not be restricted. There is clear evidence from clinical and experimental studies that a normal or high calcium supply is appropriate in calcium stone disease. Only in absorptive hypercalcuria does calcium restriction remain beneficial in combination with thiazide and citrate therapy.'

Pregnancy and breast-feeding

No problems have been reported. Calcium supplements may be required during pregnancy and breast-feeding. Some studies have shown that the use of calcium supplements in pregnancy may lower the risk of pre-eclampsia, while another has not (see above).

Adverse effects

Reported adverse effects with supplements include nausea, constipation and flatulence (usually mild). Calcium metabolism is under such tight control that accumulation in blood or tissues from excessive intakes is almost unknown; accumulation is usually due to failure of control mechanisms. Toxic effects and hypercalcaemia are unlikely with oral doses of

<2000 mg daily. However, in young children, calcium supplements should be used under medical supervision because of a risk of bowel perforation.

Interactions

Drugs

Alcohol: excessive alcohol intake may reduce calcium absorption.

Aluminium-containing antacids: may reduce calcium absorption.

Anticonvulsants: may reduce serum calcium levels.

Bisphosphonates: calcium may reduce absorption of etidronate; give 2 h apart.

Cardiac glycosides: concurrent use with parenteral calcium preparations may increase risk of cardiac arrhythmias (ECG monitoring recommended).

Corticosteroids: may reduce serum calcium levels.

Laxatives: prolonged use of laxatives may reduce calcium absorption.

Loop diuretics: increased excretion of calcium.

4-Quinolones: may reduce absorption of 4-quinolones; give 2 h apart.

Tamoxifen: calcium supplements may increase the risk of hypercalcaemia (a rare side-effect of tamoxifen therapy); calcium supplements are best avoided.

Tetracyclines: may reduce absorption of tetracyclines; give 2 h apart.

Thiazide diuretics: may reduce calcium excretion.

Nutrients

Fluoride: may reduce absorption of fluoride and vice versa; give 2 h apart.

Iron: calcium carbonate or calcium phosphate may reduce absorption of iron; give 2 h apart (absorption of iron in multiple formulations containing iron and calcium is not significantly altered).

Vitamin D: increased absorption of calcium and increased risk of hypercalcaemia; may be advantageous in some individuals.

Zinc: may reduce absorption of zinc.

Dose

Calcium is available in the form of tablets and capsules. A review of 35 US calcium supplements showed that four brands contained lower levels of calcium than claimed on the label. However, none of the products failed testing for exceeding contamination levels for lead and other heavy metals. Another survey showed that calcium supplements may contain lead,[97] but levels were not high enough to cause concern.[98]

The dose for potential prevention of osteoporosis is 1000–1200 mg (as elemental calcium) daily with 800 units of cholecalciferol. Patients who may require supplementation include those aged 65 and over who are confined to their homes and care institutes; postmenopausal women below the age of 65, where lifestyle modification is unsustainable; secondary prevention of osteoporotic fractures in postmenopausal women (this is covered by the 2005 NICE guideline[99]); prevention of osteoporotic fractures in patients taking glucocorticoids.

Note: doses are given in terms of elemental calcium. Patients should be advised that calcium supplements are not identical; they provide different amounts of elemental calcium. The calcium content of various calcium salts commonly used in supplements is shown in Table 4. Calcium carbonate is the most cost effective form of calcium supplement.[100,101] Calcium citrate is equally well absorbed

Table 4   Calcium content of commonly used calcium salts

Calcium salt	Calcium (mg/g)	Calcium (%)
Calcium amino acid chelate	180	18
Calcium carbonate	400	40
Calcium chloride	272	27.2
Calcium glubionate	65	6.5
Calcium gluconate	90	9
Calcium lactate	130	13
Calcium lactate gluconate	129	13
Calcium orotate	210	21
Calcium phosphate (dibasic)	230	23

Note: Calcium lactate and gluconate are more efficiently absorbed than calcium carbonate (particularly in patients with achlorhydria).

(a few studies have shown it to be better absorbed than calcium carbonate[102,103]) and is the supplement of choice for individuals with achlorhydria or who are taking histamine H$_2$ antagonists or protein pump inhibitors. Calcium lactate and calcium gluconate are less concentrated forms of calcium and are not practical oral supplements.

Upper safety levels

The UK Expert Group on Vitamins and Minerals (EVM) has identified a likely safe total intake of calcium for adults from supplements alone of 1500 mg daily.

The US Tolerable Upper Intake Level (UL) for calcium, the highest total amount from diet and supplements unlikely to pose no risk for most people, is 2500 mg daily for adults and children from the age of 12 months.

References

1 Dawson-Hughes B, Dallal GE, Krall EA, et al. A controlled trial of the effect of calcium supplementation on bone density in post-menopausal women. N Engl J Med 1990; 323: 878–883.
2 Chapuy MC, Arlot ME, Duboeuf F, et al. Vitamin D and calcium to prevent hip fractures in elderly women. N Engl J Med 1992; 327: 1637–1642.
3 Johnston CC, Miller JZ, Slemenda CW, et al. Calcium supplementation and increases in bone mineral density in children. N Engl J Med 1992; 327: 82–87.
4 Lloyd T, Andon MB, Rollings N, et al. Calcium supplementation and bone mineral density in adolescent girls. JAMA 1993; 270: 841–844.
5 Reid IR, Ames RW, Evans MC, et al. Effect of calcium supplementation on bone loss in postmenopausal women. N Engl J Med 1993; 328: 460–464.
6 Chevalley T, Rizzoli R, Nydegger V, et al. The effects of calcium supplements on femoral bone mineral density and vertebral fracture rate in vitamin D-replete elderly patients. Osteoporosis Int 1994; 4: 245–252.
7 Rico H, Revilla M, Villa LF, et al. Longitudinal study of the effect of calcium pidolate on bone mass in eugonadal women. Calcif Tissue Int 1994; 54: 47–80.
8 Lee WTK, Leung SSF, Leung DMT, et al. A randomised double-blind controlled calcium supplementation trial and bone and height acquisition in children. Br J Nutr 1995; 74: 125–139.
9 Reid IR, Ames RW, Evans MC, et al. Long term effects of calcium supplementation on bone loss and fractures in postmenopausal women: a randomised controlled trial. Am J Med 1995; 98: 331–335.
10 Dawson-Hughes B, Harris SS, Krall EA, Dallal GE. Effect of calcium and vitamin D supplementation on bone density in men and women 65 years of age or older. N Engl J Med 1997; 337: 670–676.
11 Chapuy MC, Pamphile R, Paris E, et al. Combined calcium and vitamin D3 supplementation in elderly women: confirmation of reversal of secondary hyperparathyroidism and hip fracture risk: the Decalyos II study. Osteoporosis Int 2002; 13: 257–264.
12 Rozen GS, Rennert G, Dodiuk-Gad RP, et al. Calcium supplementation provides an extended window of opportunity for bone mass accretion after menarche. Am J Clin Nutr 2003; 78: 993–998.
13 DiDaniele N, Carbonelli MG, Candeloro N, et al. Effect of supplementation of calcium and vitamin D on bone density and bone mineral content in peri- and post-menopause women; a double-blind, randomized controlled trial. Pharmacol Res 2004; 50: 637–641.
14 Molgaard C, Thomsen BL, Michaelsen KF. Effect of habitual dietary calcium intake on calcium supplementation in 12–14 year old girls. Am J Clin Nutr 2004; 80: 1422–1427.
15 Shea B, Wells G, Cranney A, et al. Calcium supplementation on bone loss in postmenopausal women. Cochrane Database Syst Rev 2004; (1): CD004526.
16 Dodiuk-Gad RP, Rozen GS, Rennert G, et al. Sustained effect of short-term calcium supplementation on bone mass in adolescent girls with low calcium intake. Am J Clin Nutr 2005; 81: 168–174.
17 Matkovic V, Goel PK, Badenhop-Stevens NE. Calcium supplementation and bone mineral density in females from childhood to young adulthood: a randomized controlled trial. Am J Clin Nutr 2005; 81: 175–188.
18 Winzenberg T, Shaw K, Fryer J, Jones G. Effects of calcium supplementation on bone density in healthy children: meta-analysis of randomised controlled trials. BMJ 2006; 333: 775.
19 Jackson RD, LaCroix AZ, Gass M, et al. Calcium plus vitamin D supplementation and the risk of fractures. N Engl J Med 2006; 354: 669–683.
20 Prince RL, Devine A, Dhaliwal SS, Dick IM. Effects of bone supplementation on clinical fracture and bone structure. Arch Intern Med 2006; 166: 869–875.
21 Zhu K, Devine A, Dick IM, et al. Effects of calcium and vitamin D supplementation on hip bone mineral density and calcium-related analytes in elderly ambulatory Australian women: a 5-year randomized controlled trial. J Clin Endocrinol Metab 2007; 93: 743–749.
22 Bischoff-Ferrari HA, Dawson-Hughes B, Baron JA, et al. Calcium intake and hip fracture risk in men and women: a meta-analysis of prospective cohort studies and randomized controlled trials. Am J Clin Nutr 2007; 86(6): 1780–1790.
23 Lambert HL, Eastell R, Karnik K, et al. Calcium supplementation and bone mineral accretion in

adolescent girls: an 18-mo randomized controlled trial with 2-y follow-up. *Am J Clin Nutr* 2008; 87 (2): 455–462.

24 Lappe J, Cullen D, Haynatzki G, *et al.* Calcium and vitamin D supplementation decreases incidence of stress fractures in female navy recruits. *J Bone Mineral Res* 2008; 23(5): 741–749.

25 Bischoff-Ferrari HA, Rees JR, Grau MV, *et al.* Effect of calcium supplementation on fracture risk: a double-blind randomized controlled trial. *Am J Clin Nutr* 2008; 87(6): 1945–1951.

26 Reid IR, Ames R, Mason B, *et al.* Randomized controlled trial of calcium supplementation in healthy, nonosteoporotic, older men. *Arch Intern Med* 2008; 168(20): 2276–2282.

27 Nordin BE. The effect of calcium supplementation on bone loss in 32 controlled trials in postmenopausal women. *Osteoporos Int* 2009; 20(12): 2135–213.

28 Yin J, Zhang Q, Liu A, *et al.* Calcium supplementation for 2 years improves bone mineral accretion and lean body mass in Chinese adolescents. *Asia Pac J Clin Nutr* 2010; 19(2): 152–160.

29 Matkovik V. Calcium metabolism and calcium requirements during skeletal modelling and consolidation of bone mass. *Am J Clin Nutr* 1991; 54 (Suppl): 245S–259S.

30 Recker RR, Davies MK, Hinders SM, *et al.* Bone gain in young adult women. *JAMA* 1992; 268: 2403–2408.

31 Chan GM, Hoffman K, McMurry M. Effects of dairy produce on bone and body composition in pubertal girls. *J Pediatr* 1995; 126: 551–556.

32 Cadogan J, Eastell R, Jones M, Barker ME. A study of bone growth in adolescents: the effect of an 18-month, milk-based dietary intervention. *BMJ* 1997; 315: 1255–1260.

33 Winzenberg TM, Shaw K, Fryer J, Jones G. Calcium supplementation for improving bone mineral density in children. *Cochrane Database Syst Rev* 2006; (2): CD005119.

34 Ramsdale SJ, Bassy EJ, Pye DJ. Dietary calcium intake relates to bone mineral density in premenopausal women. *Br J Nutr* 1994; 71: 77–84.

35 Valimaki MJ, Karkkainen M, Lamberg-Allardt C, *et al.* Exercise, smoking and calcium intake during adolescence and early adulthood as determinants of peak bone mass. *BMJ* 1994; 309: 230–235.

36 New SA, Bolton-Smith C, Grubb DA, Reid DM. Nutritional influences on bone mineral density: a cross sectional study in premenopausal women. *Am J Clin Nutr* 1997; 65: 1831–1839.

37 Earnshaw SA, Worley A, Hosking DJ. Current diet does not relate to bone mineral density after the menopause. The Nottingham Early Postmenopausal Intervention Cohort (EPIC) Study Group. *Br J Nutr* 1997; 78: 65–72.

38 Chiu KM. Efficacy of calcium supplements on bone mass in postmenopausal women. *J Gerontol A Biol Med Sci* 1999; 54: M275–280.

39 Lilliu H, Pamphile R, Chapuy MC, *et al.* Calcium vitamin D$_3$ supplementation is cost-effective in hip fractures prevention. *Maturitas* 2003; 44: 299–305.

40 Tang BM, Eslick GD, Nowson C, *et al.* Use of calcium or calcium in combination with vitamin D supplementation to prevent fractures and bone loss in people aged 50 years and older: a meta-analysis. *Lancet* 2007; 370: 657–666.

41 Homik JJEH, Cranney A, Shea BJ, *et al.* Calcium and vitamin D for corticosteroid-induced osteoporosis. *Cochrane Database. Syst Rev* 1998; (2): CD000952.

42 Iso H, Terao A, Kitamura A. Calcium intake and blood pressure in seven Japanese populations. *Am J Epidemiol* 1991; 133: 776–783.

43 McCarron DA, Morris CD. The calcium deficiency hypothesis of hypertension. *Ann Intern Med* 1987; 107: 919–922.

44 Grobbee DE, Hofman A. Effect of calcium supplementation on diastolic blood pressure in young people with mild hypertension. *Lancet* 1986; 2: 703–707.

45 McCarron DA, Lipkin M, Rivlin RS, Heaney RP. Dietary calcium and chronic diseases. *Med Hypotheses* 1990; 31: 265–273.

46 Kawano Y, Yoshimi H, Matsuoka H, *et al.* Calcium supplementation in patients with essential hypertension: assessment by office, home and ambulatory blood pressure. *J Hypertens* 1998; 16: 1693–1699.

47 Galloe AM, Graudal N, Moller J, *et al.* Effect of oral calcium supplementation on blood pressure in patients with hypertension: a randomised, double blind, placebo-controlled, crossover study. *J Hum Hypertens* 1993; 7: 43–45.

48 Bucher HC, Cook RJ, Guyatt GH, *et al.* Effects of dietary calcium supplementation on blood pressure – a meta-analysis of randomized controlled trials. *JAMA* 1996; 275: 1016–1022.

49 Allender PS, Cutler JA, Follman D, *et al.* Dietary calcium and blood pressure: a meta-analysis of randomized controlled trials. *Ann Intern Med* 1996; 124: 825–831.

50 Zemel MB. Dietary calcium, calcitrophic hormones, and hypertension. *Nutr Metab Cardiovasc Dis* 1994; 4: 224–228.

51 Weinberger MH, Wagner UL, Fineberg NS, *et al.* The blood pressure effects of calcium supplementation in humans of known sodium responsiveness. *Am J Hypertens* 1993; 6: 799–805.

52 Dickinson HO, Nicolson DJ, Cook JV, *et al.* Calcium supplementation for the management of primary hypertension in adults. *Cochrane Database Syst Rev* 2006; (2): CD004639.

53 Hsia J, Heiss G, Ren H, *et al.* Calcium/vitamin D supplementation and cardiovascular events. *Circulation* 2007; 115: 846–854.

54 Bolland MJ, Barber PA, Doughty RN, *et al.* Vascular events in healthy older women receiving calcium supplementation: randomised controlled trial. *BMJ* 2008; 336(7638): 262–266.

55 Lewis JR, Calver J, Zhu K, *et al.* Calcium supplementation and the risks of atherosclerotic vascular disease in older women: results of a 5-year RCT and a 4.5-year follow-up. *J Bone Miner Res* 2010; 26(1): 35–41.

56 Shah SM, Carey IM, Harris T, *et al.* Calcium supplementation, cardiovascular disease and mortality in older women. *Pharmacoepidemiol Drug Saf* 2010; 19(1): 59–64.

57 Manson JE, Allison MA, Carr JJ, *et al.* Calcium/vitamin D supplementation and coronary artery calcification in the Women's Health Initiative. *Menopause* 2010; 17(4): 683–691.

58 Bolland MJ, Avenell A, Baron JA, *et al.* Effect of calcium supplements on risk of myocardial infarction and cardiovascular events: meta-analysis. *BMJ* 2010; 341(29): c3691.

59 Bolland M, Grey A, Avenell A, *et al.* Calcium supplements with or without vitamin D and risk of cardiovascular events: reanalysis of the Womens' Health Iniative limited access dataset and meta-analysis. *BMJ* 2011: 342: d20408.

60 Hofstad B, Almendigen K, Vatn M, *et al.* Growth and recurrence of colorectal polyps: a double-blind 3-year intervention with calcium and antioxidants. *Digestion* 1998; 59: 148–156.

61 Hyman J, Baron JA, Dain BJ, *et al.* Dietary and supplemental calcium and the recurrence of colorectal adenomas. *Cancer Epidemiol Biomarkers Prev* 1998; 7: 291–295.

62 Bonithon-Kopp C, Kronborg Ole Giacosa A, *et al.* Calcium and fibre supplementation in prevention of colorectal adenoma recurrence: randomised intervention trial. *Lancet* 2000; 356: 1300–1306.

63 Terry P, Baron JA, Bergkvist L, *et al.* Dietary calcium and vitamin D intake and risk of colorectal cancer: a prospective cohort in women. *Nutr Cancer* 2002; 43: 39–46.

64 Baron JA, Tosteson TD, Wargovich MJ, *et al.* Calcium supplementation and rectal mucosal proliferation: a randomized controlled trial. *J Natl Cancer Inst* 1995; 87: 1303–1307.

65 Weisberger UM, Boeing H, Owen RW, *et al.* Effect of long-term placebo controlled calcium supplementation on sigmoidal cell proliferation in patients with sporadic adenomatous polyps. *Gut* 1996; 38: 396–402.

66 Grau MV, Baron JA, Sandler RS, *et al.* Vitamin D, calcium supplementation, and colorectal adenoma: results of a randomized trial. *J Natl Cancer Inst* 2003; 95: 1765–1771.

67 Cho E, Smith-Warner SA, Spiegelman D, *et al.* Dairy foods, calcium, and colorectal cancer: a pooled analysis of 10 cohort studies. *J Natl Cancer Inst* 2004; 96: 1015–1022.

68 Wallace K, Baron JA, Cole BF, *et al.* Effect of calcium supplementation on the risk of large bowel polyps. *J Natl Cancer Inst* 2004; 96: 921–925.

69 Grau MV, Baron JA, Sandler RS, *et al.* Prolonged effect of calcium supplementation on risk of colorectal adenomas in a randomized trial. *J Natl Cancer Inst* 2007; 99: 129–136.

70 Hartman TJ, Albert PS, Snyder K, *et al.* The association of calcium and vitamin D with risk of colorectal adenomas. *J Nutr* 2005; 135: 252–259.

71 Weingarten MA, Zalmanovici A, Yaphe J. Dietary calcium supplementation for preventing colorectal cancer and adenomatous polyps. *Cochrane Database Syst Rev* 2005;(2): CD003548.

72 Shaukat A, Scouras N, Schunemann HJ. Role of supplemental calcium in the recurrence of colorectal adenomas: a meta-analysis of randomized controlled trials. *Am J Gastroenterol* 2005; 100: 395–396.

73 Shin A, Li H, Shu XO, Yang G, *et al.* Dietary intake of calcium, fiber and other micronutrients in relation to colorectal cancer risk: results from the Shanghai Women's Health Study. *Int J Cancer* 2006; 119: 2938–2942.

74 Park S-Y, Murphy SP, Wilkens LR, *et al.* Calcium and vitamin D intake and risk of colorectal cancer: the multiethnic cohort study. *Am J Epidemiol* 2007; 165: 784–793.

75 Carroll C, Cooper K, Papaioannou D, *et al.* Supplemental calcium in the chemoprevention of colorectal cancer: a systematic review and meta-analysis. *Clin Ther* 2010; 32(5): 789–803.

76 Chan JM, Stampfer MJ, Ma J, *et al.* Dairy products, calcium and prostate cancer risk in the Physician's Health Study. *Am J Clin Nutr* 2001; 74: 549–554.

77 Baron JA, Beach M, Wallace K, *et al.* Risk of prostate cancer in a randomized clinical trial of calcium supplementation. *Cancer Epidemiol Biomarkers Prev* 2005; 14: 586–589.

78 Gao X, LaValley MP, Tucker KL. Prospective studies of dairy product and calcium intakes and prostate cancer risk: a meta-analysis. *J Natl Cancer Inst* 2005; 97: 1768–1777.

79 Lin J, Manson JE, Lee IM, *et al.* Intakes of calcium and vitamin D and breast cancer risk in women. *Arch Intern Med* 2007; 167: 1050–1059.

80 Thys-Jacobs S, Starkey P, Bernstein D, *et al.* Calcium carbonate and the premenstrual syndrome: effects on premenstrual and menstrual symptoms (Premenstrual Syndrome Study Group). *Am J Obstet Gynecol* 1998; 179: 444–452.

81 Penland JG, Johnson PE. Dietary calcium and manganese effects on menstrual cycle symptoms. *Am J Obstet Gynecol* 1993; 168: 1417–1423.

82 Thys-Jacobs S, Ceccarelli S, Bierman A, *et al.* Calcium supplementation in premenstrual syndrome: a randomized crossover trial. *J Gen Intern Med* 1989; 4: 183–189.

83 Herrara JA, Arevala Herrara M, Herrara S, *et al.* Prevention of preeclampsia by linoleic acid and calcium supplementation: a randomized controlled trial. *Obstet Gynecol* 1998; 91: 585–590.

84 Bucher HC, Guyatt GH, Cook RJ, *et al.* Effect of calcium supplementation on pregnancy induced hypertension and preeclampsia: a meta-analysis of randomized controlled trials. *JAMA* 1996; 275: 1113–1117.

85 Atallah AN, Hofmeyr GJ, Duley L. Calcium supplementation during pregnancy for preventing hypertensive disorders and related problems. *Cochrane Database* 2000; (3): CD001059.

86 Hofmeyr GJ, Duley L, Atallah A. Dietary calcium supplementation for prevention of pre-eclampsia and related problems: a systematic review and commentary. *BJOG* 2007; 114: 933–943.

87 Zemel MB. Regulation of adiposity and obesity risk by dietary calcium: mechanisms and implications. *J Am Coll Nutr* 2002; 21: S146–S151.

88 Heaney RP, Davies KM, Barger-Lux MJ. Calcium and weight: clinical studies. *J Am Coll Nutr* 2002; 21: S152–S155.

89 Shapses SA, Heshka S, Heymsfield SB. Effect of calcium supplementation on weight and fat loss in women. *J Clin Endocrinol Metab* 2004; 89: 632–637.

90 Caan B, Neuhouser M, Aragaki A, *et al.* Calcium plus vitamin D supplementation and the risk of postmenopausal weight gain. *Arch Intern Med* 2007; 167: 893–902.

91 Taylor EN, Stampfer MJ, Curhan GC. Dietary factors and the risk of incident kidney stones in men: new insights after 14 years of follow-up. *J Am Soc Nephrol* 2004; 15: 3225–3232.

92 Curhan GC. A prospective study of dietary calcium and other nutrients and the risk of symptomatic kidney stones. *N Engl J Med* 1993; 328: 833–838.

93 Borghi L, Schianchi T, Meschi T, *et al.* Comparison of two diets for the prevention of recurrent stones in idiopathic hypercalcuria. *N Engl J Med* 2002; 346: 77–84.

94 Sowers MR, Jannausch M, Wood C, *et al.* Prevalence of renal stones in a population-based study with dietary calcium, oxalate and medication exposures. *Am J Epidemiol* 1998; 147: 914–920.

95 Curhan GC, Willett WC, Speizer FE, *et al.* Comparison of dietary calcium with supplemental calcium and other nutrients as factors affecting the risk of kidney stones in women. *Am Intern Med* 1997; 126: 497–504.

96 Straub M, Hautmann RE. Developments in stone prevention. *Curr Opin Urol* 2005; 15: 119.

97 Ross EA, Szabo NJ, Tebbett IR. Lead content of calcium supplements. *JAMA* 2000; 284: 1425–1429.

98 Heaney R. Lead in calcium supplements. Cause for alarm or celebration? *JAMA* 2000; 284: 1263–1270.

99 National Institute for Health and Clinical Excellence. *The Clinical Effectiveness and Cost Effectiveness of Technologies for the Secondary Prevention of Osteoporotic Fractures in Postmenopausal Women.* London: NICE, 2005.

100 Straub DA. Calcium supplementation in clinical practice: a review of forms, doses, and indications. *Nutr Clin Pract* 2007; 22: 286–296.

101 Heaney RP, Dowell MS, Bierman J, *et al.* Absorbability and cost effectiveness in calcium supplementation. *J Am Coll Nutr* 2001; 20: 239–246.

102 Kenny AM, Prestwood KM, Biskup B, *et al.* Comparison of the effects of calcium loading with calcium citrate or calcium carbonate on bone turnover in postmenopausal women. *Osteoporos Int* 2004; 15: 290–294.

103 Heller HJ, Stewart A, Haynes S, Pak CY. Pharmacokinetics of calcium absorption from two commercial calcium supplements. *J Clin Pharmacol* 1999; 39: 1151–1154.

Carnitine

Description

Carnitine is an amino acid derivative.

Nomenclature

Carnitine is sometimes known as vitamin B_T; it is not an officially recognised vitamin.

Constituents

Carnitine exists as two distinct isomers, L-carnitine (naturally occurring carnitine) and D-carnitine (synthetic carnitine). Dietary supplements contain L-carnitine or a DL-carnitine mixture.

Human requirements

No proof of a dietary need exists. Carnitine is synthesised in sufficient quantities to meet human requirements.

Dietary intake

The average omnivorous diet is estimated to provide 100–300 mg carnitine daily.

Dietary sources

Meat and dairy products are the best sources. Fruit, vegetables and cereals are poor sources of carnitine. Carnitine is added to infant milk formulae.

Action

Carnitine has the following physiological functions:
- regulation of long-chain fatty acid transport across cell membranes
- facilitation of beta-oxidation of long-chain fatty acids and keto acids
- transportation of acyl CoA compounds.

Metabolism

Dietary carnitine is absorbed rapidly from the intestine by both passive and active transport mechanisms. Carnitine is synthesised in the liver, brain and kidney from the essential amino acids lysine and methionine.

Deficiency

Primary carnitine deficiency is caused by impairment in the membrane transport of carnitine. Symptoms may include chronic muscle weakness (due to muscle carnitine deficiency), recurrent episodes of coma and hypoglycaemia (usually in infants and children), encephalopathy and cardiomyopathy.

Secondary carnitine deficiency occurs in several inherited disorders of metabolism (particularly organic acidurias and disorders of beta-oxidation).

Despite the fact that plant foods are poor sources of carnitine, there is no evidence that vegetarians are deficient in carnitine. Endogenous synthesis prevents deficiencies.

Possible uses

Carnitine supplementation has been investigated for its potential benefit in cardiovascular disease, exercise performance, chronic fatigue syndrome and Alzheimer's disease.

Cardiovascular disease

Carnitine may be beneficial in patients with ischaemic heart disease, but only in those who have low serum carnitine levels.

Orally administered L-carnitine (2 g daily) has been shown to improve symptoms of angina,[1] and to reduce anginal attacks and glyceryl trinitrate consumption.[2] In a dose of 900 mg daily for 12 weeks, it has also been shown to improve exercise tolerance in patients with stable angina.[3]

Carnitine supplementation (4 g daily) has also been reported to improve heart rate, arterial pressures, angina and lipid patterns in a controlled study of patients who had experienced a recent myocardial infarction.[4] Yet another study showed that L-carnitine (1 g twice daily for 45 days) may be beneficial in congestive heart failure, by reducing heart rate, dyspnoea and oedema, and increasing diuresis. Supplementation also allowed for a reduction in daily digoxin dose.[5] Improvement in vascular tone (measured according to flow mediated dilatation) following a high-fat meal has been shown to improve with L-carnitine (2 g daily) compared with placebo.[6] An 8-week study in 36 patients with coronary artery disease showed that L-carnitine in combination with alpha-lipoic acid improved vascular tone and reduced blood pressure compared with placebo.[7]

Another study has provided some evidence that L-carnitine (2 g twice a day for 3 weeks) increases walking distance in patients with intermittent claudication.[8]

Hyperlipidaemias

Preliminary studies have shown that L-carnitine may reduce blood cholesterol levels. Oral administration of L-carnitine (3–4 g daily) significantly reduced serum levels of total cholesterol or triglyceride or both, and increased those of HDL cholesterol.[9–11] A trial in 30 healthy subjects found that carnitine supplementation combined with 8 weeks of aerobic exercise decreased lipid peroxidation and elevated nitrous oxide but did not further improve lipid profiles in subjects with normal lipid levels.[12]

The influence of carnitine supplementation on lipids has also been evaluated in patients with type 2 diabetes. One double-blind RCT in 12 subjects with type 2 diabetes found that L-carnitine 1 g three times a day for a period of 4 weeks did not improve lipid profile or modify insulin sensitivity.[13] In a 3-month RCT among 81 patients with diabetes comparing carnitine (2 g daily) with placebo, carnitine significantly reduced oxidised LDL levels, LDL cholesterol, triglycerides, apolipoprotein A1, apolipoprotein B-100, thiobarbituric acid-reactive substance concentrations and conjugated diene concentrations, indicating that carnitine favourably modulated the oxidative stress, including LDL oxidation, to which patients with diabetes are prone.[14] In a double-blind RCT in 75 patients with type 2 diabetes, the coadministration of carnitine and simvastatin resulted in a significant reduction in lipoprotein(a) and apoprotein(a), both of which are markers for cardiovascular risk. There was also a significant reduction in glycaemia ($P < 0.001$) and triglycerides ($P < 0.001$) while HDL cholesterol was significantly increased ($P < 0.05$).[15] Oral L-carnitine supplementation has also been shown to reduce the degree of insulin resistance in patients with impaired fasting glucose or diabetes mellitus.[16,17]

Exercise performance

Carnitine has been evaluated for an influence on athletic performance, possibly resulting from changes in metabolism of lipids and carbohydrate, but study findings have not been consistent. Data from a recent study suggest that 2 weeks of L-carnitine supplementation does not affect fat, carbohydrate or protein contribution to metabolism during prolonged moderate-intensity cycling exercise, but suppressed ammonia accumulation indicating that L-carnitine might have the potential to reduce the metabolic stress of exercise.[18] L-Carnitine (1.8 g daily) did not induce significant changes in caloric intake, body composition, resting metabolic rate, respiratory exchange ratio at rest and exercise compared with placebo in 21 overweight active volunteers.[19] In a double-blind, placebo-controlled, crossover trial in 18 healthy middle-aged men and women, L-carnitine supplementation reduced chemical damage to tissues after exercise and optimised the processes of muscle tissue repair and remodelling.[20] L-Carnitine has also been shown to up-regulate androgen receptor response, which might promote recovery from resistance exercise.[21] Doses of 1 g and 2 g L-carnitine daily have been effective in reducing muscle soreness and attenuating muscle stress after exercise.[22] An increase in maximal aerobic power was observed in subjects who received L-carnitine 2 g daily[23] and 4 g daily.[24,25] Other studies have shown no effect of supplemental carnitine on muscle carnitine and exercise performance.[26–28]

Double-blind placebo-controlled trials have shown no benefit of oral carnitine 2 g,[29] 3 g[30] or 4 g[31] on exercise performance in healthy subjects.

Fatigue

Patients with chronic fatigue syndrome have been reported to have low carnitine levels. One crossover (not blinded) parallel-design study randomised 30 patients with chronic fatigue syndrome to either 3 g L-carnitine or 100 mg amantadine.[32] At the end of the 2-month study, the carnitine group experienced clinical improvement in 12 out of the 18 studied parameters. However, no statistical comparison between carnitine and amantadine was conducted.

Carnitine makes an important contribution to cellular energy metabolism and has been investigated in trials involving subjects with mental and physical fatigue. In a placebo-controlled, double-blind RCT involving 84 elderly people, L-carnitine 2 g twice daily or placebo was given for 30 days. At the end of the study, compared with placebo, the patients treated with L-carnitine showed significant improvements in the following parameters: total fat mass (−3.1 vs −0.5 kg), total muscle mass (+2.1 vs +0.2 kg), total cholesterol (−1.2 vs +0.1 mmol/L), LDL cholesterol (−1.1 vs −0.2 mmol/L), HDL cholesterol (+0.2 vs +0.01 mmol/L), triglycerides (−0.3 vs 0.0 mmol/L), apolipoprotein A1 (−0.2 vs 0.0 g/L), and apolipoprotein B (−0.3 vs −0.1 g/L). Wessely and Powell scores decreased significantly by 40% (physical fatigue) and 45% (mental fatigue) in subjects taking L-carnitine, compared with 11% and 8%, respectively, in the placebo group ($P < 0.001$ vs placebo for both parameters). No adverse events were reported in any treatment group. The authors concluded that administration of L-carnitine to healthy elderly subjects resulted in a reduction of total fat mass, an increase of total muscle mass, and appeared to exert a favourable effect on fatigue and serum lipids.[33]

In a further placebo-controlled, randomised, double-blind trial, 66 centenarians with onset of fatigue after even slight physical activity received either 2 g L-carnitine once daily ($n = 32$) or placebo ($n = 34$). Efficacy measures included changes in total fat mass, total muscle mass, serum triacylglycerol, total cholesterol, HDL cholesterol, LDL cholesterol, Mini-Mental State Examination (MMSE), activities of daily living, and a 6-min walking corridor test. At the end of the study period, the L-carnitine-treated subjects, compared with the placebo group, showed significant improvements in the following markers: total fat mass (−1.8 vs 0.6 kg; $P < 0.01$), total muscle mass (3.8 vs 0.8 kg; $P < 0.01$), and plasma concentrations of total carnitine (12.6 vs −1.7 μmol; $P < 0.05$), plasma long-chain acyl-carnitine (1.5 vs −0.1 μmol; $P < 0.001$), and plasma short-chain acylcarnitine (6.0 vs −1.5 μmol; $P < 0.001$). Significant differences were also found in physical fatigue (−4.1 vs −1.1; $P < 0.01$), mental fatigue (−2.7 vs 0.3; $P < 0.001$), fatigue severity (−23.6 vs 1.9; $P < 0.001$) and MMSE (4.1 vs 0.6; $P < 0.001$). The authors concluded that oral administration of L-carnitine produced a reduction of total fat mass, increased total muscular mass and facilitated an increased capacity for physical and cognitive activity by reducing fatigue and improving cognitive functions.[34]

A further trial in 96 people over the age of 70 years found that L-carnitine supplementation reduced physical and mental fatigue and improved cognitive function. Muscle pain, prolonged fatigue after exercise and sleep disorders also improved significantly.[35]

Patients with coeliac disease often suffer from fatigue and carnitine has been investigated in this patient group. In a randomised double-blind versus placebo parallel study, 30 patients with coeliac disease received carnitine 2 g daily while 30 received placebo (both for 180 days). The patients underwent clinical investigation and questionnaires (Scott–Huskisson Visual Analogue Scale for Asthenia, Verbal Scale for Asthenia, Zung Depression Scale, SF-36 Health Status Survey, EuroQoL). Fatigue measured by the Scott–Huskisson Visual Analogue Scale for Asthenia was significantly reduced in the L-carnitine group compared with the placebo group ($P = 0.0021$). OCTN2, the specific carnitine transporter, was decreased in coeliac patients compared with normal subjects (−134.67% in jejunum), and increased after diet in both coeliac disease treatments. The other scales used did not show any significant difference between the two coeliac disease treatment groups. The authors concluded that carnitine therapy is safe and effective in ameliorating fatigue in coeliac disease. The efficacy of carnitine may be explained by the diet-induced OCTN2 increase, improving carnitine absorption.[36]

Carnitine supplementation has also been shown to improve fatigue symptoms in patients with cancer. A preliminary open-label study in 18 patients with cancer found that carnitine supplementation reduced fatigue, depression and sleep disruption, and improved performance.[37] A trial in 50 patients with chemotherapy-induced fatigue found that L-carnitine 4 g daily for 7 days improved fatigue and maintained this improvement until the next cycle of chemotherapy.[38] In a trial in 12 patients with advanced cancer, carnitine 6 g daily for 4 weeks reduced fatigue and improved quality of life in relation to measures associated with oxidative stress. Nutritional variables (lean body mass and appetite) increased significantly after L-carnitine supplementation. Levels of reactive oxygen species decreased and glutathione peroxidase increased, but not significantly. Pro-inflammatory cytokines did not change significantly.[39] In a further trial in 27 patients with advanced cancer, fatigue and carnitine deficiency, L-carnitine supplementation in successive doses of 250 to 3000 mg for 7 days improved fatigue, quality of sleep and depression, with positive results for fatigue most likely at the highest end of the dosage spectrum.[40]

Carnitine (intravenously administered) has also been associated with reduction of fatigue[41,42] and improvements in anaemia[43] in patients undergoing haemodialysis.

Alzheimer's disease

Preliminary evidence from two double-blind, placebo-controlled trials[44,45] suggests that carnitine supplementation could reduce the deterioration in some symptoms of Alzheimer's disease. A meta-analysis of 21 double-blind RCTs of acetyl-L-carnitine (ALC) versus placebo in the treatment of mild cognitive impairment and mild Alzheimer's disease concluded that ALC improved mild cognitive impairment or prevented deterioration, and was well tolerated.[46] More recent evidence from a Cochrane review of 16 trials suggests evidence of benefit for ALC on clinical global impression and on the MMSE test for Alzheimer's disease, but there is no evidence using objective assessments in any other area of outcome. In many cases, the trial methodologies were poor with vague descriptions of dementia. The Cochrane review concluded that at present there is no evidence to recommend the use of ALC in clinical practice.[47]

Miscellaneous

ALC is also a promising treatment for symptoms, particularly pain, of diabetic neuropathy.[48,49] It may support treatment for epilepsy[50] and complement antiretroviral therapy in patients with HIV,[51,52] but studies have not assessed the effect of carnitine on morbidity and mortality from AIDS.

> **Conclusion**
>
> Preliminary evidence suggests that carnitine supplementation may be of benefit in several cardiovascular disorders, such as angina, hyperlipidaemia, myocardial infarction, congestive heart failure and intermittent claudication. Evidence also exists that carnitine may be beneficial in Alzheimer's disease, chronic fatigue syndrome, fatigue in elderly people and in patients with cancer and diabetic neuropathy. Evidence of benefit from carnitine in exercise performance is inconsistent. While these results are clearly of interest, further evidence is required before the role of carnitine, if any, in the management of these conditions can be defined. Despite a theoretical rationale, there is as yet no good evidence that carnitine supplementation improves exercise performance.

Precautions/contraindications

The administration of the D-isomer (including a DL-mixture, contained in some supplements) may interfere with the normal function of the L-isomer and should not be used. Only the L-isomer has been used in studies.

Pregnancy and breast-feeding

No problems have been reported, but there have not been sufficient studies to guarantee the safety of carnitine in pregnancy and breast-feeding.

Adverse effects

Serious toxicity has not been reported. Nausea, vomiting and diarrhoea may occur with high doses. The risk of toxicity is greater with the D-isomer than with L-carnitine (see Precautions/contraindications); myasthenia has been reported with ingestion of DL-carnitine.

Use of the observed safe level (OSL) risk assessment method indicates that the evidence of safety is strong at intakes up to 2000 mg daily of L-carnitine equivalents for chronic supplementation, and this level is identified as the OSL. Although much higher dosages have been tested without adverse effects and may be safe, the data for intakes above 2000 mg per day are not sufficient for a confident conclusion of long-term safety.[53]

Interactions

Drugs

Anticonvulsants: increased excretion of carnitine.
Pivampicillin: increased excretion of carnitine.
Pivmecillinam: increased excretion of carnitine.

Dose

L-Carnitine supplements are available in the form of tablets and capsules. The dose is not established. In studies, doses of 1 to 6 g L-carnitine daily have been used.

Bioavailability

Bioavailability of an oral dose of carnitine is 5 to 20%. With an oral dose of 2 g, bioavailability is approximately 16% and with a 5 g oral dose is approximately 5%.[54–56] Supplemental carnitine raises plasma carnitine but also increases renal clearance.[57] Muscle carnitine is increased with long-term supplementation, but not after supplementation of less than 2 weeks' duration.[58]

References

1 Cherchi A, Lai C, Angelino F, *et al*. Effects of L-carnitine in exercise tolerance in chronic stable angina: a multicenter, double-blind, randomized placebo controlled crossover study. *Int J Clin Pharmacol Ther Toxicol* 1985; 23: 569–572.
2 Garyza G, Amico RM. Comparative study on the activity of racemic and laevorotatory carnitine in stable angina pectoris. *Int J Tissue Reactions* 1980; 2: 175–180.

3 Kamikawa T, Suzuki Y, Kobayashi A, *et al.* Effects of L-carnitine on exercise tolerance in patients with stable angina pectoris. *Jap Heart J* 1984; 25: 587–597.

4 Davini P, Bigalli A, Lamanna F, *et al.* Controlled study on L-carnitine therapeutic efficacy in post-infarction. *Drugs Exp Clin Res* 1992; 18: 355–365.

5 Ghidini O, Azzurro M, Vita G, *et al.* Evaluation of the therapeutic efficacy of L-carnitine in congestive heart failure. *Int J Clin Pharmacol Ther Toxicol* 1988; 26: 217–220.

6 Volek JS, Judelson DA, Silvestre R, *et al.* Effects of carnitine supplementation on flow-mediated dilation and vascular inflammatory responses to a high-fat meal in healthy young adults. *Am J Cardiol* 2008; 102(10): 1413–1417.

7 McMackin CJ, Widlansky ME, Hamburg NM, *et al.* Effect of combined treatment with alpha-lipoic acid and acetyl-L-carnitine on vascular function and blood pressure in patients with coronary artery disease. *J Clin Hypertens* 2007; 9(4): 249–255.

8 Brevetti G, Chiariello M, Ferulano G, *et al.* Increases in walking distance in patients with peripheral vascular disease treated with L-carnitine: a double-blind, cross-over study. *Circulation* 1988; 77: 767–773.

9 Pola P, Savi L, Grilli M, *et al.* Carnitine in the therapy of dyslipidemic patients. *Curr Ther Res* 1979; 27: 208–216.

10 Pola P, Tondi P, DalLago A, *et al.* Statistical evaluation of long-term l-carnitine therapy in hyperlipoproteinaemias. *Drugs Exp Clin Res* 1983; 12: 925–935.

11 Rossi CS, Silprandi N. Effect of carnitine on serum HDL-cholesterol: report of two cases. *Johns Hopkins Med J* 1982; 150: 51–54.

12 Bloomer RJ, Tschume LC, Smith WA. Glycine propionyl-L-carnitine modulates lipid peroxidation and nitric oxide in human subjects. *Int J Vitam Nutr Res* 2009; 79(3): 131–141.

13 Gonzalez-Ortiz M, Hernandez-Gonzalez SO, Hernandez-Salazar E, *et al.* Effect of oral L-carnitine administration on insulin sensitivity and lipid profile in type 2 diabetes mellitus patients. *Ann Nutr Metab* 2008; 52(4): 335–338.

14 Malaguarnera M, Vacante M, Avitabile T, *et al.* L-Carnitine supplementation reduces oxidized LDL cholesterol in patients with diabetes. *Am J Clin Nutr* 2009; 89(1): 71–76.

15 Galvano F, Li Volti G, Malaguarnera M, *et al.* Effects of simvastatin and carnitine versus simvastatin on lipoprotein(a) and apoprotein(a) in type 2 diabetes mellitus. *Expert Opin Pharmacother* 2009; 10(12): 1875–1882.

16 Molfino A, Cascino A, Conte C, *et al.* Caloric restriction and L-carnitine administration improves insulin sensitivity in patients with impaired glucose metabolism. *J Parenter Enteral Nutr* 2010; 34(3): 295–299.

17 Mingrone G, Greco AV, Capristo E. L-Carnitine improves glucose disposal in type 2 diabetic patients. *J Am Coll Nutr* 1999; 18: 77–82.

18 Broad EM, Maughan RJ, Galloway SD. Carbohydrate, protein, and fat metabolism during exercise after oral carnitine supplementation in humans. *Int J Sport Nutr Exerc Metab* 2008; 18 (6): 567–584.

19 Faria Coelho C, Mota JF, Paula Ravagnani FC, *et al.* [The supplementation of L-carnitine does not promote alterations in the resting metabolic rate and in the use of energetic substrates in physically active individuals]. *Arq Bras Endocrinol Metabol* 2010; 54(1): 37–44.

20 Ho JY, Kraemer WJ, Volek JS, *et al.* L-Carnitine L-tartrate supplementation favorably affects biochemical markers of recovery from physical exertion in middle-aged men and women. *Metabolism* 2010; 59(8): 1190–1199.

21 Kraemer WJ, Spiering BA, Volek JS, *et al.* Androgenic responses to resistance exercise: effects of feeding and L-carnitine. *Med Sci Sports Exerc* 2006; 38(7): 1288–1296.

22 Spiering BA, Kraemer WJ, Vingren JL, *et al.* Responses of criterion variables to different supplemental doses of L-carnitine L-tartrate. *J Strength Cond Res* 2007; 21(1): 259–264.

23 Swart I, Rossouw J, Loots J, *et al.* The effect of L-carnitine supplementation on plasma carnitine levels and various parameters of male marathon athletes. *Nutr Res* 1997; 17: 405–414.

24 Angelini C, Vergani L, Costa L, *et al.* Clinical study of efficacy of *l*-carnitine and metabolic observations inexercise physiology. In: Borum PR, ed. *Clinical Aspects of HumanCarnitine Deficiency*. Elmsford, NY: Pergamon Press; 1986: 36–42.

25 Marconi C, Sassi G, Carpinelli A, *et al.* Effects of L-carnitine loading on the aerobic and aerobic performance of endurance athletes. *Eur J Appl Physiol* 1985; 54: 131–135.

26 Barnett C, Costill D, Vukovitch , *et al.* Effect of L-carnitine supplementation on muscle and blood carnitine content and lactate accumulation during high-intensity spring cycling. *Int J Sport Nutr* 1994; 4: 280–288.

27 Vukovitch M, Costill D, Fink W, *et al.* Carnitine supplementation: effect on muscle carnitine and glycogen content during exercise. *Med Sci Sports Exerc* 1994; 26: 1122–1129.

28 Smith WA, Fry AC, Tschume LC, *et al.* Effect of glycine propionyl-L-carnitine on aerobic and anaerobic exercise performance. *Int J Sport Nutr Exerc Metab* 2008; 18(1): 19–36.

29 Colombani P, Wenk C, Kunz I, *et al.* Effects of L-carnitine supplementation on physical performance and energy metabolism of endurance trained athletes: a double-blind crossover filed study. *Eur J Appl Physiol* 1996; 73: 434–439.

30 Trappe SW, Costill DL, Goodpaster P, *et al.* The effects of L-carnitine on performance during interval swimming. *Int J Sports Med* 1994; 15: 181–185.

31 Giamberardino MA, Dragani L, Valente R, *et al.* Effects of prolonged L-carnitine administration on delayed muscle pain and CK release after eccentric effort. *Int J Sports Med* 1996; 17: 320–324.

32 Pliophys A, Pliophys S. Amantadine and L-carnitine treatment of chronic fatigue syndrome. *Neuropsychobiology* 1997; 35: 16–23.

33 Pistone G, Marino A, Leotta C, *et al.* Levocarnitine administration in elderly subjects with rapid muscle fatigue: effect on body composition, lipid profile and fatigue. *Drugs Aging* 2003; 20(10): 761–767.

34 Malaguarnera M, Cammalleri L, Gargante MP, *et al.* L-Carnitine treatment reduces severity of physical and mental fatigue and increases cognitive functions in centenarians: a randomized and controlled clinical trial. *Am J Clin Nutr* 2007; 86(6): 1738–1744.

35 Malaguarnera M, Gargante MP, Cristaldi E, *et al.* Acetyl L-carnitine (ALC) treatment in elderly patients with fatigue. *Arch Gerontol Geriatr* 2008; 46(2): 181–190.

36 Ciacci C, Peluso G, Iannoni E, *et al.* L-Carnitine in the treatment of fatigue in adult celiac disease patients: a pilot study. *Dig Liver Dis* 2007; 39 (10): 922–928.

37 Cruciani RA, Dvorkin E, Homel P, *et al.* L-Carnitine supplementation for the treatment of fatigue and depressed mood in cancer patients with carnitine deficiency: a preliminary analysis. *Ann NY Acad Sci* 2004; 1033: 168–76.

38 Graziano F, Bisonni R, Catalano V, *et al.* Potential role of levocarnitine supplementation for the treatment of chemotherapy-induced fatigue in non-anaemic cancer patients. *Br J Cancer* 2002; 86 (12): 1854–1857.

39 Gramignano G, Lusso MR, Madeddu C, *et al.* Efficacy of L-carnitine administration on fatigue, nutritional status, oxidative stress, and related quality of life in 12 advanced cancer patients undergoing anti-cancer therapy. *Nutrition* 2006; 22(2): 136–145.

40 Cruciani RA, Dvorkin E, Homel P, *et al.* Safety, tolerability and symptom outcomes associated with L-carnitine supplementation in patients with cancer, fatigue, and carnitine deficiency: a phase I/II study. *J Pain Symptom Manag* 2006; 32(6): 551–559.

41 Brass EP, Adler S, Sietsema KE, *et al.* Intravenous L-carnitine increases plasma carnitine, reduces fatigue, and may preserve exercise capacity in hemodialysis patients. *Am J Kidney Dis* 2001; 37 (5): 1018–1028.

42 Rathod R, Baig MS, Khandelwal PN, *et al.* Results of a single blind, randomized, placebo-controlled clinical trial to study the effect of intravenous L-carnitine supplementation on health-related quality of life in Indian patients on maintenance hemodialysis. *Indian J Med Sci* 2006; 60(4): 143–153.

43 Kadiroglu AK, Yilmaz ME, Sit D, *et al.* The evaluation of postdialysis L-carnitine administration and its effect on weekly requiring doses of rHuEPO in hemodialysis patients. *Ren Fail* 2005; 27(4): 367–372.

44 Spagnoli A, Lucca U, Menasce G, *et al.* Long term acetyl-L-carnitine treatment in Alzheimer's disease. *Neurology* 1991; 41: 1726–1732.

45 Sano M, Bell K, Cote L, *et al.* Double-blind parallel design pilot study of acetyl levocarnitine in patients with Alzheimer's disease. *Arch Neurol* 1992; 49: 1137–1141.

46 Montgomery SA, Thal LJ, Amrein R, *et al.* Meta-analysis of double blind randomized controlled clinical trials of acetyl-L-carnitine versus placebo in the treatment of mild cognitive impairment and mild Alzheimer's disease. *Int Clin Psychopharmacol* 2003; 18: 61–71.

47 Hudson S, Tabet N. Acetyl-L-carnitine for dementia (Cochrane Review). *Cochrane Database Syst Rev* 2003; (2): CD003158.

48 DeGrandis D, Minardi C. Acetyl-L-carnitine in the treatment of diabetic neuropathy. A long-term, randomised, double-blind, placebo-controlled study. *Drugs RD* 2002; 3(4): 223–231.

49 Sima AA, Calvani M, Mehra M, *et al.* Acetyl-L-carnitine improves pain, nerve regeneration, and vibratory perception in patients with chronic diabetic neuropathy: an analysis of two randomized placebo-controlled trials. *Diabetes Care* 2005; 28: 89–94.

50 Shuper A, Gutman A, Mimouni M. Intractable epilepsy. *Lancet* 1999; 353: 1238.

51 Moretti S, Alesse E, DiMarzio L. Effect of L-carnitine on human immunodeficiency virus-1 infection-associated apoptosis: a pilot study. *Blood* 1998; 91: 3817–3824.

52 DeSimone C, Tzantzoglou S, Famularo G. High dose L-carnitine improves immunologic and metabolic parameters in AIDS patients. *Immunopharmacol Immunotoxicol* 1993; 15: 1–12.

53 Hathcock JN, Shao A. Risk assessment for carnitine. *Regul Toxicol Pharmacol* 2006; 46(1): 23–28.

54 Harper P, Elwin CE, Cederblad G. Pharmacokinetics of intravenous and oral bolus doses of L-carnitine in healthy subjects. *Eur J Clin Pharmacol* 1988; 35(5): 555–562.

55 Evans AM, Fornasini G. Pharmacokinetics of L-carnitine. *Clin Pharmacokinet* 2003; 42(11): 941–967.

56 Rebouche CJ. Kinetics, pharmacokinetics, and regulation of L-carnitine and acetyl-L-carnitine metabolism. *Ann N Y Acad Sci* 2004; 1033: 30–41.

57 Bain MA, Milne RW, Evans AM. Disposition and metabolite kinetics of oral L-carnitine in humans. *J Clin Pharmacol* 2006; 46(10): 1163–1170.

58 Kanter MM, Williams MH. Antioxidants, carnitine, and choline as putative ergogenic aids. *Int J Sport Nutr* 1995; 5(Suppl): S120–S131.

Carotenoids

Description

Carotenoids are natural pigments found in plants, including fruit and vegetables, giving them their bright colour. About 600 carotenoids have been identified, of which about six appear to be used in significant ways by the blood or other tissues. About 50 have pro-vitamin A activity, and of these, all-*trans* beta-carotene is the most active on a weight basis and makes the most important quantitative contribution to human nutrition. Beta-carotene is fat soluble. Apart from beta-carotene, other significant carotenoids (according to research conducted so far) are alpha-carotene, astaxanthin, cryptoxanthin, lycopene, lutein and zeaxanthin.

Units

The bioavailability of those carotenoids with pro-vitamin A activity (e.g. alpha-carotene, beta-carotene, cryptoxanthin) is less than that of retinol (preformed vitamin A).

The absorption and utilisation of carotenoids varies, but the generally accepted relationship in the UK is that 1 µg retinol is equivalent to 6 µg beta-carotene or 12 µg of other pro-vitamin A carotenoids. (Other carotenoids with pro-vitamin A activity are not converted to vitamin to the same extent as is beta-carotene.) However, the bioactivity of carotenoids in foods is now known to be less than was previously thought and there is much debate about the conversion factors. The US Food and Nutrition Board revised its conversion factors in 2001 such that 1 µg retinol is equivalent to 12 µg beta-carotene or 24 µg of other provitamin A carotenoids.

The amount of beta-carotene in dietary supplements may be expressed in terms of micrograms or international units. One unit of beta-carotene is defined as the activity of 0.6 µg beta-carotene. Thus:

- 1 IU beta-carotene = 0.6 µg beta-carotene; and
- 1 µg beta-carotene = 1.67 IU beta-carotene.

Human requirements

There is currently no UK Dietary Reference Value for beta-carotene (or any other carotenoids). This is because, until recently, its only role has been considered to be as a precursor of vitamin A. Some authorities are starting to make recommendations for beta-carotene, e.g. 6 mg daily (Finland); 4 mg daily (France); 2 mg daily (Germany).

Dietary intake

In the UK, the average adult diet provides 2.28 mg (beta-carotene) daily.

Action

Carotenoids have the following functions. They:

- quench singlet oxygen and prevent the formation of free radicals. *Note*: natural beta-carotene (*cis* form) acts as an antioxidant, while the synthetic (*trans*) form has been suggested to be pro-oxidant;[1]
- react with or scavenge free radicals directly and thus act as an antioxidant;
- enhance some aspects of immune function; and
- act as precursors for vitamin A (e.g. alpha-carotene, beta-carotene, cryptoxanthin).

Dietary sources

Carotenoids are found in a wide variety of fruits and vegetables, although they may not be the ones commonly consumed. Alpha-carotene is found in palm oil, maize, carrots and pumpkin. Lycopene is concentrated in red fruits, such as tomatoes (particularly cooked and pureed tomatoes), guava, watermelon, apricots, peaches and red grapefruit. Lutein and zeaxanthin are found in dark green vegetables, red pepper and pumpkin. Cryptoxanthin is present in mangoes, oranges and peaches. The carotenoid content of various fruits and vegetables is shown in Table 1.

Table 1 Carotenoid composition of typical fruits and vegetables (μg/100 g portion)

Food	Alpha-carotene	Beta-carotene	Beta-cryptoxanthin	Lutein + zeaxanthin	Lycopene
Apricots, dried	0	17 600	0	0	864
Beet greens	3	2 560	0	7 700	0
Broccoli, boiled	0	1 042	0	2 226	0
Brussels sprouts, boiled	0	465	0	1 290	0
Cantaloupe melon	27	1 595	0	40	0
Carrots, cooked	3 700	9 800	0	260	0
Grapefruit, pink	5	603	12	13	1 462
Kale, cooked	0	6 202	0	15 798	0
Lettuce, cos	0	1 272	0	2 635	0
Mandarin orange	14	71	485	243	0
Mango, raw	17	445	11	–	–
Mango, canned, drained	–	13 120	1 550	–	–
Orange juice	2	4	15	36	0
Oranges	16	51	122	187	0
Papaya	0	276	761	75	0
Pasta with tomato sauce	0	127	0	0	3 162
Peppers, red, raw	59	2 379	2 205	–	–
Pizza, with tomato sauce	0	170	0	20	2 071
Spinach, cooked	0	5 242	0	7 043	0
Sweetcorn, canned	33	30	0	884	0
Sweet potato, cooked	0	9 488	0	0	0
Tomato soup, canned	0	235	0	90	10 920
Tomato, raw	0	520	0	100	3 100

Data from USDA-NCC Carotenoid Database for US Foods, 1998.

Metabolism

Although there are a huge number of carotenoids, most research has been conducted on beta-carotene, and less is known about the others, particularly in terms of metabolism. Hence, only the metabolism of beta-carotene is described here.

Absorption

Beta-carotene consists of two molecules of vitamin A, which are hydrolysed in the gastrointestinal tract. It is absorbed into the mucosal cells of the small intestine and converted to retinol. The efficiency of absorption is usually 20–50%, but can be as low as 10% when intake is high. The conversion of beta-carotene to retinol is regulated by the vitamin A stores of the individual and by the amount ingested; conversion efficiency varies from 2 : 1 at low intakes to 12 : 1 at higher intakes. On average, 25% of absorbed beta-carotene appears to remain intact and 75% is converted to retinol.

Distribution

Intact beta-carotene is transported in VLDL or LDL cholesterol. Blood levels, unlike those of retinol, are not maintained constant but vary roughly in proportion to the amounts ingested. Increased blood levels (hypercarotenaemia) are sometimes associated (as a secondary condition) with hypothyroidism, diabetes mellitus, and hepatic and renal disease. Hypercarotenaemia can also be caused by a rare genetic inability to convert beta-carotene to vitamin A.

All carotenoids are deposited in the liver to a lesser extent than is vitamin A. Most are stored in the adipose tissue, epidermal and dermal layers of the skin and the adrenals; there are high levels in the corpus luteum and in colostrum.

Elimination

Beta-carotene is eliminated mainly in the faeces.

Bioavailability

Beta-carotene is not very stable, and potency is lost if it is exposed to oxygen. Mild cooking processes can improve bioavailability, e.g. absorption from raw carrot can be as low as 1%, but this figure increases dramatically when carrots are subject to short periods of boiling. However, overcooking reduces bioavailability. Significant losses can also occur during frying, freezing and canning.

Deficiency

No specific symptoms have been defined.

Possible uses

Carotenoids are being investigated in a variety of conditions, particularly cancer, cardiovascular disease (CVD) and cataract.

Beta-carotene

Cancer
Epidemiological studies More than 50 epidemiological studies have demonstrated that a high intake of foods rich in carotenoids (i.e. fruit and vegetables) and high serum levels of beta-carotene are associated with reduced risk of certain cancers, especially lung cancer, but also cancers of the cervix, endometrium, breast, oesophagus, mouth and stomach.[2] High consumption of carotenoids may reduce the risk of pre-menopausal but not postmenopausal breast cancer, particularly among smokers[3] and may also increase breast cancer-free survival among women previously diagnosed with early-stage breast cancer.[4] However, in the European Prospective Investigation into Cancer and Nutrition, overall dietary intake of beta-carotene and vitamins C and E was not related to breast cancer risk in either pre- or postmenopausal women. However, in subgroups of post-menopausal women, a weak protective effect between beta-carotene and vitamin E from food and breast cancer risk could not be excluded.[5]

Fruit and vegetables contain several types of carotenoids in addition to beta-carotene, and it is incorrect to assume that beta-carotene is responsible for all the preventive effects of fruit and vegetables. For example, increased alpha-carotene intakes from diet have been associated with a reduced risk of lung cancer,[6,7] with suggestive inverse associations for other carotenoids also.

However, serum analysis has also shown an association between low serum beta-carotene levels and increased overall cancer risk, possibly indicating a more specific link. Serum alpha-tocopherol, but not beta-carotene or vitamin A, has been associated with increased prostate cancer survival.[8] Postmenopausal breast cancer has been associated with a tendency to lower levels of plasma carotenoids and tocopherols.

Intervention studies published so far have provided very little evidence for a beneficial effect of beta-carotene supplementation on cancer risk; indeed, some have indicated that there may be an increased risk.

Intervention trials A 12-year US study involving 22 071 male physicians randomly allocated to 50 mg beta-carotene every other day or placebo did not demonstrate any statistically significant benefit or harm from supplementation. In the beta-carotene group, 1273 subjects developed malignant neoplasms compared with 1293 in the placebo group. No serious adverse effects were noted in the study.[9]

In a double-blind, placebo-controlled Finnish intervention trial, known as the Alpha-Tocopherol, Beta-Carotene Prevention (ATBC) Study,[10] 29 000 male smokers were randomised to receive beta-carotene 20 mg daily, alpha-tocopherol 50 mg daily, both beta-carotene and alpha-tocopherol, or placebo. Lung cancer incidence increased in all the groups receiving beta-carotene, but the effect was stronger in those who smoked heavily, a finding consistent with the CARET study (see below). However, lung cancer incidence was not correlated with serum beta-carotene, suggesting that this was not a direct effect of beta-carotene.[11] There was also no significant effect on incidence or mortality of cancer of the pancreas,[12] nor on the incidence of colorectal adenomas.[13]

Another US study (the beta-Carotene and Retinol Efficacy Trial – CARET) in 4060 subjects with substantial work-related exposure to asbestos and also 14 254 heavy smokers, showed that beta-carotene 30 mg with vitamin

A 25 000 IU increased the risk of lung cancer compared with placebo. Mortality was also 17% higher. As a consequence, this trial was stopped prematurely.[14] Findings from a 2008 systematic review of 25 prospective observational studies assessing the associations between carotenoids and lung cancer suggest inverse associations between carotenoids and lung cancer but the decreases in risk were generally small and not statistically significant. In this review, beta-carotene supplementation was not associated with reduced lung cancer risk.[15] A further systematic review of four studies indicated that high-dose beta-carotene appears to increase the risk of lung cancer but only in current smokers.[16] A 2010 meta-analysis has also indicated that high-dose beta-carotene increases the risk of lung cancer and also gastric cancer (at 20–30 mg daily).[17]

These unexpected results were reviewed extensively and numerous possible explanations were proposed. One possible explanation for the negative results of the human beta-carotene intervention trials is that the positive effects of beta-carotene shown in case-control studies were instead the results of other nutrients that co-vary with carotenoids and carotenoids are only one of several factors in fruits and vegetables that must be consumed together to be effective. Carotenoids could also be a marker for a generally healthy lifestyle that includes a diet low in fat and high in fruits and vegetables.[18]

Another hypothesis is that a large dose of beta-carotene, such as was used in these trials, is metabolised differently than a smaller dietary dose, resulting in adverse effects. The idea was tested experimentally in a model of smoke-exposed, beta-carotene-treated ferrets. In the lungs of these animals, retinoid oxidative enzymes were elevated and retinoid levels were reduced.[19] This was found, in part, to be the result of enhanced oxidative excentric cleaving of beta-carotene to produce various beta-carotene metabolites (e.g. beta-apo-carotenals). However, when alpha-tocopherol and ascorbic acid were added to beta-carotene in ferrets exposed to cigarette smoke, the production of beta-apo-carotenals was inhibited, while the production of retinoids was increased. When either alpha-tocopherol or vitamin C alone was added, the production of retinoids was not affected, suggesting that alpha-tocopherol and

ascorbic acid may act synergistically in preventing the enhanced oxidative cleavage of beta-carotene induced by smoking exposure.[20] A more recent study in a ferret lung cancer model indicates that combined antioxidative supplementation could be a useful chemopreventive strategy against lung carcinogenesis through maintaining tissue retinoid levels and inhibiting cell proliferation and other potential carcinogenesis pathways in the lung.[21]

In patients with documented cervical dysplasia given either beta-carotene 30 mg or placebo for 9 months, complete remission occurred in 23% of the supplemented group and 47% of the placebo group, showing that beta-carotene had no beneficial effect on resolution of cervical dysplasia.[22] However, in another study there was an inverse relationship between breast cancer and beta-carotene intake in pre-menopausal women.[23]

In a further study, beta-carotene was neither beneficial nor harmful in reducing the risk of developing skin cancer. A total of 1621 subjects aged 20 to 69 were randomised into four groups – beta-carotene and sunscreen, sunscreen and placebo, beta-carotene and no sunscreen, and no sunscreen and placebo. Sunscreen was applied daily to all exposed areas of the head, neck, arms and hands, with re-application after swimming or increased perspiration. No dosing details were given for beta-carotene. At the end of the study, there were no statistically significant differences in development of basal or squamous cell carcinoma between the beta-carotene and placebo groups.[24] A lack of effect of beta-carotene supplementation in non-melanoma skin cancer was observed among men with low baseline plasma beta-carotene.[25]

More recent trials continue to show mixed results with beta-carotene alone. One RCT in 264 patients who had been treated for a recent early-stage squamous cell carcinoma of the oral cavity, pharynx or larynx found that beta-carotene 50 mg daily had no significant effect on second cancers of the head and neck (relative risk (RR), 0.69; 5% confidence interval (CI), 0.39 to 1.25) or lung cancer (RR, 1.44; 5% CI, 0.62 to 3.39) and total mortality was not affected. However, in this study the point estimates suggested a possible decrease in second head and neck cancer risk but a possible increase in lung cancer risk.[26] In a further trial involving patients treated for head and neck cancer, beta-carotene (75 mg daily) had no significant effect on the incidence of second primary tumours, but there was a statistically non-significant 40% reduction in the risk of death among subjects assigned to beta-carotene and no increase in death from CVD.[27] In patients with early-stage head and neck cancer, supplemental beta-carotene did not have pro-oxidant effects in either smokers or non-smokers.[28]

Beta-carotene has been shown in one RCT to be protective of colorectal adenoma recurrence among subjects who neither smoked cigarettes nor drank alcohol. A total of 864 subjects who had had an adenoma removed and were polyp-free were randomised to receive beta-carotene (25 mg) and/or vitamins C and E in combination (1000 mg and 400 mg, respectively) or placebo. They were followed at 1 and 4 years for adenoma recurrence. Among subjects who did not smoke or drink, beta-carotene was associated with a marked decrease in risk of one or more recurrent adenomas (RR, 0.56; 95% CI, 0.35 to 0.89), but beta-carotene supplementation conferred a modest increase in the risk of recurrence in those who smoked or drank. For people who smoked and drank more than one alcoholic drink a day, beta-carotene doubled the risk of adenoma recurrence, suggesting that both alcohol and smoking modify the effect of beta-carotene supplementation on the risk of colorectal adenoma recurrence.[29] Vitamin A and alpha-carotene have also been found to protect against recurrence of adenomatous polyps in non-smokers and non-drinkers.[30]

Cardiovascular disease

Diets rich in fruit and vegetables are generally associated with a lower risk of CVD, but evidence for a direct protective effect of beta-carotene was reported from the US Physicians' Health Study.[30] In an analysis of a subgroup of volunteers who had previously had stable angina or coronary revascularisation, 50 mg beta-carotene on alternate days reduced subsequent coronary events by 50% compared with placebo.

However, in a large placebo-controlled trial involving men between 50 and 69 who smoked five or more cigarettes a day, supplementation with beta-carotene was not helpful in angina

pectoris and may have slightly increased the incidence of the condition.[31] In this study, 5602 patients received beta-carotene 20 mg daily, 5570 patients received alpha-tocopherol 50 mg daily, 5548 patients received alpha-tocopherol 50 mg and beta-carotene 20 mg daily, and 5549 received placebo. Follow-up continued for a maximum of 7 years. Patients taking vitamin E alone or in combination with beta-carotene showed a minor decrease in angina pectoris, but beta-carotene alone was associated with a slight increase in angina incidence.

Incidence of myocardial infarction was not reduced by beta-carotene supplementation (50 mg daily) in US male physicians.[32] Beta-carotene was not effective in the treatment of increased serum triglycerides or cholesterol levels,[33] and was not shown to reduce the risk of stroke.[34]

A meta-analysis looked at the effect of antioxidant vitamins on long-term CVD outcomes included 12 RCTs, of which eight involved beta-carotene.[35] Beta-carotene was associated with a slight statistically significant increase in all-cause mortality and cardiovascular death compared with the control. The authors concluded that the use of supplements containing beta-carotene should be actively discouraged.

Eye disease

Beta-carotene may protect against cataract formation. In a retrospective study,[36] the group with the lowest serum beta-carotene levels had over five times the risk of developing cataract as the group with the highest serum levels. Two RCTs have evaluated the influence of beta-carotene supplements in age-related cataract. In the US Physicians' Health Study, 22 071 men aged 40–84 were randomly assigned to receive either beta-carotene 50 mg on alternate days or placebo for 12 years. There was no difference between the beta-carotene and placebo groups in the overall incidence of cataract, RR of cataract or cataract extraction. In smokers, however, beta-carotene appeared to attenuate excess risk of cataract by about 25%.[37] In the Women's Health Study, 39 867 female health professionals aged 45 or older were randomised to receive beta-carotene 50 mg on alternate days, vitamin E and aspirin for the prevention of cancer and CVD. The beta-carotene arm was terminated early and the main outcome measures were visually significant cataract and cataract extraction. However, 2 years of beta-carotene treatment had no large beneficial (or harmful) effect on the development of cataract.[38]

Carotenoids have also been studied for an influence on age-related macular degeneration (ARMD). A 12-year RCT among 22 071 apparently healthy US male physicians aged 40 to 84 years found that beta-carotene (50 mg every other day) had no beneficial or harmful effect on the incidence of ARMD.[39]

Diabetes

Serum beta-carotene levels may be reduced in diabetic patients, and one case-control study has shown a negative correlation between beta-carotene and glycaemic control.[40] Low concentrations of serum alpha-carotene, beta-carotene and the sum of five carotenoids also appear to be associated with increased risk of metabolic syndrome.[41] However, in the US Physicians' Health Study, beta-carotene supplementation (50 mg daily) was ineffective in reducing the risk of developing type 2 diabetes.[42]

Immune function

Data on beta-carotene's influence on the immune system are conflicting. One study showed that supplementation (beta-carotene 15 mg daily for 26 days) resulted in a significant increase in the proportion of monocytes involved in initiating immune responses.[43] However, in other studies, T-cell immunity was unaffected by beta-carotene supplementation.[44]

Lutein

Lutein is a carotenoid found in high concentrations in the eye, where it filters out blue light, and it may have a protective role in the visual apparatus and its vascular supply. There is evidence that lutein may help to prevent ARMD[45] and cataracts.[46] Supplements may also help to improve visual function in patients with retinal degeneration.[47]

A study in Miami tested the effects of 30 mg of lutein on eye pigment in two people for a period of 140 days. The results showed that 20–40 days after starting the lutein supplement, the density of the pigment in the subject's eyes

started to increase. The amount of blue light reaching the photoreceptors, Bruch's membrane and the retinal pigment epithelium (vulnerable eye tissues affected in macular degeneration) was reduced by 30–40%.[48] Another carotenoid, lycopene, appears to confer protection against oxidative changes in the epithelial cells of the lens.[49]

Dietary intake of lutein and its isomer zeaxanthin may reduce the risk of developing both cataract and macular degeneration.[50] In the US Nurses' Health Study, those in the highest quintile for consumption of lutein and zeaxanthin had a 22% reduced risk of cataract extraction compared with those in the lowest quintile.[51] In the US Physicians' Health Study, those in the highest quintile for lutein and zeaxanthin intake had a 19% reduction in risk for cataract extraction when smoking, age and other risk factors were controlled for.[52] Other carotenoids (alpha-carotene, beta-carotene, beta-cryptoxanthin, lycopene) were not associated with a reduced risk of cataract.

Similarly, in the US Beaver Dam Eye Study, lutein and zeaxanthin were the only carotenoids of those examined associated with reduction in cataracts – in this case, nuclear cataracts. People in the highest quintile of lutein intake in the distant past were half as likely to have an incidence of cataract as those in the lowest quintile.[46] As part of the same study, 252 subjects were followed over a 5-year period. Only a trend towards an inverse relationship between serum lutein and cryptoxanthin and risk of cataract development was noted.[53]

In a UK cross-sectional survey, the risk of posterior subscapular cataract was lowest in those with higher plasma concentrations of lutein and the risk of cortical cataract was lowest in people with the highest plasma concentrations of lycopene. However, the risk of nuclear cataract was lowest in people with the highest plasma concentrations of alpha- or beta-carotene.[54]

In the Carotenoids in Age-Related Eye Disease Study (CAREDS), which recruited women aged 50–79 years with intakes of lutein plus zeaxanthin outside the 78th (high) and 28th (low) percentiles, the prevalence of ARMD did not differ between the high and low intake groups when adjusted for age. However, in women under the age of 75 years without a history of chronic disease, higher intake of lutein plus zeaxathain was found to be significantly protective.[55]

In a large US prospective trial, involving 71 494 women and 41 564 men aged 50 years or over, lutein/zeaxanthin intake was not associated with the risk of self-reported early AMRD over 18 years of follow-up. However, there was a statistically non-significant and non-linear inverse association between lutein/zeaxanthin intake and neovascular AMD risk.[56]

In the first published intervention trial involving lutein, 17 patients with age-related cataracts were randomised in a double-blind study involving dietary supplementation with lutein 15 mg, alpha-tocopherol 100 mg or placebo three times a week for up to 2 years. Visual performance (visual acuity and glare sensitivity) improved in the lutein group but not with alpha-tocopherol or placebo.[57]

The second trial was a 21-month randomised, double-masked, placebo-controlled trial that involved 90 patients with atrophic ARMD. One group of patients received lutein 10 mg daily, another group received lutein 10 mg with antioxidants and vitamins and minerals, while the third group received a placebo. Visual function (as measured by macular pigment optical density, Snellen equivalent visual acuity and contrast sensitivity) improved with both lutein alone and lutein together with the other nutrients compared with placebo.[58] The authors concluded that lutein or lutein together with antioxidant vitamins was not a cure for ARMD but could reverse various symptoms of the condition and improve visual function.

Further supplementation trials have evaluated the effect of lutein supplementation on macular pigment optical density (MPOD). European[59,60] and US[61–63] trials have shown that lutein supplementation is capable of raising MPOD, which may provide protection against ARMD.

Another UK supplementation study evaluated the effect on contrast sensitivity of 6 mg lutein (with vitamins and minerals) each day in a 9-month RCT among patients with ARMD. At the end of the study, the scores for contrast sensitivity were not significantly different, suggesting that 6 mg lutein is not beneficial for this group.[64] In a Chinese study, both 6 mg and 12 mg lutein daily improved contrast sensitivity in young healthy adults.[65] A Japanese study in

13 participants found that lutein supplementation reduced visual fatigue associated with proof reading.[66]

Lycopene

Lycopene is a carotenoid pigment that functions as a free radical scavenger and antioxidant. Supplementation has been reported to protect against macular degeneration,[67] atherosclerosis,[68] and cancer, especially prostate cancer.[69,70]

Intervention trials have begun to evaluate the effects of lycopene supplements in prostate cancer. In a pilot trial, 26 men with newly diagnosed, clinically localised prostate cancer were randomised to receive 15 mg of lycopene twice daily or no supplementation for 3 weeks before radical prostatectomy. The results suggested that lycopene supplementation may reduce the growth of prostate cancer, but the authors emphasised that no firm conclusions could be reached because of the small sample size.[71]

The same research group conducted a further pilot trial involving the use of a tomato extract containing 30 mg lycopene each day in 26 men – again for 3 weeks before radical prostatectomy. After intervention, subjects in the intervention group had smaller tumours, less involvement of extra-prostatic tissue with cancer and less diffuse involvement of the prostate by high-grade prostatic intraepithelial neoplasia. Mean prostate-specific antigen (PSA) was lower in the intervention group than the placebo group. The authors concluded that this pilot study suggests that lycopene may have beneficial effects in prostate cancer, although large trials are warranted to investigate the potential preventive and/or therapeutic role of lycopene in the disease.[72]

In another trial, 54 men with prostate cancer were assigned to receive orchidectomy alone or orchidectomy plus lycopene (2 mg twice daily). At 6 months there was a significant reduction in PSA in both treatment arms, but this was more marked in the lycopene group. This change was more consistent after 2 years. Adding lycopene to orchidectomy produced a more reliable and consistent reduction in PSA, shrinking the primary tumour, diminishing secondary tumours, providing better relief from bone pain and lower urinary tract symptoms and improving survival compared with orchidectomy alone.[73] A further trial using a supplement containing lycopene, isoflavones, silymarin and antioxidants found that this supplement delayed PSA progression after potentially curative treatment (radical prostatectomy),[74] while a trial among men with advanced prostate cancer found no benefit of lycopene supplementation.[75]

A meta-analysis of 11 case-control studies and 10 cohort studies or nested case-control studies involving tomato, tomato products or lycopene concluded that tomato products may play a role in the prevention of prostate cancer, but the effect is small.[76]

Conclusion

Diets rich in carotenoids are protective against various conditions, particularly cancer and CVD. However, evidence that beta-carotene supplements are beneficial for this purpose is lacking. Other carotenoids, such as lycopene and lutein, are now being studied. Preliminary evidence suggests that lutein may be protective in cataract and macular degeneration, while lycopene may be protective against macular degeneration and prostate cancer.

Precautions/contraindications

No serious problems have been reported. Supplements should be avoided by people with known hypersensitivity to carotenoids.

Pregnancy and breast-feeding

No problems have been reported.

Adverse effects

Unlike retinol, carotenoids are generally non-toxic. Even when ingested in large amounts, they are not known to cause birth defects or to cause hypervitaminosis A, primarily because efficiency of absorption decreases rapidly as the dose increases and because conversion to vitamin A is not sufficiently rapid to induce toxicity.

Intake of >30 mg daily (either from commercial supplements or tomato or carrot juice) may lead to hypercarotenaemia, which is characterised by a yellowish coloration of the skin (including the palms of the hands and soles of the feet), and a very high concentration of carotenoids in the plasma. This is harmless and reversible and gradually disappears when excessive intake of carotenoids is corrected.

Hypercarotenaemia is clearly differentiated from jaundice by the appearance of the whites of the eyes (yellow in hypercarotenaemia but not in jaundice).

Diarrhoea, dizziness and arthralgia may occur occasionally with carotene supplements. Allergic reactions (hay fever and facial swelling), amenorrhoea and leucopenia have been reported rarely.

According to FAO/WHO, intakes of beta-carotene up to 5 mg/kg body weight are acceptable.

The only serious toxic manifestation of carotenoid intake is canthaxanthin retinopathy, which can develop in patients with erythropoietic protoporphyria and related disorders who are treated with large daily doses (50–100 mg) of canthaxanthin (a derivative of beta-carotene) for long periods.

Interactions

None specifically established (see also Vitamin A).

Dose

Beta-carotene, lutein, lycopene and mixed carotenoids are available in the form of tablets and capsules.

Beta-carotene as a single supplement should not be recommended.

References

1   Levin G, Yeshurun M, Mockady S. In vitro antiperoxidative effect of 9-*cis* beta-carotene compared with that of the all-*trans* isomer. *J Nutr Cancer* 1997; 27: 293–297.
2   Gaby SK, Singh VN. Betacarotene. In: Gaby SK, Bendich A, Singh VN, Machlin LJ, eds. *Vitamin Intake and Health. A Scientific Review*. New York: Marcel Dekker, 1991: 89–106.
3   Mignone LI, Giovannucci E, Newcomb PA, *et al*. Dietary carotenoids and the risk of invasive breast cancer. *Int J Cancer* 2009; 124(12): 2929–2937.
4   Rock CL, Natarajan L, Pu M, *et al*. Longitudinal biological exposure to carotenoids is associated with breast cancer-free survival in the Women's Healthy Eating and Living Study. *Cancer Epidemiol Biomarkers Prev* 2009; 18(2): 486–494.

5   Nagel G, Linseisen J, vanGils CH, *et al.* Dietary beta-carotene, vitamin C and E intake and breast cancer risk in the European Prospective Investigation into Cancer and Nutrition (EPIC). *Breast Cancer Res Treat* 2009; 119(3): 753–765.

6   Michaud DS, Feskanich D, Rimm EB, *et al.* Intake of specific carotenoids and risk of lung cancer in 2 prospective US cohorts. *Am J Clin Nutr* 2000; 72: 990–997.

7   Knekt P, Jarvinen R, Tempo , *et al.* Role of various carotenoids in lung cancer prevention. *J Natl Cancer Inst* 1999; 91: 182–184.

8   Watters JL, Gail MH, Weinstein SJ, *et al.* Associations between alpha-tocopherol, beta-carotene, and retinol and prostate cancer survival. *Cancer Res* 2009; 69(9): 3833–3841.

9   Hennekens CH, Buring JE, Manson JE, *et al.* Lack of effect of long-term supplementation with beta-carotene on the incidence of malignant neoplasms and cardiovascular disease. *N Engl J Med* 1996; 334: 1145–1149.

10 The Alpha-Tocopherol, Beta-Carotene Cancer Prevention Study Group. The effect of vitamin E and beta carotene on the incidence of lung cancer in male smokers. *N Engl J Med* 1994; 330: 1029–1035.

11 Albanes E, Heinonen OP, Taylor PR, *et al.* Alpha-tocopherol and beta-carotene supplements and lung cancer incidence in the alpha-tocopherol, beta-carotene cancer prevention study: effects of baseline characteristics and study compliance. *J Natl Cancer Inst* 1996; 88: 1560–1570.

12 Rautalahti MT, Virtamo JRK, Taylor PR, *et al.* The effects of supplementation with alpha-tocopherol and beta-carotene on the incidence and mortality of carcinoma of the pancreas in a randomised, controlled trial. *Cancer* 1999; 86: 37–42.

13 Maliula N, Virtamo J, Virtanen M, *et al.* The effect of alpha-tocopherol and β-carotene supplementation on colorectal adenomas in middle-aged male smokers. *Cancer Epidemiol Biomarkers Prev* 1999; 8: 489–493.

14 Omenn GS, Goodman GE, Thornquist MD, *et al.* Effects of a combination of betacarotene and vitamin A on lung cancer and cardiovascular disease. *N Engl J Med* 1996; 334: 1150–1155.

15 Gallicchio L, Boyd K, Matanoski G, *et al.* Carotenoids and the risk of developing lung cancer: a systematic review. *Am J Clin Nutr* 2008; 88(2): 372–383.

16 Tanvetyanon T, Bepler G. Beta-carotene in multivitamins and the possible risk of lung cancer among smokers versus former smokers: a meta-analysis and evaluation of national brands. *Cancer* 2008; 113(1): 150–157.

17 Druesne-Pecollo N, Latino-Martel P, Norat T, *et al.* Beta-carotene supplementation and cancer risk: a systematic review and metaanalysis of randomized controlled trials. *Int J Cancer* 2010; 127(1): 172–184.

18 Mayne ST. Antioxidant nutrients and chronic disease: use of biomarkers of exposure and oxidative stress status in epidemiologic research. *J Nutr* 2003; 33(Suppl): S933–940.

19 Liu C, Russell RM, Wang XD. Exposing ferrets to cigarette smoke and a pharmacological dose of β-carotene supplementation enhance in vitro retinoic acid catabolism in lungs via induction of cytochrome P450 enzymes. *J Nutr* 2003; 133: 173–179.

20 Liu C, Russell RM, Wang XD. Alpha-tocopherol and ascorbic acid decrease the production of beta-apo-carotenals and increase the formation of retinoids from β-carotene in the lung tissues of cigarette smoke-exposed ferrets in vitro. *J Nutr* 2004; 134: 426–430.

21 Kim Y, Chongviriyaphan N, Liu C, *et al.* Combined antioxidant (beta-carotene, alpha-tocopherol and ascorbic acid) supplementation increases the levels of lung retinoic acid and inhibits the activation of mitogen-activated protein kinase in the ferret lung cancer model. *Carcinogenesis* 2006; 27: 1410–1419.

22 Romney SL, Ho GYF, Palan PR, *et al.* Effects of betacarotene and other factors on outcome of cervical dysplasia and human papillomavirus infection. *Gynecol Oncol* 1997; 65: 483–492.

23 Bohlke K, Spiegelman D, Trichopoulou A, *et al.* Vitamins A, C and E and the risk of breast cancer: results from a case control study in Greece. *Br J Cancer* 1999; 79: 23–29.

24 Green A, Williams G, Neale R, *et al.* Daily sunscreen application and betacarotene supplementation in prevention of basal cell and squamous cell carcinomas of the skin. *Lancet* 1999; 354: 723–729.

25 Schaumberg DA, Frieling UM, Rifai N, Cook N. No effect of beta-carotene supplementation on risk of nonmelanoma skin cancer among men with low baseline plasma beta-carotene. *Cancer Epidemiol Biomarkers Prev* 2004; 6: 1079–1080.

26 Mayne ST, Cartmel B, Baum M, *et al.* Randomized trial of supplemental beta-carotene to prevent second head and neck cancer. *Cancer Res* 2001; 61: 1457–1463.

27 Toma S, Bonelli L, Sartoris A, *et al.* Beta-carotene supplementation in patients radically treated for stage I–II head and neck cancer: results of a randomized trial. *Oncol Rep* 2003; 10: 1895–1901.

28 Mayne ST, Walter M, Cartmel B, *et al.* Supplemental beta-carotene, smoking, and urinary F2-isoprostane excretion in patients with prior early stage head and neck cancer. *Nutr Cancer* 2004; 49: 1–6.

29 Baron JA, Cole BF, Mott L, *et al.* Neoplastic and antineoplastic effects of beta-carotene on colorectal adenoma recurrence: results of a randomized trial. *J Natl Cancer Inst* 2003; 95: 717–722.

30 Steck-Stott S, Forman MR, Sowell A, *et al.* Carotenoids, vitamin A and risk of adenomatous polyp recurrence in the polyp prevention trial. *Int J Cancer* 2004; 112: 295–305.

31 Gaziano JM, Manson JE, Ridker PM, *et al.* Beta-carotene supplementation for chronic stable angina. *Circulation* 1990; 82(Suppl III): 201.

32 Rapola JM, Virtamo J, Haukka JK, *et al.* Effect of vitamin E and betacarotene on the incidence of angina pectoris: a randomized, double-blind, controlled trial. *JAMA* 1996; 275: 693–698.

33 Redlich C, Chung J, Cullen M, *et al*. Effect of long-term betacarotene and vitamin A on serum cholesterol and triglycerides among participants in the Carotene and Retinol Efficacy Trial (CARET). *Atherosclerosis* 1999; 145: 425–432.

34 Ascherio A, Rimm E, Hernan MA, *et al*. Relation of consumption of vitamin E, vitamin C and carotenoids to risk for stroke among men in the United States. *Ann Intern Med* 1999; 130: 963–970.

35 Vivekananthan DP, Penn MS, Sapp SK, *et al*. Use of antioxidant vitamins for the prevention of cardiovascular disease: meta-analysis of randomized trials. *Lancet* 2003; 361: 2017–2023.

36 Jacques PF, Hartz SC, Chylack LT, *et al*. Nutritional status in persons with and without senile cataract: blood vitamin and mineral levels. *Am J Clin Nutr* 1988; 48: 152–158.

37 Christen WG, Manson JE, Glynn RJ, *et al*. A randomized trial of beta carotene and age-related cataract in US physicians. *Arch Ophthalmol* 2003; 121: 372–378.

38 Christen W, Glynn R, Sperduto R, *et al*. Age-related cataract in a randomized trial of beta-carotene in women. *Ophthalmic Epidemiol* 2004; 11: 401–412.

39 Christen WG, Manson JE, Glynn RJ, *et al*. Beta carotene supplementation and age-related maculopathy in a randomized trial of US physicians. *Arch Ophthalmol* 2007; 125(3): 333–339.

40 Abahusain MA, Wright J, Dickerson JWT, *et al*. Retinol, alpha-tocopherol and carotenoids in diabetes. *Eur J Clin Nutr* 1999; 53: 630–635.

41 Coyne T, Ibiebele TI, Baade PD, *et al*. Metabolic syndrome and serum carotenoids: findings of a cross-sectional study in Queensland, Australia. *Br J Nutr* 2009; 102(11): 1668–1677.

42 Liu S, Ajanu U, Chae C, *et al*. Long-term β-carotene supplementation and risk of type 2 diabetes mellitus. *JAMA* 1999; 282: 1073–1075.

43 Hughes DA, Wright AJA, Finglas PM, *et al*. The effect of beta-carotene supplementation on the immune function of blood monocytes from healthy male non-smokers. *J Lab Clin Med* 1997; 129: 309–317.

44 Santos MS, Leka LS, Ribaya-Mercado D, *et al*. Short and long-term beta-carotene supplementation do not influence T cell-mediated immunity in healthy elderly persons. *Am J Clin Nutr* 1997; 66: 917–924.

45 Hammond BR,Jr Johnson EJ, Russell RM, *et al*. Dietary modification of human macular pigment density. *Invest Ophthalmol Vis Sci* 1997; 38: 1795–1801.

46 Lyle BJ, Mares-Perlman JA, Klein BE, *et al*. Antioxidant intake and risk of incident age related nuclear cataracts in the Beaver Dam Eye Study. *Am J Epidemiol* 1999; 149: 801–809.

47 Dagnelie G, Zorge IS, McDonald TM. Lutein improves visual function in some patients with retinal degeneration: a pilot study via the Internet. *Optometry* 2000; 7: 147–164.

48 Landrum JT, Bone RA, Joa H, *et al*. A one year study of the macular pigment: the effect of 140 days of a lutein supplement. *Exp Eye Res* 1997; 65: 57–62.

49 Mohanty I, Joshi S, Trivedi D, *et al*. Lycopene prevents sugar-induced morphological changes

and modulates antioxidant status of human lens epithelial cells. *Br J Nutr* 2002; 88: 347–354.

50 Mares-Perlman JA, Millen AE, Ficek TL, Hankinson SE. The body of evidence to support a protective role for lutein and zeaxanthin in delaying chronic disease. *J Nutr* 2002; 132(Suppl): S518–S524.

51 Chasan-Taber L, Willett WC, Seddon JM, *et al*. A prospective study of carotenoid and vitamin A status and risk of cataract extraction in US women. *Am J Clin Nutr* 1999; 70: 509–516.

52 Brown L, Rimm EB, Seddon JM, *et al*. A prospective study of carotenoid extraction in US men. *Am J Clin Nutr* 1999; 70: 517–524.

53 Lyle BJ, Mares-Perlman JA, Klein BE, *et al*. Serum carotenoids and tocopherols and incidence of age-related nuclear cataract. *Am J Clin Nutr* 1999; 69: 272–277.

54 Gale CR, Hall NF, Phillips DIW, Martyn C. Plasma antioxidant vitamins and carotenoids and age-related cataract. *Ophthalmology* 2001; 108: 1992–1998.

55 Moeller SM, Parekh N, Tinker L, *et al*. Associations between intermediate age-related macular degeneration and lutein and zeaxanthin in the Carotenoids in Age-related Eye Disease Study (CAREDS): ancillary study of the Women's Health Initiative. *Arch Ophthalmol* 2006; 124(8): 1151–1162.

56 Cho E, Hankinson SE, Rosner B, *et al*. Prospective study of lutein/zeaxanthin intake and risk of age-related macular degeneration. *Am J Clin Nutr* 2008; 87(6): 1837–1843.

57 Olmedilla B, Granado F, Blanco I, Vaquero M. Lutein, but not alpha-tocopherol, supplementation improves visual function in patients with age-related cataracts: a 2-y double-blind, placebo-controlled pilot study. *Nutrition* 2003; 19: 21–4.

58 Richer S, Stiles W, Statuke L, *et al*. Double-masked, placebo-controlled, randomized trial of lutein antioxidant supplementation in the intervention of atrophic age-related macular degeneration: the Veterans LAST study (Lutein Antioxidant Supplementation Trial). *Optometry* 2004; 75: 216–230.

59 Kvansakul J, Rodriguez-Carmona M, Edgar DF, *et al*. Supplementation with the carotenoids lutein or zeaxanthin improves human visual performance. *Ophthalmic Physiol Opt* 2006; 26(4): 362–371.

60 Zeimer M, Hense HW, Heimes B, *et al*. The macular pigment: short- and intermediate-term changes of macular pigment optical density following supplementation with lutein and zeaxanthin and co-antioxidants. The LUNA Study. *Ophthalmologe* 2009; 106(1): 29–36.

61 Bone RA, Landrum JT, Cao Y, *et al*. Macular pigment response to a supplement containing meso-zeaxanthin, lutein and zeaxanthin. *Nutr Metab (Lond)* 2007; 4: 12.

62 Johnson EJ, Chung HY, Caldarella SM, *et al*. The influence of supplemental lutein and docosahexaenoic acid on serum, lipoproteins, and macular pigmentation. *Am J Clin Nutr* 2008; 87(5): 1521–1529.

63 Bone RA, Landrum JT. Dose-dependent response of serum lutein and macular pigment optical density

to supplementation with lutein esters. *Arch Biochem Biophys* 2010; 504(1): 50–55.

64   Bartlett HE, Eperjesi F. Effect of lutein and antioxidant dietary supplementation on contrast sensitivity in age-related macular disease: a randomized controlled trial. *Eur J Clin Nutr* 2007; 61(9): 1121–1127.

65   Ma L, Lin XM, Zou ZY, *et al*. A 12-week lutein supplementation improves visual function in Chinese people with long-term computer display light exposure. *Br J Nutr* 2009; 102(2): 186–190.

66   Yagi A, Fujimoto K, Michihiro K, *et al*. The effect of lutein supplementation on visual fatigue: a psychophysiological analysis. *Appl Ergon* 2009; 40(6): 1047–1054.

67   Mares-Perlman JA, Brady WE, Klein R, *et al*. Serum antioxidants and age related macular degeneration in a population-based case-control study. *Arch Ophthalmol* 1995; 113: 1518–1523.

68   Agarwal S, Rao AV. Tomato lycopene and low density lipoprotein oxidation: a human dietary intervention study. *Lipids* 1998; 33: 981–984.

69   Giovanucci E. Tomatoes, tomato-based products, lycopene and cancer. Review of the epidemiologic literature. *J Natl Cancer Inst* 1999; 91: 317–331.

70   Gann PH, Ma J, Giovannucci E, *et al*. Lower prostate cancer risk in men with elevated plasma lycopene levels: results of a prospective analysis. *Cancer Res* 1999; 59: 1225–1230.

71   Kucuk O, Sarkar FH, Sakr W, *et al*. Phase II randomized clinical trial of lycopene supplementation before radical prostatectomy. *Cancer Epidemiol Biomarkers Prev* 2001; 8: 861–868.

72   Kucuk O, Sarkar FH, Djuric Z, *et al*. Effects of lycopene supplementation in patients with localized prostate cancer. *Exp Biol Med* 2002; 227: 881–885.

73   Ansari MS, Gupta NP. A comparison of lycopene and orchidectomy vs orchidectomy alone in the management of advanced prostate cancer. *BJU Int* 2003; 92: 375–378.

74   Schroder FH, Roobol MJ, Boeve ER, *et al*. Randomized, double-blind, placebo-controlled crossover study in men with prostate cancer and rising PSA: effectiveness of a dietary supplement. *Eur Urol* 2005; 48: 922–930.

75   Schwenke C, Ubrig B, Thurmann P, *et al*. Lycopene for advanced hormone refractory prostate cancer: a prospective, open phase II pilot study. *J Urol* 2009; 181(3): 1098–1103.

76   Etminan M, Takkouche B, Caamano-Isorna F. The role of tomato products and lycopene in the prevention of prostate cancer: a meta-analysis of observational studies. *Cancer Epidemiol Biomarkers Prev* 2004; 3: 340–345.

Cetylated fatty acids

Description

Cetylated fatty acids (CFA) are a group of esterified fatty acids including cetyl myristoleate (CM), cetyl myristate, cetyl palmitoleate, cetyl laureate, cetyl palmitate, and cetyl oleate. CM is the main cetyl fatty acid in many supplements, though most contain a mixture of cetylated fatty acids. It is the cetyl alcohol ester of myristoleic acid, which is an omega-5 monounsaturated fatty acid, and has been isolated from mice that are immune to chemically induced arthritis.[1]

Action

The precise mechanism of action of CFA is unknown. However, they may act as surfactants, to lubricate the joints and muscles and improve the pliability of the muscles and tissues. They may also be mediators of inflammatory processes. CM possibly modulates the effects of pro-inflammatory cytokines. It has also been suggested that omega-5 fatty acids may form oxygenated metabolites through transcellular processing, and that these metabolites exert anti-inflammatory effects distinct from eicosanoids. Results from another study suggest that CM may act through inhibition of 5-lipoxygenase, a potent mediator of inflammation.[2,3] It is also thought that CFA may modulate the immune system through a programming of T cells. However, all these suggested mechanisms are putative.

Possible uses

CFA are used principally in arthritic conditions. Three small double-blind, placebo-controlled trials have evaluated CFA in osteoarthritis. One used an oral preparation, two used topical preparations.

In the trial involving the oral preparation, 64 patients with chronic knee osteoarthritis were evaluated at baseline and at 30 and 68 days after consuming either a vegetable oil placebo or CFA. Evaluations included physician assessment, knee range of motion and the Lequesne Algofunctional Index (LAI). After 68 days, patients treated with CFA exhibited significant ($P < 0.001$) increase in knee flexion compared to patients given placebo. Neither group reported improvement in knee extension. Patient responses to the LAI indicated a significant ($P < 0.001$) shift towards functional improvement for the CFA group (-5.4 points) after 68 days compared to a modest improvement in the placebo group (-2.1 points).[2]

One of the studies evaluating a topical CFA cream randomly assigned 40 patients with osteoarthritis of one or both knees to either CFA cream or placebo. Patients were tested at baseline, 30 minutes after initial treatment and after 30-day treatment of cream applied twice a day. Assessments included knee range of motion (ROM), timed 'up-and-go' from a chair and stair climbing, medial step-down test, and the unilateral anterior reach. For stair climbing ability and the up-and-go test, significant decreases in time were observed at both 30 minutes after treatment and following 30 days of treatment in the CFA group only. These differences were significant between groups. Supine ROM of the knees increased in the CFA group, whereas no difference was observed in the placebo group. For the medial step-down test, significant improvement was observed after treatment with CFA compared with baseline. For the unilateral anterior reach, significant improvement was observed for both legs in the CFA group and in only the left leg in the placebo group. However, the improvements observed in the CFA group were significantly greater than placebo group for both legs.[3] In an extension of this study, administration of CFA improved static postural stability, suggesting improved pain relief and the potential for improving exercise training following CFA.[4]

Conclusion

Cetyl fatty acids have been evaluated for arthritic conditions in three controlled trials. Preliminary results are promising and further research would help their precise role in these conditions.

Precautions/contraindications

None known.

Pregnancy and breastfeeding

Insufficient data; avoid in pregnancy and breastfeeding.

Adverse effects

CFA has been used safely when taken orally for 68 days[2] and when used topically as a cream for 30 days.[3,4] No adverse effects have been reported.

Interactions

None reported.

Dose

In trials to date, a specific blend of CFA (350 mg) with soya lecithin (50 mg) and fish oil (75 mg) has been used.

References

1 Diehl HW, May EL. Cetyl myristoleate isolated from Swiss albino mice: an apparent protective agent against adjuvant arthritis in rats. *J Pharm Sci* 1994; 83(3): 296–299.
2 Hesslink R, Jr. Armstrong D, 3rd. Nagendran MV, *et al.* Cetylated fatty acids improve knee function in patients with osteoarthritis. *J Rheumatol* 2002; 29 (8): 1708–1712.
3 Kraemer WJ, Ratamess NA, Anderson JM, *et al.* Effect of a cetylated fatty acid topical cream on functional mobility and quality of life of patients with osteoarthritis. *J Rheumatol* 2004; 31(4): 767–774.
4 Kraemer WJ, Ratamess NA, Maresh CM, *et al.* Effects of treatment with a cetylated fatty acid topical cream on static postural stability and plantar pressure distribution in patients with knee osteoarthritis. *J Strength Cond Res* 2005; 19(1): 115–121.

Chitosan

Description

Chitosan is a fibre extracted from chitin, which is a structural component of crustacean shells, crabs, shrimps and lobsters. Chitin is de-acetylated to produce chitosan.

Constituents

Chitosan is a polysaccharide containing numerous acetyl groups.

Action

Chitosan binds fat molecules as a result of its ionic nature. When taken orally, chitosan has been reported to be able to bind 8–10 times its own weight in fat from food that has been consumed. This prevents fat from being absorbed and the body then has to burn stored fat, which may lead to reductions in body fat and body weight.

Possible uses

Weight loss

In mice treated with chitosan and given a high-fat diet, chitosan prevented the increase in body weight, hyperlipidaemia and fatty liver normally induced by such a diet.[1]

In a randomised, placebo-controlled, double-blind study, 34 overweight human volunteers were given four capsules of chitosan or placebo for 28 consecutive days. Subjects maintained their normal diet and documented their food intake. After 4 weeks of treatment, body mass index, serum cholesterol, triglycerides, vitamins A, D and E and beta-carotene were not significantly different in the two groups. The results suggest that chitosan in the dose given had no effect on body weight in overweight subjects. No serious adverse effects were reported.[2]

In another placebo-controlled, double-blind study, 51 healthy obese women were given chitosan 1200 mg twice a day for 8 weeks. No reductions in weight were observed in any

treatment group. LDL cholesterol fell to a greater extent in the chitosan group than the placebo group, but there was no significant change in HDL cholesterol and triglycerides were slightly increased.[3]

A 24-week randomised, double-blind, placebo-controlled trial involving 250 obese women found that the chitosan group lost more weight than the placebo group but the effects were very small.[4] A systematic review of 15 RCTs involving a total of 1291 participants found that chitosan preparations result in a significantly greater weight loss (weighted mean difference −1.7 kg; 95% confidence interval (CI), −2.1 to −1.3; $P < 0.00001$), decrease in total cholesterol (−0.2 mmol/L; 95% CI, −0.3 to −0.1; $P < 0.00001$), and a decrease in systolic and diastolic blood pressure compared with placebo. There were no clear differences between intervention and control groups in terms of frequency of adverse events or in faecal fat excretion. However, the quality of many studies was suboptimal and analyses restricted to studies that met allocation concealment criteria, were larger, or of longer duration showed that such trials produced substantially smaller decreases in weight and total cholesterol.[5] The review concluded that the effect of chitosan on body weight is minimal and unlikely to be of clinical significance.

Cholesterol

Two double-blind RCTs in humans investigating the effect of chitosan on plasma cholesterol have shown conflicting results. One was a Japanese study involving 90 women with mild to moderate hypercholesterolaemia, which found that chitosan significantly reduced cholesterol although the effect was small.[6] The second was a Finnish study in 130 men and women with moderately increased plasma cholesterol, which found that chitosan had no effect on the concentrations of plasma lipids or glucose.[7] A meta-analysis of six studies found that the use of chitosan significantly lowered total cholesterol but not LDL cholesterol, HDL cholesterol or triglycerides. The authors' conclusion was that, based upon the currently available literature, they could only say that chitosan beneficially affects total cholesterol with 95% confidence. Additional, larger RCTs are needed to better characterise the effect of chitosan on other lipoproteins.[8]

Blood glucose

Chitosan has been shown to reduce blood glucose and cholesterol in an animal model of lean-type non-insulin-dependent diabetes mellitus with hypoinsulinaemia,[9] but had no effect in an animal model of obese-type non-insulin-dependent diabetes mellitus (NIDDM) with hyperinsulinaemia.[10] The authors concluded that chitosan could be a useful treatment for lean-type NIDDM with hypoinsulinaemia.[9] A more recent randomised double-blind trial in 12 obese subjects demonstrated that administration of chitosan for 3 months increased insulin sensitivity in obese patients, with a decrease in weight, body mass index, waist circumference and serum triglycerides.[11]

Conclusion

Chitosan is promoted for weight loss, but there have been few trials, and results have been conflicting. Any effect of chitosan on body weight is likely to be small. Chitosan has also been investigated for an effect on plasma cholesterol and blood glucose. Positive effects have been shown but as the studies have been small, recommendations for use of chitosan must await the findings of larger studies.

Precautions/contraindications

Chitosan should be avoided in patients with gastrointestinal malabsorption conditions.

Pregnancy and breast-feeding

No problems have been reported, but weight loss should not be attempted during pregnancy.

Adverse effects

There are no long-term studies assessing the safety of chitosan. However, chitosan may reduce the absorption of fat-soluble vitamins (A, D, E and K). This has been shown in animals,[10] but not

in humans.[2,3] A parallel, placebo-controlled, single blind study was completed in 56 out of 65 subjects who consumed 0, 4.5, 6.75 g per day of chitosan or 6.75 g per day glucomannan for 8 weeks. No differences were detected among the treatments in serum vitamins (vitamin A, vitamin E, 25-hydroxyvitamin D), carotenes (alpha- and beta-carotene), clinical chemistry or haematology measurements. However, the changes in the total and LDL cholesterol concentrations among the study groups were not statist'-ically significant.[12]

Interactions

The anticoagulant effect of warfarin may be potentiated by chitosan. An 83-year-old male with hypertensive cardiovascular disease, type 2 diabetes mellitus, and chronic atrial fibrillation complicated by left atrial thrombus formation was maintained on warfarin 2.5 mg daily. Marked elevation of the international normalised ratio (INR) was noticed after he self-medicated with chitosan 1200 mg twice daily. He denied taking any other drugs, natural substances, herbal medicines or nutritional supplements, and stated that he had not changed his dietary habits. After parenteral administration of vitamin K and discontinuation of chitosan, the INR returned to within the target range. However, the patient took chitosan again, and the INR increased to well above the target range. Following strong medical advice, the patient stopped taking chitosan, and the INR remained stable thereafter.[13]

Dose

Chitosan is available in the form of tablets and capsules.

The dose is not established. Dietary supplements provide 1500–3000 mg per daily dose.

Bioavailability

Chitosan cannot be hydrolysed by human digestive enzymes. In the acidic environment of the upper gastrointestinal tract, chitosan is solubilised and has a positive charge, so binds with negatively-charged molecules such as fat and bile.

References

1 Han LK, Kimura Y, Okuda H. Reduction in fat storage during chitin–chitosan treatment in mice fed a high-fat diet. *Int J Obes Relat Metab Disord* 1999; 23(2): 174–179.
2 Pittler MH, Abbott NC, Harkness EF, *et al*. Randomized, double-blind trial of chitosan for body weight reduction. *Eur J Clin Nutr* 1999; 53: 379–381.
3 Wuolijoki E, Hirvela T, Ylitalo P. Decrease in serum LDL cholesterol with microcrystalline chitosan. *Meth Find Exp Clin Pharmacol* 1999; 21: 357–361.
4 Mhurchu CN, Poppitt SD, McGill AT, *et al*. The effect of the dietary supplement, chitosan, on body weight: a randomised controlled trial in 250 over-weight and obese adults. *Int J Obes Relat Metab Disord* 2004; 28(9): 1149–1156.
5 Jull AB, Ni Mhurchu C, Bennett DA, *et al*. Chitosan for overweight or obesity. *Cochrane Database Syst Rev* 2008;(3): CD003892.
6 Bokura H, Kobayashi S. Chitosan decreases total cholesterol in women: a randomized, double-blind, placebo-controlled trial. *Eur J Clin Nutr* 2003; 57: 721–725.
7 Metso S, Ylitalo R, Nikkila M, *et al*. The effect of long-term microcrystalline chitosan therapy on plasma lipids and glucose concentrations in subjects with increased plasma total cholesterol: a random-ised placebo-controlled double-blind crossover trial in healthy men and women. *Eur J Clin Pharmacol* 2003; 59: 741–746.
8 Baker WL, Tercius A, Anglade M, *et al*. A meta-analysis evaluating the impact of chitosan on serum lipids in hypercholesterolemic patients. *Ann Nutr Metab* 2009; 55(4): 368–374.
9 Miura T, Usami M, Tsuura Y, *et al*. Hypoglycemic and hypolipidemic effect of chitosan in normal and neonatal sterptozotocin-induced diabetic mice. *Biol Pharm Bull* 1995; 18: 1623–1625.
10 Deuchi K, Kanauchi O, Shizukuishi M, *et al*. Continuous and massive intake of chitosan affects soluble vitamin status in rats fed on a high fat diet. *Biosci Biotech Biochem* 1995; 59: 1211–1216.
11 Hernandez-Gonzalez SO, Gonzalez-Ortiz M, Martinez-Abundis E, *et al*. Chitosan improves insu-lin sensitivity as determined by the euglycemic-hyperinsulinemic clamp technique in obese sub-jects. *Nutr Res* 2010; 30(6): 392–395.
12 Tapola NS, Lyyra ML, Kolehmainen RM, *et al*. Safety aspects and cholesterol-lowering efficacy of chitosan tablets. *J Am Coll Nutr* 2008; 27(1): 22–30.
13 Huang SS, Sung SH, Chiang CE. Chitosan poten-tiation of warfarin effect. *Ann Pharmacother* 2007; 41(11): 1912–1914.

Chlorella

Description

Chlorella is a single-celled freshwater alga.

Constituents

Chlorella is rich in chlorophyll. Manufacturers claim that it is a source of amino acids, nucleic acids, fatty acids, vitamins and minerals. However, content varies with conditions of growing, harvesting and processing. *Chlorella* is claimed to contain a unique substance called Chlorella Growth Factor. The claimed nutrient content of *Chlorella* is shown in Table 1.

Action

Chlorella may have antitumour and antiviral activities, and may also be able to stimulate the immune system, but these effects have not been clarified in human studies. Some research indicates that it has antioxidant activity.[1]

Possible uses

Chlorella is promoted as a tonic for general health maintenance; it is a useful source of some nutrients (e.g. beta-carotene, riboflavin, vitamin B_{12}, iron and zinc; see Constituents). One study has shown that *Chlorella* can reduce anaemia of pregnancy, probably through its iron content.[2]

In addition, *Chlorella* is claimed to be useful in: accelerating the healing of wounds and ulcers; improving digestion and bowel function; stimu-lating growth and repair of tissues; slowing down ageing; strengthening the immune system; improving the condition of the hair, skin, teeth and nails; treating colds and respiratory infect-ions; and removing poisonous substances from the body. These claims are based largely on

Table 1 Claimed[1] nutrient content of *Chlorella*

Nutrient	Per 100 g	Per typical dose (3 g)	RNI (%)[2]
Protein (g)	66	2	–
Fat (g)	9	0.3	–
Carbohydrate (g)	11	0.3	–
Vitamin A (μg), (as beta-carotene)	5500	165	28
Thiamine (mg)	2.0	0.06	8
Riboflavin (mg)	7.0	0.2	24
Niacin (mg)	30	0.9	6
Vitamin B_6 (mg)	1.5	0.05	4
Vitamin B_{12} (μg)	134	4	270
Folic acid (μg)	25	0.75	0.4
Pantothenic acid (mg)	3.0	0.09	–
Biotin (μg)	190	6	–
Vitamin C (mg)	60	1.8	5
Vitamin E (mg)	17	0.5	–
Choline (mg)	270	8.1	–
Inositol (mg)	190	5.7	–
Calcium (mg)	500	15	2
Magnesium (mg)	300	9	3
Potassium (mg)	700	21	0.6
Phosphorus (mg)	1200	36	6.5
Iron (mg)	260	8	80
Zinc (mg)	70	2	26
Copper (μg)	80	2.4	0.2
Iodine (μg)	600	18	13

[1] Reported on a product label.
[2] Reference Nutrient Intake for men aged 19–50 years.

anecdote; *Chlorella* has no proven efficacy for these conditions.

Preliminary evidence from an uncontrolled study in 20 patients over a period of 2 months showed that *Chlorella* supplementation may help relieve the symptoms of fibromyalgia.[3] However, the authors concluded that a larger, more comprehensive double-blind, placebo-controlled trial in these patients was warranted. Further work by this research group in 55 patients with fibromyalgia, 33 patients with hypertension and 9 patients with ulcerative colitis found that daily dietary supplementation with *Chlorella* may reduce high blood pressure, lower serum cholesterol levels, accelerate wound healing and enhance immune functions. The authors concluded that the potential of *Chlorella* to relieve symptoms, improve quality of life and normalise

body functions in patients with fibromyalgia, hypertension or ulcerative colitis suggests that larger, more comprehensive clinical trials of *Chlorella* are warranted.[4] More recent work has shown that a gamma-aminobutyric acid-rich *Chlorella* preparation is capable of reducing high blood pressure and borderline hypertension.[5]

Chlorella has been investigated for an influence on immune function. A community-based RCT in 124 healthy people who had received influenza vaccine showed that a *Chlorella*-derived dietary supplement did not have any effect in increasing the antibody response to influenza vaccine in the overall study population, although there was an increase in antibody response among participants aged 50–55 years. Adverse events were similar among those receiving the supplement and the placebo.[6] A study investigating immunoglobulin A concentrations in breast milk found that these were significantly higher in a group of women consuming a *Chlorella*-based supplement than in the placebo group.[7]

Chlorella intake has also been associated with altered gene expression. In a small study involving 17 healthy subjects and 17 subjects with high risk factors for lifestyle-related diseases, *Chlorella* intake resulted in noticeable reductions in body fat percentage, serum total cholesterol and fasting blood glucose levels. Through gene expression analysis, gene expression profiles were found to vary with *Chlorella* intake, with many of the genes that exhibited such behaviour returning to pre-intake expression levels after the end of the intake period. Among these were genes related to signal transduction molecules, metabolic enzymes, receptors, transporters and cytokines. A difference in expression levels was found between the two subject groups at the start of the tests, and genes with noticeable variance in expression level during *Chlorella* intake were identified in the high-risk factor group. These included genes involved in fat metabolism and insulin-signalling pathways, which suggests that these pathways could be physiologically affected by *Chlorella* intake. There were clear variations in the expression profiles of genes directly related to uptake of glucose during *Chlorella* intake, indicating that the activation of insulin-signalling pathways could be the reason for the hypoglycaemic effects of *Chlorella*.[8]

Other preliminary evidence suggests that *Chlorella* could help patients with brain tumours to better tolerate chemotherapy and radiotherapy. However, there appears to be no effect on tumour progression or survival.[9]

> **Conclusion**
> *Chlorella* has been studied in various conditions such as fibromyalgia, hypertension, ulcerative colitis and also in immune function and gene expression. Although these trials are interesting, there is insufficient reliable information to recommend the use of *Chlorella* for any indication.

Precautions/contraindications

No problems have been reported.

Pregnancy and breast-feeding

No problems have been reported.

Adverse effects

None reported, but *Chlorella* may provoke allergic reactions.

Interactions

None reported, but *Chlorella* may contain significant amounts of vitamin K. This could inhibit the activity of warfarin and other anticoagulants.

Dose

Chlorella is available in the form of tablets, capsules, liquid extracts and powder.

The dose is not established. Dietary supplements provide 500–3000 mg of the intact organism per daily dose.

References

1 Lee SH, Kang HJ, Lee HJ, *et al*. Six-week supplementation with *Chlorella* has favorable impact on antioxidant status in Korean male smokers. *Nutrition* 2009; 26(2): 175–183.
2 Nakano S, Takekoshi H, Nakano M. *Chlorella pyrenoidosa* supplementation reduces the risk of anemia, proteinuria and edema in pregnant women. *Plant Foods Hum Nutr* 2010; 65(1): 25–30.
3 Merchant RE, Carmack CA, Wise CM. Nutritional supplementation with *Chlorella pyrenoidosa* for patients with fibromyalgia syndrome: a pilot study. *Phytother Res* 2000; 14: 167–173.
4 Merchant RE, Andre CA. A review of recent clinical trials of the nutritional supplement *Chlorella pyrenoidosa* in the treatment of fibromyalgia, hypertension, and ulcerative colitis. *Altern Ther Health Med* 2001; 7(3): 79–91.
5 Shimada M, Hasegawa T, Nishimura C, *et al*. Antihypertensive effect of gamma-aminobutyric acid (GABA)-rich *Chlorella* on high-normal blood pressure and borderline hypertension in placebo-controlled double blind study. *Clin Exp Hypertens* 2009; 31(4): 342–354.
6 Halperin SA, Smith B, Nolan C, *et al*. Safety and immunoenhancing effect of a *Chlorella*-derived dietary supplement in healthy adults undergoing influenza vaccination: randomized, double-blind, placebo-controlled trial. *CMAJ* 2003; 169(2): 111–117.
7 Nakano S, Takekoshi H, Nakano M. Chlorella (*Chlorella pyrenoidosa*) supplementation decreases dioxin and increases immunoglobulin A concentrations in breast milk. *J Med Food* 2007; 10(1): 134–142.
8 Mizoguchi T, Takehara I, Masuzawa T, *et al*. Nutrigenomic studies of effects of *Chlorella* on subjects with high-risk factors for lifestyle-related disease. *J Med Food* 2008; 11(3): 395–404.
9 Merchant RE, Rice CD, Young HF. Dietary *Chlorella pyrenoidosa* for patients with malignant glioma: effects on immunocompetence, quality of life and survival. *Phytother Res* 1990; 4: 220–231.

Choline

Description

Choline is associated with the vitamin B complex; it is not an officially recognised vitamin. Choline is a component of phosphatidylcholine and an active constituent of dietary lecithin, but the two substances are not synonymous.

Human requirements

Choline is an essential nutrient for several mammalian organisms, but there is no agreement over its essentiality as a vitamin for humans. However, the US Food and Nutrition Board of the National Institute of Medicine has established a Dietary Reference Intake for adults of 550 mg a day for men and 425 mg a day for women, with lower amounts for children, together with an upper intake level of 3.5 g daily for adults over 18 years.

Dietary intake

Estimated dietary intake in the UK is 250–500 mg daily. Choline can also be synthesised in the body from phosphatidylethanolamine. Phosphatidylcholine is catalysed by the enzyme phosphatidylethanolamine-N-methyltransferase, which is induced by oestrogen. Because of their lower oestrogen concentrations, postmenopausal women have a higher dietary requirement for choline than do pre-menopausal women.[1]

Action

Choline serves as a source of labile methyl groups for transmethylation reactions. It functions as a component of other molecules such as the neurotransmitter acetylcholine, phosphatidylcholine (lecithin) and sphingomyelin, structural constituents of cell membranes and plasma lipoproteins, platelet activating factor and plasmalogen (a phospholipid found in highest concentrations in cardiac muscle membranes).

Lecithin and sphingomyelin participate in signal transduction,[2] an essential process for cell growth, regulation and function. Animal studies suggest that choline or lecithin deficiency may interfere with this critical process and that alterations in signal transduction may lead to abnormalities such as cancer and Alzheimer's disease.

Dietary sources

Choline is widely distributed in foods (mainly in the form of lecithin). The richest sources of choline are brewer's yeast, egg yolk, liver, wheatgerm, soya beans, kidney and brain. Oats, peanuts, beans and cauliflower contain significant amounts.

Metabolism

Absorption

Some choline is absorbed intact, probably by a carrier-mediated mechanism; some is metabolised by the gastrointestinal flora to trimethylamine (which produces a fishy odour).

Distribution

Choline is stored in the brain, kidney and liver, primarily as phosphatidylcholine (lecithin) and sphingomyelin. Total intake of choline and genotype can influence the concentrations of choline and its metabolites in the breast milk and blood of lactating women and thereby affect the amount of choline available to the developing infant.[3]

Elimination

Elimination of choline occurs mainly via the urine.

Deficiency

Dietary choline deficiency occurs in animals, and abnormal liver function, liver cirrhosis and fatty liver may be associated with choline deficiency in humans. Observations in patients on total parenteral nutrition have shown a choline-deficient diet to result in fatty infiltration of the liver, hepatocellular damage and liver dysfunction.[4,5] The influence of choline deficiency varies with hormone status. When deprived of dietary choline, 77% of men and 80% of postmenopausal women developed fatty liver or muscle damage, whereas only 44% of premenopausal women developed such signs of organ dysfunction. Moreover, six men developed these signs while consuming 550 mg choline daily (the AI for choline).[6] A choline-deficient diet in humans has also been associated with DNA damage. A trial in 51 adults found that subjects in whom choline-deficient diets induced liver or muscle dysfunction also had higher rates of apoptosis in their peripheral lymphocytes than did subjects who did not develop organ dysfunction.[7] Increased choline intake has been shown to attenuate DNA damage in a specific subgroup of folate-deficient men.[8]

Possible uses

As a precursor of acetylcholine, it has been suggested that choline could increase the concentration of acetylcholine in the brain. It has been suggested, therefore, that choline could be beneficial in patients with disease related to impaired cholinergic transmission (e.g. tardive dyskinesia, Huntington's chorea, Alzheimer's disease, Gilles de la Tourette, mania, memory impairment and ataxia). However, experimental evidence suggests that oral choline has no effect on choline metabolites in the brain.[9]

Comparison of studies involving choline is often complicated by lack of standardisation of doses used. However, clinical trials with tardive dyskinesia patients using choline have met with some success.[9–12]

Choline has also been suggested to improve performance in athletes. This idea arose because of findings that plasma choline concentrations were reduced in trained runners[13] and athletes[14] after sporting events. However, a double-blind crossover study in 20 cyclists showed that choline supplementation did not delay fatigue during brief or prolonged exercise.[15]

Claims have been made for the value of choline in the prevention of cardiovascular disease, including angina, atherosclerosis, hypertension, stroke and thrombosis. However, scientific evidence for these claims from RCTs is lacking. Interest has recently focused on the potential for choline (as a precursor of betaine) to reduce plasma homocysteine. One crossover study showed that phosphatidylcholine supplementation (2.6 g choline daily for 2 weeks) lowers fasting as well as post-methionine-loading plasma homocysteine concentrations in healthy men with mildly elevated homocysteine concentrations.[16] Choline (in conjunction with carnitine) supplementation has also been shown to lower lipid peroxidation and promote conservation of antioxidants (e.g. retinol and alpha-tocopherol) in women.[17] In a cross-sectional survey in 3042 adults with no history of cardiovascular disease, compared with the lowest tertile of choline intake (<250 mg daily), participants who consumed >310 mg daily had, on average, 22% lower concentrations of C-reactive protein ($P < 0.05$), 26% lower concentrations of interleukin-6 ($P < 0.05$) and 6% lower concentrations of tumour necrosis factor-alpha ($P < 0.01$), suggesting an inverse association between choline and the inflammatory process.[18] However, higher intakes of choline and betaine have not been associated with reduced risk of cardiovascular disease.[19]

Choline has also been claimed to prevent and/or treat Alzheimer's disease, senile dementia and memory loss. A Cochrane review of 14 studies found some evidence that cytidinediphosphocholine has a positive effect on memory and behaviour at least in the short to medium term, but evidence is limited by the quality of the studies.[20]

> **Conclusion**
> Research on choline supplementation is limited and studies are generally very poorly controlled. The limited research shows that choline does not appear to improve athletic performance. Very preliminary evidence suggests choline might be beneficial in poor memory and tardive dyskinesia, but evidence is not sufficient to recommend supplementation.

Precautions/contraindications

Increasing choline intake has been associated with an elevated risk of colorectal adenoma in US women enrolled in the Nurses' Health Study.[21] The authors suggested that this finding could reflect the presence of other components in the foods from which choline is derived.

Pregnancy and breast-feeding

No problems have been reported.

Adverse effects

Fishy odour; more severe symptoms relate to excessive cholinergic transmission (doses of 10 g daily or more) and include diarrhoea, nausea, dizziness, sweating, salivation, depression and a longer P-R interval in electrocardiograms.

Interactions

None established.

Dose

Choline is available in the form of tablets and capsules.

The dose is not established. Dietary supplements generally provide 250–500 mg per dose (choline chloride provides 80% choline and choline tartrate 50% choline).

References

1 Fischer LM, daCosta KA, Kwock L, *et al*. Dietary choline requirements of women: effects of estrogen and genetic variation. *Am J Clin Nutr* 2010; 92(5): 1113–1119.

2 Canty DJ, Zeisel SH. Lecithin and choline in human health and disease. *Nutr Rev* 1994; 52(10): 327–339.

3 Fischer LM, daCosta KA, Galanko J, *et al*. Choline intake and genetic polymorphisms influence choline metabolite concentrations in human breast milk and plasma. *Am J Clin Nutr* 2010; 92 (2): 336–346.

4 Zeisel SH, daCosta KA. Choline: an essential nutrient for public health. *Nutr Rev* 2009; 67(11): 615–623.

5 Sheard NF, Tayek JA, Bistrian BR, *et al*. Plasma choline concentration in humans fed parenterally. *Am J Clin Nutr* 1986; 43(2): 219–224.

6 Fischer LM, daCosta KA, Kwock L, *et al*. Sex and menopausal status influence human dietary requirements for the nutrient choline. *Am J Clin Nutr* 2007; 85(5): 1275–1285.

7 daCosta K-A, Niculescu MD, Craciunescu CN, *et al*. Choline deficiency increases lymphocyte apoptosis and DNA damage in humans. *Am J Clin Nutr* 2006; 84(1): 88–94.

8 Shin W, Yan J, Abratte CM, *et al*. Choline intake exceeding current dietary recommendations preserves markers of cellular methylation in a genetic subgroup of folate-compromised men. *J Nutr* 2010; 140(5): 975–980.

9 Davis KL, Berger PA, Hollister LE. Letter: Choline for tardive dyskinesia. *N Engl J Med* 1975; 293(3): 152.

10 Tamminga CA, Smith RC, Ericksen SE, *et al*. Cholinergic influences in tardive dyskinesia. *Am J Psychiatry* 1977; 134(7): 769–774.

11 Growdon JH, Hirsch MJ, Wurtman RJ, *et al*. Oral choline administration to patients with tardive dyskinesia. *N Engl J Med* 1977; 297(10): 524–527.

12 Gelenberg AJ, Doller-Wojcik JC, Growdon JH. Choline and lecithin in the treatment of tardive dyskinesia: preliminary results from a pilot study. *Am J Psychiatry* 1979; 136(6): 772–776.

13 Conlay LA, Sabounjian LA, Wurtman RJ. Exercise and neuromodulators: choline and acetylcholine in marathon runners. *Int J Sports Med* 1992; 13 (Suppl1): S141–S142.

14 vonAllworden HN, Horn S, Kahl J, *et al*. The influence of lecithin on plasma choline concentrations in triathletes and adolescent runners during exercise. *Eur J Appl Physiol Occup Physiol* 1993; 67(1): 87–91.

15 Spector SA, Jackman MR, Sabounjian LA, *et al*. Effect of choline supplementation on fatigue in trained cyclists. *Med Sci Sports Exerc* 1995; 27(5): 668–673.

16 Olthof MR, Brink EJ, Katan MB, *et al*. Choline supplemented as phosphatidylcholine decreases fasting and postmethionine-loading plasma homocysteine concentrations in healthy men. *Am J Clin Nutr* 2005; 82(1): 111–117.

17 Sachan DS, Hongu N, Johnsen M. Decreasing oxidative stress with choline and carnitine in women. *J Am Coll Nutr* 2005; 24(3): 172–176.

18 Detopoulou P, Panagiotakos DB, Antonopoulou S, *et al*. Dietary choline and betaine intakes in relation to concentrations of inflammatory markers in healthy adults: the ATTICA study. *Am J Clin Nutr* 2008; 87(2): 424–430.

19 Bidulescu A, Chambless LE, Siega-Riz AM, *et al*. Usual choline and betaine dietary intake and incident coronary heart disease: the Atherosclerosis Risk in Communities (ARIC) study. *BMC Cardiovasc Disord* 2007; 7(20): 20.

20 Fioravanti M, Yanagi M. Cytidinediphosphocholine (CDP-choline) for cognitive and behavioural disturbances associated with chronic cerebral disorders in the elderly. *Cochrane Database Syst Rev* 2005; 18 (2): CD000269.

21 Cho E, Willett WC, Colditz GA, *et al*. Dietary choline and betaine and the risk of distal colorectal adenoma in women. *J Natl Cancer Inst* 2007; 99 (16): 1224–1231.

Chondroitin

Description

Chondroitin is a natural physiological compound that is synthesised endogenously and secreted by the chondrocytes. It is found in joint cartilage and connective tissue (including vessel walls).

Constituents

Chondroitin is a mixture of high molecular weight glycosaminoglycans and disaccharide polymers composed of equimolar amounts of D-glucuronic acid, D-acetylgalactosamine and sulphates in 10–30 disaccharide units. (Glycosaminoglycans are the substances in which collagen fibres are embedded in cartilage.)

Action

Chondroitin absorbs water, adding to the thickness and elasticity of cartilage and its ability to absorb and distribute compressive forces. It also appears to control the formation of new cartilage matrix, by stimulating chondrocyte metabolism and synthesis of collagen and proteoglycan. Chondroitin also inhibits degradative enzymes (elastase and hyaluronidase), which break down cartilage matrix and synovial fluid, contributing to cartilage destruction and loss of joint function. Recent studies have assessed chondroitin sulphate for its influence on joint friction[1,2] and joint lubrication[3] with equivocal results.

Possible uses

Osteoarthritis

Chondroitin is claimed to be useful as a dietary supplement in combination with glucosamine in osteoarthritis and related disorders. There is some evidence to suggest that chondroitin reduces the pain of osteoarthritis in the knee compared with placebo. Chondroitin has also been shown to improve the symptoms of osteoarthritis associated with psoriasis.[4]

In a multicentre, double-blind RCT, involving 127 patients with osteoarthritis of the knee, 40 were treated with chondroitin sulphate oral gel 1200 mg daily, capsules 1200 mg daily or placebo for 3 months. Chondroitin (both formulations) significantly improved subjective symptoms, including joint mobility.[5]

In a randomised, double-blind, placebo-controlled study, 80 patients with knee osteoarthritis participated in a 6-month study and received either 2×400 mg chondroitin capsules twice a day or placebo. Symptoms of joint pain and time to perform a 20-metre walk were significantly reduced in the treated group, and there was a non-significant trend for the placebo group to use more paracetamol.[6]

A 1-year, randomised, double-blind, controlled pilot study included 42 patients with symptomatic knee osteoarthritis. Patients were treated orally with 800 mg chondroitin sulphate

or placebo. Chondroitin sulphate was well tolerated and significantly reduced pain and increased overall mobility. In addition, bone and joint metabolism stabilised in the treated patients, but not in those on placebo.[7]

A meta-analysis that included seven trials of 372 patients taking chondroitin found that, over 120 days or longer, chondroitin was significantly superior to placebo with respect to the Lesquesne index and pain rating on a visual analogue scale (VAS). Pooling the data confirmed these results, and showed at least 50% improvement in the treated versus the placebo patients. The authors concluded that further investigations using larger cohorts of patients for longer time periods were needed to prove the usefulness of chondroitin as a symptom-modifying agent in osteoarthritis.[8]

A randomised, double-blind, double-dummy study compared the efficacy of chondroitin with diclofenac in 146 patients with knee osteoarthritis. During the first month, patients received either 3×50 mg diclofenac tablets daily plus 3×400 mg placebo sachets, or 3×400 mg chondroitin sachets daily plus 3×50 mg placebo tablets. From months two to three, the diclofenac patients were given placebo sachets alone, and the chondroitin patients were given chondroitin sachets. Both groups were treated with placebo sachets from months four to six. The diclofenac group showed prompt pain reduction, which disappeared after the end of treatment. In the chondroitin group, the therapeutic response appeared later but lasted for up to 3 months after the end of treatment.[9]

Chondroitin sulphate 1 g daily was investigated in a prospective, double-blind, placebo-controlled, multicentre clinical study in patients with femorotibial osteoarthritis. Treatment continued for 3 months and there was a 3-month post-treatment period. There was a trend towards efficacy, with good tolerability after 3 months' treatment, and persistent efficacy 1 month post-treatment.[10]

In a further randomised, double-blind trial, 120 patients with symptomatic knee osteoarthritis were randomised into two groups receiving either 800 mg chodroitin sulphate or placebo daily for two periods of 3 months during 1 year. Intention-to-treat analysis included 110 patients. Various measures of pain, mobility and function, including Lequesne's algofunctional index (AFI),

VAS, walking time, global judgment and use of paracetamol significantly improved compared with placebo. Radiological progression at 12 months showed significantly decreased joint space in the placebo group with no change in the chondroitin sulphate group. Tolerability was good, with identical minor adverse events observed in both groups.[11] In a further controlled trial in 300 patients with knee osteoarthritis conducted by the same research group, placebo was associated with progressive and significant joint space narrowing while chondroitin sulphate 800 mg daily resulted in no change in mean joint space width. The differences in mean joint space width change between the two groups were significantly different. However, there was no significant change in osteoarthritic symptoms in this study.[12]

The Glucosamine/chondroitin Arthritis Intervention Trial (GAIT), a multicentre, double-blind, placebo- and celecoxib-controlled trial evaluated the efficacy of glucosamine 1500 mg daily, chondroitin sulphate 1200 mg daily, both glucosamine and chondroitin, celecoxib 200 mg daily or placebo for 24 weeks as a treatment for knee pain from osteoarthritis. A total of 1583 patients with osteoarthritis of the knee were randomly assigned to the five study arms and the primary outcome measure was a 20% decrease in knee pain from baseline to week 24. Overall, neither chondroitin nor glucosamine, nor chondroitin/glucosamine combined, had a significant effect on overall pain in this group of patients. Exploratory analysis suggested that the combination of glucosamine/chondroitin may be effective in a subgroup of patients with mild–moderate knee pain.[13] In addition, patients taking chondroitin sulphate were noted to have a statistically significant improvement in knee joint swelling. An exploratory post-hoc analysis suggested the effect of chondroitin sulphate on joint swelling occurred more often in patients with milder pain and lower Kellgren–Lawrence (K/L) grade (a type of arthritic score) at entry.[14] A subgroup of 572 patients who satisfied K/L grade 2 or 3 changes and joint space width of at least 2 mm at baseline continued in the five study arms for 24 months. No significant change in joint space width compared with placebo was found. Treatment effects on K/L grade 2, but not K/L grade 3 knees,

showed a trend toward improvement relative to the placebo group. The power of this study was diminished by the limited sample size, variance of the joint space width measurement and a smaller than expected loss in joint space width.[15]

A 2007 meta-analysis of 20 trials (3846 patients) found a high degree of heterogeneity and poor methodology among the trials, including small trials, trials with unclear concealment of allocation and also trials not analysed according to the intention-to-treat principle, which showed larger effects in favour of chondroitin. Analysis restricted to three trials with large sample sizes and intention-to-treat analysis excluded 40% of patients in the original 20 trials and indicated that the symptomatic benefit of chondroitin is minimal or non-existent.[16] A paper which reviewed five meta-analyses of RCTs (including the 2007 meta-analysis) stated that the other four meta-analyses showed significant clinical effects of chondroitin sulphate compared with placebo for pain and function measures while observing that the 2007 meta-analysis was based on 3 out of the 20 identified trials.[17]

The 2007 meta-analysis has been updated to include data from one new trial and final data from a second trial. This meta-analysis was limited to three RCTs, each over a 2-year period. Pooled results demonstrated a small significant effect of chondroitin sulfate in reducing the rate of decline in minimum joint space width 0.13 mm over 2 years (95% confidence interval (CI), 0.06 to 0.19; $P = 0.0002$), which corresponded to an effect size of 0.23 (95% CI, 0.11 to 0.35; $P = 0.0001$). These results indicate that chondroitin sulfate is effective for reducing the rate of decline in minimum joint space width in patients with knee osteoarthritis.[18] A further meta-analysis of six studies looked at the effect of both glucosamine and chondroitin on joint space narrowing in knee osteoarthritis. Both had a small but significant protective effect on minimum joint space narrowing after 2 years, suggesting that they may delay the progression of osteoarthritis of the knee.[19] A more recent analysis of 10 studies concluded that glucosamine and chondroitin, alone or in combination, do not reduce joint pain or have an impact on narrowing of joint space. The authors concluded that health authorities and health insurers should not cover the costs of these preparations.[20]

> **Conclusion**
> Chondroitin appears to offer only slight efficacy in function and pain relief in osteoarthritis. However, the large GAIT trial indicated that chondroitin sulphate could reduce joint swelling and in patients with mild to moderate osteoarthritis may reduce joint space narrowing compared with placebo.

Precautions/contraindications

No problems have been reported.

Pregnancy and breast-feeding

No problems have been reported but there have not been sufficient studies to guarantee the safety of chondroitin in pregnancy and breast-feeding. Chondroitin is probably best avoided.

Adverse effects

There are no known serious side-effects. However, there are no long term studies assessing the safety of chondroitin. Rarely, gastrointestinal effects and headache have been reported. However, studies in animals have found significantly decreased haematocrit, haemoglobin, white blood cells and platelet count, and the risk of internal bleeding has been suggested.[21] However, there are no reports of bleeding as a result of chondroitin use in humans.

Interactions

Drugs

Anticoagulants: Theoretically, chondroitin could potentiate the effects of anticoagulants.

Dose

Chondroitin is available in the form of capsules, typically containing 250–750 mg, often in combination with glucosamine. A review of two US products containing chondroitin showed that both had lower chondroitin levels than declared on the labels; this was also found for 6 out of 13 glucosamine and chondroitin combination products, all due to low chondroitin levels.[22]

The dose is not established. Manufacturers tend to recommend 400–1200 mg daily.

References

1 Basalo IM, Chahine NO, Kaplun M, *et al.* Chondroitin sulfate reduces the friction coefficient of articular cartilage. *J Biomech* 2007; 40(8): 1847–1854.

2 Bian L, Kaplun M, Williams DY, *et al.* Influence of chondroitin sulfate on the biochemical, mechanical and frictional properties of cartilage explants in long-term culture. *J Biomech* 2009; 42(3): 286–290.

3 Katta J, Jin Z, Ingham E, *et al.* Chondroitin sulphate: an effective joint lubricant? *Osteoarthritis Cartilage* 2009; 17(8): 1001–1008.

4 Moller I, Perez M, Monfort J, *et al.* Effectiveness of chondroitin sulphate in patients with concomitant knee osteoarthritis and psoriasis: a randomized, double-blind, placebo-controlled study. *Osteoarthritis Cartilage* 2010; 18(Suppl 1): S32–S40.

5 Bourgeois P, Chales G, Dehais J, *et al.* Efficacy and tolerability of chondroitin sulfate 1200 mg/day vs chondroitin sulfate 3 × 400 mg/day vs placebo. *Osteoarthritis Cartilage* 1998; 6(Suppl A): 25–30.

6 Bucsi L, Poor G. Efficacy and tolerability of oral chondroitin sulfate as a symptomatic slow-acting drug for osteoarthritis (SYSADOA) in the treatment of knee osteoarthritis. *Osteoarthritis Cartilage* 1998; 6(Suppl A): 31–36.

7 Uebelhart D, Thonar EJ, Delmas PD, *et al.* Effects of oral chondroitin sulfate on the progression of knee osteoarthritis: a pilot study. *Osteoarthritis Cartilage* 1998; 6(Suppl A): 39–46.

8 Leeb BF, Schweitzer H, Montag K, *et al.* A meta-analysis of chondroitin sulfate in the treatment of osteoarthritis. *J Rheumatol* 2000; 27(1): 205–211.

9 Morreale P, Manopulo R, Galati M, *et al.* Comparison of the anti-inflammatory efficacy of chondroitin sulfate and diclofenac sodium in patients with knee osteoarthritis. *J Rheumatol* 1996; 23(8): 1385–1391.

10 Mazieres B, Combe B, Phan Van A, *et al.* Chondroitin sulfate in osteoarthritis of the knee: a prospective, double-blind, placebo-controlled multicenter clinical study. *J Rheumatol* 2001; 28(1): 173–181.

11 Uebelhart D, Malaise M, Marcolongo R, *et al.* Intermittent treatment of knee osteoarthritis with oral chondroitin sulfate: a one-year, randomized, double-blind, multicenter study versus placebo. *Osteoarthritis Cartilage* 2004; 12(4): 269–276.

12 Michel BA, Stucki G, Frey D, *et al.* Chondroitins 4 and 6 sulfate in osteoarthritis of the knee: a randomized, controlled trial. *Arthritis Rheum* 2005; 52(3): 779–786.

13 Clegg DO, Reda DJ, Harris CL, *et al.* Glucosamine, chondroitin sulfate, and the two in combination for

painful knee osteoarthritis. *N Engl J Med* 2006; 354 (8): 795–808.

14 Hochberg MC, Clegg DO. Potential effects of chondroitin sulfate on joint swelling: a GAIT report. *Osteoarthritis Cartilage* 2008; 16(Suppl 3): S22–S24.

15 Sawitzke AD, Shi H, Finco MF, *et al*. The effect of glucosamine and/or chondroitin sulfate on the progression of knee osteoarthritis: a report from the glucosamine/chondroitin arthritis intervention trial. *Arthritis Rheum* 2008; 58(10): 3183–3191.

16 Reichenbach S, Sterchi R, Scherer M, *et al*. Meta-analysis: chondroitin for osteoarthritis of the knee or hip. *Ann Intern Med* 2007; 146(8): 580–590.

17 Monfort J, Martel-Pelletier J, Pelletier JP. Chondroitin sulphate for symptomatic osteoarthritis: critical appraisal of meta-analyses. *Curr Med Res Opin* 2008; 24(5): 1303–1308.

18 Hochberg MC. Structure-modifying effects of chondroitin sulfate in knee osteoarthritis: an updated meta-analysis of randomized placebo-controlled trials of 2-year duration. *Osteoarthritis Cartilage* 2010; 18(Suppl 1): S28–S31.

19 Lee YH, Woo JH, Choi SJ, *et al*. Effect of glucosamine or chondroitin sulfate on the osteoarthritis progression: a meta-analysis. *Rheumatol Int* 2009; 30(3): 357–363.

20 Wandel S, Juni P, Tendal B, *et al*. Effects of glucosamine, chondroitin, or placebo in patients with osteoarthritis of hip or knee: network meta-analysis. *BMJ* 2010; 341(16): c4675.

21 McNamara PS, Barr SC, Erb HN. Hematologic, hemostatic, and biochemical effects in dogs receiving an oral chondroprotective agent for thirty days. *Am J Vet Res* 1996; 57(9): 1390–1394.

22 Consumerlab. Product review. Glucosamine and Chondroitin. http://www.consumerlab.com (accessed 12 Novemeber 2006).

Chromium

Description

Chromium is an essential trace mineral.

Human requirements

In the UK, no Reference Nutrient Intake or Estimated Average Requirement has been set. A safe and adequate intake is, for adults, 50–400 µg daily; for children and adolescents, 0.1–1.0 µg/kg daily.

In the USA, the daily Adequate Intake for those aged 19–50 years is 35 µg for men and 25 µg for women; for those over 51 years, it is 30 µg for men and 20 µg for women.

Dietary intake

In the UK, the average adult diet provides 13.6–47.7 µg daily.

Action

Chromium functions as an organic complex known as glucose tolerance factor, which is thought to be a complex of chromium, nicotinic acid and amino acids. It potentiates the action of insulin and thus influences carbohydrate, fat and protein metabolism. Chromium also appears to influence nucleic acid synthesis and to play a role in gene expression.

Dietary sources

Wholegrain cereals (including bran cereals), brewer's yeast, broccoli, processed meats and spices are the best sources. Dairy products and most fruits and vegetables are poor sources.

Metabolism

Absorption

Chromium is poorly absorbed (0.5–2% of intake); absorption occurs in the small intestine by mechanisms that have not been clearly elucidated but which appear to involve processes other than simple diffusion.

Distribution

Chromium is transported in the serum or plasma bound to transferrin and albumin. It is widely distributed in the tissues.

Elimination

Absorbed chromium is excreted mainly by the kidneys, with small amounts lost in hair, sweat and bile.

Bioavailability

Absorption of chromium is increased by oxalate and by iron deficiency, and reduced by phytate. Diets high in simple sugars (glucose, fructose, sucrose) increase urinary chromium losses. Absorption is also increased in patients with diabetes mellitus, and depressed in the elderly. Stress and increased physical activity appear to increase urinary losses.

Deficiency

Gross chromium deficiency is rarely seen in humans, but signs and symptoms of marginal deficiency include impaired glucose tolerance, fasting hyperglycaemia, raised circulating insulin levels, glycosuria, decreased insulin binding, reduced number of insulin receptors, elevated serum cholesterol, elevated serum triglycerides, and central and peripheral neuropathy.

Possible uses

Because of its effects on insulin, chromium has been investigated for a potential role in diabetes mellitus, and it has also been promoted for body building in athletes. It has also been investigated for a potential role in cholesterol lowering and reducing the risk of cardiovascular disease.

Diabetes mellitus

Chromium deficiency may result in insulin resistance,[1] although other researchers have concluded that low-chromium diets have no effect on either insulin or blood glucose.[2] Chromium supplementation may improve glycaemic control in some patients with type 1 and 2 diabetes and gestational diabetes, but relatively high doses (e.g. 1000 µg daily) may be needed. Serum lipid fractions may also be reduced by chromium in patients with diabetes.

Chromium picolinate (200 µg three times a day) reduced glycosylated haemoglobin in a woman with type 1 diabetes mellitus, and the patient also reported improved blood glucose values.[3] Chromium picolinate (200 µg daily) increased insulin sensitivity in patients with type 1 and type 2 diabetes, allowing for a reduction in dose of insulin or hypoglycaemic drugs without compromising glucose control.[4] Steroid-induced diabetes was improved after supplementation with chromium 200 µg three times a day, and chromium 200 µg daily was sufficient to maintain normal blood glucose thereafter.[5]

In a double-blind, placebo-controlled trial, 180 patients with type 2 diabetes were randomised to receive 250 µg chromium twice a day, 100 µg chromium twice a day, or placebo. After 2 months, glycosylated haemoglobin levels were significantly lower in the high-dose chromium group and after 4 months were lower in both chromium groups compared with placebo. Fasting and 2-hour insulin levels were significantly lower in both chromium groups at 2 and 4 months, but significantly lower glucose values and lower plasma cholesterol were found only in the high-dose chromium group.[6]

In a prospective, double-blind, placebo-controlled, crossover study in 28 subjects with type 2 diabetes, serum triglycerides were significantly reduced by chromium (200 µg daily for 2 months).[7] However, there was no change in fasting glucose, or plasma LDL or HDL levels.

In a double-blind, placebo-controlled, crossover study, 78 patients with type 2 diabetes in Saudi Arabia received in random order brewer's yeast (23 µg chromium) and 200 µg chromium from chromium chloride for 4 weeks each. Mean HDL cholesterol and serum and urinary chromium were all raised by chromium intake. After each chromium phase, mean drug dosage tended to decrease, but was not significant except in the case of glibenclamide. There was no change in dietary intakes or body mass index. Overall, brewer's yeast was associated with better chromium retention and more positive effects than chromium chloride.[8]

Supplementation of nicotinic acid together with chromium may increase its effectiveness. In a study involving 16 healthy elderly volunteers, neither chromium 200 µg daily nor nicotinic acid 100 mg daily affected fasting glucose or glucose tolerance. However, chromium administered with nicotinic acid resulted in a 15% decrease in the area under the glucose curve and a 7% decrease in fasting glucose.[9]

A systematic review and meta-analysis of 15 RCTs involving 618 participants, of whom 193 had type 2 diabetes and 425 were in good health or had impaired glucose tolerance, showed that there was no effect of chromium on glucose or insulin concentrations in non-diabetic subjects and the data for people with diabetes were inconclusive.[10] Only one of the studies in the meta-analysis, involving 155 subjects in China, showed that chromium reduced glucose and insulin concentrations and haemoglobin A1c (HbA1c).

Further studies have investigated other potential effects of chromium in patients with diabetes. Chromium supplementation has been found to minimise increased oxidative stress in patients with type 2 diabetes mellitus and high HbA1c levels.[11] Chromium supplementation (400 or 800 µg) improved glucose tolerance in 10 out of 13 subjects in a randomised crossover study.[12] Short-term chromium supplementation (1000 µg) has also been found to shorten QTc interval in patients with type 2 diabetes mellitus.[13]

A 12-week placebo-controlled trial in 36 patients with type 2 diabetes found that chromium 400 µg (as chromium-enriched yeast) was associated with a significant decrease in fasting serum glucose compared with placebo. Blood markers of oxidative stress – glutathione peroxidase activity and levels of reduced glutathione – were unchanged in the chromium group but decreased significantly in the placebo group, while serum HbA1c and glycated protein (fructosamine) increased in the placebo group but were unchanged in the chromium group. Fasting serum insulin decreased in both groups with a greater tendency in the chromium group.[14]

However, a randomised, double-blind, placebo-controlled trial of high-dose chromium supplementation (500 or 1000 µg daily) in obese patients with type 2 diabetes found no differences in HbA1c reduction across the two doses of chromium and placebo. There were no significant differences in lipid profile, blood pressure, insulin requirements and body mass index. The authors concluded that there is no evidence that high-dose chromium treatment is effective in obese Western patients with type 2 diabetes.[15] A further trial with chromium yeast by the same research group, in this case using a dose of 400 µg daily in patients being treated with oral hypoglycaemic agents, found no difference between chromium yeast and placebo in terms of change in HbA1c, lipid

profile, body mass index, blood pressure, body fat and insulin resistance.[16]

Patient phenotype may be important in relation to the clinical response to chromium in diabetes. A RCT in 73 subjects with type 2 diabetes found that 63% of the patients responded to chromium supplementation (1000 µg daily) in relation to parameters of improved glycaemic control compared with 30% with placebo. The only subject variable significantly associated with the clinical response to chromium was the baseline insulin sensitivity. The authors suggest that, because baseline insulin sensitivity accounted for nearly 40% of the variance in clinical response to chromium, subject phenotype appears to be important in assessing clinical response to chromium.[17]

More recently, trials have evaluated the combination of chromium and biotin in glucose control. Both nutrients play roles in regulating carbohydrate metabolism. All four trials to date have used a dose of 600 µg chromium with 2 mg biotin. This combination has been shown to reduce the area under the glucose curve, fructosamine, triglycerides and triglyceride/HDL cholesterol ratio;[18] to lower HbA1c and blood glucose;[19] and to reduce triglycerides, the ratio of LDL to HDL cholesterol, blood glucose, fructosamine and the area under the glucose curve.[20] In patients with type 2 diabetes and dyslipidaemia, the chromium/biotin combination was associated with significant reduction in total cholesterol, LDL cholesterol and atherogenic index. Significant decreases in LDL cholesterol, total cholesterol, HbA1c and VLDL cholesterol were observed in patients who were also taking statins.[19] Improvements in glycaemic control seem to be most pronounced in poorly controlled diabetic patients on oral therapy.[21]

Multiple drug regimens in HIV are associated with an increased incidence of insulin resistance. Based on associations between chromium supplementation and improved insulin sensitivity in some studies, eight patients with HIV on antiretroviral therapy were given high-dose chromium picolinate 1000 µg daily for 8 weeks. Glucose disposal and insulin resistance improved during the course of the study with no changes in other blood or HIV parameters. However, two subjects experienced abnormalities of liver function during the study, while another experienced an elevation in blood urea nitrogen.[22] A further controlled trial in 52 HIV-positive subjects with elevated glucose or lipids, or evidence of body fat redistribution, and who had insulin resistance showed that chromium nicotinate 400 µg daily improved insulin resistance, metabolic abnormalities and body composition, suggesting that chromium supplements alleviate some of the antiretroviral-associated metabolic abnormalities.[23]

Obesity

In some controlled human studies, chromium has been reported to reduce body fat,[24, 25] and increase fat-free mass,[26] but to have no effect in others.[27] A recent RCT showed that chromium supplementation did not improve key features of the metabolic syndrome in obese non-diabetic patients.[28] A meta-analysis of 10 trials found that chromium picolinate had a favourable effect on body weight. However, sensitivity analysis suggested that this effect was largely dependent on the results of a single trial. The authors concluded that the effect of chromium is likely to be small and its clinical relevance debatable.[29] A more recent trial in 83 women found that chromium picolinate 200 µg daily did not affect body weight or body fat.[30] A placebo-controlled trial in 42 overweight women found that chromium picolinate 1000 µg daily significantly reduced food intake, hunger levels and fat cravings compared with placebo, and there was a tendency (non-significant) to lose weight.[31] Supplementation of 1000 µg of chromium picolinate alone, and in combination with nutritional education, did not affect weight loss in a recent study among a population of overweight adults.[32]

Body-building

Chromium supplements are claimed to influence body composition during body-building programmes, although there is little evidence for this. In a study involving 36 men on a weight-training programme, chromium supplementation had no effect on strength, fat-free mass or muscle mass.[33] Chromium picolinate (200 µg a day) did not alter body fat, lean body mass and skin-fold thickness in untrained young men on an exercise programme.[34] Neither body composition nor strength changed as a result of chromium picolinate supplementation (200 µg daily) in football players during a 9-week training programme.[35] Young women on a weight-training programme taking chromium picolinate (200 µg daily for

12 weeks) gained significantly more weight than those taking a placebo, and there was a nonsignificant increase in lean body mass.[36] However, there were no effects on body composition or strength in the young men on the same programme. In moderately obese women placed on an exercise programme, 12 weeks of chromium supplementation (400 µg daily) did not significantly affect body composition, resting metabolic rate, plasma glucose, serum insulin, plasma glucagons, serum C-peptide and serum lipid concentrations.[37] Moreover, the use of combined chromium picolinate with conjugated linoleic acid supplementation over 3 months did not affect diet and exercise induced changes in weight and body composition or improve indices of metabolic and cardiovascular health in a trial in 35 overweight young women.[38] In a study in 16 overweight men, chromium picolinate supplementation (600 µg daily) did not augment glycogen synthesis during recovery from high-intensity exercise and high-carbohydrate feeding.[39]

Cardiovascular disease

Chromium supplements have been claimed to reduce serum cholesterol levels, and there is some evidence for this.

Two placebo-controlled trials, one in 76 men on beta-blockers (a double-blind study)[40] the other in 76 patients with atherosclerosis (not blinded),[41] showed a significant increase in serum HDL cholesterol with chromium (300 µg daily in the first study, 200 µg daily in the second). In a double-blind, placebo-controlled, crossover study in 28 healthy subjects,[42] chromium supplementation (200 µg daily) resulted in a statistically significant reduction in total and LDL cholesterol. HDL was not raised significantly, although apolipoprotein A1 (the principal protein in HDL) was increased.

Depression

Patients with depression may respond to chromium. In a double-blind RCT, 113 adults with atypical depression, most of whom were obese, were randomised to receive 600 µg elemental chromium or placebo. Chromium produced an improvement in reducing carbohydrate craving and appetite increase and diurnal variation in feelings. The results suggested that the main benefit of chromium was in depressed patients with high carbohydrate craving. The authors concluded that further research is needed in depressed patients specifically selected for symptoms of increased appetite and carbohydrate craving.[43]

Polycystic ovary syndrome

Polycystic ovary syndrome (POS) is associated with glucose intolerance and, on the basis of its association with improved glucose metabolism in some studies, chromium has been investigated in this condition. In one pilot study, chromium picolinate 200 µg daily improved glucose tolerance compared with placebo but did not improve ovulatory frequency or hormonal parameters.[44] A further trial in five obese subjects with POS found that chromium 1000 µg daily was associated with a 38% mean improvement in glucose disposal rate.[45]

> ### Conclusion
> Preliminary evidence suggests that chromium may improve insulin resistance and glucose control in diabetes, although not all studies have reached this conclusion. Preliminary evidence also suggests that chromium may improve serum lipid levels. However, there is no good evidence that chromium reduces body weight or body fat. Despite claims made for chromium in sports, there is no evidence that it has body-building effects in athletes. Preliminary evidence suggests that chromium may be helpful in depression with carbohydrate craving.

Precautions/contraindications

Chromium supplements containing yeast should be avoided by patients taking monoamine oxidase inhibitors. Patients with diabetes mellitus should not take chromium supplements unless medically supervised (chromium may potentiate insulin).

Pregnancy and breast-feeding

No problems reported at normal dietary intakes.

Adverse effects

Trivalent chromium (Cr(III)) compounds have been associated with genotoxicity. In 2005, the UK Committee on Mutagenicity (COM) reviewed the available evidence and concluded that the balance of evidence suggested that chromium picolinate was not genotoxic. However, reports in the literature continue to raise this issue. An Australian review suggested that the potential for genotoxic side-effects of Cr(III) complexes may outweigh possible benefits in insulin control and that recommendations for their use as either nutritional supplements or antidiabetic drugs should be reconsidered.[46] A US report, however, suggested that genotoxic effects of Cr(III) had been demonstrated *in vitro* under high-exposure conditions and that nutritional benefits appear to outweigh the theoretical risk of genotoxic effects *in vivo* at normal or modestly elevated physiological intake levels.[47]

Industrial exposure to high amounts of chromate dust is associated with an increased incidence of lung cancer and may cause allergic dermatitis and skin ulcers. The hexavalent form (not found in food or supplements) can cause renal and hepatic necrosis.

Interactions

Drugs

Insulin: may reduce insulin requirements in diabetes mellitus (monitor blood glucose).
Oral hypoglycaemics: may potentiate effects of oral hypoglycaemics.

Dose

Chromium is available in the form of chromium picolinate, chromium nicotinic acid, chromium chloride or as an organic complex in brewer's yeast. It is available in tablet and capsule form and is present in multivitamin/mineral preparations.

The dose is not established. Studies have been conducted with 200 to 500 µg elemental chromium daily. Dietary supplements provide, on average, 200 µg in a daily dose.

References

1   Mertz W. Chromium in human nutrition: a review. *J Nutr* 1993; 123: 626–633.
2   Anderson R. Nutritional factors influencing the glucose/insulin system: chromium. *J Am Coll Nutr* 1997; 16: 404–410.

3 Fox G, Sabovic Z. Chromium picolinate supplementation for diabetes mellitus. *J Fam Pract* 1998; 46: 83–86.

4 Ravina A, Slezak L, Rubal A. Clinical use of the trace element chromium (III) in the treatment of diabetes mellitus. *J Trace Elem Exper Med* 1995; 8: 183–190.

5 Ravina A, Slezak L, Mirsky N, *et al.* Reversal of corticosteroid-induced diabetes mellitus with supplemental chromium. *Diabet Med* 1999; 16(2): 164–167.

6 Anderson R, Cheng N, Bryden N. Elevated intakes of supplemental chromium improve glucose and insulin variables in individuals with type 2 diabetes. *Diabetes* 1997; 46: 1786–1791.

7 Lee N, Reasner C. Beneficial effect of chromium supplementation on serum triglyceride levels in NIDDM. *Diabetes Care* 1994; 17: 1449–1452.

8 Bahijiri SM, Mira SA, Mufti AM, *et al.* The effects of inorganic chromium and brewer's yeast supplementation on glucose tolerance, serum lipids and drug dosage in individuals with type 2 diabetes. *Saudi Med J* 2000; 21(9): 831–837.

9 Urberg M, Zemel M. Evidence for synergism between chromium and nicotinic acid in the control of glucose tolerance in elderly humans. *Metabolism* 1987; 36: 896–899.

10 Althuis M, Jordan N, Ludington E, *et al.* Glucose and insulin responses to dietary chromium supplements: a meta-analysis. *Am J Clin Nutr* 2002; 76: 148–155.

11 Cheng H, Lai M, Hou W, *et al.* Antioxidant effects of chromium supplementation with type 2 diabetes mellitus and euglycemic subjects. *J Agric Food Chem* 2004; 52: 1385–1389.

12 Frauchiger M, Wenk C, Colombani P. Effects of acute chromium supplementation on postprandial metabolism in healthy young men. *J Am Coll Nutr* 2004; 23: 351–357.

13 Vrtovec M, Vrtovec B, Briski A, *et al.* Chromium supplementation shortens QTc interval duration in patients with type 2 diabetes mellitus. *Am Heart J* 2005; 149(4): 632–636.

14 Racek J, Trefil L, Rajdl D, *et al.* Influence of chromium-enriched yeast on blood glucose and insulin variables, blood lipids, and markers of oxidative stress in subjects with type 2 diabetes mellitus. *Biol Trace Elem Res* 2006; 109(3): 215–230.

15 Kleefstra N, Houweling ST, Jansman FG, *et al.* Chromium treatment has no effect in patients with poorly controlled, insulin-treated type 2 diabetes in an obese Western population: a randomized, double-blind, placebo-controlled trial. *Diabetes Care* 2006; 29(3): 521–525.

16 Kleefstra N, Houweling ST, Bakker SJ, *et al.* Chromium treatment has no effect in patients with type 2 diabetes in a Western population: a randomized, double-blind, placebo-controlled trial. *Diabetes Care* 2007; 30(5): 1092–1096.

17 Wang CZ, Aung HH, Zhang B, *et al.* Chemopreventive effects of heat-processed *Panax quinquefolius* root on human breast cancer cells. *Anticancer Res* 2008; 28 2008;(5A): 2545–2551.

18 Singer GM, Geohas J. The effect of chromium picolinate and biotin supplementation on glycemic control in poorly controlled patients with type 2 diabetes mellitus: a placebo-controlled, double-blinded, randomized trial. *Diabetes Technol Ther* 2006; 8(6): 636–643.

19 Albarracin C, Fuqua B, Geohas J, *et al.* Combination of chromium and biotin improves coronary risk factors in hypercholesterolemic type 2 diabetes mellitus: a placebo-controlled, double-blind randomized clinical trial. *J Cardiometab Syndr* 2007; 2(2): 91–97.

20 Geohas J, Daly A, Juturu V, *et al.* Chromium picolinate and biotin combination reduces atherogenic index of plasma in patients with type 2 diabetes mellitus: a placebo-controlled, double-blinded, randomized clinical trial. *Am J Med Sci* 2007; 333(3): 145–153.

21 Albarracin CA, Fuqua BC, Evans JL, *et al.* Chromium picolinate and biotin combination improves glucose metabolism in treated, uncontrolled overweight to obese patients with type 2 diabetes. *Diabetes Metab Res Rev* 2008; 24(1): 41–51.

22 Feiner JJ, McNurlan MA, Ferris RE, *et al.* Chromium picolinate for insulin resistance in subjects with HIV disease: a pilot study. *Diabetes Obes Metab* 2008; 10(2): 151–158.

23 Aghdassi E, Arendt BM, Salit IE, *et al.* In patients with HIV-infection, chromium supplementation improves insulin resistance and other metabolic abnormalities: a randomized, double-blind, placebo controlled trial. *Curr HIV Res* 2010; 8(2): 113–120.

24 Kaats G, Blum K, Fisher J. Effects of chromium picolinate supplementation on body composition: a randomized, double-masked, placebo-controlled study. *Curr Ther Res* 1996; 57: 747–756.

25 Kaats G, Blum K, Pullin D. A randomized double-masked, placebo-controlled study of the effects of chromium picolinate supplementation on body composition: a replication and extension of a previous study. *Curr Ther Res* 1998; 59: 379–388.

26 Cefalu W, Bell-Farrow A, Wang Z. The effect of chromium supplementation on carbohydrate metabolism and body fat distribution. *Diabetes* 1997; 46(Suppl 1): 55A.

27 Trent L, Thieding-Cancel D. Effects of chromium picolinate on body composition. *J Sports Med Phys Fitness* 1995; 35: 273–280.

28 Iqbal N, Cardillo S, Volger S, *et al.* Chromium picolinate does not improve key features of metabolic syndrome in obese nondiabetic adults. *Metab Syndr Relat Disord* 2009; 7(2): 143–150.

29 Lukaski HC, Bolonchuk WW, Siders WA, *et al.* Chromium supplementation and resistance training: effects on body composition, strength, and trace element status of men. *Am J Clin Nutr* 1996; 63(6): 954–965.

30 Lukaski HC, Siders WA, Penland JG. Chromium picolinate supplementation in women: effects on body weight, composition, and iron status. *Nutrition* 2007; 23(3): 187–195.

31 Anton SD, Morrison CD, Cefalu WT, *et al.* Effects of chromium picolinate on food intake and satiety. *Diabetes Technol Ther* 2008; 10(5): 405–412.

32 Yazaki Y, Faridi Z, Ma Y, *et al.* A pilot study of chromium picolinate for weight loss. *J Altern Complement Med* 2010; 16(3): 291–299.

33 Pittler M, Stevinson C, Ernst E. Chromium picolinate for reducing body weight: meta-analyisis of randomized trials. *Int J Obes Relat Metab Disord* 2003; 27: 522–529.

34 Hallmark MA, Reynolds TH, DeSouza CA, *et al.* Effects of chromium and resistive training on muscle strength and body composition. *Med Sci Sports Exerc* 1996; 28 1996;(1): 139–144.

35 Clancy SP, Clarkson PM, DeCheke ME, *et al.* Effects of chromium picolinate supplementation on body composition, strength, and urinary chromium loss in football players. *Int J Sport Nutr* 1994; 4 1994;(2): 142–153.

36 Hasten DL, Rome EP, Franks BD, *et al.* Effects of chromium picolinate on beginning weight training students. *Int J Sport Nutr* 1992; 2(4): 343–350.

37 Roeback JR,Jr Hla KM, Chambless LE, *et al.* Effects of chromium supplementation on serum high-density lipoprotein cholesterol levels in men taking beta-blockers. A randomized, controlled trial. *Ann Intern Med* 1991; 115(12): 917–924.

38 Diaz ML, Watkins BA, Li Y, *et al.* Chromium picolinate and conjugated linoleic acid do not synergistically influence diet- and exercise-induced changes in body composition and health indexes in overweight women. *J Nutr Biochem* 2008; 19(1): 61–68.

39 Volek JS, Silvestre R, Kirwan JP, *et al.* Effects of chromium supplementation on glycogen synthesis after high-intensity exercise. *Med Sci Sports Exerc* 2006; 38(12): 2102–2109.

40 Volpe S, Huang H, Larpadisorn K, *et al.* Effect of chromium supplementation and exercise on body composition, resting metabolic rate and selected biochemical parameters in moderately obese women following an exercise program. *J Am Coll Nutr* 2001; 20: 293–306.

41 Abraham A, Brooks B, Eylath U. The effect of chromium supplementation on serum glucose and lipids in patients with and without non-insulin dependent diabetes. *Metabolism* 1992; 41: 768–771.

42 Press R, Geller J, Evans G. The effect of chromium picolinate on serum cholesterol and apolipoprotein fractions in human subjects. *West J Med* 1990; 152: 41–45.

43 Docherty JP, Sack DA, Roffman M, *et al.* A double-blind, placebo-controlled, exploratory trial of chromium picolinate in atypical depression: effect on carbohydrate craving. *J Psychiatr Pract* 2005; 11 (5): 302–314.

44 Lucidi RS, Thyer AC, Easton CA, *et al.* Effect of chromium supplementation on insulin resistance and ovarian and menstrual cyclicity in women with polycystic ovary syndrome. *Fertil Steril* 2005; 84 (6): 1755–1757.

45 Lydic ML, McNurlan M, Bembo S, *et al.* Chromium picolinate improves insulin sensitivity in obese subjects with polycystic ovary syndrome. *Fertil Steril* 2006; 86 2006;(1): 243–246.

46 Levina A, Lay PA. Chemical properties and toxicity of chromium(III) nutritional supplements. *Chem Res Toxicol* 2008; 21(3): 563–571.

47 Eastmond DA, Macgregor JT, Slesinski RS. Trivalent chromium: assessing the genotoxic risk of an essential trace element and widely used human and animal nutritional supplement. *Crit Rev Toxicol* 2008; 38(3): 173–190.

Cinnamon

Description

Cinnamon is a spice that has been used for thousands of years both for its enhancement of taste and for its potential medicinal benefits. It is derived from the dried inner bark of evergreen trees grown in South Asia (Ceylon cinnamon) and Southeast Asia (Chinese cinnamon).

The constituents of cinnamon include cinnamaldehyde (cinnamic aldehyde, 3-phenyl-2-propenal) as the major constituent from the bark and eugenol (2-methoxy-4-(2-propenyl) phenol) as the primary component in extracts from the leaf. Other constituents in cinnamon include cinnamyl alcohol, coumarin, phenolic acids, terpenes, carbohydrates and tannins.

Action

Cinnamon bark appears to have antibacterial activity,[1] but there is a lack of evidence of antimicrobial benefit in humans. One study evaluated the capacity of cinnamon to inhibit *Helicobacter pylori* in the stomach and demonstrated no benefit.[2] There is some limited evidence of anti-cancer activity.[3–5]

An antioxidant activity of cinnamon has been identified. Reports from cell culture models and studies in rats show that cinnamon and cinnamaldehyde have antioxidant activity and scavenge free radicals.[6–8] Limited evidence suggests that cinnamon can suppress inflammatory processes.[2,9]

Much recent research has focused on the potential for cinnamon bark to influence glucose and insulin metabolism. Cinnamon polyphenols have been shown to have insulin-like activity,[10,11] enhance insulin activity,[12] improve insulin sensitivity[13] and improve glucose uptake into cells.[14–16]

Possible uses

Orally, cinnamon has been used for type 2 diabetes, gas (flatulence), muscle and gastrointestinal spasms, preventing nausea and vomiting, diarrhoea, infections, the common cold and loss of appetite.

Cinnamon has attracted interest for a potential role in diabetes. Evidence for an antidiabetic action of cinnamon constituents in humans is inconsistent but suggestive of a possible modest action in lowering blood glucose levels. In two studies, cinnamon ingestion improved *in vivo* glucose tolerance in healthy human subjects.[17,18] A crossover trial in 15 healthy subjects found that ingestion of 3 g cinnamon reduced postprandial serum insulin and increased glucagon-like peptide 1 (GLP-1) concentrations without significantly affecting blood glucose, glucose-dependent insulinotropic polypeptide (GIP), ghrelin concentration, satiety or gastric emptying rate. The results indicate a relation between the amount of cinnamon consumed and the decrease in insulin concentration.[19]

Several intervention studies have evaluated cinnamon in patients with diabetes. A 40-day trial in 60 patients with type 2 diabetes found that intake of 1, 3 or 6 g cinnamon per day reduced serum glucose, triglyceride, low-density lipoprotein cholesterol and total cholesterol, and it suggested that the inclusion of cinnamon in the diet of people with type 2 diabetes would reduce

risk factors associated with diabetes and cardiovascular diseases.[20] A trial of 120-days duration in 65 patients with type 2 diabetes found that cinnamon 3 g daily decreased fasting blood glucose levels but did not affect haemoglobin (Hb) A1c or blood lipids.[21]

A 42-day trial in 25 postmenopausal women with type 2 diabetes showed no effect of cinnamon 1.5 g daily on fasting blood glucose, HbA1c or blood lipid profile.[22] Another trial using the same 1.5 g dose of cinnamon, but in 60 male and female patients with diabetes, again found no effect on fasting blood glucose, HbA1c or blood lipid profile.[23] Lower doses also had no effects on diabetes parameters. One trial in 57 adolescents with type 1 diabetes found no effect of cinnamon 1 g daily over 90 days on HbA1c, total daily insulin use or number of hypoglycaemic episodes,[24] while a 90-day trial in 43 patients with type 2 diabetes found no effect of the same dose on fasting blood glucose, HbA1c, insulin levels and blood lipids.[25]

Though cinnamon can improve fasting glucose in humans, data on insulin sensitivity are limited and controversial. A trial in eight male volunteers who underwent two 14-day interventions involving cinnamon or placebo supplementation (3 g/day) found that cinnamon ingestion reduced the glucose response to an oral glucose tolerance test (OGTT) on day 1 and day 14. Cinnamon ingestion also reduced insulin responses to OGTT on day 14 as well as improving insulin sensitivity on day 14. These effects were lost following cessation of cinnamon feeding, indicating that cinnamon may improve glycaemic control and insulin sensitivity, but the effects are quickly reversed.[26]

A meta-analysis[27] and four recent reviews[28–31] have evaluated and summarised the evidence for an effect of cinnamon on diabetes parameters, indicating that studies are inconsistent but that the antidiabetic action of cinnamon warrants further study.

Precautions/contraindications

There is insufficient reliable information; caution is required in liver disease.

Pregnancy and breast-feeding

Insufficient data.

Adverse effects

Cinnamon has been well tolerated in clinical trials. Concern exists about the coumarin content, particularly in patients with liver disease.

Interactions

Potential exacerbation of antidiabetes drug action.

Dose

Cinnamon intakes in studies are considerably greater than levels consumed in a typical diet, with amounts ranging from 1 to 6 g daily for periods of time ranging from 6 weeks to 4 months.

Conclusion

There is suggestive evidence from human studies that cinnamon can lower blood glucose and modulate insulin levels associated with type 2 diabetes. However, the data are as yet weak and inconclusive. Evidence that cinnamon lowers diabetes-related blood cholesterol and improves lipid profile is inconclusive. The antidiabetic action of cinnamon warrants further study.

References

1 Lee HS, Ahn YJ. Growth-inhibiting effects of *Cinnamomum cassia* bark-derived materials on human intestinal bacteria. *J Agric Food Chem* 1998; 46: 8–12.

2 Nir Y, Potasman I, Stermer E, Tabak M, Neeman I. Controlled trial of the effect of cinnamon extract on *Helicobacter pylori*. *Helicobacter* 2000; 5: 94–97.

3 Kwon BM, Lee SH, Choi SU, et al. Synthesis and in vitro cytotoxicity of cinnamaldehydes to human solid tumor cells. *Arch Pharm Res* 1998; 21: 147–152.

4 Schoene NW, Kelly MA, Polansky MM, Anderson RA. A polyphenol mixture from cinnamon targets p38 MAP kinase-regulated signaling pathways to produce G2/M arrest. *J Nutr Biochem* 2009; 20: 614–620.

5 Schoene NW, Kelly MA, Polansky MM, Anderson RA. Water-soluble polymeric polyphenols from cinnamon inhibit proliferation and alter cell cycle distribution patterns of hematologic tumor cell lines. *Cancer Lett* 2005; 230: 134–140.

6 Singh G, Maurya S, DeLampasona MP, Catalan CA. A comparison of chemical, antioxidant and antimicrobial studies of cinnamon leaf and bark volatile oils, oleoresins and their constituents. *Food Chem Toxicol* 2007; 45: 1650–1661.

7 Jayaprakasha GK, Ohnishi-Kameyama M, Ono H, Yoshida M, Jaganmohan Rao L. Phenolic constituents in the fruits of *Cinnamomum zeylanicum* and their antioxidant activity. *J Agric Food Chem* 2006; 54: 1672–1679.

8 Ranjbar A, Ghasmeinezhad S, Zamani H, et al. Antioxidative stress potential of *Cinnamomum zeylanicum* in humans: a comparative cross-sectional clinical study. *Therapy* 2006; 3: 113–117.

9 Youn HS, Lee JK, Choi YJ, et al. Cinnamaldehyde suppresses Toll-like receptor 4 activation mediated through the inhibition of receptor oligomerization. *Biochem Pharmacol* 2008; 75: 494–502.

10 Anderson RA, Broadhurst CL, Polansky MM, et al. Isolation and characterization of polyphenol type-A polymers from cinnamon with insulin-like biological activity. *J Agric Food Chem* 2004; 52: 65–70.

11 Jarvill-Taylor KJ, Anderson RA, Graves DJ. A hydroxychalcone derived from cinnamon functions as a mimetic for insulin in 3T3-L1 adipocytes. *J Am Coll Nutr* 2001; 20: 327–336.

12 Imparl-Radosevich J, Deas S, Polansky MM, et al. Regulation of PTP-1 and insulin receptor kinase by fractions from cinnamon: implications for cinnamon regulation of insulin signalling. *Horm Res* 1998; 50: 177–182.

13 Anderson RA. Chromium and polyphenols from cinnamon improve insulin sensitivity. *Proc Nutr Soc* 2008; 67: 48–53.

14 Roffey B, Atwal A, Kubow S. Cinnamon water extracts increase glucose uptake but inhibit adiponectin secretion in 3T3-L1 adipose cells. *Mol Nutr Food Res* 2006; 50: 739–745.

15 Verspohl EJ, Bauer K, Neddermann E. Antidiabetic effect of *Cinnamomum cassia* and *Cinnamomum zeylanicum* in vivo and in vitro. *Phytother Res* 2005; 19: 203–206.

16 Qin B, Nagasaki M, Ren M, et al. Cinnamon extract (traditional herb) potentiates in vivo insulin-regulated glucose utilization via enhancing insulin signaling in rats. *Diabetes Res Clin Pract* 2003; 62: 139–148.

17 Solomon TP, Blannin AK. Effects of short-term cinnamon ingestion on in vivo glucose tolerance. *Diabetes Obes Metab* 2007; 9: 895–901.

18 Hlebowicz J, Darwiche G, Bjorgell O, Almer LO. Effect of cinnamon on postprandial blood glucose, gastric emptying, and satiety in healthy subjects. *Am J Clin Nutr* 2007; 85: 1552–1556.

19 Hlebowicz J, Hlebowicz A, Lindstedt S, et al. Effects of 1 and 3 g cinnamon on gastric emptying, satiety,

and postprandial blood glucose, insulin, glucose-dependent insulinotropic polypeptide, glucagon-like peptide 1, and ghrelin concentrations in healthy subjects. *Am J Clin Nutr* 2009; 89: 815–821.

20 Khan A, Safdar M, Ali Khan MM, Khattak KN, Anderson RA. Cinnamon improves glucose and lipids of people with type 2 diabetes. *Diabetes Care* 2003; 26: 3215–3218.

21 Mang B, Wolters M, Schmitt B, *et al.* Effects of a cinnamon extract on plasma glucose, HbA, and serum lipids in diabetes mellitus type 2. *Eur J Clin Invest* 2006; 36: 340–344.

22 Vanschoonbeek K, Thomassen BJ, Senden JM, Wodzig WK, van Loon LJ. Cinnamon supplementation does not improve glycemic control in postmenopausal type 2 diabetes patients. *J Nutr* 2006; 136: 977–980.

23 Suppapitiporn S, Kanpaksi N, Suppapitiporn S. The effect of cinnamon cassia powder in type 2 diabetes mellitus. *J Med Assoc Thai* 2006; 89 (Suppl 3): S200–S205.

24 Altschuler JA, Casella SJ, MacKenzie TA, Curtis KM. The effect of cinnamon on A1C among adolescents with type 1 diabetes. *Diabetes Care* 2007; 30: 813–816.

25 Blevins SM, Leyva MJ, Brown J, *et al.* Effect of cinnamon on glucose and lipid levels in non insulin-dependent type 2 diabetes. *Diabetes Care* 2007; 30: 2236–2237.

26 Solomon TP, Blannin AK. Changes in glucose tolerance and insulin sensitivity following 2 weeks of daily cinnamon ingestion in healthy humans. *Eur J Appl Physiol* 2009; 105: 969–976.

27 Pham AQ, Kourlas H, Pham DQ. Cinnamon supplementation in patients with type 2 diabetes mellitus. *Pharmacotherapy* 2007; 27: 595–599.

28 Chase CK, McQueen CE. Cinnamon in diabetes mellitus. *Am J Health Syst Pharm* 2007; 64: 1033–1035.

29 Baker WL, Gutierrez-Williams G, White CM, Kluger J, Coleman CI. Effect of cinnamon on glucose control and lipid parameters. *Diabetes Care* 2008; 31: 41–43.

30 Dugoua JJ, Seely D, Perri D, *et al.* From type 2 diabetes to antioxidant activity: a systematic review of the safety and efficacy of common and cassia cinnamon bark. *Can J Physiol Pharmacol* 2007; 85: 837–847.

31 Singletary K. Cinnamon. Overview of health benefits. *Nutrition Today* 2008; 43: 263–266.

Coenzyme Q

Description

Coenzyme Q is a naturally occurring enzyme cofactor found in the mitochondria of the body cells.

Nomenclature

Several types of coenzyme Q have been identified and numbered from zero upwards. The variety found in human tissue is coenzyme Q_{10} (ubiquinone) and so is the term used here.

Action

Coenzyme Q_{10} has the following functions:

- It is involved in electron transport and supports the synthesis of adenosine triphosphate (ATP) in the mitochondrial membrane.
- It plays a vital role in intracellular energy production.
- It is a fat-soluble antioxidant that helps to stabilise cell membranes, preserving cellular integrity and function. It also helps to regenerate vitamin E to its antioxidant form.
- It is essential for normal myocardial function.
- It has immunostimulant activity.
- It may be obtained from the diet or a food supplement, but it is also produced endogenously.

Dietary sources

Meat and fatty fish products are the most concentrated sources, although smaller quantities are found in wholegrain cereals, soya beans, nuts and vegetables, particularly spinach and broccoli. The relative importance of endogenous synthesis and dietary intake to coenzyme Q_{10} status has not been established. Coenzyme Q_{10} is also found in a number of food supplements, either as the sole active ingredient or in combination with vitamins and/or minerals, especially magnesium.

Metabolism

Absorption of coenzyme Q_{10} from the diet or a supplement occurs in the small intestine and is influenced by the presence of food and drink. It is better absorbed in the presence of a fatty meal. After absorption, it is transported to the liver where it is incorporated into lipoproteins and bound principally to VLDL and LDL cholesterol. It is then concentrated in the tissues. One study found that coenzyme Q_{10} from both foods and supplements significantly raised serum concentrations.[1] Animal data show that coenzyme Q_{10} in large doses is taken up by all tissues including heart and brain mitochondria.[2]

A study evaluating plasma coenzyme Q_{10} response to oral ingestion of various formulations found that both total plasma coenzyme Q_{10} and net increase over baseline concentrations show a gradual increase with increasing doses of coenzyme Q_{10}. Plasma coenzyme Q_{10} concentrations plateau at a dose of 2400 mg using one specific chewable tablet formulation. The efficiency of absorption decreases as the dose increases. About 95% of circulating coenzyme Q_{10} occurs as ubiquinol, with no appreciable change in the ratio following coenzyme Q_{10} ingestion. Higher plasma coenzyme Q_{10} concentrations are necessary to facilitate uptake by peripheral tissues and also the brain.[3] Solubilised formulations of coenzyme Q_{10} (both ubiquinone and ubiquinol) have superior bioavailability as evidenced by their enhanced plasma coenzyme Q_{10} responses[2,3]

Coenzyme Q_{10} is produced endogenously from tyrosine within all cells of the body, but specifically in the heart, liver, kidney and pancreas, where it plays an indispensable role in intracellular energy production. Several cofactors are involved in its synthesis, including riboflavin, pyridoxine, folic acid, vitamin B_{12}, niacin, pantothenic acid and vitamin C. The ability to synthesise coenzyme Q_{10} decreases as people get older. The concentration of coenzyme Q_{10} in human tissue appears to be related to age, peaking at age 20 and declining after that.[4]

Deficiency

Because coenzyme Q_{10} is not an essential nutrient in the same way as a vitamin or mineral, no Dietary Reference Values or RDAs have been established. However, there is increasing speculation based on serum and/or biopsy samples that certain signs and symptoms are associated with a lack of coenzyme Q_{10}.

Deficiency has been linked to:

- congestive heart failure (CHF)[5]
- ischaemic heart disease[6]
- cardiomyopathy[7]
- hypertension[6]
- use of HMG-CoA reductase inhibitors[8]
- hyperthyroidism[9]
- breast cancer.[10]

Whether the observed lack of coenzyme Q_{10} in these conditions is a true deficiency that contributes to the development of the disease or is caused by the disease itself is unclear. In heart failure, those with the most advanced disease have lower coenzyme Q_{10} levels than those with less advanced disease.[11] Low serum coenzyme Q_{10} levels are also associated with a significant risk of heart failure or increased mortality.[12]

Deficiency may occur as a result of:

- inadequate intake or production, particularly if requirements are increased because of disease
- inadequate production caused by older age or by deficiencies of nutrients required for its synthesis
- genetic or acquired defects in synthesis or metabolism
- interactions with medicines: beta-blockers, clonidine, gemfibrozil, hydralazine, hydrochlorothiazide, methyldopa, statins and tricyclic antidepressants may reduce levels of coenzyme Q_{10}.

Possible uses

Cardiovascular disease

The potential role of coenzyme Q_{10} in CVD has been studied over more than 30 years. Studies increasingly look at its role in specific cardiovascular conditions but an open study in 424 patients published in 1994 indicated that coenzyme Q_{10} supplementation may have benefits in cardiac function in patients with a range of cardiovascular disorders, including ischaemic cardiomyopathy, dilated cardiomyopathy, primary diastolic dysfunction, hypertension, valvular heart disease and mitral valve prolapse.[13]

More recent trials have indicated that coenzyme Q_{10} can improve endothelial function and extracellular superoxide dismutase in patients with ischaemic heart disease[14] and improve functional capacity, endothelial function and left ventricular contractility in patients with CHF.[14]

Congestive heart failure

There is substantive evidence suggesting a role for coenzyme Q_{10} in CHF. Oxidative stress is believed to play a role in the aetiology of CHF. It has been suggested that low coenzyme Q_{10} levels found in patients with CHF contribute to the disease while supplementation with preparations that include coenzyme Q_{10} may produce an improvement.[5]

A double-blind, placebo-controlled study investigated 322 patients with CHF who were randomly assigned to receive 2 mg/kg coenzyme Q_{10} daily or a placebo for 1 year. The number of episodes of pulmonary oedema or cardiac asthma was significantly fewer in the intervention group than the placebo group. The supplemented patients also had fewer hospitalisations.[15] A meta-analysis of eight clinical trials of coenzyme Q_{10} in patients with CHF found that supplemental treatment of CHF was significant, with significant improvement in stroke volume, ejection fraction, cardiac output, cardiac index and diastolic volume index.[16]

A more recent meta-analysis including 11 trials in patients with chronic heart failure found a net improvement in ejection fraction with a more profound effect in patients not receiving angiotensin-converting enzyme inhibitors. Cardiac output also increased significantly. Doses used across the trials ranged from 60 to 200 mg daily with treatment periods ranging from 1 to 6 months. [17]

Not all clinical trials have produced positive results. In a double-blind, placebo-controlled, crossover study, 30 patients with chronic left ventricular dysfunction were randomised to receive coenzyme Q_{10} or a placebo for 3 months each. Plasma levels of coenzyme Q_{10} increased to more than twice baseline values, but there were no significant differences between treatments in left ventricular ejection fraction, cardiac volumes, haemodynamic indices or quality of life measures.[18] In another RCT, 55 patients with CHF were randomly assigned to receive 200 mg coenzyme Q_{10} or a placebo daily for 6 months. Patients receiving the supplement had higher serum concentrations of coenzyme Q_{10}, but there were no differences in cardiac performance, peak oxygen consumption and exercise duration between the treated group and the placebo group.[19]

Angina

Coenzyme Q_{10} levels tend to be low in patients with ischaemic heart disease and several clinical trials have been conducted in patients with angina. Overall, coenzyme Q_{10} appears to delay onset of angina and increases patients' stamina on a treadmill. In one RCT, 144 patients with acute myocardial infarction were given 120 mg coenzyme Q_{10} or a placebo daily for 28 days, starting within 3 days of the heart attack. There was a significant improvement in angina pectoris, total arrhythmias and poor left ventricular function in the intervention group. Total cardiac events, including cardiac deaths and non-fatal infarction, were also significantly lower in the supplemented group than the placebo group.[20]

Hypertension

Coenzyme Q_{10} has been investigated for hypertension both as a stand-alone treatment and as an adjunct to conventional anti-hypertensive medication. In one randomised double-blind study involving 83 patients, an oral dose of 60 mg taken twice a day over 12 weeks was found to produce a mean reduction in systolic blood pressure of 17.8 ± 7.3 mmHg.[21] Another double-blind study in 59 patients with hypertension found that adding 120 mg coenzyme Q_{10} daily to existing anti-hypertensive medication causes an additional reduction in systolic and diastolic blood pressure after 8 weeks of treatment.[22]

A Cochrane review including three placebo-controlled clinical trials with a total of 96 participants found that treatment with coenzyme Q_{10} in subjects with systolic blood pressure (SBP) >140 mmHg or diastolic blood pressure (DBP) >90 mmHg resulted in mean decreases in SBP of 11 mmHg (95% confidence interval (CI), 8 to 14) and DBP of 7 mmHg (95% CI, 5 to 8). The authors conclusion was that, because of the possible unreliability of some of the included studies, it is uncertain whether or not coenzyme Q_{10} reduces blood pressure in the long-term management of primary hypertension.[23]

Cardiac surgery

Studies have looked at the use of coenzyme Q_{10} supplements before cardiac surgery. Oral supplementation with coenzyme Q_{10} for 2 weeks before cardiac surgery has been shown to improve post-operative heart function and shorten hospital stays.[24,25] However, supplementation with 600 mg coenzyme Q_{10} 12 h before surgery did not improve myocardial protection in patients undergoing coronary revascularisation.[26]

Exercise performance

Coenzyme Q_{10} is essential in energy metabolism and has, therefore, been investigated for athletic performance. Controlled trials using doses of 60–150 mg daily over 4 to 8 weeks have generally shown no improvements in physical performance. However, in one double-blind crossover trial, there were positive results on both objective and subjective parameters of physical performance. In this study, 94% of athletes felt that coenzyme Q_{10} improved their performance and recovery times, compared with 33% taking a placebo.[27]

A study in 17 healthy volunteers evaluated the effect of oral coenzyme Q_{10} (100 or 300 mg daily) or placebo for 8 days on physical fatigue during exercise. Subjective fatigue sensation, physical performance and recovery period were improved in the group taking 300 mg coenzyme Q compared with placebo.[28]

More recent trials evaluating the role of coenzyme Q_{10} supplementation in physical exercise have continued to generate positive, albeit minor benefits. For example, acute supplementation with coenzyme Q_{10} resulted in higher muscle coenzyme Q_{10} concentration, lower serum superoxide dismutase and oxidative stress, and higher malondialdehyde levels during and following exercise, while chronic coenzyme Q_{10} supplementation increased plasma coenzyme Q_{10} concentrations and tended to increase time to exhaustion.[29] Coenzyme Q_{10} may increase fat oxidation, with augmented autonomic nervous activity during low intensity exercise.[30] Treatment with moderate- to high-dose coenzyme Q_{10} for 60 days had minor effects on cycle exercise aerobic capacity and post-exercise lactate but did not affect other clinically relevant variables such as strength or resting lactate.[31] In a trial looking at the influence of coenzyme Q_{10} on several muscle power tests, power increased only with coenzyme Q_{10} supplementation during one of the tests. Fatigue indices decreased with coenzyme Q_{10} supplementation, but these decreases did not differ from those seen with placebo supplementation.[32]

Parkinson's disease

Studies suggest that oxidative damage, inflammation and mitochondrial impairment may play a role in the aetiology of Parkinson's disease.[33] In a multicentre, placebo-controlled, double-blind study comparing three different doses of coenzyme Q_{10} (300, 600, and 1200 mg) in 80 patients with early Parkinson's disease, significant improvements were reported after 9 months in the group taking 1200 mg daily.[34]

A further trial evaluated the effects of coenzyme Q_{10} on symptoms of patients with midstage Parkinson's disease (without motor fluctuations). The study involved 131 patients stabilized on anti-parkinsonian treatment. They were randomly assigned to coenzyme Q_{10} 100 mg three times a day or placebo for 3 months. In this study, there were no significant changes in the primary outcome variable (the change of the sum score of the Unified Parkison's Disease Rating Scale parts II and III). No secondary outcome measure showed a significant change between placebo and the coenzyme Q_{10} group. The frequency and quality of adverse events was similar in both treatment groups.[35]

Huntington's chorea

A randomised double-blind study involving 347 patients with early Huntington's chorea showed that a dose of coenzyme Q_{10} 600 mg daily taken over 30 months produced a trend towards slow decline and beneficial improvements in some parameters. However, changes were not significant.[36]

Cancer

Observational studies of women diagnosed with breast cancer have reported reduced blood coenzyme Q_{10} concentrations. There have also been several case reports of remissions or partial remissions in patients with tumours. A pilot study evaluated the survival of patients with end-stage cancer who received supplements of coenzyme Q_{10} and a mixture of other antioxidants (e.g. vitamin C, selenium, folic acid and beta-carotene). During a period of 9 years, 41 patients who had end-stage cancer were included. Forty patients were followed until death and one patient was lost to follow-up and presumed dead. Primary cancers were located in the breast, brain, lungs, kidneys, pancreas, oesophagus, stomach, colon, prostate, ovaries and skin. Median predicted survival was 12 months (range 3 to 9 months), whereas median actual survival was 17 months (1 to 120 months), which is over 40% longer than the median predicted survival. Mean actual survival was 28.8 months, compared with 11.9 months for mean predicted survival. Ten patients (24%) survived for less time than predicted, whereas 31 (76%) survived for longer. Treatments were very well tolerated with few adverse effects.[37]

Suggestions that coenzyme Q_{10} might reduce the toxicity of cancer treatments has been tested in several (poor quality) trials. A systematic review of six studies concluded that coenzyme Q_{10} provides some protection against cardiotoxicity or liver toxicity during cancer treatment. However, the authors concluded that rigorous trials are needed to determine the efficacy of coenzyme Q_{10} for improving cancer treatment tolerability.[38]

Migraine
An open trial investigated the effects of coenzyme Q_{10} 150 mg daily for 3 months in 32 individuals with a history of migraine. Coenzyme Q_{10} was associated with a significant reduction in both the frequency of attacks and the number of days with migraine.[39] Low levels of coenzyme Q_{10} have been found in paediatric and adolescent patients suffering from migraine. A study in which youngsters with low coenzyme Q_{10} levels were advised to take a supplement showed that those who returned for follow-up had decreased headache frequency and disability.[40]

Male infertility
Coenzyme Q_{10} supplementation has been evaluated for an effect on semen parameters, sperm function and reproductive hormone profiles in infertile men. A 26-week RCT in 212 infertile men with idiopathic oligoasthenoteratospermia found a significant improvement in sperm density, morphology and motility with coenzyme

Q_{10} therapy (each $P = 0.01$). The coenzyme Q_{10} group had a significant decrease in serum follicle-stimulating hormone and luteinising hormone at the end of the 26-week treatment. However, further studies are needed to draw a final conclusion and evaluate the effect of coenzyme Q_{10} supplementation on the pregnancy rate.[41]

> **Conclusion**
> Results from preliminary studies with coenzyme Q_{10} suggest that it may help to improve symptoms of CHF, and may help to protect against myocardial infarction. Studies in angina and hypertension are inconclusive. Studies conducted so far do not justify the use of coenzyme Q_{10} in cancer, athletes and sports people and AIDS, though some of the preliminary research justifies more rigorous trials to investigate potential benefits. Preliminary evidence from the use of coenzyme Q_{10} in Parkinson's disease is promising. However, there is insufficient evidence to make definite recommendations for coenzyme Q_{10} as a dietary supplement.

Pregnancy and breast-feeding

Safety in pregnancy has not been established.

Adverse effects

Coenzyme Q_{10} seems to be safe and relatively well tolerated in doses of up to 1200 mg daily.[42] There are occasional reports of gastrointestinal discomfort, dizziness and skin rash, but these tend to occur with doses over 200 mg daily.

Interactions

Drugs
Statins: Simvastatin, pravastatin and lovastatin reduce endogenous synthesis of coenzyme Q_{10}.[8] The mechanism of action of statins is inhibition of HMG-CoA reductase. Inhibition of this enzyme appears to inhibit the intrinsic biosynthesis of coenzyme Q_{10} at the same time. This reduces coenzyme Q_{10} concentrations, so constituting a new risk for cardiovascular disease. However, different statins many produce

different effects, with some evidence, for example, that atoravastatin reduces tissue levels of coenzyme Q_{10} but pitavastatin does not.[43] A systematic review of trials evaluating the role of coenzyme Q_{10} in patients taking statins concluded that statin treatment reduces plasma coenzyme Q_{10} levels and that a supplement of coenzyme Q_{10} increases plasma levels. However, the authors concluded that there is insufficient evidence that supplementation might improve symptoms of statin-associated myopathy because data on coenzyme Q_{10} supplementation on myopathic symptoms were scarce and contradictory. They suggested that the routine use of coenzyme Q_{10} cannot be recommended in patients treated with statins, but that coenzyme Q_{10} can be tested in patients who develop statin-related myalgia and who cannot be treated successfully with other agents.[44] Trials published since this systematic review have produced conflicting data, with some showing that coenzyme Q_{10} supplementation improves statin related myopathy[45] while others showed that it did not improve symptoms,[46] influence liver enzyme levels in those taking statins,[47] or increase tissue levels of coenzyme Q_{10}.[48] Coenzyme Q_{10} supplementation has also been shown to improve endothelial dysfunction in statin-treated patients with type 2 diabetes.[49] Plasma levels of coenzyme Q_{10} do not appear to influence clinical outcomes with rovustatin.[50]

Warfarin: Case reports suggest that coenzyme Q_{10} may decrease International Normalised Ratio (INR) in patients previously stabilised on anticoagulants. However, a double-blind crossover study in 24 patients on long-term warfarin found that oral coenzyme Q_{10} 100 mg daily had no significant effect on INR or warfarin levels.[51] In patients on warfarin, high doses of coenzyme Q_{10} should be used with caution.

Treatment of cardiovascular disorders: Coenzyme Q_{10} should not be used to treat cardiovascular disorders without medical supervision.

Dose

Coenzyme Q_{10} is sold in capsules and tablets in strengths of 10–150 mg. Doses used in studies investigating cardiovascular disease and prevention of migraine have ranged from 100 to 150 mg daily. However, higher doses have been used in angina (150–600 mg daily) and Parkinson's disease (up to 1200 mg daily). Doses used to prepare for heart surgery have varied between 30 and 100 mg daily for 1 to 2 weeks before surgery and a month afterwards.

People who wish to try coenzyme Q_{10} for cardiovascular conditions or migraine prevention should be advised it may take 10–12 weeks to have an effect. However, all patients with cardiovascular conditions should take medical advice before taking coenzyme Q_{10}.

References

1 Weber C, Bysted A, Holmer G. Coenzyme Q_{10} in the diet: daily intake and relative bioavailability. *Mol Aspects Med* 1997; 18: S251–S254.

2 Bhagavan HN, Chopra RK. Coenzyme Q_{10}: absorption, tissue uptake, metabolism and pharmacokinetics. *Free Radic Res* 2006; 40(5): 445–453.

3 Bhagavan HN, Chopra RK. Plasma coenzyme Q_{10} response to oral ingestion of coenzyme Q_{10} formulations. *Mitochondrion* 2007; 7(Suppl 1): S78–S88.

4 Kalen A, Appelkvist EL, Dallner G. Age-related changes in the lipid composition of rat and human tissue. *Lipids* 1989; 24: 579–584.

5 Sole MJ, Jeejeebhoy KN. Conditioned nutritional requirements: therapeutic relevance to heart failure. *Herz* 2002; 27: 174–178.

6 Karlsson J, Diamant B, Folkers K, *et al.* Muscle fibre types, ubiquinone content and exercise capacity in hypertension and effort angina. *Ann Med* 1991; 23: 339–344.

7 Mortensen SA, Vadhanavikit S, Muratsu K, *et al.* Coenzyme Q_{10}: clinical benefits with biochemical correlates suggesting a scientific breakthrough in the management of chronic heart failure. *Int J Tissue React* 1990; 12: 155–162.

8 Overvard K, Diamant B, Holm L, *et al.* Coenzyme Q_{10} in health and disease. *Eur J Clin Nutr* 1999; 53: 764–770.

9 Bianchi G, Solaroli E, Zaccheroni V, *et al.* Oxidative stress and antioxidant metabolites in patients with hyperthyroidism: effect of treatment. *Horm Metab Res* 1999; 31: 620–624.

10 Folkers K, Osterborg A, Nylander M, *et al.* Activities of vitamin Q_{10} in animal models and a serious deficiency in patients with cancer. *Biochem Biophys Res Commun* 1997; 234: 296–299.

11 Mortensen SA. Perspectives on therapy of cardiovascular diseases with coenzyme Q (ubiquinone). *Clin Invest* 1993; 71: S116–S123.

12 Jameson S. Statistical data support prediction of death within 6 months on low levels of coenzyme

Q_{10} and other entities. *Clinical Invest* 1993; 71: S137–S139.

13 Langsjoen H, Langsjoen P, Langsjoen P, *et al.* Usefulness of coenzyme Q10 in clinical cardiology: a long term study. *Mol Aspects Med* 1994; (Suppl 15): S165–S175.

14 Belardinelli R, Mucaj A, Lacalaprice F, *et al.* Coenzyme Q_{10} and exercise training in chronic heart failure. *Eur Heart J* 2006; ehl158.

15 Morisco C, Trimarco B, Condorelli M. Effect of coenzyme Q_{10} therapy in patients with congestive heart failure: a long term multicenter randomized study. *Clinical Invest* 1993; 71: S134–S136.

16 Soja AM, Mortensen SA. Treatment of congestive heart failure with coenzyme Q_{10} illustrated by meta-analyses of clinical trials. *Mol Aspects Med* 1997; 18: S159–S168.

17 Sander S, Coleman CI, Patel AA, *et al.* The impact of coenzyme Q_{10} on systolic function in patients with chronic heart failure. *J Card Fail* 2006; 12 (6): 464–472.

18 Watson PS, Scalia GM, Galbraith A, *et al.* Lack of effect of coenzyme Q on left ventricular function in patients with congestive heart failure. *J Am Coll Cardiol* 1999; 33: 1549–1552.

19 Khatta M, Alexander BS, Krichten CM, *et al.* The effect of coenzyme Q_{10} with congestive heart failure. *Ann Intern Med* 2000; 132: 636–640.

20 Singh RB, Wander GS, Rastogi A, *et al.* Randomized, double-blind, placebo-controlled trial of coenzyme Q_{10} in patients with acute myocardial infarction. *Cardiovasc Drugs Ther* 1998; 12: 347–353.

21 Burke BE, Neuenschwander R, Olson RD. Randomized, double-blind, placebo-controlled trial of coenzyme Q_{10} in isolated systolic hypertension. *South Med J* 2001; 94: 1112–1117.

22 Singh RB, Niaz MA, Rastogi SS, *et al.* Effect of hydrosoluble coenzyme Q_{10} on blood pressures and insulin resistance in hypertensive patients with coronary artery disease. *J Hum Hypertens* 1999; 13: 203–208.

23 Ho MJ, Bellusci A, Wright JM. Blood pressure lowering efficacy of coenzyme Q_{10} for primary hypertension. *Cochrane Database Syst Rev* 2009; 7(4): CD007435.

24 Rosenfeldt FL, Pepe S, Linnane A, *et al.* The effects of ageing on the response to cardiac surgery: protective strategies for the ageing myocardium. *Biogerontology* 2002; 3: 37–40.

25 Makhija N, Sendasgupta C, Kiran U, *et al.* The role of oral coenzyme Q_{10} in patients undergoing coronary artery bypass graft surgery. *J Cardiothorac Vasc Anesth* 2008; 22(6): 832–839.

26 Taggart DP, Jenkins M, Hooper J, *et al.* Effects of short term supplementation with coenzyme Q_{10} on myocardial protection during cardiac operations. *Ann Thorac Surg* 1996; 61: 829–833.

27 Ylikoski T, Piirainen J, Hanninen O, *et al.* The effect of coenzyme Q_{10} on the exercise performance of cross-country skiers. *Mol Aspects Med* 1997; 18: S283–S290.

28 Mizuno K, Tanaka M, Nozaki S, *et al.* Antifatigue effects of coenzyme Q10 during physical fatigue. *Nutrition* 2008; 24: 293–299.

29 Cooke M, Iosia M, Buford T, *et al.* Effects of acute and 14-day coenzyme Q_{10} supplementation on exercise performance in both trained and untrained individuals. *J Int Soc Sports Nutr* 2008; 5: 8.

30 Zheng A, Moritani T. Influence of CoQ10 on autonomic nervous activity and energy metabolism during exercise in healthy subjects. *J Nutr Sci Vitaminol (Tokyo)* 2008; 54(4): 286–290.

31 Glover EI, Martin J, Maher A, *et al.* A randomized trial of coenzyme Q_{10} in mitochondrial disorders. *Muscle Nerve* 2010; 42(5): 739–748.

32 Gokbel H, Gul I, Belviranl M, *et al.* The effects of coenzyme Q_{10} supplementation on performance during repeated bouts of supramaximal exercise in sedentary men. *J Strength Cond Res* 2010; 24(1): 97–102.

33 Ebadi M, Govitrapong P, Sharma S, *et al.* Ubiquinone (coenzyme Q_{10}) and mitochondria in oxidative stress in Parkinson's disease. *Biol Signals Recept* 2001; 10: 224–253.

34 Shults CW, Oakes D, Kieburtz K, *et al.* Effects of coenzyme Q_{10} in early Parkinson disease: evidence of slowing of the functional decline. *Arch Neurol* 2002; 59: 1541–1550.

35 Storch A, Jost WH, Vieregge P, *et al.* Randomized, double-blind, placebo-controlled trial on symptomatic effects of coenzyme Q_{10} in Parkinson disease. *Arch Neurol* 2007; 64: 938–944.

36 Huntingdon's Study Group A randomized, placebo-controlled trial of coenzyme Q_{10} and remacemide in Huntingdon's disease. *Neurology* 2001; 57: 397–404.

37 Hertz N, Lister RE. Improved survival in patients with end-stage cancer treated with coenzyme Q(10) and other antioxidants: a pilot study. *J Int Med Res* 2009; 37(6): 1961–1971.

38 Roffe L, Schmidt K, Ernst E. Efficacy of coenzyme Q_{10} for improved tolerability of cancer treatments: a systematic review. *J Clin Oncol* 2004; 22(21): 4418–4424.

39 Rozen TD, Oshinsky ML, Gebeline CA, *et al.* Open label trial of coenzyme Q_{10} as a migraine preventive. *Cephalgia* 2002; 22: 137–141.

40 Hershey AD, Powers SW, Vockell AL, *et al.* Coenzyme Q_{10} deficiency and response to supplementation in pediatric and adolescent migraine. *Headache* 2007; 47(1): 73–80.

41 Safarinejad MR. Efficacy of coenzyme Q_{10} on semen parameters, sperm function and reproductive hormones in infertile men. *J Urol* 2009; 182(1): 237–248.

42 Hathcock JN, Shao A. Risk assessment for coenzyme Q_{10} (ubiquinone). *Regul Toxicol Pharmacol* 2006; 45(3): 282–288.

43 Kawashiri MA, Nohara A, Tada H, *et al.* Comparison of effects of pitavastatin and atorvastatin on plasma coenzyme Q_{10} in heterozygous familial

hypercholesterolemia: results from a crossover study. *Clin Pharmacol Ther* 2008; 83(5): 731–739.

44   Marcoff L, Thompson PD. The role of coenzyme Q_{10} in statin-associated myopathy: a systematic review. *J Am Coll Cardiol* 2007; 49(23): 2231–2237.

45   Caso G, Kelly P, McNurlan MA, *et al.* Effect of coenzyme Q_{10} on myopathic symptoms in patients treated with statins. *Am J Cardiol* 2007; 99(10): 1409–1412.

46   Young JM, Florkowski CM, Molyneux SL, *et al.* Effect of coenzyme Q(10) supplementation on simvastatin-induced myalgia. *Am J Cardiol* 2007; 100 (9): 1400–1403.

47   Mabuchi H, Nohara A, Kobayashi J, *et al.* Effects of CoQ_{10} supplementation on plasma lipoprotein lipid, CoQ_{10} and liver and muscle enzyme levels in hypercholesterolemic patients treated with atorvastatin: a randomized double-blind study. *Atherosclerosis* 2007; 195(2): e182–189.

48   Keith M, Mazer CD, Mikhail P, *et al.* Coenzyme Q_{10} in patients undergoing CABG: effect of statins and nutritional supplementation. *Nutr Metab Cardiovasc Dis* 2008; 18(2): 105–111.

49   Hamilton SJ, Chew GT, Watts GF. Coenzyme Q_{10} improves endothelial dysfunction in statin-treated type 2 diabetic patients. *Diabetes Care* 2009; 32(5): 810–812.

50   McMurray JJ, Dunselman P, Wedel H, *et al.* Coenzyme Q_{10}, rosuvastatin, and clinical outcomes in heart failure: a pre-specified substudy of CORONA (controlled rosuvastatin multinational study in heart failure). *J Am Coll Cardiol* 2010; 56(15): 1196–1204.

51   Engelson J, Nielson JD, Hansen KF. Effect of coenzyme Q_{10} and *Ginkgo biloba* on warfarin dosage in patients on long-term warfarin treatment. A randomized, double-blind, placebo-controlled crossover trial. *Ugeskr Laeger* 2003; 165: 1868–1871.

Collagen hydrolysate

Description

Collagen hydrolysate (also known as hydrolysed collagen, gelatine hydrolysate, hydrolysed gelatine) is a bioavailable form of collagen, prepared by enzymatic hydrolysis of collagenous tissue. Collagen is a major constituent of connective tissue and a protein component of articular cartilage, which is a part of the joint. However, the absorption of orally ingested coll agen that has not been hydrolysed is poor. Products available as food supplements therefore generally contain collagen hydrolysate.

Constituents

Collagen hydrolysate provides high levels of amino acids. Among these are glycine and proline, two amino acids essential for the stability and regeneration of cartilage. A single pictogram of type II collagen contains more than 1 billion glycine molecules and 620 million proline molecules.[1]

Action

Collagen hydrolysate can stimulate collagen synthesis in the chondrocytes. (Chondrocytes are the cells responsible for maintenance of the connective tissue in the joints.) Treatment of cultured chondrocytes with collagen hydrolysate increases synthesis of type II collagen[2,3] and proteoglycans.[3,4] In addition, the presence of collagen fractions in cultures of osteoclasts inhibits bone resorption while concomitantly stimulating collagen synthesis.[5] Evidence also suggests that collagen hydrolysate can increase both firmness and flexibility in connective tissue[6] and increase cartilage mass.[7]

Two hypotheses have been developed to explain why collagen hydrolysate stimulates the chondrocytes to synthesise collagen. Firstly, although the amino acids present in collagen are not 'essential', as they can be synthesised by the body, the regular intake of collagen hydrolysate could supply the required amounts of the amino acids glycine, proline and hydroxyproline in a readily bioavailable form to joint tissue subject to ongoing wear and tear, so compensating for any lack of such amino acids in collagen-rich tissues. Secondly, the presence of collagen peptides could be recognised and understood by the chondrocytes as a sign of degradation of the proper collagen. This could lead the chondrocytes to synthesise collagen to compensate for this effect.[2]

Preliminary research in animal models of rheumatoid arthritis suggests that gelatine in combination with the antioxidant enzyme superoxide dismutase might suppress joint inflammation.[8]

Collagen hydrolysate may also inhibit bone collagen breakdown in people with osteoporosis[9] and inhibit bone resorption while concomitantly stimulating collagen synthesis.[5]

Dietary source

Collagen can be synthesised in the body from amino acids, but it is also obtained from the diet. As a constituent of connective tissue, collagen hydrolysate is found principally in meats where gristle or connective tissue is still intact. The quantity of collagen in food varies and depends on several factors such as animal species, breed, genetics, age, nutritional status and anatomical area of the animal. Good sources include well-cooked meat dishes (e.g. stews of beef, pork, veal, lamb, oxtail), offal (e.g. pig's foot, brain, tongue, marrowbones), minced beef, cooked pork meats (e.g. sausage, boiled ham, shoulder), meat stock (e.g. veal, chicken or beef), fish (particularly small fish, such as sardines, where the bones are consumed). Collagen can also be found in processed foods containing gelatine such as processed cheeses, instant soups, sauces, ice cream, jellies, milk jellies, sweets (e.g. marshmallows) and all gelatine products.

Metabolism

Following oral administration, collagen hydrolysate is hydrolysed, absorbed in the gastrointestinal tract and transported in the bloodstream in the form of peptides and amino acids (proline, hydroxyproline, glycine) to the articular cartilage.[10,11]

Possible uses

Osteoarthritis

There is clinical evidence that collagen hydrolysate can improve joint function and reduce pain in osteoarthritis.

One of the earliest trials was an open-label study involving 56 patients with osteoarthritis of the femur, knee or tibia, or degenerative disc disease of the spine. Administration of collagen hydrolysate 5–7 g daily was associated with reduced pain or general improvement in condition in 67% of patients.[12]

Further open-label trials in subjects with osteoarthritis or painful joints treated with collagen hydrolysate 10 g daily showed similar trends (i.e. pain reduction and improved joint function).[6,7,13–19]

The earliest placebo-controlled trial evaluated 81 patients with osteoarthritis of the hip or knee and used a crossover design to compare four different nutritional supplements, including collagen hydrolysate 10 g daily. Of the patients taking collagen hydrolysate, 81% achieved a meaningful reduction in joint pain compared with 23% taking egg albumin. In addition, 69% of the patients taking collagen hydrolysate had a ≥50% reduced use of analgesics compared with 35% of those taking egg albumin. The authors concluded that collagen hydrolysate can substantially reduce symptoms of joint discomfort and suggested that administration of this ingredient provides a set of amino acids which improve the structure of cartilage.[20]

Another placebo-controlled trial in 175 patients (40–80 years) with mild osteoarthritis of the knee evaluated the effect of gelatine hydrolysate 10 g daily (with calcium and vitamin C) over 14 weeks. There was an improvement in pain, stiffness and mobility measures compared with placebo. The gelatine hydrolysate group showed significant improvement compared with placebo on certain strength and work performance tests, especially tests that challenged the joint structure. A subgroup of patients with severe osteoarthritis showed that those in the gelatine group had more extensive improvement in leg strength and function compared with placebo.[21]

A further placebo-controlled trial investigated 92 patients with a variety of arthritic conditions who ingested gelatine hydrolysate 10 g daily over 6 months. At baseline and after 6 months of treatment, mobility and pain both improved according to subjectively assessed criteria. Furthermore, the patients who took gelatine hydrolysate had higher blood levels of hydroxyproline than placebo, confirming the delivery of an important component of collagen to the bloodstream.[22]

A more recent randomised, placebo-controlled, double-blind study recruited 250 patients with mild osteoarthritis of the knee (based on American College of Rheumatology criteria) and gave them either collagen hydrolysate 10 g daily or placebo for 14 weeks.[23] A total of 190 patients (88 treatment and 102 placebo patients) completed the study. After 14 weeks of treatment, the collagen hydrolysate group showed statistically significant ($P < 0.05$) improvement in three out of six isokinetic leg strength measures compared with placebo, particularly in tests presenting the greatest challenges of stress to joint structure. Improvement in a wider range of leg strength measures was confirmed in further publications by this same research group,[24,25] who concluded that these beneficial findings could be the result of early changes in articular cartilage. This suggestion is also consistent with data from animals.[10]

A large multi-centre, randomised, double-blind, placebo-controlled trial recruited 389 patients with knee osteoarthritis. This study included 20 sites in Germany, the UK and the USA. Patients were randomised to receive either 10 g collagen hydrolysate per day or placebo by mouth for 24 weeks.[9] Primary outcome measures were the Western Ontario McMaster University Osteoarthritis Index (WOMAC) pain score, function score and patient global assessment. The overall results did not detect statistically significant differences for pain in patients treated with collagen vs placebo. Interestingly, the level of symptom reduction was different between the three countries. In German patients ($n = 112$), there was a statistically significant reduction in pain with collagen hydrolysate ($P = 0.016$), and functional improvement ($P = 0.007$), but not patient global evaluation ($P = 0.074$). However drop-out rates, which were higher in the UK and USA (37 and 42%, respectively) than in Germany (6%) were a strong prognostic factor for all the primary end points. Paracetamol intake was also a significant prognostic factor.[26] The reasons for the differences in the effects of collagen hydrolysate between the patients in Germany and those in the UK and the USA are unclear, but the author suggested that differences in dietary collagen could explain the differences between the three countries, with collagen hydrolysate having less effect in countries where dietary collagen is greater.

A randomised, double-blind, placebo-controlled trial of 24 weeks' duration involving 147 athletes with no evidence of joint disease investigated the effect of collagen hydrolysate 10 g daily in joint pain, inflammation and mobility using the visual analogue scale.[27] When data from all subjects were evaluated, six parameters showed statistically significant changes with the dietary supplement collagen hydrolysate compared with placebo. These were joint pain at rest, assessed by the physician ($P = 0.025$), and five parameters assessed by study participants: joint pain when walking ($P = 0.007$), joint pain when standing ($P = 0.011$), joint pain at rest ($P = 0.039$), joint pain when carrying objects ($P = 0.014$) and joint pain when lifting ($P = 0.018$). When a subgroup analysis of subjects with knee arthralgia ($n = 63$) was performed, the difference between the effect of collagen hydrolysate vs placebo was more pronounced. The parameter joint pain at rest, assessed by the physician, had a statistical significance level of $P = 0.001$, while the other five parameters based on the participants' assessments were also statistically significant: joint pain when walking ($P = 0.003$), joint pain when standing ($P = 0.015$), joint pain at rest ($P = 0.021$), joint pain when running in a straight line ($P = 0.027$) and joint pain when changing direction ($P = 0.026$). The authors concluded that the results of this study have implications for the use of collagen hydrolysate to support joint health and possibly reduce the risk of joint deterioration in a high-risk group and suggest that athletes consuming collagen hydrolysate can reduce parameters (such as pain) that have a negative impact on athletic performance.

Conclusion

Results from several clinical trials suggest that collagen hydrolysate at a dose of 10 g daily may help to improve joint function and reduce pain in people with osteoarthritis. Further controlled trials are required to confirm these promising findings.

Pregnancy and breast-feeding

Safety in pregnancy and breast-feeding has not been established. However, collagen is a natural constituent of an omniverous diet.

Adverse effects

Evidence suggests that collagen hydrolysate in doses of up to 10 g daily for 6 months is safe.[9] Because collagen hydrolysate may be derived from beef bones and skin, concern has been expressed about contamination with diseased animal parts. To date, there are no reports of disease transmission to humans from contaminated collagen sources. Allergic reactions to collagen may occur.

Dose

Most clinical trials have used a dose of 10 g collagen hydrolysate daily. Food supplements provide doses of 5–10 g collagen hydrolysate.

Bioavailability

Studies have shown that a high percentage of an oral dose of collagen hydrolysate is absorbed. A Dutch trial using a simulated gastrointestinal tract model showed that 82% of an orally administered dose of collagen hydrolysate passes through the intestinal mucosa[28] while results from another study indicated that 90% of an oral dose of collagen hydrolysate is absorbed within approximately 6 hours.[10]

Post-prandial plasma concentrations of the amino acids proline, hydroxyproline and glycine increased significantly in rats fed with collagen hydrolysate compared with a control group.[11] In a placebo-controlled study in humans in which collagen hydrolysate 10 g daily was given for 44$\frac{1}{2}$ months, plasma concentrations of proline, hydroxyproline and glycine increased significantly in comparison with those of the control group.[29]

References

1   Clark KL. Nutritional considerations in joint health. *Clin Sports Med* 2007; 26: 101–118.
2   Oesser S, Seifert J. Stimulation of type II collagen biosynthesis and secretion in bovine chondrocytes cultured with degraded collagen. *Cell Tissue Res* 2003; 311: 393–399.
3   Oesser S, Haggenmuller D, Schulze C. Collagen hydrolysate modulates the extracellular matrix metabolism of human chondrocytes. *Ann Rheum Dis* 2006; 65(Suppl. II): 401.
4   Benito-Ruiz P, Camacho Zambrano MM, Carrillo Arcentales JN, *et al.* A randomized controlled trial on the efficacy and safety of a food ingredient, collagen hydrolysate, for improving joint comfort. *Int J Food Sci Nutr* 2009; 60(Suppl 2): 99–113.
5   Takada Y, Aoe S, Kato K, *et al.* Collagen containingpreparations for strengthening bone. European Patent Application No.EP 0798 001 A2 (1.10.97).
6   Weh L, Petau C. Change in the properties of tissue through the administration of gelatine. *Extracta Orthopaedica* 2001; 4: 12–16.
7   Fernandez J, Perez O. Effects of gelatine hydrolysates in the prevention of athletic injuries. *Archivos de Medicina del Deporte* 1998; 15(66): 277–282.
8   Kakimoto K, Kojima Y, Ishii K, *et al.* The suppressive effect of gelatin-conjugated superoxide dismutase on disease development and severity of collagen-induced arthritis in mice. *Clin Exp Immunol* 1993; 94: 241–246.
9   Moskowitz RW. Role of collagen hydrolysate in bone and joint disease. *Semin Arthritis Rheum* 2000; 30: 87–99.
10 Oesser S, Adam M, Babel W, Seifert J. Oral administration of (14)C labeled gelatin hydrolysate leads to an accumulation of radioactivity in cartilage of mice (C57/BL). *J Nutr* 1999; 129: 1891–1895.
11 Lohmann M. Untersuchungen zur Bedeutung von Gelatine AlsProteinbestandteil Inagurldissertation. Agrarwissenschaftliche Fakultat. Universitat Kiel 1994.
12 Krug E. Zur unterstutzenden Therapie bei Osteo- und Chondropathien (On supportive therapy for osteo- and chondropathy). *Z Erfahrungsheikunde* 1979; 11: 930–938.
13 Banzer W, Ziesing A, Dietmar A. Results of a clinical surveillance on collagen hydrolysate consumption in arthritis. *Med Sci Sports Exerc* 2006; 38: S438.
14 Beuker F, Rosenfeld J. Die Wirkung regelmassigergelatine-substitution auf die funktionalitat arthrotisch veranderter kniegelenke. Proceedings, Fourth International Congress Physical Activity, Aging and Sports, Heidelberg, Germany. 27–31 August 1996.
15 Fleschenhar K, Alf D. Ergebnisse einer Anwendungsbeobachtung zu Kollagen-Hydrolysat. CH-Alpha. *Orthopaedische Praxis* 2005; 9: 486–494.
16 Gotz B. Well nourished cartilage does not grind. *Artzliche Praxis* 1982; 34:.
17 Oberschelp U. Individuelle Arthrosetherapie ist moglich. *Therapie Woche* 1985; 44: 5094–5097.
18 Seeligmuller K, Bonn K, Happel H. Dem Knorpel auf die Sprunge helfen (Help and support for cartilage). *Europaische Pharmatforschung* 1993; 43: 1810–1813.
19 Seeligmuller K, Heppel KH. Kann eine Gelatine/L-Cystine-Mischung die Kollagen und Proteoglykansynthese stimulieren? *Arthrostherapie* 1989; 39: 3153–3157.

20 Adam M. Welche Wirkung haben Gelatinepreparate? (What effects do gelatin preparations have?) *Therapie Woche* 1991; 41: 2456–2461.

21 McCarthy S, Carpenter MR, Barrell M *et al*. The effectiveness of gelatine supplementation treatment in individuals with symptoms of mild osteoarthritis. A randomized, double-blind, placebo-controlled study. Presented at the 2000 Annual Meeting of the American Academy of Family Physicians, Dallas, Texas, 22 September 2000. (Report of study in US Family Practice News, Dec 1, 2000.)

22 Beuker F, Eck T, Rosenfeld J. Biochemical and clinical examinations on the effects of regular applications of gelatin on degenerative changes of the motoric system (abstract). *Int J Sports Med* 1996; 17(Suppl. 1): S67–70.

23 Zuckley L, Angelopoulou K, Carpenter M, *et al*. Collagen hydrolysate improves joint function in adults with mild symptoms of osteoarthritis of the knee. Annual meeting abstracts: D24. *Med Sci Sports Exerc* 2004; 36: S153–154.

24 Carpenter MR, Carpenter RL, McCarthy S, *et al*. Collagen hydrolysate supplementation improves symptoms in patients with severe osteoarthritis. *Med Sci Sports Exerc* 2005; 37: S91.

25 Carpenter RL, Peel JB, Carpenter MR, *et al*. Effectiveness of a collagen hydrolysate-based supplement on joint pain, range of motion and muscle function in individuals with mild osteoarthritis of the knee: a randomized clinical trial. *Ann Rheum Dis* 2005; 64(Suppl. 3): 1544–1545.

26 Selbmann HC, Fischer IU, Moskowitz R. Collagen hydrolysate in osteoarthritis of the knee. Analysis of country specific responses. *J Bone Joint Surg Br* 2006; 88-B: 104–105.

27 Clark KL, Sebastianelli W, Flechsenhar KR, *et al*. 24-Week study on the use of collagen hydrolysate as a dietary supplement in athletes with activity-related joint pain. *Curr Med Res Opin* 2008; 24: 1485–1496.

28 Zeijdner E. Digestibility of collagen hydrolysate during passage through a dynamic gastric and small intestinal model (TIM-1). TNO Nutrition and Food Research Report, 24 June 2002.

29 Beuker F. Ernahrungs-Umschau 70. *Heft 2* 1993; 64.

Conjugated linoleic acid

Description

Conjugated linoleic acid (CLA) is a naturally occurring polyunsaturated fatty acid. Nine different isomers of CLA have been identified, and their double bonds are conjugated at carbons 9 and 11 or 10 and 12 in the *cis* and *trans* configuration. CLA is found in low concentrations in blood and tissues, although the body does not synthesise CLA endogenously. CLA is readily absorbed from food and supplements.

Dietary sources

CLA is present in small quantities in many foods, especially beef and dairy produce. Cooking has been shown to increase the CLA content of meat. Changes in the way beef and dairy animals have been reared in the past decade have reduced the amount of CLA in the diet.

Action

CLA is essential for the delivery of dietary fat into cells. It transports glucose into cells, and helps glucose to be used to provide energy and build muscle rather than being converted to fat. It is this effect that lies behind the claims that CLA is useful for promoting weight loss. CLA is also an antioxidant and enhances the immune system.

Possible uses

CLA is being marketed for loss of body weight, and is also being investigated for prevention of cancer.

Body weight and energy expenditure

CLA is being promoted for control of body weight, and early evidence from animal studies was promising. In mice, CLA has been shown to reduce fat accumulation and increase protein accumulation without any change in food intake,[1] to reduce energy intake, increase metabolism and reduce body fat,[2] to reduce body fat and increase lean body mass without affecting body weight,[3] and to reduce body fat and increase energy expenditure.[4]

Human clinical data are now appearing in the literature, but with somewhat conflicting results. A 12-week randomised double-blind study including 60 overweight or obese volunteers given various doses of CLA from 1.7 to 6.8 g daily found that CLA was associated with a significantly higher reduction in body fat mass than placebo. The reduction in body fat was significant for the groups taking 3.4 and 6.8 g CLA.[5] A 4-week double-blind RCT in 25 obese men aged 39–64 with metabolic disorder found that CLA 4.2 g daily was associated with a significant reduction in abdominal fat but with no concomitant effects on overall obesity and other cardiovascular risk factors.[6]

A Dutch RCT in 54 men and women involved subjects being put on a very low-calorie diet (2.1 MJ daily) for 3 weeks, followed by 13 weeks on either low- or high-dose CLA (1.8 or 3.6 g daily) or placebo. Weight regain after the low-calorie diet was not significantly different between the active and placebo groups, but subjects on CLA did gain a significantly greater proportion of that weight as fat-free mass (4.6% vs 3.4%). The effect was similar for the low- and high-dose CLA.[7] As part of this study, appetite and food intake was also measured. Appetite (hunger, satiety and fullness) was favourably, dose dependently affected by consumption of both 1.8 and 3.6 g CLA daily. However, this did not affect energy intake at breakfast and did not improve body weight maintenance.[8]

A 12-month study investigated the effect of CLA in 180 healthy overweight adults. Body fat mass was significantly reduced in the CLA groups.[9] As part of the same study, 134 of the participants were included in an open study for a further 12 months to evaluate the safety of CLA and assess its effect on body composition. The extended study found that CLA 3.4 g daily decreases body fat mass and may help to maintain initial reductions in body fat mass and weight in the long term. The supplement was well tolerated.[10]

CLA has also been investigated in people who are exercising. A human study showed that 5.6–7.2 g CLA daily produced non-significant gains in muscle size and strength in experienced and inexperienced training men.[11] A double-blind 12-week RCT in 20 healthy people with body mass index (BMI) <25 who did standardised exercise in a gym for 90 min three times weekly

found that CLA 1.8 g daily reduced body fat but not body weight.[12]

A further study investigated the effect of CLA 6 g daily in 23 resistance-trained subjects. Results showed some statistical trends, but CLA did not significantly affect changes in total body mass, percentage body fat, bone mass or fat-free mass, indicating that CLA does not appear to possess significant ergogenic value for experienced resistance-trained athletes.[13]

A longer term trial (6 months) in 40 healthy overweight adults (age 18–44 years) found that a supplement of CLA (3.2 g daily) significantly reduced body fat, and prevented weight gain during the holiday season.[14] A further 6-month trial in 118 overweight adults found that CLA (3.4 g daily) significantly decreased body fat mass compared with placebo. The reduction in body fat mass was located mostly in the legs, and in women. Waist–hip ratio decreased significantly and lean body mass increased. All changes were independent of diet and physical activity.[15] Another study assessed the effect of 12-month supplementation of CLA (3.4 g) on body fat and body weight regain in moderately obese people (BMI >28) who had previously lost 8% of their body weight. No significant difference in body weight or fat regain was observed between the CLA group and placebo.[16]

There is some evidence that a specific isomer of CLA may be the bioactive component in relation to weight change. A US study in 21 adults with type 2 diabetes found that a CLA mixture of predominantly two isomers (c9t11 and t10c12) resulted in an increase in plasma CLA that was inversely correlated with body weight and serum leptin levels. However, these significant correlations were only seen with the t10c12-CLA.[17]

A further study involved healthy subjects who were given a 50:50 mixture of the two key isomers (c9t11 and t10c12) added to flavoured yoghurt for 14 weeks. In this study, there was a significant increase in resting metabolic rate with the CLA product vs placebo, but there was no change in body composition.[18]

A more recent study evaluated a similar CLA isomer mixture (3.9 g daily) for 12 weeks (compared with a high oleic acid sunflower oil) in 62 non-obese exercising adults. There were no significant effects of CLA on body composition or distribution, energy metabolism or appetite.

Serum total cholesterol and LDL cholesterol decreased in both groups. However, CLA had a favourable effect on plasma insulin and serum non-esterified fatty acid concentration.[19]

A 6-month trial involving 23 subjects evaluated the influence of CLA (3.2 g daily; mixed isomers: c9t11 and t10c12) on fat oxidation and energy expenditure during sleep. The study detected a positive difference in fat utilisation, fat oxidation and energy expenditure during sleep.[20]

A further RCT employing a 50:50 ratio of c9t11 and t10c12 isomers 3.2 g daily or 6.4 g CLA daily for 12 weeks in 48 otherwise healthy obese humans found that lean body mass increased by 0.64 kg in the group receiving 6.4 g CLA daily ($P < 0.05$) after 12 weeks of intervention. However, there were significant decreases in serum HDL cholesterol and significant increases in certain inflammatory markers (C-reactive protein, interlukin-6) in this group, although all values remained within normal limits. The intervention was well tolerated and no severe adverse events were reported, although mild gastrointestinal adverse events were reported in all treatment groups.[21] A 98-day supplementation trial with a 50:50 mixture of the two isomers in a dairy product was unable to alter body composition, although a significant increase in the resting metabolic rate was induced.[18]

A recent meta-analysis of 18 studies in which CLA was given to test its efficacy in reducing fat mass found that a dose of 3.2 g daily of CLA produces a modest loss of body fat in humans.[22] A similar meta-analysis of the same 18 studies found fat-free mass increases in humans during CLA treatment, but the onset of the increase was rapid and the total increase was small (<1%).[23] A trial published since this meta-analysis in which 55 obese postmenopausal women with diabetes supplemented their diet with CLA for 36 weeks (35 women completed the trial) also showed that CLA reduced BMI ($P = 0.0022$) and total adipose mass ($P = 0.0187$) without altering lean mass.[24]

Cardiovascular disease

Animal research suggests an effect of CLA supplementation on preventing atherosclerosis,[25,26] but one study has shown that CLA does not produce beneficial lipid profiles.[27] One human study in 17 healthy female volunteers found that CLA 3.9 g daily for 2 months did not alter blood cholesterol or lipoprotein levels.[28] In the same study, there were no effects of CLA on blood coagulation and platelet function.[29] Another human RCT in 51 normolipidaemic patients found that an isomeric blend of CLA significantly reduced plasma triglycerides and VLDL cholesterol concentrations.[30] A double-blind RCT in 401 subjects (aged 40–70 years) with a BMI >25 showed that 4 g CLA daily had no effect on pulse wave velocity (a marker of atherosclerosis) or on blood pressure, body composition, insulin resistance, or concentrations of lipid, glucose and C-reactive protein.[31]

An 8-week supplementation of CLA enhanced the effect of ramipril on blood pressure reduction in treated obese hypertensive patients. It also increased plasma adiponectin concentration ($P < 0.05$) and decreased plasma concentrations of leptin and angiotensinogen ($P < 0.05$); however, significant change was not observed in angiotensin-converting enzyme activity. The antihypertensive effect of CLA might be related to the changed secretion of hypertensive adipocytokines in plasma.[32]

Insulin sensitivity

Based on preliminary work in animals,[33] there has been some hope that CLA could improve insulin resistance. An 8-week Canadian RCT in 16 normal weight, healthy young adults living a sedentary lifestyle found that an isomeric blend of CLA 4 g daily significantly improved insulin sensitivity by 27% compared with the control group. Insulin sensitivity improved in 6 out of 10 of the treated group while two deteriorated and two had no change.[34]

An Irish RCT in 32 overweight diabetic subjects found the opposite. Treatment consisted of 8 weeks of either placebo or an isomeric blend of CLA (3 g daily). CLA produced a 6.3% significant increase in fasting glucose concentration and a reduction in insulin sensitivity.[35] Two further studies from the same research group found that both of the common CLA isomers have a negative effect on insulin resistance in obese non-diabetics.[36,37]

A Norwegian RCT evaluated the effect of a mixture of the main isomers (c9t11 and t10c12) on insulin resistance in 188 healthy overweight and obese male and female adults.

The methodology involved use of the euglycae-mic hyperinsulinaemic clamp, which is consid-ered the standard for measuring insulin resistance (and which few other CLA studies have used). No significant differences were found in lean body mass and CLA did not affect glucose metabolism or insulin sensitiv-ity.[38] Another recent trial suggests that CLA may attenuate the proinflammatory state in adipose tissue that predisposes to obesity-induced insulin secretion.[39]

Cancer

Preliminary evidence from *in vitro* work and animals suggests that CLA may reduce the risk of cancer,[40–42] but other studies have not con-firmed this.[43] In experimental cancer studies, diets containing 0.1% c9t11 and t10c12 CLA have been found to inhibit colon cancer cell metastasis *in vivo*. However, *in vitro*, only the c9t11 isomer, not t10c12, inhibited colon can-cer cell migration.[44]

Miscellaneous

Based on findings in experimental animals and cells in culture that CLA can positively influence calcium and bone metabolism, research is now being conducted in humans. However, one dou-ble-blind RCT in 60 healthy adult men aged 39–64 found that CLA 3 g daily for 6 weeks had no significant effect on markers of bone formation or bone resorption or on serum or urinary cal-cium levels.[45]

CLA has also been investigated for effects on immune function. One study in humans found that CLA supplementation resulted in a dose-dependent reduction in mitogen-induced T-lymphocyte activation,[46] while other studies have shown that CLA had a minimal effect on the markers of human immune function.[47,48] A study in 50 volunteers showed that CLA dietary supplementation had no consistent effects on the virological or clinical course of experimental human rhinovirus in colds.[49]

Conclusion

Studies with CLA in humans have not been able to show a significant effect on body weight, body composition or weight regain related to either of the CLA isomers. Some studies suggest a tendency towards a decrease in body fat mass and an increase in body lean mass, while some others raise con-cern about the possibility of deleterious effects of *trans*-10,*cis*-12 CLA on lipid profile, glucose metabolism and insulin sensitivity. Animal studies suggest that CLA may have beneficial effects on atherosclerosis, bone metabolism and immune function, but prelim-inary human studies have not demonstrated such beneficial effects.

Precautions/contraindications

Until more is known, caution should be exer-cised in the use of CLA supplements because of potential problems with insulin resistance. Although this is not proven, people likely to use CLA will be overweight and most likely to suffer from insulin resistance.

Pregnancy and breast-feeding

No problems have been reported, but there have not been sufficient studies to guarantee the safety of CLA in pregnancy and breast-feeding.

Adverse effects

A 12-week study in 60 healthy overweight Japanese volunteers found the the occurrence of adverse events tended to be higher in the two groups given CLA (3.4 g daily or 6.8 g daily) than in the placebo group, but all of the adverse events were mild to moderate, within normal ranges and temporary. Serum aspartate aminotransferase (AST) activity did not differ significantly between the groups at 12 weeks, but in the higher-dose CLA group it was slightly increased from the baseline. Serum alanine aminotransferase (ALT) activity was higher in the higher-dose CLA group than in the placebo group after 12 weeks and was higher than at the baseline in both CLA groups. However, statistical analysis of the population of apparently healthy volunteers who had normal blood parameters at the base-line revealed that AST and ALT levels did not differ significantly among the three groups at 12 weeks. Moreover, no clinically significant changes in vital signs were observed in any of the groups. These results indicate that CLA at a daily dose of 3.4 g is a safe dietary level in healthy Japanese populations in terms of the parameters examined.[50]

CLA consumption is associated with hepatomegaly in animals. A daily intake of 19.3 g CLA for 3 weeks did not produce clinically relevant effects on markers of liver and kidney function in healthy volunteers.[51]

Interactions

None reported.

Dose

CLA is produced for supplements from sunflower oil and is available in the form of capsules.

The dose is not established. Animal research has used large doses, equivalent to several grams a day for humans. However, dietary supplements tend to provide a dose of 1–4 g daily.

References

1 DeLany JP, Blohm F, Truett AA, *et al.* Conjugated linoleic acid rapidly reduces body fat content in mice without affecting energy intake. *Am J Physiol* 1999; 276(Pt2): R1172–R1179.

2 West DB, DeLany JP, Camet PM, *et al.* Effects of conjugated linoleic acid on body fat and energy metabolism in the mouse. *Am J Physiol* 1998; 275 (Pt2): R667–R672.

3 Park Y, Allbright KJ, Liu W, *et al.* Effect of conjugated linoleic acid on body composition in mice. *Lipids* 1997; 32: 853–858.

4 West DB, Blohm FY, Truett AA, *et al.* Conjugated linoleic acid persistently increases total energy expenditure in AKR/J mice without uncoupling protein gene expression. *J Nutr* 2000; 130(10): 2471–2477.

5 Blankson H, Stakkestad JA, Fagertun H, *et al.* Conjugated linoleic acid reduces body fat mass in overweight and obese humans. *J Nutr* 2000; 130: 2943–2948.

6 Riserus U, Berglund L, Vessby B. Conjugated linoleic acid reduced abdominal adipose tissue in obese middle-aged men with signs of the metabolic syndrome: a randomised controlled trial. *Int J Obes Relat Metab Disord* 2001; 25: 1129–1135.

7 Kamphuis MM, Lejeune MP, Saris WH, *et al.* The effect of conjugated linoleic acid supplementation after weight loss on body weight regain, body composition and resting metabolic rate in overweight subjects. *Int J Obes Relat Metab Disord* 2003; 27: 840–847.

8 Kamphuis MM, Lejeune MP, Saris WH, *et al.* Effect of conjugated linoleic acid supplementation after weight loss on appetite and food intake in overweight subjects. *Eur J Clin Nutr* 2003; 57: 1268–1274.

9 Gaullier JM, Halse J, Hoye K, *et al.* Conjugated linoleic acid supplementation for 1 y reduces body fat mass in healthy overweight humans. *Am J Clin Nutr* 2004; 79: 1118–1125.

10 Gaullier JM, Halse J, Hoyce K, *et al.* Supplementation with conjugated linoleic acid for 24 months is well tolerated by and reduces body fat mass in healthy, overweight humans. *J Nutr* 2005; 135: 778–784.

11 Ferreira M, Krieder R, Wilson M. Effects of CLA supplementation during resistance training on body muscle and strength. *J Strength Conditioning Res* 1998; 11: 280.

12 Thom E, Wadstein J, Gudmundsen O. Conjugated linoleic acid reduces body fat in healthy exercising humans. *J Int Med Res* 2001; 29: 392–396.

13 Kreider RB, Ferreira MP, Greenwood M, *et al.* Effects of conjugated linoleic acid supplementation during resistance training on body composition, bone density, strength and selected haematological markers. *J Strength Cond Res* 2002; 16: 325–334.

14 Watras AC, Buchholz AC, Close RN, *et al.* The role of conjugated linoleic acid in reducing body fat and preventing holiday weight gain. *Int J Obes* 2007; 31 (3): 481–487.

15 Gaullier JM, Halse J, Hoivik HO, *et al.* Six months supplementation with conjugated linoleic acid induces regional-specific fat mass decreases in overweight and obese. *Br J Nutr* 2007; 97(3): 550–560.

16 Larsen TM, Toubro S, Gudmundsen O, *et al.* Conjugated linoleic acid supplementation for 1 y does not prevent weight or body fat regain. *Am J Clin Nutr* 2006; 83(3): 606–612.

17 Belury MA, Mahon A, Banni S. The conjugated linoleic acid (CLA) isomer, t10c12-CLA, is inversely associated with changes in body weight and serum leptin in subjects with type 2 diabetes mellitus. *J Nutr* 2003; 133: 257S–260S.

18 Nazare JA, de laPerriere AB, Bonnet F, *et al.* Daily intake of conjugated linoleic acid-enriched yoghurts: effects on energy metabolism and adipose tissue gene expression in healthy subjects. *Br J Nutr* 2007; 97(2): 273–280.

19 Lambert EV, Goedecke JH, Bluett K, *et al.* Conjugated linoleic acid versus high-oleic acid sunflower oil: effects on energy metabolism, glucose tolerance, blood lipids, appetite and body composition in regularly exercising individuals. *Br J Nutr* 2007; 97(5): 1001–1011.

20 Close RN, Schoeller DA, Watras AC, *et al.* Conjugated linoleic acid supplementation alters the 6-mo change in fat oxidation during sleep. *Am J Clin Nutr* 2007; 86(3): 797–804.

21 Steck SE, Chalecki AM, Miller P, *et al.* Conjugated linoleic acid supplementation for twelve weeks

increases lean body mass in obese humans. *J Nutr* 2007; 137(5): 1188–1193.

22 Whigham LD, Watras AC, Schoeller DA. Efficacy of conjugated linoleic acid for reducing fat mass: a meta-analysis in humans. *Am J Clin Nutr* 2007; 85 (5): 1203–1211.

23 Schoeller DA, Watras AC, Whigham LD. A meta-analysis of the effects of conjugated linoleic acid on fat-free mass in humans. *Appl Physiol Nutr Metab* 2009; 34(5): 975–978.

24 Norris LE, Collene AL, Asp ML, *et al.* Comparison of dietary conjugated linoleic acid with safflower oil on body composition in obese postmenopausal women with type 2 diabetes mellitus. *Am J Clin Nutr* 2009; 90(3): 468–476.

25 Lee KN, Kritchevsky D, Pariza MW. Conjugated linoleic acid and atherosclerosis in rabbits. *Atherosclerosis* 1994; 108: 19–25.

26 Nicolosi RJ, Rogers EJ, Kritchevsky D, *et al.* Dietary conjugated linoleic acid reduces plasma lipoproteins and early aortic atherosclerosis in hypercholesterolemic hamsters. *Artery* 1997; 22: 266–277.

27 Kritchevsky D, Tepper SA, Wright S, *et al.* Influence of conjugated linoleic acid (CLA) on establishment and progression of atherosclerosis in rabbits. *J Am Coll Nutr* 2000; 19: 472S– 2000; 477S.

28 Benito P, Nelson GJ, Kelley DS, *et al.* The effect of conjugated linoleic acid on plasma lipoproteins and tissue fatty acid composition in humans. *Lipids* 2001; 36: 229–236.

29 Benito P, Nelson GJ, Kelley DS, *et al.* The effect of conjugated linoleic acid on platelet function, platelet fatty acid composition and blood coagulation in humans. *Lipids* 2001; 36: 221–227.

30 Noone EJ, Roche HM, Nugent AP, *et al.* The effect of dietary suppelementation using isomeric blends of conjugated linoleic acid on lipid metabolism in healthy human subjects. *Br J Nutr* 2002; 88: 243–251.

31 Sluijs I, Plantinga Y, deRoos B, *et al.* Dietary supplementation with *cis*-9, *trans*-11 conjugated linoleic acid and aortic stiffness in overweight and obese adults. *Am J Clin Nutr* 2009; 91(1): 175–183.

32 Zhao WS, Zhai JJ, Wang YH, *et al.* Conjugated linoleic acid supplementation enhances antihypertensive effect of ramipril in Chinese patients with obesity-related hypertension. *Am J Hypertens* 2009; 22(6): 680–686.

33 Houseknecht KL, van denHeuvel JP, Moya-Camarena SY, *et al.* Dietary conjugated linoleic acid normalises impaired glucose tolerance in the Zucker diabetic fatty fa/fa rat. *Biochem Biophys Res Commun* 1998; 244: 678–682.

34 Eyjolfson V, Spriet LL, Dyck DJ. Conjugated linoleic acid improves insulin sensitivity in young, sedentary humans. *Med Sci Sports Exerc* 2004; 36: 814–820.

35 Moloney F, Yeow TP, Mullen A, *et al.* Conjugated linoleic acid supplementation, insulin sensitivity, and lipoprotein metabolism in patients with type 2 diabetes mellitus. *Am J Clin Nutr* 2004; 80: 887–895.

36 Riserus U, Vessby B, Amlov J, *et al.* Supplementation with *trans*10,*cis*12-conjugated linoleic acid induces hyperproinsulinaemia in obese men: close association with impaired insulin sensitivity. *Diabetologia* 2004; 47: 1016–1019.

37 Riserus U, Vesby B, Amer P, *et al.* Effects of *cis*-9, *trans*-11-conjugated linoleic acid supplementation on insulin sensitivity, lipid peroxidation and pro-inflammatory markers in obese men. *Am J Clin Nutr* 2004; 80: 279–283.

38 Syvertsen C, Halse J, Hoivik HO, *et al.* The effect of 6 months supplementation with conjugated linoleic acid on insulin resistance in overweight and obese. *Int J Obes* 2007; 31: 1148–1154.

39 Moloney F, Toomey S, Noone E, *et al.* Antidiabetic effects of *cis*-9, *trans*-11-conjugated linoleic acid may be mediated via anti-inflammatory effects in white adipose tissue. *Diabetes* 2007; 56(3): 574–582.

40 Cesano A, Visonneau S, Scimeca JA, *et al.* Opposite effects of linoleic acid and conjugated linolenic acid on human prostatic cancer in SCID mice. *Anticancer Res* 1998; 18(Suppl 3A): 1429–1434.

41 Thompson H, Zhu Z, Banni S, *et al.* Morphological and biochemical status of the mammary gland influenced by conjugated linoleic acid: implication for a reduction in mammary cancer risk. *Cancer Res* 1997; 57: 5067–5072.

42 Parodi PW. Cow's milk fat components as potential carcinogenic agents. *J Nutr* 1997; 127: 1055–1060.

43 Petrik MB, McEntee MF, Johnson BT, *et al.* Highly unsaturated (n-3) fatty acids, but not alpha linolenic, conjugated linoleic or gamma-linolenic acids, reduce tumourigenesis in Apc(−/+) mice. *J Nutr* 2000; 130: 2434–2443.

44 Soel SM, Choi OS, Bang MH, *et al.* Influence of conjugated linoleic acid isomers on the metastasis of colon cancer cells in vitro and in vivo. *J Nutr Biochem* 2007; 18(10): 650–657.

45 Doyle C, Jewell C, Mullen A, *et al.* Effect of dietary supplementation with conjugated linoleic acid on markers of calcium and bone metabolism in healthy adult men. *Eur J Clin Nutr* 2005; 59: 432–440.

46 Tricon S, Burdge GC, Kew S, *et al.* Effects of *cis*-9, *trans*-11 and *trans*-10, *cis*-12 conjugated linoleic acid on immune cell function in healthy humans. *Am J Clin Nutr* 2004; 80: 1626–1633.

47 Nugent AP, Roche HM, Noone EJ, *et al.* The effects of conjugated linoleic acid supplementation on immune function in healthy volunteers. *Eur J Clin Nutr* 2005; 59: 742–750.

48 Mullen A, Moloney F, Nugent AP, *et al.* Conjugated linoleic acid supplementation reduces peripheral blood mononuclear cell interleukin-2 production in healthy middle-aged males. *J Nutr Biochem* 2007; 18(10): 658–666.

49 Peterson KM, O'Shea M, Stam W, *et al.* Effects of dietary supplementation with conjugated linoleic acid on experimental human rhinovirus infection and illness. *Antivir Ther* 2009; 14(1): 33–43.

50   Iwata T, Kamegai T, Yamauchi-Sato Y, *et al.* Safety of dietary conjugated linoleic acid (CLA) in a 12-weeks trial in healthy overweight Japanese male volunteers. *J Oleo Sci* 2007; 56(10): 517–525.

51   Wanders AJ, Leder L, Banga JD, *et al.* A high intake of conjugated linoleic acid does not affect liver and kidney function tests in healthy human subjects. *Food Chem Toxicol* 2009; 48(2): 587–590.

Copper

Description

Copper is an essential trace mineral.

Human requirements

See Table 1 for Dietary Reference Values for copper.

Dietary intake

In the UK, the average adult diet provides: for men, 1.82 mg daily; for women, 1.31 mg.

Action

Copper functions as an essential component of several enzymes (e.g. superoxide dismutase) and other proteins. It plays a role in bone formation and mineralisation, and in the integrity of the connective tissue of the cardiovascular system. Copper promotes iron absorption and is required for the synthesis of haemoglobin. It is involved in melanin pigment formation, cholesterol metabolism and glucose metabolism. In the central nervous system, it is required for the formation of myelin and is important for normal neurotransmission. Copper has prooxidant effects *in vitro* but antioxidant effects *in vivo*; there is accumulating evidence that adequate copper is required to maintain antioxidant effects within the body.[1]

Dietary sources

See Table 2 for dietary sources of copper.

Table 1   Dietary Reference Values for copper (mg/day)

Age	UK		USA	
			EU RDA = none	
	RNI	EVM	Safe intake	TUL
0–3 months	0.3		0.2	–
4–6 months	0.3		0.22	–
7–12 months	0.3		0.22	–
1–3 years	0.4		0.34	1.0
4–6 years	0.6		1.0–1.5	–
4–8 years	–		0.44	3.0
7–10 years	0.7		–	–
9–13 years	–		0.7	5.0
14–18 years	–		0.89	8.0
Males				
11–14 years	0.8		–	–
15–18 years	1.0		–	–
19–50+ years	1.2	5	0.9	10.0
Females				
11–14 years	0.8		–	–
15–18 years	1.0		–	–
19–50+ years	1.2	5	0.9	10.0
Pregnancy	*		1.0	10.0[2]
Lactation	+0.3		1.0[1]	10.0[2]

* No increment.
[1] ≤18 years, 1.3 mg.
[2] ≤18 years, 8.0 mg.
Note: No EAR, LRNI or FAO/WHO RNIs have been derived for copper.
EVM, safe upper level from supplements alone;
RNI, Reference Nutrient Intake;
TUL, Tolerable Upper Intake Level from diet and supplements.

Table 2 Dietary sources of copper

Food portion	Copper content (mg)
Breakfast cereals	
1 bowl *All-Bran* (45 g)	0.2
1 bowl Bran Flakes (45 g)	0.1
1 bowl *muesli* (95 g)	0.3
2 pieces *Shredded Wheat*	0.2
2 *Weetabix*	0.2
Cereal products	
Bread, brown, 2 slices	0.1
white, 2 slices	0.1
wholemeal, 2 slices	0.2
1 chapati	0.1
Pasta, brown, boiled (150 g)	0.3
white, boiled (150 g)	0.1
Rice, brown, boiled (165 g)	0.5
white, boiled (165 g)	0.2
Meat	
Meat, average, cooked (100 g)	0.2
Liver, lambs, cooked (90 g)	9.0
calf, cooked (90 g)	11.0
Kidney, lambs, cooked (75 g)	0.4
Vegetables	
Chick peas, lentils, or red kidney beans, cooked (105 g)	0.2
Potatoes, boiled (150 g)	0.1
Mushrooms, cooked (100 g)	0.4
Green vegetables (100 g)	0.02
Fruit	
1 banana	0.3
1 orange	0.1
2 handfuls raisins	0.1
8 *dried apricots*	0.2
Nuts	
20 almonds	0.2
10 Brazil nuts	0.4
30 hazelnuts	0.4
30 peanuts	0.3
Milk chocolate (100 g)	0.3
Plain chocolate (100 g)	0.7

[a] Excellent sources (**bold**); good sources (*italic*).

Metabolism

Absorption

Copper is absorbed mainly in the small intestine, with a small amount absorbed in the stomach; absorption is probably by a saturable carrier-mediated mechanism at low levels of intake, and by passive diffusion at high levels of intake.

Distribution

Copper is rapidly taken up by the liver and incorporated into caeruloplasmin. It is stored primarily in the liver. Copper is transported bound to caeruloplasmin.

Elimination

Elimination is mainly via bile into the faeces; small amounts are excreted in the urine, sweat and via epidermal shedding.

Bioavailability

Absorption may be reduced by phytate (present in bran and high-fibre foods) and non-starch polysaccharides (dietary fibre), but recommended intakes of fibre-containing foods are unlikely to compromise copper status.

Deficiency

Deficiency of copper is rare, but may lead to hypochromic and microcytic anaemias, leucopenia, neutropenia, impaired immunity and bone demineralisation. However, copper supplementation of the usual diet (3 or 6 mg daily) in healthy young adult females, while apparently improving copper status, had no effect on biochemical markers of bone formation or bone resorption over 4-week periods.[2] By contrast, copper supplementation (2 mg daily) in eight college women improved copper status, reduced plasma $F_{2\alpha}$-isoprostanes (a marker of oxidant stress) and gave a 62% increase in the urine ratio of collagen crosslinks to a measure of total collagen. None of these effects were observed in women given placebo.[3]

Deficiency may also be caused by Menke's syndrome (an X-linked genetic disorder in which copper absorption is defective); this disease is characterised by a reduced level of copper in the blood, liver and hair, progressive mental deterioration, defective keratinisation of the hair and hypothermia.

Marginal deficiency may result in elevated cholesterol levels, impaired glucose tolerance, defects in pigmentation and structure of the hair, and demyelination and degeneration of the nervous system. In infants and children, copper deficiency can lead to skeletal fragility and increased susceptibility to infections, especially those of the respiratory tract.

Copper deficiency has been linked to many of the processes, including atherosclerosis and thrombosis, associated with ischaemic heart disease. Whether this relationship is important in humans remains unanswered. More information is required concerning possible mild copper deficiency in human populations.

Possible uses

Copper has been claimed to be protective against hypercholesterolaemia. In various animal species, it has been demonstrated that feeding a copper-deficient diet results in increased serum cholesterol levels,[1] but studies in humans have shown inconsistent results.[1,4,5] A recent study in 16 young women (mean age 24 years) found that copper supplementation 3 or 6 mg daily improved copper status and that the concentration of fibrinolytic factor plasminogen activator inhibitor type 1 was significantly reduced by about 30% after supplementation with copper 6 mg daily.[6]

Disturbed copper homeostasis has been associated with pathological processes in Alzheimer's disease. However, a randomized controlled trial involving 68 patients with mild Alzheimer's disease showed that copper supplementation (8 mg daily) had no influence on progression of the disease.[7] Claims for the value of copper supplements in rheumatoid arthritis and psoriasis have not been proved.

> **Conclusion**
> There are no proven benefits in taking copper supplements unless there is a proven deficiency, which should be treated under medical supervision.

Precautions/contraindications

Copper should not be used in Wilson's disease (the disorder may be exacerbated); or hepatic and biliary disease.

Pregnancy and breast-feeding

No problems have been reported with normal intakes.

Adverse effects

Excessive doses (unlikely from supplements) can cause epigastric pain, anorexia, nausea, vomiting and diarrhoea, hepatic toxicity and jaundice, hypotension, haematuria (blood in urine, pain on urination, lower back pain), metallic taste, convulsions and coma.

Copper toxicity may also occur in patients with Wilson's disease (an inherited disorder in which patients exhibit a deficiency of plasma caeruloplasmin and an excess of copper in the liver and bloodstream). There is a theoretical possibility of copper toxicity in women who use copper-containing intrauterine contraceptive devices (further studies required).

Interactions

Drugs

Penicillamine: reduces absorption of copper and vice versa; give 2 h apart.
Trientine: reduces absorption of copper and vice versa; give 2 h apart.

Nutrients

Iron: large doses of iron may reduce copper status and vice versa; give 2 h apart. However, a recent study suggests that copper does not influence the bioavailability of iron in aqueous solution.[8]
Vitamin C: large doses of vitamin C (>1 g daily) may reduce copper status.
Zinc: large doses of zinc may reduce absorption of copper and vice versa; give 2 h apart.

Dose

Copper supplements are available in the form of tablets and capsules, but mostly they are found in multivitamin and mineral supplements. The copper content of various commonly used salts is: copper amino acid chelate (20 mg/g); copper gluconate (140 mg/g); copper sulphate (254 mg/g).

There is no established use or dose for copper as an isolated supplement.

Upper safety levels

The UK Expert Group on Vitamins and Minerals (EVM) has identified a safe total intake of copper for adults from supplements alone of 5 mg daily.

The US Tolerable Upper Intake Level for copper, the highest total amount from diet and supplements unlikely to pose no risk for most people, is 10 mg daily for adults, 8 mg daily for youngsters aged 14–18 years, 5 mg daily for youngsters aged 9–13 years, 3 mg daily for children aged 4–8 years and 1 mg daily for children aged 1–3 years.

References

1 Klevay LM, Inman L, Johnson LK, *et al.* Increased cholesterol in plasma in a young man during experimental copper depletion. *Metabolism* 1984; 33: 1112–1118.
2 Cashman KD, Baker A, Ginty F, *et al.* No effect of copper supplementation on biochemical markers of bone metabolism in healthy young adult females despite apparently improved copper status. *Eur J Clin Nutr* 2001; 55(7): 525–531.
3 DiSilvestro RA, Selsby J, Siefker K. A pilot study of copper supplementation effects on plasma F2alpha isoprostanes and urinary collagen crosslinks in young adult women. *J Trace Elem Med Biol* 2010; 24(3): 165–168.
4 Medeiros D, Pellum L, Brown B. Serum lipids and glucose as associated with haemoglobin levels and copper and zinc intake in young adults. *Life Sci* 1983; 32: 1897–1904.
5 Shapcott D, Vobecky JS, Vobecky J, Demers PP. Plasma cholesterol and the plasma copper/zinc ratio in young children. *Sci Total Environ* 1985; 42: 197–200.
6 Bugel S, Harper A, Rock E, *et al.* Effect of copper supplementation on indices of copper status and certain CVD risk markers in young healthy women. *Br J Nutr* 2005; 94: 231–236.
7 Kessler H, Bayer TA, Bach D, *et al.* Intake of copper has no effect on cognition in patients with mild Alzheimer's disease: a pilot phase 2 clinical trial. *J Neural Transm* 2008; 115(8): 1181–1187.
8 Olivares M, Pizarro F, deRomana DL, *et al.* Acute copper supplementation does not inhibit non-heme iron bioavailability in humans. *Biol Trace Elem Res* 2009; 136(2): 180–186.

Creatine

Description

Creatine is an amino acid synthesised from the amino acid precursors arginine, glycine and methionine. The kidneys use arginine and glycine to make guanidinoacetate, which the liver methylates to form creatine. The highest concentrations of creatine are found in skeletal muscle, but high concentrations are also found in heart and smooth muscle, as well as brain, kidney and spermatozoa.

Action

Creatine combines readily with phosphate to form creatine phosphate, which is a source of high-energy phosphate that is released during the anaerobic phase of muscle contraction. The phosphorus from creatine phosphate is transferred to adenosine diphosphate (ADP), creating adenosine triphosphate (ATP) and releasing creatine. Stored creatine phosphate can fuel the first 4–5 s of a sprint, but another fuel must provide the energy to sustain the activity.

Creatine supplements increase the storage of creatine phosphate, thus making more ATP available for the working muscles and enabling them to work harder before becoming fatigued. There appears to be an upper limit for creatine storage in muscle, and supplementation increases levels most in athletes with low stores of creatine, rather than those with high levels.

Dietary sources

Creatine is found in food, and the average omnivorous diet supplies about 1–2 g creatinine daily, although vegetarians consume less. This is because creatine is found principally in animal foods, such as fish and meat. Only trace amounts are found in plant foods. If the dietary supply is limited, creatine can be synthesised endogenously.

Possible uses

Creatine has been investigated for a possible role in sports and athletics.

Exercise performance

Supplementation increases levels of creatine in plasma and skeletal muscle, and it is used to enhance exercise performance. A study in 1992 was the first to show that creatine supplementation (5 g four to six times a day) for several consecutive days increased the creatine concentration of skeletal muscle; the authors concluded that creatine supplementation might enhance exercise performance in humans.[1]

The first published investigation into the effect of oral creatine supplementation on exercise performance in humans showed that ingestion of creatine (20 g daily for 5 days) was found to improve performance during repeated bouts of maximal isokinetic knee-extensor exercise, reducing fatigue by 6%.[2] Several studies since this time have confirmed the ability of creatine to improve sports performance in a variety of settings and sports.[3–11] However, several studies have reported no effects of creatine supplementation on exercise performance.[12–15] These trials have also reported changes in body mass and fat-free mass with creatine (Table 1).[16–58]

Miscellaneous

There is preliminary evidence that creatine may improve strength in people with chronic heart failure,[59] chronic obstructive pulmonary disease (COPD),[60] (although two trials have shown no benefit in COPD[61,62]) and in neuromuscular diseases.[63–65] A Cochrane systematic review including 12 RCTs concluded that short- and medium-term creatine treatment improves muscle strength in people with muscular dystrophies, and is well tolerated.[66] Evidence from RCTs does not show significant improvement in muscle strength in metabolic myopathies.[67] A recent trial found that creatine (20 g daily for 5 days, 5 g daily thereafter) improved muscle strength in people with Parkinson's disease.[68] Creatine supplements may also be an effective adjunct to vitamin supplements for lowering plasma homocysteine.[69] A study evaluating creatine in schizophrenia found no benefit.[70] Creatine has been shown to improve cognitive function in older adults[71] but not in young adults.[72]

Preliminary evidence suggests that supplementation may be a useful therapeutic strategy for older adults to attenuate loss in muscle strength and performance in functional living tasks.[73] In addition, when combined with resistance training, creatine supplementation has been shown to increase lean tissue mass and improves leg strength, endurance, and average power in older men.[24]

Precautions/contraindications

Creatine should be used with caution in renal or hepatic disease. However, the increase in urinary excretion of creatinine observed with creatine supplementation does not indicate renal impairment. Rather, it correlates with the increase in muscle creatine storage and the increased rate of muscle creatine degradation to creatinine.

Creatine is not on the International Olympic Committee Drug List, but some consider it to be in the 'grey zone' between doping and substances allowed to enhance performance.

Conclusion

Despite a large number of clinical trials, there remains a dearth of high-quality research on creatine supplementation. Investigations of the effect of creatine on performance, strength and endurance in laboratory studies have yielded roughly equal numbers of studies showing positive effects and no effect. Field studies (i.e. of individuals participating in normal sports activities) have shown less impressive results than laboratory studies.

Creatine supplementation improves performance during exercise of high to maximal intensity, and its use could potentially benefit sports involving either single bouts of high-intensity exercise (e.g. sprint running, swimming, rowing, cycling) or multiple bouts (e.g. soccer, rugby, hockey). It also has the potential to benefit an athlete involved in training that involves repetitive bouts of high-intensity exercise. However, there is no evidence that creatine can benefit prolonged, submaximal exercise (e.g. middle- or long-distance running), and it may impair endurance exercise by contributing to weight gain.

Pregnancy and breast-feeding

No problems have been reported. However, there have not been sufficient studies to

Table 1 Clinical trials evaluating creatine supplementation in sports and athletics

Reference	Duration and type of trial	Study group	Dose of creatine	Outcome measures	Observed effects
Armentano et al. (2007)[16]	7 day placebo-controlled	35 US Army volunteers (20 men and 15 women; age, 22–36 years)	20 g/day for 7 day	Exercise performance, blood pressure, renal function	No significant difference in 2-min push-up counts; no adverse changes in blood pressure, body composition, body weight, or serum creatine phosphokinase
Banerjee et al. (2010)[17]	8-week randomised, placebo-controlled single-blind study	33 steroid-naive, ambulatory boys with Duchenne muscular dystrophy	5 g/day	Cellular energetics, manual muscle test score and functional status	Oral creatine significantly improved the muscle phosphocreatine/inorganic phosphate ratio and preserved the muscle strength short term
Bassit et al. (2008)[18]	5-day randomised, placebo-controlled double-blind study	11 triathletes, each with at least 3 years' experience of participation in this sport (following a half ironman competition)	20 g/day	Inflammatory response: interleukin-1β, interleukin-6, tumour necrosis factor-α, interferon-α, prostaglandin E_2	Reduction in inflammatory response with creatine after competition
Bemben et al. (2010)[19]	14-week double-blind, randomised, placebo-controlled study	42 middle-aged men in a resistance training programme	5 g/day vs protein vs creatine + protein vs placebo	Strength and lean body mass	Resistance training in middle-aged and older men significantly increased muscular strength and added muscle mass with no additional benefits from creatine and/or protein supplementation
Brose et al. (2003)[20]	14-week double-blind, randomised, placebo-controlled study	28 healthy men and women >65 years in a whole body resistance exercise programme	5 g/day	Total body mass, fat-free mass, measures of muscle strength and functional capacity	Addition of creatine to the exercise stimulus enhanced the increase in total and fat-free mass, and gains in several indices of isometric muscle strength

(Continued)

Table 1 *(continued)*

Reference	Duration and type of trial	Study group	Dose of creatine	Outcome measures	Observed effects
Burke *et al.* (2008)[21]	8-week randomised, placebo-controlled study	24 men and 18 women with minimal resistance exercise training experience (1 year) who were participating in at least 30 min of structured physical activity (i.e., walking, jogging, cycling) 3–5 times per week for 49 days	Creatine: 0.25 g/kg lean-tissue mass for 7 days; 0.06 g/kg lean tissue mass	Changes in muscle insulin-like growth factor-1 (IGF-1)	Creatine increased the accumulation of muscle IGF-1 during resistance training
Candow *et al.* (2008)[22]	10-week randomised placebo-controlled study	Older men (59–77 years) during resistance training	0.1 g/kg creatine + 0.3 g/kg protein (n = 10), creatine (n = 13), or placebo (n = 12) on training days	Lean tissue mass, muscle thickness, measures of muscle strength, urinary indicators of cytotoxicity (formaldehyde), myofibrillar protein degradation and bone resorption	Creatine combined with protein increased lean tissue mass and resulted in a greater relative increase in bench press but not leg press strength; creatine reduced muscle protein degradation and bone resorption without increasing formaldehyde production
Casey *et al.* (1996)[11]	5-day uncontrolled study	9 subjects	20 g/day (after and before bouts of 30-s maximal isokinetic cycling	Work production and ATP synthesis	Increased work production and reduction in loss of ATP with creatine
Chilibeck *et al.* (2007)[23]	8-week randomised, placebo-controlled study	18 Rugby Union football players	0.1 g/kg per day	Body composition, muscular endurance, aerobic endurance	Creatine increased muscular endurance but had no effect on body composition or aerobic endurance

Study	Study design	Subjects	Dose	Outcomes measured	Results
Chrusch et al. (2001)[24]	Randomised, placebo-controlled study	30 men, average age 70 years	0.3 g/kg for the first 5 days (loading phase) and 0.07 g/kg thereafter combined with resistance training	Muscular strength, muscular endurance, power, lean tissue, fat mass	Creatine supplementation, when combined with resistance training, increased lean tissue mass and improved leg strength, endurance and average power
Cooke et al. (1997)[14]	5-day, randomised placebo-controlled study	80 healthy active men	20 g/day with two bouts of high-intensity cycle sprinting	Maximal peak power output, absolute time to fatigue	No effect on ability to reproduce or maintain a high percentage of peak power during the second bout of exercise
Cooke et al. (1995)[15]	5-day, randomised placebo-controlled study	12 healthy untrained men	20 g/day with two bouts of high-intensity cycle sprinting	Maximal peak power output, absolute time to fatigue	No effect of creatine on peak power or fatigue
Cramer et al. (2007)[25]	9-day, randomised placebo-controlled study	25 men	10.5 g/day with isokinetic resistance training	Measures of muscular strength	Non-significant improvement in muscular strength with creatine
Cribb et al. (2007)[26]	10-week randomised, placebo-controlled study	Resistance-trained men	0.1 g/kg creatine daily + protein + carbohydrate vs protein + carbohydrate during resistance exercise	Strength, body composition, muscle structure	Creatine produced greater lean body mass
Eckerson et al. (2008)[27]	30-day double-blind placebo-controlled study	32 men	5 g/day creatine	Body weight and anaerobic working capacity	Body weight increased; no effect on anaerobic working capacity
Ferguson & Syrotuik (2006)[28]	10-week randomised, placebo-controlled study	26 female trainees	0.3 g/kg per day + resistance training	Body composition and strength	No greater increase in strength or lean body mass beyond training only
Fukuda et al. (2010)[29]	5-day, randomised placebo-controlled study	50 moderately trained men and women	5 g four times daily for 5 days	Anaerobic running capacity	Significantly increased anaerobic running capacity in men but not women; non-significant increase in body weight
Gotshalk et al. (2008)[30]	7-day, randomised placebo-controlled study	30 women (58–71 years)	0.3 g/kg per day	Body composition, muscular strength and lower-body motor functional performance	Increase in strength, power and lower-body motor functional performance with creatine
Gotshalk et al. (2002)[31]	7-day, randomised placebo-controlled study	18 active men (59–72 years)	0.3 g/kg per day	Muscle performance and functional capacity	Creatine improved muscle strength and performance

(Continued)

Table 1 *(continued)*

Reference	Duration and type of trial	Study group	Dose of creatine	Outcome measures	Observed effects
Greenhaff *et al.* (1993)[32]	5-day, randomised placebo-controlled study	12 subjects	4 × 5 g creatine/day	Muscle torque production and plasma ammonia and blood lactate accumulation during 5 bouts of exercise	Muscle peak torque production was greater and plasma ammonia accumulation was lower with creatine; no differences were found when comparing blood lactate levels
Gualano *et al.* (2008)[33]	3-month randomised placebo-controlled study	22 healthy sedentary men	10 g/day + moderate aerobic training	Plasma insulin, oral glucose tolerance test	Creatine improved glucose tolerance but had no effect on insulin sensitivity
Herda *et al.* (2009)[34]	30-day randomised placebo-controlled study	58 healthy men	5 g/day creatine monohydrate vs 2.5 g polyethylene glycosylated (PEG) creatine vs 1.25 g PEG creatine vs placebo	Muscular strength, endurance and power output	Smaller doses of PEG creatine increased muscle strength to the same extent as 5 g creatine monohydrate, but lower doses did not alter body mass, power output or endurance; compared with placebo, none of the supplements improved peak power output or muscle endurance
Hoffman *et al.* (2006)[35]	10-week randomised placebo-controlled study	33 men	Creatine vs creatine + beta-alanine vs placebo + resistance training	Muscle strength, power, body composition, plasma testosterone, cortisol, growth hormone, sex hormone-binding globulin	Changes in lean body mass and per cent body fat were greater ($P < 0.05$) with creatine + beta-alanine than creatine alone or placebo; significantly greater strength improvements were seen in both treated groups compared with placebo; resting testosterone concentrations were elevated with creatine but no other significant endocrine changes were noted
Johnston *et al.* (2009)[36]	Single-blind, crossover design	7 men (18–25 years)	Placebo on days 1–7, creatine 4 × 5 g daily on days 15–21	Lean tissue mass, strength and endurance	During immobilization, creatine supplementation better maintained lean tissue mass, elbow flexor strength and endurance and elbow extensor strength and endurance than did placebo

Study	Study design	Subjects	Regimen	Measures	Results
Jones et al. (1999)[6]	10 days + 10 weeks randomised double-blind placebo-controlled study	16 elite ice hockey players	5 g four times a day for 5 days followed by 5 g/day for 10 weeks, followed by 5 cycle sprints and 6 skating sprints	Measures of performance on the cycle and skating sprints	No changes in the placebo group; with creatine average mean power output over the 5 sprints was significantly higher at 10 days and 10 weeks; average peak power output over the 5 sprints improved significantly from baseline; average on-ice sprint performance was significantly faster at 10 days and 10 weeks
Jones et al. (2002)[37]	Uncontrolled study	7 men, 2 women	20 g/day for 5 days, 5 g/day thereafter	Oxygen-uptake kinetics during cycling	With moderate exercise, no change in oxygen uptake with creatine, but a reduction in oxygen uptake with creatine loading in heavy exercise
Jones et al. (2009)[38]	5 day (subjects act as own controls)	7 healthy men	4 × 5 g/day	Phosphocreatine kinetics	Creatine results in slowing of phosphocreatine kinetics in exercise and subsequent recovery
Juhasz et al. (2009)[39]	5-day, randomised placebo-controlled study	16 male competitive swimmers (mean age 15.9 years)	4 × 5g daily + swimming sprints	Swimming performance	Compared with placebo, creatine reduced swimming time
Kerksick et al. (2009)[40]	28-day randomised double-blind controlled study	24 resistance-trained men	20 g/day creatine for 5 days, 5 g/day for remaining 23 days vs same regimen with creatine + pinitol	Performance measures and body mass	Significant improvements in upper- and lower-body strength and body composition occurred in both groups; however, significantly greater increases in lean mass and fat-free mass occurred in the creatine group than in the creatine + pinitol group
Kingsley et al. (2009)[41]	5-day, randomised placebo-controlled study	18 active men	20 g/day (in between 2 cycling trials)	Markers of oxidative stress and antioxidant defences	Creatine did not enhance non-enzymatic antioxidant defence or protect against lipid peroxidation
Koenig et al. (2008)[42]	5-day, randomised placebo-controlled study	60 active men (mean age 22 years)	25 g/day creatine vs 100 kcal carbohydrate vs 250 kcal carbohydrate vs placebo, in between 2 sets of 10 jumps	Jump height	Creatine and carbohydrate were better for sustaining jump height than placebo; 250 kcal carbohydrate was as effective as creatine
Law et al. (2009)[43]	2- or 5-day, randomised placebo-controlled study	17 trained men	4 × 5 g/day + resistance loading	Muscular strength and anaerobic performance	5-day supplementation improved performance but 2-day supplementation did not

(Continued)

Table 1 *(continued)*

Reference	Duration and type of trial	Study group	Dose of creatine	Outcome measures	Observed effects
McNaughton *et al.* (1998)[10]	5-day, randomised placebo-controlled study	16 men (mean age 21 years)	20 g/day	Kayak ergometer performances	Creatine improved work performance
Mujika *et al.* (1996)[12]	7-day, randomised placebo-controlled study	20 highly trained swimmers	4 × 5 g/day	Sprint swimming performance and energy metabolism	No significant differences in performance times
Mujika *et al.* (2000)[4]	7-day, randomised placebo-controlled study	17 highly trained male soccer players	4 × 5 g/day	Jump, sprint and endurance tests	Creatine favourably affected repeated sprint performance and limited the decay in jumping ability after the intensive endurance test; intermittent endurance performance was not affected by creatine
Odland *et al.* (1997)[44]	3-day, randomised placebo-controlled study	9 men	20 g/day in between cycling tests 14 days apart	Power output, fatigue, post-exercise blood lactate	No effect on cycling performance
Pluim *et al.* (2006)[45]	4 weeks and 6 days randomised placebo-controlled study	36 competitive male tennis players (mean age 23 years)	6 days creatine loading, maintenance phase of 4 weeks	Tennis performance (e.g. stroke velocity)	Creatine was not effective in improving selected indicators of tennis performance
Rawson *et al.* (2007)[46]	10-day, randomised placebo-controlled study	22 healthy, weight-trained men (19–27 years)	Creatine (no dose given) or a placebo for 10 days; assessment from 5 to 10 days	Markers of muscle damage following a hypoxic resistance test	Creatine did not reduce skeletal damage or enhance recovery
Rici-Sanz *et al.* (2008)[47]	5-day, randomised placebo-controlled study	20 trained men	21 g creatine vs 250 g carbohydrate vs placebo	Resting myocellular glycogen and phosphocreatine	Creatine loading did not increase muscle glycogen storage
Romer *et al.* (2001)[3]	5-day double-blind crossover study	9 male squash players	0.075 g/kg 4 times daily	Exercise performance	Creatine improved high intensity, intermittent exercise performance
Safdar *et al.* (2008)[48]	2 × 20 days randomised, placebo-controlled, crossover, double-blind design,	12 young, healthy, non-obese men	20 g/day for 3 days, 5 g/day for 7 days; placebo for 10 days	mRNA expression and protein content in human skeletal muscle	Creatine increased fat-free mass, total body water, and body weight; up-regulated the expression of mRNA from certain genes and the protein content of kinases involved in cell function

Reference	Study design	Subjects	Dosage	Outcomes measured	Results
Sculthorpe et al. (2010)[49]	8-day, randomised placebo-controlled study	40 men (mean age 24 years)	25 g/day for 5 days, 5 g/day for 3 days	Range of movement of ankle and shoulder	Creatine reduced range of movement for ankle and shoulder and increased body mass
Sewell et al. (2008)[50]	2 × 5 day randomised crossover study	Six healthy men	Creatine vs carbohydrate (with cycling)	Glycogen content of skeletal muscle	Creatine had no effect on muscle glycogen either at rest or after strenuous exercise
Silva et al. (2007)[51]	21-day randomised placebo-controlled study	16 female swimmers	20 g/day	Swimming velocity, body composition and hydrodynamic variables	Creatine produced significant effects on gross and/or propelling efficiency during swimming in female athletes; however, it did not influence performance, body weight or body composition
Snow et al. (1998)[13]	5-day, randomised placebo-controlled study	8 active untrained men	30 g/day	Sprint exercise performance and skeletal muscle anaerobic metabolism	No effect of creatine on sprint exercise performance or muscle aerobic metabolism
Spillane et al. (2009)[52]	47-day, randomised placebo-controlled study	30 non-resistance-trained men	Creatine monohydrate vs creatine ethyl ester vs placebo: 20 g/day for 5 days followed by 5 g/day for 42 days; combined with resistance training	Body composition, muscle mass, muscle strength and power, serum and muscle creatine, and serum creatinine	Compared with creatine monohydrate, creatine ethyl ester was not as effective at increasing serum and muscle creatine levels or in improving body composition or muscle mass, strength and power
Stout et al. (2007)[53]	14-day double-blind crossover design	15 men and women (mean age 74 years)	20 g/day for 1 week, 10 g/day for 1 week	Physical working capacity at fatigue threshold, maximal isometric grip strength, sit-to-stand and body weight	Creatine increased grip strength and working capacity but no effect on sit-to-stand or body weight
Tarnopalsky et al. (2001)[54]	8-week double-blind randomised study	19 young healthy men	10 g/day + glucose vs protein + glucose	Fat-free mass, strength, muscle fibre area	Compared with protein, creatine produced increased fat-free mass, but no difference in strength
Theodorou et al. (2005)[55]	4-day double-blind randomised study	10 swimmers (mean age 17.8 years)	5 × 5 g/day creatine vs creatine + glucose	Swimming performance	Both interventions produced faster swims but there was no difference between the intervention groups
Thompson et al. (1996)[56]	6-week, randomised placebo-controlled study	10 female swimmers	2 g/day	Skeletal muscle metabolism and oxygen supply	No effect of creatine on muscle creatine concentration, muscle oxygen supply or muscle aerobic or anaerobic metabolism

(Continued)

Table 1 *(continued)*

Reference	Duration and type of trial	Study group	Dose of creatine	Outcome measures	Observed effects
Urbanski et al. (1999)[8]	5-day double-blind, randomised, balanced, crossover design	10 physically active, untrained, college-aged males (mean age 26.4 years)	4×5 g/day	Maximal strength and time to fatigue during isometric exercise	Creatine improved maximal strength and time to fatigue, but improved strength was restricted to movements performed with a large muscle mass
Vandebuerie et al. (1998)[9]	Double-blind crossover design	12 elite cyclists	Creatine 25 g/day for 5 days vs 25 g/day for 5 days + 5 g/h during exercise vs placebo	Sprint power, endurance time to fatigue	Compared with placebo, creatine, but not CC, increased peak and mean sprint power output by 8–9% for all 5 sprints; endurance time to exhaustion was not affected by either creatine regimens
Volek et al. (1999)[7]	12-week randomised placebo-controlled study	19 healthy resistance trained men	25 g/day for 1 week followed by 5 g/day combined with heavy resistance training	Fat-free mass, physical performance, muscle morphology	Creatine supplementation enhanced fat-free mass, physical performance and muscle morphology
Volek et al. (2004)[57]	4-week randomised placebo-controlled study	17 men	0.3 g/kg per day combined with resistance exercise	Performance, body composition, hormone concentration	Performance and body mass increased to a greater extent with creatine; changes in some hormones
Walter et al. (2008)[58]	5-day week randomised placebo-controlled study	16 college age men	20 g/day	Electromyographic fatigue threshold on cycle ergometer test	Non-significant influence of creatine on threshold

guarantee the safety of creatine in pregnancy and breast-feeding. Creatine is best avoided.

Adverse effects

No serious toxic effects have been documented. In a survey of 52 college athletes supplementing with creatine, 16 reported diarrhoea, 13 reported muscle cramps and seven dehydration.[74] Another survey, which involved 28 male baseball players and 24 male football players aged 18–23, found that 16 (31%) experienced diarrhoea, 13 (25%) experienced muscle cramps, 7 (13%) reported unwanted weight gain, 7 (13%) reported dehydration and 12 reported various other side-effects.[75] In the same survey, 39 (75%) exceeded the maintenance dose of 2–5 g daily.

In a placebo-controlled trial involving 175 subjects and lasting 310 days, creatine monohydrate supplementation 10 g daily did not result in significant differences in adverse effects compared with placebo. Occurrence of nausea, gastrointestinal discomfort and diarrhoea was similar in both groups. After 2 months of treatment, oedematous limbs were seen more often in subjects using creatine, probably because of water retention. Severe diarrhoea and severe nausea caused three subjects in the creatine group to stop taking it, after which these adverse events subsided.[76]

In another report a patient with nephrotic syndrome who had been supplementing with creatine experienced deterioration in renal function,[77] and a previously healthy 20-year-old man developed interstitial nephritis after taking creatine (20 g daily) for 4 weeks.[78]

Chronic administration of a large quantity of creatine can increase the production of formaldehyde. Formaldehyde is well known to cross-link proteins and DNA, and may cause potentially serious side-effects.[79]

Creatine supplementation often causes weight gain, which can be mistaken for increase in muscle mass. Increasing intracellular creatine may cause an osmotic influx of water into the cell because creatine is an osmotically active substance. It is, therefore, possible that the weight gained is due to water retention and not increased muscle.

The safety of prolonged use of creatine is of concern. Individuals should be advised not to take the loading dose of 20 g daily for more than 5 days and not to supplement for a total period of longer than 30 days until effects are better known. Evidence is not robust enough to set a safe upper level for creatine. Evidence of safety is strong at intakes up to 5 g daily for chronic supplementation, and this level is identified as the Observed Safe Level. Although much higher levels have been tested under acute conditions without adverse effects and may be safe, the data for intakes above 5 g daily are not sufficient for a confident conclusion of long-term safety.[80]

Interactions

No known drug interactions. Caffeine may reduce or abolish the ergogenic effects of creatine.

Dose

Creatine is available mainly in the form of powder. A review of 13 US products showed that 11 of them contained the weight of creatine claimed. One of the products was found to contain less than the claimed amount and one failed to meet its claim of being free from the impurity dicyandiamide.

The usual dose regimen used in studies is 5 g creatine monohydrate four times a day for the first 5 days as a loading dose, then 2–5 g daily as maintenance. These doses should not be exceeded because of the risk of adverse effects (see above).

References

1 Harris RC, Soderlund K, Hultman E. Elevation of creatine in resting and exercised muscle of normal subjects by creatine supplementation. *Clin Sci* 1992; 83: 367–374.
2 Greenhaff PL, Casey A, Short AH, *et al*. Influence of oral creatine supplementation on muscle torque during repeated bouts of maximal voluntary exercise in man. *Clin Sci* 1993; 84: 565–571.
3 Romer LM, Barrington JP, Jeukendrup AE. Effects of oral creatine supplementation on high intensity, intermittent exercise performance in competitive squash players. *Int J Sports Med* 2001; 22(8): 546–552.
4 Mujika I, Padilla S, Ibanez J, *et al*. Creatine supplementation and sprint performance in soccer players. *Med Sci Sports Exerc* 2000; 32(2): 518–525.

5   Rici-Sanz J, Mendez Marco MT. Creatine enhances oxygen uptake and performance during alternating intensity exercise. *Med Sci Sports Exerc* 2000; 32: 379–385.

6   Jones AM, Atter T, Georg KP. Oral creatine supplementation improves multiple sprint performance in elite ice-hockey players. *J Sports Med Phys Fitness* 1999; 39(3): 189–196.

7   Volek JS, Duncan ND, Mazzetti SA, *et al.* Performance and muscle fiber adaptations to creatine supplementation and heavy resistance training. *Med Sci Sports Exerc* 1999; 31(8): 1147–1156.

8   Urbanski RL, Vincent WJ, Yaspelkis BB. 3rd Creatine supplementation differentially affects maximal isometric strength and time to fatigue in large and small muscle groups. *Int J Sport Nutr* 1999; 9(2): 136–145.

9   Vandebuerie F, Vanden Eynde B, Vandenberghe K, *et al.* Effect of creatine loading on endurance capacity and sprint power in cyclists. *Int J Sports Med* 1998; 19(7): 490–495.

10   McNaughton LR, Dalton B, Tarr J. The effects of creatine supplementation on high-intensity exercise performance in elite performers. *Eur J Appl Physiol Occup Physiol* 1998; 78(3): 236–240.

11   Casey A, Constantin-Teodosiu D, Howell S, *et al.* Creatine ingestion favorably affects performance and muscle metabolism during maximal exercise in humans. *Am J Physiol* 1996; 271(Pt1): E31–E37.

12   Mujika I, Chatard JC, Lacoste L, *et al.* Creatine supplementation does not improve sprint performance in competitive swimmers. *Med Sci Sports Exerc* 1996; 28(11): 1435–1441.

13   Snow RJ, McKenna MJ, Selig SE, *et al.* Effect of creatine supplementation on sprint exercise performance and muscle metabolism. *J Appl Physiol* 1998; 84(5): 1667–1673.

14   Cooke WH, Barnes WS. The influence of recovery duration on high-intensity exercise performance after oral creatine supplementation. *Can J Appl Physiol* 1997; 22(5): 454–267.

15   Cooke WH, Grandjean PW, Barnes WS. Effect of oral creatine supplementation on power output and fatigue during bicycle ergometry. *J Appl Physiol* 1995; 78(2): 670–673.

16   Armentano MJ, Brenner AK, Hedman TL, *et al.* The effect and safety of short-term creatine supplementation on performance of push-ups. *Mil Med* 2007; 172(3): 312–317.

17   Banerjee B, Sharma U, Balasubramanian K, *et al.* Effect of creatine monohydrate in improving cellular energetics and muscle strength in ambulatory Duchenne muscular dystrophy patients: a randomized, placebo-controlled 31P MRS study. *Magn Reson Imaging* 2010; 28(5): 698–707.

18   Bassit RA, Curi R, Costa Rosa LF. Creatine supplementation reduces plasma levels of pro-inflammatory cytokines and PGE2 after a half-ironman competition. *Amino Acids* 2008; 35(2): 425–431.

19   Bemben MG, Witten MS, Carter JM, *et al.* The effects of supplementation with creatine and protein on muscle strength following a traditional resistance training program in middle-aged and older men. *J Nutr Health Aging* 2010; 14(2): 155–159.

20   Brose A, Parise G, Tarnopolsky MA. Creatine supplementation enhances isometric strength and body composition improvements following strength exercise training in older adults. *J Gerontol A Biol Sci Med Sci* 2003; 58(1): 11–19.

21   Burke DG, Candow DG, Chilibeck PD, *et al.* Effect of creatine supplementation and resistance-exercise training on muscle insulin-like growth factor in young adults. *Int J Sport Nutr Exerc Metab* 2008; 18(4): 389–398.

22   Candow DG, Little JP, Chilibeck PD, *et al.* Low-dose creatine combined with protein during resistance training in older men. *Med Sci Sports Exerc* 2008; 40(9): 1645–1652.

23   Chilibeck PD, Magnus C, Anderson M. Effect of in-season creatine supplementation on body composition and performance in rugby union football players. *Appl Physiol Nutr Metab* 2007; 32(6): 1052–1057.

24   Chrusch MJ, Chilibeck PD, Chad KE, *et al.* Creatine supplementation combined with resistance training in older men. *Med Sci Sports Exerc* 2001; 33: 2111–2117.

25   Cramer JT, Stout JR, Culbertson JY, *et al.* Effects of creatine supplementation and three days of resistance training on muscle strength, power output, and neuromuscular function. *J Strength Cond Res* 2007; 21(3): 668–677.

26   Cribb PJ, Williams AD, Hayes A. A creatine-protein-carbohydrate supplement enhances responses to resistance training. *Med Sci Sports Exerc* 2007; 39(11): 1960–1968.

27   Eckerson JM, Bull AA, Moore GA. Effect of thirty days of creatine supplementation with phosphate salts on anaerobic working capacity and body weight in men. *J Strength Cond Res* 2008; 22(3): 826–832.

28   Ferguson TB, Syrotuik DG. Effects of creatine monohydrate supplementation on body composition and strength indices in experienced resistance trained women. *J Strength Cond Res* 2006; 20(4): 939–946.

29   Fukuda DH, Smith AE, Kendall KL, *et al.* The effects of creatine loading and gender on anaerobic running capacity. *J Strength Cond Res* 2010; 24(7): 1826–1833.

30   Gotshalk LA, Kraemer WJ, Mendonca MA, *et al.* Creatine supplementation improves muscular performance in older women. *Eur J Appl Physiol* 2008; 102(2): 223–231.

31   Gotshalk LA, Volek JS, Staron RS, *et al.* Creatine supplementation improves muscular performance in older men. *Med Sci Sports Exerc* 2002; 34(3): 537–543.

32   Greenhaff PL, Casey A, Short AH, *et al.* Influence of oral creatine supplementation of muscle torque

during repeated bouts of maximal voluntary exercise in man. *Clin Sci (Lond)* 1993; 84(5): 565–571.

33 Gualano B, Novaes RB, Artioli GG, *et al.* Effects of creatine supplementation on glucose tolerance and insulin sensitivity in sedentary healthy males undergoing aerobic training. *Amino Acids* 34(2): 245–250.

34 Herda TJ, Beck TW, Ryan ED, *et al.* Effects of creatine monohydrate and polyethylene glycosylated creatine supplementation on muscular strength, endurance, and power output. *J Strength Cond Res* 2009; 23(3): 818–826.

35 Hoffman J, Ratamess N, Kang J, *et al.* Effect of creatine and beta-alanine supplementation on performance and endocrine responses in strength/power athletes. *Int J Sport Nutr Exerc Metab* 2006; 16(4): 430–446.

36 Johnston AP, Burke DG, MacNeil LG, *et al.* Effect of creatine supplementation during cast-induced immobilization on the preservation of muscle mass, strength, and endurance. *J Strength Cond Res* 2009; 23(1): 116–120.

37 Jones AM, Carter H, Pringle JS, *et al.* Effect of creatine supplementation on oxygen uptake kinetics during submaximal cycle exercise. *J Appl Physiol* 2002; 92(6): 2571–2577.

38 Jones AM, Wilkerson DP, Fulford J. Influence of dietary creatine supplementation on muscle phosphocreatine kinetics during knee-extensor exercise in humans. *Am J Physiol Regul Integr Comp Physiol* 2009; 296(4): R1078–R1087.

39 Juhasz I, Gyore I, Csende Z, *et al.* Creatine supplementation improves the anaerobic performance of elite junior fin swimmers. *Acta Physiol Hung* 2009; 96(3): 325–336.

40 Kerksick CM, Wilborn CD, Campbell WI, *et al.* The effects of creatine monohydrate supplementation with and without D-pinitol on resistance training adaptations. *J Strength Cond Res* 2009; 23(9): 2673–2682.

41 Kingsley M, Cunningham D, Mason L, *et al.* Role of creatine supplementation on exercise-induced cardiovascular function and oxidative stress. *Oxid Med Cell Longev* 2009; 2(4): 247–254.

42 Koenig CA, Benardot D, Cody M, *et al.* Comparison of creatine monohydrate and carbohydrate supplementation on repeated jump height performance. *J Strength Cond Res* 2008; 22(4): 1081–1086.

43 Law YL, Ong WS, Gillian Yap TL, *et al.* Effects of two and five days of creatine loading on muscular strength and anerobic power in trained athletes. *J Strength Cond Res* 2009; 23: 906–914.

44 Odland LM, MacDougall JD, Tarnopolsky MA, *et al.* Effect of oral creatine supplementation on muscle [PCr] and short-term maximum power output. *Med Sci Sports Exerc* 1997; 29(2): 216–219.

45 Pluim BM, Ferrauti A, Broekhof F, *et al.* The effects of creatine supplementation on selected factors of tennis specific training. *Br J Sports Med* 2006; 40(6): 507–511; discussion 511–512.

46 Rawson ES, Conti MP, Miles MP. Creatine supplementation does not reduce muscle damage or enhance recovery from resistance exercise. *J Strength Cond Res* 2007; 21(4): 1208–1213.

47 Rico-Sanz J, Zehnder M, Buchli R, *et al.* Creatine feeding does not enhance intramyocellular glycogen concentration during carbohydrate loading: an in vivo study by ^{31}P- and ^{13}C-MRS. *J Physiol Biochem* 2008; 64(3): 189–196.

48 Safdar A, Yardley NJ, Snow R, *et al.* Global and targeted gene expression and protein content in skeletal muscle of young men following short-term creatine monohydrate supplementation. *Physiol Genom* 2008; 32(2): 219–228.

49 Sculthorpe N, Grace F, Jones P, *et al.* The effect of short-term creatine loading on active range of movement. *Appl Physiol Nutr Metab* 2010; 35(4): 507–511.

50 Sewell DA, Robinson TM, Greenhaff PL. Creatine supplementation does not affect human skeletal muscle glycogen content in the absence of prior exercise. *J Appl Physiol* 2008; 104(2): 508–512.

51 Silva AJ, Machado Reis V, Guidetti L, *et al.* Effect of creatine on swimming velocity, body composition and hydrodynamic variables. *J Sports Med Phys Fitness* 2007; 47(1): 58–64.

52 Spillane M, Schoch R, Cooke M, *et al.* The effects of creatine ethyl ester supplementation combined with heavy resistance training on body composition, muscle performance, and serum and muscle creatine levels. *J Int Soc Sports Nutr* 2009; 6(6): 6.

53 Stout JR, Sue Graves B, Cramer JT, *et al.* Effects of creatine supplementation on the onset of neuromuscular fatigue threshold and muscle strength in elderly men and women (64–86 years). *J Nutr Health Aging* 2007; 11(6): 459–464.

54 Tarnopolsky MA, Parise G, Yardley NJ, *et al.* Creatine-dextrose and protein-dextrose induce similar strength gains during training. *Med Sci Sports Exerc* 2001; 33(12): 2044–2052.

55 Theodorou AS, Havenetidis K, Zanker CL, *et al.* Effects of acute creatine loading with or without carbohydrate on repeated bouts of maximal swimming in high-performance swimmers. *J Strength Cond Res* 2005; 19(2): 265–269.

56 Thompson CH, Kemp GJ, Sanderson AL, *et al.* Effect of creatine on aerobic and anaerobic metabolism in skeletal muscle in swimmers. *Br J Sports Med* 1996; 30(3): 222–225.

57 Volek JS, Ratamess NA, Rubin MR, *et al.* The effects of creatine supplementation on muscular performance and body composition responses to short-term resistance training overreaching. *Eur J Appl Physiol* 2004; 91: 628–637.

58 Walter AA, Smith AE, Herda TJ, *et al.* Effects of creatine loading on electromyographic fatigue threshold in cycle ergometry in college-age men. *Int J Sport Nutr Exerc Metab* 2008; 18(2): 142–151.

59 Andrews R, Greenhaff P, Curtis S, *et al.* The effect of dietary creatine supplementation on skeletal muscle metabolism in congestive heart failure. *Eur Heart J* 1998; 19: 617–622.

60　Fuld JP, Kilduff LP, Neder JA, *et al.* Creatine supplementation during pulmonary rehabilitation in chronic obstructive pulmonary disease. *Thorax* 2005; 60: 531–537.

61　Deacon SJ, Vincent EE, Greenhaff PL, *et al.* Randomized controlled trial of dietary creatine as an adjunct therapy to physical training in chronic obstructive pulmonary disease. *Am J Respir Crit Care Med* 2008; 178(3): 233–239.

62　Al-Ghimlas F, Todd DC. Creatine supplementation for patients with COPD receiving pulmonary rehabilitation: a systematic review and meta-analysis. *Respirology* 2010; 15(5): 785–795.

63　Tarnoplosky M, Martin J. Creatine monohydrate increases strength in patients with neuromuscular disease. *Neurology* 1999; 52: 854–857.

64　Chung YL, Alexanderson H, Pipitone N, *et al.* Creatine supplements in patients with idiopathic inflammatory myopathies who are clinically weak after conventional pharmacologic treatment: six-month, double-blind, randomized, placebo-controlled trial. *Arthritis Rheum* 2007; 57(4): 694–702.

65　Rosenfeld J, King RM, Jackson CE, *et al.* Creatine monohydrate in ALS: effects on strength, fatigue, respiratory status and ALSFRS. *Amyotroph Lateral Scler* 2008; 9(5): 266–272.

66　Kley R, Vorgerd M, Tarnopolsky M. Creatine for treating muscle disorders. *Cochrane Database Syst Rev* 2007;(1): CD004760.

67　Pastula DM, Moore DH, Bedlack RS. Creatine for amyotrophic lateral sclerosis/motor neuron disease. *Cochrane Database Syst Rev* 2010; 16(6): CD005225.

68　Hass CJ, Collins MA, Juncos JL. Resistance training with creatine monohydrate improves upper-body strength in patients with Parkinson disease: a randomized trial. *Neurorehabil Neural Repair* 2007; 21(2): 107–115.

69　Korzun WJ. Oral creatine supplements lower plasma homocysteine concentrations in humans. *Clin Lab Sci* 2004; 17: 102–106.

70　Kaptsan A, Odessky A, Osher Y, *et al.* Lack of efficacy of 5 grams daily of creatine in schizophrenia: a randomized, double-blind, placebo-controlledtrial. *J Clin Psychiatry* 2007; 68(6): 881–884.

71　McMorris T, Mielcarz G, Harris RC, *et al.* Creatine supplementation and cognitive performance in elderly individuals. *Neuropsychol Dev Cogn B Aging Neuropsychol Cogn* 2007; 14(5): 517–528.

72　Rawson ES, Lieberman HR, Walsh TM, *et al.* Creatine supplementation does not improve cognitive function in young adults. *Physiol Behav* 2008; 95(12): 130–134.

73　Gotshalk LA, Volek JS, Staron RS, *et al.* Creatine supplementation improves muscular performance in older men. *Med Sci Sports Exerc* 2002; 34: 537–543.

74　Juhn MS, Tarnopolsky M. Potential side effects of oral creatine supplementation: a critical review. *J Am Diet Ass* 1998; 8: 298–304.

75　Juhn MS, O'Kane JW, Vinci DM. Oral creatine supplementation in male college athletes: a survey of dosing habits and side effects. *J Am Diet Assoc* 1999; 99: 593–595.

76　Groenveld GJ, Beijer C, Veldink JH, *et al.* Few adverse effects of long-term creatine supplementation in a placebo-controlled trial. *Int J Sports Med* 2005; 26: 307–13.

77　Pritchard NR, Kalra PA. Renal dysfunction accompanying oral creatine supplements. *Lancet* 1998; 351: 1252–1253.

78　Koshy KM, Griswold E, Schneeberger EE. Interstitial nephritis in a patient taking creatine. *N Engl J Med* 1999; 340: 814–815.

79　Yu PH, Deng Y. Potential cytotoxic effect of chronic administration of creatine, a nutrition supplement to augment athletic performance. *Med Hypotheses* 2000; 54: 726–728.

80　Shao A, Hathcock JN. Risk assessment for creatine monohydrate. *Regul Toxicol Pharmacol* 2006; 45(3): 242–251.

Curcumin

Description

Curcumin is one of three curcuminoids in the spice turmeric, and the one responsible for the spice's vibrant yellow colour. Turmeric is used in traditional Ayurvedic medicine, but modern interest in it began in 1971 when curcumin was suggested to have anti-inflammatory and anti-oxidant properties.[1]

Action

Curcumin modulates the inflammatory response by down-regulating the activity of cyclooxygenase (COX) 2,[2] lipoxygenase[3] and inducible nitric oxide synthase (iNOS) enzymes[4] and by inhibiting the production of the inflammatory cytokines tumour necrosis factor-alpha (TNF-α) and interleukin (IL)-1, -2, -6, -8 and -12.[5]

COX 2 and iNOS inhibition are probably accomplished via curcumin's suppression of nuclear factor kappa B, which is involved in regulation of inflammation, cellular inflammation and tumorigenesis.[4]

Curcumin may have antithrombotic effects. Preliminary research suggests it might inhibit platelet-activating factor and arachidonic acid platelet aggregation, possibly by interfering with thromboxane synthesis.[6] Curcumin also exhibits growth inhibitory activity against several tumour cell lines.[5] Curcumin seems to induce apoptosis in cancer cells and may inhibit angiogenesis.[7,8] Curcumin also has antioxidant[9] and immunomodulatory[10] effects.

Possible uses

Curcumin has been evaluated as a treatment for dyspepsia. A double-blind placebo-controlled study performed in Thailand compared the effects of 500 mg curcumin four times daily against placebo, as well as against a locally popular over-the-counter treatment. A total of 116 people were enrolled in the study. After 7 days, 87% of the curcumin group experienced full or partial symptom relief from dyspepsia, compared with 53% of the placebo group; this difference was statistically significant.[11]

Curcumin has shown some promise for helping to maintain remission and prevent relapse in ulcerative colitis. In a double-blind placebo-controlled study, 89 people with quiescent ulcerative colitis were given either placebo or curcumin (1 g twice daily) along with standard treatment. Over the 6-month treatment period, the relapse rate was significantly lower in the treatment group compared with the placebo group.[12]

Other proposed uses of turmeric or curcumin have less supporting evidence. Based on *in vitro* and animal studies, and on preliminary human trials, curcumin is recommended for the treatment of such conditions as osteoarthritis, menstrual pain and irritable bowel syndrome,[13] with some evidence that it may improve gall bladder function.[14] There is also preliminary evidence that curcumin might have activity in Alzheimer's disease. In animal models, curcumin caused disaggregation of amyloid beta, and decreased brain amyloid, plaque and oxidised protein levels.[15]

Bioavailability

The bioavailability of oral curcumin is low[16,17] due to a combination of efficient first-pass metabolism, poor gastrointestinal absorption, rapid elimination and poor aqueous solubility.

Conclusion
Curcumin has been extensively evaluated in *in vitro* studies for anti-inflammatory, antioxidant and anti-tumour effects. Preliminary trials in humans suggest it may be useful in the treatment of dyspepsia and ulcerative colitis, but these findings require confirmation in double-blind trials.

Precautions/contraindications

Insufficient reliable information. There is some evidence that curcumin can be toxic to the liver when taken in high doses or for a prolonged period of time. Curcumin should probably be avoided by people with liver disease.

Pregnancy and breast-feeding

Insufficient data. Avoid.

Adverse effects

In human trials, only minor side-effects of curcumin, namely diarrhoea,[18] have been reported, and it is considered safe and well tolerated at doses up to 12 g daily[19]. As a caveat, however, these trials have usually examined short-term outcomes. There is some evidence that long-term high-dose curcumin administration in rodents can be tumorigenic.[20] It has also been shown that curcumin's predominant activity switches from antioxidant to pro-oxidant with increasing concentration.[21]

Interactions

None reported.

Dose

Not established, but complementary practitioners often recommend a dose that provides 400–600 mg of curcumin three times daily.

References

1 Sreejayan N, Rao MN. Free radical scavenging activity of curcuminoids. *Arzneimittelforschung* 1996; 46: 169–171.

2 Zhang F, Altorki NK, Mestre JR, Subbaramaiah K, Dannenberg AJ. Curcumin inhibits cyclooxygenase-2 transcription in bile acid- and phorbol ester-treated human gastrointestinal epithelial cells. *Carcinogenesis* 1999; 20: 445–451.

3 Rao CV. Regulation of COX and LOX by curcumin. *Adv Exp Med Biol* 2007; 595: 213–226.

4 Surh YJ, Chun KS, Cha HH, *et al.* Molecular mechanisms underlying chemopreventive activities of anti-inflammatory phytochemicals: down-regulation of COX-2 and iNOS through suppression of NF-kappa B activation. *Mutat Res* 2001; 480481: 243–68.

5 Deeb D, Xu YX, Jiang H, *et al.* Curcumin (diferuloyl-methane) enhances tumor necrosis factor-related apoptosis-inducing ligand-induced apoptosis in LNCaP prostate cancer cells. *Mol Cancer Ther* 2003; 2: 95–103.

6 Shah BH, Nawaz Z, Pertani SA, *et al.* Inhibitory effect of curcumin, a food spice from turmeric, on platelet-activating factor- and arachidonic acid-mediated platelet aggregation through inhibition of thromboxane formation and Ca^{2+} signaling. *Biochem Pharmacol* 1999; 58: 1167–1172.

7 Chen QY, Lu GH, Wu YQ, *et al.* Curcumin induces mitochondria pathway mediated cell apoptosis in A549 lung adenocarcinoma cells. *Oncol Rep* 2010; 23: 1285–1292.

8 Zhang J, Du Y, Wu C, *et al.* Curcumin promotes apoptosis in human lung adenocarcinoma cells through miR-186* signaling pathway. *Oncol Rep* 2010; 24: 1217–1223.

9 Menon VP, Sudheer AR. Antioxidant and anti-inflammatory properties of curcumin. *Adv Exp Med Biol* 2007; 595: 105–125.

10 Srivastava RM, Singh S, Dubey SK, Misra K, Khar A. Immunomodulatory and therapeutic activity of curcumin. *Int Immunopharmacol* 2011; 11(3): 331–341.

11 Thamlikitkul V, Bunyapraphatsara N, Dechatiwongse T, *et al.* Randomized double blind study of *Curcuma domestica* Val. for dyspepsia. *J Med Assoc Thai* 1989; 72: 613–620.

12 Hanai H, Iida T, Takeuchi K, *et al.* Curcumin maintenance therapy for ulcerative colitis: randomized, multicenter, double-blind, placebo-controlled trial. *Clin Gastroenterol Hepatol* 2006; 4: 1502–1506.

13 Bundy R, Walker AF, Middleton RW, Booth J. Turmeric extract may improve irritable bowel syndrome symptomology in otherwise healthy adults: a pilot study. *J Altern Complement Med* 2004; 10: 1015–1018.

14 Rasyid A, Rahman AR, Jaalam K, Lelo A. Effect of different curcumin dosages on human gall bladder. *Asia Pac J Clin Nutr* 2002; 11: 314–318.

15 Baum L, Lam CW, Cheung SK, *et al.* Six-month randomized, placebo-controlled, double-blind, pilot clinical trial of curcumin in patients with Alzheimer disease. *J Clin Psychopharmacol* 2008; 28: 110–113.

16 Anand P, Kunnumakkara AB, Newman RA, Aggarwal BB. Bioavailability of curcumin: problems and promises. *Mol Pharm* 2007; 4: 807–818.

17 Sharma RA, McLelland HR, Hill KA, *et al.* Pharmacodynamic and pharmacokinetic study of oral *Curcuma* extract in patients with colorectal cancer. *Clin Cancer Res* 2001; 7: 1894–1900.

18 Sharma RA, Euden SA, Platton SL, *et al.* Phase I clinical trial of oral curcumin: biomarkers of systemic activity and compliance. *Clin Cancer Res* 2004; 10: 6847–6854.

19 Lao CD, Ruffin MT,4th Normolle D, *et al.* Dose escalation of a curcuminoid formulation. *BMC Complement Altern Med* 2006; 6: 10.

20 Somasundaram S, Edmund NA, Moore DT, *et al.* Dietary curcumin inhibits chemotherapy-induced apoptosis in models of human breast cancer. *Cancer Res* 2002; 62: 3868–3875.

21 Sandur SK, Ichikawa H, Pandey MK, *et al.* Role of pro-oxidants and antioxidants in the anti-inflammatory and apoptotic effects of curcumin (diferuloylmethane). *Free Radic Biol Med* 2007; 43: 568–580.

Dehydroepiandrosterone

Description

Dehydroepiandrosterone (DHEA) is the most abundant hormone secreted by the adrenal glands. It is a steroid hormone and secreted by the zona reticularis of the adrenals. DHEA circulates in the blood as dehydroepiandrosterone-3-sulphate (DHEAS), which is converted as required to DHEA. Production of DHEA in humans normally peaks between the ages of 20 and 30 years, and then begins a steady progressive decline.[1]

Action

DHEA and DHEAS are the precursors for other hormones, including oestrogens and androgens. The degree of androgenic versus oestrogenic effect of DHEA may depend on the individual's hormonal status. For example, there is some evidence that DHEA has different effects in pre-menopausal and postmenopausal women.[2]

DHEA has also been shown to stimulate insulin growth factor-1 (IGF-1),[3] a hormone that stimulates anabolic metabolism, enhances insulin sensitivity, accelerates muscle growth and enhances energy production.

Possible uses

Supplementation with DHEA has been claimed to produce several health benefits including enhancement of immune function, increased muscle mass, improvements in memory and mood, improvement in symptoms of autoimmune disorders such as lupus erythematosus, and to have a general anti-ageing effect. However, evidence for a beneficial effect of DHEA supplements in all these conditions is inconclusive.

Immunity

The first *in vivo* evidence of an immunomodulatory effect of DHEA came from a prospective, randomised, double-blind, crossover study involving 11 postmenopausal women with 3-week treatment arms. Results showed that DHEA supplementation reduced T helper cell populations and increased natural killer cell populations.[4]

In a single-blind, placebo-controlled study, nine healthy men (mean age 63 years) were supplemented with a placebo for 2 weeks, followed by DHEA 50 mg daily for 20 weeks.[5] DHEA stimulated immune function by significantly increasing the number of monocyte and B-cells, stimulating B- and T-cell mitogenic response, interleukin-2 secretion and the number and cytotoxicity of natural killer cells. The authors acknowledged that the results of this study had limited application because post-treatment immune response was not measured.

However, in two other studies,[6,7] DHEA produced no significant effects on antibody response to influenza vaccine.

In a placebo-controlled trial among 40 stable, treated patients with human HIV infection, no significant immune effects were observed with DHEA. There appeared to be no benefit with regard to lean muscle mass or bone density in the DHEA recipients. DHEA treatment had a positive impact on overall quality of life. DHEA supplementation in patients with fully suppressed HIV was associated with an improvement in quality of life but appeared to have no beneficial antiviral, immunomodulatory, hormonal or body composition effects, suggesting that it should not be used routinely as an adjunctive therapy in this population.[8]

Body composition

In a double-blind, placebo-controlled study, 10 healthy men were randomised to receive either 1600 mg DHEA or placebo daily for 28 days. Compared with placebo, body fat was reduced significantly, by 31% in the supplemented group, but there was no change in body weight. There was also a 7.5% reduction in LDL cholesterol.[9] Furthermore, in another randomised, double-blind, placebo-controlled study in morbidly obese adolescents,[10] 40 mg DHEA twice a day had no effect on body weight. In two other studies,[11,12] DHEA 1600 mg daily for 4 weeks had no significant effect on body weight or lean body mass.

Cognitive function, mood and depression

In a double-blind, placebo-controlled crossover study, 30 healthy subjects aged 40–70 years were randomised to receive in random order either 50 mg DHEA or placebo daily for 3 months each. During DHEA supplementation there was a significant increase in perceived physical and psychological well-being. There was no effect on insulin sensitivity, body fat or libido.[13]

In a double-blind, placebo-controlled crossover study, 17 healthy, elderly male subjects received 50 mg DHEA daily or a placebo for 2 weeks. There was no change in memory or mood in the supplemented group.[14]

In a small double-blind RCT, DHEA (50 mg twice a day) did not significantly improve cognitive performance or overall ratings of change in severity. A transient effect on cognitive performance may have been seen at month 3, but this narrowly missed significance.[15] A more recent trial in 110 men and 115 women (aged 55–85 years) also found that DHEA supplementation had no benefit on cognitive performance or well-being in this population group.[16]

A Cochrane systematic review[17] investigating the effect of DHEA supplementation on cognition and well-being in people aged over 50 years found three RCTs matching its criteria. The review concluded that the evidence does not support a beneficial effect of DHEA supplementation on cognitive function of non-demented middle-aged or elderly people. The authors stated that 'There is no consistent evidence from the controlled trials that DHEA produces any adverse effects'. In view of growing public enthusiasm for DHEA supplementation, particularly in the USA, and the theoretical possibility of long-term neuroprotective effects of DHEA/S, they added that 'there is a need for further high quality trials in which the duration of DHEA treatment is longer than one year, and the number of participants is large enough to provide adequate statistical power'.

A trial published since the Cochrane review evaluated 27 women aged 65–90 years with mild to moderate cognitive impairment and living in a long-term care facility in Japan. Twelve women were assigned to receive oral DHEA 25 mg daily for 6 months. The control group of 15 women were matched for age and cognitive function and were followed without hormone replacement. Cognitive function and basic activities of daily living (ADL) scores were assessed at at baseline and at 3 and 6 months. Plasma hormone levels including testosterone, DHEA, DHEAS and oestradiol were also followed up. After 6 months, DHEA treatment significantly increased plasma testosterone, DHEA and DHEAS levels by two- to three-fold compared with baseline, but had no effect on oestradiol. DHEA administration increased cognitive scores and maintained basic ADL score, while cognition and basic ADL deteriorated in the control group. Among the cognitive domains, DHEA treatment improved verbal fluency.[18]

In a double-blind, placebo-controlled study,[19] 32 patients with severe depression, either medication-free or stabilised on antidepressants, received either DHEA (maximum dose 90 mg daily) or placebo for 6 weeks. DHEA was associated with a significantly greater decrease in the Hamilton Depression Rating Scale than placebo, and 5 of the 11 patients treated with DHEA compared with none of the 11 subjects in the placebo group showed a 50% or greater reduction in symptoms of depression.

A study in patients with schizophrenia found that DHEA (up to 100 mg daily) was associated with significant improvement in negative symptoms as well as in depressive and anxiety symptoms in individuals receiving DHA.[20]

Plasma levels of DHEA fall with the progression of HIV diseases and DHEA is being investigated for potential benefit. A study in 32 patients with advanced HIV disease found improved mental function scores with DHEA 50 mg daily for 4 months,[21] while another study in 40 HIV-positive patients demonstrated improvements in quality of life with DHEA.[8]

Systemic lupus erythematosus

In a double-blind, placebo-controlled study,[22] 28 women with mild to moderate systemic lupus erythematosus (SLE) were randomised to receive 200 mg DHEA or placebo daily for 3 months. In the supplemented group, there were insignificant improvements in SLE Disease Activity Index scores, physicians' assessment of disease activity and a reduction in the dose of prednisone used. There was a significant improvement in patients' assessment of disease activity with DHEA compared with placebo.

In an open study, 50 women with mild to moderate SLE were treated with 50–200 mg DHEA daily for 6–12 months. Supplementation was associated with a significant reduction in disease activity and significant improvement in patient and physician assessment compared with baseline.[23]

In a double-blind RCT, 120 adult women with active SLE received oral DHEA (200 mg daily) or placebo for 24 weeks. DHEA treatment was well tolerated, significantly reduced the number of SLE flares and improved patients' global assessment of disease activity.[24]

Sports performance

It is often claimed that individuals can enhance their muscle capacity by boosting DHEA levels through oral supplementation. A 12-month study in 280 healthy men and women (aged 60–89 years) found that the supplement restored DHEA levels to the normal range for young adults. However, there were no beneficial effects on muscle state.[25]

A 12-week randomised, placebo-controlled trial in 31 sedentary, postmenopausal women found that combined endurance and resistance training significantly improved body composition, physical performance, insulin sensitivity and LDL cholesterol particle number and size, whereas DHEA (50 mg daily) had no additional benefits.[26]

In a 6-month trial among 99 frail elderly women, involved in a gentle exercise programme of chair aerobics or yoga, DHEA supplementation (50 mg daily) improved lower extremity strength and function. No changes were found in bone mineral density.[27] A further trial among 87 elderly men (with low testosterone) and 57 elderly women (both with low levels of DHEA) showed that neither DHEA nor low-dose testosterone replacement in elderly people had physiologically relevant beneficial effects on body composition, physical performance, insulin sensitivity, or quality of life.[28]

Bone turnover

DHEA has been investigated for an effect on bone turnover. An RCT in young women with anorexia nervosa compared the effects of DHEA with hormone replacement therapy (HRT). In initial analyses, total hip bone mineral density (BMD) increased significantly and similarly in both treatment groups. Bone formation markers increased transiently at 6–9 months in the DHEA group compared with the HRT group, and both treatments significantly reduced bone resorption markers. However, both groups gained weight and there was no treatment effect after correcting for weight gain. In addition, DHEA was associated with improvement in specific psychological parameters.[29] In another study in middle-aged to elderly men, oral DHEA did not affect bone turnover when used for a 6-month period.[30] In a further trial among 225 healthy adults aged 55–85 years, daily administration of 50 mg DHEA had a modest and selective beneficial effect on BMD and bone resorption in women, but provided no bone benefit for men.[31] A similar trial in 55 men and 58 women aged 65–75 years again showed a selective benefit of DHEA (combined with calcium and vitamin D) in elderly women but not men.[29]

Miscellaneous

There is no evidence that DHEA supplements prevent ageing in humans. However, chronic DHEA administration has been shown to be capable of modifying circulating levels of androgens and progestins in both early and late postmenopausal women by modulating the age-related changes in adrenal function.[32]

Reports have suggested that DHEA might reduce the risk of heart disease. Epidemiological studies have been conflicting, and although some animal and human studies have shown that DHEA may reduce LDL cholesterol and platelet aggregation, controlled trials are needed to assess the effects of DHEA supplementation on cardiovascular risk. A controlled trial in 40 subjects with Addison's disease showed that short-term DHEA supplementation did not significantly affect measures of arterial stiffness or endothelial function in patients with adrenal insufficiency.[33]

DHEA has also been reported to improve insulin sensitivity and reduce blood glucose levels, but again results from studies have been conflicting. One small study in 24 men found that DHEA 25 mg daily improved insulin sensitivity and vascular endothelial function and decreased the plasma activator inhibitor type 1 concentration. The authors concluded that these beneficial changes have the potential to attenuate the development of age-related disorders such as cardiovascular disease.[34]

> **Conclusion**
>
> The role of DHEA supplements in all conditions studied is inconclusive. Some studies have shown that DHEA improves the immune response while others have not. There is no good evidence that DHEA helps to reduce body weight. There is limited evidence that it may improve well-being and reduce symptoms of depression, but it seems to have no effect on memory or cognition. Preliminary evidence suggests that DHEA could improve symptoms of SLE.

Precautions/contraindications

DHEA is contraindicated in individuals who have (or have a history of) prostate cancer or oestrogen-dependent tumours (e.g. breast or uterine cancer). It should be used with caution in patients with diabetes mellitus (because it may alter blood glucose regulation). Blood glucose and doses of insulin and oral hypoglycaemics should be monitored in patients with diabetes.

Pregnancy and breast-feeding

The effects of DHEA in pregnancy and breast-feeding are unknown. It is probably best avoided.

Adverse effects

There is no known toxicity or serious side-effects. However, the safety of long-term administration is unknown. DHEA alters the levels of other hormones, and has both oestrogenic and androgenic activity. Potential side-effects in women are therefore increased facial hair and increased loss of head hair, menstrual irregularities and deepening of the voice. The risk of breast cancer may also be increased, but results from studies are conflicting, with some showing that DHEA may reduce risk while others show that it may increase risk. A review concluded that

prolonged intake of DHEA may promote breast cancer in postmenopausal women.[35] Potential side-effects in men include an increased risk of prostate cancer.

A study in 22 healthy men[36] suggested that doses up to 200 mg daily for 4 weeks were safe and well tolerated. Another study in 24 healthy elderly men and women (67.8 ± 4.3 years) suggested that daily doses of 25 or 50 mg DHEA are safe in elderly subjects.[37] There were no large increases in blood levels of androgens and oestrogens in this study.

Interactions

Theoretically DHEA could interact with insulin, oral hypoglycaemic agents, oestrogens (including HRT) and androgens.

In one study, DHEA appeared to demonstrate an influence on antipsychotic extrapyramidal symptoms, with improvement observed particularly in parkinsonian symptoms.[38] However, in another study, DHEA was not an effective adjunct in the treatment of antipsychotic side-effects, symptoms and quality-of-life impairment in schizophrenia, but it did appear to improve sustained attention and visual and movement skills.[39] A further trial in 40 patients treated with olanzapine demonstrated that DHEA produced some improvement in parkinsonism and akathisia but there was no change in psychosis. Patients receiving DHEA appeared to demonstrate relatively stable glucose levels compared with controls at the end of the study. An improvement in cognitive performance (most notably memory), which did not reach significance owing to low sample number, was observed following DHEA administration.[40]

Bioavailability

Administration of DHEA 200 mg (for research purposes) resulted in higher DHEA C_{max}, AUC and overall concentrations in women than in men ($P < 0.03$); DHEAS parameter estimates were similar between men and women. Following a single dose of DHEA 200 mg, DHEA concentrations increased five- to six-fold in both men and women, and DHEAS concentrations increased five-fold in men and 21-fold in women relative to endogenous concentrations. The results of this study indicate that the pharmacokinetics of DHEA differ between older men and women.[41]

Dose

DHEA is available in the form of tablets and capsules.

The dose is not established. Dietary supplements tend to provide 5–50 mg daily.

References

1   Nafziger AN, Bowlin SJ, Jenkins PL, *et al*. Longitudinal changes in dihydroepiandrosterone sulfate and concentrations in men and women. *J Lab Clin Med* 1998; 131: 316–323.
2   Ebeling P, Koivisto VA. Physiological importance of dehydroepiandrosterone. *Lancet* 1994; 343: 1479–1481.
3   Casson PR, Santoro N, Elkind-Hirsch K, *et al*. Postmenopausal dehydroepiandrosterone administration increases free insulin-like growth factor-1 and decreases high density lipoprotein: a six-month trial. *Fertil Steril* 1998; 70: 107–110.
4   Casson PR, Andersen RN, Herrod HG, *et al*. Oral dehydroepiandrosterone in physiologic doses modulates immune function in postmenopausal women. *Am J Obstet Gynecol* 1993; 169: 1536–1539.
5   Khorram O, Vu L, Yen SS. Activation of immune function by dehydroepiandrosterone (DHEA) in age-advanced men. *J Gerontol A Biol Sci Med Sci* 1997; 52: M1–M7.
6   Degelau J, Guay D, Hallgren H. The effect of DHEAS on influenza vaccine in aging adults. *J Am Geriatr Soc* 1997; 45: 747–751.
7   Ben-Yehuda A, Daneberg HD, Zakay-Rones Z, *et al*. The influence of sequential annual vaccination and of DHEA administration on the efficacy of the immune response to influenza vaccine in the elderly. *Mech Ageing Dev* 1998; 102: 299–306.
8   Abrams DI, Shade SB, Couey P, *et al*. Dehydroepiandrosterone (DHEA) effects on HIV replication and host immunity: a randomized placebo-controlled study. *AIDS Res Hum Retroviruses* 2007; 23(1): 77–859.
9   Nestler JE, Barlascini CO, Clore JN, *et al*. Dehydroepiandrosterone reduces serum low density lipoprotein levels and body fat but does not alter insulin sensitivity in normal men. *J Clin Endocrinol Metab* 1988; 66: 57–61.
10 Vogiatzi MG, Boeck MA, Vlachopapadopoulou E, *et al*. Dehydroepiandrosterone in morbidly obese adolescents: effects on weight, body composition, lipids and insulin resistance. *Metabolism* 1996; 45: 1011–1015.
11 Welle S, Jozefowicz R, Statt M. Failure of dehydroepiandrosterone to influence energy and protein metabolism in humans. *J Clin Endocrinol Metab* 1990; 71: 1259–1264.
12 Usiskin KS, Butterworth S, Clore JN, *et al*. Lack of effect of dehydroepiandrosterone in obese men. *Int J Obes* 1990; 14: 457–463.
13 Morales AJ, Nolan JJ, Nelson JC, *et al*. Effects of replacement dose of DHEA in men and women of advancing age. *J Clin Endocrinol Metab* 1994; 78: 1360–1367.
14 Wolf OT, Naumann E, Helhammer DH, *et al*. Effects of dehydroepiandrosterone replacement in elderly men on event-related potentials, memory and well being. *J Gerontol A Biol Med Sci Med Sci* 1998; 53: M385–M3990.
15 Wolkowitz OM, Kramer JH, Reus VI, *et al*. DHEA treatment of Alzheimer's disease: a randomized, double-blind, placebo-controlled study. *Neurology* 2003; 60(7): 1071–1076.
16 Kritz-Silverstein D, vonMuhlen D, Laughlin GA, *et al*. Effects of dehydroepiandrosterone supplementation on cognitive function and quality of life: the DHEA and Well-Ness (DAWN) Trial. *J Am Geriatr Soc* 2008; 56(7): 1292–1298.
17 Grimley Evans J, Malouf R, Huppert F, *et al*. Dehydroepiandrosterone (DHEA) supplementation for cognitive function in healthy elderly people. *Cochrane Database Syst Rev* 2006; (4): CD006221.
18 Yamada S, Akishita M, Fukai S, *et al*. Effects of dehydroepiandrosterone supplementation on cognitive function and activities of daily living in older women with mild to moderate cognitive impairment. *Geriatr Gerontol Int* 2010; 10(4): 280–28719.
19 Wolkowitz OM, Reus VI, Keebler A, *et al*. Double-blind treatment of major depression with dehydroepiandrosterone. *Am J Psychiatry* 1999; 156: 646–649.
20 Strous RD, Maayan R, Lapidus R, *et al*. Dehydroepiandrosterone augmentation in the management of negative, depressive, and anxiety symptoms in schizophrenia. *Arch Gen Psychiatry* 2003; 60: 133–141.
21 Piketty C, Jayle D, Leplege A, *et al*. Double-blind placebo-controlled trial of oral dehydroepiandrosterone in patients with advanced HIV disease. *Clin Endocrinol* 2001; 55: 325–330.
22 Van Vollenhoven RF, Engleman EG, McGuire GL, *et al*. Dehydroepiandrosterone in systemic lupus erythematosus. Results of a double-blind, placebo-controlled, randomised clinical trial. *Arthritis Rheum* 1995; 38: 1826–1831.
23 Van Vollenhoven RF, Morabito LM, Engleman EG, *et al*. Treatment of systemic lupus erythematosus with dehydroepiandrosterone: 50 patients treated up to 12 months. *J Rheumatol* 1998; 25: 285–289.
24 Chang DM, Lan JL, Lin HY, Luo SF. Dehydroepiandrosterone treatment of women with mild-to-moderate systemic lupus erythmatosus:

a multicenter, randomized, double-blind, placebo-controlled trial. *Arthritis Rheum* 2002; 46: 2924–2927.

25 Percheron G, Hogrel JY, Denot-Ledunois S, *et al.* Effect of 1-year oral administration of dehydroepiandrosterone to 60- to 80-year-old individuals on muscle function and cross-sectional area: a double-blind placebo-controlled trial. *Arch Intern Med* 2003; 163(6): 720–727.

26 Igwebuike A, Irving BA, Bigelow ML, *et al.* Lack of dehydroepiandrosterone effect on a combined endurance and resistance exercise program in post-menopausal women. *J Clin Endocrinol Metab* 2008; 93(2): 534–538.

27 Kenny AM, Boxer RS, Kleppinger A, *et al.* Dehydroepiandrosterone combined with exercise improves muscle strength and physical function in frail older women. *J Am Geriatr Soc* 2010; 58(9): 1707–1714.

28 Nair KS, Rizza RA, O'Brien P, *et al.* DHEA in elderly women and DHEA or testosterone in elderly men. *N Engl J Med* 2006; 355(16): 1647–1659.

29 Gordon CM, Grace E, Emans SJ, *et al.* Effects of oral dehydroepiandrosterone on bone density in young women with anorexia nervosa: a randomized trial. *J Clin Endocrinol Metab* 2002; 87(11): 4935–4941.

30 Kahn AJ, Halloran B, Wolkowitz O, *et al.* Dehydroepiandrosterone supplementation and bone turnover in middle-aged to elderly men. *J Clin Endocrinol Metab* 2002; 87: 1544–1549.

31 von Muhlen D, Laughlin GA, Kritz-Silverstein D, *et al.* Effect of dehydroepiandrosterone supplementation on bone mineral density, bone markers, and body composition in older adults: the DAWN trial. *Osteoporos Int* 2008; 19(5): 699–707.

32 Genazzani AR, Pluchino N, Begliuomini S, *et al.* Long-term low-dose oral administration of dehydroepiandrosterone modulates adrenal response to adrenocorticotropic hormone in early and late post-menopausal women. *Gynecol Endocrinol* 2006; 22(11): 627–635.

33 Rice SP, Agarwal N, Bolusani H, *et al.* Effects of dehydroepiandrosterone replacement on vascular function in primary and secondary adrenal insufficiency: a randomized crossover trial. *J Clin Endocrinol Metab* 2009; 94(6): 1966–1972.

34 Kawano H, Yasue H, Kitagawa A, *et al.* Dehydroepiandrosterone supplementation improves endothelial function and insulin sensitivity in men. *J Clin Endocrinol Metab* 2003; 88: 3190–3195.

35 Stoll BA. Dietary supplements of dehydroepiandrosterone in relation to breast cancer risk. *Eur J Clin Nutr* 1999; 53: 771–775.

36 Davidson M, Marwah A, Sawchuk RJ, *et al.* Safety and pharmacokinetic study with escalating doses of 3-acetyl-7-oxo-dehydroepiandrosterone in healthy male volunteers. *Clin Invest Med* 2000; 23: 300–310.

37 Legrain S, Massien C, Lahlou N, *et al.* Dehydroepiandrosterone replacement administration: pharmacokinetic and pharmacodynamic studies in healthy elderly subjects. *J Clin Endocrinol Metab* 2000; 85: 3208–3217.

38 Nachshoni T, Ebert T, Abramovitch Y, *et al.* Improvement of extrapyramidal symptoms following dehydroepiandrosterone (DHEA) administration in antipsychotic treated schizophrenia patients: a randomized, double-blind placebo controlled trial. *Schizophr Res* 2005; 79(23): 251–256.

39 Ritsner MS, Gibel A, Ratner Y, *et al.* Improvement of sustained attention and visual and movement skills, but not clinical symptoms, after dehydroepiandrosterone augmentation in schizophrenia: a randomized, double-blind, placebo-controlled, crossover trial. *J Clin Psychopharmacol* 2006; 26(5): 495–499.

40 Strous RD, Stryjer R, Maayan R, *et al.* Analysis of clinical symptomatology, extrapyramidal symptoms and neurocognitive dysfunction following dehydroepiandrosterone (DHEA) administration in olanzapine treated schizophrenia patients: a randomized, double-blind placebo controlled trial. *Psychoneuroendocrinology* 2007; 32(2): 96–105.

41 Frye RF, Kroboth PD, Kroboth FJ, *et al.* Sex differences in the pharmacokinetics of dehydroepiandrosterone (DHEA) after single- and multiple-dose administration in healthy older adults. *J Clin Pharmacol* 2000; 40(6): 596–605.

Dong quai

Description

Dong quai (*Angelica sinensis*) is a plant that grows at high altitudes in the cold, damp, mountainous regions of China, Korea and Japan. It takes 3 years for the plant to reach maturity, after which the root is harvested and dried to produce food supplements and herbal remedies. Dong quai has been used for more than 2000 years in traditional Chinese medicine (TCM) as a spice, tonic and medicine.

Constituents

Dong quai root contains several active constituents, the chief of which are:[1,2] ferulic acid, Z-ligustilide, *n*-butylidenephthalide, *n*-butylphthalide, nicotinic acid and succinic acid. It also contains significant amounts of vitamin A, carotenoids, vitamin B_{12}, vitamin E, ascorbic acid, folinic acid, biotin, various phytosterols (e.g. beta-sitosterol), calcium, magnesium and other minerals. Other constituents include *n*-valerophenone-O-carboxylic acid, delta-2,4-dihydrophthalic anhydride, uracil, adenine, carvacrol, safrole, isosafrole, sesquiterpenes, beta-cadinene, *n*-dodecanol, *n*-tetradecanol, palmitic acid, angelic acid, myristic acid, sucrose and a polysaccharide with a molecular weight of approximately 3000.

Dong quai also contains natural coumarin derivatives: angelol, angelicone, bergapten, oxypeucedanin, osthole, psoralen, and 7-desmethylsuberosin.

Action

Dong quai potentially has anticoagulant, anti-platelet, haematopoietic, antispasmodic activity (against uterine contractions)[3] and immuno-stimulatory activity.[2] It also has antioxidant activity.[4] It possibly has oestrogenic activity,[5,6] although this is controversial.

Possible uses

In TCM, dong quai is used (usually in combination with three or more other herbs) for various purposes including reproductive (e.g. menstrual cramps and irregularity, menopausal symptoms including hot flushes and infertility), circulatory (e.g. anaemia, hypertension and as a 'blood purifier'), respiratory and allergic conditions.

Studies in animals suggest that dong quai may be helpful in cardiac arrhythmia, prevent plaque formation and atherosclerosis,[7] promote sleep, prevent infection, promote urination, soothe ulcers, lower blood pressure and act as a mild laxative.[2]

Evidence in humans is weak and much of the research is available only in Chinese languages. Studies available in the English language have evaluated dong quai in menopausal symptoms, premenstrual syndrome and heart disease.

Menopausal symptoms

In a double-blind, placebo-controlled study, 71 postmenopausal women were randomised to receive 4.5 g dong quai root in capsules or placebo daily for 24 weeks. The women had elevated follicle stimulating hormone (FSH) levels and complained of hot flushes. At the end of the study period, there were no significant differences in menopausal symptoms or in the number of hot flushes, with both treatment and placebo arms noting improved symptoms. Serum levels of oestradiol, oestrone, sex-hormone-binding globulin, and blood pressure and weight did not differ between groups. Endometrial thickness increased by 2.3 mm in the placebo group and 0.3 mm in the dong quai group, suggesting that dong quai has no oestrogenic effects, and the authors could not explain why endometrial thickness increased in the placebo group. The authors concluded that dong quai administered alone does not produce oestrogen-like responses in the endometrium and is no more effective than placebo at relieving hot flushes.[5]

Premenstrual syndrome

A review has suggested that there is a pharmacological basis for using dong quai in premenstrual syndrome.[8] This refers to Chinese studies that have reported the use of intravenous dong quai in animal studies and found increased contractility of the uterus.

Cardiovascular disease

A review of sodium ferulate (an active principle of dong quai) states that sodium ferulate is approved by State Drugs Administration of China as a drug for treatment of cardiovascular and cerebrovascular diseases and that it has antithrombotic, platelet aggregation inhibitory and antioxidant activities in animals and humans. The review adds that sodium ferulate has been widely used in China to treat cardiovascular and cerebrovascular diseases and to prevent thrombosis and concludes that *in vitro* and *in vivo* data support the view that sodium ferulate is a useful substance for the treatment of cardiovascular diseases.[9]

Precautions/contraindications

Dong quai has been used safely in a clinical trial lasting up to 24 weeks.[5] There are no long-term safety data in humans. Because of the possible oestrogenic effects, dong quai is best avoided in hormone sensitive conditions such as breast, ovarian and endometrial cancer, endometriosis and uterine fibroids. Some of the constituents of dong quai may be carcinogenic.

Pregnancy and breast-feeding

Dong quai has uterine stimulant effects so is potentially unsafe in pregnancy. There is evidence to suggest that it could cause congenital malformations if taken during the first trimester.[10] Dong quai is best avoided in pregnancy and lactation.

Adverse effects

Dong quai is well tolerated when taken orally, but see precautions above; may also cause photosensitivity. There is one case report of gynaecomastia with dong quai.[11]

Interactions

Warfarin, anticoagulants and anti-platelet drugs: increased anticoagulant effects of warfarin and increased risk of bleeding;[12] in one case, after 4 weeks of dong quai 565 mg once or twice daily, the international normalised ratio (INR) increased to 4.9 INR normalised 4 weeks after discontinuation of dong quai; dong quai is thought to inhibit platelet activation and aggregation; given these data, dong quai should not be taken by patients on warfarin.[13,14]

References

1 Zhao KJ, Dong TT, Tu PF, *et al.* Molecular genetic and chemical assessment of radix *Angelica* (Dangqui) in China. *J Agric Food Chem* 2003; 51: 2576–2583.

2 Monograph. *Angelica sinensis. Altern Med Rev* 2004; 9: 429–433.

3 Shi M, Chang L, He G. [Stimulating action of *Carthamus tinctorius* L., *Angelica sinensis* (Oliv.) Diels and *Leonurus sibiricus* L. on the uterus]. *Zhongguo Zhong Yao Za Zhi* 1995; 20: 173–175, 192.

4 Jia M, Yang TH, Yao XJ, *et al.* [Anti-oxidative effect of *Angelica* polysaccharide sulphate]. *Zhong Yao Cai* 2007; 30: 185–188.

5 Hirata JD, Swiersz LM, Zell B, *et al.* Does dong quai have estrogenic effects in postmenopausal women? A double-blind, placebo-controlled trial *Fertil Steril* 1997; 68: 981–986.

6 Liu J, Burdette JE, Xu H, *et al.* Evaluation of estrogenic activity of plant extracts for the potential treatment of menopausal symptoms. *J Agric Food Chem* 2001; 49: 2472–2479.

7 Yim TK, Wu WK, Pak WF, *et al.* Myocardial protection against ischaemia-reperfusion injury by a *Polygonum multiflorum* extract supplemented 'Dang-Gui decoction for enriching blood', a compound formulation, ex vivo. *Phytother Res* 2000; 14: 195–199.

8 Zhu DP. Dong quai. *Am J Chin Med* 1987; 15: 117–125.

9 Wang BH, Ou-Yang JP. Pharmacological actions of sodium ferulate in cardiovascular system. *Cardiovasc Drug Rev* 2005; 23: 161–172.

10 Chuang CH, Doyle P, Wang JD, *et al.* Herbal medicines used during the first trimester and major congenital malformations: an analysis of data from a pregnancy cohort study. *Drug Saf* 2006; 29: 537–548.

11 Goh SY, Loh KC. Gynaecomastia and the herbal tonic 'Dong Quai'. *Singapore Med J* 2001; 42: 115–116.

12 Page RL, 2nd, Lawrence JD. Potentiation of warfarin by dong quai. *Pharmacotherapy* 1999; 19: 870–876.

13 Heck AM, DeWitt BA, Lukes AL. Potential interactions between alternative therapies and warfarin. *Am J Health Syst Pharm* 2000; 57: 1221–1227; quiz, 1228–1230.

14 Fugh-Berman A. Herb-drug interactions. *Lancet* 2000; 355: 134–138.

Evening primrose oil

Description

Evening primrose oil is derived from the seeds of *Oenothera biennis* and other species.

Constituents

Evening primrose oil contains gamma-linolenic acid (GLA) and linoleic acid. Starflower oil (borage oil) and blackcurrant oil are also used as sources of GLA in dietary supplements. Evening primrose oil contains 8–11% GLA. Starflower oil contains 20–25% GLA, but the biological activity of starflower oil may be no greater than that of evening primrose oil, i.e. on a weight-for-weight basis, starflower oil has not been proved to be twice as active as evening primrose oil. Blackcurrant oil contains 15–25% GLA.

Action

GLA is not an essential dietary component. It is normally synthesised in the body by the action of delta-6-desaturase on linoleic acid (obtained in the diet from vegetable and seed oils, e.g. sunflower oil).

GLA is a precursor of dihomogamma-linolenic acid (DGLA) and the series 1 prostaglandins (PG), and also of arachidonic acid (see Figure 1). Most of the DGLA formed from GLA is metabolised to PG1s; conversion of DGLA to arachidonic acid is very slow. Arachidonic acid is normally obtained from meat in the diet.

Supplementation with GLA increases the ratio of DGLA to arachidonic acid. DGLA levels are elevated to a greater extent by the administration of GLA than by the administration of linoleic acid (for reasons that are not entirely clear).

Prostaglandin PGE_1 (produced from DGLA) inhibits platelet aggregation and is also a vasodilator; it has less potent inflammatory effects than prostaglandins of the PG2 series, thromboxane A_2 and series 4 leukotrienes (produced from arachidonic acid).

The efficacy of GLA is thus thought to be due, in part, to the increased production of PG1 series prostaglandins at the expense of PG2 series prostaglandins, thromboxane A_2 and series 4 leukotrienes.

Deficiency

Patients with diabetes mellitus or eczema may be at risk of GLA deficiency. Despite some claims, there is little evidence that foods rich in saturated fat and sugar, drinking alcohol, stress, pollution, high blood cholesterol, ageing, viral infections and hormone imbalances lead to GLA deficiency.

Possible uses

Evening primrose oil is used widely as a dietary supplement for various disorders, including premenstrual syndrome (PMS), hypertension, asthma and angina. It is claimed to reduce blood cholesterol levels and to act as a slimming aid.

Disorders for which evening primrose oil has been tested in controlled clinical trials include atopic dermatitis, diabetic neuropathy, mastalgia and breast cysts, menopausal flushing, Reynaud's phenomenon, rheumatoid arthritis, schizophrenia, Sjogren's syndrome, ulcerative colitis and various cancers. Evening primrose oil is being investigated in a range of other disorders including multiple sclerosis and hyperactivity in children.

Skin conditions

The efficacy of evening primrose oil in inflammatory skin conditions such as eczema is difficult to judge, because several trials have shown improvements in both the treatment and placebo groups. However, results indicate that for efficacy, high doses and long-term treatment are necessary. Evening primrose oil may work in these conditions not only by supplying

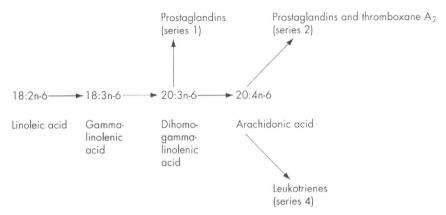

Figure 1 Metabolism of gamma-linolenic acid and arachidonic acid.

precursors of prostaglandins but also by supplying the essential fatty acids to maintain cell membranes.

A double-blind crossover study involving 99 patients showed improvement in symptoms of eczema with doses of 4–6 g daily of evening primrose oil in adults and 2 g daily in children.[1] Another trial involving 25 patients showed that evening primrose oil (45 mg GLA per capsule) improved symptoms of eczema. Although there was also an improvement in the placebo group, this was not as great as in the evening primrose oil group.[2] A further double-blind crossover study showed no clinical benefit in the use of evening primrose oil for atopic eczema in a mixed group of adults and children.[3] Adult doses in this study were 12 or 16 500-mg capsules each day. Another study in patients with chronic dermatitis of the hands[3] showed no difference between the effects of evening primrose oil (12 500-mg capsules each day) or placebo (sunflower oil capsules). Similarly conflicting results have been found in studies in children.[4,5]

A double-blind RCT investigated the possible preventive effect of GLA supplementation on the development of atopic dermatitis in infants at risk. One hundred and eighteen formula-fed infants with a maternal history of atopic disease received borage oil supplement (100 mg GLA) or sunflower oil supplement for the first 6 months of life. The intention-to-treat analysis showed a favourable trend for severity of atopic dermatitis associated with GLA supplementation, but no significant effects in the other atopic outcomes, including serum immunoglobulin E

(IgE). The authors concluded that early supplementation with GLA in children at high familial risk does not prevent the expression of atopy, but it tends to alleviate the severity of atopic dermatitis in later infancy in these children.[6]

A meta-analysis conducted by authors from Wassen International of 26 clinical studies, including 1207 patients with atopic eczema, concluded that Efamol evening primrose oil has a simultaneous, beneficial effect on itch/pruritis, crusting, oedema and redness (erythema) that becomes apparent between 4 and 8 weeks after treatment is initiated. However, the magnitude of this effect is reduced in association with increasing frequency of potent steroid use. The authors suggest that this and other confounding factors may account for the inconsistent responses reported in the literature and that there may be 'responders' and 'non-responders' to GLA.[7]

A trial in a hospital in India randomised patients diagnosed with atopic dermatitis to 500 mg evening primrose oil or placebo capsules for 5 months. At the end of the fifth month, 24 (96%) patients in the treatment group and 8 (32%) patients in the placebo group showed improvement, with no significant adverse effects reported.[8]

Premenstrual syndrome and the menopause

Evening primrose oil has been studied for its effect on the physical and psychological symptoms of PMS in some women. However, few good studies have been carried out. A review of four studies[9] concluded that evening primrose oil is effective for the treatment of PMS. However, another study in 38 women[10] showed no differences between the effect of placebo and evening primrose oil on symptoms such as fluid retention, breast pain or swelling or mood changes.

Some trials with evening primrose oil in cyclical mastalgia and breast tenderness have shown positive results.[11,12] However, the response can be slow, and it can take several months to decide whether or not treatment is successful. A recent study in 555 women with moderate to severe mastalgia found that GLA (Efamast) efficacy did not differ from that of placebo fatty acids and the presence or absence of antioxidant vitamins made no difference.[13]

Trial data on the effects of evening primrose oil during the menopause are conflicting. In one of the most recent studies,[14] involving 56 post-menopausal women suffering hot flushes, GLA offered no benefit over placebo.

Rheumatoid arthritis

Results from trials with evening primrose oil in rheumatoid arthritis have been mixed. In one study of 20 patients, treatment with non-steroidal anti-inflammatory drugs (NSAIDs) was stopped and administration of evening primrose oil resulted in no significant changes in symptoms of arthritis.[15] In another study involving 49 patients,[16] treatment with evening primrose oil (equivalent to 540 mg GLA daily) or a combination of evening primrose oil and fish oil (450 mg GLA plus 240 mg eicosapentaenoic acid) allowed for a significant reduction in dose of NSAIDs. However, another study in 20 patients[17] who received either evening primrose oil or olive oil twice daily for 12 weeks, showed no significant differences in terms of prostaglandin levels, therapeutic response or laboratory parameters. However, those individuals whose pro-inflammatory prostaglandin and thromboxane levels were reduced tended to have better therapeutic responses.

Asthma

GLA has also been investigated in asthma, with mixed results. Two trials showed negative results.[18,19] However, a placebo-controlled trial in 35 atopic subjects with mild to moderate asthma found that a combination of GLA and eicosapentaenoic acid reduced blood leukotrienes, improved self-reported asthma status and reduced bronchodilator use.[20]

Obesity

GLA has recently been investigated as an adjunct in the treatment of human obesity. This research arose out of an observation of distorted essential fatty acid distribution in obese human beings that persisted after major weight loss. In this study, 50 formerly obese subjects were randomised into a double-blind study and given either 890 mg of GLA daily (5 g borage oil daily) or 5 g olive oil daily for 1 year. After 12 subjects in each group had completed 1 year of supplementation, weight regain differed between the GLA (2.17 ± 1.78 kg) and control (8.78 ± 2.78 kg) groups ($P < 0.03$). The initial study was terminated, and all remaining subjects were assessed over a 6-week period. Unblinding revealed weight regains of 1.8 ± 1.6 kg in the GLA group and 7.6 ± 2.1 kg in controls for the 13 and 17 subjects, respectively, who completed a minimum of 50 weeks in the study. Weight regain did not differ in the remaining 10 GLA and 5 control subjects who completed <50 weeks in the study. In a follow-up study, a subgroup from both the original GLA (GLA-GLA, $n = 9$) and the original control (control-GLA, $n = 14$) populations either continued or crossed over to GLA supplementation for an additional 21 months. Interim weight regains between 15 and 33 months were 6.48 ± 1.79 kg and 6.04 ± 2.52 kg for the GLA-GLA and control-GLA groups, respectively. Adipose triglyceride GLA levels increased by 152% ($P < 0.0001$) in the GLA group at 12 months, but did not increase further after 33 months of GLA administration. In conclusion, GLA reduced weight regain in humans following major weight loss, suggesting a role for essential fatty acids in fuel partitioning in humans prone to obesity.[21]

Miscellaneous

Encouraging findings have been reported with trials of evening primrose oil in diabetic neuropathy,[22,23] hypercholesterolaemia,[24,25] or obesity.[26]

Recent studies have also been conducted into the potential benefit of GLA in dry eye syndrome and periodontal disease. A preliminary study in 26 patients found that GLA, or linoleic acid, or tear substitutes reduced ocular surface inflammation and improved dry eye syndrome.[27] A study among 76 contact lens wearers found that an evening primrose oil supplement was effective in alleviating dry eye symptoms and improving overall lens comfort in patients suffering from contact lens-associated dry eye.[28]

In a small study involving 30 adults with periodontitis, GLA was found to have beneficial effects, which were more impressive than those for omega-3 fatty acids and lower doses of the two supplements in combination.[29] Further studies will be necessary to more fully assess the potential of GLA in these conditions.

Conclusion

Results of clinical studies with GLA in skin conditions, including atopic dermatitis, as well as PMS and rheumatoid arthritis, have produced conflicting results. However, some individuals with these conditions do appear to benefit. Preliminary research indicates that GLA may be beneficial in diabetic neuropathy.

Precautions/contraindications

Evening primrose oil should be avoided in patients with epilepsy and in those taking epileptogenic drugs, e.g. phenothiazines. There is some evidence that GLA may increase the risk of seizures in these patients.[30]

Pregnancy and breast-feeding

Caution should be used in pregnancy (because of possible hormonal effects). No problems have been reported in breast-feeding.

Adverse effects

Toxicity appears to be low. Reported adverse effects include nausea, diarrhoea and headache. One report[30] has warned of a potential risk of

inflammation, thrombosis and immunosuppression due to slow accumulation of tissue arachidonic acid after prolonged use of GLA for more than 1 year. A further article reported the case of a 50-year-old female with a productive cough who was initially diagnosed with bronchial hyperresponsiveness and gastroesophageal reflux disease (GERD). The patient was treated for GERD. Because the productive cough persisted, the patient underwent chest CT, fibreoptic bronchoscopy and open lung biopsy. She was diagnosed with lipoid pneumonia. The patient was questioned regarding the use of lipid substances, and she reported the chronic use of evening primrose oil. After the discontinuation of the substance and the maintenance of GERD treatment, her condition improved.[31]

Interactions

Drugs

Phenothiazines: increased risk (small) of epileptic fits.

Dose

Evening primrose oil and other supplements containing GLA are generally available in the form of capsules. A US review of nine evening primrose oil products, three borage oil products and four blackcurrant seed oil products (all containing GLA) found that all products apart from one met their label claim.

Symptomatic relief of eczema: 320–480 mg (as GLA) daily; child 1–12 years, 160–320 mg daily.

Symptomatic relief of cyclical and non-cyclical mastalgia: 240–320 mg (as GLA) daily for 12 weeks (then stopped if no improvement).

Dietary supplements provide 40–300 mg (as GLA) per daily dose.

Note: doses are given in terms of GLA; evening primrose oil supplements are not identical; they provide different amounts of GLA.

References

1 Wright S, Burton JL. Oral evening primrose seed oil improves atopic eczema. *Lancet* 1982; 2: 1120–1122.
2 Schalin-Karrila M, Mattila L, Jansen CT. Evening primrose oil in the treatment of atopic eczema: effect on clinical status, plasma phospholipid fatty acids

and circulating blood prostaglandins. *Br J Dermatol* 1987; 117: 11–19.

3   Bamford JT, Gibson RW, Renier CM. Atopic eczema unresponsive to evening primrose oil. *J Am Acad Dermatol* 1985; 13: 959–965.

4   Hederos CA, Berg A. Epogam evening primrose oil treatment in atopic dermatitis and asthma. *Arch Dis Child* 1996; 75: 494–497.

5   Biagi PL, Bordoni A, Masi M. A long-term study on the use of evening primrose oil (Efamol) in atopic children. *Drugs Exp Clin Res* 1988; 14: 285–90.

6   vanGool CJ, Thijs C, Henquet CJ, *et al.* Gamma-linolenic acid supplementation for prophylaxis of atopic dermatitis – a randomized controlled trial in infants at high familial risk. *Am J Clin Nutr* 2003; 77: 943–951.

7   Morse NL, Clough PM. A meta-analysis of randomized, placebo-controlled clinical trials of Efamol evening primrose oil in atopic eczema. Where do we go from here in light of more recent discoveries? *Curr Pharm Biotechnol* 2006; 7: 503–524.

8   Senapati S, Banerjee S, Gangopadhyay DN. Evening primrose oil is effective in atopic dermatitis: a randomized placebo-controlled trial. *Indian J Dermatol Venereol Leprol* 2008; 74(5): 447–452.

9   Horrobin DF. The role of essential fatty acids and prostaglandins in the premenstrual syndrome. *J Reprod Med* 1983; 28: 465–468.

10   Khoo SK, Munro C, Battistutta D. Evening primrose oil and treatment of pre-menstrual syndrome. *Med J Aust* 1990; 153: 189–192.

11   McFayden IJ, Forrest AP, Chetty U. Cyclical breast pain – some observations and the difficulties in treatment. *Br J Gen Pract* 1992; 46: 161–164.

12   Steinbrunn BS, Zera RT, Rodriguez JL. Mastalgia – tailoring treatment to type of breast pain. *Postgrad Med* 1997; 102: 183–188.

13   Goyal A, Mansel RE. A randomized multicenter study of gamolenic acid (Efamast) with and without antioxidant vitamins and minerals in the management of mastalgia. *Breast J* 2005; 11: 41–47.

14   Chenoy S, Hussain S, Tayob Y, *et al.* Effect of oral gamolenic acid from evening primrose oil on menopausal flushing. *BMJ* 1994; 308: 501–503.

15   Belch JJ, Ansell D, Madhock R, *et al.* The effects of altering dietary essential fatty acids on requirements for non-steroidal anti-inflammatory drugs in patients with rheumatoid arthritis. *Ann Rheum Dis* 1988; 47: 96–104.

16   Hansen TM, Lerche A, Kassis V, *et al.* Treatment of rheumatoid arthritis with prostaglandin E1 precursors *cis*-linoleic acid and gamma-linolenic acid. *Scand J Rheumatol* 1983; 12: 85–88.

17   Jannti J, Seppala E, Vapaatalo H. Evening primrose oil and olive oil in the treatment of rheumatoid arthritis. *Clin Rheumatol* 1989; 8: 238–244.

18   Ebden P, Bevan C, Banks J. A study of evening primrose seed oil in atopic asthma. *Prostaglandins Leukot Essent Fatty Acids* 1989; 35: 69–72.

19   Stenius-Aarniala B, Aro A, Hakulinen A. Evening primrose and fish oil are ineffective as supplementary treatment of bronchial asthma. *Ann Allergy* 1989; 62: 534–537.

20   Surette ME, Stull D, Lindemann J. The impact of a medical food containing gammalinolenic and eicosapentaenoic acids on asthma management and the quality of life of adult asthma patients. *Curr Med Res Opin* 2008; 24: 559–567.

21   Schirmer MA, Phinney SD. Gamma-linolenate reduces weight regain in formerly obese humans. *J Nutr* 2007; 137: 1430–1435.

22   Gamma-Linolenic Acid Multicenter Trial Group. Treatment of diabetic neuropathy with gamma-linolenic acid. *Diabetes Care* 1993; 16: 8–15.

23   Jamal GA, Carmichael H. The effect of gamma-linolenic acid on human diabetic peripheral neuropathy: a double-blind placebo-controlled trial. *Diabetic Med* 1990; 7: 319–323.

24   Viikari J, Lehtonen A. Effect of evening primrose oil on serum lipids and blood pressure in hyperlipidemic subjects. *Int J Clin Pharmacol Ther Toxicol* 1986; 24: 668–670.

25   Boberg M, Vessby B, Selenius I. Effects of dietary supplementation with *n*-6 and *n*-3 long-chain polyunsaturated fatty acids on serum lipoproteins and platelet function in hypertriglyceridaemic patients. *Acta Med Scand* 1986; 220: 153–160.

26   Haslett C, Douglas JG, Chalmers SR. A double-blind evaluation of evening primrose oil as an anti-obesity agent. *Int J Obesity* 1983; 7: 549–553.

27   Barabino S, Rolando M, Camicione P, *et al.* Systemic linoleic acid and gamma-linolenic acid therapy in dry eye syndrome with an inflammatory component. *Cornea* 2003; 22: 77–101.

28   Kokke KH, Morris JA, Lawrenson JG. Oral omega-6 essential fatty acid treatment in contact lens associated dry eye. *Cont Lens Anterior Eye* 2008; 31(3): 141–146; quiz 170.

29   Rosenstein ED, Kushner LJ, Kramer N, Kazandijan G. Pilot study of dietary fatty acid supplementation in the treatment of adult periodontitis. *Prostaglandins Leukot Essent Fatty Acids* 2003; 68: 213–218.

30   Phinney S. Potential risk of prolonged gamma-linolenic acid use. *Ann Intern Med* 1994; 120: 692.

31   Rabahi MF, Ferreira AA, Madeira JG, *et al.* Lipoid pneumonia secondary to long-term use of evening primrose oil. *J Bras Pneumol* 2010; 36(5): 657–661.

Fish oils

Description

There are two types of fish oil supplements:

- fish liver oil: this is generally obtained from the liver of the cod, halibut or shark; and
- fish body oil: this is normally derived from the flesh of the herring, sardine or anchovy.

Constituents

Fish liver oil is a rich source of vitamins A and D; concentrations in cod liver oil liquids normally range between 750 and 1200 μg (2500–4000 IU) vitamin A per 10 mL and 2.5–10 μg (100–400 IU) vitamin D per 10 mL; halibut and shark liver oils are more concentrated sources of these vitamins. Fish body oil is low in vitamins A and D. Vitamin E is also present in both types of fish oil and extra vitamin E is normally added to supplements.

Fish liver oil and fish body oil are sources of polyunsaturated fatty acids (PUFAs) of the omega-3 series (eicosapentaenoic acid (EPA) and docosahexaenoic acid (DHA).

Human requirements

EPA and DHA can be synthesised in the body (in small amounts) from alpha-linolenic acid (contained in vegetable oils, e.g. soya bean, linseed and rapeseed oils). However, this conversion may be inefficient in some individuals.

Recommended intakes

Various recommendations, both in the UK and elsewhere, have been made for the intake of very-long-chain n-3 fatty acids (EPA/DHA) (Table 1).

Dietary intake

The National Diet and Nutrition Survey in British adults found that mean intake of omega-3 fatty acids is 270 mg daily, half of which comes from oily fish. However, oily fish is consumed by only 27% of the population. For the other 73% of the population, mean intake is 147 mg daily. Most oily fish is consumed by older people: among 50–64 year olds, 42% of women and 36% of men eat fish while in the 19–24 age group, only 13% of women and 3% of men eat fish.[1]

Dietary sources

Oily fish is the best source, but some so-called 'functional foods' including eggs, bread, margarines and milk are fortified with EPA/DHA. Algae are good sources of EPA/DHA and are being investigated as sources for supplements and functional foods (Table 1). However, the technological expertise is not yet available.

Action

Fish oils have several effects.

- Alteration of lipoprotein metabolism. Fish oils reduce both fasting and post-prandial plasma triacylglycerols and VLDL cholesterol. With moderate intakes of fish oils, both HDL and LDL cholesterol tend to increase. High intakes reduce HDL cholesterol and may increase LDL in some patients. A meta-analysis of published human trials (that each provided 7 g daily of fish oils for at least 2 weeks) showed that serum cholesterol is unaffected by long-chain n-3 fatty acid consumption. However, triacylglycerols fell by 25–30%, LDL increased by 5–10% and HDL fell by 1–3%.[2] Fish oil supplementation has also been shown to reduce triacylglycerols in HIV-infected hypertriglyceridaemic patients.[3] Another RCT found that DHA (1 g daily) reduced triacylglycerols by 21.8% while DHA plus EPA (total: 1.252 mg daily) reduced triacylglycerols by 18.3%; this difference was not significant.[4] Another RCT found that DHA (3 g daily) reduced

Table 1 Recommended intakes of fish oils

Organisation	Recommended intake
UK Food Standards Agency (FSA)	2 portions of fish/week (including one oily); equivalent to 450 mg omega-3 LCPUFAs daily
British Dietetic Association	
People with heart disease	2–3 portions of high omega-3 (oily) fish/week *or* 0.5–1 g omega-3s (EPA and DHA) daily
Everyone else	Follow FSA recommendation
National Institute for Health and Clinical Excellence (NICE): secondary prevention following a heart attack	7 g omega-3 fatty acids each week from 2–4 portions of oily fish; if this is unachievable from diet, take 1 g daily of omega-3 fatty acids
American Heart Association	
People without documented CHD	Eat a variety of fish (preferably oily) fish at least twice a week
People with documented CHD	1 g EPA/DHA/daily preferably from fatty fish *or* consider supplement 1 g EPA+DHA/daily (with medical advice)
People with raised triglycerides	2–4 g/daily of EPA+DHA (with medical advice)
International Society for the Study of Fatty Acids and Lipids (ISSFAL)	Minimum of 500 mg daily EPA+DHA for cardiovascular health
World Health Organization (WHO)	2 portions of fish/week; equivalent to 250–500 mg/daily EPA+DHA

triacylyglycerols, and small, dense LDL particles.[5] A further RCT in patients with type 2 diabetes mellitus found that fish oil (5.9 g daily), compared with corn oil, increased HDL size and small LDL concentration.[6]

- Inhibition of atherosclerosis. Fish oils reduce the plasma concentrations of several atherogenic lipoproteins (see above), but other mechanisms may be important. Thus, these effects may be associated with reduced synthesis of cytokines and interleukin 1α and through stimulation of the endothelial production of nitric oxide.[7] Preliminary research has shown a non-significant favourable effect of n-3 fatty acid supplementation (6 g daily) on carotid intima thickness and progression, but more studies are needed to confirm this.[8]
- Prevention of thrombosis. Thrombosis is a major complication of coronary atherosclerosis, which can lead to myocardial infarction. The n-3 fatty acids have anti-thrombotic actions through inhibiting the synthesis of thromboxane A_2 from arachidonic acids in platelets.[9] Thromboxane A_2 causes platelet aggregation and vasoconstriction, and as a

result fish oil increases bleeding time and reduces the 'stickiness' of the platelets. Fish oil also enhances the production of prostacyclin, which leads to vasodilatation and less 'sticky' platelets. These effects help to reduce the risk of thrombosis.

- Hypocoagulant effect. Dietary n-3 fatty acids appear to provoke a hypocoagulant, vitamin K-independent effect in humans, the degree of which may depend on fibrinogen level.[10]
- Improved arterial vasodilatation. Fish oil supplementation has been shown to improve endothelium-dependent vasodilatation (in addition to other cardiovascular risk factors such as lowering triacylglycerols, increasing HDL cholesterol).[11] An RCT in overweight hypertensive patients with 8-week follow-up demonstrated significant improvement in large artery elasticity with fish oil (3 g daily) compared with placebo.[12]
- Inhibition of inflammation. Diets rich in omega-3 fatty acids appear to reduce the inflammatory response.[13] Fish oil supplementation (in combination with exercise) has also been shown to counteract inflammation.[14]

- Inhibition of the immune response. Immune reactivity is generally reduced by omega-3 fatty acids.[15,16]
- Reduction in heart rate. A meta-analysis of 30 RCTs found that fish oil decreased heart rate by 1.6 beats per minute compared with placebo. In trials where initial heart beat was high and/or the study period was long, reduction in heart rate averaged 2.5 beats/min. Heart rate reduction did not significantly vary with dosage of fish oil.[17]
- Influence on arrhythmias. Fish oil may reduce the incidence of lethal myocardial infarction and sudden death. This may be due to the prevention of fatal cardiac arrhythmias. Evidence from some studies indicates an anti-arrhythmic action of fish oil,[18] while evidence from other studies does not.[19–21] In patients undergoing coronary artery bypass surgery, omega-3 fatty acids (2 g daily) substantially reduced the incidence of post-operative atrial fibrillation.[22] In a further study in patients with a recent episode of sustained ventricular arrhythmia and an implantable cardioverter defibrillator (ICD), fish oil did not reduce the risk of ventricular tachycardia and ventricular fibrillation and there was evidence of a pro-arrhythmic effect in some patients.[23] A review confirmed the impact on the fundamental elements (ion channels, exchangers and modulators) of n-3 fatty acids on cardiac electrical activity, but cautioned the translation of this understanding into evidence-based policy for reduction of cardiac arrhythmia.[24]

Mechanism of action
Fish oils appear to act by:

- modulation of pro-inflammatory and pro-thrombotic eicosanoid (prostaglandin, thromboaxone and leukotriene) production; and
- reduction in interleukin-1 and other cytokines.

Eicosanoid production
The effects of omega-3 fatty acids are thought to be due to the partial replacement of arachidonic acid with EPA in cell membrane lipids. This leads to increased production of PG3 series prostaglandins, thromboxane A_3 and series 5 leukotrienes at the expense of PG2 series prostaglandins, thromboxane A_2 and series 4 leukotrienes (see Figure 1).

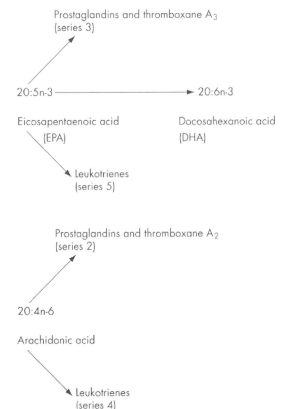

Figure 1   Metabolism of eicosapentaenoic acid and arachidonic acid.

Thromboxane A_3 (produced from EPA) is less effective at stimulating platelet aggregation than thromboxane A_2 (produced from arachidonic acid). Prostaglandins of the PG3 series have less potent inflammatory effects than prostaglandins of the PG2 series. In addition, DHA inhibits the formation of the more inflammatory prostaglandins of the PG2 series, while EPA acts as a substrate for the synthesis of the less inflammatory prostaglandins of the PG3 series.

Series 5 leukotrienes (produced by EPA) have weaker inflammatory effects than series 4 leukotrienes (produced by arachidonic acid).

Possible uses

Fish liver oils are used as a source of vitamins A and D. Both fish liver oils and fish body oils are used as a source of EPA and DHA.

In addition, fish oils appear to have a role in the prevention and management of certain

Table 2 Typical very-long-chain n-3 fatty acid (EPA and DHA) content of fish and fish oils

Food	Average serving (g)	Total EPA/ DHA per serving[1]
Kippers	130	3.37
Mackerel	160	3.09
Pilchards (canned in tomato sauce)	110	2.86
Trout	230	2.65
Salmon (fresh)	100	2.7
Sardines (canned in tomato sauce)	100	1.67
Herring	119	1.56
Salmon (canned or smoked)	100	1.55
Crab (canned)	85	0.85
Plaice	130	0.39
Tuna, fresh	120	1.8
Cod	120	0.30
Mussels	40	0.24
Haddock	120	0.19
Tuna (canned in oil, drained)	45	0.17
Tuna (canned in brine, drained)	45	0.08
Prawns	60	0.06
Cod liver oil liquid[2]	10 mL	1.5–3.0
Cod liver oil capsules[2]	Varies	0.1–0.4
Fish oil capsules[2]	Varies	0.1–0.4

[1] Source (except 2): Holland B, Brown J, Buss DH. Fish and fish products; the third supplement to *McCance & Widdowson's The Composition of Food*, 5th edn. London: HMSO, 1993.
[2] Source: product labels. Doses and amounts of EPA/DHA vary between products.

conditions such as coronary heart disease (CHD) and stroke, rheumatoid arthritis, inflammatory bowel disease, psoriasis and asthma, mental disorders such as depression, schizophrenia and Alzheimer's disease (AD), nephropathy, various cancers and diabetes mellitus.

Cardiovascular disease

The consumption of fish is associated with lower rates of CHD in many epidemiological studies. Seminal findings in Eskimos have been confirmed and extended to Western populations, and in most studies there is an inverse relationship between the intake of fish or n-3 fatty acids and total mortality or cardiovascular mortality.[25–29] However, some studies,[30,31] have not shown any benefit, possibly because fish intake was higher in the studied population as a whole.

Intervention studies, in which the intake of fish or fish oil was increased, have also shown beneficial effects (see Table 3). One classic study[58] investigated 2000 Welsh men who had just recovered from their first heart attack. The men were randomised to a 'fish advice group', in which they were asked to eat at least two portions of oily fish a week, or failing this fish oil in capsule form, or a 'no fish advice group'. After 2 years, there was a 29% reduction in mortality in the fish/fish oil group, which was attributable to a reduction in CHD deaths. However, although there were fewer fatal heart attacks in the fish group, the total number of heart attacks did not decrease.

The GISSI Prevenzione trial[59] investigated the effects of n-3 PUFAs (1 g daily), vitamin E (300 mg daily) or both as supplements in a study involving 11 324 patients surviving recent myocardial infarction. Treatment with n-3 PUFAs, but not vitamin E, reduced total deaths and cardiovascular deaths, and the effect of the combined treatment was similar to that for n-3 PUFAs alone.

Overall, a consistent body of evidence derived from several hundred studies has indicated that a daily ingestion of at least 1 g of EPA and DHA results in a reduction in total mortality, cardiovascular mortality and morbidity.[60] The American Heart Association recommends that patients with CHD should consume 1 g EPA + DHA per day, preferably from oily fish, although if this is difficult to achieve from diet alone, a fish oil supplement may form part of the dietary and lifestyle change.

However, a more recent large trial involving 3114 men with angina found a higher risk of cardiac death in men consuming fish oil. Subjects in the trial were allocated to four groups: (i) advised to eat two portions of oily fish each week or take fish oil capsules; (ii) advised to eat more fruit, vegetables and oats; (iii) advised to eat oily fish and more fruit, vegetables and oats; and (iv) no specific dietary advice. Mortality was evaluated after 3–9 years. All-cause mortality

Table 3 Clinical trials and systematic reviews evaluating the effect of fish oils on cardiovascular disease and cognitive/mental health

Reference	Duration and type of trial	Dose of fishoil/omega-3	Study group	Outcome measures	Observed effects
Cardiovascular disease					
Bucher et al. (2002)[32]	Meta-analysis	Trials comparing dietary or non-dietary n-3 PUFAs with placebo	11 trials (7951 intervention patients; 7855 control patients; all with CHD)	Risk of myocardial infarction and overall mortality in patients with CHD	Both dietary and non-dietary intake of n-3 polyunsaturated fatty acids reduced overall mortality, mortality from myocardial infarction, and sudden death in patients with CHD
Wang et al. (2004)[33]	Systematic review	Omega-3 supplements or oily fish or alpha-linolenic acid	11 prospective studies and 1 randomised controlled trial in patients with CVD	CVD outcomes	Consumption of omega-3 fatty acids from fish or from supplements of fish oil reduced all-cause mortality and various CVD outcomes
Balk et al. (2004)[34]	Systematic review	Omega-3 supplements or oily fish or alpha-linolenic acid	123 studies	CVD risk factors and intermediate markers of CVD	A large consistent effect was found only for triglycerides
Vanschoonbeek et al. (2004)[10]	4-week open trial (Netherlands)	3 g omega-3 fatty acids	25 healthy males (borderline overweight)	Thrombin generation	Fish oil reduced fibrinogen and factor V levels as well as thrombin generation in plasma
Hooper et al. (2004)[35]	Meta-analysis	Various	48 randomised controlled trials (36 913 participants)	Total mortality, cardiovascular events or cancers	Influence of dietary and supplemental omega 3s on cardiovascular events, mortality and cancer was unclear
Mozaffarian et al. (2005)[17]	Meta-analysis	Fish oil	30 randomised controlled trials	Heart rate	Fish oil reduced heart rate, particularly in those with high heart rate
Geelen et al. (2005)[21]	14-week placebo-controlled trial (Netherlands)	1.5 g n-3 fatty acids daily or placebo	74 patients with frequent premature ventricular complexes	ECG measures: heart-rate-corrected QT interval, T-loop width, spatial QRS-T angle and spatial U-wave amplitude	None of the ECG measures were affected by n-3 fatty acids
Geelen et al. (2005)[20]	14-week randomised controlled trial (Netherlands)	1.5 g/day of either n-3 fatty acids or placebo	84 patients with ≥ 1440 premature ventricular complexes/24 h	Heart rate and premature ventricular complexes (common form of arrhythmia that may trigger arrhythmias that are more life threatening)	Treatment did not significantly affect the number of premature ventricular complexes but decreased heart rate
Wang et al. (2006)[36]	Meta-analysis	Various	14 randomised controlled trials	Cardiovascular outcomes	Increased consumption of n-3 PUFAs from fish or fish-oil supplements, but not of alpha-linolenic acid, reduced the rates of all-cause mortality, cardiac and sudden death, and possibly stroke

Reference	Study design	Dose	Participants	Outcome measured	Results
Schwellenbach et al. (2006)[4]	8-week randomised controlled trial	1000 mg DHA or 1252 mg DHA + EPA	116 patients with coronary artery disease and raised triglycerides	Triglycerides	Triglycerides decreased by an average of 21.8% in the DHA group and 18.3% in the DHA + EPA group, but no difference between the two groups
Hooper et al. (2006)[37]	Meta-analysis	Various	48 randomised controlled trials (36 913 participants) and 41 cohort studies	Total mortality, cardiovascular events, or cancer	No clear effect on total mortality, combined cardiovascular events, or cancer
Theobald et al. (2007)[38]	Randomised controlled trial	0.7 g DHA	38 healthy men and women (40–65 years)	Vascular function and biochemical indices of endothelial dysfunction	Moderate dose DHA lowered diastolic blood pressure but did not influence indices of endothelial function or arterial stiffness in the short term
Hill et al. (2007)[11]	Randomised controlled trial (Australia)	6 g tuna fish oil (1.9 g n-3 PUFA) + exercise vs placebo vs placebo + exercise	Overweight volunteers with high blood pressure, cholesterol or triacylglycerols	Plasma lipids, blood pressure, arterial function	Fish oil supplementation lowered triacylglycerols, increased HDL cholesterol, and improved endothelium-dependent arterial vasodilatation; both fish oil and exercise reduced body fat
Hartweg et al. (2007)[39]	Meta-analysis	Various	23 randomised controlled trials in patients with type 2 diabetes	Lipid risk factors	Fish oil reduced triacylglycerols and VLDL cholesterol, but may have an adverse effect on LDL cholesterol
Kelley et al. (2007)[5]	90-day double-blind, randomised, placebo parallel study	3 g DHA/day	34 men (39–66 years) with hypertriglyceridaemia	Lipid risk factors	n-3 PUFA supplementation reduced triacylglycerol but may increase LDL cholesterol
Tavazzi et al. (2008)[40]	Randomised controlled trial (Italy)	1 g daily n-3 PUFA	3494 patients with symptomatic heart failure randomised to intervention group; 3494 patients to placebo group	Morbidity and mortality	Treatment with n-3 PUFA may provide a small beneficial advantage in terms of mortality and admission to hospital for cardiovascular reasons in patients with heart failure in a context of usual care
Yusof et al. (2008)[41]	8-week randomised controlled trial (UK)	1.8 g EPA + 0.3 g DHA	Healthy middle-aged men with cardiovascular risk factors	Plasma lipids and inflammatory markers	No significant effect of fish oil
Sjoberg et al. (2009)[42]	Randomised controlled trial (Australia)	Fish oil (1 g containing 260 mg DHA + 60 mg EPA) at daily doses of 2 g (n=16), 4 g (n=17) or 6 g (n=17)	67 overweight or obese adults	Blood pressure, heart rate and compliance of large and small arteries	No effect of fish oil on any measure
Poppitt et al. (2009)[43]	12-week randomised controlled trial	3 g/day encapsulated fish oil containing approximately 1.2 g total omega-3 (0.7 g DHA; 0.3 g EPA) or placebo oil	122 patients with stroke	Cardiovascular biomarkers	No effect of fish oil on any cardiovascular biomarkers

(Continued)

Table 3 (continued)

Reference	Duration and type of trial	Dose of fishoil/ omega-3	Study group	Outcome measures	Observed effects
Finzi et al. (2010)[44]	The GISSI-HF trial	n3-PUFAs	566 patients with heart failure enrolled in the GISSI-HF trial who received an implantable cardioverter defibrillator for secondary or primary prevention of ventricular fibrillation or tachycardia	Arrhythmia	Tendency towards an anti-arrhythmic effect with fish oil
Nodari et al. (2010)[45]	12-month randomised controlled trial (Italy)	2 g n-3 PUFAs or placebo	133 patients with non-ischaemic dilated cardiomyopathy	Left ventricular systolic function and functional capacity	n-3 PUFAs increased left ventricular systolic function and functional capacity and may reduce hospitalisations for heart failure
Kromhout et al. (2010)[46]	40-month randomised controlled trial (Netherlands)	Trial margarines with four supplements: (i) EPA + DHA (targeted additional daily intake 400 mg EPA–DHA), (ii) alpha-linolenic acid (ALA; targeted additional daily intake 2 g ALA), (iii) EPA + DHA + ALA, or (iv) no supplement (placebo)	4837 patients who had had a myocardial infarction and were receiving state-of-the-art antihypertensive, antithrombotic, and lipid-modifying therapy (60–80 years; 78% men)	Rate of major cardiovascular events	Low-dose supplementation with EPA–DHA or ALA did not significantly reduce the rate of major cardiovascular events
Einvik et al. (2010)[47]	A 3-year 2 × 2 factorial designed clinical trial (Norway)	Diet counselling and/or 2.4 g n-3 PUFA supplementation	563 Norwegian men, 72% without overt cardiovascular disease (64–76 years)	All-cause mortality and cardiovascular events	A tendency toward reduction in all-cause mortality in the n-3 PUFA groups
Wong et al. (2010)[48]	Randomised controlled trial (Hong Kong)	4 g fish oil/day or placebo	97 patients with type 2 diabetes and without prior CV disease	Vascular function and metabolic profile	Fish-oil supplement had no significant beneficial effect on vascular endothelial function, but improved renal function without changes in endothelial function, metabolic profiles, blood pressure, inflammation or oxidative stress

Cognitive function and depression

Study	Study type	Intervention	Participants	Outcome	Findings
Silvers et al. (2005)[49]	12-week randomised controlled trial (New Zealand)	8 g fish oil or placebo plus existing therapy for depression	77 participants	Mood and depression	Mood improved in both groups but there was no difference between fish oil and placebo
Nemets et al. (2006)[50]	Pilot trial	Omega-3 PUFAs	28 children	Depression	Fish oil improved symptoms of depression
Freund et al. (2006)[51]	6-month randomised controlled trial	1.7 g DHA + 0.6 g EPA	204 patients with Alzheimer's disease	Cognition	Omega-3 did not delay the rate of cognitive decline
Appleton et al. (2006)[52]	Meta-analysis	Various	12 randomised controlled trials	Depressed mood	Limited effect of omega-3 PUFAs on depressed mood
Rogers et al. (2008)[53]	12-week randomised controlled trial (UK)	1.5 g/day EPA + DHA supplementation	218 mild to moderately depressed individuals	Mood and depression	No effects of n-3 PUFAs on mood and depression
van de Rest et al. (2008)[54]	26-week randomised controlled trial	400 or 1800 mg/day EPA + DHA, or placebo capsules	302 elderly people (> 65 years)	Mental well-being, cognitive performance	No effect on mental well-being or cognitive performance
Martins et al. (2009)[55]	Meta-analysis	Various	28 randomised controlled trials	Depression	EPA may be more efficacious than DHA in treating depression
Dangour et al. (2010)[56]	24 month randomised controlled trial (UK)	Daily capsules providing 200 mg EPA + 500 mg DHA or olive oil	867 cognitively healthy adults (70–79 years)	Cognitive function	No decline in either arm of the study
Appleton et al. (2010)[57]	Meta-analysis	Various	35 randomised controlled trials	Depressed mood	The evidence available provides some support for a benefit of n-3 PUFAs in individuals with diagnosed depressive illness but no evidence of any benefit in individuals without a diagnosis of depressive illness

CHD, coronary heart disease; CVD, cardiovascular disease; DHA, docosahexaenoic acid; EPA, eicosapentaenoic acid; PUFA, polyunsaturated fatty acids; PVC, premature ventricular complexes.

was not reduced by any form of advice. Risk of cardiac death was higher among subjects advised to take oily fish than among those not so advised. The excess risk was largely found in those taking fish oil capsules. The authors concluded that the result is unexplained; that it may arise from risk compensation or some other effect on the behaviour of patients or doctors.[61]

Recent meta-analyses and systematic reviews have considered this issue. A meta-analysis of 11 RCTs that compared dietary or non-dietary intake of n-3 fatty acids with placebo in patients with CHD found that dietary and non-dietary intake of n-3 fatty acids reduces overall mortality, mortality due to myocardial infarction and sudden death in patients with CHD.[32]

A systematic review[35,37] investigated the role of omega-3 fatty acids for prevention and treatment of CVD using both RCT and cohort studies. RCTs were included where omega-3 intake or advice was randomised and unconfounded and study duration was at least 6 months. Cohort studies were included where a cohort was followed up for at least 6 months and omega-3 intake estimated. Forty-eight RCTs and 41 cohort studies were included. Pooled trial results did not show a reduction in the risk of total mortality or combined cardiovascular events in those taking additional omega-3 fats (with significant statistical heterogeneity). Sensitivity analysis, retaining only studies at low risk of bias, reduced heterogeneity and again suggested no significant effect of omega-3 fats. Restricting analysis to trials increasing fish-based omega-3 fats, or those increasing short-chain omega-3s, did not suggest significant effects on mortality or cardiovascular events in either group. Subgroup analysis by dietary advice or supplementation, baseline risk of CVD or omega-3 dose suggested no clear effects of these factors on primary outcomes. The reviewers concluded that: 'It is not clear that dietary or supplemental omega-3 fats alter total mortality, or combined cardiovascular events in people with, or at high risk of, CVD in the general population. There is no evidence that people should be advised to stop taking rich sources of omega-3 fats, but further high-quality trials are needed to confirm suggestions of a protective effect of omega-3 fats on CV health. There is no clear evidence that omega-3 fats differ in effectiveness according to fish or plant sources, dietary or supplemental sources, dose or presence of placebo.'

These results are discussed in a further paper where the suggestion is made that fish oil could have either anti- or pro-arrhythmic effects depending on the medical status of the individual, and that this could explain conflicting results.[62] However, this systematic review has attracted criticism on the basis that it did not include several cohort trials, it analysed primary and secondary prevention trials together and included studies involving alpha-linolenic acid and fish oils.

A second review of the effects of omega-3 fatty acids on CVD[33] includes prevention studies, including 11 RCTs and one prospective cohort study that reported outcomes on CVD populations ($n = 16\,000$ patients). Trials lasted from 1.5 to 5 years. Eleven secondary prevention studies were considered in this review. Four trials used fish oil (EPA + DHA) supplements in doses of 0.27–4.8 g daily and were of good methodological quality. The largest trial reported that fish oil supplements reduce all-cause mortality and CVD outcomes but do not affect stroke. Six trials reported contradictory data on stroke, with three trials using omega-3 supplements reporting increased strokes and three diet/dietary advice trials reporting reduced strokes. One study, which randomised a total of 300 patients to 1.7 g daily of EPA and DHA or an equivalent amount of corn oil for 1.5 years, reported no beneficial effect of omega-3 fats on any CVD outcomes.

Primary prevention studies considered in this review included 22 prospective cohort studies, four case–control studies, one cross-sectional study and one RCT, which reported data on outcomes in the general population. These studies were conducted in many parts of the world, the methodological quality was generally good, most of the cohort studies had several thousand subjects and study duration ranged from 4 to 30 years. Most of the large cohort studies reported that fish consumption reduces all-cause mortality and CVD events, although some studies reported no significant or negative effects. Benefits in primary prevention of stroke were not clearly seen. The review also indicated that the relative effect of alpha-linolenic acid versus fish oil is not clear and that there are few data concerning the needs of different high-risk populations.

A further US systematic review[34] looked at the effect of omega-3 fatty acids on cardiovascular risk factors. The strongest and most consistent effect of omega-3 fatty acids was found on lowering triglyceride levels. The effect of omega-3 fatty acids on other lipids was weaker. In general, LDL cholesterol and HDL cholesterol were found to rise to a small extent. No consistent effect was found on levels of lipoprotein A. Total apolipoprotein B and apolipoprotein B-100 levels fell, while LDL apolipoprotein B levels increased. There was no consistent effect on markers of inflammation and thrombosis, including C-reactive protein, fibrinogen, factor VII, factor VIII and platelet aggregation. There was an overall trend towards a net reduction of relative risk of 14% in coronary artery restenosis, while data on the effect of omega-3 fatty acids on carotid artery intima-media thickness were found to be conflicting. The review suggested that fish oil consumption may benefit exercise capacity and heart rate variability (which may reduce the incidence of ventricular arrhythmias) among people with coronary artery disease.

A large Japanese trial in 18 645 patients with a totalcholesterol of 6.5 mmol/L or greater, randomised patients toreceive either EPA 1.8 g daily with a statin or a statincontrol with a 5-year follow-up.[63] The primary end point was any major coronary event, including sudden cardiac death, fatal and non-fatal myocardial infarction and other non-fatal events, including unstable angina pectoris, angioplasty, stenting or coronary artery bypass grafting. Analysis was by intention to treat. After follow-up, there was a 19% relative reduction ($P = 0.011$) in major coronary events in the EPA group compared to the statin control group. Unstable angina and non-fatal coronary events were also significantly reduced in the EPA group. The benefits were in addition to statin treatment. However, sudden cardiac death and coronary death did not differ between the two groups. The authors concluded that EPA is a promising treatment for prevention of major coronary events, especially non-fatal coronary events, in this group of patients who had dyslipidaemia and were treated with a statin.

Sudden death due to heart disease imposes a significant population burden throughout the world. A US analysis considered a hypothetical population and calculated the estimated impact of three interventions to prevent sudden death: raising blood n-3 fatty acids, distributing automated external defibrillators (AEDs) and implanting cardioverter defibrillators (ICDs) in appropriate candidates. Raising n-3 fatty acids would be expected to reduce total mortality by 6.4%, distributing AEDs would be expected to reduce total mortality by 0.8%, and implanting ICDs would be expected to lower total mortality by 3.3%. According to the authors, raising n-3 fatty acids could potentially have eight times the impact of distributing AEDs and twice the impact of implanting ICDs.[64]

More recent trials and meta-analyses have continued to generate positive or neutral findings in relation to fish oil and cardiovascular health. In an Italian trial, n-3 PUFAs 1 g daily was found to provide a small beneficial advantage in terms of mortality and admission to hospital for cardiovascular issues in patients with heart failure.[40] Further analysis of the GISSI trial among a subgroup of patients with heart failure showed a tendency towards an anti-arrhythmic effect with fish oil supplementation.[44] Another Italian trial showed that n-3 PUFAs (2 g daily) improved left ventricular systolic function and functional capacity among patients with heart failure. Other controlled trials have found no influence of fish oil on cardiovascular markers, including plasma lipids,[41] blood pressure[42] and vascular endothelial function.[48] Among two Norwegian trials, low-dose supplementation with EPA and DHA did not significantly reduce the rate of major cardiovascular events[46] but higher doses produced a tendency towards a reduction in all-cause mortality.[47]

Rheumatoid arthritis

Fish oils appear to alleviate the symptoms of rheumatoid arthritis, and this is commensurate with the role of n-3 fatty acids in suppression of the production of inflammatory eicosanoids. Overall, the evidence for use of fish oil as an adjunctive treatment in rheumatoid arthritis is quite strong.[65]

Several studies have shown that very-long-chain n-3 fatty acids reduce pain and morning stiffness,[66] decrease the need for non-steroidal anti-inflammatory drugs (NSAIDs),[67–70] and increase the cyclo-oxygenase inhibitory activity of paracetamol.[71] Moreover, a meta-analysis of 10 double-blind, placebo-controlled randomised trials in 395 patients showed that fish oil taken for 3 months was associated with a statistically significant reduction in joint tenderness and morning stiffness, but no significant improvements in joint swelling, grip strength or erythrocyte sedimentation rate (ESR, a marker of inflammation).[72]

However, a US review conducted for the Office of Dietary Supplements, National Institutes of Health, on the effects of omega-3 fatty acids on rheumatoid arthritis concluded that from nine studies reporting outcomes in patients with rheumatoid arthritis, omega-3 fatty acids had no effect on patient reports of pain, swollen joint count, ESR and patients' global assessment by meta-analysis.[73]

A meta-analysis of 17 RCTs assessing the pain relieving effects of omega-3 PUFAs in patients with rheumatoid arthritis or joint pain secondary to inflammatory bowel disease showed that supplementation with omega-3 PUFAs for 3–4 months reduced patient-reported joint pain intensity, minutes of morning stiffness, number of painful and/or tender joints and NSAID consumption, but significant effects were not noted for physician-assessed pain.[74]

A Dutch double-blind, placebo-controlled, parallel-group study in 66 patients with rheumatoid arthritis using 1.4 g EPA, 0.211 g DHA and 0.5 g gamma-linolenic acid with micronutrients found no significant change from baseline in tender joint count, swollen joint count, visual analogue scales for pain and disease activity, grip strength, functionality scores and morning stiffness. The conclusion was that this study adds information regarding doses of omega-3 fatty acids below which anti-inflammatory effects in rheumatoid arthritis are not seen.[75]

Inflammatory bowel disease

Fish oil has been found to have some benefits in patients with Crohn's disease or ulcerative colitis, but no real conclusions can be drawn. A review of five studies[76] investigating the effect of n-3 fatty acids in Crohn's disease was inconclusive, but a later study showed that an enteric-coated preparation of very-long-chain n-3 fatty acids significantly reduced the rate of relapse in patients with Crohn's disease in remission.[77]

In patients with ulcerative colitis, fish oil supplements have been found to reduce corticosteroid requirements,[78] improve gastrointestinal histology,[79] and reduce disease activity index.[80]

A systematic review of 13 controlled trials assessed the effects of n-3 fatty acids on clinical, sigmoidoscopic or histological scores, rates of remission or relapse, or requirements for steroids and other immunosuppressive agents in Crohn's disease or ulcerative colitis. Most clinical trials were of good quality. Fewer than six were identified that assessed the effects of n-3 fatty acids on any single outcome of clinical, endoscopic or histological scores or remission or relapse rates. Consistent across three studies was the finding that n-3 fatty acids reduce corticosteroid requirements, although statistical significance was shown in only one of these studies. The conclusion of the review was that the available data are insufficient to draw conclusions about the effects of n-3 fatty acids on clinical, endoscopic or histologic scores or remission or relapse rate.[81]

A Cochrane review of six studies evaluating the efficacy of fish oil for the maintenance of remission in ulcerative colitis could not pool data as the methodology and outcomes were so different, and hence concluded that no definitive conclusion relating to fish oil could be made.[82] A Cochrane analysis evaluating trials of fish oil for maintenance of remission in Crohn's disease concluded that the existing data do not support use of fish oils for this purpose.[83]

Psoriasis

Fish oils have been claimed to be beneficial in some individuals with psoriasis, leading to reduced itching and erythema. However, six RCTs[84–89] produced inconclusive results.

Asthma

Because asthma is an inflammatory condition which appears to involve eicosanoids, it is biologically plausible that fish oil could be of benefit. However, results of studies have been discouraging and there is no clear evidence that fish oils are beneficial in asthma. One study has suggested that fish oil could be protective in suppressing exercise-induced bronchoconstriction in athletes,[90] and another that fish oil may be beneficial in children with bronchial asthma.[91]

A US systematic review including 31 reports (describing 26 unique studies) stated that it is impossible to conclude anything with respect to the value of using omega-3 fatty acid supplementation in the management and/or prevention of asthma for adults or children either in or beyond North America. This is due to the lack of sufficiently consistent evidence, as well as the paucity of evidence from well-designed, well-conducted and adequately powered studies. Further research is needed to establish or refute the value of omega-3 fatty acids to prevent or treat asthma in children and adults.[92]

A Cochrane review assessed the effect of omega-3 fatty acids in asthma. Nine RCTs were included. There was no consistent effect on any of the analysable outcomes: FEV_1, peak flow rate, asthma symptoms, asthma medication use or bronchial hyper-reactivity. One of the trials in children, which combined dietary manipulation with fish oil supplementation, showed improved peak flow and reduced asthma medication use. There were no adverse effects associated with fish oil supplements. The authors concluded that there is little evidence to recommend that people with asthma supplement or modify dietary intake of marine omega-3 fatty acids in order to improve their asthma control. Equally there is no evidence that they are at risk if they do so.[93]

Diabetes

Although fish oil has been linked with deterioration in glucose and insulin control in patients with diabetes mellitus, results from studies with fish oil in such patients have been inconsistent. Treatment with n-3 fatty acids led to a moderate increase in blood glucose levels in patients with diabetes in two studies,[94,95] but not in another.[96] Reduced insulin sensitivity has also been observed.[95] However, a meta-analysis concluded that fish oil has no adverse effects on glucose or insulin metabolism in patients with diabetes, and lowers triacylglycerol levels effectively by 30%.[97] A further meta-analysis involving patients with type 2 diabetes concluded that n-3 PUFA decreases diastolic blood pressure (by a mean of 1.8 mmHg) and appears to increase factor VII. The reviewers concluded that more rigorously conducted trials are required to establish conclusively the role of n-3 PUFA in cardiovascular risk markers and clinical outcomes in type 2 diabetes.[39]

A US systematic review[73] including 18 studies of type 2 diabetes or the metabolic syndrome concluded that omega-3 fatty acids had a favourable effect on triglyceride levels, but had no effect on total cholesterol, HDL cholesterol, LDL cholesterol, fasting blood sugar, or glycosylated haemoglobin (HbA1c), by meta-analysis. Omega-3 fatty acids had no effect on plasma insulin or insulin resistance in patients with type 2 diabetes or the metabolic syndrome.

A Cochrane review looked at 18 trials and 823 participants followed for a mean of 8.9 weeks with a mean dose of omega-3 PUFA of 3.5 g daily. Outcomes studied were glycaemic control and lipid levels. Meta-analysis of pooled data demonstrated a significant effect of fish oil on lowering triglycerides by 0.45 mmol/L (95% confidence interval (CI), 0.58 to 0.32) and raising LDL cholesterol by 0.11 mmol/L (95% CI, 0.00 to 0.22). No statistically significant effect was observed for fasting glucose, HbA1c, total or HDL cholesterol. The triglyceride lowering effect and the elevation in LDL cholesterol were most marked in those trials that recruited people with hypertriglyceridaemia and used higher doses of fish oil. No adverse effects were reported. The reviewers concluded that fish oil supplementation in type 2 diabetes lowers triglycerides, may raise LDL cholesterol (especially in hypertriglyceridaemic patients on high doses of fish oil) and has no significant effect on glycaemic control.[98]

A further review and statement by the American Diabetes Association[99] made several provisional conclusions about the role of n-3 fatty acids in diabetes: they are effective in reducing plasma triacylglycerols and platelet reactivity in patients with diabetes; whether they reduce arrhythmias and blood pressure in these patients remains to be established; evidence suggests no clinically meaningful effects (adverse or favourable) on insulin sensitivity and glucose tolerance at doses of 1–6 g daily. Whether diabetic individuals derive specific benefit from the administration of n-3 fatty acids in long-term trials with hard end points, such as death, myocardial infarction and stroke is still unanswered. Currently there is some expectation of benefit and a reasonable certainty of no harm.

Mental health

The potential role of fish oil in mental disorders is now being investigated. A number of studies have found low levels of n-3 fatty acids in cell membranes of patients with depression, schizophrenia and Alzheimer's disease, and it has been suggested that low dietary intakes of n-3 fatty acids or an imbalance in the n-6:n-3 ratio might be associated with these conditions. Use of cod liver oil has been associated with reduced prevalence of depression in Norway.[100] A preliminary RCT in 49 patients who repeatedly self-harmed found that EPA (1.2 g daily) plus DHA (0.9 g daily) for 12 weeks significantly improved scores for depression, suicidal feelings and stress, but had no effect on scores for impulsivity, aggression and hostility.[101]

A Cochrane review including five short, small trials concluded that there are no clear effects of omega-3 fatty acids in schizophrenia and that large, well-conducted trials are needed.[102] A US systematic review of the effects of omega-3 fats on mental health found that evidence was somewhat suggestive of benefit for omega-3 fatty acids as a short-term intervention for schizophrenia. However, the trials need replication with better methodology. One of the included trials demonstrated a clinical effect in depressive symptoms (rather than depressive disorders) and should not be taken to support the idea that omega-3 fatty acids are beneficial for depressive disorders. The review concluded that there is insufficient evidence to recommend omega-3 fatty acids as a supplemental treatment for any other psychiatric disorders or as a primary treatment for any of the conditions considered in the review (i.e. mainly schizophrenia and depression).[103]

A double-blind, placebo-controlled trial in 28 patients with major depressive disorder found that omega-3 PUFAs (6.6 g daily) significantly decreased the score on the 21-item Hamilton Rating Scale for Depression. The authors concluded that from the preliminary findings in this study, omega-3 PUFAs could improve the short-term course of illness and were well tolerated in patients with major depressive disorder.[104]

A further double-blind, placebo-controlled trial of fish oil involved 77 participants who were randomly allocated to receive 8 g of either fish oil or olive oil per day for 12 weeks in addition to their existing antidepressant therapy.[49] Mood increased significantly in both groups within the first 2 weeks of the study and this improvement was sustained throughout. However, there was no evidence that fish oil improved mood when compared with placebo oil, despite an increase in circulating omega-3 polyunsaturated fatty acids.

A systematic review of 18 RCTs investigating the effects of n-3 PUFAs on depressed mood concluded that the effects are limited but are difficult to evaluate because of study heterogeneity.[52] More recent trials have no influence of omega-3 PUFA supplementation on depression[53] and mental well being.[105] However, EPA may been more effective than DHA in depression.[55] A meta-analysis of 35 RCTs concluded that the available evidence provides some support of a benefit of n-3 PUFAs in individuals with diagnosed depression, but no evidence of benefit in individuals without a diagnosis of depressive illness.[57]

Cognitive function and neurological conditions

A US systematic review that included 12 articles concluded that fish consumption was only weakly associated with a reduced risk of cognitive impairment and had no association with cognitive decline. Fish consumption was associated with a reduced risk of Alzheimer's disease (which was significant in only one of the included studies), while omega-3 consumption and consumption of DHA (but not ALA or EPA) were associated with a significant reduction in the incidence of Alzheimer's. There were no significant associations for Parkinson's disease and effects in multiple sclerosis varied considerably from no benefit to increased disability with omega-3 fatty acids.[106]

A Cochrane review of omega-3 fatty acids for prevention of dementia found that a growing body of evidence from biological, observational and epidemiological studies suggests a protective effect of omega-3 fatty acids against dementia.[107] However, the reviewers found no randomised trials that met their selection criteria and they concluded there is no good evidence to support the use of dietary or supplemental omega-3 fatty acids for the prevention of cognitive impairment or dementia.

More recent trials have also shown mixed outcomes. The Swedish OmegAD study, involving 174 patients with Alzheimer's disease, found that administration of omega-3 fatty acids (2.3 g daily) did not delay the rate of cognitive decline. However, positive effects were observed in a small group of patients with mild Alzheimer's disease.[51] Moreover, in this study supplementation did not result in marked effects in neuropsychiatric symptoms, except for possible effects on depressive symptoms.[108]

A Japanese study[109] involving 21 patients with mild cognitive dysfunction found that supplementation with DHA and arachidonic acid improved memory and attention in those with organic brain lesions butnot in those with Alzheimer's disease. In the prospective Atherosclerosis Risk in Communities Study, higher plasma n-3 PUFA levels were associated with reduced risk of decline in verbalfluency, particularly in hypertensive and dyslipidaemic subjects.[110] In the Dutch Zutphen Elderly Study, a moderate intake of EPA plus DHA from fish was associated with less 5-year subsequent cognitivedecline than no fish intake.[111] Neither a Dutch trial employing daily dosesof 400 or 1800 mg omega PUFAs[54] nor a UK trial employing 700 mg omega 3 PUFAs,[57] both trials in elderly people, found any improvement in cognitive function.

Child and maternal health

Claims are increasingly made that an increase in maternal omega-3 fatty acid intake has the potential to influence both maternal health during pregnancy and also foetal health and birth weight. Results of studies conducted in the Faroe Islands suggest that marine diets, which contain omega-3 fatty acids, increase birth weight either by prolonging pregnancy or by increasing foetal growth rate. In addition it has been hypothesised that marine oils may reduce the risks of certain pregnancy complications, including pre-term delivery, intrauterine growth retardation, pre-eclampsia and gestational diabetes.

Similarly, it has also been suggested that accumulation of omega-3 fatty acids in the child post-delivery can affect the development and health of the child. Infants fed with human milk have improved neurocognitive development compared to formula-fed infants and it has been suggested that one of the contributing factors may be the availability of long-chain derivatives of linoleic acid and alpha-linolenic acid, which are present naturally only in human milk. Infant formulae containing omega-3 long-chain PUFAs are now on the UK market.

A US systematic review has addressed these issues.[112] Various outcomes, including pregnancy outcomes, growth pattern outcomes, neurological development outcomes, visual function outcomes and cognitive development outcomes were considered. Fifteen RCTs, all poor quality, addressed pregnancy outcomes in relation to omega-3 intake in the mother. No difference was found in duration of gestation in 10 studies, while four very poor-quality studies found that omega-3 fatty acids increased the duration of gestation compared with placebo. There was no significant effect on the proportion of premature deliveries in 10 studies. Meta-analysis of the incidence of premature deliveries showed inconsistent evidence of the use of omega-3 fatty acid supplements during the second or third trimester of pregnancy to reduce the incidence of premature pregnancies in both high- and low-risk populations. No significant effects were found for omega-3 fatty acids on the incidence of gestational hypertension and pre-eclampsia. There were no significant differences in birth weight between supplemented and non-supplemented groups of mothers.

A Polish meta-analysis concluded that n-3 long chain PUFA supplementation during pregnancy may enhance pregnancy duration and head circumference, but that mean effect size is small. There were no significant differences in birth weight and birth length.[113]

Maternal intake of omega-3 fatty acids was also investigated for an effect on growth pattern outcomes in the infant. Overall effects on infant growth patterns were found to be non-significant in infants from birth to 12 months of age. Analysis of studies in which pre-term infants were fed formula milk containing omega-3 fatty acids resulted in non-significant findings for growth parameters. In formula-fed term infants, meta-analysis demonstrated a non-significant overall effect of formulae containing DHA and arachidonic acid compared with control formula on growth patterns at 4 and 12 months.

Neurological development outcomes from studies included in the review were not significantly affected by maternal intake during pregnancy or the omega-3 content of breast milk. No significant differences in neurological outcomes were found in either pre-term infants or term infants fed supplemented formula milk compared with control formula.

According to this review, visual function in the infant was not significantly affected by either maternal intake during pregnancy or the omega-3 content of breast milk. Variable results in visual function according to formula intake in both pre-term and term infants have been found. Better or faster maturation of visual acuity has been found in some studies but not all.

Effects on cognitive development in infants according to maternal intake of omega-3 during pregnancy, the omega-3 content of maternal breast milk, and whether pre-term and term formulae were supplemented with omega-3 were also inconsistent.

In summary, this systematic review concluded that pregnancy outcomes were either unaffected by omega-3 fatty acid supplementation or the results were inconclusive. Results suggested an absence of effects with respect to the impact of supplementation on gestational hypertension, pre-eclampsia or eclampsia. Results concerning the impact of the intake of omega-3 fatty acids on the development of infants are primarily, although not uniformly, inconclusive.

More recent trials have shown: a small effect of DHA levels in breast milk on early language development in breast-fed infants;[114] a positive effect of maternal n-3 supplementation on child growth at 2.5 years;[115] a positive effect of DHA supplementation in mothers on child neuro-development, as measured by the Bayley Psychomotor Development Index at 30 months of age (but with no other advantages before, at or after this age);[116] a positive effect of formula supplemented with long-chain PUFAs on visual acuity;[117] and a beneficial effect of maternal fish oil supplementation on child eye and hand co-ordination at age 2½ years.[118,119] However, the use of DHA-rich fish oil capsules during pregnancy in a trial involving 2399 women did not result in improved cognitive and language development in the 766 offspring who were followed up during early childhood, nor did it lower levels of postpartum depression in mothers.[120]

There is also some evidence that maternal dietary n-3 PUFA intake can reduce the risk of development of allergy in the infant.[121,122]

Behavioural problems

Fatty acids have been the subject of a great deal of attention over their potential benefit in children with various behavioural disorders. There is growing evidence that a relative lack of certain polyunsaturated fatty acids may contribute to related neurodevelopmental and psychiatric disorders such as dyslexia and attention deficit hyperactivity disorder (ADHD).

An RCT in 117 children with developmental coordination disorder found that supplementation with omega-3 and omega-6 fatty acids resulted in significant improvements in reading, spelling and behaviour over 3 months of treatment. No effect on motor skills was apparent in this study.[123]

In a study involving 40 children (aged 6–12 years) with ADHD, DHA supplementation (3.6 g/week) for 2 months did not improve ADHD-related symptoms.[124] A further study in 60 children with ADHD found that DHA supplementation (345 mg daily) did not reduce symptoms of ADHD[125]

A recent 15-week RCT in 132 Australian children aged 7–12 years with high ADHD scores found medium to strong positive treatment effect on parental ratings of core ADHD symptoms (inattention, hyperactivity/impulsivity) in two groups given supplements containing n-3 PUFAs and n-3 PUFAs plus micronutrients. No additional effects were found with the micronutrients. Supplementation for a further 15 weeks was associated with significant improvements on the parent ratings. No significant effects were found on the teacher rating scales.[126]

An 8-week open-label pilot study in nine children with ADHD supplemented with 16.2 g EPA/DHA daily reported significant improvement in behaviour (inattention, hyperactivity, oppositional/defiant behaviour and conduct disorder).[127]

Fish oil (providing 3600 mg DHA + 840 mg EPA per week) for 3 months was associated in one study with reduced physical aggression, particularly in girls.[128] A 16-week RCT among 450 children aged 8–10 years in a mainstream school population found no clear benefit of a supplement containing DHA and EPA on children's behaviour and learning.[129] However, EPA may be more effective than DHA in behavioural problems among children. A 15-week RCT among 92 children with ADHD aged 7–12 years found that two ADHD subgroups (oppositional and less-hyperactive/impulsive children) improved after 15-week EPA treatment. Increasing EPA and decreasing omega-6 fatty acid concentrations in phospholipids were also related to clinical improvement.[130]

Renal disease

Fish oil has been investigated for potential benefit in kidney disease. In a placebo-controlled, multicentre trial, 106 patients were randomised to receive either 12 g of fish oil daily over a period of 2 years or placebo.[131] The rate of loss of kidney function was retarded in the supplemented group and the beneficial effect was suggested to be due to the impact of n-3 fatty acids on eicosanoid production and other factors. However, other studies have shown no such benefits and more work is needed. A more recent RCT investigated the effect of low-dose omega-3 PUFAs (0.85 g EPA and 0.57 g DHA) in 14 patients with IgA nephropathy. The supplement was effective in slowing renal progression in these high-risk patients.[132]

A US systematic review, which included nine studies assessing the effect of omega-3 fatty acids in renal disease, found there were varying effects on serum creatinine and creatinine clearance and no effect on progression to end-stage renal disease. In a single study that assessed the effect on haemodialysis graft patency, graft patency was better with fish oil than with placebo. No studies in this review assessed the effects of omega-3 fatty acids on requirements for corticosteroids.[73]

Cancers

In animal studies, fish oils have been shown to reduce cell proliferation and pre-cancerous cell changes, and some epidemiological studies in humans have suggested that fish oils might be protective against cancer. A US systematic review concluded that evidence from the large body of literature does not suggest a significant association between omega-3 fatty acids and cancer incidence. From a small body of literature no significant association was found between omega-3 fatty acids and clinical outcomes after tumour surgery.[133] Another systematic review of 38 papers (published between 1966 and October 2005) did not provide any evidence to suggest a significant association between omega-3 fatty acids and cancer incidence.[134]

A systematic review evaluating the effects of n-3 fatty acid administration in cancer cachexia concluded that doses of at least 1.5 g daily for a prolonged period of time to patients with advanced cancer is associated with improvement in clinical, biological and quality of life parameters.[135]

Miscellaneous

A US systematic review consideredthe role of omega-3 fatty acids in systemic lupus erythematosus (SLE). Among the three studies included in the review, variable effects on SLE were found. Omega-3 fatty acids had no effect on corticosteroid requirements in one study. No studies were identified that assessed the effects of omega-3 fatty acids on requirements for other immunosuppressive drugs for SLE. None of the studies used a measure of disease activity that incorporates both subjective and objective measures of disease activity.[73]

A 12-month double-blind RCT in 31 patients with multiple sclerosis found that a low-fat diet supplemented with omega-3 PUFA can have moderate benefits in patients with relapse-remitting multiple sclerosis who are taking concurrent disease-modifying therapies.[136]

Omega-3 fatty acids have also been investigated for a role in prevention of osteoporosis. A review that included five reviews and 11 *in vivo* studies (eight in animals and three RCTs in humans) found that two of the human RCTs showed a positive effect of a low n-6:n-3 ratio on bone, while the third human study showed no effect. The authors concluded that these data, though preliminary, suggest that a diet with a low n-6:n-3 ratio may have beneficial effects on bone mineral density.[137] A US systematic review[68] including five human studies concluded that the effect of omega-3 fatty acids on bone was variable.

A US systematic review has lookedat the effects of omega-3 fatty acids in eye health. Sixteenstudies were identified, of which only two were RCTs. The reviewconcluded that from the studies identified, no conclusions could bereached about the effect of omega-3 fatty acids as a primaryor secondary prevention in eye health, including age related macular degeneration, retinitis pigmentosa, cataract, and also vascular disease of the retina in patients with and without diabetes.[138]

There is also growing interest in the role of n-3 fattyacids in other conditions affecting respiration, including hay fever, chronic obstructive pulmonary disease and cystic fibrosis.

> **Conclusion**
>
> Fish oil appears to reduce the risk of CHD. It may help to: reduce the risk of thrombosis by increasing bleeding tendency; reduce blood levels of triacylglycerols; prevent atherosclerosis and arrhythmias; and reduce blood pressure. Fish oil could have beneficial effects in inflammatory conditions such as rheumatoid arthritis, Crohn's disease and inflammatory bowel disorders, but evidence of benefit in asthma and psoriasis is poor. Fish oil may have a role in various mental disorders, such as depression, schizophrenia and Alzheimer's disease, but research in this area is in its infancy. Evidence of benefit of fish oil in maternal and child health, including child development and visual acuity, is conflicting. Evidence of value of omega-3 fatty acids in childhood behavioural disorders, such as developmental coordination disorder, is increasing.

Precautions/contraindications

Patients with blood clotting disorders or those taking anticoagulants should be monitored while taking fish oils.

Pregnancy and breast-feeding

Use in pregnancy should be supervised (because of the potential for vitamin A toxicity with excessive intakes of fish liver oil).

Adverse effects

Vitamin A and D toxicity (fish liver oil only). The unpleasant taste of fish liver oil liquids may be masked by mixing with fruit juice or milk.

Fish oil supplements are generally safe, and in one prospective study involving 295 people aged 18–76 years,[139] 10–20 mL of fish oil providing 1.8–3.6 g EPA/DHA for 7 years was not associated with any serious adverse effects. The safety of n-3 fatty acids from fish oil (derived from menhaden) was reviewed by the US Food and Drug Administration (FDA) in 1997. After reviewing more than 2600 articles, the FDA concluded that dietary intakes of up to 3 g daily of EPA/DHA from menhaden oil were generally regarded as safe (GRAS).[140] The FDA came to this conclusion after considering three main issues related to the safety of fish oils: firstly, the risk of deteriorating glycaemic control in type 2 diabetes; secondly, prolonged bleeding times; thirdly, the risk of increasing LDL levels in patients with hypertriglyceridaemia.

Many fish oil supplements (e.g. cod liver oil, halibut liver oil) contain vitamin A and vitamin D – fat-soluble vitamins that can be toxic in excessive amounts. However, the amount of these vitamins contained, for example, in an average multivitamin supplement containing no more than 100% of the RDAs together with the amounts in a recommended dose of, say, ordinary cod liver oil are unlikely to be harmful. However, care should be taken in pregnancy not to take excessive amounts of vitamin A, and product labels should be checked.

Other safety concerns expressed in relation to fish oils include the potential to increase bleeding time (a beneficial effect in relation to prevention of CHD) and the possibly of altering glycaemic control in diabetes. However, it is unlikely that any of these effects is a problem, particularly with intakes of < 3 g EPA/DHA daily. Nevertheless, patients taking anticoagulant medication or those with blood clotting disorders should be monitored while taking fish oils. This does not mean that such patients have to avoid fish oils – just that their doctor should be aware of it.

There is also concern about industrial contaminants in fish oil supplements. These include dioxins and polychlorinated biphenyls (PCBs). There is no immediate danger to health, but risks come from long exposure to high levels. In 2001, the UK Committee on Toxicity (COT) set a tolerable daily intake for dioxins and dioxin-like PCBs of 2 pg toxicity equivalence (TEQ) per kg body weight daily. (For comparison the EU Scientific Committee on Food (SCF) set a tolerable weekly intake of 14 pg/kg body weight.) Since July 2002 it has been an offence to place on the market any fish oil supplements containing higher contaminant levels.

Interactions

Drugs

Anticoagulants: may increase the risk of bleeding; use of fish oils should be medically supervised, but fish oils need not be avoided in patients taking anticoagulants. One RCT involving 260 patients who had undergone coronary bypass surgery found that fish oil (4 g daily) resulted in no long-term effects on parameters of fibrinolysis and coagulation and was not additive with warfarin or aspirin in producing bleeding tendency.[141] A further trial in 16 subjects found that fish oil supplementation (3–6 g daily) did not result in significant change on the anticoagulation status of patients receiving warfarin.[142] However a single case study in a 67-year-old woman found that increase in fish oil dose from 1 g to 2 g daily resulted in an increase in the international normalised ratio (INR) from 2.8 to 4.3 in one month; the INR decreased to 1.6 one week after subsequent fish oil reduction, necessitating a return to the original warfarin dosing regimen.[143]

Aspirin: may increase the risk of bleeding; use of fish oils in patients on long-term treatment with aspirin should be medically supervised.

Dipyridamole: may increase the risk of bleeding; use of fish oils should be medically supervised.

Nutrients

Vitamin E: fish oils increase the requirement for vitamin E (absolute additional requirements not established, but 3–4 mg vitamin E per gram of total EPA/DHA appears to be adequate; sufficient amounts of vitamin E are added to most fish oil supplements; there is unlikely to be a need for any extra). Theoretically, vitamin E may be synergistic in increasing the bleeding tendency with fish oil, although there is no evidence for this.

Supplements

Gingko biloba: may increase the bleeding tendency with fish oils, although there is no evidence for this.

Ginseng: may increase the bleeding tendency with fish oils, although there is no evidence for this.

Dose

Fish oil supplements are available in the form of capsules and liquids.

The dose is not established. Dietary supplements provide 100–1500 mg combined EPA/DHA per dose; clinical trials of fish oil supplements showing beneficial effects have often used 3–4 g daily (combined EPA/DHA), but doses of 1–2 g daily may be adequate.

Note 1: Intake of cod liver oil should not be increased above the doses recommended on the product label to achieve higher intakes of EPA/DHA (risk of vitamin A and D toxicity). Several capsules of cod liver oil could be required to provide the same amount of EPA/DHA as a single dose of cod liver oil liquid. There is no risk of vitamin toxicity with one dose of cod liver oil liquid, but toxicity is likely if several capsules are ingested (vitamin concentration is usually higher in capsules).

Note 2: Fish oil supplements are not identical; they provide different amounts of EPA/DHA.

References

1 Department of Health. *The National Diet and Nutrition Survey: Adults aged 19 to 64 Years*. Vol. 3: *Vitamin and Mineral Intake and Urinary Analysis*. London: The Stationery Office, 2003.

2 Harris WS. n-3 Fatty acids and serum lipoproteins: human studies. *Am J Clin Nutr* 1997; 65 (Suppl): 1645S–1654S.

3 DeTruchis P, Kirstetter M, Perier A, *et al.* Reduction in triglyceride level with n-3 polyunsaturated fatty acids in HIV-infected patients taking potent antiretroviral therapy: a randomized prospective study. *J Acquir Immune Defic Syndr* 2007; 44(3): 278–285.

4 Schwellenbach LJ, Olson KL, McConnell KJ, *et al.* The triglyceride-lowering effects of a modest dose of docosahexaenoic acid alone versus in combination with low dose eicosapentaenoic acid in patients with coronary artery disease and elevated triglycerides. *J Am Coll Nutr* 2006; 25(6): 480–485.

5 Kelley DS, Siegel D, Vemuri M, *et al.* Docosahexaenoic acid supplementation improves fasting and postprandial lipid profiles in hypertriglyceridemic men. *Am J Clin Nutr* 2007; 86(2): 324–333.

6 Mostad IL, Bjerve KS, Lydersen S, *et al.* Effects of marine n-3 fatty acid supplementation on lipoprotein subclasses measured by nuclear magnetic resonance in subjects with type II diabetes. *Eur J Clin Nutr* 2008; 62(3): 419–429.

7 Shimokawa H, Vanhoutte PM. Dietary omega-3 fatty acids and endothelium-dependent relaxations in porcine coronary arteries. *Am J Physiol* 1989; 256: H968–H973.

8 Baldassarre D, Amato M, Eligini S, et al. Effect of n-3 fatty acids on carotid atherosclerosis and haemostasis in patients with combined hyperlipoproteinemia: a double-blind pilot study in primary prevention. *Ann Med* 2006; 38(5): 367–375.

9 Goodnight SH,Jr Harris WS, Connor WE, et al. Polyunsaturated fatty acids, hyperlipidaemia and thrombosis. *Arteriosclerosis* 1982; 2: 87–113.

10 Vanschoonbeek K, Feijge MA, Paquay M, et al. Variable hypocoagulant effect of fish oil intake in humans: modulation of fibrinogen level and thrombin generation. *Arterioscler Thromb Vasc Biol* 2004; 24(9): 1734–1740.

11 Hill AM, Buckley JD, Murphy KJ, et al. Combining fish-oil supplements with regular aerobic exercise improves body composition and cardiovascular disease risk factors. *Am J Clin Nutr* 2007; 85(5): 1267–1274.

12 Wang S, Ma AQ, Song SW, et al. Fish oil supplementation improves large arterial elasticity in overweight hypertensive patients. *Eur J Clin Nutr* 2008; 62(12): 1426–1431.

13 Terano T, Salmon JA, Higg GA, et al. Eicosapentaenoic acid as a modulator of inflammation. Effect on prostaglandin and leukotriene synthesis. *Biochem Pharmacol* 1986; 35: 779–785.

14 Hill AM, Worthley C, Murphy KJ, et al. n-3 Fatty acid supplementation and regular moderate exercise: differential effects of a combined intervention on neutrophil function. *Br J Nutr* 2007; 98(2): 300–309.

15 Endres S, Ghorbani R, Kelley VE. The effect of dietary supplementation with n-3 polyunsaturated fatty acids on the synthesis of interleukin-1 and tumour necrosis factor by mononuclear cells. *N Engl J Med* 1989; 320: 265–271.

16 Meydani SN, Lichtenstein AH, Colwell S. Immunologic effects of national cholesterol education panel step-2 diets with and without fish-derived n-3 fatty acid enrichment. *J Clin Invest* 1993; 92: 105–113.

17 Mozaffarian D, Geelen A, Brouwer IA, et al. Effect of fish oil on heart rate in humans: a meta-analysis of randomized controlled trials. *Circulation* 2005; 112: 1945–1952.

18 Singer P, Wirth M. Can n-3 PUFA reduce cardiac arrhythmias? Results of a clinical trial. *Prostaglandins Leukot Essent Fatty Acids* 2004; 71: 153–159.

19 Geelen A, Brouwer IA, Zock PL, et al. n-3 Fatty acids do not affect electrocardiographic characteristics of healthy men and women. *J Nutr* 2002; 132: 3051–3054.

20 Geelen A, Brouwer IA, Schouten EG, et al. Effects of n-3 fatty acids from fish on premature ventricular complexes and heart rate in humans. *Am J Clin Nutr* 2005; 81: 416–420.

21 Geelen A, Zock PL, Brouwer IA, et al. Effect of n-3 fatty acids from fish oil on electrocardiographic characteristics in patients with frequent premature ventricular complexes. *Br J Nutr* 2005; 93: 787–790.

22 Calo L, Bianconi L, Colivicchi F, et al. n-3 Fatty acids for the prevention of atrial fibrillation after coronary artery bypass surgery: a randomized controlled trial. *J Am Coll Cardiol* 2005; 45: 1723–1728.

23 Raitt MH, Connor WE, Morris C, et al. Fish oil supplementation and risk of ventricular tachycardia and ventricular fibrillation in patients with implantable defibrillators: a randomized controlled trial. *JAMA* 2005; 293: 2884–2891.

24 London B, Albert C, Anderson ME, et al. Omega-3 fatty acids and cardiac arrhythmias: prior studies and recommendations for future research: a report from the National Heart, Lung, and Blood Institute and Office of Dietary Supplements Omega-3 Fatty Acids and Their Role in Cardiac Arrhythmogenesis Workshop. *Circulation* 2007; 116(10): e320–e335.

25 Dolecek TA. Epidemiological evidence of relationships between dietary polyunsaturated fatty acids and mortality in the multiple risk factor intervention trial. *Proc Soc Exp Biol Med* 1992; 200: 177–182.

26 Ascherio A, Rimm RB, Stampfer MJ, et al. Dietary intake of marine n-3 fatty acids, fish intake and the risk of coronary disease among men. *N Engl J Med* 1995; 332: 997–982.

27 Siscovick DS, Raghunathan TE, King I, et al. Dietary intake and cell membrane levels of long chain fatty acids and the risk of primary cardiac arrest. *JAMA* 1995; 274: 1363–1367.

28 Daviglus ML, Stamler J, Orencia AJ, et al. Fish consumption and the 30-year risk of fatal myocardial infarction. *N Engl J Med* 1997; 336: 1046–1052.

29 Albert CM, Hennekens CH, O'Donnell CJ, et al. Fish consumption and risk of sudden cardiac death. *JAMA* 1998; 279: 23–28.

30 Lapidus L, Andersson H, Bengtsson C, et al. Dietary habits in relation to incidence of cardiovascular disease and death in women: a 12-year follow-up of participants in the population study of women in Gothenburg, Sweden. *Am J Clin Nutr* 1986; 44: 444–448.

31 Morris MC, Mason JE, Rosner B, et al. Fish consumption and cardiovascular disease in the Physicians' Health Study: a prospective study. *Am J Epidemiol* 1995; 142: 166–175.

32 Bucher HC, Hengstler P, Schindler C, et al. n-3 Polyunsaturated fatty acids in coronary heart disease: a meta-analysis of randomized controlled trials. *Am J Med* 2002; 112(4): 298–304.

33 Wang C, Chung M, Lichtenstein A, et al. Effects of Omega-3 Fatty Acids on Cardiovascular Disease [Evidence Report/Technology Assessment 94]. Rockville, MD: Agency for Healthcare Research and Quality, 2004. http://www.ahcpr.

gov/clinic/epcsums/o3cardsum.htm (accessed 9 May 2011).

34 Balk E, Chung M, Lichenstein A, *et al.* Effects of Omega-3 Fatty Acids on Cardiovascular Risk Factors and Intermediate Markers of Cardiovascular Disease [Evidence Report/Technology Assessment 93]. Rockville, MD: Agency for Healthcare Research and Quality, 2004. http://www.ahrq.gov/clinic/epcsums/o3cardrisksum.htm (accessed 30 October 2006).

35 Hooper L, Thompson RL, Harrison RA, *et al.* Omega 3 fatty acids for prevention and treatment of cardiovascular disease. *Cochrane Database Syst Rev* 2004; 18(4): CD003177.

36 Wang C, Harris WS, Chung M, *et al.* n-3 Fatty acids from fish or fish-oil supplements, but not α-linolenic acid, benefit cardiovascular disease outcomes in primary- and secondary-prevention studies: a systematic review. *Am J Clin Nutr* 2006; 84(1): 5–17.

37 Hooper L, Thompson RL, Harrison RA, *et al.* Risks and benefits of omega 3 fats for mortality, cardiovascular disease, and cancer: systematic review. *BMJ* 2006; 332(7544): 752–760.

38 Theobald HE, Goodall AH, Sattar N, *et al.* Low-dose docosahexaenoic acid lowers diastolic blood pressure in middle-aged men and women. *J. Nutr* 2007; 137(4): 973–978.

39 Hartweg J, Farmer AJ, Holman RR, *et al.* Meta-analysis of the effects of n-3 polyunsaturated fatty acids on haematological and thrombogenic factors in type 2 diabetes. *Diabetologia* 2007; 50(2): 250–258.

40 Tavazzi L, Maggioni AP, Marchioli R, *et al.* Effect of n-3 polyunsaturated fatty acids in patients with chronic heart failure (the GISSI-HF trial): a randomised, double-blind, placebo-controlled trial. *Lancet* 2008; 372(9645): 1223–1230.

41 Yusof HM, Miles EA, Calder P. Influence of very long-chain n-3 fatty acids on plasma markers of inflammation in middle-aged men. *Prostaglandins Leukot Essent Fatty Acids* 2008; 78(3): 219–228.

42 Sjoberg NJ, Milte CM, Buckley JD, *et al.* Dose-dependent increases in heart rate variability and arterial compliance in overweight and obese adults with DHA-rich fish oil supplementation. *Br J Nutr* 2009; 103(2): 243–248.

43 Poppitt SD, Howe CA, Lithander FE, *et al.* Effects of moderate-dose omega-3 fish oil on cardiovascular risk factors and mood after ischemic stroke: a randomized, controlled trial. *Stroke* 2009; 40(11): 3485–3492.

44 Finzi AA, Latini R, Barlera S, *et al.* Effects of n-3 polyunsaturated fatty acids on malignant ventricular arrhythmias in patients with chronic heart failure and implantable cardioverter-defibrillators: a substudy of the Gruppo Italiano per lo Studio della Sopravvivenza nell'Insufficienza Cardiaca (GISSI-HF) trial. *Am Heart J* 2010; 161 (2): 338–343.

45 Nodari S, Triggiani M, Campia U, *et al.* Effects of n-3 polyunsaturated fatty acids on left ventricular function and functional capacity in patients with dilated cardiomyopathy. *J Am Coll Cardiol* 2010; 57(7): 870–879.

46 Kromhout D, Giltay EJ, Geleijnse JM. n-3 fatty acids and cardiovascular events after myocardial infarction. *N Engl J Med* 2010; 363(21): 2015–2026.

47 Einvik G, Klemsdal TO, Sandvik L, *et al.* A randomized clinical trial on n-3 polyunsaturated fatty acids supplementation and all-cause mortality in elderly men at high cardiovascular risk. *Eur J Cardiovasc Prev Rehabil* 2010; 17(5): 588–592.

48 Wong CY, Yiu KH, Li SW, *et al.* Fish-oil supplement has neutral effects on vascular and metabolic function but improves renal function in patients with type 2 diabetes mellitus. *Diabet Med* 2010; 27(1): 54–60.

49 Silvers KM, Woolley CC, Hamilton FC, *et al.* Randomised double-blind placebo-controlled trial of fish oil in the treatment of depression. *Prostaglandins Leukot Essent Fatty Acids* 2005; 72(3): 211–218.

50 Nemets H, Nemets B, Apter A, *et al.* Omega-3 treatment of childhood depression: a controlled, double-blind pilot study. *Am J Psychiatry* 2006; 163(6): 1098–1100.

51 Freund-Levi Y, Eriksdotter-Jonhagen M, Cederholm T, *et al.* Omega-3 fatty acid treatment in 174 patients with mild to moderate Alzheimer disease: OmegAD study: a randomized double-blind trial. *Arch Neurol* 2006; 63(10): 1402–1408.

52 Appleton KM, Hayward RC, Gunnell D, *et al.* Effects of n-3 long-chain polyunsaturated fatty acids on depressed mood: systematic review of published trials. *Am J Clin Nutr* 2006; 84(6): 1308–1316.

53 Rogers PJ, Appleton KM, Kessler D, *et al.* No effect of n-3 long-chain polyunsaturated fatty acid (EPA and DHA) supplementation on depressed mood and cognitive function: a randomised controlled trial. *Br J Nutr* 2008; 99(2): 421–431.

54 van de Rest O, Geleijnse JM, Kok FJ, *et al.* Effect of fish oil on cognitive performance in older subjects: a randomized, controlled trial. *Neurology* 2008; 71(6): 430–438.

55 Martins JG. EPA but not DHA appears to be responsible for the efficacy of omega-3 long chain polyunsaturated fatty acid supplementation in depression: evidence from a meta-analysis of randomized controlled trials. *J Am Coll Nutr* 2009; 28(5): 525–542.

56 Dangour AD, Allen E, Elbourne D, *et al.* Effect of 2-y n-3 long-chain polyunsaturated fatty acid supplementation on cognitive function in older people: a randomised, double-blind, controlled trial. *Am J Clin Nutr* 2010; 91(6): 1725–1732.

57 Appleton KM, Rogers PJ, Ness AR. Updated systematic review and meta-analysis of the effects of

n-3 long-chain polyunsaturated fatty acids on depressed mood. *Am J Clin Nutr* 2010; 91(3): 757–770.

58   Burr ML, Fehily AM, Gilbert JF, *et al.* Effects of changes in fat, fish and fibre intakes on death and myocardial infarction: diet and reinfarction trial (DART). *Lancet* 1989; ii: 757–761.

59   Gruppo Italiano per lo Studio della Sopravvivenza nell'Infarto miocardico. Dietary supplementation with n-3 polyunsaturated fatty acids and vitamin E after myocardial infarction: results of the GISSI-Prevenzione trial. *Lancet* 1999; 354: 447–455.

60   von Schacky C. The role of omega-3 fatty acids in cardiovascular disease. *Curr Atheroscler Rep* 2003; 52: 139–145.

61   Burr ML, Asffield-Watt PA, Dunstan FD, *et al.* Lack of benefit of dietary advice to men with angina: results of a controlled trial. *Eur J Clin Nutr* 2003; 57: 193–200.

62   Burr M, Dunstan FDJ, George CH. Is fish oil good or bad for heart disease? Two trials with apparently conflicting results *J Membrane Biol* 2005; 206: 155–163.

63   Yokoyama M, Origasa H, Matsuzaki M, *et al.* Effects of eicosapentaenoic acid on major coronary events in hypercholesterolaemic patients (JELIS): a randomised open-label, blinded endpoint analysis. *Lancet* 2007; 369(9567): 1090–1098.

64   Kottke T, Wu LA, Brekke LN, *et al.* Preventing sudden death with n-3 (omega-3) fatty acids and defibrillators. *Am J Prevent Med* 2006; 31(4): 316–323.

65   James M, Proudman S, Cleland L. Fish oil and rheumatoid arthritis: past, present and future. *Proc Nutr Soc* 2010; 69(3): 316–323.

66   Kremer J. Effects of modulation of inflammatory and immune parameters in patients with rheumatic and inflammatory disease receiving dietary supplements of n-3 and n-6 fatty acids. *Lipids* 1996; 31: S243–S247.

67   Lau C, Morely KD, Belch JJ. Effects of fish oil supplementation on non-steroidal anti-inflammatory drug requirements in patients with mild rheumatoid arthritis – a double blind placebo-controlled study. *Br J Rheumatol* 1993; 32: 982–989.

68   Geusens P, Wouters C, Nijs J, *et al.* Long term effect of omega-3 fatty acid supplementation in active rheumatoid arthritis. *Arthritis Rheum* 1994; 37: 824–829.

69   Fortin P, Lew RA, Liang MH, *et al.* Validation of a meta-analysis: the effects of fish oil on rheumatoid arthritis. *J Clin Epidemiol* 1995; 48: 1379–1390.

70   Galarraga B, Ho M, Youssef HM, *et al.* Cod liver oil (n-3 fatty acids) as an non-steroidal anti-inflammatory drug sparing agent in rheumatoid arthritis. *Rheumatology* 2008; 47(5): 665–669.

71   Caughey GE, James MJ, Proudman SM, *et al.* Fish oil supplementation increases the cyclooxygenase

inhibitory activity of paracetamol in rheumatoid arthritis patients. *Complement Ther Med* 2010; 18 (34): 171–174.

72   Kremer JM, Lawrence DA, Petrillo GF, *et al.* Effects of high-dose fish oil on rheumatoid arthritis after stopping nonsteroidal antiinflammatory drugs. Clinical and immune correlates. *Arthritis Rheum* 1995; 38(8): 1107–1114.

73   MacLean C, Mojica WA, Morton SC, *et al.* Effects of Omega-3 Fatty Acids on Lipids and Glycemic Control in Type II Diabetes and the Metabolic Syndrome and on Inflammatory Bowel Disease, Rheumatoid Arthritis, Renal Disease, Systemic Lupus Erythematosus and Osteoporosis [Evidence Reports/Technology Assessment 89]. Rockville, MD: Agency for Healthcare Research and Quality, 2005. http://www.ncbi.nlm.nih.gov/books/NBK37146/ (accessed 1 May 2011).

74   Goldberg RJ, Katz J. A meta-analysis of the analgesic effects of omega-3 polyunsaturated fatty acid supplementation for inflammatory joint pain. *Pain* 2007; 129(12): 210–223.

75   Remans PH, Sont JK, Wagenaar LW, *et al.* Nutrient supplementation with polyunsaturated fatty acids and micronutrients in rheumatoid arthritis: clinical and biochemical effects. *Eur J Clin Nutr* 2004; 58(6): 839–845.

76   Young-In K. Can fish oil maintains Crohn's disease in remission? *Nutr Rev* 1996; 54: 248–257.

77   Belluzzi A, Brignola C, Campieri M, *et al.* Effect of enteric-coated fish oil preparation on relapses in Crohn's disease. *N Engl J Med* 1996; 334: 1557–1560.

78   Hawthorne A, Daneshmend TK, Hawkey CJ, *et al.* Treatment of ulcerative colitis with fish oil supplementation: a prospective 12-month randomized controlled trial. *Gut* 1992; 33: 922–928.

79   Stenson WF, Cort D, Rodgers J, *et al.* Dietary supplementation with fish oil in ulcerative colitis. *Ann Intern Med* 1992; 116(8): 609–614.

80   Aslan A, Triadafilopoulos G. Fish oil fatty acid supplementation in active ulcerative colitis: a double-blind, placebo-controlled, crossover study. *Am J Gastroenterol* 1992; 87: 432–437.

81   MacLean CH, Mojca WA, Newberry SJ, *et al.* Systematic review of the effects of n-3 fatty acids in inflammatory bowel disease. *Am J Clin Nutr* 2005; 82: 611–619.

82   De Ley M, de Vos R, Hommes DW, *et al.* Fish oil for induction of remission in ulcerative colitis. *Cochrane Database Syst Rev* 2007; (4): CD005986.

83   Turner D, Zlotkin SH, Shah PS, *et al.* Omega 3 fatty acids (fish oil) for maintenance of remission in Crohn's disease. *Cochrane Database Syst Rev* 2009; 21(1): CD006320.

84   Mayser P, Mrowietz U, Arenberger P, *et al.* Omega-3 fatty acid-based lipid infusion in patients with chronic plaque psoriasis: results of a double-blind, randomized, placebo-controlled, multicenter trial. *J Am Acad Dermatol* 1998; 38(4): 539–547.

85 Veale D, Torley HI, Richards IM, *et al*. A double-blind placebo controlled trial of Efamol Marine on skin and joint symptoms of psoriatic arthritis. *Br J Rheumatol* 1994; 33: 954–958.

86 Soyland E, Funk J, Rajka G, *et al*. Effect of dietary supplementation with very-long-chain n-3 fatty acids in patients with psoriasis. *N Engl J Med* 1993; 328(25): 1812–1816.

87 Gupta AK, Ellis CN, Tellner DC, *et al*. Double-blind, placebo-controlled study to evaluate the efficacy of fish oil and low-dose UVB in the treatment of psoriasis. *Br J Dermatol* 1989; 120(6): 801–807.

88 Gupta AK, Ellis CN, Goldfarb MT, *et al*. The role of fish oil in psoriasis. A randomized, double-blind, placebo-controlled study to evaluate the effect of fish oil and topical corticosteroid therapy in psoriasis. *Int J Dermatol* 1990; 29(8): 591–595.

89 Bjorneboe A, Smith AK, Bjorneboe GE, *et al*. Effect of dietary supplementation with n-3 fatty acids on clinical manifestations of psoriasis. *Br J Dermatol* 1988; 118(1): 77–83.

90 Mickleborough T, Murray RL, Inoescu AA, Lindley MR, *et al*. Fish oil supplementation reduces severity of exercise-induced bronchoconstriction in elite athletes. *Am J Respire Crit Care Med* 2003; 168: 1181–1189.

91 Nagakura T, Matsuda S, Shichijyo K, *et al*. Dietary supplementation with fish oil rich in omega-3 polyunsaturated fatty acids in children with bronchial asthma. *Eur Respir J* 2000; 16(5): 861–865.

92 Schachter H, Reisman J, Tran K, *et al*. Health Effects of Omega-3 Fatty Acids on Asthma [Evidence Report/Technology Assessment 91]. Rockville, MD: Agency forHealthcare Research and Quality, 2004. http://www.ncbi.nlm.nih.gov/books/NBK37196/ (accessed 1 May 2011).

93 Thien F, DeLuca S, Woods R, *et al*. Cochrane review. Dietary marine fatty acids (fish oil) for asthma in adults and children. *Evidence-Based Child Health* 2011; 6: 984–1012.

94 Vessby B, Karlstrom B, Boberg M, *et al*. Polyunsaturated fatty acids may impair blood glucose control in type 2 diabetic patients. *Diabetic Med* 1992; 9: 126–133.

95 Mostad IL, Bjerve KS, Bjorgaas MR, *et al*. Effects of n-3 fatty acids in subjects with type 2 diabetes: reduction of insulin sensitivity and time-dependent alteration from carbohydrate to fat oxidation. *Am J Clin Nutr* 2006; 84(3): 540–550.

96 Toft I, Bonaa KH, Ingebretsen OC, *et al*. Effects of n-3 polyunsaturated fatty acids on glucose homeostasis and blood pressure in essential hypertension. A randomized, controlled trial. *Ann Intern Med* 1995; 123: 911–918.

97 Friedberg C, Janssen MJ, Heine RJ, *et al*. Fish oil and glycaemic control in diabetes. *Diabetes Care* 1998; 21: 494–500.

98 Hartweg J, Perera R, Montori V, *et al*. Omega-3 polyunsaturated fatty acids (PUFA) for type 2 diabetes mellitus. *Cochrane Database Syst Rev* 2008; 23(1): CD003205.

99 DeCaterina R, Madonna R, Bertolotto A, *et al*. n-3 Fatty acids in the treatment of diabetic patients: biological rationale and clinical data. *Diabetes Care* 2007; 30(4): 1012–1026.

100 Raeder MB, Steen VM, Vollset SE, *et al*. Associations between cod liver oil use and symptoms of depression: the Hordaland Health Study. *J Affect Disord* 2007; 101(13): 245–249.

101 Hallahan B, Hibbeln JR, Davis JM, *et al*. Omega-3 fatty acid supplementation in patients with recurrent self-harm: single-centre double-blind randomised controlled trial. *Br J Psychiatry* 2007; 190(2): 118–122.

102 Joy C, Mumby-Croft R, Joy LA. Polyunsaturated fatty acid supplementation for schizophrenia. *Cochrane Database Syst Rev* 2006; (3): CD001257.

103 Schachter H, Reisman J, Tran K, *et al*. Effects of Omega-3 Fatty Acids on Mental Health [Evidence Report/Technology Assessment 116]. Rockville, MD: Agency for Healthcare Research and Quality, 2005. http://www.ncbi.nlm.nih.gov/books/NBK37689/ (accessed 1 May 2011).

104 Su K, Huang SY, Chiu CC, *et al*. Omega-3 fatty acids in major depressive disorder. A preliminary double-blind, placebo-controlled trial. *Eur Neuropsychopharmacol* 2003; 13: 267–271.

105 van deRest O, Geleijnse JM, Kok FJ, *et al*. Effect of fish-oil supplementation on mental well-being in older subjects: a randomized, double-blind, placebo-controlled trial. *Am J Clin Nutr* 2008; 88(3): 706–713.

106 MacLean C, Issa AM, Newberry SJ, *et al*. Effects of Omega-3 Fatty Acids on Cognitive Function with Aging, Dementia and Neurological Diseases [Evidence Report/Technology Assessment 114] Rockville, MD: Agency for Healthcare Research and Quality, 2005. http://www.ncbi.nlm.nih.gov/books/NBK37650/ (accessed 1 May 2011).

107 Lim WS, Gammack JK, VanNiekerk J, *et al*. Omega 3 fatty acid for the prevention of dementia. *Cochrane Database Syst Rev* 2006; 25(1): CD005379.

108 Freund-Levi Y, Basun H, Cederholm T, *et al*. Omega-3 supplementation in mild to moderate Alzheimer's disease: effects on neuropsychiatric symptoms. *Int J Geriatr Psychiatry* 2008; 23(2): 161–169.

109 Kotani S, Sakaguchi E, Warashina S, *et al*. Dietary supplementation of arachidonic and docosahexaenoic acids improves cognitive dysfunction. *Neurosci Res* 2006; 56(2): 159–164.

110 Beydoun MA, Kaufman JS, Satia JA, *et al*. Plasma n-3 fatty acids and the risk of cognitive decline in older adults: the Atherosclerosis Risk in Communities Study. *Am J Clin Nutr* 2007; 85 (4): 1103–1111.

111 van Gelder BM, Tijhuis M, Kalmijn S, *et al*. Fish consumption, n-3 fatty acids, and subsequent 5-y

cognitive decline in elderly men: the Zutphen Elderly Study. *Am J Clin Nutr* 2007; 85(4): 1142–1147.

112 Lewin G, Schachter HM, Yuen D, *et al*. Effects of Omega-3 Fatty Acids on Child and Maternal Health [Evidence Report/Technology Assessment 118]. Rockville, MD: Agency for Healthcare Research and Quality, 2005. http://www.ahrq.gov/clinic/epcsums/o3mchsum.htm (accessed 9 May 2011).

113 Szajewska H, Horvath A, Koletzko B. Effect of n-3 long-chain polyunsaturated fatty acid supplementation of women with low-risk pregnancies on pregnancy outcomes and growth measures at birth: a meta-analysis of randomized controlled trials. *Am J Clin Nutr* 2006; 83(6): 1337–1344.

114 Lauritzen L, Jorgensen MH, Olsen SE, *et al*. Maternal fish oil supplementation in lactation: effect on developmental outcomes in breast fed infants. *Reprod Nutr Dev* 2005; 45: 535–547.

115 Lauritzen L, Hoppe C, Straarup EM, *et al*. Maternal fish oil supplementation in lactation and growth during the first 2.5 years of life. *Pediatr Res* 2005; 58(2): 235–242.

116 Jensen CL, Voigt RG, Prager TC, *et al*. Effects of maternal docosahexaenoic acid intake on visual function and neurodevelopment in breastfed term infants. *Am J Clin Nutr* 2005; 82(1): 125–132.

117 Birch EE, Castaneda YS, Wheaton DH, *et al*. Visual maturation of term infants fed long-chain polyunsaturated fatty acid-supplemented or control formula for 12 mo. *Am J Clin Nutr* 2005; 81(4): 871–879.

118 Dunstan JA, Simmer K, Dixon G, *et al*. Cognitive assessment at 2½ years following fish oil supplementation in pregnancy: a randomized controlled trial. *Arch Dis Child Fetal Neonatal Ed* 2008; 93 (1): F45–F50.

119 Dunstan JA, Simmer K, Dixon G, Prescott SL. Cognitive assessment at 2½ years following fish oil supplementation in pregnancy: a randomized controlled trial. *Arch. Dis. Child. Fetal Neonatal Ed.* 2006:adc.2006.099085.

120 Makrides M, Gibson RA, McPhee AJ, *et al*. Effect of DHA supplementation during pregnancy on maternal depression and neurodevelopment of young children: a randomized controlled trial. *JAMA* 2010; 304(15): 1675–1683.

121 Denburg JA, Hatfield HM, Cyr MM, *et al*. Fish oil supplementation in pregnancy modifies neonatal progenitors at birth in infants at risk of atopy. *Pediatr Res* 2005; 57(2): 276–281.

122 Dunstan JA, Mori TA, Barden A, *et al*. Fish oil supplementation in pregnancy modifies neonatal allergen-specific immune responses and clinical outcomes in infants at high risk of atopy: a randomized, controlled trial. *J Allergy Clin Immunol* 2003; 112(6): 1178–1184.

123 Richardson A, Montgomery P. The Oxford–Durham study: a randomized, controlled trial of dietary supplementation with fatty acids in children with developmental disorder. *Pediatrics* 2005; 115: 1360–1366.

124 Hirayama S, Hamazaki T, Terasawa K. Effect of docosahexaenoic acid-containing food administration on symptoms of attention-deficit/hyperactivity disorder — a placebo-controlled double-blind study. *Eur J Clin Nutr* 2004; 58: 467–473.

125 Voigt RG, Llorente AM, Jensen CL, *et al*. A randomized, double-blind, placebo-controlled trial of docosahexaenoic acid supplementation in children with attention-deficit/hyperactivity disorder. *J Pediatr* 2001; 139(2): 189–196.

126 Sinn N, Bryan J. Effect of supplementation with polyunsaturated fatty acids and micronutrients on learning and behavior problems associated with child ADHD. *J Dev Behav Pediatr* 2007; 28(2): 82–91.

127 Sorgi PJ, Hallowell EM, Hutchins HL, *et al*. Effects of an open-label pilot study with high-dose EPA/DHA concentrates on plasma phospholipids and behavior in children with attention deficit hyperactivity disorder. *Nutr J* 2007; 6(1): 16.

128 Itomura M, Hamazaki K, Sawazaki S, *et al*. The effect of fish oil on physical aggression in schoolchildren — a randomized, double-blind, placebo-controlled trial. *J Nutr Biochem* 2005; 16: 163–171.

129 Kirby A, Woodward A, Jackson S, *et al*. A double-blind, placebo-controlled study investigating the effects of omega-3 supplementation in children aged 8–10 years from a mainstream school population. *Res Dev Disabil* 2010; 31(3): 718–730.

130 Gustafsson PA, Birberg-Thornberg U, Duchen K, *et al*. EPA supplementation improves teacher-rated behaviour and oppositional symptoms in children with ADHD. *Acta Paediatr* 2010; 99 (10): 1540–1549.

131 Donadio J, Bergstralh EJ, Offord KP, *et al*. A controlled trial of fish oil in IgA nephropathy. Mayo Nephrology Collaborative Group. *N Engl J Med* 1994; 331: 1194–1199.

132 Alexopoulos E, Stangou M, Pantzaki A, *et al*. Treatment of severe IgA nephropathy with omega-3 fatty acids: the effect of a 'very low dose' regimen. *Ren Fail* 2004; 26(4): 453–459.

133 MacLean C, Newberry SJ, Mojica WA, *et al*. Effects of Omega-3 Fatty Acids on Cancer [Evidence Report/Technology Assessment 191]. Rockville, MD: Agency for Healthcare Research and Quality, 2005. http://www.ahcpr.gov/clinic/epcsums/o3cansum.htm (accessed 9 May 2011).

134 MacLean CH, Newberry SJ, Mojica WA, *et al*. Effects of omega-3 fatty acids on cancer risk. *JAMA* 2006; 295: 403–415.

135 Colomer R, Moreno-Nogueira JM, Garcia-Luna PP, *et al*. n-3 Fatty acids, cancer and cachexia: a systematic review of the literature. *Br J Nutr* 2007; 97(5): 823–831.

136 Albertazzi P, Coupland K. Polyunsaturated fatty acids. Is there a role in postmenopausal osteoporosis prevention? *Maturitas* 2002; 42: 13–22.

137 Weinstock-Guttman B, Baier M, Park Y, *et al.*
Low fat dietary intervention with omega-3 fatty
acid supplementation in multiple sclerosis
patients. *Prostaglandins Leukot Essent Fatty
Acids* 2005; 73(5): 397–404.

138 Hodge W, Barnes D, Schachter HM, *et al.* Effects
of Omega-3 Fatty Acids on Eye Health [Evidence
Report/Technology Assessment 117]. Rockville,
MD: Agency for Healthcare Research and
Quality, 2005. http://www.ahrq.gov/clinic/epc-
sums/o3eyesum.htm (accessed 9 May 2011).

139 Saynor R, Gillott T. Changes in blood lipids and
fibrinogen with a note on safety in a long term
study on the effects of n-3 fatty acids in subjects
receiving fish oil supplements and followed for
seven years. *Lipids* 1992; 27: 533–538.

140 Food and Drug Administration. Final Rule.
Substances affirmed as generally recognized as
safe: menhaden oil. *Fed Reg* 1997; 62: 30750–
30757.

141 Eritsland J, Arnesen H, Seljeflot I, *et al.* Long-term
effects of n-3 polyunsaturated fatty acids on
haemostatic variables and bleeding episodes in
patients with coronary artery disease. *Blood
Coagul Fibrinol* 1995; 6(1): 17–22.

142 Bender NK, Kraynak MA, Chiquette E, *et al.*
Effects of marine fish oils on the anticoagulation
status of patients receiving chronic warfarin therapy. *J Thromb Thrombolysis* 1998; 5(3): 257–261.

143 Buckley MS, Goff AD, Knapp WE. Fish oil interaction with warfarin. *Ann Pharmacother* 2004; 38
(1): 50–52.

Flavonoids

Description

Flavonoids (or bioflavonoids) are a large group of polyphenolic compounds, ubiquitously present in foods of plant origin. Some flavonoids (e.g. quercetin, rutin) are available as dietary supplements.

Constituents

Bioflavonoids are a group of polyphenolic anti-oxidants, which often occur as glycosides. Flavonoids can be further subdivided into five main groups:

- flavonols (e.g. kaempferol, quercetin and myricetin);
- flavones (e.g. apigenin and luteolin);
- flavonones (e.g. hesperetin, naringenin, eriodictyol);
- flavan-3-ols (e.g. (+)-catechin, (+)-gallo-catechin, (−)-epicatechin, (−)-epigallocate-chin);
- anthocyanins (e.g. cyanidin, delphinidin, mal-vidin, pelargonidin, peonidin, petunidin); and
- proanthocyanidins.

More than 4000 flavonoids have been identi-fied, and many have been studied in the labora-tory and in animal studies, but apart from quercetin, few have been studied in humans.

Most flavonoids are colourless but some are responsible for the bright colours of many fruit and vegetables. Flavonoids are distinguished from the carotenoids (see Carotenoids), which are the red, yellow and orange pigments found in fruit and vegetables. Unlike carotenoids, flavonoids are water soluble.

Action

Flavonoids appear to display several effects.[1] They:

- act as scavengers of free radicals, including superoxide anions, singlet oxygen and lipid peroxyl radicals (they have antioxidant properties);
- sequester metal ions;
- inhibit *in vitro* oxidation of LDL cholesterol;
- inhibit cyclo-oxygenase, leading to lower platelet aggregation, decreased thrombotic tendency and reduced anti-inflammatory activity;
- inhibit histamine release;
- improve capillary function by reducing fragil-ity of capillary walls and thus preventing abnormal leakage; and
- inhibit various stages of tumour development (animal studies only).

The activities of flavonoids are dependent on their chemical structure.

Human requirements

No proof of a dietary need exists.

Dietary intake

Estimates of dietary flavonoid intake vary from 10 to 100 mg daily, depending on the population studied, the technique used and the number and identity of flavonoids measured. If all flavonoids are included, intake may be several hundreds of milligrams a day, particularly if red wine is consumed in large amounts. Estimated mean daily total flavonoid intake among US adults is 189.7 mg, mainly from flavan-3-ols (83.5%), followed by flavanones (7.6%), flavonols (6.8%), anthocyanidins (1.6%), flavones (0.8%) and isoflavones (0.6%). The greatest daily mean intake of flavonoids was from the following foods: tea (157 mg), citrus fruit juices (8 mg), wine (4 mg) and citrus fruits (3 mg).[2]

Dietary sources

Flavonoids are found in the white segment or ring of fruit (especially citrus fruit) and vegetables, and also in tea and red wine. In the UK, tea, apples and onions seem to be major sources. Flavonoid content of foods varies widely (see Table 1). Cherry tomatoes contain higher concentrations than normal-sized tomatoes, and Lollo Rosso lettuce more than iceberg lettuce.[1] The flavonoid content of red wine may also vary widely, depending on the source, growing conditions and harvesting of the grapes.[3] Chocolate is also a good source of flavonoids (including flavonols, flavanols, catechins, epicatechins and proanthocyanidins).

Possible uses

Flavonoids have been investigated for a potential role in the prevention of cardiovascular disease (CVD), cancer and cataracts. The totality of evidence suggests a role for flavonoids in prevention of CVD, cancer and possibly other chronic diseases.[4,5]

Cardiovascular disease

Epidemiological studies have suggested that consumption of fruit and vegetables may protect against CVD. That such a benefit could occur as a result of dietary antioxidant vitamins is well known, but the presence of flavonoids in these foods may also account for these findings. Research interest in specific flavonoid-rich foods (mostly cocoa, tea, red wine and soya) has also developed in relation to CVD, with mixed findings.[6]

Flavonoids may help to reduce the risk of heart disease (possibly by helping to dilate the coronary arteries and by preventing atherosclerosis). The Zutphen study from the Netherlands[7] demonstrated a reduced risk of coronary heart disease (CHD) and a reduced incidence of myocardial infarction in men aged 65–84 years associated with increased ingestion of dietary flavonoids. The major dietary sources of flavonoids in this study were tea (61%), onions (13%) and apples (10%). Flavonoid intake was inversely associated with CHD mortality, with a 68% reduction in risk for intake > 19 mg daily. There was, however, no correlation between flavonoid intake and CHD incidence among those with no history of myocardial infarction. The researchers later updated their results,[8] extending follow-up to 10 years. Similar results for CHD mortality were found, but a smaller risk reduction and a borderline significant trend ($P = 0.08$) for the incidence of CHD existed.

Another part of the Zutphen study[9] investigated a cohort of men aged 50–69 years, following them up for 15 years. Dietary flavonoids (mainly quercetin) were inversely associated with stroke incidence after adjustment for potential confounders, including antioxidant vitamins. The relative risk (RR) of stroke for the highest versus the lowest quartile of flavonoid intake was 0.27. A lower stroke risk was also observed for the highest quartile of beta-carotene intake, but vitamins C and E were not associated with stroke risk. Black tea contributed about 70% to flavonoid intake. The RR for daily consumption of 4.7 cups or more of tea versus less than 2.6 cups of tea was 0.31 (95% confidence interval (CI), 0.12 to 0.84).

However, the Caerphilly study in Wales showed no reduced risk of heart disease with increasing flavonoid consumption.[10] This

Table 1 Flavonoid content of selected foods (mg/100 g)

Food	Flavonols	Flavones	Flavanones	Flavan-3-ols	Anthocyanidins	Pro-anthocyanidins
Apples	4.42	0	–	9.09	–	80–130
Bananas	–	–	–	0	–	3.37
Beans, kidney	–	–	–	2.01	–	510
Blackberries	–	–	–	–	–	23.31
Blackcurrants	13.50	–	–	1.17		149.7
Blueberries	3.93	–	–	1.11	112.55	176.49
Broccoli, cooked	2.44	–	–	–	–	0
Cherries, raw	1.25	0	–	11.70	117.42	19.13
Chocolate bar, dark	–	–	–	53.49	–	170
Chocolate bar, milk	–	–	–	13.45	–	70
Elderberry, raw	42.00	–	–	–	749.24	–
Grapefruit juice	0.1	–	24.13	–	–	0
Grapes, black	2.8	0	–	20.9	–	–
Grapes, green	1.32	0	–	4.92	–	81.54
Kale, raw	34.45	0	–	–	–	–
Kiwi	–	–	–	0.45	–	1.83
Lemon juice, raw	–	0	18.33	–	–	–
Nectarines	–	–	–	2.74	–	29.36
Onions, cooked	19.71	–	–	–	–	0
Onions, red, raw	37.87	0	–	–	13.14	–
Orange juice	–	–	5.08	–	–	0
Orange	–	–	43.88	–	–	0
Parsley, raw	8.85	303.24	0	–	–	0
Peaches	0	0	0	2.33	–	71.75
Pears	0.3	0	–	3.53	–	42.3
Plums, black	1.2	0	–	6.19	–	220.66
Pomegranate	–	–	–	–	–	1.10
Raspberries	0.83	–	–	9.23	47.6	25.07
Strawberries	1.44	0	–	4.47	–	141.67
Tea, black, brewed	3.86	0	–	73.44	–	13.34
Tea, green, brewed	5.21	0.34	–	132.43	–	–
Tomato, cherry	2.87	–	–	–	–	0
Tomato, raw	0.64	0	–	–	–	0
Thyme, fresh	–	56.00	–	–	–	–
Wine, table red	1.64	0	–	11.9	9.19	61.63
Wine, table white	0.06	0	–	1.38	0.06	0.81

USDA database: http://www.nal.usda.gov/fnic/foodcomp
–, Not analysed to date.

investigation involved 1900 men aged 45–59 years who were studied for up to 14 years. Tea provided 82% of the flavonoid intake, and was strongly and positively associated with risk of CHD.

Baseline flavonoid intake was estimated in 16 cohorts of the Seven Countries Study,[11] and mortality from CHD, cancer and all causes was investigated after 25 years of follow-up. Average intake of flavonoids was inversely associated with mortality from CHD and explained about 25% of the variance in CHD rates in the 16 cohorts. Flavonoid intake was not independently associated with mortality from other causes, including cancer.

Two studies used data from American cohorts of men and women. One study investigated the relationship between flavonoid intake and CHD risk in 34 789 men aged 40–75 years in 1986 with a follow-up of 6 years.[12] The main sources of flavonoids were tea and onions. Flavonoid intake > 40 mg daily was not associated with reduced CHD risk. The Iowa Womens' Health Study[13] investigated 34 492 postmenopausal women aged 55–69 for subsequent risk of CHD over a 10-year follow-up period. Compared with women in the lowest quintile (< 5.8 mg daily) of flavonoid intake, those in the highest quintile (18.7 mg daily) had a significant 32% reduced risk of CHD death.

The association of tea intake with aortic atherosclerosis has also been investigated in a Dutch study.[14] In a prospective study of 3454 men and women aged 55 and older, who were free of CVD at baseline, tea intake was inversely correlated with severe (but not mild or moderate) aortic atherosclerosis.

A meta-analysis of seven prospective cohort studies published before 2001 included 2087 fatal CHD events. Comparison of those in the top third with those in the bottom third of dietary flavonol intake yielded a combined RR of 0.8 (95% CI, 0.69 to 0.93) after adjustment for known CHD risk factors and other dietary components. The authors concluded that high dietary intakes of flavonols from a small number of fruits and vegetables, tea and red wine may be associated with reduced risk of CHD mortality in free-living populations.[15]

A prospective study in 38 445 women (free of CVD and cancer) with a mean follow-up period of 6.9 years found no significant linear trend for CVD and important vascular events across quintiles of flavonoid intake. No individual flavonol or flavone was associated with CVD. Broccoli and apple consumption were associated with non-significant reductions in CVD risk. A small proportion of women (1185) consuming four or more cups of tea a day had a reduction in the risk of important vascular events but with a non-significant linear trend. In this study flavonoid intake was not strongly associated with risk of CVD.[16]

In the SU.VI.MAX study (an 8-year trial evaluating the effect of antioxidant supplementation on the incidence of major chronic disease), flavonoid-rich food in women was inversely associated with systolic blood pressure. No such relationship was seen in men. Women in the highest tertile of flavonoid-rich food consumption were at lower risk for CVD (odds ratio (OR), 0.31; 95% CI, 0.14 to 0.68), while a positive tendency was observed in men. In this study, a high consumption of flavonoid-rich food appeared to reduce cardiovascular risk in women.[17]

The Iowa Womens' Health Study, an epidemiological study in 34 489 postmenopausal women, evaluated the intake of flavonoids through a food frequency questionnaire. The findings were that dietary intakes of flavanones, anthocyanidins and certain foods rich in flavonoids (e.g. bran, apples, pears, strawberries, chocolate, red wine) were associated with reduced risk of death from CHD, CVD and all causes.[18] However, epidemiological data from the US Nurses' Health Study did not support an inverse association between either flavanol or flavone intake and CHD risk.[19]

In the Kuopio (Finnish) Ischaemic Heart Disease Risk Factor Study, higher intakes of flavonoids were associated with reduced risk of stroke. Men in the highest quartile of flavonol and flavan-3-ol intakes, respectively, had RR values of 0.55 (95% CI, 0.31 to 0.99) and 0.59 (95% CI, 0.30 to 1.14) for ischaemic stroke compared with the lowest quartile. After multivariate adjustment, the RR for CVD death in the highest quartile of flavanone and flavone intakes were 0.54 (95% CI, 0.32 to 0.92) and 0.65 (95% CI, 0.40 to 1.05), respectively.[20] A meta-analysis of prospective studies suggested that a high intake of flavonols, compared with a low intake, was inversely associated with non-fatal and fatal stroke with a pooled RR of 0.80 (95% CI, 0.65 to 0.98).[21]

Chocolate has attracted attention for its possible role in preventing CVD. A systematic review of 136 publications, mainly short-term feeding trials, suggested that cocoa and chocolate may exert benefit on cardiovascular risk via lowering blood pressure, anti-inflammatory effects, anti-platelet function, raised HDL and decreased LDL oxidation. An associated meta-analysis of flavonoid intake suggests that these compounds may lower cardiovascular mortality.[22]

Intervention trials have shown that flavonoids can reverse endothelial dysfunction. Endothelial dysfunction appears to be important in the pathogenesis of CVD so any improvement could reduce the risk of coronary events. However, there is considerable variation in the response in endothelial function to flavonoids and this may be related to inter-individual differences in flavonoid metabolism.[23–25] Evidence also suggests an inverse relationship between dietary flavonoids and carotid artery intima-media thickness, which could also contribute to the reduced CVD risk with higher flavonoid intake.[26]

Cancer

Activity of flavonoids against malignant cells has been demonstrated *in vitro*,[27–29] and there is much current interest in the potential use of bioflavonoids in the prevention and treatment of cancer.

In a Finnish study involving 9959 men and women (initially cancer free) aged from 15 to 99, high dietary flavonoid intake was shown to reduce the risk of cancer.[30] Researchers involved in the Iowa Women's Health Study showed that in 35 000 postmenopausal women, those who drank more than two cups of tea a day were 32% less likely to have cancers of the mouth, oesophagus, stomach, colon and rectum. Risk of urinary tract cancer was reduced by 60%. In those who drank more than four cups of tea a day, the risk of cancer was lowered by 63%.[31] Onions are high in flavonoids, which might explain the reduced risk of stomach cancer among those with a high intake of onions in a group of 120 852 men and women aged 55 to 69 years.[32] In another US study among middle-aged and older women, there was no evidence of a major role for five common flavonols and

flavones or selected flavonoid-rich foods in cancer prevention.[33]

A review of data from four cohort studies and six case-control studies examining associations between flavonoid intake and cancer risk found consistent evidence that flavonoids, especially quercetin, may reduce the risk of lung cancer.[34]

In the Nurses' Health Study II, validated food frequency questionnaires from 90 630 women showed no associations between flavonols and breast cancer risk and there were no associations between individual flavonols such as kaempferol, quercetin and myricetin and breast cancer risk. However, there was a significant inverse association between breast cancer and beans and lentils.[35]

The risk of colorectal cancer in relation to flavonoid intake was evaluated in a Scottish prospective case–control study. Increased consumption of flavonols, quercetin, catechin and epicatechin were associated with reduced colorectal cancer risk even after controlling for fruit and vegetable consumption. No risk reductions were observed with intake of flavones, flavonones and phytoestrogens.[36] Further analysis of data from the same study showed that flavonols, specifically quercetin, obtained from non-tea components of the diet may be linked with reduced risk of developing colon cancer.[37] However, findings from a Dutch case–control study did not support an association of dietary flavonol, flavone and catechin intake with colorectal cancer.[38]

A high intake of flavonoids was also associated with a reduced incidence of lung cancer in middle-aged Finnish men who smoked.[39] The conclusion of a meta-analysis, which included eight prospective studies and four case–control studies, was that the highest intake of flavonoids was significantly associated with decreased lung cancer risk in prospective studies, studies conducted in Finnish population, studies without adjustment for fruits and vegetables or vitamins, men, smokers and studies using dietary history interview for flavonoids intake estimation.[40]

Ovarian cancer risk has aslso been studied. In an Italian prospective study, there was a significant trend towards reduced risk between ovarian cancer and flavonols (OR, 0.63; 95% CI, 0.47 to 0.84) as well as isoflavones (OR, 0.51; 95% CI, 0.37 to0.69), comparing the highest with the lowest quintile.[41]

Cataract

There may be a role for flavonoids in preventing diabetes-related cataract formation. In diabetes mellitus, excess sorbitol or dulcitol is produced by the conversion of glucose by aldose reductase. The dulcitol cannot be further metabolised and therefore forms a hard crystalline layer in the lens, which forms the cataract. Flavonoids are potent inhibitors of the enzyme,[42] but further studies are required before flavonoids could be recommended for cataract prevention.

Miscellaneous

Experimental studies have demonstrated that some flavonoids prevent ulcer formation,[43] and that they may be useful in treating ulcers. Dietary flavonoid intake may contribute to maintaining healthy body weight.[44] Diets high in some flavonoid-rich foods have been associated with better cognitive performance in older people.[45]

Flavonoids have been investigated for potential anti-viral activity. *In vitro* tests have shown some activity against rhinovirus (responsible for 50% of common colds), but little activity against herpes simplex and influenza virus.[46]

Many claims have been made for the usefulness of bioflavonoids in a range of disorders, including haemorrhoids, allergy, asthma, menopausal symptoms and the prevention of habitual abortion, but scientific studies are required to investigate these claims.

The suggestion has been made that flavonoids may reduce the occurrence of type 2 diabetes. However, a prospective study in 38 018 women aged over 45 and free of CVD, cancer and diabetes with an average 8.8-year follow-up found that total flavonols, flavones or individual compounds were associated with risk of type 2 diabetes, although apple and tea consumption was inversely associated with diabetes risk.[47]

Quercetin

As a dietary supplement, quercetin is promoted for prevention and treatment of atherosclerosis and hyperlipidaemia, diabetes, cataracts, hay fever, peptic ulcer, inflammation, prevention of cancer and for treating prostatitis. A preliminary, double-blind, placebo-controlled trial in chronic non-bacterial prostatitis showed that quercetin reduced pain and improved quality of life, but had no effect on voiding dysfunction.[48] However, there is insufficient reliable information about the effectiveness of quercetin for other indications.

Rutin

As a dietary supplement, rutin is used to reduce capillary permeability and treat symptoms of varicose veins. In combination with bromelain and trypsin, rutin is used to treat osteoarthritis. In one double-blind trial, 73 patients with osteoarthritis of the knee were randomly assigned to a combination enzyme product (containing rutin, bromelain and trypsin) or diclofenac. The enzyme product had a similar effect on reducing pain and mobility of the knee to diclofenac.[49] However, there is insufficient reliable information about the effectiveness of rutin for other indications.

> **Conclusion**
> High dietary intakes of flavonoids have been linked with a reduced risk of CHD, cancer and cataracts. However, although a number of supplements (e.g. quercetin, rutin) are now available, there is currently only limited evidence that supplements are beneficial in any condition.

Pregnancy and breast-feeding

No problems have been reported.

Adverse effects

None reported. However, there are no long-term studies assessing the safety of flavonoid supplements.

Interactions

None reported.

Dose

Flavonoids (e.g. quercetin, rutin) are available in the form of tablets and capsules.

The dose is not established; dietary supplements of quercetin and rutin provide around 500 mg in a single dose.

References

1 Crozier A, McDonald MS, Lean MEJ, Black C. Quantitative analysis of the flavonoid content of tomatoes, onions, lettuce and celery. *J Agric Food Chem* 1997; 45: 590–595.

2 Chun OK, Chung SJ, Song WO. Estimateddietary flavonoid intake and major food sources of U.S. adults. *J Nutr* 2007; 137(5): 1244–1252.

3 McDonald MS, Hughes M, Burns J, *et al.* A survey of the free and conjugated flavonol content of sixty five red wines of different geographical origin. *J Agric Food Chem* 1998; 46: 368–375.

4 Knekt P, Kumpulainen J, Jarvinen R, *et al.* Flavonoid intake and risk of chronic diseases. *Am J Clin Nutr* 2002; 76: 560–568.

5 Graf BA, Milbury PE, Blumberg JB. Flavonols, flavones, flavonones and human health. *J Med Food* 2005; 8: 281–290.

6 Hooper L, Kroon PA, Rimm EB, *et al.* Flavonoids, flavonoid-rich foods, and cardiovascular risk: a meta-analysis of randomized controlled trials. *Am J Clin Nutr* 2008; 88(1): 38–50.

7 Hertog MGL, Feskens EJM, Hollman PCH, *et al.* Dietary antioxidant flavonoids and risk of coronary heart disease: the Zutphen elderly study. *Lancet* 1993; 342: 1007–1011.

8 Hertog MG, Feskens EJ, Hollman PC, *et al.* Antioxidant flavonols and coronary heart disease risk (letter). *Lancet* 1997; 349: 699.

9 Keli SO, Hertog MG, Feskens EJ. Dietary flavonoids, antioxidant vitamins and the incidence of stroke; the Zutphen study. *Arch Intern Med* 1996; 156: 637–642.

10 Hertog MG, Sweetman PM, Fehily AM, *et al.* Antioxidant flavonols and ischaemic heart disease in a Welsh population of men: the Caerphilly Study. *Am J Clin Nutr* 1997; 65: 1489–1494.

11 Hertog MG, Kromhout D, Aravanis C, *et al.* Flavonoid intake and long-term risk of coronary heart disease and cancer in the seven countries study. *Arch Intern Med* 1995; 155: 381–386.

12 Rimm EB, Katam MB, Ascherio A, *et al.* Relation between intakes of flavonoids and risk for coronary heart disease in male health professionals. *Ann Intern Med* 1996; 125: 384–389.

13 Yochum L, Kushi LH, Meyer K, Folsom AR. Dietary flavonoid intake and risk of cardiovascular disease in postmenopausal women. *Am J Epidemiol* 1999; 149: 943–949.

14 Geleijinse JM, Launer LJ, Hofman A, *et al.* Tea flavonoids may protect against atherosclerosis. *Arch Intern Med* 1999; 159: 2170–2174.

15 Huxley RR, Neil HA. The relation between dietary flavonol intake and coronary heart disease mortality: a meta-analysis of prospective cohort studies. *Eur J Clin Nutr* 2003; 57: 904–908.

16 Sesso HD, Gaziano JM, Liu S, Buring JE. Flavonoid intake and the risk of cardiovascular disease in women. *Am J Clin Nutr* 2003; 77: 1440–1448.

17 Mennen LI, Saphino D, deBree A, *et al.* Consumption of foods rich in flavonoids is related to a decreased cardiovascular risk in apparently healthy women. *J Nutr* 2004; 134: 923–926.

18 Mink PJ, Scrafford CG, Barraj LM, *et al.* Flavonoid intake and cardiovascular disease mortality: a prospective study in postmenopausal women. *Am J Clin Nutr* 2007; 85(3): 895–909.

19 Lin J, Rexrode KM, Hu F, *et al.* Dietary intakes of flavonols and flavones and coronary heart disease in US women. *Am J Epidemiol* 2007; 165(11): 1305–1313.

20 Mursu J, Voutilainen S, Nurmi T, *et al.* Flavonoid intake and the risk of ischaemic stroke and CVD mortality in middle-aged Finnish men: the Kuopio Ischaemic Heart Disease Risk Factor Study. *Br J Nutr* 2008; 100(4): 890–895.

21 Hollman PC, Geelen A, Kromhout D. Dietary flavonol intake may lower stroke risk in men and women. *J Nutr* 2010; 140(3): 600–604.

22 Ding EL, Hutfless SM, Ding X, Girotra S. Chocolate and prevention of cardiovascular disease: a systematic review. *Nutr Metab* 2006; 3: 2.

23 Hodgson J, Puddey IB, Burke V, Croft KD. Is reversal of endothelial dysfunction by tea related to flavonoid metabolism? *Br J Nutr* 2006; 95: 14–17.

24 Geraets L, Moonen HJJ, Brauers K, *et al.* Dietary flavones and flavonoles are inhibitors of poly(ADP-ribose)polymerase-1 in pulmonary epithelial cells. *J. Nutr* 2007; 137(10): 2190–2195.

25 Loke WM, Hodgson JM, Proudfoot JM, *et al.* Pure dietary flavonoids quercetin and (−)-epicatechin augment nitric oxide products and reduce endothelin-1 acutely in healthy men. *Am J Clin Nutr* 2008; 88(4): 1018–1025.

26 Mursu J, Nurmi T, Tuomainen TP, *et al.* The intake of flavonoids and carotid atherosclerosis: the Kuopio Ischaemic Heart Disease Risk Factor Study. *Br J Nutr* 2007; 98(4): 814–818.

27 Havsteen B. Flavonoids. A class of natural products of high pharmacological potency. *Biochem Pharmacol* 1983; 32: 1141.

28 Tripathi VD, Rastogi RP. Flavonoids in biology and medicine. *J Sci Ind Res* 1981; 40: 116.

29 Kandaswami C, Perkins E, Soloniuk DS, *et al.* Antiproliferative effects of citrus flavonoids on a human squamous cell carcinoma *in vitro. Cancer Lett* 1991; 56: 147–152.

30 Knekt P, Jarvinen R, Seppanen R, *et al.* Dietary flavonoids and the risk of lung cancer and other malignant neoplasms. *Am J Epidemiol* 1997; 146: 223–230.

31 Zheng W, Doyle TJ, Kushi LH. Tea consumption and cancer incidence in a prospective cohort study of postmenopausal women. *Am J Epidemiol* 1996; 144: 175–182.

32 Dorant E, van denBrandt PA, Goldbohm RA. Consumption of onions and a reduced risk of stomach carcinoma. *Gastroenterology* 1996; 110: 12–20.

33 Wang L, Lee IM, Zhang SM, *et al*. Dietary intake of selected flavonols, flavones, and flavonoid-rich foods and risk of cancer in middle-aged and older women. *Am J Clin Nutr* 2009; 89(3): 905–912.

34 Neuhouser ML. Dietary flavonoids and cancer risk: evidence from human population studies. *Nutr Cancer* 2004; 50: 1–7.

35 Adebamowo CA, Cho E, Sampson L, *et al*. Dietary flavonol-rich foods intake and the risk of breast cancer. *Int J Cancer* 2005; 114: 628–633.

36 Theodoratou E, Kyle J, Cetnarskyj R, *et al*. Dietary flavonoids and the risk of colorectal cancer. *Cancer Epidemiol Biomarkers Prev* 2007; 16(4): 684–693.

37 Kyle JA, Sharp L, Little J, *et al*. Dietary flavonoid intake and colorectal cancer: a case-control study. *Br J Nutr* 2009; 103(3): 429–436.

38 Simons CC, Hughes LA, Arts IC, *et al*. Dietary flavonol, flavone and catechin intake and risk of colorectal cancer in the Netherlands Cohort Study. *Int J Cancer* 2009; 125(12): 2945–2952.

39 Mursu J, Nurmi T, Tuomainen TP, *et al*. Intake of flavonoids and risk of cancer in Finnish men: the Kuopio Ischaemic Heart Disease Risk Factor Study. *Int J Cancer* 2008; 123(3): 660–663.

40 Tang NP, Zhou B, Wang B, *et al*. Flavonoids intake and risk of lung cancer: a meta-analysis. *Jpn J Clin Oncol* 2009; 39(6): 352–359.

41 Rossi M, Negri E, Lagiou P, *et al*. Flavonoids and ovarian cancer risk: a case–control study in Italy. *Int J Cancer* 2008; 123(4): 895–898.

42 Wagner H. Phenolic compounds ofpharmaceutical interest. In: Swain T, Harborne JB, Van Sumere CF (eds). *Biochemistry of Plant Phenolics*. New York: Plenum Press, 1979; 604–605.

43 Farkas L, Gabor M, Kallay F, Wagner H. Flavonoids and bioflavonoids. In *Proceedings, International Bioflavonoid Symposium, Munich*. Amsterdam: Elsevier,1977.

44 Hughes LA, Arts IC, Ambergen T, *et al*. Higher dietary flavone, flavonol, and catechin intakes are associated with less of an increase in BMI over time in women: a longitudinal analysis from the Netherlands Cohort Study. *Am J Clin Nutr* 2008; 88(5): 1341–1352.

45 Nurk E, Refsum H, Drevon CA, *et al*. Intake of flavonoid-rich wine, tea, and chocolate by elderly men and women is associated with better cognitive test performance. *J Nutr* 2009; 139(1): 120–127.

46 Tshuiya Y, Shimuzu M, Hiyama Y, *et al*. Antiviral activity of naturally occurring flavonoids *in vitro*. *Chem Pharm Bull* 1985; 33: 3881.

47 Song Y, Manson JE, Buring JE, *et al*. Associations of dietary flavonoids with risk of type 2 diabetes and markers of insulin resistance and systemic inflammation in women: a prospective study and cross-sectional analysis. *J Am Coll Nutr* 2005; 24: 376–384.

48 Shoskes DA, Zeitlin SI, Shahed A, Rajfer A. Quercetin in men with category III chronic prostatitis: a preliminary prospective, double-blind, placebo-controlled trial. *Urology* 1999; 54: 960–963.

49 Klein G, Kullich W. Short-term treatment of painful osteoarthritis of the knee with oral enzymes. *Clin Drug Invest* 2000; 19: 15–23.

Flaxseed oil

Description

Flaxseed is the soluble fibre mucilage obtained from the fully developed seed of *Linus usitatissimum*.

Constituents

Flaxseed is a rich source of alpha-linolenic acid (ALA) and lignans. ALA is the parent polyunsaturated fatty acid (PUFA) of the n-3 (omega-3) series. ALA should not be confused with linoleic acid (LA), which is the parent PUFA of the n-6 (omega-6) series of PUFAs. It has been estimated that the ratio of n-3 to n-6 fatty acids in the diet of early humans was 1 : 1,[1] but the ratio in the typical Western diet is now around 1 : 10 due to increased use of vegetable oils rich in LA as well as reduced fish consumption.[2]

Action

Flaxseed oil, which contains approximately three times more n-3 than n-6 fatty acids, may help to reverse the imbalance between n-3 and n-6 fats.

ALA is converted to longer-chain PUFAs such as eicosapentaenoic acid (EPA) and docosahexaenoic acid (DHA) through a series of elongation and desaturation reactions. However, studies suggest that conversion of ALA to longer-chain PUFAs, particularly DHA, in human beings is limited.[3,4] One small study showed that flaxseed oil supplementation could elevate levels of EPA (but not DHA) in tissues to concentrations comparable with those associated with fish oil supplementation.[5] Dietary flaxseed oil supplementation in lactating women increased breast milk, plasma and erythrocyte content of ALA, EPA and docosapentaenoic acid (DPA), but had no effect on breast milk, plasma or erythrocyte DHA content.[6] There is also evidence that ALA conversion can be down-regulated by increased availability of EPA and DHA, but is not up-regulated by increased ALA consumption.[7]

Preliminary data suggest that men and women differ in their ability to convert ALA to EPA and DHA. Studies of ALA metabolism in healthy young men indicate that approximately 8% of dietary ALA is converted to EPA and 0–4% is converted to DHA.[8] In healthy young women, approximately 21% of dietary ALA is converted to EPA and 9% is converted to DHA.[9] The increased conversion efficiency of young women compared to men appears to be related to the effects of oestrogen.[10,11]

LA is also converted to longer-chain PUFAs, such as dihomo-gamma-linolenic acid (DGLA) and arachidonic acid (AA). ALA and LA compete for the same elongase and desaturase enzymes in the synthesis of longer-chain PUFA. Although ALA is the preferred substrate of the delta-6 desaturase enzyme, an excess of dietary LA compared with ALA results in a greater proportion of AA relative to EPA formation.[10,12] With a diet rich in LA, conversion of ALA to its longer-chain derivatives has been shown to be reduced by 40–50%.[3] Reducing intake of n-6 from vegetable oils and increasing intake of n-3 rich flaxseed oil has been shown to maximise EPA levels.[5]

Lignans are a type of phytoestrogen. They are digested in the colon to produce enterodiol and enterolactone, lignans that are thought to be protective against cancer.

Bioavailability

Consumption of 2.4 or 3.6 g flaxseed oil daily (in capsules) has been shown to be sufficient to significantly increase erythrocyte ALA, EPA and DPA, but unlike fish oil (0.6 or 1.2 g daily) did not raise erythrocyte DHA.[13] A study using whole or milled flaxseed (30 g) or flaxseed oil (containing 6 g ALA) baked into muffins and tested in healthy men and women over 3 months found that flaxseed oil and milled flaxseed delivered significant levels of ALA into plasma while whole flaxseed did not. No significant changes were detected in either plasma EPA or DHA.[14] A study testing the bioavailability of 50 g flaxseed flour and 20 g flaxseed oil in healthy subjects found plasma n-3 fatty acids were raised only after 2 and 4 weeks of supplementation, respectively.[15] Consumption of raw ground flaxseed (5–25 g) for 7 days raised urinary lignan (enterolactone and enterodiol) levels in a dose-dependent manner in healthy, young women. There were no differences in total urinary lignan excretion with the raw compared to the processed forms of flaxseed at an intake of 25 g.[16]

Possible uses

Traditionally, flaxseed has been used for constipation and other bowel disorders such as diverticulitis and irritable bowel syndrome (IBS). In theory, it may also be useful as a source of n-3 fatty acids for the same conditions (e.g. cardiovascular disease and other inflammatory disorders) where fish oil has benefit. It is also a useful oil for vegetarians, to help improve the balance between omega-3 and omega-6 fatty acids, because vegetarians tend to consume significant quantities of omega-6 fatty acids.

Cardiovascular disease
Several human trials (Table 1) have evaluated the effect of flaxseed on cardiovascular disease, cardiovascular mortality and cardiovascular risk markers. There is some evidence that flaxseed can favourably influence blood lipids and markers of inflammation, but the trials have employed disparate, and in some cases poor, methodology, making it difficult to conclude that flaxseed is of benefit. Findings in these trials depend on the duration of the trial, the types of subject, the dose and the food or capsule vehicle for flaxseed.

Cancer
There is some evidence from animal studies that flaxseed inhibits tumour growth, particularly mammary tumours.[42,43]. Evidence from a

Table 1 Human studies evaluating flaxseed in cardiovascular disease and its risk factors

Reference	Duration and type of trial	Dose of flaxseed	Study group	Outcome measures	Observed effects
Allman et al. (1995)[17]	Prospective study with random allocation	Flaxseed oil vs sunflower seed oil	11 healthy young men	Platelet fatty acids, platelet aggregation	Platelet EPA:arachidonic acid ratio (considered a marker for reduced thromboxane production and platelet aggregation potential) increased in the flaxseed group ($P < 0.05$); platelet aggregation response decreased in those taking flaxseed oil ($P < 0.05$)
Bloedon et al. 2008[18]	10-week placebo-controlled randomised trial	40 g/day flaxseed in baked products vs wheat bran baked products with low-fat diet	62 men and postmenopausal women with dyslipidaemia	Fasting lipoproteins, measures of insulin resistance, inflammation, oxidative stress, safety	Compared with wheat, flaxseed significantly reduced LDL cholesterol at 5 but not 10 weeks; flaxseed reduced lipoprotein(a) by a net of 14% ($P = 0.02$), and reduced insulin resistance compared with wheat at 10 weeks, but did not affect markers of inflammation (IL-6, CRP) or oxidative stress (oxidized LDL, urinary isoprostanes) at any time points; in men, flaxseed reduced plasma HDL cholesterol by a net of 16% ($P = 0.03$) and 9% ($P = 0.05$) at 5 and 10 weeks, respectively
Brouwer et al. (2004)[19]	Meta-analysis	Flaxseed oil	5 prospective cohort studies and 3 clinical trials	Mortality from heart disease	Reduced mortality but increased risk of prostate cancer
Coulman et al. (2009)[20]	Randomised crossover study	25 g flaxseed vs 25 g sesame seed vs 12.5 g flaxseed + 12.5 g sesame seed	16 postmenopausal women	Plasma lipids	Plasma lipids unaffected by all treatments
Dodin et al. (2005, 2008)[21,22]	12-month randomised controlled study	40 g/day flaxseed vs wheatgerm	191 women	Fatty acids, apoA1, apoB, lipoprotein(a), cholesterol, LDL particle size, fibrinogen, CRP, insulin, glucose	Flaxseed had a limited effect on lipoprotein metabolism; it reduced total serum and HDL cholesterol compared with wheatgerm
Finnegan et al. (2003)[23]	6-month placebo-controlled, parallel study	0.8 or 1.7 g/day EPA + DHA, 4.5 or 9.5 g ALA/day, or an n-6 PUFA control	150 moderately hyperlipidaemic study	Atherogenic risk factors	Change in fasting or postprandial lipid, glucose, or insulin concentrations or blood pressure was not significantly different after any of the n-3 PUFA interventions compared with the n-6 PUFA control; EPA + DHA reduced triacylglycerol to a greater extent than ALA; susceptibility to LDL oxidation was higher after EPA + DHA than control or ALA
Fukumitsu et al. (2010)[24]	12-week double-blind, randomised, placebo-controlled study	Flaxseed lignan capsules vs placebo	30 moderately hypercholesterolaemic men	Plasma cholesterol and liver disease risk factors	Significant reduction in the LDL/HDL cholesterol ratio with flaxseed; improvement in liver enzyme levels

Reference	Study design	Intervention	Subjects	Outcome measures	Results
Goyens & Mensink (2006)[25]	9-week randomised double-blind study	ALA-rich diet (6.8 g/day) vs EPA/DHA-rich diet (1.05 g EPA/day + 0.55 g DHA/day) vs control (oleic acid-rich diet)	37 mildly hypercholesterolaemic subjects, 14 men and 23 women aged 60–78 years	Cardiovascular risk markers	ALA influenced LDL cholesterol and apoB levels more favourably than did EPA/DHA
Hallund et al. (2006)[26]	2 × 6-week randomised double-blind, placebo-controlled crossover study	Low-fat muffin with and without flaxseed lignan	22 healthy postmenopausal women	Flow-mediated, endothelium-dependent vasodilatation and nitroglycerin-mediated, endothelium-independent vasodilatation	No effect of flaxseed lignan on endothelial function
Hallund et al. (2008)[27]	2 × 6-week randomised double-blind, placebo-controlled crossover study	Low-fat muffin with and without flaxseed lignan	22 healthy postmenopausal women	CRP, IL6, tumour necrosis factor-alpha, soluble intracellular adhesion molecule-1, soluble vascular cell adhesion molecule-1, monocyte chemoattractant protein-1	Reduction in CRP with lignan; no effect on the other inflammatory markers
Harper et al. (2006)[28]	26-week randomised double-blind trial	3 g ALA from flaxseed vs olive oil placebo	56 participants	Plasma LDL cholesterol, HDL cholesterol, intermediate density lipoprotein cholesterol, lipid particle sizes	No changes in lipoprotein particle size or plasma lipoprotein concentration with ALA
Jenkins et al. (1999)[29]	2 × 3-week treatment periods in a randomised, crossover trial	Muffins containing flaxseed or wheatbran	29 hyperlipidaemic subjects (22 men and 7 postmenopausal women)	Plasma cholesterol, apolipoproteins	Flaxseed reduced total cholesterol, LDL cholesterol, but had no effects on lipoprotein ratios and increase oxidation of protein thiol groups
Kaul et al. (2008)[30]	12-week double-blinded, placebo-controlled, clinical trial	Two 1 g capsules of placebo, fish oil, flaxseed oil or hempseed oil per day	86 healthy male and female volunteers	Blood lipids, LDL oxidation, platelet aggregation	No changes with any of the treatments
Layne et al. (1996)[31]	3-month randomised controlled trial	Flaxseed oil, fish oil or olive oil (35mg/kg per day)	Normal healthy volunteers	Plasma triacylglycerol; total, LDL and HDL cholesterol	Fish oil reduced triacylglycerol while flaxseed did not
Lemay et al. (2002)[32]	2 × 2-month treatment periods in a randomised, crossover trial	40 g/day flaxseed vs HRT (with and without progestogen)	25 menopausal women with dyslipidaemia	Blood lipids	Only HRT improved blood lipid profile and markers for cardiovascular health
Lucas et al. (2002)[33]	3-month double-blind randomised study	40 g/day flaxseed vs wheat control (with calcium and vitamin D)	Postmenopausal women not on HRT	Lipid profiles	Flaxseed reduced LDL, HDL and total cholesterol and triacylglycerol compared with control
Pan et al. (2009)[34]	Meta-analysis	Various	28 studies	Blood lipid profiles	Flaxseed significantly reduced circulating total and LDL cholesterol, but the changes were dependent on the type of intervention, sex and initial lipid profiles of the subjects
Paschos et al. (2007)[35]	12-week prospective, two-group, parallel-arm design	Flaxseed oil, rich in ALA (8 g/day) vs safflower oil (11 g/day linoleic acid)	59 middle-aged dyslipidaemic men	Blood pressure	Supplementation with ALA resulted in significantly lower systolic and diastolic blood pressure levels compared with linoleic acid

(Continued)

Table 1 (continued)

Reference	Duration and type of trial	Dose of flaxseed	Study group	Outcome measures	Observed effects
Paschos et al. (2007)[36]	12-week prospective, two-group, parallel-arm design	Flaxseed oil, rich in ALA (8 g/day) vs safflower oil (11 g/day linoleic acid)	35 non-diabetic, dyslipidaemic men, aged 38–71 years	Plasma adiponectin	No change with flaxseed oil
Patade et al. (2008)[37]	3-month randomised controlled trial	Flaxseed vs flaxseed + oatbran vs control	55 Native American postmenopausal women with mild to moderately hypercholesterolaemia (5.1–9.8 mmol/L)	Blood lipids	Reduced total and LDL cholesterol with flaxseed; no change in HDL cholesterol or triacylglycerols
Schwab et al. (2006)[38]	2 × 4- week randomised, double-blind crossover design	Flaxseed oil vs hempseed oil (30 ml/day)	14 healthy volunteers	Blood lipids, glucose, insulin, haemostatic factors	Minor (but different) effects on concentrations of fasting serum total or lipoprotein lipids between hemp and flaxseed oils; no significant changes in plasma glucose or insulin or in haemostatic factors
Wendland et al. (2006)[39]	Meta-analysis	Various	14 studies (minimum duration 4 weeks)	Changes in plasma concentrations of total cholesterol, LDL cholesterol, HDL cholesterol, VLDL cholesterol, triglyceride, fibrinogen, and fasting glucose; changes in body mass index, weight, and systolic and diastolic blood pressure	Fibrinogen and fasting plasma glucose were reduced; treatment with ALA did not significantly modify total cholesterol, triglycerides, weight, body mass index, LDL cholesterol, VLDL cholesterol, apoB, diastolic or systolic blood pressure
Wilkinson et al. (2005)[40]	12-week randomised controlled diet	Flaxseed oil, sunflower oil or sunflower oil + fish oil	57 men expressing an atherogenic lipoprotein phenotype	Plasma lipids	No significant influence of flaxseed on plasma lipids compared with fish oil
Zhang et al. (2008)[41]	8-week, randomised, double-blind, placebo-controlled study	Placebo vs 2 doses of flaxseed extract	55 hypercholesterolaemic subjects	Blood lipids, glucose	Flaxseed lignan extract decreased plasma cholesterol and glucose concentrations in a dose-dependent manner

ALA, alpha-linolenic acid; apo, apolipoprotein; CRP, C-reactive protein; DHA, docosahexaenoic acid; EPA, eicosapentaenoic acid; HRT, hormone-replacement therapy; IL, interleukin; PUFA, polyunsaturated fatty acid.

clinical trial involving 161 patients with prostate cancer suggests that flaxseed (30 g daily) was associated with biological alterations that may be protective for prostate cancer with proliferation rates significantly lower among men assigned to flaxseed supplementation.[44]

Three recent meta-analyses have examined the relationship between ALA acid and prostate cancer. One pooled observational data from nine studies,[19] another pooled observational data from five studies,[45] and both reported that high intakes of ALA were associated with an increased risk of prostate cancer. The most recent meta-analysis pooled data from eight case-control and eight prospective studies. The summary estimate revealed that high ALA dietary intakes or tissue concentrations are weakly associated with prostate cancer risk (relative risk (RR), 1.20; 95% confidence interval (CI) 1.01 to 1.43). When examined by study type (i.e. retrospective compared with prospective or dietary ALA compared with tissue concentration) or by decade of publication, only the six studies examining blood or tissue ALA concentrations revealed a statistically significant association. With the exception of these studies, there was significant heterogeneity and evidence of publication bias. After adjustment for publication bias, there was no association between ALA and prostate cancer (RR, 0.96; 95% CI, 0.79 to 1.17).[46]

Benign prostatic hyperplasia

In a preliminary trial, flaxseed has been shown to improve lower urinary tract symptoms in men with benign prostatic hyperplasia (BPH). This 4-month Chinese study involved 87 subjects with BPH, 78 of whom completed the trial. The authors concluded that the therapeutic efficacy of flaxseed appeared comparable to that of medication used in BPH such as alpha-adrenoceptor blockers and 5-alpha reductase inhibitors.[41]

Diabetes

Flaxseed supplementation has been studied for effects on glucose and insulin control in patients with type 2 diabetes. A Chinese trial in 73 type 2 diabetic patients with mild hypercholesterolaemia found that flaxseed derived lignan capsules (360 mg lignan daily) resulted in modest yet statistically significant improvements in glycaemic control.[47] A Canadian study in 32 type 2 diabetic patients found that high-dose flaxseed oil (5.5 g daily ALA) had no impact on fasting blood serum glucose, insulin or HbA1c levels, suggesting in this study that flaxseed oil had no effect on glycaemic control.[48] A further Canadian trial in 34 participants with well-controlled type 2 diabetes found that neither flaxseed nor flaxseed oil influenced glycaemic control.[49]

Autoimmune disorders

In a double-blind, placebo-controlled study involving 22 patients with rheumatoid arthritis, 30 g flaxseed powder daily for 3 months had no effect on clinical subjective parameters of the disorder compared with sunflower oil.[50]

A small study in eight patients with systemic lupus erythematosus (SLE), present as lupus nephritis, found that flaxseed in a dose of 30 g daily improved renal function and inflammatory mediators and was well tolerated.[51] A further study of 24 months duration, by the same research group recruited 23 of 40 patients asked to participate. These 23 patients were randomised to receive 30 g ground flaxseed daily or control. In the 15 patients who finished the study, serum creatinine declined in the patients who took flaxseed compared to placebo. The nine patients who best adhered to the treatment had lower creatinine levels than the 17/40 patients who did not participate. This study suggests that flaxseed could be renoprotective in lupus nephritis, but poor adherence makes the findings somewhat uncertain.[52]

Another trial in 38 women with SLE or rheumatoid arthritis associated with dry eye Sjogren's syndrome found that flaxseed oil capsules 1 g or 2 g daily reduced eye inflammation and ameliorated the symptoms of keratoconjunctivitis sicca.[53]

Hot flushes

A pilot trial in 28 women who experienced at least 14 hot flushes a week for at least 1 month found that crushed flaxseed 40 g daily was associated with reduced hot flush activity in women not taking oestrogen therapy. This reduction was greater than would be expected with placebo.[54] However, a double-blind, placebo-controlled trial in 38 women who had been postmenopausal for 1 to 10 years showed that flaxseed 25 g daily was no more effective than placebo at reducing hot flushes.[55]

Conclusion

Theoretically, flaxseed as a source of n-3 fatty acids could benefit the same conditions as those indicated for fish oil. However, conversion of ALA to EPA and particularly DHA is poor and is also limited by high LA intakes. Moreover, research data are derived largely from poor quality studies and are currently insufficient to make recommendations for supplements for reduction in risk of heart disease and cancer or management of rheumatoid arthritis and other inflammatory conditions. Flaxseed has promising future use, but the available literature does not support its use as a supplement for any condition at this time.[56]

Precautions/contraindications

No problems have been reported.

Pregnancy and breast-feeding

No problems have been reported, but there have not been sufficient studies to guarantee the safety of flaxseed in pregnancy and breast-feeding.

Adverse effects

There are no known toxicity or serious side-effects, but no long-term studies have assessed the safety of flaxseed. Flaxseed contains cyanogenic glycosides, which are naturally-occurring toxicants. The long-term effects of these compounds are unknown, but high doses could increase plasma thiocyanate levels.

Interactions

None reported.

Dose

Flaxseed oil is available in the form of a liquid and in capsules.

The dose is not established. Manufacturers suggest one tablespoon of flaxseed oil daily.

References

1 Simopoulos AP, Leaf A, Salem N. Jr. Workshop statement on the essentiality of and recommended dietary intakes for omega-6 and omega-3 fatty acids. *Prostaglandins Leukot Essent Fatty Acids* 2000; 63(3): 119–121.

2 Kris-Etherton PM, Harris WS, Appel LJ. Fish consumption, fish oil, omega-3 fatty acids, and cardiovascular disease. *Circulation* 2002; 106(21): 2747–2757.

3 Gerster H. Can adults adequately convert alpha-linolenic acid (18:3n-3) to eicosapentaenoic acid (20:5n-3) and docosahexaenoic acid (22:6n-3)? *Int J Vitam Nutr Res* 1998; 68(3): 159–173.

4 Pawlosky RJ, Hibbeln JR, Novotny JA, *et al.* Physiological compartmental analysis of alpha-linolenic acid metabolism in adult humans. *J Lipid Res* 2001; 42(8): 1257–1265.

5 Mantzioris E, James MJ, Gibson RA, *et al.* Dietary substitution with an alpha-linolenic acid-rich vegetable oil increases eicosapentaenoic acid concentrations in tissues. *Am J Clin Nutr* 1994; 59(6): 1304–1309.

6 Francois CA, Connor SL, Bolewicz LC, *et al.* Supplementing lactating women with flaxseed oil does not increase docosahexaenoic acid in their milk. *Am J Clin Nutr* 2003; 77(1): 226–233.

7 Burdge GC, Finnegan YE, Minihane AM, *et al.* Effect of altered dietary n-3 fatty acid intake upon plasma lipid fatty acid composition, conversion of [13C]alpha-linolenic acid to longer-chain fatty acids and partitioning towards beta-oxidation in older men. *Br J Nutr* 2003; 90(2): 311–321.

8 Burdge GC, Jones AE, Wootton SA. Eicosapentaenoic and docosapentaenoic acids are the principal products of alpha-linolenic acid metabolism in young men. *Br J Nutr* 2002; 88(4): 355–363.

9 Burdge GC, Wootton SA. Conversion of alpha-linolenic acid to eicosapentaenoic, docosapentaenoic and docosahexaenoic acids in young women. *Br J Nutr* 2002; 88(4): 411–420.

10 Burdge G. Alpha-linolenic acid metabolism in men and women: nutritional and biological implications. *Curr Opin Clin Nutr Metab Care* 2004; 7 (2): 137–144.

11 Giltay EJ, Gooren LJ, Toorians AW, *et al.* Docosahexaenoic acid concentrations are higher in women than in men because of estrogenic effects. *Am J Clin Nutr* 2004; 80(5): 1167–174.

12 Liou YA, King DJ, Zibrik D, *et al.* Decreasing linoleic acid with constant alpha-linolenic acid in dietary fats increases (n-3) eicosapentaenoic acid in plasma phospholipids in healthy men. *J Nutr* 2007; 137(4): 945–952.

13 Barcelo-Coblijn G, Murphy EJ, Othman R, *et al.* Flaxseed oil and fish-oil capsule consumption alters human red blood cell n-3 fatty acid composition: a multiple-dosing trial comparing 2 sources of n-3 fatty acid. *Am J Clin Nutr* 2008; 88(3): 801–809.

14 Austria JA, Richard MN, Chahine MN, *et al.* Bioavailability of alpha-linolenic acid in subjects

after ingestion of three different forms of flaxseed. *J Am Coll Nutr* 2008; 27(2): 214–221.

15 Cunnane SC, Ganguli S, Menard C, *et al.* High alpha-linolenic acid flaxseed (*Linum usitatissimum*): some nutritional properties in humans. *Br J Nutr* 1993; 69(2): 443–453.

16 Nesbitt PD, Lam Y, Thompson LU. Human metabolism of mammalian lignan precursors in raw and processed flaxseed. *Am J Clin Nutr* 1999; 69(3): 549–555.

17 Allman MA, Pena MM, Pang D. Supplementation with flaxseed oil versus sunflowerseed oil in healthy young men consuming a low fat diet: effects on platelet composition and function. *Eur J Clin Nutr* 1995; 49(3): 169–178.

18 Bloedon LT, Balikai S, Chittams J, *et al.* Flaxseed and cardiovascular risk factors: results from a double blind, randomized, controlled clinical trial. *J Am Coll Nutr* 2008; 27(1): 65–74.

19 Brouwer I, Katan MB, Zock PL. Dietary alpha-linolenic acid is associated with reduced risk of fatal coronary heart disease, but increased prostate cancer: a meta-analysis. *J Nutr* 2004; 134: 919–922.

20 Coulman KD, Liu Z, Michaelides J, *et al.* Fatty acids and lignans in unground whole flaxseed and sesame seed are bioavailable but have minimal antioxidant and lipid-lowering effects in postmenopausal women. *Mol Nutr Food Res* 2009; 53(11): 1366–1375.

21 Dodin S, Cunnane SC, Masse B, *et al.* Flaxseed on cardiovascular disease markers in healthy menopausal women: a randomized, double-blind, placebo-controlled trial. *Nutrition* 2008; 24(1): 23–30.

22 Dodin S, Lemay A, Jacques H, *et al.* The effects of flaxseed dietary supplement on lipid profile, bone mineral density, and symptoms in menopausal women: a randomized, double-blind, wheat germ placebo-controlled clinical trial. *J Clin Endocrinol Metab* 2005; 90(3): 1390–1397.

23 Finnegan YE, Minihane AM, Leigh-Firbank EC, *et al.* Plant- and marine-derived n-3 polyunsaturated fatty acids have differential effects on fasting and postprandial blood lipid concentrations and on the susceptibility of LDL to oxidative modification in moderately hyperlipidemic subjects. *Am J Clin Nutr* 2003; 77(4): 783–795.

24 Fukumitsu S, Aida K, Shimizu H, *et al.* Flaxseed lignan lowers blood cholesterol and decreases liver disease risk factors in moderately hypercholesterolemic men. *Nutr Res* 2010; 30(7): 441–446.

25 Goyens P, Mensink RP. Effects of alpha-linolenic acid versus those of EPA/DHA on cardiovascular risk markers in healthy elderly subjects. *Eur J Clin Nutr* 2006; 60: 978–984.

26 Hallund J, Tetens I, Bugel S, *et al.* Daily consumption for six weeks of a lignan complex isolated from flaxseed does not affect endothelial function in healthy postmenopausal women. *J Nutr* 2006; 136(9): 2314–2318.

27 Hallund J, Tetens I, Bugel S, *et al.* The effect of a lignan complex isolated from flaxseed on inflammation markers in healthy postmenopausal women. *Nutr Metab Cardiovasc Dis* 2008; 18(7): 497–502.

28 Harper CR, Edwards MC, Jacobson TA. Flaxseed oil supplementation does not affect plasma lipoprotein concentration or particle size in human subjects. *J Nutr* 2006; 136(11): 2844–2848.

29 Jenkins DJ, Kendall CW, Vidgen E, *et al.* Health aspects of partially defatted flaxseed, including effects on serum lipids, oxidative measures, and ex vivo androgen and progestin activity: a controlled cross-over trial. *Am J Clin Nutr* 1999; 69(3): 395–402.

30 Kaul N, Kreml R, Austria JA, *et al.* A comparison of fish oil, flaxseed oil and hempseed oil supplementation on selected parameters of cardiovascular health in healthy volunteers. *J Am Coll Nutr* 2008; 27(1): 51–58.

31 Layne KS, Goh YK, Jumpsen JA, *et al.* Normal subjects consuming physiological levels of 18:3(n-3) and 20:5(n-3) from flaxseed or fish oils have characteristic differences in plasma lipid and lipoprotein fatty acid levels. *J Nutr* 1996; 126(9): 2130–2140.

32 Lemay A, Dodin S, Kadri N, *et al.* Flaxseed dietary supplement versus hormone replacement therapy in hypercholesterolemic menopausal women. *Obstet Gynecol* 2002; 100(3): 495–504.

33 Lucas EA, Wild RD, Hammond LJ, *et al.* Flaxseed improves lipid profile without altering biomarkers of bone metabolism in postmenopausal women. *J Clin Endocrinol Metab* 2002; 87(4): 1527–1532.

34 Pan A, Yu D, Demark-Wahnefried W, *et al.* Meta-analysis of the effects of flaxseed interventions on blood lipids. *Am J Clin Nutr* 2009; 90(2): 288–297.

35 Paschos GK, Magkos F, Panagiotakos DB, *et al.* Dietary supplementation with flaxseed oil lowers blood pressure in dyslipidaemic patients. *Eur J Clin Nutr* 2007; 61(10): 1201–1206.

36 Paschos GK, Zampelas A, Panagiotakos DB, *et al.* Effects of flaxseed oil supplementation on plasma adiponectin levels in dyslipidemic men. *Eur J Nutr* 2007; 46(6): 315–320.

37 Patade A, Devareddy L, Lucas EA, *et al.* Flaxseed reduces total and LDL cholesterol concentrations in Native American postmenopausal women. *J Womens Health (Larchmt)* 2008; 17(3): 355–366.

38 Schwab US, Callaway JC, Erkkila AT, *et al.* Effects of hempseed and flaxseed oils on the profile of serum lipids, serum total and lipoprotein lipid concentrations and haemostatic factors. *Eur J Nutr* 2006; 45(8): 470–477.

39 Wendland E, Farmer A, Glasziou P, *et al.* Effect of alpha linolenic acid on cardiovascular risk markers: a systematic review. *Heart* 2006; 92: 166–169.

40 Wilkinson P, Leach C, Ah-Sing EE, *et al.* Influence of alpha-linolenic acid and fish-oil on markers of cardiovascular risk in subjects with an atherogenic lipoprotein phenotype. *Atherosclerosis* 2005; 181 (1): 115–124.

41 Zhang W, Wang X, Liu Y, *et al.* Effects of dietary flaxseed lignan extract on symptoms of benign prostatic hyperplasia. *J Med Food* 2008; 11(2): 207–214.

42 Serraino M, Thompson LU. The effect of flaxseed supplementation on the initiation and promotional stages of mammary tumorigenesis. *Nutr Cancer* 1992; 17: 153–159.

43 Thompson LU, Rickard SE, Orcheson LJ, *et al.* Flaxseed and its lignan and oil components reduce mammary tumor growth at a late stage of carcinogenesis. *Carcinogenesis* 1996; 17(6): 1373–1376.

44 Demark-Wahnefried W, Polascik TJ, George SL, *et al.* Flaxseed supplementation (not dietary fat restriction) reduces prostate cancer proliferation rates in men presurgery. *Cancer Epidemiol Biomarkers Prev* 2008; 17(12): 3577–3587.

45 Dennis L, Snetselaar L, Smith BJ, *et al.* Problems with the assessment of dietary fat in prostate cancer studies. *Am J Epidemiol* 2004; 160: 436–444.

46 Simon JA, Chen Y-H, Bent S. The relation of α-linolenic acid to the risk of prostate cancer: a systematic review and meta-analysis. *Am J Clin Nutr* 2009; 89(5): 1558S–1564S.

47 Pan A, Sun J, Chen Y, *et al.* Effects of a flaxseed-derived lignan supplement in type 2 diabetic patients: a randomized, double-blind, cross-over trial. *PLoS ONE* 2007; 2(11): e1148.

48 Barre DE, Mizier-Barre KA, Griscti O, *et al.* High dose flaxseed oil supplementation may affect fasting blood serum glucose management in human type 2 diabetics. *J Oleo Sci* 2008; 57(5): 269–273.

49 Taylor CG, Noto AD, Stringer DM, *et al.* Dietary milled flaxseed and flaxseed oil improve n-3 fatty acid status and do not affect glycemic control in individuals with well-controlled type 2 diabetes. *J Am Coll Nutr* 2010; 29(1): 72–80.

50 Nordstrom DC, Honkanen VE, Nasu Y, *et al.* Alpha-linolenic acid in the treatment of rheumatoid arthritis. A double-blind, placebo-controlled and randomized study: flaxseed vs. safflower seed. *Rheumatol Int* 1995; 14(6): 231–234.

51 Clark WF, Parbtani A, Huff MW, *et al.* Flaxseed: a potential treatment for lupus nephritis. *Kidney Int* 1995; 48(2): 475–480.

52 Clark WF, Kortas C, Heidenheim AP, *et al.* Flaxseed in lupus nephritis: a two-year nonplacebo-controlled crossover study. *J Am Coll Nutr* 2001; 20(2Suppl): 143–148.

53 Pinheiro MN,Jr dosSantos PM, dosSantos RC, *et al.* Oral flaxseed oil (*Linum usitatissimum*) in the treatment for dry-eye Sjogren's syndrome patients. *Arq Bras Oftalmol* 2007; 70(4): 649–655.

54 Pruthi S, Thompson SL, Novotny PJ, *et al.* Pilot evaluation of flaxseed for the management of hot flashes. *J Soc Integr Oncol* 2007; 5(3): 106–112.

55 Simbalista RL, Sauerbronn AV, Aldrighi JM, *et al.* Consumption of a flaxseed-rich food is not more effective than a placebo in alleviating the climacteric symptoms of postmenopausal women. *J Nutr* 2009; 140(2): 293–297.

56 Basch E, Bent S, Collins J, *et al.* Flax and flaxseed oil (*Linum usitatissimum*): a review by the Natural Standard Research Collaboration. *J Soc Integr Oncol* 2007; 5(3): 92–105.

Fluoride

Description

Fluoride is a trace element.

Human requirements

There does not appear to be a physiological requirement for fluoride and, in the UK, no Reference Nutrient Intake has been set, but a safe and adequate intake, for infants only, is 0.05 mg/kg daily.

Action

Fluoride has a marked affinity for hard tissues, and forms calcium fluorapatite in teeth and bone. It protects against dental caries and may have a role in bone mineralisation. It helps remineralisation of bone in pathological conditions of demineralisation.

Dietary sources

Foods high in fluoride include seafoods and tea. Cereals and milk are poorer sources. An important source of fluoride is fluoridated drinking water. In the UK, tea provides 70% of the total intake; if the water is fluoridated, consumption of large volumes of tea can result in fluoride intakes of 4–12 mg daily.

Metabolism

Absorption
Oral fluoride is rapidly absorbed by passive transport from the gastrointestinal tract; some is absorbed from the stomach, and some from the small intestine.

Distribution
Fluoride is found principally in bones and teeth.

Elimination
Elimination is mainly via the urine, with small amounts lost in sweat (especially in warm climates) and bile.

Deficiency

No essential function has been clearly established; low levels of fluoride in drinking water are associated with dental caries.

Possible uses

Dental caries
Fluoride is recommended for the prophylaxis of dental caries in infants and children (see Dose, below).

Osteoporosis
Evidence for a role of fluoride in osteoporosis and prevention of fracture is conflicting. In one study,[1] there was a higher incidence of fractures in an area of Italy with a lower concentration of fluoride in the water than in another area. In another study,[2] women with continuous exposure to fluoridated water for 20 years were compared with those with no exposure. In those with exposure, BMD was 2.6% higher at the femoral neck, 2.5% higher at the lumbar spine and 1.9% lower at the distal radius. In addition, the risk of hip fracture was slightly reduced, as was the risk of vertebral fracture. However, there was no difference in the risk of humerus fracture and a non-significant trend towards an increased risk of wrist fracture.

In an intervention study,[3] sodium fluoride (75 mg daily) was no more effective than placebo in retarding progression of spinal osteoporosis. Another study in 202 post-menopausal women[4] with vertebral fractures showed that sodium fluoride 75 mg daily was not an effective treatment. Yet another intervention study[5] showed that fluoride (as sodium fluoride 50 mg daily or monofluorophosphate 200 mg or 150 mg daily) was no more effective than calcium and vitamin D in preventing new vertebral fractures in women with post-menopausal osteoporosis. A trial comparing etidronate with fluoride[6] in the treatment of post-menopausal osteoporosis showed that although fluoride was more effective at increasing lumbar bone mass, there were no differences in fracture incidence.

Precautions/contraindications

The British Association for Community Dentistry advises that fluoride is unnecessary for infants under 6 months and that fluoride should not be given in areas where the drinking water contains fluoride levels that exceed 700 µg/L.

Adverse effects

Chalky white patches on the surface of the teeth (may occur with recommended doses); yellow-brown staining of teeth, stiffness and aching of bones (with chronic excessive intake). Symptoms of acute overdose include diarrhoea, nausea, gastrointestinal cramp, bloody vomit, black stools, drowsiness, weakness, faintness, shallow breathing, tremors and increased watering of mouth and eyes.

Interactions

None reported.

Dose

Systemic fluoride supplements should not be prescribed without reference to the fluoride content of the local water supply (information available from the local Water Board). See Table 1 for daily fluoride doses in infants and children.

Table 1 Daily doses[1] of fluoride (expressed as fluoride ion) in infants and children

Fluoride content of water	Under 6 months	6 months–3 years	3–6 years	Over 6 years
<300 µg	none	250 µg	500 µg	1 mg
300–700 µg	none	none	250 µg	500 µg
>700 µg	none	none	none	none

[1] Recommended by the British Dental Association, the British Society of Paediatric Dentistry and the British Association for the Study of Community Dentistry (*Br Dent J* 1997; 182: 6–7).

References

1   Fabiani L, Leoni V, Vitali M. Bone-fracture incidence rate in two Italian regions with different fluoride concentration levels in drinking water. *J Trace Elem Med Biol* 1999; 13: 232–237.

2   Phipps KR, Orwoll ES, Mason JD, Cauley JA. Community water fluoridation, bone mineral density, and fractures: prospective study of effects in older women. *BMJ* 2000; 321: 860–864.

3   Kleerekoper M, Peterson EL, Nelson DA, *et al*. A randomized trial of sodium fluoride as a treatment for osteoporosis. *Osteoporosis Int* 1991; 1: 155–161.

4   Riggs BL, Hodgson SF, O'Fallon M, *et al*. Effect of fluoride treatment on the fracture rate in postmenopausal women with osteoporosis. *N Engl J Med* 1990; 322: 802–809.

5   Meunier PJ, Sebert JL, Reginster JY, *et al*. Fluoride salts are no better at preventing new vertebral fractures than calcium-vitamin D in postmenopausal osteoporosis; the FAVO study. *Osteoporosis Int* 1998; 8: 4–12.

6   Guanabens N, Farrerons J, Perez-Edo L, *et al*. Cyclical etidronate versus sodium fluoride in established postmenopausal osteoporosis: a randomized 3 year trial. *Bone* 2000; 27: 123–128.

Folic acid

Description

Folic acid is a water-soluble vitamin of the vitamin B complex.

Nomenclature

Folic acid (pteroylglutamic acid) is the parent compound for a large number of derivatives collectively known as folates. Folate is the generic term used to describe the compounds that exhibit the biological activity of folic acid; it is the preferred term for the vitamin present in foods that represents a mixture of related compounds (folates).

Human requirements

See Table 1 for Dietary Reference Values for folic acid.

Dietary intake

In the UK, the average adult diet provides: for men, 322 µg daily; for women, 224 µg daily.

Action

Folates are involved in a number of single carbon transfer reactions, especially in the synthesis of purines and pyrimidines (and hence the

Table 1 Dietary Reference Values for folic acid (µg/day)

							EU RDA = 200 µg
Age		UK				USA		FAO/WHO RNI
	LRNI	EAR	RNI	EVM	RDA	TUL	
0–3 months	30	40	50		65	–	80
4–6 months	30	40	50		65	–	80
7–12 months	30	40	50		80	–	80
1–3 years	35	50	70		150	300	150
4–6 years	50	75	100		–	–	200
4–8 years	–	–	–		200	400	–
7–10 years	75	110	150		–	–	300[1]
9–13 years	–	–	–		300	600	400
14–18 years	–	–	–		400	800	400
Males							
11–14 years	100	150	200		–	–	–
15–50+ years	100	150	200	1000	400	1000	400
Females							
11–14 years	100	150	200		–	–	–
15–50+ years	100	150	200	1000	400	1000	400
Pregnancy			+100[2]		600	1000[3]	600
Lactation			+60		500	1000[3]	600

[1] 7–9 years;
[2] The Department of Health recommends that all women who are pregnant or planning a pregnancy should take a folic acid supplement (see dose);
[3] ≤ 18 years, 800 µg daily.
EAR = Estimated Average Requirement.
EVM = Likely safe daily intake from supplements alone.
LRNI = Lowest Reference Nutrient Intake.
RNI = Reference Nutrient Intake.
TUL = Tolerable Upper Intake Level (not determined for thiamine).

synthesis of DNA), glycine and methionine. They are also involved in some amino acid conversions and the formation and utilisation of formate. Deficiency leads to impaired cell division (effects most noticeable in rapidly regenerating tissues).

Dietary sources

See Table 2 for dietary sources of folic acid.

Metabolism

Absorption
Absorption of folate takes place mainly in the jejunum.

Distribution
Folate is stored mainly in the liver. Enterohepatic recycling is important for maintaining serum levels.

Table 2　Dietary sources of folic acid

Food portion	Folate content (µg)
Breakfast cereals	
1 bowl All-Bran (45 g)	*80*
1 bowl Bran Flakes (45 g)	**110**
1 bowl Corn Flakes (30 g)	*70*
1 bowl muesli (95 g)	**130**
1 bowl Start (40 g)	**140**
Cereal products	
Bread, brown, 2 slices	*30*
white, 2 slices	*25*
wholemeal 2 slices	*30*
fortified, 2 slices	**70**
1 chapati	*10*
Milk and dairy products	
Milk, whole,semi-skimmed, or skimmed (284 ml; ½ pint)	*15*
Soya milk (284 ml; ½ pint)	*50*
1 pot yoghurt (150 g)	*25*
Cheese, average (50 g)	*15*
Camembert (50 g)	*50*
Meat	
Liver, lambs, cooked (90 g)	**220**
Kidney, lambs, cooked (75 g)	*60*
Vegetables	
Broccoli, boiled (100 g)	*65*
Brussels sprouts, boiled (100 g)	**110**
Cabbage, boiled (100 g)	*30*
Cauliflower, boiled (100 g)	*50*
Kale, boiled (100 g)	*90*
Lettuce (30 g)	*20*
Peas, boiled (100 g)	*50*
Potatoes, boiled (150 g)	**145**
Spinach, boiled (100 g)	**100**
1 small can baked beans (200 g)	*45*
Chickpeas, cooked (105 g)	**110**
Red kidney beans (105 g)	*90*
Fruit	
1 orange	*45*
1 large glass orange juice	*40*
Half a grapefruit	*20*
Yeast	
Brewer's yeast (10 g)	**400**
Marmite, spread on 1 slice bread	*50*

Excellent source (**bold**); good source (*italics*).

Elimination

Excretion of folate is largely renal, but folates may also be eliminated in the faeces (mainly as a result of folate synthesis by the gut microflora). Folates are also found in breast milk.

Bioavailability

Folates leach into cooking water and are destroyed by cooking or food processing at high temperatures.

Deficiency

Folate deficiency results in reduction of DNA synthesis and hence in reduction of cell division. While DNA synthesis occurs in all dividing cells, deficiency is most easily seen in tissues with high rates of cell turnover such as erythrocytes (red blood cells). The main clinical observation associated with folate deficiency is, therefore, megaloblastic anaemia.

The main causes of folate deficiency are as follows:

- Decreased dietary intake. This occurs in people eating inadequate diets, such as some elderly people, those on low incomes, and alcoholics who substitute alcoholic drinks for good sources of nutrition.
- Decreased intestinal absorption. Patients with disorders of malabsorption (e.g. coeliac disease) may suffer folate deficiency.
- Increased requirements. Increased requirement for folate, and hence an increased risk of deficiency, can occur in pregnancy, during breast-feeding, in haemolytic anaemia and leukaemia.
- Alcoholism. Chronic alcoholism is a common cause of folate deficiency. This may occur as a result of poor dietary intake, reduced absorption or increased excretion by the kidney. The presence of alcoholic liver disease increases the likelihood of folate deficiency.
- Drugs. Long-term use of certain drugs (e.g. phenytoin, sulfasalazine) is associated with folate deficiency.
- Signs and symptoms include megaloblastic, macrocytic anaemia, weakness, tiredness,

irritability, forgetfulness, dyspnoea, anorexia, diarrhoea, weight loss, headache, syncope, palpitations and glossitis. In babies and young children, growth may be affected.

Possible uses

Pregnancy and pre-pregnancy

The risk of neural tube defects (NTDs) can be reduced by increased folic acid intake during the periconceptual period.[1–5] These findings gave rise to recommendations in several countries that women intending to become pregnant should consume additional folic acid. The reason for the beneficial effect of folic acid is unclear. Although it may be a result of deficiency, a genetic defect in the gene for methylene tetrahydrofolate reductase (MTHFR), estimated to occur in about 5–15% of white populations, appears to result in an increased requirement for folates and an increased risk of recurrent early pregnancy loss and NTDs.[6,7] In addition, elevated levels of plasma homocysteine have been observed in mothers producing offspring with NTDs,[8] and the possibility that this factor could have toxic effects on the foetus at the time of neural tube closure is currently under further investigation.

Whether folic acid taken throughout pregnancy has any benefit on birth outcome is unclear. Re-analysis of data from a large randomised trial, combined with trials from an updated Cochrane review, found no association between folic acid supplementation and birth weight, placental weight or gestational age. Folic acid at high dose (5 mg daily) was associated with reduced risk of low birth weight (pooled relative risk (RR, 0.73; 95% confidence interval (CI), 0.53 to 0.99). Overall there was no conclusive evidence of benefit for folic acid supplementation in pregnant women given from time of booking onwards.[9] However, a Norwegian trial exploring the role of folic acid supplements, dietary folates and multivitamins, found that folic acid supplements given early in pregnancy seem to reduce the risk of cleft lip (with or without cleft palate) by about one third.[10]

Results from some trials have suggested that folic acid is associated with an increase in twin pregnancies. A Hungarian study involving 38 151 women found that both pre- and post-conceptual supplementation of a high dose of folic acid and multivitamins are associated with a slight increase in the incidence of twin pregnancies.[11] A British prospective cohort study involving 602 women undergoing fertility treatment found that the likelihood of a twin birth after *in vitro* fertilisation rose with increased concentrations of plasma folate and red-cell folate. There was no association between folate and vitamin B_{12} levels and the likelihood of a successful pregnancy, but the *MTHFR* genotype was associated with the women's potential to produce healthy embryos.[12]

Cardiovascular disease

Marginal folate status is also associated with elevated plasma homocysteine levels, a known risk factor for cardiovascular disease (CVD) mortality.[13–15] Mechanisms by which plasma homocysteine may be associated with increased risk of CVD have not been clearly established, but possibilities include:[16]

- oxidative damage to the vascular endothelium;
- inhibition of endothelial anticoagulant factors, resulting in increased clot formation;
- increased platelet aggregation; and
- proliferation of smooth muscle cells, resulting in increased vulnerability of the arteries to obstruction.

Homocysteine is derived from dietary methionine, and it is removed by conversion to cystathionine, cysteine and pyruvate, or by remethylation to methionine. Rare inborn errors of metabolism can cause severe elevations in plasma homocysteine levels. One example is homocystinuria, which occurs as a result of a genetic defect in the enzyme cystathione beta-synthase. Genetic changes in the enzymes involved in the remethylation pathway, including MTHFR and methionine synthase, are also associated with increase in plasma homocysteine concentrations. All such cases are associated with premature vascular disease, thrombosis and early death.

However, such genetic disorders are rare and cannot account for the raised homocysteine levels observed in many patients with CVD. However, attention is now being given to the possibility that deficiency of the various vitamins that act as cofactors for the enzymes involved in homocysteine metabolism could result in increased homocysteine concentrations. In particular, folate is required for the normal function of MTHFR, vitamin B_{12} for methionine synthase and vitamin B_6 for cystathione beta-synthase.

In theory, lack of any one of these three vitamins could cause hyperhomocysteinaemia, and could therefore increase the risk of CVD. In the Framingham Heart Study,[17] a cohort study on vascular disease, it was shown that folic acid, vitamin B_6 and vitamin B_{12} are determinants of plasma homocysteine levels, with folic acid showing the strongest association.

The question of whether increased vitamin intake can reduce cardiovascular risk was examined in the Nurses' Health Study,[18] which showed that those with the highest intake of folate had a 31% lower incidence of heart disease than those with the lowest intake. For vitamin B_6, those with the highest intake had a 33% lower risk of heart disease, while in those with the highest intake of both folate and vitamin B_6, the risk of heart disease was reduced by 45%. The risk of heart disease was reduced by 24% in those who regularly used multivitamins. In a large Australian study involving 1419 men and 1531 women aged 20–90, the risk of fatal CVD was not associated with serum folate and serum B_{12} concentrations.[19]

Another question is whether homocysteine levels can be lowered with folate and other B vitamins. Folic acid (250 μg daily), in addition to usual dietary intakes of folate, significantly decreased plasma homocysteine concentrations in healthy young women,[20] and breakfast cereal fortified with folic acid reduced plasma homocysteine in men and women with coronary artery disease.[21] Another study has demonstrated that the addition of vitamin B_{12} to folic acid supplements or enriched foods (400 μg folic acid daily) maximises the reduction of homocysteine.[22] Furthermore, two meta-analyses[23–25] suggest that administration of folic acid reduces plasma homocysteine concentrations and that vitamin B_{12} but not vitamin B_6 may have an additional effect.[24] Vitamin B_6 alone also seems to be less effective than a combination of folic acid and B_{12} in lowering plasma homocysteine concentrations in patients with coronary artery disease.[25,26]

A meta-analysis of 25 RCTs involving 2595 subjects found that the proportional reductions in plasma homocysteine concentrations produced by folic acid were greater at higher homocysteine and lower folate pretreatment concentrations.[27] They were also greater in women than men. Vitamin B_{12} produced further reduction in homocysteine, but vitamin B_6 had no significant effect. The conclusion of this meta-analysis was that daily doses of ≥ 0.8 mg folic acid are required to achieve maximal reduction in homocysteine concentrations produced by folic acid. Doses of 0.2 mg and 0.4 mg were associated with 60% and 90%, respectively, of this maximal effect.[27] A more recent RCT also found that the homocysteine lowering effect of B vitamins (folate, B_6 and B_{12}) was maximal in those with high homocysteine and low B_{12} levels.[28]

Although high homocysteine levels are associated with CVD, the question as to whether lowering homocysteine reduces cardiovascular risk has not been clearly answered. A meta-analysis in 2002[29] found strong evidence that the association between homocysteine and CVD is causal, and calculated that lowering homocysteine concentrations by 3 μmol/L (achievable by increasing folic acid intake) would reduce the risk of ischaemic heart disease by 16%, deep vein thrombosis by 25% and stroke by 24%.

However, a more recent meta-analysis that investigated the association between the gene *MTHFR* and coronary heart disease (CHD) found no strong evidence to support this association, concluding that the possible benefit of folic acid in preventing CVD, through lowering homocysteine, is in some doubt.[30]

In addition, an RCT in Singaporean stroke patients found that the a *MTHFR* polymorphism (C677T) did not significantly influence the effect of vitamin therapy on homocysteine levels. In this study, the magnitude of the reduction in homocysteine levels at 12 months was similar, irrespective of *MTHFR* genotype.[31] However, a more recent trial in Taiwan found that low-dose folic acid supplementation (400 μg daily) significantly reduced homocysteine by 1.8 (mol/L after 8 weeks, for those with hyperhomocystinaemia, especially for carriers of *MTHFR* C677T.

In another trial, moderate reduction of total homocysteine after non-disabling cerebral infarction had no effect on vascular outcomes during 2 years of follow-up.[32] Further trials of homocysteine lowering with folic acid either alone or in combination with other B vitamins have shown no significant effects on biomarkers of inflammation, endothelial dysfunction and hypercoagulablity,[33–35] or inflammatory and thrombogenic markers in smokers.[36] One trial found that folate (5 mg daily) and B_{12} (500 μg daily) improved insulin resistance and endothelial dysfunction in patients with metabolic syndrome.[37] Another study showed no improvement in markers of endothelial dysfunction and low-grade inflammation in patients with type 2 diabetes,[38] while another found that short-term folic acid supplementation (5 mg daily) significantly enhances endothelial function in type 2 diabetes.[39]

Two large RCTs (the Heart Outcomes Prevention Evaluation (HOPE)[40] and the NORVIT Trial[41]) found that B_{12}, folic acid and B_6 in combination reduced plasma homocysteine, but did not reduce the risk of major cardiovascular events in patients with CVD,[40] and did not reduce the risk of recurrent CVD after acute myocardial infarction.[41] Secondary analysis from HOPE-2 found that decreasing homocysteine levels did not alter the risk for symptomatic venous thromboembolism.[42]

A Dutch trial in 701 patients (20–80 years) with diagnosed recurrent deep vein thrombosis (DVT) or pulmonary embolism evaluated the potential for secondary prevention of DVT with folic acid, B_{12} and B_6 combined compared with placebo over a period of 2.5 years. Patients with high homocysteine levels and normal homocysteine levels were evaluated compared with placebo in two different studies. The hazard ratio (HR) associated with B vitamin treatment was 0.84 (95% CI, 0.56 to 1.26); in the group with high homocysteine, HR was 1.14 (95% CI, 0.65 to 1.98) and in the group with normal homocysteine HR was 0.58 (95% CI, 0.31 to 1.07). The results of this study, therefore, showed no benefit of B vitamins in the prevention of recurrent venous thrombosis.[43] A further study among 3096 participants in Norway, undergoing coronary angiography, found no effect of treatment with folic acid/vitamin B_{12} or vitamin B_6 on total mortality or cardiovascular events.[44]

Observational data suggest that benefits of folic acid with other B vitamins may be greater in women. However, in the US Women and Folic Acid Cardiovascular Study (WAFACS) a combination pill of folic acid 2.5 mg, vitamin B_6 50 mg and vitamin B_{12} 1 mg failed to reduce total cardiovascular events in high-risk women after 7.3 years of treatment and follow-up.[45]

A meta-analysis which included 16 958 participants with pre-existing vascular disease concluded that folic acid supplementation has not been shown to reduce risk of CVD or all-cause mortality among people with prior history of vascular disease.[46] Interestingly, a trial in 90 people which looked at the effect of folic acid, vitamins B_6 and B_{12} on inflammatory markers of atherosclerosis found that in patients with stable coronary artery disease, folic acid with vitamins B_6 and B_{12} does not affect these inflammatory markers.[47] This failure to reverse inflammatory markers may help to explain the negative results in clinical secondary B vitamin trials.

Folic acid intervention has also been evaluated in endothelial function. A small 2-week trial in which folic acid (10 mg daily) was given to 19 patients with type 2 diabetes found that folic acid improved endothelial dysfunction but did not alter inflammatory markers.[48] An 8-week RCT in 124 children with type 1 diabetes found that, compared with placebo, folic acid 5 mg with vitamin B_6 100 mg improved endothelial dysfunction as demonstrated by improved flow-mediated dilatation (FMD).[49] A meta-analysis of 14 studies involving 732 people found that folic acid improved endothelial function (as measured with the use of FMD), which could potentially reduce the risk of CVD.[50] A more recently published paper described a substudy from the Australian VITATOPS trial, designed to test the efficacy of long-term B vitamin supplementation (folic acid 2 mg, vitamin B_6 25 mg, vitamin B_{12} 0.5 mg) in the prevention of vascular events in patients with stroke. This paper also described a meta-analysis of studies designed to test the effect of B vitamin treatment on carotid intima-media thickness and FMD in patients with stroke. Overall conclusions were that short-term treatment with B vitamins was associated with increased FMD but longer term therapy did not improve carotid intima-media thickness or FMD in people with a history of stroke.[51] A further RCT by the same research group found that the same B vitamin combination had no effect on arterial wall inflammation.[52]

Trials with folic acid evaluating other disorders of the cardiovascular system have also shown mixed results. A Swiss RCT involving 553 patients who had undergone percutaneous coronary intervention were randomised to receive a combination of vitamin B_6 (10 mg daily), vitamin B_{12} (400 µg daily) and folic acid 1 mg daily. This vitamin combination was found to significantly reduce the incidence of major adverse events after percutaneous coronary intervention.[53]

A 2-year trial in 276 healthy older participants with hyperhomocystinaemia showed that folic acid (1 mg) with vitamin B_{12} (500 µg) and vitamin B_6 (10 mg) reduced homocysteine but had no influence on blood pressure.[54] In a 3.2 year trial involving 2056 participants with advanced chronic kidney disease or end-stage renal disease and high homocysteine levels, a daily capsule containing folic acid (40 mg) vitamin B_6 (100 mg) and vitamin B_{12} (2 mg) did not improve survival or reduce the incidence of vascular disease.[55]

However, a recent meta-analysis which assessed the efficacy of folic acid in the prevention of stroke found that supplementation significantly reduced the risk of stroke in primary prevention.[56] Stroke outcome has also been measured in the Heart Outcomes Prevention Evaluation 2 (HOPE-2) trial, which randomised 5522 participants with known CVD to a daily combination of folic acid 2.5 mg, vitamin B_6 50 mg and vitamin B_{12} 1 mg or placebo for 5 years. Vitamin therapy reduced the incidence of overall stroke and non-fatal stroke, but had no significant effect on stroke severity or disability. Patients aged under 69 years from regions without folic acid food fortification, with higher baseline cholesterol and homocysteine levels and those not receiving antiplatelet or lipid-lowering drugs had a larger treatment benefit.[57] Participants with chronic kidney disease within the HOPE-2 study were evaluated separately for cardiovascular risk. However, there were no significant treatment benefits with the B vitamin combination on death from cardiovascular causes, myocardial infarction and stroke. More patients in the treatment group were hospitalised for heart failure and unstable angina.[58]

Debate continues over whether raised serum homocysteine concentrations cause ischaemic heart disease and stroke and whether folic acid, with or without other B vitamins, which lowers homocysteine, will reduce the risk of these disorders. Different researchers have produced different findings, often as a result of variation in experimental design and have also reached opposite conclusions from similar evidence. A British analysis concluded that, despite these differences, evidence supports a modest protective effect for folic acid.[59] However, the current balance of evidence is not in favour of high-dose folic acid with vitamins B_6 and B_{12} in the secondary prevention of CVD. A Cochrane analysis of eight RCTs found no evidence that, compared with placebo or standard care, homocysteine-lowering interventions in the form of folic acid, vitamin B_6 or B_{12}, given alone or in combination, at any dosage prevents myocardial infarction, stroke or reduces total mortality in patients at risk or with established CVD.[60] Similar conclusions have also been drawn from further RCTs and reviews.[61–66] Table 3 summarises the RCTs and meta-analyses involving folic acid and cardiovascular outcomes.

Cancer

Colon cancer

Marginal folate status also appears to be associated with certain cancers,[88] notably colon cancer, although it is at present unclear as to whether it is folate or some other nutritional factors that could be involved. Various mechanisms for this protective effect have been proposed, but folate seems to be inversely associated with tumour promoter methylation.[89] However, supplementation with high doses of folic acid and vitamin B_{12} did not favourably influence promoter methylation and/or also uracil incorporation in people with previous colorectal tumours.[90] Data, including those from two prospective studies[91,92] and four case–control studies,[93–96] indicate that inadequate intake of folate may increase risk of colon cancer. However, a recent prospective study has indicated that low plasma folate concentrations may protect against colorectal cancer. A bell-shaped curve was observed between plasma folate and colorectal cancer risk. The MTHFR C677T polymorphism was associated with a reduced risk of colorectal cancer that was independent of folate status.[97]

There is some evidence – albeit limited – that use of supplements containing folic acid could reduce the risk of colon cancer.[98,99] More recent studies have also found a lower incidence of colorectal adenomas in people with higher

Table 3 Clinical trials and systematic reviews evaluating the effect of folic acid on cardiovascular disease, cancer and cognitive health

Reference	Duration and type of trial	Dose of folic acid	Study group	Outcome measures	Observed effects
Cardiovascular disease					
Spoelstra-de et al. (2004)[38]	6-month placebo-controlled trial (Netherlands)	5 mg daily	41 patients with type diabetes and mild hyperhomocystinaemia	Biochemical markers of endothelial dysfunction and low-grade inflammation (e.g. C-reactive protein)	Improvement in markers of endothelial dysfunction and low-grade inflammation
Toole et al. (2004)[32]	2-year double-blind randomised controlled trial (US)	High-dose (25 mg pyridoxine, 0.4 mg cobalamin, 2.5 mg folic acid) or low-dose (200 µg pyridoxine, 6 µg cobalamin, 20 µg folic acid) formulation	3680 adults with non-disabling cerebral infarction	Risk of recurrent stroke	No effect of either treatment on vascular outcomes
Setola et al. (2004)[37]	2 month double-blind, parallel, identical placebo–drug, randomised study (Italy)	Folic acid 5 mg + vitamin B$_{12}$ 500 µg or placebo	50 patients with metabolic syndrome	Insulin resistance and endothelial function	Folate and vitamin B$_{12}$ treatment improved insulin resistance and endothelial dysfunction
Dusitanond et al. (2005)[34]	Randomised controlled trial (Australia)	Folic acid 2 mg, vitamin B$_{12}$ 0.5 mg, and vitamin B$_6$ 25 mg	285 patients with recent transient ischaemic attack or stroke	Markers of vascular inflammation, endothelial dysfunction, and hypercoagulability	B vitamins did not significantly reduce blood concentrations of biomarkers of inflammation, endothelial dysfunction, or hypercoagulability
Mangoni et al. (2005)[39]	4 week double-blind, randomised controlled, parallel group trial (Australia)	Folic acid 5 mg/day	26 patients with type 2 diabetes	Endothelial function	Folic acid significantly improved endothelial function
Lonn et al. (2006)[40]	5-year randomised controlled trial (Canada)	2.5 mg folic acid, 50 mg vitamin B$_6$, and 1 mg of vitamin B$_{12}$	5522 patients with CVD or diabetes (≥ 55 years)	Major cardiovascular events	No reduction in major cardiovascular events
Bonaa et al. (2006)[41]	2 × 2 factorial randomised controlled trial (Norway)	Daily treatment: (i) 0.8 mg folic acid, 0.4 mg vitamin B$_{12}$ and 40 mg vitamin B$_6$; (ii) 0.8 mg folic acid and 0.4 mg vitamin B$_{12}$; (iii) 40 mg vitamin B$_6$; or (iv) placebo	3749 men and women who had had an acute myocardial infarction within 7 days before randomisation	Secondary prevention of CVD	No reduction in recurrent CVD
Namazi et al. (2006)[67]	6-month randomised controlled trial (Iran)	Folic acid 1 mg daily	200 patients for 3 months after successful coronary angioplasty	Restenosis within 6 months	Folic acid did not decrease the rate of restenosis and need for revascularisation after coronary angioplasty

(Continued)

Table 3 (continued)

Reference	Duration and type of trial	Dose of folic acid	Study group	Outcome measures	Observed effects
Bazzano et al. (2006)[46]	Meta-analysis	Folic acid (with CVD as end point)	12 randomised controlled trials	Risk of CVD and all-cause mortality in persons with pre-existing vascular disease or renal disease	Folic acid not shown to reduce risk of CVD or all-cause mortality among participants with prior history of vascular disease
Bleys et al. (2006)[68]	Meta-analysis	Folic acid, B_{12} and B_6	Randomised controlled trial	Progression of atherosclerosis	No evidence of a protective effect of B vitamins on atherosclerosis
McMahon et al. (2007)[54]	2-year randomised controlled trial (US)	Folate (1 mg), vitamin B_{12} (500 µg), and vitamin B-6 (10 mg), or a placebo	267 healthy older subjects	Blood pressure	No effect
Ray et al. (2007)[42]	5-year randomised controlled trial (Canada)	2.5 mg folic acid, 50 mg vitamin B_6 and 1 mg vitamin B_{12} or matching placebo	5522 persons with known CVD or diabetes mellitus and at least one other risk factor for vascular disease diagnosed and confirmed symptomatic deep vein thrombosis or pulmonary embolism (≥ 55 years)	Venous thromboembolism	No reduction in risk for symptomatic venous thromboembolism
De Bree et al. (2007)[50]	Meta-analysis	Various	14 randomised controlled trials (732 subjects)	Endothelial function	Improved endothelial function with folic acid
Wang et al. (2007)[56]	Meta-analysis	Various	8 randomised controlled trials	Stroke prevention	Folic acid reduced risk of stroke
Bleie et al. (2007)[47]	Single centre, prospective double-blind clinical interventional study, randomised in a 2 × 2 factorial design	Four groups: (i) folic acid 0.8 mg, vitamin B_{12} 0.4 mg and vitamin B_6 40 mg; (ii) folic acid and vitamin B_{12}; (iii) vitamin B_6 alone; or (iv) placebo	90 patients with suspected coronary artery disease (38–80 years; 21 female)	Inflammatory markers associated with atherosclerosis	Folic acid had no effect
Albert et al. (2008)[45]	7.3 year randomised controlled trial	Combination pill of 2.5 mg folic acid, 50 mg vitamin B_6, and 1 mg vitamin B_{12}	5442 women who were US health professionals aged 42 years or older, with either a history of CVD or three or more coronary risk factors	A composite outcome of myocardial infarction, stroke, coronary revascularisation or CVD mortality	No reduction in combined endpoint
Ebbing et al. (2008)[44]	Randomised controlled trial 2 × 2 factorial design (Norway)	Daily: (i) 0.8 mg folic acid, 0.4 mg vitamin B_{12} and 40 mg vitamin B_6; (n = 772); (ii) 0.8 mg folic acid and 0.4 mg vitamin B_{12} (n = 772); (iii) 40 mg vitamin B_6; (n = 772); or placebo (n = 780)	3096 adults	A composite of all-cause death, non-fatal acute myocardial infarction, acute hospitalisation for unstable angina pectoris, and non-fatal thromboembolic stroke	No effect on total mortality or cardiovascular events

(Continued)

Study	Study type	Intervention	Participants	Outcome	Results
Song et al. (2009)[69]	7.3 years randomised controlled trial (US)	Combination pill of 2.5 mg folic acid, 50 mg vitamin B6 and 1 mg vitamin B12	5442 female health professionals with a history of CVD or three or more CVD risk factors, included 4252 women free of diabetes at baseline (≥ 40 years)	Diabetes risk	No significant effect on diabetes risk
Hodis et al. (2009)[70]	3.1 year randomised controlled trial (US)	5 mg folic acid, 0.4 mg vitamin B12 and 50 mg vitamin B6	506 participants with an initial raised homocysteine level without diabetes and CVD (40–89 years)	Atherosclerosis progression	B vitamins significantly reduced progression of early-stage subclinical atherosclerosis (carotid intima-media thickness)
Marti-Carvajal et al. (2009)[60]	Meta-analysis	Various	8 randomised controlled trials (24 210 participants)	CV events	Folic acid and B vitamins did not reduce the risk of non-fatal or fatal myocardial infarction, stroke, or all-cause death
Ntaios et al. (2009)[71]	18 month randomised controlled trial (Greece)	Folic acid 5 mg	103 patients with at least one cardiovascular risk factor	Carotid IMT	Folic acid resulted in significant intima-media thickness reduction
Armitage et al. (2010)[61]	Randomised controlled trial (UK) (6.7 years follow-up)	2 mg folic acid + 1 mg vitamin B12 daily or matching placebo	12 064 survivors of myocardial infarction in secondary care hospitals in the UK	First major vascular event, defined as major coronary event (coronary death, myocardial infarction, or coronary revascularization), fatal or non-fatal stroke, or non-coronary revascularization.	No beneficial effects on vascular outcomes
Heinz et al. (2010)[62]	2-year randomised controlled trail (Germany)	5 mg folic acid, 50 μg vitamin B12 and 20 mg vitamin B6 (active treatment) or 0.2 mg folic acid, 4 μg vitamin B12 and 1.0 mg vitamin B6 (placebo) given 3 times per week	650 patients with end-stage renal disease who were undergoing haemodialysis	Primary outcome total mortality; secondary outcome fatal and non-fatal cardiovascular events	B vitamins did not reduce total mortality and had no significant effect on the risk of cardiovascular events in patients with end-stage renal disease
Clarke et al. (2010)[63]	Meta-analysis	Various	8 large, randomised, placebo-controlled trials of folic acid supplementation involving 37 485 individuals at increased risk of CVD	Cardiovascular events	No significant effects within 5 years on cardiovascular events
Ebbing et al. (2010)[64]	Pooling of data from 2 randomised controlled trails with extended post-trial observational follow-up	(i) 0.8 mg folic acid, 0.4 mg vitamin B12 and 40 mg vitamin B6; (ii) 0.8 mg folic acid and 0.4 mg vitamin B12; (iii) 40 mg vitamin B6; or (iv) placebo	6837 patients with ischaemic heart disease	Cardiovascular outcomes	No short- or long-term benefit of folic acid plus vitamin B12 on cardiovascular outcomes
Kurt et al. (2010)[72]	8-week randomised controlled trail (Turkey)	Folate (5 mg) and vitamin B12 (500 μg)	44 elderly people with vitamin B12 deficiency	Coronary flow reserve	Significant improvement in coronary flow reserve with folate and B12

Table 3 *(continued)*

Reference	Duration and type of trial	Dose of folic acid	Study group	Outcome measures	Observed effects
Miller et al. (2010)[65]	Meta-analysis	Various	Randomised controlled trials	CVD and stroke	No influence on primary CVD outcomes or stroke
Vitatops Trial Study Group (2010)[66]	Randomised, double-blind, parallel, placebo-controlled trial	2 mg folic acid, 25 mg vitamin B_6 and 0.5 mg vitamin B_{12}	8164 patients with recent stroke or transient ischaemic attack (within the past 7 months) from 123 medical centres in 20 countries	Composite of stroke, myocardial infarction, or vascular death	No reduced incidence of major vascular events
Cancer					
Cole et al. (2007)[73]	A double-blind, placebo-controlled, 2-factor, phase III, randomised clinical trial	1 mg folic acid, or placebo; or aspirin 81 mg or 325 mg or placebo	1021 men and women with a recent history of colorectal adenomas and no previous invasive large intestine carcinoma	Primary outcome measure occurrence of at least 1 colorectal adenoma; secondary outcomes occurrence of advanced lesions and adenoma multiplicity	Folic acid was associated with higher risks of having three or more adenomas and of non-colorectal cancers; no benefit of folic acid supplementation
Zhang et al. (2008)[74]	Randomised controlled trial (US)	2.5 mg folic acid, 50 mg vitamin B_6 and 1 mg vitamin B_{12}	5442 US female health professionals with pre-existing CVD or three or more coronary risk factors ($\geq$ 42 years)	Confirmed newly diagnosed total invasive cancer or breast cancer	No significant effect of B vitamins on overall risk of total invasive cancer or breast cancer
Jaszewski et al. (2008)[75]	3-year randomised controlled trial	5 mg folic acid	137 patients with colorectal adenomas	Recurrence of colonic adenomas	Significant reduction in the recurrence of colonic adenomas
Carroll et al. (2010)[76]	Meta-analysis	Various	6 randomised controlled trials	Colorectal cancer	No evidence that folic acid is effective in the chemoprevention of colorectal adenomas or colorectal cancer for any population
Cognitive function					
Stott et al. (2005)[26]	A factorial 2 × 2 × 2 randomised controlled trial (UK)	3 active treatments: (i) folic acid 2.5 mg plus vitamin B_{12} 500 µg; (ii) vitamin B_6 25 mg; (iii) riboflavin 25 mg	185 patients	Cognitive function	No significant effect on cognitive function
McMahon et al. (2006)[77]	2-year randomised controlled trial	Folate 1 mg, vitamin B_{12} 0.5 mg and vitamin B_6 10 mg	276 healthy participants, ($\geq$ 65 years)	Cognitive performance	No effect

Study	Study type	Intervention	Participants	Outcome	Result
Balk et al. (2007)[78]	Meta-analysis	Various	14 trials	Cognitive function	No evidence of benefit from folic acid, B6, B12
Durga et al. (2007)[79]	Randomised, double blind, controlled trial (Netherlands)	0.8 mg folic acid or placebo	818 participants	Cognitive performance	The 3-year change in memory, information processing speed and sensorimotor speed were significantly better in the folic acid group than in the placebo group
Kang et al. (2008)[80]	Randomised controlled trial (US)	Daily folic acid 2.5 mg, vitamin B6 50 mg and vitamin B12 1 mg	2009 health professionals with CVD or three or more risk factors (>65 years)	Cognitive change	No effect on decline in cognitive function; benefit in those with low B vitamin intake
Jia et al. (2008)[81]	Systematic review	Various	22 trials (3442 participants)	Cognitive function	No effect
Ford et al. (2010)[82]	Randomised controlled trial (Australia)	0.4 mg vitamin B12, 2 mg folic acid and 25 mg B6	299 men with hypertension (>75 years)	Cognitive function	No effect
Wald et al. (2010)[83]	Meta-analysis	Various	9 randomised controlled trials (2835 participants)	Cognitive function	No effect of folic acid, with or without other B vitamins, on cognitive function within 3 years of the start of treatment
Smith et al. (2010)[84]	2-year randomised controlled trial	Daily folic acid 0.8 mg, vitamin B12 0.5 mg and vitamin B6 20 mg	271 patients with mild cognitive impairment	Change in the rate of atrophy of the whole brain	Slowing of brain atrophy with B vitamins
Depression					
Taylor et al. (2004)[85]	Meta-analysis	Various	3 randomised controlled trials (247 participants)	Depression	Some evidence of a role for folate in treating depression
Ford et al. (2008)[86]	2-year randomised controlled trial (Australia)	0.4 mg B12, 2 mg folic acid and 25 mg B6 per day (n = 150) or placebo (n = 149)	299 men free of depression (>75 years)	Depression	B vitamins were no better than placebo at reducing incidence of depression and severity of depressive symptoms
Almeida et al. (2010)[87]	Randomised controlled trial (Australia)	Folic acid 2 mg, vitamin B6 25 mg and vitamin B12 0.5 mg	273 people with stroke	Onset of major depression; prevalence of depression at the end of treatment	Reduction in major depression

CVD, cardiovascular disease; IMT, intima-media thickness.

intakes of and plasma concentrations of folate and lower homocysteine.[100]

A meta-analysis of seven cohort and nine case–control studies also added support for the hypothesis that folate has a small protective effect against colorectal cancer.[101] However, a further meta-analysis of six RCTS found no evidence that folic acid supplementation had any preventive effect against colorectal adenomas and colorectal cancers.[76]

There is some evidence that high folate intake may have a particular effect in reducing colorectal cancer risk in people with high alcohol intake,[102,103] or in smokers.[104] In women with high alcohol intake, there is also a strong inverse relationship between dietary folate intake and ovarian cancer risk.[74,105]

Breast cancer

Higher folate intake has also been shown to reduce breast cancer risk in women with loss of expression of the gene for the oestrogen receptor, but not in those with such expression (ER+).[106] High folate intake has also been associated with a lower incidence of postmenopausal breast cancer in a cohort of Swedish women.[107] A meta-analysis of observational studies (13 case–control studies and 9 cohort studies) of folate and breast cancer risk found severe methodological problems with the studies assessed and concluded that evidence is currently insufficient to say that a lack of dietary folate is associated with the risk of breast cancer. The same authors evaluated the association between the common polymorphism of *MTHFR* and breast cancer risk from 17 studies. No difference in breast cancer risk and *MTHFR* C677T genotype was found, and there was no evidence of an interaction between folate intake and *MTHFR* genotype on breast cancer risk.[108]

A study investigating the effect of folate taken in pregnancy on breast cancer found that women taking high doses of folate throughout pregnancy may be more likely to die of breast cancer in later life than women taking no folate. The authors suggested that this could be a chance finding, so further studies should be conducted.[109]

Miscellaneous cancer

Folate intake has been inversely associated with endometrial cancer[110] and for dietary folate (but not supplement use) with prostate cancer.[105]

WAFACS, designed to evaluate the effect of combined folic acid, vitamin B_6 and B_{12} in the secondary prevention of CVD, has also evaluated outcomes in terms of cancer risk. In this group of 5442 health professionals, aged 42 years or over, a total of 379 developed invasive cancer (187 in the B vitamin group, 192 in the placebo group). Compared with women in the placebo group, those receiving B vitamins had a similar risk of developing total invasive cancer (HR, 0.97; 95% CI, 0.79 to 1.18; $P = 0.75$) breast cancer (HR, 0.83; 95% CI, 0.6 to 1.14; $P = 0.24$) and death from any cancer (HR, 0.82; 95% CI, 0.56 to 1.21; $P = 0.32$).[74]

WAFACS also evaluated the risk of developing type 2 diabetes mellitus in this group of women with cardiovascular disease or risk factors. There was no significant difference between the B vitamin group and placebo, and no evidence for modification of effect by baseline intakes of dietary folate, vitamin B_6 and vitamin B_{12}.[69]

Cognitive impairment

There is an apparent increase in mental disorders associated with reduced folate status.[111] A double-blind RCT in 818 men and women aged 50–70 years found that folic acid 800 µg daily for 3 years significantly improved domains of cognitive function including memory, information processing speed and sensorimotor speed compared with placebo.[79] As part of the same trial, folic acid was also found to slow age-related decline in hearing.[112]

Studies have found that cognitive impairment and Alzheimer's disease are also associated with low blood levels of folate and vitamin B_{12} and elevated homocysteine levels.[113–124] However, an observational study evaluating dietary folate intakes found that dietary intakes of folate, with or without vitamin B_{12} and B_6 does not appear to be associated with the development of Alzheimer's disease.[125] In older people with low vitamin B_{12} status, high serum folate has been associated with cognitive impairment, but when B_{12} status was normal, high serum folate was associated with protection against cognitive impairment.[126]

A meta-analysis of four randomised controlled intervention trials provide no evidence that folic acid, with or without vitamin B_{12}, has a beneficial effect on cognitive function or mood in cognitively impaired older people.[127] A systematic review of 14 RCTs (mostly of low quality and limited applicability) concluded that there is not yet adequate evidence of an effect of folic acid, vitamin B_6 or B_{12}, alone or in combination, on cognitive function testing in people with either normal or impaired cognitive function.[78]

Further RCTs have continued to show no significant benefits for combination folic acid, vitamin B_6 and vitamin B_{12} in relation to cognition. WAFACS, which was designed to test a combination of folic acid 2.5 mg, vitamin B_6 50 mg and vitamin B_{12} 1 mg on secondary prevention of CVD in female health professionals, found that the vitamin intervention did not delay cognitive decline in these women with CVD or cardiovascular risk factors.[80]

A Dutch study compared the effects of walking or combined folic acid 5 mg, vitamin B_{12} 0.4 mg and vitamin B_6 50 mg or placebo for 1 year in 152 people aged 70–80 years. Neither the walking programme nor the vitamin intervention was effective in improving cognition. The walking programme, however, was effective in improving memory in men and attention in women (in those with good adherence).[128]

An Australian trial in 299 elderly men with hypertension found no evidence that a combination of folic acid 2 mg, vitamin B_6 25 mg and vitamin B_{12} 400 μg could improve cognitive function in this population group.[82]

Two trials in people with mild to moderate Alzheimer's disease also reported no benefit of combined B vitamin therapy. One was a study in Taiwan in which 89 patients received an anticholinesterase inhibitor plus folic acid 1 mg, vitamin B_6 5 mg, mecobalamin 500 mg with other vitamins and iron or an anticholinesterase inhibitor plus placebo. No significant benefits were found on cognition and activities of daily living scores between vitamins and placebo at 26 weeks.[129] A US trial evaluated an intervention comprising folic acid 5 mg, vitamin B_6 25 mg and vitamin B_{12} 1 mg or placebo in 409 individuals with Alzheimer's disease. The B vitamin supplement did not slow cognitive decline and was associated with greater incidence of depression.[130]

A recent meta-analysis of nine RCTs found no benefit of folic acid with or without other B vitamins on cognitive function within 3 years of starting treatment.[83] Whether longer trials would show benefit is not known.

Depression

Evidence exists of a link between depression and low folate levels, and some RCTs have found folate supplements helpful when added to conventional antidepressants. A recent US study amongst 110 patients with major depressive disorder compared levels of folate, B_{12} and homocysteine with the time taken to respond to the antidepressant fluoxetine. The 15% of patients who initially had low folate levels took longer to onset of clinical improvement than those with normal folate. Initial levels of B_{12} and homocysteine had no relationship to response onset.[131]

A systematic review of three RCTs of folate supplementation suggests that folate may have a potential role as a supplement to other treatments for depression. Patients with low folate intake given extra folate had reduced Hamilton Depression Rating Scale scores and increased odds of a 50% score improvement compared to placebo. Folate given to patients with initially normal folate had no significant impact.[85] Two other recent RCTs in which average folate status was normal or not measured also found no evidence that folate supplements helped depression.[132,133] A Cochrane review also concluded that there is limited evidence for folic acid supplementation in depression,[134] but a further meta-analysis concluded that folic acid could reduce the risk of depression after stroke.[87]

An Australian trial has evaluated the potential for combined folic acid, vitamin B_6 and B_{12} intervention in depression. This two-year placebo-controlled trial involved 299 men aged 75 years and older who were free of clinically significant depression. They were randomly assigned to be treated with 2 mg folic acid, 400 μg vitamin B_{12} and 25 mg vitamin B_6 or placebo. At the end of the trial, 84.3% of men treated with vitamins and 79.1% of those treated with placebo remained free of clinically significant depression. This difference was not statistically significant.[86]

A UK study has investigated a genetic factor in the link between folate and depression. A cross-sectional observational study of 3478 women (from a heart health study) compared the presence of the *MTHFR* C677T genotype with the presence of depressive symptoms. Eight other similar studies were meta-analysed together with the new results. Depression was found to be associated with the C677T genotype.[108]

In summary, it is clear that a proportion of depressed patients have low folate status and that this can be associated with a worse response to antidepressants. Whether low folate is the cause or effect of depression in these patients is less clear. Evidence to date from RCTs of folate supplementation in depression is minimal but positive. Patients with depression should be tested for red cell folate and supplemented when folate is low, particularly if they are elderly or have co-existing nutritional risk.

Hip fracture

Preliminary evidence from one RCT in 628 patients in Japan aged 65 or older with stroke found that daily oral treatment with folic acid 5 mg and mecobalamin 1500 µg reduced plasma homocysteine and the risk of hip fracture.[135] However, a two-year New Zealand trial in 276 healthy patients aged ≥ 65 years found that supplementation with folic acid 1 mg, vitamin B_{12} 500 µg, and vitamin B_6 10 mg produced no significant benefit on markers of bone turnover (bone-specific alkaline phosphatase, bone-derived collagen fragments).[136]

Miscellaneous

Homocysteine-lowering therapy with B vitamins has been evaluated in other conditions. Preliminary evidence of benefit in migraine has been obtained from a 6-month RCT in 52 patients diagnosed with migraine with aura. Supplementation with folic acid 2 mg, vitamin B_6 25 mg and vitamin B_{12} 400 µg reduced migraine disability, headache frequency and pain severity compared with placebo. In this study, the treatment effect was associated with the *MTHFR* C677T genotype.[137]

The WAFACS has also looked at outcomes for age-related macular degeneration (ARMD). Findings in these women at high risk of CVD were that B vitamin combination reduced the risk of ARMD compared with placebo (RR, 0.66; 95% CI, 0.47 to 0.93). For visually significant ARMD, the RR was 0.59 (CI, 0.36 to 0.95).[138]

A Swedish study has evaluated B vitamin supplementation in 65 patients with long-standing coeliac disease. Folic acid 0.8 mg, cyanocobalamin 0.5 mg and pyridoxine 3 mg or placebo were given for 6 months. Following B vitamin supplementation, plasma homocysteine fell by a median of 34%, accompanied by significant

improvement in well-being, notably anxiety and depressed mood for patients with poor well-being.[139]

Conclusion

There is good evidence that folic acid reduces the risk of neural tube defects, and supplementation is recommended pre-conceptually and during the first 12 weeks of pregnancy. Folic acid reduces elevated plasma homocysteine levels, a risk factor for CVD, particularly for secondary CVD events in patients with pre-existing CVD. However, evidence from a growing number of trials suggests that potentially pharmacological doses of folic acid, with or without other B vitamins, do not appear to reduce the risk of CVD. This may be confused by *MTHFR* polymorphisms, which may influence the effect of folic acid. Moreover, the link between homocysteine and CVD may be weaker than previously thought. Epidemiological studies have shown an inverse relationship between serum folate levels and colon cancer and breast cancer. However, there is no robust evidence of benefit from folic acid supplementation in any type of cancer. Poor folate status has also been demonstrated in some people with depression or poor cognitive function, but supplementation with folic acid and other B vitamins has not been shown to improve cognition or delay cognitive decline in elderly people. Depressed patients should be tested for folate and supplemented when folate is low. A recent large trial has shown that folic acid supplementation can slow the decline in cognitive impairment in old age, and further trials are ongoing.

Precautions/contraindications

In pernicious anaemia, folic acid will correct the haematological abnormalities, but neuropathy may be precipitated. Doses of folic acid of >400 µg daily are not recommended until pernicious anaemia has been ruled out.

Pregnancy and breast-feeding

No problems have been reported. Supplements are required during pregnancy and when planning a pregnancy (see Dose).

Adverse effects

Folic acid is generally considered to be safe even in high doses, but it may lead to convulsions in patients taking anticonvulsants and may precipitate neuropathy in pernicious anaemia. Some gastrointestinal disturbance and altered sleep pattern has been reported at doses of 15 mg daily. Allergic reactions (shortness of breath, wheezing, fever, erythema, skin rash, itching) have been reported rarely.

Interactions

Drugs

Anticonvulsants: requirements for folic acid may be increased, but concurrent use of folic acid may antagonise the effects of anticonvulsants; an increase in anticonvulsant dose may be necessary in patients who receive supplementary folic acid (monitoring required).

Antibiotics: may interfere with the microbiological assay for serum and erythrocyte folic acid (falsely low results).

Colestyramine: may reduce the absorption of folic acid; patients on prolonged colestyramine therapy should take a folic acid supplement 1 h before colestyramine administration.

Methotrexate: acts as a folic acid antagonist; risk significant with high dose and/or prolonged use.

Oestrogens (including oral contraceptives): may reduce blood levels of folic acid.

Pyrimethamine: acts as a folic acid antagonist; risk significant with high dose and/or prolonged use; folic acid supplements should be given in pregnancy.

Sulfasalazine: may reduce the absorption of folic acid; requirements for folic acid may be increased; may compromise the efficacy of sulfasalazine.[140]

Trimethoprim: acts as a folic acid antagonist; risk significant with high dose and/or prolonged use.

Nutrients

Adequate amounts of all B vitamins are required for optimal functioning; deficiency or excess of one B vitamin may lead to abnormalities in the metabolism of another.

Zinc: folic acid may reduce the absorption of zinc.

Dose

Folic acid is available in the form of tablets.

For prevention of first occurrence of NTDs in women who are planning a pregnancy, oral, 400 µg daily before conception until 12th week of pregnancy.

For prevention of recurrence of NTDs, oral, 5 mg daily before conception until 12th week of pregnancy.

For prophylaxis during pregnancy (after 12th week), oral, 200–500 µg daily. A Cochrane review concluded that folate supplementation in pregnancy appears to improve haemoglobin status and folate status.[141]

In women with diabetes mellitus, oral, 5 mg daily before conception until the 12th week. This is because women with diabetes are at significantly increased risk of having a baby with NTDs. This dose has been recommended by Diabetes UK (2005), the British Medical Association (2004) and the Society of Obstetricians and Gynaecologists (2003).

As a dietary supplement, oral, 100–500 µg daily.

When co-prescribed with methotrexate, in patients who suffer mucosal or gastrointestinal side-effects with this drug, folic acid 5 mg each week may help to reduce the frequency of such side-effects. This dose has been recommended by ATTRACT, the *British National Formulary* and PRODIGY.

Upper safety levels

The UK Expert Group on Vitamins and Minerals (EVM) has identified a likely safe total intake of folic acid for adults from supplements alone of 1000 µg daily.

References

1 Laurence KM, James N, Miller MH, *et al*. Double-blind randomised controlled trial of folate treatment before conception to prevent recurrence of neural tube defects. *BMJ* 1981; 282: 1509–1511.

2 Smithells RW, Seller MJ, Harris R, *et al*. Further experience of vitamin supplementation for prevention of neural tube defect recurrences. *Lancet* 1983; i: 1027–1031.

3 Medical Research Council Vitamin Study Research Group. Prevention of neural tube defects: results of the Medical Research Council Vitamin Study. *Lancet* 1991; 338: 131–137.

4 Czeizel AE, Dudas I. Prevention of the first occurrence of neural tube defects by periconceptual

vitamin supplementation. *New Engl J Med* 1992; 327: 1832–1835.

5 Weller MM, Shapiro S, Mitchel AA, *et al.* Periconceptual folic acid exposure and risk of occurrent neural tube defects. *JAMA* 1993; 269: 1257–1261.

6 Molloy AM, Daly S, Mills JL, *et al.* Thermolabile variant of 5,10 methylenetetrahydrofolate reductase associated with low red cell folates: implications for folate intake recommendations. *Lancet* 1997; 349: 1591–1593.

7 Nelen WLDM, Van derMolen EF, Blom HJ, *et al.* Recurrent early pregnancy loss and genetic related disturbances in folate and homocysteine metabolism. *Br J Hosp Med* 1997; 58: 511–513.

8 Mills JL, McPartlin P, Kirke PM, *et al.* Homocysteine metabolism in pregnancies complicated by neural tube defects. *Lancet* 1995; 345: 149–151.

9 Charles DH, Ness AR, Campbell D, *et al.* Folic acid supplements in pregnancy and birth outcome: re-analysis of a large randomised controlled trial and update of Cochrane review. *Paediatr Perinat Epidemiol* 2005; 19: 112–124.

10 Wilcox AJ, Lie RT, Solvoll K, *et al.* Folic acid supplements and risk of facial clefts: national population based case-control study. *BMJ* 2007; 334: 464.

11 Czeizel AE, Vargha P. Preconceptual folic acid/multivitamin supplementation and twin pregnancy. *Am J Obstet Gynecol* 2004; 191: 790–794.

12 Haggarty P, McCallum H, McBain H, *et al.* Effect of B vitamins and genetics on success of in-vitro fertilisation: prospective cohort study. *Lancet* 2006; 367: 1513–1539.

13 Alfthan G, Aro A, Gey KF. Plasma homocysteine and cardiovascular disease mortality. *Lancet* 1997; 349: 397.

14 Nygard O, Nordrehaug JE, Refsum H, *et al.* Plasma homocysteine levels and mortality in patients with coronary artery disease. *New Engl J Med* 1997; 337: 230–236.

15 Wald NJ, Watt HC, Law MR, *et al.* Homocysteine and ischaemic heart disease: results of a prospective study with implications on prevention. *Arch Int Med* 1998; 158: 862–867.

16 Weir DG, Scott JM. Homocysteine as a risk factor for cardiovascular and related disease: nutritional implications. *Nutr Res Rev* 1998; 11: 311–338.

17 Selhub J, Jacques PF, Wilson PWF, *et al.* Vitamin status and intake as primary determinants of homocysteinaemia in an elderly population. *JAMA* 1993; 270: 2693–2698.

18 Rimm EB, Willett WC, Hu FB, *et al.* Folate and vitamin B_6 from diet and supplements in relation to risk of coronary heart disease among women. *JAMA* 1998; 279: 359–364.

19 Hung J, Beilby JP, Knuiman MW, *et al.* Folate and vitamin B-12 and risk of fatal cardiovascular disease: cohort study from Busselton, Western Australia. *BMJ* 2003; 326: 131–135.

20 Brouwer IA, vanDusseldorp M, Thomas CMG, *et al.* Low-dose folic caid supplementation decreases plasma homocysteine concentrations: a randomized trial. *Am J Clin Nutr* 1999; 69: 99–104.

21 Malinow MR, Duell PB, Hess DL, *et al.* Reduction of plasma homocysteine levels by breakfast cereal fortified with folic acid in patients with coronary heart disease. *New Engl J Med* 1998; 338: 1009–1015.

22 Bronstrup A, Hages M, Prinz-Langenohl R, *et al.* Effects of folic acid and combinations of folic acid and vitamin B-12 on plasma homocysteine concentrations in healthy young women. *Am J Clin Nutr* 1998; 68: 1104–1110.

23 Boushey CJ, Beresford SAA, Omenn GS, *et al.* A quantitative assessmemt of plasma homocysteine as a risk factor for vascular disease: probable benefits of increasing folic acid intake. *JAMA* 1995; 274: 1049–1057.

24 Homocysteine Lowering Trialists' Collaboration. Lowering blood homocysteine with folic acid based supplements: meta-analysis of randomised trials. *BMJ* 1998; 316: 894–898.

25 Lee BJ, Huang MC, Chung LJ, *et al.* Folic acid and vitamin B_{12} are more effective than vitamin B_6 in lowering fasting plasma homocysteine concentration in patients with coronary artery disease. *Eur J Clin Nutr* 2004; 58: 481–487.

26 Stott DJ, MacIntosh G, Lowe GD, *et al.* Randomized controlled trial of homocysteine-lowering vitamin treatment in elderly patients with vascular disease. *Am J Clin Nutr* 2005; 82: 1320–1326.

27 Homocysteine Lowering Trialists' Collaboration. Dose-dependent effects of folic acid on blood concentrations of homocysteine: a meta-analysis of the randomized trials. *Am J Clin Nutr* 2005; 82: 806–812.

28 Flicker L, Vasikaran SD, Thomas J, *et al.* Efficacy of B vitamins in lowering homocysteine in older men. *Stroke* 2006; 37: 547.

29 Wald DS, Law M, Morris JK. Homocysteine and cardiovascular disease: evidence on causality from a meta-analysis. *BMJ* 2002; 325: 1202–1204.

30 Lewis SJ, Ebrahim S, Davey Smith G. Meta-analysis of *MTHFR* → T polymorphism and coronary heart disease: does totality of evidence support a causal role for homocysteine and preventive potential of folate? *BMJ* 2005; 331: 1053–1058.

31 Ho GYH, Eikelboom JW, Hankey GJ, *et al.* Methylenetetrahydrofolate reductase polymorphisms and homocysteine-lowering effect of vitamin therapy in Singaporean stroke patients. *Stroke* 2006; 37: 456.

32 Toole JF, Malinow MR, Chambless LE, *et al.* Lowering homocysteine in patients with ischemic stroke to prevent recurrent stroke, myocardial infarction, and death: the Vitamin Intervention for Stroke Prevention (VISP) randomized controlled trial. *JAMA* 2004; 291: 565–575.

33 Peeters AC, van der Molen EF, Blom HJ, *et al.* The effect of homcysteine reduction by B-vitamin

supplementation on markers of endothelial dysfunction. *Throm Haemostat* 2004; 92: 1086–1091.

34 Dusitanond P, Eikelboom JW, Hankey JG, *et al.* Homocysteine-lowering treatment with folic acid, cobalamin, and pyridoxine does not reduce blood markers of inflammation, endothelial dysfunction, or hypercoagulability in patients with previous transient ischaemic attack or stroke: a randomized substudy of the VITATOPS trial. *Stroke* 2005; 36: 144–146.

35 Durga J, vanTits LJ, Schouten EG, *et al.* Effect of lowering of homocysteine levels on inflammatory markers: a randomized controlled trial. *Arch Intern Med* 2005; 165: 1388–1394.

36 Mangoni AA, Arya R, Ford E, *et al.* Effects of folic acid supplementation on inflammatory and thrombogenic markers in chronic smokers. A randomised controlled trial. *Thromb Res* 2003; 110: 13–17.

37 Setola A, Mont LD, Galluccio E, *et al.* Insulin resistance and endothelial function are improved after folate and vitamin B_{12} therapy in patients with metabolic syndrome: relationship between homocysteine levels and hyperinsulinaemia. *Eur J Endocrinol* 2004; 151: 483–489.

38 de Spoelstra MA, Brouwer CB, Terheggen F, *et al.* No effect of folic acid on markers of endothelial dysfunction or inflammation in patients with type 2 diabetes mellitus and mild hyperhomocysteinaemia. *Neth J Med* 2004; 62(7): 246–253.

39 Mangoni AA, Sherwood RA, Asonganyi B, *et al.* Short-term oral folic acid supplementation enhances endothelial function in patients with type 2 diabetes. *Am J Hypertens* 2005; 18(2Pt1): 220–226.

40 Lonn E, Yusuf S, Arnold MJ, *et al.* Homocysteine lowering with folic acid and B vitamins in vascular disease. *N Engl J Med* 2006; 354(15): 1567–1577.

41 Bonaa KH, Njolstad I, Ueland PM, *et al.* Homocysteine lowering and cardiovascular events after acute myocardial infarction. *N Engl J Med* 2006; 354(15): 1578–1588.

42 Ray JG, Kearon C, Yi Q, *et al.* Homocysteine-lowering therapy and risk for venous thromboembolism: a randomized trial. *Ann Intern Med* 2007; 146(11): 761–767.

43 den Heijer M, Willems HP, Blom HJ, *et al.* Homocysteine lowering by B vitamins and the secondary prevention of deep vein thrombosis and pulmonary embolism: a randomized, placebo-controlled, double-blind trial. *Blood* 2007; 109 (1): 139–144.

44 Ebbing M, Bleie O, Ueland PM, *et al.* Mortality and cardiovascular events in patients treated with homocysteine-lowering B vitamins after coronary angiography: a randomized controlled trial. *JAMA* 2008; 300(7): 795–804.

45 Albert CM, Cook NR, Gaziano JM, *et al.* Effect of folic acid and B vitamins on risk of cardiovascular events and total mortality among women at high risk for cardiovascular disease: a randomized trial. *JAMA* 2008; 299(17): 2027–2036.

46 Bazzano LA, Reynolds K, Holder KN, *et al.* Effect of folic acid supplementation on risk of cardiovascular diseases: a meta-analysis of randomized controlled trials. *JAMA* 2006; 296(22): 2720–2726.

47 Bleie Ø, Semb AG, Grundt H, *et al.* Homocysteine-lowering therapy does not affect inflammatory markers of atherosclerosis in patients with stable coronary artery disease. *J Intern Med* 2007; 262(2): 244–253.

48 Title LM, Ur E, Giddens K, *et al.* Folic acid improves endothelial dysfunction in type 2 diabetes–an effect independent of homocysteine-lowering. *Vasc Med* 2006; 11(2): 101–109.

49 MacKenzie KE, Wiltshire EJ, Gent R, *et al.* Folate and vitamin B_6 rapidly normalize endothelial dysfunction in children with type 1 diabetes mellitus. *Pediatrics* 2006; 118(1): 242–253.

50 de Bree A, van Mierlo LA, Draijer R. Folic acid improves vascular reactivity in humans: a meta-analysis of randomized controlled trials. *Am J Clin Nutr* 2007; 86(3): 610–617.

51 Potter K, Hankey GJ, Green DJ, *et al.* The effect of long-term homocysteine-lowering on carotid intima-media thickness and flow-mediated vasodilation in stroke patients: a randomized controlled trial and meta-analysis. *BMC Cardiovasc Disord* 2008; 8: 24.

52 Potter K, Lenzo N, Eikelboom JW, *et al.* Effect of long-term homocysteine reduction with B vitamins on arterial wall inflammation assessed by fluoro-deoxyglucose positron emission tomography: a randomised double-blind, placebo-controlled trial. *Cerebrovasc Dis* 2009; 27(3): 259–265.

53 Schnyder G, Roffi M, Flammer Y, *et al.* Effect of homocysteine-lowering therapy with folic acid, vitamin B_{12}, and vitamin B_6 on clinical outcome after percutaneous coronary intervention: the Swiss Heart study: a randomized controlled trial. *JAMA* 2002; 288(8): 973–979.

54 McMahon JA, Skeaff CM, Williams SM, *et al.* Lowering homocysteine with B vitamins has no effect on blood pressure in older adults. *J Nutr* 2007; 137(5): 1183–1187.

55 Jamison RL, Hartigan P, Kaufman JS, *et al.* Effect of homocysteine lowering on mortality and vascular disease in advanced chronic kidney disease and end-stage renal disease: a randomized controlled trial. *JAMA* 2007; 298(10): 1163–1170.

56 Wang X, Qin X, Demirtas H, *et al.* Efficacy of folic acid supplementation in stroke prevention: a meta-analysis. *Lancet* 2007; 369(9576): 1876–1882.

57 Saposnik G, Ray JG, Sheridan P, *et al.* Homocysteine-lowering therapy and stroke risk, severity, and disability: additional findings from the HOPE 2 trial. *Stroke* 2009; 40(4): 1365–1372.

58 Mann JF, Sheridan P, McQueen MJ, *et al.* Homocysteine lowering with folic acid and B vitamins in people with chronic kidney disease: results of the renal HOPE-2 study. *Nephrol Dial Transplant* 2008; 23(2): 645–653.

59 Wald DS, Wald NJ, Morris JK, *et al.* Folic acid, homocysteine, and cardiovascular disease: judging causality in the face of inconclusive trial evidence. *BMJ* 2006; 333(7578): 1114–1117.

60 Marti-Carvajal A, Sola I, Lathyris D, *et al.* Homocysteine lowering interventions for preventing cardiovascular events. *Cochrane Database Syst Rev* 2009; (4): CD006612.

61 Armitage JM, Bowman L, Clarke RJ, *et al.* Effects of homocysteine-lowering with folic acid plus vitamin B_{12} vs placebo on mortality and major morbidity in myocardial infarction survivors: a randomized trial. *JAMA* 2010; 303(24): 2486–2494.

62 Heinz J, Kropf S, Domröse U, *et al.* B vitamins and the risk of total mortality and cardiovascular disease in end-stage renal disease: results of a randomized controlled trial. *Circulation* 2010; 121(12): 1432–1438.

63 Clarke R, Halsey J, Lewington S, *et al.* Effects of lowering homocysteine levels with B vitamins on cardiovascular disease, cancer, and cause-specific mortality: meta-analysis of 8 randomized trials involving 37 485 individuals. *Arch Intern Med* 2010; 170(18): 1622–1631.

64 Ebbing M, Bønaa KH, Arnesen E, *et al.* Combined analyses and extended follow-up of two randomized controlled homocysteine-lowering B-vitamin trials. *J Intern Med* 2010; 268(4): 367–382.

65 Miller ER, 3rd Juraschek S, Pastor-Barriuso R, *et al.* Meta-analysis of folic acid supplementation trials on risk of cardiovascular disease and risk interaction with baseline homocysteine levels. *Am J Cardiol* 2010; 106(4): 517–527.

66 VITATOPS Trial Study Group. B vitamins in patients with recent transient ischaemic attack or stroke in the VITAmins TO Prevent Stroke (VITATOPS) trial: a randomised, double-blind, parallel, placebo-controlled trial. *Lancet Neurol* 2010; 9(9): 855–865

67 Namazi MH, Motamedi MR, Safi M, *et al.* Efficacy of folic acid therapy for prevention of in-stent restenosis: a randomized clinical trial. *Arch Iran Med* 2006; 9(2): 108–110.

68 Bleys J, Miller ER,3rd Pastor BR, *et al.* Vitamin-mineral supplementation and the progression of atherosclerosis: a meta-analysis of randomized controlled trials. *Am J Clin Nutr* 2006; 84(4): 880–887 quiz 954955.

69 Song Y, Cook NR, Albert CM, *et al.* Effect of homocysteine-lowering treatment with folic acid and B vitamins on risk of type 2 diabetes in women: a randomized, controlled trial. *Diabetes* 2009; 58(8): 1921–1928.

70 Hodis HN, Mack WJ, Dustin L, *et al.* High-dose B vitamin supplementation and progression of subclinical atherosclerosis: a randomized controlled trial. *Stroke* 2009; 40(3): 730–736.

71 Ntaios G, Savopoulos C, Karamitsos D, *et al.* The effect of folic acid supplementation on carotid intima-media thickness in patients with cardiovascular risk: a randomized, placebo-controlled trial. *Int J Cardiol* 2009; 143(1): 16–19.

72 Kurt R, Yilmaz Y, Ermis F, *et al.* Folic acid and vitamin B_{12} supplementation improves coronary flow reserve in elderly subjects with vitamin B_{12} deficiency. *Arch Med Res* 2010; 41(5): 369–372.

73 Cole BF, Baron JA, Sandler RS, *et al.* Folic acid for the prevention of colorectal adenomas: a randomized clinical trial. *JAMA* 2007; 297(21): 2351–2359.

74 Zhang SM, Cook NR, Albert CM, *et al.* Effect of combined folic acid, vitamin B_6, and vitamin B_{12} on cancer risk in women: a randomized trial. *JAMA* 2008; 300(17): 2012–2021.

75 Jaszewski R, Misra S, Tobi M, *et al.* Folic acid supplementation inhibits recurrence of colorectal adenomas: a randomized chemoprevention trial. *World J Gastroenterol* 2008; 14(28): 4492–4498.

76 Carroll C, Cooper K, Papaioannou D, *et al.* Meta-analysis: folic acid in the chemoprevention of colorectal adenomas and colorectal cancer. *Aliment Pharmacol Ther* 2010; 31(7): 708–718.

77 McMahon JA, Green TJ, Skeaff CM, *et al.* A controlled trial of homocysteine lowering and cognitive performance. *N Engl J Med* 2006; 354(26): 2764–2772.

78 Balk EM, Raman G, Tatsioni A, *et al.* Vitamin B_6, B_{12}, and folic acid supplementation and cognitive function: a systematic review of randomized trials. *Arch Intern Med* 2007; 167(1): 21–30.

79 Durga J, van Boxtel MP, Schouten EG, *et al.* Effect of 3-year folic acid supplementation on cognitive function in older adults in the FACIT trial: a randomised, double blind, controlled trial. *Lancet* 2007; 369(9557): 208–216.

80 Kang JH, Cook N, Manson J, *et al.* A trial of B vitamins and cognitive function among women at high risk of cardiovascular disease. *Am J Clin Nutr* 2008; 88(6): 1602–1610.

81 Jia X, McNeill G, Avenell A. Does taking vitamin, mineral and fatty acid supplements prevent cognitive decline? A systematic review of randomized controlled trials *J Hum Nutr Diet* 2008; 21(4): 317–336.

82 Ford AH, Flicker L, Alfonso H, *et al.* Vitamins B (12), B(6), and folic acid for cognition in older men. *Neurology* 2010; 75(17): 1540–1547.

83 Wald DS, Kasturiratne A, Simmonds M. Effect of folic acid, with or without other B vitamins, on cognitive decline: meta-analysis of randomized trials. *Am J Med* 2010; 123(6): 522–527.

84 Smith AD, Smith SM, deJager CA, *et al.* Homocysteine-lowering by B vitamins slows the rate of accelerated brain atrophy in mild cognitive impairment: a randomized controlled trial. *PLoS One* 2010; 5(9): e12244.

85 Taylor M, Carney SM, Goodwin GM, *et al.* Folate for depressive disorders: systematic review and meta-analysis of randomized controlled trials. *J Psychopharmacol* 2004; 18: 251–256.

86 Ford AH, Flicker L, Thomas J, *et al.* Vitamins B_{12}, B_6, and folic acid for onset of depressive symptoms in older men: results from a 2-year placebo-controlled randomized trial. *J Clin Psychiatry* 2008; 69(8): 1203–1209.

87 Almeida OP, Marsh K, Alfonso H, *et al.* B-vitamins reduce the long-term risk of depression after stroke: the VITATOPS-DEP trial. *Ann Neurol* 2010; 68(4): 503–510.

88 Mason JB. Folate status: effects on carcinogenesis. In: Bailey LB (ed.), *Folates in Health and Disease*. New York: Marcel Dekker, 1995: 361–378.

89 van den Donk M, vanEngeland M, Pellis L, *et al.* Dietary folate intake in combination with *MTHFR* C677T genotype and promoter methylation of tumor suppressor and DNA repair genes in sporadic colorectal adenomas. *Cancer Epidemiol Biomarkers Prev* 2007; 16(2): 327–333.

90 van den Donk M, Pellis L, Crott JW, *et al.* Folic acid and vitamin B-12 supplementation does not favorably influence uracil incorporation and promoter methylation in rectal mucosa DNA of subjects with previous colorectal adenomas. *J Nutr* 2007; 137(9): 2114–2120.

91 Giovannucci E, Rimm EB, Ascherio A, *et al.* Alcohol, low methionine, low folate diets and risk of colon cancer in men. *J Natl Cancer Inst* 1995; 87: 265–273.

92 Glynn SA, Albanes D, Pietinen P, *et al.* Colorectal cancer and folate status: a nested case-control study among male smokers. *Cancer Epidemiol Biomarkers Prev* 1996; 5: 487–494.

93 Benito E, Stigglebout A, Bosch FX, *et al.* Nutritional factors in colorectal cancer risk: a case-control study in Majorca. *Int J Cancer* 1991; 49: 161–167.

94 Meyer F, White E. Alcohol and nutrients in relation to colon cancer in middle-aged adults. *Am J Epidemiol* 1993; 138: 225–236.

95 Ferraroni M, La Vecchia C, D'Avanzo B, *et al.* Selected micronutrient intake and the role of colon cancer. *Br J Cancer* 1994; 70: 1150–1155.

96 Freudenheim JL, Graham S, Marshall JR, *et al.* Folate intake and carcinogenesis of the colon and rectum. *Int J Epidemiol* 1991; 20: 368–374.

97 Van Guelpen B, Hultdin J, Johansson I, *et al.* Low folate levels may protect against colorectal cancer. *Gut* 2006; 55(10): 1461–1466.

98 White E, Shannon JS, Patterson RE. Relationship between vitamin and calcium supplement use and colon cancer. *Cancer Epidemiol Biomarkers Prev* 1997; 6: 769–774.

99 Giovannucci E, Stampfer MJ, Colditz GA, *et al.* Multivitamin use, folate and colon cancer in women in the Nurses' Health Study. *Ann Intern Med* 1998; 129: 517–524.

100 Martinez ME, Henning SM, Alberts DS. Folate and colorectal neoplasia: relation between plasma and dietary markers of folate and adenoma recurrence. *Am J Clin Nutr* 2004; 79: 691–697.

101 Sanjoaquin MA, Allen N, Couto E, *et al.* Folate intake and colorectal cancer risk: a meta-analytical approach. *Int J Cancer* 2005; 113: 825–828.

102 Boyapati SM, Bostick RM, McGlynn KA, *et al.* Folate intake, *MTHFR* C677T polymorphism, alcohol consumption, and risk for sporadic colorectal adenoma (United States). *Cancer Causes Control* 2004; 15: 493–501.

103 Le Marchand L, Wilkens LR, Kolonel LN, *et al.* The *MTHFR* C677T polymorphism and colorectal cancer: the multiethnic cohort study. *Cancer Epidemiol Biomarkers Prev* 2005; 14: 198–203.

104 Larrson SC, Giovannucci E, Wolk A. A prospective study of dietary folate intake and risk of colorectal cancer: modification by caffeine intake and cigarette smoking. *Epdemiol Biomarkers Prev Cancer* 2005; 14: 740–743.

105 Schernhammer E, Wolpin B, Rifai N, *et al.* Plasma folate, vitamin B_6, vitamin B_{12}, and homocysteine and pancreatic cancer risk in four large cohorts. *Cancer Res* 2007; 67(11): 5553–5560.

106 Zhang SM, Hankinson SE, Hunter DJ, *et al.* Folate intake and risk of breast cancer characterized by hormone receptor status. *Cancer Epidemiol Biomarkers Prev* 2005; 14: 2004–2008.

107 Ericson U, Sonestedt E, Gullberg B, *et al.* High folate intake is associated with lower breast cancer incidence in postmenopausal women in the Malmo Diet and Cancer cohort. *Am J Clin Nutr* 2007; 86(2): 434–443.

108 Lewis SJ, Harbord RM, Harris R, *et al.* Meta-analyses of observational and genetic association studies of folate intakes or levels and breast cancer risk. *J Natl Cancer Inst* 2006; 98(22): 1607–1622.

109 Charles D, Ness AR, Campbell D, *et al.* Taking folate in pregnancy and risk of maternal breast cancer. *BMJ* 2004; 329: 1375–1376.

110 Xu W-H, Shrubsole MJ, Xiang Y-B, *et al.* Dietary folate intake, *MTHFR* genetic polymorphisms, and the risk of endometrial cancer among Chinese women. *Cancer Epidemiol Biomarkers Prev* 2007; 16(2): 281–287.

111 Bottiglieri E, Crellin RF, Reynolds EH. Folates and neuropsychiatry. In Bailey L (ed.), *Folate in Health and Disease*. New York: Marcel Dekker 1995; 435–462.

112 Durga J, Verhoef P, Anteunis LJ, *et al.* Effects of folic acid supplementation on hearing in older adults: a randomized, controlled trial. *Ann Intern Med* 2007; 146(1): 1–9.

113 Luchsinger JA, Tang M-X, Miller J, *et al.* Relation of higher folate intake to lower risk of Alzheimer disease in the elderly. *Arch Neurol* 2007; 64(1): 86–92.

114 Haan MN, Miller JW, Aiello AE, *et al.* Homocysteine, B vitamins, and the incidence of dementia and cognitive impairment: results from the Sacramento Area Latino Study on Aging. *Am J Clin Nutr* 2007; 85(2): 511–517.

115 Tucker KL, Qiao N, Scott T, *et al.* High homocysteine and low B vitamins predict cognitive

decline in aging men: the Veterans Affairs Normative Aging Study. *Am J Clin Nutr* 2005; 82(3): 627–635.

116 Ravaglia G, Forti P, Maioli F, *et al.* Homocysteine and folate as risk factors for dementia and Alzheimer disease. *Am J Clin Nutr* 2005; 82(3): 636–643.

117 Kado DM, Karlamangla AS, Huang MH, *et al.* Homocysteine versus the vitamins folate, B$_6$, and B$_{12}$ as predictors of cognitive function and decline in older high-functioning adults: MacArthur Studies of Successful Aging. *Am J Med* 2005; 118(2): 161–167.

118 Ellinson M, Thomas J, Patterson A. A critical evaluation of the relationship between serum vitamin B, folate and total homocysteine with cognitive impairment in the elderly. *J Hum Nutr Diet* 2004; 17: 371–383.

119 Quadri P, Fragiacomo C, Pezzati R, *et al.* Homocysteine, folate, and vitamin B-12 in mild cognitive impairment, Alzheimer disease, and vascular dementia. *Am J Clin Nutr* 2004; 80(1): 114–122.

120 Luchsinger JA, Tang MX, Shea S, *et al.* Plasma homocysteine levels and risk of Alzheimer disease. *Neurology* 2004; 62(11): 1972–1976.

121 Wang HX, Wahlin A, Basun H, *et al.* Vitamin B (12) and folate in relation to the development of Alzheimer's disease. *Neurology* 2001; 56(9): 1188–1194.

122 Clarke R. Vitamin B$_{12}$, folic acid, and the prevention of dementia. *N Engl J Med* 2006; 354(26): 2817–2819.

123 Joosten E, Lesaffre E, Riezler R, *et al.* Is metabolic evidence for vitamin B-12 and folate deficiency more frequent in elderly patients with Alzheimer's disease? *J Gerontol A Biol Sci Med Sci* 1997; 52(2): M76–M79.

124 Feng L, Ng TP, Chuah L, *et al.* Homocysteine, folate, and vitamin B-12 and cognitive performance in older Chinese adults: findings from the Singapore Longitudinal Ageing Study. *Am J Clin Nutr* 2006; 84(6): 1506–1512.

125 Morris MC, Evans DA, Schneider JA, *et al.* Dietary folate and vitamins B-12 and B-6 not associated with incident Alzheimer's disease. *J Alzheimers Dis* 2006; 9(4): 435–443.

126 Morris MS, Jacques PF, Rosenberg IH, *et al.* Folate and vitamin B-12 status in relation to anemia, macrocytosis, and cognitive impairment in older Americans in the age of folic acid fortification. *Am J Clin Nutr* 2007; 85(1): 193–200.

127 Malouf R, Grimley Evans J, Areosa Sastre A. Folic acid with or without vitamin B$_{12}$ for cognition and dementia. *Cochrane Database Syst Rev* 2003; (4): CD004514.

128 van Uffelen JG, Chinapaw MJ, van Mechelen W, *et al.* Walking or vitamin B for cognition in older adults with mild cognitive impairment? A randomised controlled trial *Br J Sports Med* 2008; 42(5): 344–351.

129 Sun Y, Lu CJ, Chien KL, *et al.* Efficacy of multivitamin supplementation containing vitamins B$_6$ and B$_{12}$ and folic acid as adjunctive treatment with a cholinesterase inhibitor in Alzheimer's disease: a 26-week, randomized, double-blind, placebo-controlled study in Taiwanese patients. *Clin Ther* 2007; 29(10): 2204–2214.

130 Aisen PS, Schneider LS, Sano M, *et al.* High-dose B vitamin supplementation and cognitive decline in Alzheimer disease: a randomized controlled trial. *JAMA* 2008; 300(15): 1774–1783.

131 Papakostas GI, Petersen T, Lebowitz BD, *et al.* The relationship between serum folate, vitamin B$_{12}$, and homocysteine levels in major depressive disorder and the timing of improvement with fluoxetine. *Int J Neuropsychopharmacol* 2005; 8(4): 523–528.

132 Williams E, Stewart-Knox B, Bradbury I, *et al.* Effect of folic acid supplementation on mood and serotonin response in healthy males. *Br J Nutr* 2005; 94(4): 602–608.

133 Bryan J, Calvaresi E. Association between dietary intake of folate and vitamins B-12 and B-6 and self-reported psychological well-being in Australian men and women in midlife. *J Nutr Health Aging* 2004; 8: 226–232.

134 Taylor M, Carney S, Geddes J, *et al.* Folate for depressive disorders. *Cochrane Database Syst Rev* 2003; (2): CD003390.

135 Sato Y, Honda Y, Iwamoto J, *et al.* Effect of folate and mecobalamin on hip fractures in patients with stroke: a randomized controlled trial. *JAMA* 2005; 293(9): 1082–1088.

136 Green TJ, McMahon JA, Skeaff CM, *et al.* Lowering homocysteine with B vitamins has no effect on biomarkers of bone turnover in older persons: a 2-y randomized controlled trial. *Am J Clin Nutr* 2007; 85(2): 460–464.

137 Lea R, Colson N, Quinlan S, *et al.* The effects of vitamin supplementation and *MTHFR* (C677T) genotype on homocysteine-lowering and migraine disability. *Pharmacogenet Genomics* 2009; 19(6): 422–428.

138 Christen WG, Glynn RJ, Chew EY, *et al.* Folic acid, pyridoxine, and cyanocobalamin combination treatment and age-related macular degeneration in women: the Women's Antioxidant and Folic Acid Cardiovascular Study. *Arch Intern Med* 2009; 169(4): 335–341.

139 Hallert C, Svensson M, Tholstrup J, *et al.* Clinical trial: B vitamins improve health in patients with coeliac disease living on a gluten-free diet. *Aliment Pharmacol Ther* 2009; 29(8): 811–816.

140 Ouma P, Parise ME, Hamel MJ, *et al.* A randomized controlled trial of folate supplementation when treating malaria in pregnancy with sulfadoxine-pyrimethamine. *PLOS Clin Trials* 2006; 1(6): e28.

141 Mahomed K. Folate supplementation in pregnancy. *Cochrane Database Syst Rev* 1997; (3): CD000183.

Gamma-oryzanol

Description

Gamma-oryzanol is one of several lipid fractions obtained from rice bran oil.

Constituents

Gamma-oryzanol is a mixture of phytosterols (plant sterols), including campesterol, cycloartanol, cycloartenol, beta-sitosterol, stigmasterol, and also ferulic acid.

Action

Phytosterols appear to reduce lipid levels and ferulic acid has antioxidant properties. Gamma-oryzanol has also been suggested to have anabolic properties, but evidence is conflicting.

Possible uses

Gamma-oryzanol has been investigated for a role in lipid lowering and improving exercise performance.

Lipid lowering

Several animal studies[1-4] have shown a lipid-lowering effect with gamma-oryzanol supplementation, but one study did not.[5]

In two uncontrolled studies in humans with hyperlipidaemia, gamma-oryzanol was shown to reduce serum cholesterol levels. One study involved 80 patients with hyperlipidaemia who were given gamma-oryzanol for 6 months. In those with type IIa and IIb hypercholesterolaemia, serum cholesterol fell by 12% and 13%, respectively, but the reduction was significant only after 3 months. Plasma triglycerides reduced significantly after 3 months and there was a non-significant increase in HDL cholesterol.[6] In the other study, 20 patients with chronic schizophrenia with dyslipidaemia were given 300 mg gamma-oryzanol daily for 16 weeks. Both total and LDL cholesterol fell significantly, but there was no significant change in HDL levels.[7]

More recent trials have continued to show an influence of gamma-oryzanol on blood lipids. Rice bran oil with varied amounts of gamma-oryzanol improved lipoprotein pattern in mildly hypercholesterolaemic men.[8] A trial of a combined dietary supplementation with gamma-oryzanol, n-3 polyunsaturated fatty acids, vitamin E and niacin in 57 dyslipidaemic men showed that this supplement, compared with placebo and a supplement without gamma-oryzanol, significantly improved lipid levels and also improved inflammatory status.[9]

Exercise

In a double-blind, placebo-controlled study, 22 weight-trained men were given 500 mg gamma-oryzanol daily or placebo for 9 weeks. There were no differences between the groups for measures of circulating concentrations of testosterone, cortisol, oestradiol, growth hormone, insulin or beta-endorphin, blood lipids, calcium, magnesium and albumin. Resting cardiovascular variables decreased in both groups and vertical jump power and one-repetition maximum muscle strength (bench press and squat) increased in both groups. The authors concluded that gamma-oryzanol 500 mg for 9 weeks did not influence either performance or physiological parameters in moderately weight-trained men.[10]

> ### Conclusion
> Preliminary evidence from animal studies and uncontrolled studies indicates that gamma-oryzanol may reduce serum cholesterol levels. There is no good evidence that it improves exercise performance. Further research is required.

Precautions/contraindications

None have been reported.

Pregnancy and breast-feeding

No problems have been reported, but there have not been sufficient studies to guarantee the safety of gamma-oryzanol in pregnancy and breast-feeding.

Adverse effects

There are no long-term studies assessing the safety of gamma-oryzanol in humans. There is some evidence from a Japanese study that doses up to 600 mg daily cause dry mouth, somnolence, hot flushes, irritability and headaches.[11]

Interactions

None reported.

The effects of gamma-oryzanol on several cytochrome P450 (CYP) specific reactions in human liver microsomes have been investigated to predict drug interactions with gamma-oryzanol *in vivo* from *in vitro* data. In this study, gamma-oryzanol had little inhibitory effects on CYP activities, indicating that this compound would not be expected to cause clinically significant interactions with other CYP-metabolised drugs at expected therapeutic concentrations.[12]

Dose

Gamma-oryzanol is available in the form of tablets and capsules.

The dose is not established. Dietary supplements provide 100–500 mg daily.

References

1 Seetharamaiah GS, Chandrasekhara N. Studies on hypercholesterolemic activity of rice bran oil. *Atherosclerosis* 1989; 78: 219–223.
2 Rukmini C, Raghuram TC. Nutritional and biochemical aspects of the hypolipidemic action of rice bran oil: a review. *J Am Coll Nutr* 1991; 10: 593–601.
3 Rong N, Ausman LM, Nicolosi RJ. Oryzanol decreases cholesterol absorption and fatty streaks in hamsters. *Lipids* 1997; 32: 303–309.
4 Cheng HH, Ma CY, Chou TW, *et al.* Gamma-oryzanol ameliorates insulin resistance and hyperlipidemia in rats with streptozotocin/nicotinamide-induced type 2 diabetes. *Int J Vitam Nutr Res* 2010; 80(1): 45–53.
5 Sugano M, Tsuji E. Rice bran oil and cholesterol metabolism. *J Nutr* 1997; 127: S521S–S524.
6 Yoshino G, Kazumi T, Amano M, *et al.* Effects of gamma-oryzanol and probucol on hyperlipidemia. *Curr Ther Res* 1989; 45: 975–982.
7 Sasaki J, Takada Y, Handa K, *et al.* Effects of gamma-oryzanol on serum lipids and apolipoproteins in dyslipidemic schizophrenics receiving major tranquillisers. *Clin Ther* 1990; 12: 263–268.
8 Berger A, Rein D, Schafer A, *et al.* Similar cholesterol-lowering properties of rice bran oil, with varied gamma-oryzanol, in mildly hypercholesterolemic men. *Eur J Nutr* 2005; 44(3): 163–173.
9 Accinni R, Rosina M, Bamonti F, *et al.* Effects of combined dietary supplementation on oxidative and inflammatory status in dyslipidemic subjects. *Nutr Metab Cardiovasc Dis* 2006; 16(2): 121–127.
10 Fry AC, Bonner E, Lewis DL, *et al.* The effects of gamma-oryzanol supplementation during resistance exercise training. *Int J Sport Nutr* 1997; 7: 318–329.
11 Takemoto T. Clinical trial of Hi-Z fine granules (gamma-oryzanol) on gastrointestinal symptoms at 375 hospitals. *Shinyaku To Rinsho* 1977; 26.
12 Umehara K, Shimokawa Y, Miyamoto G. Effect of gamma-oryzanol on cytochrome P450 activities in human liver microsomes. *Biol Pharm Bull* 2004; 27 (7): 1151–1153.

Garlic

Description

Garlic is the fresh bulb of *Allium sativum*, which is related to the lily family (Liliaceae).

Constituents

The major constituents of garlic include alliin, allicin, diallyl disulphide and ajoene, but these compounds form only a small proportion of the compounds that have been isolated from crushed, cooked and dried garlic.

Alliin, present in fresh garlic, is converted by the enzyme allinase into allicin when the garlic bulb is crushed. Allicin can be converted (by heat) into diallyldisulphide, which in turn is converted into various sulphide-containing substances that cause the typical smell of garlic. Allicin and diallyldisulphide combine to form ajoene.

Possible uses

Garlic has been cultivated for thousands of years for medicinal purposes, such as bites, tumours, wounds, headache, cancer and heart disease, and but has also been used as a pungent flavouring agent for cooking.

Evidence for the beneficial effects of garlic is accumulating but is still incomplete. Interpretation of trials is made difficult by the fact that different forms of garlic are used and that active ingredients may be lost in processing.[1] The use of standardised dried garlic preparations or fresh garlic appears to provide the most beneficial effects. Extracts or oils prepared by steam distillation or organic solvents, or 'odourless' garlic preparations, may have little activity.[2,3] Any preparation that produces no odour whatsoever may be clinically ineffective, because release of the biologically active allicin has not occurred. However, allicin is rapidly destroyed even by crushing the fresh bulb, and some suggest that although allicin may be important for cholesterol lowering, it may not be important for protecting against cancer.

Cardiovascular disease

Hyperlipidaemia

Many studies have looked at the potential effects of garlic on serum lipid levels. In a placebo-controlled, double-blind study of 40 patients with hypercholesterolaemia,[3] total cholesterol, triglycerides and blood pressure decreased significantly in the group receiving garlic. Daily doses of 900 mg of a garlic powder preparation (equivalent to 2700 mg fresh garlic) were administered over 16 weeks, and differences were significant after 4 weeks of treatment.

In a randomised, double-blind, placebo-controlled study of 42 healthy adults, 300 mg of a standardised garlic preparation three times daily showed a significantly greater reduction in total and LDL cholesterol than placebo.[4] In a study of eight healthy males, ingestion of a garlic clove (approximately 3 g a day for 16 weeks) resulted in an approximately 20% reduction in serum cholesterol.[5]

In another study, serum levels of total cholesterol, LDL cholesterol and triglycerides decreased significantly after administration of 400 mg garlic three times a day for a month.[5] In a study involving 56 men, administration of an aged garlic extract (AGE, 7.2 g daily) resulted in a 7% reduction in total cholesterol compared with baseline and a 6% reduction compared with placebo.[6] In a multicentre, placebo-controlled, double-blind study carried out in Germany[7] using standardised dried garlic tablets, total cholesterol fell by 11%.

In 35 renal transplant patients, garlic 680 mg twice daily (equivalent to 4080 µg allicin) or placebo was administered over 12 weeks.[8] After 6 weeks, total and LDL cholesterol had fallen, changes that were maintained at 12 weeks. Garlic had no effect on triglyceride or HDL levels. Yet other studies using garlic 700 mg daily for 8 weeks,[9] 200 mg three times a day for 12 weeks,[10] or 1000 mg a day for 24 weeks[11] have resulted in 12–14% reductions in serum cholesterol. Other studies[12–15] demonstrated no effect of garlic on hyperlipidaemia, however.

A meta-analysis of studies[16] evaluating the effect of garlic on serum cholesterol included five of the above studies.[3,7,9–11] The garlic dose was 600–1000 mg daily for 8–24 weeks. The pooled results of the meta-analysis indicated that patients treated with garlic achieved mean total serum cholesterol concentrations 230–290 mg/L lower than patients in placebo groups. Since the investigators used a range of dose regimens, the optimum dose for garlic could not be identified.

More recently another meta-analysis,[17] which included 13 trials, found that garlic reduced total cholesterol level from baseline significantly more than placebo. The weighted mean difference was 0.41 mmol/L (157 mg/L). However, when the trials with the highest scores for methodological quality were analysed alone, the differences in cholesterol levels between garlic and placebo were non-significant. The authors concluded that garlic is superior to placebo in reducing cholesterol levels, but the robustness of the data is questionable and any effect likely to be small. The use of garlic for hypercholesterolaemia was, therefore, debatable.

A double-blind, randomised, placebo-controlled trial in 90 overweight normolipidaemic subjects aged 40–75 years who smoked >10 cigarettes/day compared the effect of a well-characterised garlic powder (2.1 g/day), atorvastatin (40 mg/day) and placebo on plasma lipids and C-reactive protein. None of the variables showed significant differences between the garlic-treated and the placebo groups. In contrast, compared with the placebo group, atorvastatin treatment resulted in significantly lower plasma concentrations of C-reactive protein, total cholesterol, LDL cholesterol, triacylglycerols and tumour necrosis factor-alpha.[18]

A more recent RCT evaluated the effect of raw garlic and two commonly used garlic supplements (powdered garlic, AGE) on cholesterol concentrations in 192 adults with moderate hypercholesterolaemia. Garlic product doses equivalent to an average-sized garlic clove (4-g clove) were consumed on 6 days a week for 6 months. There were no statistically significant effects of the three forms of garlic on LDL cholesterol concentrations. The 6-month mean changes in LDL cholesterol concentrations were raw garlic +0.01 mmol/L (SD, 0.50), powdered supplement +0.08 mmol/L (SD, 0.44), AGE supplement +0.005 mmol/L (SD, 0.46) and placebo −0.10 mmol/L (SD, 0.43). There were no statistically significant effects on HDL cholesterol, triglyceride levels, or total cholesterol: HDL cholesterol ratio.[19]

A further RCT that employed a well-characterised time-release garlic preparation (Allicor 600 mg daily) in 42 men with mild hypercholesterolaemia found that Allicor produced a significant 7.6% decrease in total blood cholesterol compared with baseline in the treated patients by the end of the 12-week study, which was 11.5% lower than in the placebo group. LDL cholesterol in Allicor-treated patients fell by 11.8% and 13.8% at 8 and 12 weeks, respectively. HDL cholesterol had increased by 11.5% by the end of the study. A time-release garlic preparation may be beneficial in providing a prolonged effect on blood lipid fractions.[20]

Evidence from two further meta-analyses is somewhat inconsistent and to a considerable extent related to the heterogeneity of the studies. In a meta-analysis of 29 trials, garlic was found to significantly lower total cholesterol and triacylglycerol but exhibited no significant effect on LDL or HDL cholesterol.[21] A meta-analysis of 13 trials including 1056 subjects concluded that garlic produced no significant lowering of serum cholesterol, LDL cholesterol, triacylglycerol or apolipoprotein B and no significant effect on HDL cholesterol.[22]

Garlic has been evaluated for an effect in various psychopathological parameters in patients with hypercholesterolaemia. In a 16-week prospective, double-blind, placebo-controlled trial, 33 patients with hypercholesterolaemia and no evidence of CVD were randomly assigned to receive garlic or placebo. Garlic in the form of alliin 22.4 mg daily was given to 13 patients and placebo to 20. Both groups received dietary counselling. No significant changes were observed in levels of total cholesterol, LDL, HDL and triglycerides, or in the psychopathologic parameters evaluated.[23]

An RCT in 15 men with angiographically proven coronary artery disease (CAD) investigated the role of aged garlic in endothelial function. Aged garlic was used because it contains antioxidant compounds that increase nitric oxide production and decrease the output of inflammatory cytokines from cultured cells. Oxidative stress and increased systemic inflammation may contribute to endothelial dysfunction. During supplementation, flow-mediated endothelium-dependent dilatation (FMD) increased significantly from the baseline and mainly in those men with lower baseline FMD. Markers of oxidant stress (plasma oxidised LDL and peroxides), systemic inflammation (plasma C-reactive protein and interleukin-6) and endothelial activation did not change significantly during the study. The authors concluded that short-term treatment with AGE may improve endothelial function in men with CAD treated with aspirin and a statin.[24]

An RCT in 65 patients at intermediate risk of cardiovascular disease (CVD) evaluated an aged garlic preparation combined with B vitamins against placebo for progression of atherosclerosis, vascular function and oxidative and inflammatory biomarkers. At 12 months, progression of atherosclerosis was significantly lower in the aged garlic/B vitamin group than the placebo group. Total and LDL cholesterol were also decreased and there was an improvement in vascular function and oxidative biomarkers.[25]

A systematic review of garlic's effects on cardiovascular risk concluded that there are insufficient data to draw conclusions regarding garlic's effects on clinical cardiovascular outcomes such as claudication and myocardial infarction. Garlic preparations may have a small positive short-term effect on lipids. Whether effects are sustainable beyond 3 months is unclear.[26]

Hypertension

Several studies have evaluated the efficacy of garlic in hypertension. In a multicentre, randomised, placebo-controlled, double-blind study of 47 patients with mild hypertension, garlic powder tablets, 200 mg three times a day for 12 weeks, produced significant reductions in blood pressure as well as total cholesterol and triglycerides.[10] In an acute pilot study of nine patients with severe hypertension, single doses of 2400 mg of a garlic powder preparation (standardised to release 0.6% allicin) produced a significant reduction in diastolic blood pressure 5–14 h after administration.[27]

A meta-analysis of studies[28] evaluated the efficacy of garlic on blood pressure. Only prospective, randomised studies with two or more treatment group comparisons and a duration of at least 4 weeks were included, and eight studies met the defined criteria. Six of the studies were placebo-controlled, one compared garlic with a diuretic and reserpine, and another compared garlic with bezafibrate. All but one of the studies were supposedly double-blind, but with the odour of garlic being difficult to mask, it is not clear whether the studies really were blinded. All eight studies used the same dried garlic powder in doses of 600–900 mg daily (equivalent to 1.8–2.7 g fresh garlic daily) for 1–12 months. The pooled mean reduction in systolic blood pressure was 7.7 mmHg and the pooled mean diastolic pressure 5.0 mmHg more with garlic. However, there have not been enough trials with different garlic doses for the optimum dose to be defined.

In a systematic review,[26] consistent reductions in blood pressure with garlic were not found and no effects on glucose or insulin sensitivity were found.

A meta-analysis of 11 RCTs showed a mean decrease of 4.6 ± 2.8 mmHg for systolic blood pressure (SBP) in the garlic group compared to placebo ($n = 10$; $P = 0.001$). Subgroup meta-analysis by baseline blood pressure found the mean decrease in subjects with hypertension was 8.4 ± 2.8 mmHg for SBP ($n = 4$; $P < 0.001$), and 7.3 ± 1.5 mmHg for diastolic blood pressure (DBP) ($n = 3$; $P < 0.001$). Regression analysis revealed a significant association between blood pressure at the start of the intervention and the level of blood pressure reduction (SBP: $R = 0.057$; $P = 0.03$; DBP: $r = -0.315$; $P = 0.02$). The authors concluded that this meta-analysis suggests that garlic preparations are superior to placebo in reducing blood pressure in individuals with hypertension.[29] A further meta-analysis of 10 trials confirmed the main benefits of garlic in blood pressure to be in patients with elevated blood pressure. No blood pressure reductions with garlic were observed in those without hypertension.[30] A further RCT added weight to this conclusion and also showed that time-released garlic powder tablets are more effective for the treatment of mild and moderate hypertension than are regular garlic supplements.[31] Yet another trial showed that aged garlic is superior to placebo in lowering SBP and similarly to current first-line medications in patients with treated but uncontrolled hypertension.[32]

Peripheral artery disease

A Cochrane review assessed the effects of garlic for the treatment of peripheral arterial occlusive disease. One eligible trial (small, of short duration) found no statistically significant effect of garlic on walking distance.[33]

Platelet aggregation

Suggested benefits of garlic in CVD could be related to reduction in platelet aggregation, but studies of garlic on platelet aggregation have shown inconsistent results, possibly related to differences in study design and doses used. A preliminary trial in healthy men found no significant effect of garlic extract on platelet aggregation.[34]

A 10-month placebo-controlled intervention trial found that AGE produced a significant reduction of epinephrine- and, to a lesser degree, collagen-induced platelet aggregation but failed to demonstrate an inhibition of adenosine diphosphate (ADP)-induced aggregation. Platelet adhesion to fibrinogen, measured in a laminar flow chamber at moderately high shear rate, was reduced by approximately 30% in subjects taking AGE compared with placebo supplement.[35]

A 13-week study in normolipidaemic subjects who took AGE (Kyolic) found that it significantly inhibited both the total percentage and the initial rate of platelet aggregation at concentrations of ADP up to 10 μmol/L, but the maximum rate of aggregation was unaffected.[36]

In a further trial, the effect of AGE was evaluated in doses between 2.4 and 7.2 g daily vs equal amounts of placebo. The trial was a randomised double-blind study and included 34 normal healthy men and women. Platelet aggregation and adhesion were measured at 2-week intervals throughout the study. Threshold concentrations for epinephrine and collagen increased moderately during AGE administration compared with the placebo and baseline periods. Only at the highest supplementation level did AGE show a slight increase in the threshold level of ADP-induced aggregation. Platelet adhesion to collagen, fibrinogen and von Willebrand factor was investigated by perfusing whole blood through a laminar flow chamber under controlled flow conditions. Adherence of platelets was inhibited by AGE in a dose-dependent manner when collagen was the adhesive surface perfused at low shear rates (approximately $30 \, s^{-1}$). At high shear rates ($1200 \, s^{-1}$), AGE also inhibited platelet adhesion to collagen but only at higher intake levels. Adhesion to von Willebrand factor was reduced only at 7.2 g AGE daily, but adherence to fibrinogen was potently inhibited at all levels of supplementation. In this study, AGE exerted selective inhibition on platelet aggregation and adhesion, platelet functions that may be important for the development of cardiovascular events such as myocardial infarction and ischaemic stroke.[37]

A small controlled trial involving five healthy volunteers found that a daily dose of 4.2 g raw garlic has no effect on platelet aggregation.[38] A placebo-controlled trial involving the administration of garlic oil in 14 healthy volunteers found that platelet aggregation was induced *ex vivo* by adrenaline, collagen or ADP. Four hours after consuming one large dose of oil derived from 9.9 g garlic, there was little or no effect in the reduction of platelet aggregation. Platelet aggregation induced by adrenaline was reduced slightly but significantly (12% reduction; $P < 0.05$). The oil had no effect on collagen- or ADP-induced aggregation. The authors concluded that the results of this controlled trial indicate that this type of garlic oil should not be relied on in persons with conditions in which reductions in platelet aggregation are desired or necessary.[39]

Diabetes mellitus

A specific garlic preparation (Allicor) has been investigated in a Russian study for an influence on metabolic effects in diabetes mellitus. The 4-week double-blind placebo-controlled study involved 60 type 2 diabetic patients. Fasting blood glucose was measured daily, and serum fructosamine as well as cholesterol and triglyceride levels were determined at baseline, and after 1, 2, 3 and 4 weeks. Treatment with Allicor resulted in better metabolic control due to the lowering of fasting blood glucose, serum fructosamine and serum triglyceride levels.[40]

Cancer

Preliminary data from *in vitro* animal and epidemiological studies suggest that garlic may have a protective effect in cancer development and progression. Results of epidemiological case-control studies in China[41] and Italy[42] suggest that garlic may reduce the risk of gastric cancer. Epidemiological studies cannot by themselves establish causal relationships and prospective data on this possible effect of garlic on cancer risk are required.

Garlic consumption has been associated with a reduced risk of colon cancer in some studies,[43,44] but not others.[45] However, in other studies, garlic consumption was not associated with reduced risk of stomach cancer,[46] breast cancer[47] or prostate cancer.[48] A meta-analysis of the relation between cooked garlic, raw garlic or both raw and cooked garlic on the risk of colorectal and stomach cancers showed that garlic may be associated with a protective effect against both types of cancer.[49]

A systematic review[26] found that garlic supplementation for less than 3–5 years was not associated with decreased risk of breast, lung, gastric, colon or rectal cancer. Some case-control studies suggest that high dietary garlic consumption may be associated with decreased risks of laryngeal, gastric, colorectal and endometrial cancers and adenomatous colorectal polyps.

Antioxidant activity

Reduced peroxidation may play a part in some of garlic's suggested beneficial effects. A controlled trial in 22 subjects (11 of whom had atherosclerosis and 11 acted as healthy controls) found that garlic extract 1 mL/kg daily over 6 months significantly lowered plasma and erythrocyte malondialdehyde (MDA), an oxidant.[50] A further trial from the same research group in 13 elderly subjects found that ingestion of garlic led to significantly lowered plasma and erythrocyte MDA levels and to increased activities of some antioxidant enzymes, indicating that consumption of garlic can decrease oxidation reactions.[51]

Antimicrobial activity

Garlic is being investigated for antibacterial, antifungal and antiviral activity, but current evidence is too limited to recommend garlic for the prevention of infections.

Conclusion

Garlic has been evaluated for an influence on blood lipids in many studies and an increasing number of meta-analyses. Though some studies show favourable effects on blood lipids, evidence remains inconsistent because of study heterogeneity, poor methodology, short duration and small numbers of subjects in some trials. There is some evidence from small trials that garlic supplements reduce blood pressure in those with high blood pressure. There is preliminary evidence that garlic

reduces platelet aggregation and may reduce the risk of cancer, but controlled clinical trials are needed to confirm this. Garlic has been used for centuries for antibacterial and antiviral effects. Although such effects have been demonstrated *in vitro*, controlled clinical studies are needed to confirm these findings. Where benefits have been seen, they have often occurred with standardised preparations of garlic, including slow-release garlic and aged garlic.

Precautions/contraindications

Hypersensitivity to garlic.

Pregnancy and breast-feeding

No problems have been reported. However, there have not been sufficient studies to guarantee the safety of garlic supplements in pregnancy and breast-feeding.

Adverse effects

Unpleasant breath odour; indigestion; hypersensitivity reactions including contact dermatitis and asthma have been reported occasionally. A spinal haematoma (isolated report) has been attributed to the antiplatelet effects of garlic.

Interactions

None reported. Theoretically, garlic could increase bleeding with anticoagulants, aspirin and antiplatelet drugs.

Dose

Garlic supplements are available in the form of tablets and capsules. A US review of 18 products found that 10 products met the label claim for content, while eight products did not.

The dose is not established, but 400–1000 mg (equivalent to 2–5 g fresh garlic or one to two cloves) daily of a standardised garlic product has been used in several studies. Dietary supplements provide 400–1000 mg dried garlic daily. Some products state their alliin concentration. Alliin is converted to allicin, but the amount converted can be as little as 10% to over 50%. Conversion depends on the amount and activity of the converting enzyme alliinase. The allicin yield of garlic, fresh or dried, can vary by more than threefold depending on the garlic used. One gram of fresh garlic should yield about 1000 to 3333 µg of allicin. Because garlic is two-thirds water, dried garlic should yield about three times as much allicin as an equal weight of fresh garlic, but this can vary depending on how well the garlic has been dried. One gram of well-dried powdered garlic bulb should yield about 3000–10 000 µg of allicin, but can be higher or lower based on the garlic and its processing. A garlic 'extract' is supposed to be more concentrated than fresh or dried garlic. However, unless a product states its level of concentration, the extract may not be much different from regular dried powder (about three times the strength of fresh garlic). In garlic oils, allicin is converted into allyl sulphides that are also thought to have biological activity. Aged garlic does not have the characteristic odour of garlic because it does not produce allicin. However, it does contain allicin-related compounds that may have clinical effect. AGE should be standardised to contain not less than 0.05% S-allyl-L-cysteine (SAC). The amount of SAC in a 1400-mg daily dose of AGE powder would be about 700 µg.

References

1 Kleijnen J, Knipschild P, TerRiet G. Garlic, onions and cardiovascular risk factors. A review of the evidence from human experiments with emphasis on commercially available preparations. *Br J Clin Pharmacol* 1989; 28: 533–544.
2 Mansell P, Reckless JP. Garlic. *BMJ* 1991; 303: 379–380.
3 Vorberg G, Schneider B. Therapy with garlic: results of a placebo-controlled, double-blind study. *Br J Clin Pract* 1990; 44(Suppl 69): 7–11.
4 Jain AK, Vargas R, Gotzkowsky S, McMahon FG. Can garlic reduce levels of serum lipids? A controlled clinical study *Am J Med* 1993; 94: 632–635.
5 Ali M, Thompson M. Consumption of a garlic clove a day could be beneficial in preventing thrombosis. *Prostaglandins Leukot Essent Fatty Acids* 1995; 53: 211–212.
6 Steiner M, Khan AH, Holberd D, *et al.* A doubleblind crossover study in moderately hypercholesterolemic men that compared the effect of aged garlic extract and placebo administration on blood lipids. *Am J Clin Nutr* 1996; 64: 866–870.
7 Mader FH. Treatment of hyperlipidaemia with garlic-powder tablets. *Arzneimittelforschung* 1990; 40: 1111–1116.
8 Silagy S, Neil A. Garlic as a lipid lowering agent – a meta-analysis. *J R Coll Physicians London* 1994; 28: 39–45.
9 Plengvidhya C, Chinayon S, Sitprija S, *et al.* Effects of spray dried garlic preparation on primary hyperlipoproteinaemia. *J Med Ass Thai* 1988; 71: 248–252.
10 Auer W, Eiber A, Hertkorn E, *et al.* Hypertension and hyperlipidaemia: garlic helps in mild cases. *Br J Clin Pract* 1990; 44(Suppl 69): 3–6.
11 Lau BH, Lam F, Wang-Chen R. Effect of an odor modified garlic preparation on blood lipids. *Nutr Res* 1987; 7: 139–149.
12 Simons LA, Balasubramaniam S, von Konigsmark M, *et al.* On the effect of garlic on plasma lipids and lipoproteins in mild hypercholesterolaemia. *Atherosclerosis* 1995; 113: 219–225.
13 Isaacsohn JL, Moser M, Stein EA, *et al.* Garlic powder and plasma lipids and lipoproteins: a multicenter, randomized, placebo-controlled trial. *Arch Intern Med* 1998; 158: 1189–1194.
14 Berthold HK, Sudhop T, vonBergmann K. Effect of a garlic oil preparation on serum lipoproteins and cholesterol metabolism: a randomized controlled trial. *JAMA* 1998; 279: 1900–1902.
15 Luley C, Lehmann-Leo W, Moeller B, *et al.* Lack of efficacy of dried garlic in patients with hyperlipoproteinaemia. *Arzneimittelforschung* 1986; 36: 766–768.
16 Warshafsky S, Kamer RS, Sivak SL. Effect of garlic on total serum cholesterol: a meta-analysis. *Ann Intern Med* 1993; 119: 599–605.
17 Stevinson C, Pittler M, Ernst E. Garlic for treating hypercholesterolaemia. *Ann Intern Med* 2000; 133: 420–429.
18 van Doorn MB, Espirito Santo SM, Meijer P, *et al.* Effect of garlic powder on C-reactive protein and plasma lipids in overweight and smoking subjects. *Am J Clin Nutr* 2006; 84: 1324–1329.
19 Gardner CD, Lawson LD, Block E, *et al.* Effect of raw garlic vs commercial garlic supplements on plasma lipid concentrations in adults with moderate hypercholesterolemia: a randomized clinical trial. *Arch Intern Med* 2007; 167: 346–353.
20 Sobenin IA, Andrianova IV, Demidova ON, *et al.* Lipid-lowering effects of time-released garlic powder tablets in double-blinded placebo-controlled randomized study. *J Atheroscler Thromb* 2008; 15 (6): 334–338.
21 Reinhart KM, Talati R, White CM, *et al.* The impact of garlic on lipid parameters: a systematic review and meta-analysis. *Nutr Res Rev* 2009; 22 (1): 39–48.
22 Khoo YS, Aziz Z. Garlic supplementation and serum cholesterol: a meta-analysis. *J Clin Pharm Ther* 2009; 34(2): 133–145.
23 Peleg A, Hershcovici T, Lipa R, *et al.* Effect of garlic on lipid profile and psychpathologic parameters in

people with mild to moderate hypercholesterol-aemia. *Isr Med Ass J* 2003; 5: 637–640.

24 Williams MJ, Sutherland WH, McCormick MP, *et al*. Aged extract improves endothelial function in men with coronary artery disease. *Phytother Res* 2005; 19: 314–319.

25 Budoff MJ, Ahmadi N, Gul KM, *et al*. Aged garlic extract supplemented with B vitamins, folic acid and L-arginine retards the progression of subclinical atherosclerosis: a randomized clinical trial. *Prev Med* 2009; 49(23): 101–107.

26 Mulrow C, Lawrence V, Ackermann A, *et al*. *Garlic: Effects on Cardiovascular Risks and Disease, Protective Effects Against Cancer, and Clinical Adverse Effects*. [Evidence Report/ Technology Assessment, 20]. Washington, DC: US Department of Health & Human Services; 2000, http://www.ncbi.nlm.nih.gov/books/NBK33263/ (accessed 13 April 2011).

27 McMahon GF, Vargas R. Can garlic lower blood pressure? A pilot study *Pharmacotherapy* 1993; 13: 406–407.

28 Silagy CA, Neil HAW. A meta-analysis of the effect of garlic on blood pressure. *J Hypertens* 1994; 12: 463–468.

29 Ried K, Frank OR, Stocks NP, Fakler P, Sullivan T. Effect of garlic on blood pressure: a systematic review and meta-analysis. *BMC Cardiovasc Disord* 2008; 8: 13.

30 Reinhart KM, Coleman CI, Teevan C, *et al*. Effects of garlic on blood pressure in patients with and without systolic hypertension: a meta-analysis. *Ann Pharmacother* 2008; 42(12): 1766–1771.

31 Sobenin IA, Andrianova IV, Fomchenkov IV, *et al*. Time-released garlic powder tablets lower systolic and diastolic blood pressure in men with mild and moderate arterial hypertension. *Hypertens Res* 2009; 32(6): 433–437.

32 Ried K, Frank OR, Stocks NP. Aged garlic extract lowers blood pressure in patients with treated but uncontrolled hypertension: a randomised controlled trial. *Maturitas* 2010; 67(2): 144–150.

33 Jepson RG, Kleijnen J, Leng GC. Garlic for peripheral arterial occlusive disease. *Cochrane Database Syst Rev* 2005;(2): CD000095.

34 Morris J, Burke V, Mori TA, *et al*. Effects of garlic extract on platelet aggregation: a randomized placebo-controlled double-blind study. *Clin Exp Pharmacol Physiol* 1995; 22: 414–417.

35 Steiner M, Lin RS. Changes in platelet function and susceptibility of lipoproteins to oxidation associated with administration of aged garlic extract. *J Cardiovasc Pharmacol* 1998; 31: 904–908.

36 Rahman K, Billington D. Dietary supplementation with aged garlic extract inhibits ADP-induced platelet aggregation in humans. *J Nutr* 2000; 130: 2662–2665.

37 Steiner M, Li W. Aged garlic extract, a modulator of cardiovascular risk factors: a dose-finding study on the effects of AGE on platelet functions. *J Nutr* 2001; 131: S980–S984.

38 Scharbert G, Kalb ML, Duris M, *et al*. Garlic at dietary doses does not impair platelet function. *Anesth Analg* 2007; 105: 1214–1218.

39 Wojcikowski K, Myers S, Brooks L. Effects of garlic oil on platelet aggregation: a double-blind placebo-controlled crossover study. *Platelets* 2007; 18: 29–34.

40 Sobenin IA, Nedosugova LV, Filatova LV, *et al*. Metabolic effects of time-released garlic powder tablets in type 2 diabetes mellitus: the results of double-blinded placebo-controlled study. *Acta Diabetol* 2008; 45: 1–6.

41 You WC, Blot WJ, Chang YS. Allium vegetables and reduced risk of stomach cancer. *J Natl Cancer Inst* 1989; 81: 162–164.

42 Buiatti E, Palli D, Declari A. A case control study of gastric cancer and diet in Italy. *Int J Cancer* 1989; 44: 611–616.

43 Steinmetz KA, Kushi LH, Bostick RM, *et al*. Vegetables, fruit, and colon cancer in the Iowa Women's Health Study. *Am J Epidemiol* 1994; 139: 1–15.

44 Witte JS, Longnecker MP, Bird CL, *et al*. Relation of vegetable, fruit, and grain consumption to colorectal adenomatous polyps. *Am J Epidemiol* 1996; 144: 1015–1025.

45 LeMarchand L, Hankin JH, Wilkens LR, *et al*. Dietary fiber and colorectal cancer risk. *Epidemiology* 1997; 8: 658–665.

46 Dorant E, van denBrandt PA, Goldbohm RA. Allium vegetable consumption, garlic supplement intake, and female breast carcinoma incidence. *Breast Cancer Res Treat* 1995; 33: 163–170.

47 Dorant E, van den Brandt PA, Goldbohm RA, *et al*. Consumption of onions and a reduced risk of stomach carcinoma. *Gastroeneterology* 1996; 110: 12–20.

48 Key TJA, Silcocks PB, Davey GK, *et al*. A case-control study of diet and prostate cancer. *Br J Cancer* 1997; 76: 678–687.

49 Fleischauer AT, Poole C, Arab L. Garlic consumption and cancer prevention: meta-analyses of colorectal and stomach cancers. *Am J Clin Nutr* 2000; 72: 1047–1052.

50 Durak I, Aytac B, Atmaca Y, *et al*. Effects of garlic extract consumption on plasma and erythrocyte antioxidant parameters in atherosclerotic patients. *Life Sci* 2004; 75: 1959–1966.

51 Avci A, Atli T, Erguder IB, *et al*. Effects of garlic consumption on plasma and erythrocyte antioxidant parameters in elderly subjects. *Gerontology* 2008; 54: 173–176.

Ginkgo biloba

Description

Ginkgo biloba is an extract from the dried leaves of *Ginkgo biloba* (maidenhair tree). In Germany, it is one of the most frequently prescribed supplements for cognitive disorders.

Constituents

The leaf contains amino acids, flavonoids and terpenoids (including bilobalide and ginkgolides A, B, C, J and M).

Action

The pharmacological properties of ginkgo biloba have been reviewed.[1,2] Ginkgo biloba extract has the following properties. It:

- antagonises platelet activating factor, reducing platelet aggregation and decreasing the production of oxygen free radicals[3,4]
- increases blood flow, produces arterial vasodilatation and reduces blood viscosity[5]
- has free radical scavenging properties[6,7]
- may influence neurotransmitter metabolism.[8]

These effects are probably due to stimulation of prostaglandin biosynthesis or by direct vasoregulatory effects on catecholamines.[6,9] In addition, ginkgo biloba acts as an antioxidant.[10]

Possible uses

Ginkgo biloba has been studied for the treatment of cerebrovascular disease and peripheral vascular insufficiency.

Memory and cognitive function

The main interest in ginkgo has focused on its use in patients with poor memory and poor cognitive function due to cerebral insufficiency, and it is licensed for this indication in Germany. A review of over 40 European clinical trials evaluated ginkgo's efficacy in the treatment of cerebral and peripheral insufficiency.[2,11] All 40 trials showed positive effects, and the authors concluded that there may have been publication bias. Of the 40 trials, eight were judged to be of good quality. The majority of studies evaluated 12 symptoms: difficulty in concentration; difficulty in memory; absent-mindedness; confusion; lack of energy; tiredness; decreased physical performance; depression; anxiety; dizziness; tinnitus and headaches. Seven of the eight trials showed statistically and clinically significant positive effects of ginkgo compared with placebo. No serious adverse effects were reported.

A meta-analysis of 11 placebo-controlled, randomised, double-blind studies (which included six of the studies) showed that ginkgo was significantly better than placebo for all symptoms associated with cerebrovascular insufficiency of old age. Of the 11 studies, one study was inconclusive, but all the rest showed positive effects.[12]

In a double-blind, placebo-controlled study, 31 patients over the age of 50 years were randomised to receive gingko biloba 40 mg or placebo three times a day. Using a range of psychometric tests, ginkgo was shown to produce a significant improvement in cognitive function at both 12 and 24 weeks.[13] More recent double-blind, placebo-controlled trials have confirmed the benefits of ginkgo on memory[14] and cognitive function.[15,16]

However, in a 6-week RCT, involving 98 men and 112 women over the age of 60 with no cognitive impairment, gingko biloba 40 mg three times a day did not facilitate performance on standard neuropsychological tests of learning, memory, attention and concentration, or naming and verbal fluency. The ginkgo group also did not differ from the control group in terms of self-reported memory function or global rating by spouses, friends and relatives. The authors concluded that ginkgo provides no measurable benefit in memory or related cognitive function to adults with healthy cognitive function.[17] Similarly, a trial in 90 elderly people with above average cognitive function found that ginkgo biloba did not improve cognitive function.[16,18]

A trial in 118 cognitively intact elderly people over the age of 85 evaluated the effect of ginkgo biloba extract on delaying the progression to cognitive impairment. In the intention-to-treat analysis, there was no reduced risk of progression in clinical dementia and no less of a decline in memory function among the ginkgo biloba group. In the secondary analysis, where the medication adherence was controlled, the ginkgo group had a lower risk of progression in clinical dementia and a smaller decline in memory scores. There were more ischaemic strokes and transient ischaemic attacks in the ginkgo group.[19]

Further trials have also indicated a lack of benefit for gingko biloba in reducing cognitive impairment. Gingko biloba 120 mg twice a day was not effective in reducing either the overall incidence rate of dementia or Alzheimer's disease incidence in elderly individuals with normal cognition or those with mild cognitive impairment.[20] The Ginkgo Evaluation of Memory (GEM) study, a randomised, double-blind, placebo-controlled clinical trial of 3069 community-dwelling participants aged 72 to 96 years also concluded that the use of ginkgo biloba, 120 mg twice daily, did not result in less cognitive decline in older adults with normal cognition or in those with mild cognitive impairment.

Effects of gingko biloba in young adults have been less well characterised. A double-blind, placebo-controlled trial in 19 men and 23 women (mean age 23.6 years) investigated the effect of ginkgo biloba (mean dose 184.5 mg daily) on various alertness, performance, affective state and chemosensory tests after meals over a 13-week period. Ginkgo biloba was found to be ineffective at alleviating the symptoms of post-lunch dip or at enhancing smell and taste function.[21]

A double-blind RCT in 52 students found that an acute dose of ginkgo significantly improved performance in tests of attention and memory. However, there were no effects on working memory, planning, mental flexibility or mood. Moreover, after 6 weeks of treatment, there were no significant effects of ginkgo on mood or any of the cognitive tests, suggesting that tolerance developed to the effects, at least in this young healthy population.[22]

A recent re-analysis of three trials in 78 healthy young subjects receiving 120 mg ginkgo biloba extract or placebo found that ginkgo produced a significant improvement on the 'quality of memory' factor that was most evident at 1 and 4 h after the dose had been given, but had a negative effect on performance on the 'speed of attention' factor that was most evident at 1 and 6 hours post-dose. This finding was opposite to the researchers' previous work, which found improvement in the speed of attention task performance.[23]

Ginkgo biloba has also been investigated for effects on cognition and mood in post-menopausal women. In one small controlled trial, ginkgo 120 mg daily for 7 days was associated with significantly better non-verbal memory, sustained attention and frontal lobe function than placebo. However, the two groups did not differ in tests of planning, immediate or delayed paragraph recall, delayed recall of pictures, menopausal symptoms, sleepiness, physiological symptoms or aggressive behaviour.[24] In a further trial, post-menopausal women (aged 51–67 years) were randomly allocated to receive ginkgo 120 mg daily for 6 weeks. The only significant effects of ginkgo were limited to the test of mental flexibility, and also to those with poorer performance, who were mainly in the late stages of menopause (mean age 61 years).[25]

Ginkgo biloba has been assessed for effects on cognitive function in multiple sclerosis and dyslexia. In a 12-week trial in patients with multiple sclerosis, ginkgo biloba was not associated overall with significant improvement in cognitive function. However, a treatment effect trend suggests that ginkgo biloba may have an effect on cognitive domains assessed by the Stroop test (e.g. colour word interference, word test), such as susceptibility to interference and mental flexibility.[26] An open-label trial in 15 children (5–16 years) with dyslexia found that ginkgo biloba 80 mg in a single morning dose decreased the score of the standardised tests for dyslexia. The authors highlight the need for a double-blind trial.[27]

Dementia

In a double-blind, placebo-controlled trial, 216 patients with Alzheimer's disease were randomised to receive either 240 mg ginkgo biloba EGb 761 extract or placebo for 24 weeks. In the

156 patients who completed the study, the frequency of responders in the two groups differed significantly in favour of EGb 761. Analysis of the results on an intention-to-treat basis showed similar results and the authors concluded that EGb 761 was beneficial in dementia of the Alzheimer type and in multi-infarct dementia.[28]

A 52-week, randomised, double-blind, placebo-controlled, parallel-design, multicentre study in 309 patients found that EGb 761 120 mg daily improved measures of cognitive function, daily living, and social performance and psychopathology. The authors concluded that ginkgo was safe and capable of maintaining, or in some cases improving, cognitive and social function in patients with dementia.[29] Of the 309 patients, 244 completed the study up to 26 weeks, but analysis on an intention-to-treat basis still showed significant benefits with ginkgo biloba.[30]

A review of 50 articles, of which four randomised, placebo-controlled, double-blind trials met the inclusion criteria, concluded that there is a small but significant effect of treatment for 3–6 months with 120–240 mg ginkgo biloba extract on objective measures of cognitive function in Alzheimer's disease.[31]

However, in another study of 214 elderly patients with dementia or memory impairment, who were split into three groups and given one of two different doses of ginkgo biloba extract EGb 761 or a placebo, no differences were detected in memory function after 24 weeks.[32] The authors suggested that these results came about because of the effort made to find a good placebo (ginkgo has a pronounced taste and smell). However, others have questioned the validity of the study, suggesting that a positive effect would have been unlikely in such a heterogeneous population where all types of memory loss were included.[33]

In preliminary trials, ginkgo biloba appears to show similar outcomes to those found with prescription drugs (e.g. donepezil, tacrine and possibly other cholinesterase inhibitors).[34–36]

More recent trials have shown inconsistent results. A 24-week RCT in 214 patients with dementia or age-associated memory impairment did not find a significant effect of ginkgo (special extract EGb 761) treatment. There was no dose–effect relationship and no effect of prolonged ginkgo treatment.[37] However, intention-to-treat analysis of another study concluded that ginkgo

(EGb 761) improved cognitive function in a clinically relevant manner in patients suffering from dementia.[38] A review comparing different doses of ginkgo biloba with cholinesterase inhibitors in the treatment of dementia found significant benefits on cognition with cholinesterase inhibitors, but only with ginkgo when all doses were pooled.[39] An RCT in 513 patients with dementia of the Alzheimer's type did not show efficacy of ginkgo. However, there was little cognitive and functional decline in the placebo-treated patients, which may have compromised the sensitivity of the trial to detect a treatment effect. This study was, therefore, inconclusive with respect to the efficacy of ginkgo biloba.[40,41] A commuity based RCT of 6 months' duration found no evidence that a standard dose of high purity ginkgo biloba confers benefit for treating mild–moderate dementia over 6 months.[42]

A 22-week trial in 400 patients with Alzheimer's disease or vascular dementia found that ginkgo biloba special extract EGb 761 was superior to placebo in all cognitive and non-cognitive measures made in the study.[43] Additional results from the same trial included improvements with ginkgo compared with placebo in apathy/indifference, anxiety, irritability/lability, depression/dysphoria and sleep/night-time behaviour.[44]

A Cochrane review found that ginkgo was associated with benefit in cognition after 12 weeks of use but not after 24 weeks and that doses exceeding 200 mg daily, but not lower doses, were associated with benefit. However, ginkgo was associated with benefits in daily living scores at lower rather than high doses. Overall, the analysis concluded that evidence of benefit for ginkgo in cognition and dementia is inconsistent and unconvincing. Early trials, which showed beneficial results, used unsatisfactory methodology, and more modern trials, with better methodology, show inconsistent results. There is need for a large trial using modern methodology with intention-to-treat analysis to provide robust estimates of the size and mechanism of any treatment effects.[45]

A meta-analysis of nine trials (12 to 52 weeks in duration) using the standardised extract EGb 761 concluded that ginkgo biloba appears more effective than placebo. Effect sizes were moderate, and clinical relevance difficult to determine. No consistent results were available for quality of life and neuropsychiatric symptoms, possibly because of the heterogeneity of the study populations.[46] A meta-analysis of six trials evaluating the effect of standardised ginkgo biloba extract found a significant difference in favour of gingko when taken over 6 months.[47]

Peripheral vascular disease

In the review of 40 trials mentioned above,[11] 15 controlled trials evaluated the role of ginkgo in intermittent claudication, and of these, two were judged to be of reasonable quality. One showed significant increase in walking distance tolerated before pain with ginkgo,[48] and the other showed a greater reduction in pain at rest.[49]

In a multicentre, randomised, double-blind, placebo-controlled study involving 74 patients with peripheral arterial occlusive disease, pain-free walking distance improved in patients given either 120 or 240 mg ginkgo biloba daily, with a greater improvement in the group given the higher dose.[50]

In another multicentre, double-blind, placebo-controlled trial, 111 patients with peripheral occlusive arterial disease were randomised to receive 120 mg ginkgo biloba extract or placebo for 24 weeks. Pain-free walking and maximum walking distance were significantly greater in the ginkgo group and subjective assessment by the patients showed an amelioration of complaints in both groups.[51]

A meta-analysis of eight RCTs with 415 participants concluded that ginkgo biloba extract is superior to placebo in the symptomatic treatment of intermittent claudication. However, the size of the overall treatment effect is modest and of uncertain clinical relevance.[52] A more recent double-blind trial in patients with Reynaud's disease found that ginkgo biloba reduced the number of attacks of digital ischaemia by 56% whereas placebo reduced the number by 27%.[53] Another trial found that exercise treatment combined with ginkgo treatment did not produce greater beneficial effects than exercise training alone in patients with peripheral arterial disease.[54]

In a 4-month trial involving 62 adults of mean age 70 years with peripheral arterial disease, ginkgo biloba produced a modest but insignificant increase in maximal treadmill walking time and flow-mediated vasodilation.[55] Most recently, however, a meta-analysis of 11 trials concluded that there is no evidence that Ginkgo biloba has a clinically significant benefit for patients with intermittent claudication.[56]

Tinnitus

There are many reports in the literature that ginkgo biloba may be effective in tinnitus. However, recent trials suggest there is little evidence of benefit. An RCT in 66 adults together with six further RCTs were meta-analysed, and ginkgo was found not to benefit patients with tinnitus.[57] A Cochrane review of 12 trials excluded 10 trials on methodological grounds. No trials of tinnitus in cerebral insufficiency reached a satisfactory standard for inclusion in the review and there was no evidence that ginkgo was effective for the primary complaint of tinnitus.[58]

Mountain sickness

Two trials have demonstrated that ginkgo biloba given 24 h before, and during exposure to, high altitude can reduce symptoms of acute mountain sickness.[59,60] However, trials to date suggest that ginkgo biloba is not as effective as acetazolamide.[61,62]

Cardiovascular disease

Two controlled trials have demonstrated that ginkgo biloba improves coronary blood flow in patients with coronary artery disease, which is linked to improvement in the balance of vasoactive substances such as nitric oxide and endothelin-1.[63,64]

In a further controlled trial involving 3069 patients aged over 75 years, there was no evidence that ginkgo biloba reduced total or cardiovascular mortality or cardiovascular events, but there were more peripheral vascular disease events in the placebo arm.[65] Moreover, ginkgo biloba did not reduce blood pressure or the incidence of hypertension in this group of elderly men and women.[66]

A Cochrane review of ginkgo biloba for acute ischaemic stroke concluded that the methodological quality of the trials to date had been too poor to support the routine use of ginkgo biloba to promote recovery after stroke.[67] Further research is needed in all these areas.

Miscellaneous

Ginkgo biloba has been claimed to be of value in a number of other conditions, including asthma, sexual dysfunction, premenstrual syndrome, age-related macular degeneration, migraine, schizophrenia and attention deficit hyperactivity disorder or autism.

A single blind RCT in students with premenstrual syndrome found a significant decrease in the overall severity of symptoms and physical and psychologic symptoms in both ginkgo (23.68%) and placebo (8.74%) groups ($P < 0.001$). However, the mean decrease in the severity of symptoms was significantly more in the ginkgo group than the placebo group ($P < 0.001$).[68]

A review (which included one study) of the role of ginkgo in age-related macular degeneration concluded that, although a beneficial effect was observed, only 20 people were enrolled in the trial and assessment was not masked, thus making the results equivocal.[69]

A preliminary trial in 50 women suffering from migraine with aura showed that ginkgo biloba (ginkgolide B) was effective in reducing both the frequency and the duration of migraine.[70] A meta-analysis of six trials concluded that ginkgo as add-on therapy to conventional medicine ameliorated the symptoms of chronic schizophrenia.[71] However, ginkgo has been found to be less effective than methylphenidate in treating attention deficit hyperactivity disorder,[72] but a small trial in three patients with autistic spectrum disorder showed that ginkgo improved some behavioural symptoms.[73] Further research is needed in all these areas.

Conclusion

Some studies have shown that gingko biloba may slow the progression of dementia, particularly in Alzheimer's disease, and may be comparable in efficacy to prescription drugs. Evidence that gingko improves memory and concentration in the elderly is inconsistent as is evidence of its benefit in peripheral arterial disease. There is preliminary evidence for benefit of ginkgo in conditions such as migraine, attention deficit hyperactivity disorder and schizophrenia, but further research is needed to clarify these findings. Ginkgo should not be taken in any of these conditions without medical advice.

Precautions/contraindications

Ginkgo biloba should not be used for the treatment of disease without medical supervision. It is contraindicated in hypertension.

Ginkgo has been associated with increased bleeding tendency. However, a recent trial showed no evidence that EGb 761 inhibits blood coagulation, platelet aggregation and haemorrhagic complications.[74] In a trial in older adults with peripheral arterial disease or cardiovascular disease risk, a relatively high dose of ginkgo biloba combined with 325 mg daily aspirin did not have a clinically or statistically detectable impact on indices of coagulation examined over 4 weeks, compared with the effect of aspirin alone. No adverse bleeding events were observed, although the trial was limited to a small sample size.[75]

There is anecdotal evidence that ginkgo might be associated with seizure, so until more is known, ginkgo should be avoided in epilepsy or in patients at risk of seizure. There is also preliminary evidence that ginkgo increases insulin clearance,[76] and this should be borne in mind in monitoring blood glucose in diabetes.

Pregnancy and breast-feeding

Contraindicated in pregnancy, breast-feeding and in children.

Adverse effects

There are few reports of serious toxicity. Headache, nausea, vomiting, heartburn and diarrhoea have been reported occasionally. There have been rare reports of severe allergic reactions, including skin reactions (e.g. itching, erythema and blisters) and convulsions.

Interactions

Drugs

Anticoagulants, aspirin, antiplatelet drugs: use ginkgo biloba with caution. However, a recent study showed no effect of ginkgo on the pharmacodynamics and pharmacokinetics of warfarin in healthy patients.[77] In a small group of healthy Korean men, the addition of a single dose of ginkgo biloba extract did not prolong the bleeding time and was not associated with additional antiplatelet effects compared with the administration of ticlopidine alone. The coadministration of ginkgo biloba extract with ticlopidine was not associated with any significant changes in the pharmacokinetic profile of ticlopidine compared with ticlopidine administered alone.[78]

There is preliminary evidence that ginkgo can influence cytochrome P450, including CYP3A4 and other drug-metabolising enzymes.[79] It may alter protease inhibitor pharmacokinetics and has been shown to reduce serum midazolam concentrations.[78] In another study, midazolam clearance was reduced by ginkgo biloba[80,81] and tolbutamide blood levels were reduced.[81] Caution should be exerted in combining ginkgo with any drugs, particularly when using drugs with a narrow therapeutic margin and/or in elderly people.

Dose

Ginkgo biloba is available in the form of tablets, capsules and tincture. A review of 30 US ginkgo biloba products found that nearly one-quarter did have the expected chemical marker compounds for ginkgo biloba extract (e.g. flavone glycosides, terpene lactones).

Most clinical trials have used a 50 : 1 concentrated leaf extract (EGb 761) standardised to 24% flavone glycosides and 6% terpene glycones. (A standardised 40 mg tablet should, therefore, contain 9.6 mg flavone glycosides and 2.4 mg terpene glycones.)

A single-dose pharmacokinetic study evaluated the bioavailability of three different gingko biloba preparations. The resulting maximum plasma concentrations (median) of bilobalide, ginkgolide A and ginkgolide B after administration of the maximum daily dose of the different ginkgo products were 3.53, 3.62 and 1.38 ng/mL, respectively, after administration of Geriaforce tincture; 11.68, 7.36 and 4.18 ng/mL, respectively, after taking ginkgo fresh plant extract tablets; and 26.85, 16.44 and 9.99 ng/mL, respectively, after administration of EGb 761 tablets.[82]

Studies have used 120–240 mg daily. Dietary supplements provide 40–80 mg in a dose.

References

1 Braquet P. The ginkgolides: potent platelet activating factor antagonists isolated from *Ginkgo biloba* L.: chemistry, pharmacology and clinical applications. *Drugs Future* 1987; 12: 643–699.

2 Kleijnen J, Knipschild P. Ginkgo biloba for cerebral insufficiency. *Br J Clin Pharmacol* 1992; 34: 352–358.

3 Chung KF, Dent G, McCusker M, *et al.* Effect of a ginkgolide mixture (BN 52063) in antagonising skin and platelet responses to platelet activating factor in man. *Lancet* 1987; 1: 248–251.

4 Braquet P, Hosford D. Ethnopharmacology and the development of natural PAF antagonists as therapeutic agents. *J Ethnopharmacol* 1991; 32: 135–139.

5 Jung F, Morowietz C, Kiesewetter H, Wenzel E. Effect of ginkgo biloba on fluidity of blood and peripheral microcirculation in volunteers. *Arzneimittelforschung* 1990; 40: 589–593.

6 Pincemail J, Dupuis M, Nasr C. Superoxide anion scavenging effect and superoxide dismutase activity of Ginkgo biloba extract. *Experientia* 1989; 45: 708–712.

7 Robak J, Gryglewski RJ. Flavonoids are scavengers of superoxide anions. *Biochem Pharmacol* 1988; 37: 837–841.

8 Defeudis FG. *Ginkgo biloba Extract (EGb 761): Pharmacological Activities and Clinical Applications*. Paris: Editions Scientifiques, Elsevier, 1991: 78–84.

9 Nemecz G, Combest WL. Ginkgo biloba. *US Pharmacist* 1997; 22: 144–151.

10 Kobuchi H. Ginkgo biloba extract (EGB 761): inhibitory effect of nitric oxide production in the macrophage cell line RAW264.7. *Biochem Pharmacol* 1997; 53: 897–903.

11 Kleijnen J, Knipschild P. Ginkgo biloba. *Lancet* 1992; 340: 1136–1139.

12 Hopfenmuller W. Evidence for a therapeutic effect of Ginkgo biloba special extract. Meta-analysis of 11 clinical studies in patients with cerebrovascular insufficiency in old age. *Arzneimittelforschung* 1994; 44: 1005–1013.

13 Rai GS, Shovlin C, Wesnes KA. A double-blind, placebo-controlled study of Ginkgo biloba extract ('tanakan') in elderly outpatients with mild to moderate memory impairment. *Curr Med Res Opin* 1991; 12: 350–355.

14 Rigney U, Kimber S, Hindmarch I. The effects of acute doses of standardized Ginkgo biloba extract on memory and psychomotor performance in volunteers. *Phytother Res* 1999; 13: 408–415.

15 Mix JA, Crews WD. An examination of the efficacy of Ginkgo biloba extract Egb761 on the neuropsychologic functioning of cognitively intact older adults. *J Altern Complement Med* 2000; 6: 219–229.

16 Baurle P, Suter A, Wormstall H. Safety and effectiveness of a traditional ginkgo fresh plant extract:

results from a clinical trial. *Forsch Komplementmed* 2009; 16(3): 156–161.

17 Solomon PR, Adams F, Silver A, *et al.* Ginkgo for memory enhancement: a randomized controlled trial. *JAMA* 2002; 288: 835–840.

18 Carlson JJ, Farquhar JW, Dinucci E, *et al.* Safety and efficacy of a ginkgo biloba-containing dietary supplement on cognitive function, quality of life, and platelet function in healthy, cognitively intact older adults. *J Am Diet Assoc* 2007; 107: 422–432.

19 Dodge HH, Zitzelberger T, Oken BS, *et al.* A randomized placebo-controlled trial of Ginkgo biloba for the prevention of cognitive decline. *Neurology* 2008; 70(19Pt2): 1809–1817.

20 DeKosky ST, Williamson JD, Fitzpatrick AL, *et al.* Ginkgo biloba for prevention of dementia: a randomized controlled trial. *JAMA* 2008; 300(19): 2253–2262.

21 Mattes RD, Pawlick MK. Effects of ginkgo biloba on alertness and chemosensory function in healthy adults. *Hum Psychopharmacol* 2004; 19: 81–90.

22 Elsabagh S, Hartley DE, Ali O, *et al.* Differential cognitive effects of gingko biloba after acute and chronic treatment in healthy young volunteers. *Psychopharmacology* 2005; 179: 437–446.

23 Kennedy DO, Jackson PA, Haskell CF, Scholey AB. Modulation of cognitive performance following single doses of 120 mg Ginkgo biloba extract administered to healthy young volunteers. *Hum Psychopharmacol* 2007; 22: 559–566.

24 Hartley DE, Heinze L, Elsabagh S, File SE. Effects on cognition and mood in postmenopausal women of 1-week treatment with ginkgo biloba. *Pharmacol Biochem Behav* 2003; 75: 711–720.

25 Elsabagh S, Hartley DE, File SE. Limited cognitive benefits in Stage 2 postmenopausal women after 6 weeks of treatment with ginkgo biloba. *J Psychopharmacol* 2005; 19: 173–181.

26 Lovera J, Bagert B, Smoot K, *et al.* Ginkgo biloba for the improvement of cognitive performance in multiple sclerosis: a randomized, placebo-controlled trial. *Mult Scler* 2007; 13: 376–385.

27 Donfrancesco R, Ferrante L. Ginkgo biloba in dyslexia: a pilot study. *Phytomedicine* 2007; 14: 367–370.

28 Kanowski S. Proof of efficacy of the ginkgo biloba special extract EGB 761 in outpatients suffering mild to moderate primary degenerative dementia of the Alzheimer type of multi-infarct dementia. *Pharmacopsychiatry* 1996; 29: 47–56.

29 Le Bars PL. A placebo-controlled, double-blind, randomized trial of an extract of Ginkgo biloba for dementia. *JAMA* 1997; 278: 1327–1332.

30 LeBars PL, Kieser M, Itil KZ. A 26-week analysis of a double-blind placebo-controlled trial of the ginkgo biloba extract Egb 761 in dementia. *Dement Geriatr Cogn Disord* 2000; 11: 230–237.

31 Oken BS, Storzbach DM, Kaye JA. The efficacy of Ginkgo biloba on cognitive function in Alzheimer disease. *Arch Neurol* 1998; 55: 1409–1415.

32 van Dongen MC, van Rossum E, Kessels AG, *et al.* The efficacy of ginkgo for elderly people with dementia and age-associated memory impairment: new results of a randomized clinical trial. *J Am Geriatr Soc* 2000; 48: 1183–1194.

33 Weber W. Ginkgo not effective for memory loss in elderly. *Lancet* 2000; 356: 1389.

34 Itil TM, Eralp E, Ahmed I, *et al.* The pharmacological effects of ginkgo biloba, a plant extract, on the brain of dementia patients in comparison with tacrine. *Psychopharmacol Bull* 1998; 34: 391–397.

35 Wettstein A. Cholinesterase inhibitors and Ginkgo extracts – are they comparable in the treatment of dementia? Comparison of published placebo-controlled efficacy studies of at least six months' duration *Phytomedicine* 2000; 6: 393–401.

36 Yancheva S, Ihl R, Nikolova G, *et al.* Ginkgo biloba extract EGb 761(R), donepezil or both combined in the treatment of Alzheimer's disease with neuropsychiatric features: a randomised, double-blind, exploratory trial. *Aging Ment Health* 2009; 13(2): 183–190.

37 van Dongen M, van Rossum E, Kessels A, *et al.* Ginkgo for elderly people with dementia and age-associated memory impairment: a randomized clinical trial. *J Clin Epidemiol* 2003; 56: 367–376.

38 Kanowski S, Hoerr R. Ginkgo biloba extract EGb 761 in dementia: intent-to-treat analyses of a 24-week, multi-center, double-blind, placebo-controlled, randomized, trial. *Pharmacopsychiatry* 2003; 36: 297–303.

39 Kurz A, VanBaelen B. Ginkgo biloba compared with cholinesterase inhibitors in the treatment of dementia: a review based on meta-analyses by the Cochrane collaboration. *Dement Geriatr Cogn Disord* 2004; 18: 217–226.

40 Schneider LS, DeKosky ST, Farlow MR, *et al.* A randomized, double-blind, placebo-controlled trial of two doses of ginkgo biloba extract in dementia of the Alzheimer's type. *Curr Alzheimer Res* 2005; 2: 541–551.

41 Snitz BE, O'Meara ES, Carlson MC, *et al.* Ginkgo biloba for preventing cognitive decline in older adults: a randomized trial. *JAMA* 2009; 302(24): 2663–2670.

42 McCarney R, Fisher P, Iliffe S, *et al.* Ginkgo biloba for mild to moderate dementia in a community setting: a pragmatic, randomised, parallel-group, double-blind, placebo-controlled trial. *Int J Geriatr Psychiatry* 2008; 23(12): 1222–1230.

43 Napryeyenko O, Borzenko I. Ginkgo biloba special extract in dementia with neuropsychiatric features. A randomised, placebo-controlled, doubleblind clinical trial. *Arzneimittelforschung* 2007; 57: 4–11.

44 Scripnikov A, Khomenko A, Napryeyenko O. Effects of Ginkgo biloba extract EGb 761 on neuropsychiatric symptoms of dementia: findings from a randomised controlled trial. *Wien Med Wochenschr* 2007; 157: 295–300.

45 Birks J, Grimley Evans J. Ginkgo biloba for cognitive impairment and dementia. *Cochrane Database Syst Rev* 2009;(1): CD003120.

46 Weinmann S, Roll S, Schwarzbach C, *et al.* Effects of ginkgo biloba in dementia: systematic review and meta-analysis. *BMC Geriatr* 2010; 10(14): 14.

47 Wang BS, Wang H, Song YY, *et al.* Effectiveness of standardized ginkgo biloba extract on cognitive symptoms of dementia with a six-month treatment: a bivariate random effect meta-analysis. *Pharmacopsychiatry* 2010; 43(3): 86–91.

48 Bauer U. 6-month double-blind randomised clinical trial of Ginkgo biloba extract versus placebo in two parallel groups in patients suffering from peripheral arterial insufficiency. *Arzneimitteforschung* 1984; 34: 716–720.

49 Saudreau F, Serise JM, Pillet J, *et al.* Efficacité de l'extrait de Ginkgo biloba dans le traitement des artériopathies oblitérantes chroniques des membres inférieurs as stade III de la classification de fontaine. *J Mal Vasc* 1989; 14: 177–182.

50 Peters H, Kieser M, Holscher U. Demonstration of the efficacy of ginkgo biloba special extract EGb 761 on intermittent claudication: a placebo-controlled double-blind multicenter trial. *VASA* 1998; 27: 106–110.

51 Schweizer J, Hautmann C. Comparison of two dosages of ginkgo biloba extract EGb 761 in patients with peripheral arterial occlusive disease Fontaine's stage IIb: a randomised, double-blind, multicentric clinical trial. *Arzneimittelforschung* 1999; 49: 900–904.

52 Pittler MH, Ernst E. Ginkgo biloba extract for the treatment of intermittent claudication: a meta-analysis of randomized trials. *Am J Med* 2000; 108: 276–281.

53 Muir AH, Robb R, McLaren M, *et al.* The use of ginkgo biloba in Raynaud's disease: a double-blind placebo controlled trial. *Vasc Med* 2002; 7: 265–267.

54 Wang J, Zhou S, Bronks R, *et al.* Supervised exercise training combined with ginkgo biloba treatment for patients with peripheral arterial disease. *Clin Rehabil* 2007; 21: 579–586.

55 Gardner CD, Taylor-Piliae RE, Kiazand A, *et al.* Effect of ginkgo biloba (EGb 761) on treadmill walking time among adults with peripheral artery disease: a randomized clinical trial. *J Cardiopulm Rehabil Prev* 2008; 28(4): 258–265.

56 Nicolai SP, Gerardu VC, Kruidenier LM, *et al.* From the Cochrane library: ginkgo biloba for intermittent claudication. *VASA* 2010; 39(2): 153–158.

57 Rejali D, Sivakumar A, Balaji N. Ginkgo biloba does not benefit patients with tinnitus: a randomized placebo-controlled double-blind trial and metaanalysis of randomized trials. *Clin Otolaryngol Allied Sci* 2004; 29: 226–231.

58 Hilton M, Stuart E. Ginkgo biloba for tinnitus. *Cochrane Database Syst Rev* 2004;(2): CD003852.

59 Gertsch JH, Seto TB, Mor J, Onopa J. Ginkgo biloba for the prevention of severe acute mountain sickness (AMS) starting one day before rapid ascent. *High Alt Med Biol* 2002; 3: 29–37.

60 Moraga FA, Flores A, Serra J, *et al.* Ginkgo biloba decreases acute mountain sickness in people ascending to high altitude at Ollague (3696 m) in northern Chile. *Wilderness Environ Med* 2007; 18: 251–257.

61 Chow T, Browne V, Heileson HL, *et al.* Ginkgo biloba and acetazolamide prophylaxis for acute mountain sickness: a randomized, placebocontrolled trial. *Arch Intern Med* 2005; 165: 296–301.

62 Gertsch JH, Basnyat B, Johnson EW, *et al.* Randomised, double blind, placebo controlled comparison of ginkgo biloba and acetazolamide for prevention of acute mountain sickness among Himalayan trekkers: the prevention of high altitude illness trial (PHAIT). *BMJ* 2004; 328: 797.

63 Wu Y, Li S, Cui W, *et al.* Ginkgo biloba extract improves coronary blood flow in patients with coronary artery disease: role of endothelium-dependent vasodilation. *Planta Med* 2007; 73: 624–628.

64 Wu YZ, Li SQ, Zu XG, *et al.* Ginkgo biloba extract improves coronary artery circulation in patients with coronary artery disease: contribution of plasma nitric oxide and endothelin-1. *Phytother Res* 2008; 22: 734–739.

65 Kuller LH, Ives DG, Fitzpatrick AL, *et al.* Does Ginkgo biloba reduce the risk of cardiovascular events? *Circ Cardiovasc Qual Outcomes* 2009; 3 (1): 41–47.

66 Brinkley TE, Lovato JF, Arnold AM, *et al.* Effect of Ginkgo biloba on blood pressure and incidence of hypertension in elderly men and women. *Am J Hypertens* 2010; 23(5): 528–533.

67 Zeng X, Liu M, Yang Y, *et al.* Ginkgo biloba for acute ischaemic stroke. *Cochrane Database Syst Rev* 2005; (4): CD003691.

68 Ozgoli G, Selselei EA, Mojab F, *et al.* A randomized, placebo-controlled trial of *Ginkgo biloba* L. in treatment of premenstrual syndrome. *J Altern Complement Med* 2009; 15(8): 845–851.

69 Evans JR. Ginkgo biloba extract for age-related macular degeneration. *Cochrane Database Syst Rev* 1999;(3):CD001175.

70 D'Andrea G, Bussone G, Allais G, *et al.* Efficacy of ginkgolide B in the prophylaxis of migraine with aura. *Neurol Sci* 2009; 30(Suppl 1): S121–S124.

71 Singh V, Singh SP, Chan K. Review and meta-analysis of usage of ginkgo as an adjunct therapy in chronic schizophrenia. *Int J Neuropsychopharmacol* 2009; 13(2): 257–271.

72 Salehi B, Imani R, Mohammadi MR, *et al.* Ginkgo biloba for attention-deficit/hyperactivity disorder in children and adolescents: a double blind, randomized controlled trial. *Prog Neuropsychopharmacol Biol Psychiatry* 2009; 34(1): 76–80.

73 Niederhofer H. First preliminary results of an observation of ginkgo biloba treating patients with autistic disorder. *Phytother Res* 2009; 23(11): 1645–1646.

74 Kohler S, Funk P, Kieser M. Influence of a 7-day treatment with ginkgo biloba special extract EGb 761 on bleeding time and coagulation: a randomized, placebo-controlled, double-blind study in healthy volunteers. *Blood Coagul Fibrinolysis* 2004; 15: 303–309.

75 Gardner CD, Zehnder JL, Rigby AJ, *et al.* Effect of Ginkgo biloba (EGb 761) and aspirin on platelet aggregation and platelet function analysis among older adults at risk of cardiovascular disease: a randomized clinical trial. *Blood Coagul Fibrinolysis* 2007; 18: 787–793.

76 Kudolo GB. The effect of 3-month ingestion of Ginkgo biloba extract on pancreatic beta-cell function in response to glucose loading in normal glucose tolerant individuals. *J Clin Pharmacol* 2000; 40: 647–654.

77 Jiang X, Williams KM, Liauw WS, *et al.* Effect of ginkgo and ginger on the pharmacokinetics and pharmacodynamics of warfarin in healthy subjects. *Br J Clin Pharmacol* 2005; 59: 425–432.

78 Kim BH, Kim KP, Lim KS, *et al.* Influence of ginkgo biloba extract on the pharmacodynamic effects and pharmacokinetic properties of ticlopidine: an open-label, randomized, two-period, two-treatment, two-sequence, single-dose crossover study in healthy Korean male volunteers. *Clin Ther* 2010; 32(2): 380–390.

79 Budzinski JW, Foster BC, Vandenhoek S, *et al.* An *in vitro* evaluation of human cytochrome P450 3A4 inhibition by selected commercial herbal extracts and tinctures. *Phytomedicine* 2000; 7: 273–282.

80 Robertson SM, Davey RT, Voell J, *et al.* Effect of Ginkgo biloba extract on lopinavir, midazolam and fexofenadine pharmacokinetics in healthy subjects. *Curr Med Res Opin* 2008; 24: 591–599.

81 Uchida S, Yamada H, Li XD, *et al.* Effects of Ginkgo biloba extract on pharmacokinetics and pharmacodynamics of tolbutamide and midazolam in healthy volunteers. *J Clin Pharmacol* 2006; 46: 1290–1298.

82 Woelkart K, Feizlmayr E, Dittrich P, *et al.* Pharmacokinetics of bilobalide, ginkgolide A and B after administration of three different *Ginkgo biloba* L. preparations in humans. *Phytother Res* 2010; 24(3): 445–450.

Ginseng

Description

Ginseng is the collective term used to describe several species of plants belonging to the genus *Panax*. These include the Asian ginsengs (*Panax ginseng* and *Panax japonicus*), which have been used medicinally for more than 2000 years in China, Japan and Korea. American ginseng (*Panax quinquefolius* L) grows in North America and much of it is exported to the Far East. Siberian/Russian ginseng (*Eleuthrococcus senticosus*) is not considered to be true ginseng because it is not a species of the genus *Panax*. However, as a supplement, it is often promoted alongside Asian and American ginseng products.

Constituents

Panax ginseng contains complex mixtures of saponins known as ginsenosides, which are found in the roots. At least 20 saponins have been isolated from ginseng roots. However, species vary in composition and concentration, and varying concentrations of different saponins appear to exert opposite pharmacological effects.[1,2] This may explain the conflicting results reported in clinical studies, although issues such as type of ginseng, time of harvest, storage and lack of standardisation of active ingredients may also be important. Eleutherosides are believed to be the active ingredients in Siberian ginseng, but these have different chemical structures than the ginsenosides. Studies evaluating the effects of ginseng preparations in glucose metabolism have found different outcomes across different roots[3] and batches[4] of American ginseng. Heat processing of both Korean and American ginseng has been shown to enhance their free-radical scanning[5,6] and anti-proliferative activities.[7,8]

Action

Ginseng has a wide range of pharmacological effects, but its clinical significance in humans has not been fully investigated. Differences in composition of the different species lead to differences in activity.

Analgesic activity, anti-pyretic activity, anti-inflammatory activity, CNS-stimulating and CNS-depressant activity, hypotensive and hypertensive activity, histamine-like activity and antihistamine activity, hypoglycaemic activity and erythropoietic activity have all been reported.[2] Opposing activities such as hypertension and hypotension are thought to be a result of different ginsenosides in one preparation.

The most consistent biochemical explanation for the effects of the ginsenosides is a facilitating influence on the hypothalamic–pituitary–adrenal axis.[9,10] Interactions with central cholinergic[11] and dopaminergic mechanisms[12] have also been demonstrated.

Possible uses

Ginseng is an ancient remedy that has been used for thousands of years in the East. A number of extravagant claims have been made for it, including aphrodisiac and anti-ageing properties. It is not claimed to cure any specific disease, but to restore general vitality. Ginseng is claimed to be useful for:

- improving stamina;
- alleviating symptoms of tiredness and exhaustion;
- headaches;
- amnesia and mental function;
- improving libido and sexual vigour and preventing impotence;
- regulating blood pressure;
- preventing diabetes mellitus;
- preventing signs of old age and extending youth;
- improving immunity; and
- reducing the risk of cancer.

Available evidence for some of these claims has come mainly from animal studies, including increased adaptability to stress,[13] increasing stamina,[14] decreasing learning time,[15] reduction in blood pressure,[16] anti-inflammatory activity[17] and improved sleep.[18]

Cardiovascular function

Ginseng has been suggested to influence cardiovascular function. One double-blind RCT in healthy adults investigated the potential influence of *Panax* ginseng on electrocardiographic parameters: PR, QRS, QT, QT_c and RR intervals, and QT and QT_c interval dispersion. Effects on blood pressure and heart rate were also evaluated. Thirty subjects were randomly allocated to receive 28 days of therapy with *Panax* ginseng 200 mg or placebo. *Panax* ginseng was found to significantly increase the QT_c interval and decrease diastolic blood pressure 2 h after ingestion on the first day of therapy.[19]

North American ginseng has been evaluated for its effect on blood pressure. Sixteen individuals with hypertension were randomised to receive placebo treatment on two mornings or powdered North American ginseng on six mornings. After treatment, blood pressure was measured every 10 min for 160 min, and the mean obtained for the overall 160-min period. None of the North American ginsengs or their means differed from placebo in their overall effect on mean blood pressure change. None affected blood pressure versus placebo at 10-min intervals, but their mean versus placebo increased systolic and diastolic blood pressure at 100 min. The authors concluded that these findings together suggested that North American ginseng exerts a neutral acute effect on blood pressure in hypertensive individuals.[20]

A further study in 24 children undergoing heart surgery found that a ginsenosides compound injected intravenously may attenuate gastrointestinal mucosal injury and inhibit the systemic inflammatory response that occurs after cardiopulmonary bypass in patients with congenital heart disease.[21]

A systematic review of 34 studies investigating the influence of ginseng on blood pressure, lipids and/or blood glucose found mixed results, with current evidence not supporting the use of ginseng to treat cardiovascular risk factors. Some studies suggest a small reduction in blood pressure and some that ginseng improves blood lipid profiles and lowers blood glucose. However, the authors concluded that the overall picture is inconsistent and well-designed RCTs are lacking.[22] A recent 12-week RCT found that American ginseng had no effect on 24-h blood pressure.[23] A preliminary clinical study in 17 healthy young men and women showed that Korean red ginseng many improve arterial stiffness.[24]

Cognitive function

In an uncontrolled study in humans, ginseng has been shown to increase stamina in athletes and concentration in radio operators.[25] In a double-blind, placebo-controlled trial, 60 elderly patients received a supplement containing *Panax* ginseng and vitamins and minerals or placebo daily for 8 weeks. There was no difference in the ability of the supplement or placebo to influence the rehabilitation of these patients, and the effects of the ginseng could not be separated from the other ingredients in the product.[26]

A trial in 30 healthy young adults given ginseng G115 200 mg, ginseng G115 400 mg or placebo found notable behavioural effects during sustained mental activity, particularly with 200 mg ginseng. These included significantly improved subtraction task performance and significantly reduced mental fatigue. Both the ginseng treatments led to significant reductions in blood glucose levels and the authors suggested that the effects on mental performance may be related to the acute gluco-regulatory properties of the extract.[27]

An open-label study evaluated the efficacy of *Panax* ginseng in cognitive performance of patients with Alzheimer's disease (AD). Consecutive patients were randomly assigned to the ginseng ($n = 58$) or the control ($n = 39$) groups, and the ginseng group was treated with *Panax* ginseng powder (4.5 g daily for 12 weeks. Cognitive performances were monitored using the mini-mental state examination (MMSE) and AD assessment scale (ADAS) during 12 weeks of the ginseng treatment and at 12 weeks after the ginseng discontinuation. MMSE and ADAS scales showed no baseline difference between the groups. After ginseng treatment, the cognitive subscale of ADAS and the MMSE score began to show improvements and continued up to 12 weeks ($P = 0.029$ and $P = 0.009$ vs baseline, respectively). After discontinuing ginseng, the improved ADAS and MMSE scores declined to the levels of the control group. These results suggest that *Panax* ginseng is clinically effective in the cognitive performance of AD patients.[28]

Studies have also investigated the cognitive effects of *Panax* ginseng and ginkgo biloba in combination. In a trial involving 20 healthy young adults, receiving 320, 640 and 960 mg of the combination, the most striking result was a dose-dependent improvement in performance on the 'quality of memory' factor at the highest dose of the combination (960 mg). Further analysis revealed that this effect was differentially targeted at the secondary memory rather than the working memory component. There was also a dose-dependent decrement in performance of the 'speed of attention' factor for both the 320 and 640 mg doses.[29]

A further trial by this same group investigated the influence of ginkgo 360 mg, ginseng 400 mg, 960 mg of a ginseng/ginkgo combination and a matching placebo on both mood and cognition. All three treatments were associated with improved secondary memory performance, with the ginseng treatment showing some improvement in the speed of performing memory tasks and in the accuracy of attentional tasks. Following the combination, there was improvement in some mental arithmetic tasks. No modulation of the speed of performing attention tasks was evident. Improvements in self-rated mood were also found following ginkgo and to a lesser extent the combination product.[30]

Korean red ginseng has also been evaluated for potential benefit in patients with dementia. A 12-week randomised, controlled study enrolled 61 patients with AD into low-dose Korean red ginseng (4.5 g daily), high-dose Korean red ginseng (9 g daily) or control. The ADAS, Korean version of the MMSE (K-MMSE) and clinical dementia rating (CDR) scale were used to assess the change in cognitive and functional performance at the end of the 12-week study period. The patients in the high-dose group showed significant improvement on the ADAS and CDR after 12 weeks of Korean red ginseng therapy when compared with those in the control group ($P = 0.032$ and 0.006, respectively). Both high- and low-dose Korean red ginseng treatment groups showed improvement from baseline MMSE when compared with the control group (1.42 vs −0.48), but this improvement was not statistically significant.[31]

Diabetes

A small preliminary study[32] showed that American ginseng reduced blood sugar levels both in people who had diabetes mellitus and in healthy subjects. However, because the study looked only at a single time point, it is unclear what the results mean for real meals or prevention and treatment of diabetes. But the research suggests that ginseng may be useful in preventing sharp increases in blood sugar. A trial in 10 non-diabetic subjects studied the effect of escalating the dose and administration time of American ginseng to evaluate changes in glucose tolerance. This study found that 3, 6 or 9 g American ginseng taken 40, 80 or 120 min before a glucose challenge similarly improved glucose tolerance.[3] A further study in 10 patients with type 2 diabetes showed that American ginseng reduced postprandial glycaemia, and that no more than 3 g was required to achieve reductions.[33]

A double-blind, placebo-controlled study in 36 patients with type 2 diabetes showed that ginseng therapy (100 and 200 mg) significantly reduced fasting blood glucose and elevated mood, and the 200-mg dose resulted in a statistically significant reduction in glycated haemoglobin.[34]

Further trials have shown variable effects on blood glucose, possibly because of the variety and concentration of ginsenosides in the preparations tested. One trial showed that American ginseng reduced post-prandial glycaemia in subjects without diabetes. This reduction was time-dependent, but not dose-dependent. An effect was seen only when the ginseng was administered 40 min before the challenge. Doses within the range 1–3 g were equally effective.[35] Another trial found that American ginseng 6 g daily did not reduce post-prandial glycaemia. The authors suggested that a possible explanation for this was the reduced total ginsenosides in the product, indicating that the ginsenoside profile of American ginseng might play a role in its hypoglycaemic effects.[36]

A further study with Asian ginseng found both null and opposing effects on indices of acute post-prandial plasma glucose and insulin, with the authors concluding that this could be explained by the marked ginsenoside differences in the product.[37] The same research group went on to look at the effects of eight popular types of ginseng on acute post-prandial glycaemic indices in healthy humans to find again that there was some variability. They concluded that the ginsenoside content might be involved but that other components might also have an effect.[38]

Trials with ginseng have generally suffered from poor methodology. A recent longer term randomised, controlled trial of 12 weeks duration randomised 19 patients with well-controlled type 2 diabetes to 6 g daily Korean red ginseng or placebo. There was no change in the primary endpoint (haemoglobin A1c (HbA1c)) in this study. However, patients remained well controlled (HbA1c = 6.5%) throughout. The ginseng treatment also decreased the 75-g oral glucose tolerance test–plasma glucose indices by 8–11%, and the fasting plasma insulin and 75-g oral glucose tolerance test–plasma insulin indices fell by 33–38%. Fasting insulin sensitivity index and 75 g-oral glucose tolerance test-insulin sensitivity indices increased by 33% compared with placebo ($P < 0.05$). Safety and compliance outcomes remained unchanged.[39]

Results from a further placebo-controlled trial showed that chronic use of *Panax* ginseng by non-diabetic individuals had little long-term effect on glucose regulation.[40] The benefits to glucose regulation associated with long-term ginseng use in other research may only be present in populations with compromised glucose control.

Cancer

Case–control[41] and cohort[42] studies in Korean subjects have shown that incidence of cancer is lower in those who consume ginseng than in those who do not.

A randomised, double-blinded, placebo-controlled trial including 643 patients with chronic atrophic gastritis in four hospitals in Zhejiang Province, China, involved the administration of red ginseng extract powder (1 g) to each patient each week for 3 years with follow-up for 8 years. Twenty-four cancers of various organs were diagnosed from these subjects during the 11 years: eight lung, six stomach, two liver, two colorectal and one cancer each of the nasopharynx, oesophagus, pancreas, urinary bladder, prostate and gallbladder. The red ginseng group, which included both men and women, demonstrated a relative cancer risk of 0.54 (95% confidence interval (CI), 0.23 to 1.28; $P = 0.13$) compared with the placebo group, which was not statistically significant. Among the 24 cancer patients, 21 were male. The male red ginseng group showed a relative cancer risk of 0.35 (95% CI, 0.13 to 0.96; $P = 0.03$)

compared with the male placebo group, which was significant. The beneficial effects in this study were, therefore, seen in men but not in men and women overall.[43]

Sexual function

A placebo-controlled (not blinded study) included 90 patients with erectile dysfunction.[44] They were randomly assigned to receive *Panax* ginseng (300 mg daily), trazodone or placebo. Patient satisfaction, libido and penile rigidity and girth were greater in the ginseng group than in the other two groups, but changes in the frequency of intercourse, premature ejaculation and morning erections were not found in any group. None of the treatments resulted in complete remission of erectile dysfunction.

Korean ginseng has been investigated for a role in erectile dysfunction. A total of 45 patients with diagnosed erectile dysfunction were enrolled in a double-blind, placebo-controlled, crossover study in which the effects of Korean red ginseng (900 mg three times a day) were compared with placebo. Mean International Index of Erectile Function scores and scores on penetration and maintenance were significantly higher in patients treated with Korean red ginseng. Penile tip rigidity also showed significant improvement for ginseng versus placebo. The authors concluded that Korean red ginseng can be an effective alternative for treating male erectile dysfunction.[45]

A systematic review of seven randomised, controlled trials provided suggestive evidence for the effectiveness of red ginseng in the treatment of erectile dysfunction. However, the total number of trials included in the analysis, the total sample size and the methodological quality of the primary studies were too low for the authors to draw definitive conclusions.[46] A more recent RCT in 143 men with erectile dysfunction found that mountain ginseng (*Panax* ginseng) did improve erectile function.[47] Moreover, a placebo-controlled trial among 32 postmenopausal women found that Korean red ginseng 1 g daily significantly improved sexual arousal compared with placebo.[48]

Exercise performance

Several human studies have shown an ergogenic effect in exercise, but a review concluded that such trials have been poorly controlled and not blinded, and that there is no compelling evidence that ginseng improves exercise performance in humans.[49] Double-blind, placebo-controlled trials do not support an ergogenic effect of ginseng on exercise performance,[50–53] or on the response of anabolic hormones (growth hormone, testosterone, cortisol, insulin-like growth factor 1) following resistance status.[54]

A double-blind RCT in 38 active healthy adults investigated the effect of 400 mg daily of G115 (equivalent to 2 g *Panax* ginseng) on secretory IgA, performance and recovery after interval exercise. There was no significant change in secretory IgA (an indicator of mucosal immunity). Supplementation with ginseng failed to improve physical performance and heart rate recovery of individuals undergoing repeated bouts of exhausting exercise.[55]

A trial with *Panax* notoginseng found that a dose of 1350 mg daily for 30 days improved endurance time to exhaustion by 7 min and lowered mean blood pressure (from 113 ± 12 to 109 ± 14 mmHg) and maximum oxygen consumption at the 24th minute (from 32.5 ± 8 to 27.6 ± 8 ml/min per kg body weight) during endurance cycle exercise.[56] A trial in 13 physically active male students found that supplementation with American ginseng for 4 weeks prior to exhaustive aerobic treadmill running did not enhance aerobic work capacity but significantly reduced plasma creatine kinase during the exercise. The authors concluded that the reduction in plasma creatine kinase may be due to the fact that American ginseng is effective in decreasing skeletal muscle cell membrane damage induced by exercise during the high-intensity treadmill run.[57]

A placebo-controlled 8-week trial in 60 fit young men (17–22 years) found that 3 g ginseng daily did not affect physical performance, including exercise heart rate, total exercise time and peak power output. There were also no changes in lactate threshold and oxidation rates of fat and carbohydrate.[58] A further RCT in 10 healthy men found that 1125 mg daily North American ginseng for 5 weeks did not significantly affect exercise induced changes in plasma concentrations of lactate, insulin, cortisol, growth hormone or immune response,[59] while a placebo-controlled study among 25 postmenopausal women found that American ginseng supplementation had no effect on heart rate, blood pressure, plasma blood glucose or lactate concentration at rest or immediately after exercise tests and increased oxidative stress, as reflected by elevated oxidative damage markers and the increased erythrocyte antioxidant enzyme activity.[60]

Upper respiratory tract infections

Two trials have investigated the potential benefit of ginseng in preventing upper respiratory tract infection. In one trial, American ginseng over 8 or 12 weeks was found to be safe, well tolerated and potentially effective in preventing acute respiratory illness caused by influenza and respiratory syncytial virus.[61] A further trial with American ginseng in 323 subjects aged 18–65 years found that supplementation for 4 months reduced the mean number of colds per person, the proportion of subjects who experienced two or more colds, the severity of symptoms and the number of days on which cold symptoms were reported.[62]

Quality of life

Both *Panax* ginseng and Siberian ginseng have been found to improve aspects of mental health and social functioning after 4 weeks of therapy, although these benefits attenuate with continued use.[63,64] In another study, *Panax* ginseng had no influence on mood or affect.[65] Siberian ginseng has been shown to have potential efficacy for patients with moderate fatigue.[66] In a further study, *Panax* ginseng (G115) was found to improve aspects of working memory performance and subjective ratings of calmness in healthy young adults.[67] Yet another study identified robust working memory enhancement following administration of American ginseng.[68]

> ## Conclusion
> Ginseng has been used for thousands of years, but modern studies with ginseng in human have produced conflicting results, perhaps due to lack of standardised products, variation in dosage, differences in harvest conditions of the plants and types of ginseng used. Ginseng is taken for a range of other indications but there is little evidence that ginseng slows the ageing process, helps mental or physical functioning in the elderly, increases exercise performance or improves sexual function.

Precautions/contraindications

Ginseng should be avoided by children and used with caution by patients with CVD (including hypertension), diabetes mellitus, asthma, schizophrenia and other disorders of the nervous system. Because of a possible effect on blood glucose, the effect of ginseng on glucose measurement in diabetes should be borne in mind.

Pregnancy and breast-feeding

Ginseng should be avoided due to a lack of good quality data.[69]

Adverse effects

Ginseng is relatively non-toxic, but in high doses (>3 g ginseng root daily) can give rise to the following symptoms: insomnia, nervous excitation, euphoria; nausea and diarrhoea (especially in the morning); skin eruptions; oedema; oestrogenic effects (e.g. breast tenderness; temporary return of menstruation in post-menopausal women).[70,71]

A systematic review of the adverse effects and drug interactions of *Panax* ginseng concluded that the incidence of adverse effects with ginseng monopreparations is similar to that with placebo. The most commonly experienced adverse events are headache, sleep and gastrointestinal disorders. The possibility of more serious adverse events is indicated in isolated case reports and data from reporting schemes. However, causality is often difficult to determine from the evidence provided. Combination products containing ginseng as one of several constituents have been associated with serious adverse events and even fatalities. Possible interactions include ginseng and warfarin and ginseng and phenelzine.[72]

Interactions

Drugs

Tranquillisers: ginseng may reverse the effects of sedatives and tranquillisers.
Digoxin: ginseng may increase blood levels of digoxin.[73]
Warfarin: ginseng may influence the effect of warfarin.[74–77]

Drugs used in HIV: because ginseng use is prevalent in patients with HIV, studies have evaluated the potential for interaction; two recent trials have shown that American ginseng does not alter the pharmacokinetics of zidovudine[28] or indinavir.[78]

Dose

Ginseng is available in the form of tablets, capsules, teas, powders and tinctures. Red ginseng is derived from steam-treated ginseng roots and white ginseng from air-dried roots. Surveys have found that the ginsenoside concentrations in different products vary enormously.[1,79] A review of 21 US products found that seven had less than the required concentration of ginsenosides, two products contained lead above acceptable levels and eight contained unacceptable levels of quintozene and hexachlorobenzene.

The dose is not established. Manufacturers tend to recommend 0.5–3 g daily of the dried root or its equivalent.

References

1   Cui J, Garle M, Eneroth P, Bjorkhem L. What do commercial ginseng preparations contain? *Lancet* 1994; 344: 134.

2   Hikino H, Traditional remedies and modern assessment: the case for ginseng. In: Wijesekera ROB, ed. *The Medicinal Plant Industry*. Boca Raton, FL: CRC Press, 1991: 149–166.

3   Vuksan V, Stavro MP, Sievenpiper JL, *et al.* American ginseng improves glycemia in individuals with normal glucose tolerance: effect of dose and time escalation. *J Am Coll Nutr* 2000; 19(6): 738–744.

4   Dascalu A, Sievenpiper JL, Jenkins AL, *et al.* Five batches representative of Ontario-grown American ginseng root produce comparable reductions of postprandial glycemia in healthy individuals. *Can J Physiol Pharmacol* 2007; 85(9): 856–864.

5   Kang KS, Yamabe N, Kim HY, *et al.* Increase in the free radical scavenging activities of American ginseng by heat processing and its safety evaluation. *J Ethnopharmacol* 2007; 113(2): 225–232.

6   Kim KT, Yoo KM, Lee JW, *et al.* Protective effect of steamed American ginseng (Panax quinquefolius L.) on V79-4 cells induced by oxidative stress. *J Ethnopharmacol* 2007; 111(3): 443–450.

7   Wang CZ, Aung HH, Zhang B, *et al.* Chemopreventive effects of heat-processed *Panax quinquefolius* root on human breast cancer cells. *Anticancer Res* 2008; 28(5A): 2545–2551.

8   Wang CZ, Zhang B, Song WX, *et al.* Steamed American ginseng berry: ginsenoside analyses and anticancer activities. *J Agric Food Chem* 2006; 54 (26): 9936–9942.

9   Filaretov AA, Bogdanova TS, Podvigina TT, Bogdanov AL. Role of pituitary-adrenocortical system in body adaption possibilities. *Exp Clin Endocrinol* 1988; 92: 129–136.

10   Fulder S. Ginseng and the hypothalamic control of stress. *Am J Chinese Med* 1981; 9: 112–118.

11   Benishin CG, Lee R, Wang LCH, Liu HJ. Effects of ginsenoside Rb-1 on central cholinergic metabolism. *Pharmacology* 1991; 42: 223–229.

12   Watanebe H, Ohta-Himamura L, Asakura W, *et al.* Effect of *Panax* ginseng on age-related changes in the spontaneous motor activity and dopaminergic system in rat. *Jpn J Pharmacol* 1991; 55: 51–56.

13   Bittles AH, Fulder SJ, Grant EC, Nicholls W. The effect of ginseng on lifespan and stress response in mice. *Gerontology* 1979; 25: 125–131.

14   Brekhman II, Dardymov IV. New substances of plant origin which increase non-specific stress. *Ann Rev Pharmacol* 1969; 9: 419–430.

15   Saito H, Tschuiya M, Naka S, Takugi K. Effects of *Panax* ginseng root on conditioned avoidance response in rats. *Jpn J Pharmacol* 1977; 27: 509–516.

16   Lee DC, Lee MO, Kim CY, Clifford DH. Effect of ether, ethanol, and aqueous extracts of ginseng on cardiovascular function in dogs. *Can J Comp Med* 1981; 45: 182–185.

17   Yuan WX, Gui LH, Zhou JY, *et al.* Some pharmacological effects of ginseng saponins. *Zhongguo Yaoli Zuebo* 1983; 4: 124–128.

18   Lee SP, Honda K, Ho-Rhee Y, Inoue S. Chronic intake of *Panax* ginseng extract stabilises sleep and wakefulness in sleep-deprived rats. *Neurosci Lett* 1990; 111: 217–221.

19   Caron MF, Hotsko AL, Robertson S, *et al.* Electrocardiographic and hemodynamic effects of *Panax* ginseng. *Ann Pharmacother* 2002; 36: 758–763.

20   Stavro PM, WooM Heim TF, *et al.* North American ginseng exerts a neutral effect on blood pressure in individuals with hypertension. *Hypertension* 2005; 46: 406–411.

21   Xia ZY, Liu XY, Zhan LY, *et al.* Ginsenosides compound (shen-fu) attenuates gastrointestinal injury and inflammatory response after cardiopulmonary bypass in patients with congenital heart disease. *J Thorac Cardiovasc Surg* 2005; 130: 258–264.

22   Buettner C, Yeh GY, Phillips RS, *et al.* Systematic review of the effects of ginseng on cardiovascular risk factors. *Ann Pharmacother* 2006; 40: 83–95.

23   Stavro PM, Woo M, Leiter L, *et al.* Long-term intake of North American ginseng has no effect on 24-hour blood pressure and renal function. *Hypertension* 2006; 47: 791.

24   Jovanovski E, Jenkins A, Dias AG, *et al.* Effects of Korean red ginseng (*Panax* ginseng C.A. Mayer)

and its isolated ginsenosides and polysaccharides on arterial stiffness in healthy individuals. *Am J Hypertens* 2010; 23(5): 469–472.

25 Medvedev MA. The effect of ginseng on the working performance of radio operators. In: *Papers on the Study of Ginseng and Other Medicinal Plants of the Far East*, Vol. 5. Vladivostok: Primorskoe Knizhnoe Izdatelsvo, 1963.

26 Thommessen B, Laake K. No identifiable effect of ginseng (Gericomplex) as an adjuvant in the treatment of geriatric patients. *Aging (Milano)* 1996; 8: 417–420.

27 Reay JL, Kennedy DO, Scholey AB. Single doses of *Panax* ginseng (G115) reduce blood glucose levels and improve cognitive performance during sustained mental activity. *J Psychopharmacol* 2005; 19: 357–365.

28 Lee ST, Chu K, Sim JY, *et al.* Panax ginseng enhances cognitive performance in Alzheimer disease. *Alzheimer Dis Assoc Disord* 2008; 22(3): 222–226.

29 Kennedy DO, Scholey AB, Wesnes KA. Differential, dose dependent changes in cognitive performance following acute administration of a ginkgo biloba/panax ginseng combination to healthy young volunteers. *Nutr Neurosci* 2001; 4: 399–412.

30 Kennedy DO, Scholey AB, Wesnes KA. Modulation of cognition and mood following administration of single doses of ginkgo biloba, ginseng, and a ginkgo/ginseng combination to healthy young adults. *Physiol Behav* 2002; 75: 739–751.

31 Heo JH, Lee ST, Chu K, *et al.* An open-label trial of Korean red ginseng as an adjuvant treatment for cognitive impairment in patients with Alzheimer's disease. *Eur J Neurol* 2008; 15(8): 865–868.

32 Vuksan V, Sievenpiper JL, Koo VVY, *et al.* American ginseng (*Panax quinquefolius* L.) reduces postprandial glycemia in nondiabetic subjects and subjects with type 2 diabetes mellitus. *Arch Intern Med* 2000; 160: 1009–1013.

33 Vuksan V, Stavro MP, Sievenpiper JL, *et al.* Similar postprandial glycemic reductions with escalation of dose and administration time of American ginseng in type 2 diabetes. *Diabetes Care* 2000; 23: 1221–1226.

34 Sotaniemi EA, Haapakoski E, Rautio A. Ginseng therapy in non-insulin-dependent diabetic patients. *Diabetes Care* 1995; 18: 1373–1375.

35 Vuksan V, Sievenpiper JL, Wong J, *et al.* American ginseng (*Panax quinquefolius* L.) attenuates postprandial glycemia in a time-dependent but not dose dependent manner in healthy individuals. *Am J Clin Nutr* 2001; 73: 753–758.

36 Sievenpiper JL, Arnason JT, Leiter LA, Vuksan V. Variable effects of American ginseng: a batch of American ginseng (*Panax quinquefolius* L.) with a depressed ginsenoside profile does not affect postprandial glycemia. *Eur J Clin Nutr* 2003; 57: 243–248.

37 Sievenpiper JL, Arnason JT, Leiter LA, Vuksan V. Null and opposing effects of Asian ginseng (*Panax ginseng* C.A. Meyer) on acute glycaemia: results of two acute dose escalation studies. *J Am Coll Nutr* 2003; 22: 524–532.

38 Sievenpiper JL, Arnason JT, Leiter LA, Vuksan V. Decreasing, null and increasing effects of eight popular types of ginseng on acute postprandial glycemic indices in healthy humans: the role of ginsenosides. *J Am Coll Nutr* 2004; 23: 248–258.

39 Vuksan V, Sung MK, Sievenpiper JL, *et al.* Korean red ginseng (*Panax* ginseng) improves glucose and insulin regulation in well-controlled, type 2 diabetes: results of a randomized, double-blind, placebo-controlled study of efficacy and safety. *Nutr Metab Cardiovasc Dis* 2008; 18(1): 46–56.

40 Reay JL, Scholey AB, Milne A, *et al.* Panax ginseng has no effect on indices of glucose regulation following acute or chronic ingestion in healthy volunteers. *Br J Nutr* 2009; 101(11): 1673–1678.

41 Yun TK, Choi SY. Preventive effect of ginseng intake against various human cancers: a case-control study on 1987 matched pairs. *Cancer Epidemiol Biomarkers Prev* 1995; 4: 401–408.

42 Yun TK. Experimental and epidemiological evidence of the cancer preventive effects of *Panax* ginseng CA Meyer. *Nutr Rev* 1996; 54(11pt2): S71–S81.

43 Yun TK, Zheng S, Choi SY, *et al.* Non-organ-specific preventive effect of long-term administration of Korean red ginseng extract on incidence of human cancers. *J Med Food* 2010; 13(3): 489–494.

44 Choi HK, Seong DH, Rha KH. Clinical efficacy of Korean red ginseng for erectile dysfunction. *Int J Impot Res* 1995; 7: 181–186.

45 Hong B, Ji YH, Hong JH, *et al.* A double-blind crossover study evaluating the efficacy of Korean red ginseng in patients with erectile dysfunction: a preliminary report. *J Urol* 2002; 168: 2070–2073.

46 Jang DJ, Lee MS, Shin BC, *et al.* Red ginseng for treating erectile maximal exercise in human beings. *World J Gastroenterol* 2005; 11(34): 5327–5331.

47 Kim TH, Jeon SH, Hahn EJ, *et al.* Effects of tissue-cultured mountain ginseng (*Panax* ginseng CA Meyer) extract on male patients with erectile dysfunction. *Asian J Androl* 2009; 11(3): 356–361.

48 Oh KJ, Chae MJ, Lee HS, *et al.* Effects of Korean red ginseng on sexual arousal in menopausal women: placebo-controlled, double-blind crossover clinical study. *J Sex Med* 2011; 7(4Pt1): 1469–1477.

49 Bahrke MS, Morgan WP. Evaluation of ergogenic properties of ginseng. *Sports Med* 1994; 18: 229–248.

50 Allen JD, McLung J, Nelson AG, *et al.* Ginseng supplementation does not enhance healthy adults' peak aerobic exercise performance. *J Am Coll Nutr* 1998; 17: 462–466.

51 Engels HJ, Wirth JC. No ergogenic effects of ginseng (*Panax* ginseng CA Meyer) during graded maximal aerobic exercise. *J Am Diet Assoc* 1997; 97: 1110–1115.

52 Morris AC, Jacobs I, McLellan TM, *et al.* No ergogenic effect of ginseng ingestion. *Int J Sport Nutr* 1996; 6: 263–271.

53 Engels HJ, Kolokouri I. Cieslak TJ. Wirth JC. Effects of ginseng supplementation on supramaximal exercise performance and short-term recovery. *J Strength Cond Res* 2001; 15: 290–295.

54 Youl Kang H, Hwan Kim S, Jun Lee W, Byrne HK. Effects of ginseng ingestion on growth hormone, testosterone, cortisol, and insulin-like growth factor 1 responses to acute resistance exercise. *J Strength Cond Res* 2002; 16: 179–183.

55 Engels HJ, Fahlman MM, Wirth JC. Effects of ginseng on secretory IgA, performance and recovery from interval exercise. *Med Sci Sports Exerc* 2003; 35: 690–696.

56 Liang MT, Podolka TD, Chuang WJ. *Panax* notoginseng supplementation enhances physical performance during endurance exercise. *J Strength Cond Res* 2005; 19: 108–114.

57 Hsu CC, Ho MC, Lin LC, *et al.* American ginseng supplementation attenuates creatine kinase level induced by submaximal exercise in human beings. *World J Gastroenterol* 2005; 14: 5327–5331.

58 Kulaputana O, Thanakomsirichot S, Anomasiri W. Ginseng supplementation does not change lactate threshold and physical performances in physically active Thai men. *J Med Assoc Thai* 2007; 90(6): 1172–1179.

59 Biondo PD, Robbins SJ, Walsh JD, *et al.* A randomized controlled crossover trial of the effect of ginseng consumption on the immune response to moderate exercise in healthy sedentary men. *Appl Physiol Nutr Metab* 2008; 33(5): 966–975.

60 Dickman JR, Koenig RT, Ji LL. American ginseng supplementation induces an oxidative stress in postmenopausal women. *J Am Coll Nutr* 2009; 28(2): 219–228.

61 McElhaney JE, Gravenstein S, Cole SK, *et al.* A placebo-controlled trial of a proprietary extract of North American ginseng (CVT-E002) to prevent acute respiratory illness in institutionalized older adults. *J Am Geriatr Soc* 2004; 52: 13–19.

62 Predy GN, Goel V, Lovlin R, *et al.* Efficacy of an extract of North American ginseng containing polyfuranosyl-pyranolsylsaccharides for preventing upper respiratory tract infections: a randomized controlled trial. *CMAJ* 2005; 173: 1043–1048.

63 Ellis JM, Reddy P. Effects of *Panax* ginseng on quality of life. *Ann Pharmacother* 2002; 36: 375–379.

64 Cicero AF, Derosa G, Brilliante R, *et al.* Effects of Siberian ginseng (*Eleutherococcus senticosus* maxim.) on elderly quality of life: a randomized clinical trial. *Arch Geriatr Suppl* 2004; 9: 69–73.

65 Cardinal BJ, Engels HJ. Ginseng does not enhance psychological well-being in healthy, young adults: results of a double-blind, placebo-controlled, randomized clinical trial. *J Am Diet Assoc* 2001; 101: 655–660.

66 Hartz AJ, Bentler S, Noyes R, *et al.* Randomized controlled trial of Siberian ginseng for chronic fatigue. *Psychol Med* 2004; 34: 51–61.

67 Reay JL, Scholey AB, Kennedy DO. *Panax* ginseng (G115) improves aspects of working memory performance and subjective ratings of calmness in healthy young adults. *Hum Psychopharmacol* 2010; 25(6): 462–471.

68 Scholey A, Ossoukhova A, Owen L, *et al.* Effects of American ginseng (*Panax quinquefolius*) on neurocognitive function: an acute, randomised, double-blind, placebo-controlled, crossover study. *Psychopharmacology (Berl)* 2010; 212(3): 345–356.

69 Seely D, Dugoua JJ, Perri D, *et al.* Safety and efficacy of panax ginseng during pregnancy and lactation. *Can J Clin Pharmacol* 2008; 15(1): e87–e94.

70 Siegel RK. Ginseng abuse syndrome: problems with the panacea. *JAMA* 1979; 241: 1614–1615.

71 Greenspan EM. Ginseng and vaginal bleeding. *JAMA* 1983; 249: 2018.

72 Coon JT, Ernst E. *Panax* ginseng: a systematic review of adverse effects and drug interactions. *Drug Saf* 2002; 25: 323–344.

73 McRae S. Elevated serum digoxin levels in a patient taking digoxin and Siberian ginseng. *CMAJ* 1996; 155: 293–295.

74 Janetzky K. Probable interaction between warfarin and ginseng. *Am J Health Syst Pharm* 1997; 54: 692–693.

75 Cheng TO. Ginseng–warfarin interaction. *ACC Curr J Rev* 2000; 9: 84.

76 Palop-Larrea V, Gonzalvez-Perales JL, Catalan-Oliver C, *et al.* Metrorrhagia and ginseng. *Ann Pharmacother* 2000; 34: 1347–1348.

77 Yuan CS, Wei G, Dey L, *et al.* Brief communication: American ginseng reduces warfarin's effect in healthy patients: a randomized controlled trial. *Ann Intern Med* 2004; 141: 23–27.

78 Andrade AS, Hendrix C, Parsons TL, *et al.* Pharmacokinetic and metabolic effects of American ginseng (*Panax quinquefolius*) in healthy volunteers receiving the HIV protease inhibitor indinavir. *BMC Complement Altern Med* 2008; 8: 50.

79 American Botanical Council. Ginseng Evaluation Program. http://abc.herbalgram.org/site/DocServer/Ginseng_Evaluation_Program.pdf?docID=241 (accessed 18 April 2011).

Glucosamine

Description

Glucosamine is a natural substance found in mucopolysaccharides, mucoproteins and chitin. It is found in relatively high concentrations in the joints. Some foods, such as crabs, oysters and the shells of prawns, are relatively rich in glucosamine, but supplements are the best source of additional glucosamine. It is available as a synthetically manufactured dietary supplement in the form of glucosamine sulphate and glucosamine hydrochloride.

Constituents

Glucosamine is a hexosamine sugar and a basic building block for the biosynthesis of glycoprotein, glycolipids, hyaluronic acid, glycosaminoglycans and proteoglycans, which are important constituents of articular cartilage. Chondroitin sulphate (sometimes found together with glucosamine in supplements), which is synthesised by the chondrocytes, is one example of a glycosaminoglycan.

Action

Glucosamine is important for maintaining the elasticity, strength and resilience of cartilage in joints. This helps to reduce damage to the joints. In addition to supporting cartilage and other connective tissue, glucosamine enhances both the production of hyaluronic acid and its anti-inflammatory action.

The mechanism of action is not fully understood, but administration of glucosamine is believed to stimulate production of cartilage components and allow rebuilding of damaged cartilage. *In vitro* studies have found that glucosamine can increase mucopolysaccharide and collagen synthesis in fibroblast tissue.[1] Glucosamine also appears to activate core protein synthesis in human chondrocytes.[2]

Possible uses

Glucosamine is used to promote the maintenance of joint function and to treat pain, increase mobility, and help to repair damaged joints in individuals with osteoarthritis and other joint disorders. It is sometimes provided in supplements with chondroitin, with which it may act synergistically. Both substances have anti-inflammatory activities,[3,4] and both affect cartilage metabolism *in vitro*.[5,6] Animal studies have also demonstrated that glucosamine has anti-arthritic effects.[7,8]

Since 1990, more than 50 studies have examined the effects of glucosamine on osteoarthritis. However, many of these studies have been short, and many have major design flaws and critical problems with data analysis and interpretation of results. Some of the largest RCTs, meta-analyses and systematic reviews are shown in Table 1.

> **Conclusion**
> Glucosamine and also chondroitin are likely to be effective therapies for the symptoms of osteoarthritis, but the degree of benefit apparent in the literature is probably overestimated because of methodological flaws in the studies. Further long-term, adequately designed, rigorous controlled studies are required before the role of glucosamine in the treatment of bone and joint disorders can be fully determined. In addition, further trials are needed to determine whether glucosamine can significantly modify the radiological progression of osteoarthritis.

Precautions/contraindications

Glucosamine may alter glucose regulation and insulin sensitivity. Intravenous glucosamine induces insulin resistance in rats and mice[49–52] and in human muscle cells.[53] Research in human subjects with oral supplements is conflicting. One study reported no change in insulin

239

Table 1   Clinical trials and systematic reviews evaluating glucosamine supplementation in joint pain and arthritis

Reference	Duration and type of trial	Dose of glucosamine	Study group	Outcome measures	Observed effects
Black et al. (2009)[9]	Systematic review	Various	5 systematic reviews and 1 clinical guideline	Clinical effectiveness and cost-effectiveness of glucosamine sulphate/hydrochloride and chondroitin sulphate on progression of OA of the knee	Inconsistent effects, with modest effects on reported pain and function; reduction in joint space narrowing more consistently observed but effect small and clinical significance uncertain; cost-effectiveness was not conclusively demonstrated
			8 primary trials >12 months' duration	As above	Statistically significant improvements in joint space loss, pain and function for glucosamine sulphate, but the clinical importance of these differences was not clear. In two studies of glucosamine sulphate, the need for knee arthroplasty was reduced from 14.5% to 6.3% at 8 years of follow-up
Bruyere et al. (2003)[10]	3-year randomised, placebo-controlled, prospective study	Not defined	212 patients with knee OA	Mean joint space width	Glucosamine was associated with less joint space narrowing than placebo especially in patients with less affected joints at baseline
Bruyere et al. (2004)[11]	Two 3-year, randomised, placebo-controlled, prospective, independent studies	Not defined	414 (319 of whom were post-menopausal women) with knee OA	Symptoms and joint space width	Compared with placebo, glucosamine produced no joint space narrowing and pain symptoms improved
Bruyere et al. (2008)[12]	Follow-up (5 years) of patients in Brueyere et al. (2004)[11]	Not defined	275 (81% of trial patients with at least 13 months of treatment with glucosamine)	Total knee replacement	Total knee replacement occurred in twice as many patients in the glucosamine group as in placebo group
Christgau et al. (2004)[13]	3-year double-blind, placebo-controlled clinical trial	Not defined	212 patients with knee OA	Urinary collagen type IIC-telopeptide fragments (marker of collagen turnover); symptoms on WOMAC scale	Patients with high collagen turnover responded best to glucosamine

Study	Trial design	Dose	Participants	Outcomes	Results
Cibere et al. (2004)[14]	A 4-centre, 6-month, randomised, double-blind, placebo-controlled glucosamine discontinuation trial	1500 mg daily	137 current users of glucosamine with knee OA who had experienced at least moderate improvement in knee pain after starting glucosamine	Primary outcome: proportion of disease flares in the glucosamine and placebo groups using an intent-to-treat analysis. Secondary outcomes: time to disease flare; analgesic medication use; severity of disease flare; and change in pain, stiffness, function and quality of life in the glucosamine and placebo groups	No evidence of symptomatic benefit from continued use of glucosamine sulphate
Clegg et al. (2006)[15]	24-week, multicentre, double-blind, placebo- and celecoxib-controlled trial (GAIT)	1500 mg glucosamine daily, 1200 mg chondroitin sulphate daily, both glucosamine and chondroitin sulphate, 200 mg celecoxib daily	1583 patients with symptomatic knee OA	A 20% decrease in knee pain from baseline to week 24	Overall, glucosamine and chondroitin sulphate were not significantly better than placebo in reducing knee pain by 20%; for patients with moderate-to-severe pain at baseline, the rate of response was significantly higher with combined therapy than with placebo
Cohen et al. (2003)[16]	8-week placebo-controlled trial	Topical glucosamine and chondroitin	63 patients	Pain on WOMAC, VAS and SF scale	Topical glucosamine and chondroitin was more effective than placebo at relieving pain after 4 and 8 weeks. Reduction in symptoms was twice as great with glucosamine
Drovanti et al. (1980)[17]	30-day placebo controlled trial	1500 mg daily	80 patients with OA	Articular pain, joint tenderness and swelling, and restriction of active and passive movements	
Gruenwald et al. (2009)[18]	26-week two-centre, two-armed, randomised, double-blind, comparison study	Glucosamine sulphate 1500 mg daily + eicosapentaenoic acid and docosahexaenoic acid (group A) compared with glucosamine sulphate 1500 mg daily alone (group B)	177 patients with moderate-to-severe hip or knee OA	A 20% decrease in knee pain from baseline to week 26; pain and symptoms on WOMAC scale	OA symptoms (morning stiffness, pain in hips and knees) were reduced at the end of the study: by 48.5 to 55.6% in group A and by 41.7 to 55.3% in group B; the reduction was greater in group A than in group B

(Continued)

Table 1 (Continued)

Reference	Duration and type of trial	Dose of glucosamine	Study group	Outcome measures	Observed effects
Herrero-Beaumont et al. (2007)[19]	Randomised, placebo-controlled, double-blind trial	Glucosamine 1500 mg daily, paracetamol 3 g daily or placebo	318 patients with moderately severe knee OA	Change in the Lequesne index after 6 months; change in WOMAC scale	Glucosamine was significantly better than placebo and paracetamol at reducing Lequesne index and WOMAC scale ratings
Hughes & Carr (2002)[20]	6-month randomised, placebo-controlled, double-blind trial	1500 mg daily	80 patients with knee OA	Patients' global assessment of pain in the affected knee	No difference between placebo and glucosamine (placebo response was 33%); there was a statistically significant difference between groups in knee flexion (mean difference 13°; 95% confidence interval, −23.13 to −1.97, but this difference was small and could have been a result of measurement error
Kawasaki et al. (2008)[21]	18-month placebo controlled trial	Glucosamine hydrochloride, risedronate, or placebo	142 women with moderate knee OA, who had been recommended to undergo home exercise at the first visit to the hospital	Scales for pain evaluation and knee function	Improvement in all groups; no significant benefit of glucosamine
Kayne et al. (2000)[22]	Meta-analysis	Glucosamine vs placebo or glucosamine vs NSAID	10 trials	Symptoms of OA (scoring system)	5/10 trials passed arbitrary pass mark
Lee et al. (2009)[23]	Meta-analysis	2 studies with glucosamine, 4 with chondroitin	6 studies	Joint space narrowing	Glucosamine sulphate did not show a significant effect over controls on minimum narrowing over the first year of treatment. After 3 years of treatment, there was a small to moderate protective effect on minimum joint space narrowing. The same was observed for chondroitin sulphate, which had a small but significant protective effect on minimum narrowing after 2 years

Study	Design	Intervention	Sample	Outcome measure	Results
Marti-Bonmati et al. (2009)[24]	6-month placebo-controlled trial	Not defined	16 patients with cartilage degeneration	Pain and functional outcome on VAS and American Knee Society score, capillary permeability (vascular abnormality in OA)	Pain, functional outcomes and capillary permeability significantly improved with glucosamine
Matsuno et al. (2009)[25]	3 month clinical trial (each patient acted as own control)	Glucosamine plus chondroitin plus quercetin glucoside (GCQG) supplement	46 patients with OA and 22 with RA	Pain symptoms, daily activities, VAS, synovial fluid properties	The OA group showed a significant improvement in pain symptoms, daily activities (walking and climbing up and down stairs), and VAS; changes in the synovial fluid properties with respect to the protein concentration, molecular size of hyaluronic acid, and chondroitin 6-sulphate concentration were also observed. No such effects were observed in the RA group
McAlindon et al. (2000)[26]	Meta-analysis and systematic quality assessment	Glucosamine and/or chondroitin	15 studies	Effect in OA	Moderate to large effects were observed, but quality issues and likely publication bias suggest that these effects were exaggerated
Muller-Fassbender et al. (1994)[27]	A 4-week randomised, double-blind, parallel-group study	Glucosamine sulphate 500 mg vs ibuprofen 400 mg, both three times a day	200 hospitalised patients with active OA of the knee	A reduction in the Lequesne index by at least 2 points if the enrollment value was higher than 12 points, or by at least 1 point if the enrollment value was ≤12 points	Similar response in both groups but adverse effects were lower with glucosamine
Ng et al. (2010)[28]	24-week clinical trial (patients acted as own control)	1500 mg glucosamine daily for 6 weeks followed by 12-week progressive walking programme + glucosamine	36 low-active participants (aged 42 to 73 years) with mild to moderate knee or hip OA	Physical activity levels, physical function (self-paced step test), and the WOMAC Osteoarthritis Index for pain, stiffness and physical function	Glucosamine for 6 weeks improved all measures; measures improved further with walking programme
Noack et al. (1994)[29]	A 4-week, multicentre, randomised, placebo-controlled, double-blind, parallel-group study	Glucosamine sulphate 500 mg three times a day	252 outpatients with knee OA (Lequesne's criteria), radiological stage between I and III, Lequesne index of at least 4 points and symptoms for at least 6 months	A reduction of at least 3 points in the Lequesne index	No difference between glucosamine and placebo

(Continued)

Table 1 *(Continued)*

Reference	Duration and type of trial	Dose of glucosamine	Study group	Outcome measures	Observed effects
Pavelka et al. (2002)[30]	3-year randomised, placebo-controlled trial	Glucosamine sulphate 500 mg three times a day	222 patients with mild to moderate knee OA (using American College of Rheumatology criteria)	Minimum joint space width and symptoms on WOMAC and Lequesne index	Joint space width did not change with glucosamine, but narrowed with placebo; symptoms improved with glucosamine compared with placebo
Petersen et al. (2009)[31]	A 12-week double-blind, placebo controlled, randomised study	Glucosamine, ibuprofen or placebo combined with strength training of the legs	36 elderly patients with bilateral tibiofemoral knee OA determined by radiography	Serum cartilage oligomeric matrix protein (COMP) and urine c-telopeptide of type-2 collagen (CTX-II) as markers for cartilage turnover	Serum COMP was reduced with glucosamine compared with ibuprofen and placebo; urinary CTX-II levels did not change in any of the groups
Poolsup et al. (2005)[32]	Systematic review	Glucosamine (dose not defined)		Structural and symptom effects in knee OA	Glucosamine more effective than placebo in delaying structural progression of knee OA and reducing pain; no more adverse effects with glucosamine than placebo
Qiu et al. (2005)[33]	A 4-week multicentre, randomised, parallel-controlled clinical trial	Glucosamine hydrochloride (1440 mg daily) vs glucosamine sulphate (1500 mg daily)	142 patients with knee OA	Knee pain at rest, at movement and at pressure, knee swelling, morning stiffness and walking ability on Lequesne scale	No significant differences in efficacy and safety between the glucosamine salts
Reginster et al. (2001)[34]	3-year randomised, double-blind placebo-controlled trial	Glucosamine 1500 mg daily	212 patients with knee OA	Mean joint space width, minimum joint space width, symptoms on WOMAC scale	Mean and minimum joint space width did not change with glucosamine but reduced with placebo; WOMAC symptoms worsened with placebo and improved with glucosamine
Reichelt et al. (1994)[35]	6-week multicentre, randomised, placebo-controlled, double-blind, parallel-group study	Glucosamine sulphate 400 mg twice a week intramuscularly	155 patients with knee OA	A response of at least 3 points reduction in the Lequesne index	A significant decrease in the index was observed for glucosamine compared with placebo; responder rate was 55% with glucosamine, 31% with placebo

Study	Study type	Intervention	Population	Outcome measure	Findings
Richy et al. (2003)[36]	Meta-analysis	Oral glucosamine sulphate and chondroitin sulphate		Joint space narrowing, Lequesne index, WOMAC, VAS for pain, mobility, safety, and response to treatment	Significant efficacy of glucosamine on all outcomes, including joint space narrowing and WOMAC; chondroitin was found to be effective on Lequesne index and VAS
Rozendaal et al. (2008)[37]	2-year randomised placebo-controlled trial	Glucosamine 1500 mg daily	222 patients with hip OA	WOMAC pain and function scales, joint space narrowing	No difference in measures with glucosamine or placebo
Rozendaal et al. (2009)[38]	As above	As above	Subgroup analysis of patients based on radiographic severity and type of OA	As above	Glucosamine was no more effective than placebo in analysed subgroups
Ruane & Griffiths (2002)[39]	Mini-review	Glucosamine 1500 mg daily vs ibuprofen 1200 mg daily	2 trials in 218 adult patients with OA	Relief of joint pain	Glucosamine was of similar efficacy as ibuprofen
Sawitzke et al. (2008)[40]	A 24-month, double-blind, placebo-controlled study, conducted at 9 sites in the USA as part of GAIT	Glucosamine 500 mg three times daily, chondroitin sulphate 400 mg three times daily, a combination of glucosamine and chondroitin sulphate three times daily, celecoxib 200 mg daily, or placebo	572 patients with knee OA who satisfied radiographic criteria (Kellgren–Lawrence grade 2 or grade 3 changes and joint space width of at least 2 mm at baseline)	Mean change in joint space width from baseline	No statistically significant difference in mean joint space width loss was observed in any treatment group compared with the placebo group; treatment effects seen on knees with Kellgren–Lawrence grade 2 but not grade 3, which showed a trend toward improvement relative to the placebo group
Sawitzke et al. (2010)[41]	As above	As above	662 patients (as above)	20% reduction in WOMAC index for pain over 24 months	No treatment achieved a clinically important difference in WOMAC pain or function compared with placebo; however, glucosamine and celecoxib showed beneficial but not significant trends
Schollissen et al. (2010)[42]	6-month placebo controlled trial	Glucosamine sulphate vs paracetamol vs placebo	WOMAC index data from the Glucosamine Unum In Die (once-a-day) Efficacy trial[19]	Cost per quality adjusted life year	Glucosamine was a highly cost-effective therapy compared with paracetamol and placebo

(Continued)

Table 1 *(Continued)*

Reference	Duration and type of trial	Dose of glucosamine	Study group	Outcome measures	Observed effects
Towheed et al. (2005)[43]	Systematic review	Glucosamine vs placebo	20 studies (2570 patients)	Pain and WOMAC function	Pooled results from studies using a non-Rotta preparation or adequate allocation concealment failed to show benefit in pain and WOMAC function; studies evaluating the Rotta preparation show that glucosamine was superior to placebo in the treatment of pain and functional impairment resulting from symptomatic OA; WOMAC outcomes of pain, stiffness and function did not show a superiority of glucosamine over placebo for both Rotta and non-Rotta preparations of glucosamine; glucosamine was as safe as placebo
Vlad et al. (2007)[44]	Systematic review	Glucosamine for pain or OA	15 trials	Factors influencing heterogeneity among glucosamine trials	Heterogeneity is larger than would be expected by chance; glucosamine hydrochloride is not effective; effect sizes were consistently higher among trials with industry involvement; potential explanations include different glucosamine preparations, inadequate allocation concealment and industry bias
Wandel et al. (2010)[45]	Network meta-analysis	Glucosamine, chondroitin, or their combination with placebo or head to head	10 trials in 3803 patients	Pain intensity; change in minimal joint space width	Compared with placebo, glucosamine, chondroitin and their combination do not reduce joint pain or have an impact on narrowing of joint space

Study	Type of trial	Dose	Population	Outcomes measured	Results
Wangroongsub et al. (2010)[46]	Randomised placebo-controlled trial	Glucosamine sulphate with potassium salt 1500 mg daily or glucosamine sulphate with sodium salt 1500 mg daily	90 patients with symptomatic mild and moderate knee OA (Ahlback stage 1 to 4)	Range of motion, presence or absence of joint effusion, WOMAC and SF-36	Both groups demonstrated improvement of WOMAC score and SF-36 at final follow-up but this did not reach statistical significance; differences of WOMAC score and SF-36 between the two groups were not significant at any follow-up visit
Wilkens et al. (2010)[47]	6-month double-blind, randomised, placebo-controlled trial	1500mg glucosamine daily	250 patients >25 years with chronic low back pain (>6 months) and degenerative lumbar OA	Pain-related disability, pain, quality of life on various scales	Glucosamine compared with placebo did not result in reduced pain-related disability after the 6-month intervention and after 1-year follow-up
Yoshimura et al. (2009)[48]	3 month clinical trial	Glucosamine 1.5 g or 3 g daily	Soccer players	Biomarkers for collagen degradation and synthesis before and after glucosamine	Glucosamine prevents type II collagen degradation but maintains type II collagen synthesis

GAIT, Glucosamine/Chondroitin Arthritis Intervention Trial; OA, osteoarthritis; RA, rheumatoid arthritis; SF, short form (36) health survey; VAS, visual analogue scale; WOMAC, Western Ontario MacMaster University Osteoarthritis Index.

sensitivity in humans after 4 weeks of therapy with oral glucosamine (500 mg three times daily),[54] another no change in insulin resistance after 6 weeks of therapy with oral glucosamine (500 mg three times daily),[55] another no significant effects on haemoglobin A1c levels in patients with type 2 diabetes after 90 days of therapy (oral glucosamine 500 mg three times daily),[56] while yet another reported no effects on serum insulin, plasma glucose and glycated haemoglobin after 12 weeks (oral glucosamine 500 mg three times daily).[57]

However, a more recent study in humans found that oral glucosamine (1500 mg daily) may affect glucose levels in people with untreated diabetes or glucose intolerance.[58] Two recent systematic reviews concluded that oral glucosamine did not affect glucose control in humans,[59,60] but that data are limited in patients with diabetes and close monitoring for potential changes in glucose control is recommended in these patients.[60] A further trial concluded that glucosamine at commonly consumed doses does not have significant effects on glycaemic control, lipid profile or levels of apolipoprotein A1 in people with diabetes.[61]

A systematic review that included 11 studies (six RCTs and five prospective studies) found that four of the studies showed decreased insulin sensitivity or increased fasting glucose in subjects taking glucosamine. Three of these trials were clinical studies using oral glucosamine. Studies that included subjects with baseline impaired glucose tolerance or insulin resistance were more likely to detect an effect on glucose metabolism than studies without such subjects.[62] More studies are still needed, particularly ones including subjects at high risk for impairments in glucose homeostasis, before a definite conclusion can be made.

Pregnancy and breast-feeding

No problems have been reported, but there have not been sufficient studies to guarantee the safety of glucosamine in pregnancy and breast-feeding. Glucosamine is probably best avoided.

Adverse effects

Glucosamine is relatively non-toxic, and does not appear to be associated with serious side-effects. Side-effects reported include constipation, diarrhoea, heartburn, nausea, drowsiness, headache and rash. Risk assessment supports safety at intakes of up to 2000 mg daily of glucosamine.[63]

Interactions

Drugs

Warfarin: The Medicines and Healthcare products Regulatory Agency (MHRA) has received reports of an interaction between glucosamine and warfarin. In these cases, patients who had previously stable international normalised ratios (INRs) on warfarin had an increase in their INR after they started taking glucosamine supplements.[64] A 2008 paper[65] found 20 reports in the US Food and Drug Administration MedWatch database and 21 reports in the World Health Organization adverse drug reactions database of glucosamine or glucosamine–chondroitin sulphate use with warfarin associated with altered coagulation (manifested by increased INR or increased bleeding or bruising). Interactions resolved by stopping the supplement or in some cases by reducing the dose of either glucosamine or warfarin.[65] The mechanism of any interaction is unclear; however, patients on warfarin are recommended not to take glucosamine.

In theory insulin or oral hypoglycaemics may be less effective.

Dose

Glucosamine is available in the form of tablets, capsules and powders as glucosamine sulphate, glucosamine hydrochloride and N-acetyl-D-glucosamine. It is also available in the form of cream. A review of 10 products containing glucosamine found that all products contained the labelled amounts of glucosamine, but 6 out of 13 products containing glucosamine and chondroitin did not pass, all due to low chondroitin levels.

The dose is not definitely established. However, a dose of glucosamine sulphate 500 mg three times a day (1500 mg daily) has been used in most studies and this is the dose recommended by many manufacturers. Full therapeutic benefit may take more than 4 weeks.

References

1 McCarty MF. The neglect of glucosamine as treatment for osteoathritis. *Med Hypotheses* 1994; 42: 323–327.

2 Bassleer C, Henroitin Y, Franchimont P. In vitro evaluation of drugs proposed as chondroprotective agents. *Int J Tissue React* 1992; 14: 231–241.

3 Sentnikar I, Cereda R, Pacini MA, et al. Antireactive properties of glucosamine sulphate. *Arznemittelforschung* 1991; 41: 157–161.

4 Ronca F, Palmieri L, Panicucci P, et al. Anti-inflammatory activity of chondroitin sulphate. *Osteoarthritis Cartilage* 1998; 6(Suppl A): 14–21.

5 Bassleer CT, Combal JP, Bougaret S, et al. Effects of chondroitin sulphate and interleukin-1 beta on human articular chondrocytes cultivated in clusters. *Osteoarthritis Cartilage* 1998; 6: 196–204.

6 Bassleer CT, Rovati L, Franchimont P. Stimulation of proteoglycan production by glucosamine sulphate in chondrocytes isolated from human osteoarthritic articular cartilage in vitro. *Osteoarthritis Cartilage* 1998; 6: 196–204.

7 Setnikar I, Pacini MA, Revel L. Antiarthritic effects of glucosamine sulfate studied in animal models. *Arzneimittelforschung* 1991; 41: 542–545.

8 Uebelhart D, Thonar EJ, Zhang J, et al. Protective effect of exogenous chondroitin 4,6-sulfate in the acute degradation of articular cartilage in the rabbit. *Osteoarthritis Cartilage* 1998; 6(Suppl A): 6–13.

9 Black C, Clar C, Henderson R, et al. The clinical effectiveness of glucosamine and chondroitin supplements in slowing or arresting progression of osteoarthritis of the knee: a systematic review and economic evaluation. *Health Technol Assess* 2009; 13(52): 1–148.

10 Bruyere O, Honore A, Ethgen O, et al. Correlation between radiographic severity of knee osteoarthritis and future disease progression. Results from a 3-year prospective, placebo-controlled study evaluating the effect of glucosamine sulfate. *Osteoarthritis Cartilage* 2003; 11(1): 1–5.

11 Bruyere O, Pavelka K, Rovati LC, et al. Glucosamine sulfate reduces osteoarthritis progression in postmenopausal women with knee osteoarthritis: evidence from two 3-year studies. *Menopause* 2004; 11(2): 138–143.

12 Bruyere O, Pavelka K, Rovati LC, et al. Total joint replacement after glucosamine sulphate treatment in knee osteoarthritis: results of a mean 8-year observation of patients from two previous 3-year, randomised, placebo-controlled trials. *Osteoarthritis Cartilage* 2008; 16(2): 254–260.

13 Christgau S, Henrotin Y, Tanko LB, et al. Osteoarthritic patients with high cartilage turnover show increased responsiveness to the cartilage protecting effects of glucosamine sulphate. *Clin Exp Rheumatol* 2004; 22(1): 36–42.

14 Cibere J, Kopec JA, Thorne RA, et al. Randomized, double-blind, placebo-controlled glucosamine discontinuation trial in knee osteoarthritis. *Arthritis Rheum* 2004; 51: 738–745.

15 Clegg DO, Reda DJ, Harris CL, et al. Glucosamine, chondroitin sulfate, and the two in combination for painful knee osteoarthritis. *N Engl J Med* 2006; 354 (8): 795–808.

16 Cohen M, Wolfe R, Mai T, et al. A randomized, double blind, placebo controlled trial of a topical cream containing glucosamine sulfate, chondroitin sulfate, and camphor for osteoarthritis of the knee. *J Rheumatol* 2003; 30(3): 523–528.

17 Drovanti A, Bignamini AA, Rovati AL. Therapeutic activity of oral glucosamine sulfate in osteoarthrosis: a placebo-controlled double-blind investigation. *Clin Ther* 1980; 3(4): 260–272.

18 Gruenwald J, Petzold E, Busch R, et al. Effect of glucosamine sulfate with or without omega-3 fatty acids in patients with osteoarthritis. *Adv Ther* 2009; 26(9): 858–871.

19 Herrero-Beaumont G, Ivorra JA, DelCarmen Trabado M, et al. Glucosamine sulfate in the treatment of knee osteoarthritis symptoms: a randomized, double-blind, placebo-controlled study using acetaminophen as a side comparator. *Arthritis Rheum* 2007; 56(2): 555–567.

20 Hughes R, Carr A. A randomized, double-blind, placebo-controlled trial of glucosamine sulphate as an analgesic in osteoarthritis of the knee. *Rheumatology* 2002; 41: 279–284.

21 Kawasaki T, Kurosawa H, Ikeda H, et al. Additive effects of glucosamine or risedronate for the treatment of osteoarthritis of the knee combined with home exercise: a prospective randomized 18-month trial. *J Bone Miner Metab* 2008; 26(3): 279–287.

22 Kayne SB, Wadeson K, MacAdam A. Glucosamine: an effective treatment for osteoarthritis? A meta-analysis *Pharm J* 2000; 265: 759–763.

23 Lee YH, Woo JH, Choi SJ, et al. Effect of glucosamine or chondroitin sulfate on the osteoarthritis progression: a meta-analysis. *Rheumatol Int* 2009; 30(3): 357–363.

24 Marti-Bonmati L, Sanz-Requena R, Rodrigo JL, et al. Glucosamine sulfate effect on the degenerated patellar cartilage: preliminary findings by pharmacokinetic magnetic resonance modeling. *Eur Radiol* 2009; 19(6): 1512–1518.

25 Matsuno H, Nakamura H, Katayama K, et al. Effects of an oral administration of glucosamine-chondroitin-quercetin glucoside on the synovial fluid properties in patients with osteoarthritis and rheumatoid arthritis. *Biosci Biotechnol Biochem* 2009; 73(2): 288–292.

26 McAlindon TE, LaValley MP, Gulin JP, et al. Glucosamine and chondroitin for treatment of osteoarthritis: a systematic quality assessment and meta-analysis. *JAMA* 2000; 283(11): 1469–1475.

27 Muller-Fassbender H, Bach GL, Haase W, et al. Glucosamine sulfate compared to ibuprofen in osteoarthritis of the knee. *Osteoarthritis Cartilage* 1994; 2(1): 61–69.

28 Ng NT, Heesch KC, Brown WJ. Efficacy of a progressive walking program and glucosamine sulphate supplementation on osteoarthritic symptoms of the hip and knee: a feasibility trial. *Arthritis Res Ther* 2010; 12(1): R25.

29 Noack W, Fischer M, Forster KK, *et al.* Glucosamine sulfate in osteoarthritis of the knee. *Osteoarthritis Cartilage* 1994; 2(1): 51–59.

30 Pavelka K, Gatterova J, Olejarova M, *et al.* Glucosamine sulfate use and delay of progression of knee osteoarthritis: a 3-year, randomized, placebocontrolled, double-blind study. *Arch Intern Med* 2002; 162: 2113–2123.

31 Petersen SG, Saxne T, Heinegard D, *et al.* Glucosamine but not ibuprofen alters cartilage turnover in osteoarthritis patients in response to physical training. *Osteoarthritis Cartilage* 2009; 18(1): 34–40.

32 Poolsup N, Suthisisang C, Channark P, *et al.* Glucosamine long-term treatment and the progression of knee osteoarthritis: systematic review of randomized controlled trials. *Ann Pharmacother* 2005; 39(6): 1080–1087.

33 Qiu GX, Weng XS, Zhang K, *et al.* [A multi-central, randomized, controlled clinical trial of glucosamine hydrochloride/sulfate in the treatment of knee osteoarthritis]. *Zhonghua Yi Xue Za Zhi* 2005; 85(43): 3067–3070.

34 Reginster JY, Deroisy R, Rovati LC, *et al.* Long-term effects of glucosamine sulphate on osteoarthritis progression: a randomised, placebo-controlled clinical trial. *Lancet* 2001; 357(9252): 251–256.

35 Reichelt A, Forster KK, Fischer M, *et al.* Efficacy and safety of intramuscular glucosamine sulfate in osteoarthritis of the knee. A randomised, placebo-controlled, double-blind study. *Arzneimittelforschung* 1994; 44(1): 75–80.

36 Richy F, Bruyere O, Ethgen O, *et al.* Structural and symptomatic efficacy of glucosamine and chondroitin in knee osteoarthritis: a comprehensive meta-analysis. *Arch Intern Med* 2003; 163(13): 1514–1522.

37 Rozendaal RM, Koes BW, van Osch GJVM, *et al.* Effect of glucosamine sulfate on hip osteoarthritis: a randomized trial. *Ann Intern Med* 2008; 148(4): 268–277.

38 Rozendaal RM, Uitterlinden EJ, van Osch GJ, *et al.* Effect of glucosamine sulphate on joint space narrowing, pain and function in patients with hip osteoarthritis; subgroup analyses of a randomized controlled trial. *Osteoarthritis Cartilage* 2009; 17 (4): 427–432.

39 Ruane R, Griffiths P. Glucosamine therapy compared to ibuprofen for joint pain. *Br J Community Nursing* 2002; 7: 148–152.

40 Sawitzke AD, Shi H, Finco MF, *et al.* The effect of glucosamine and/or chondroitin sulfate on the progression of knee osteoarthritis: a report from the Glucosamine/chondroitin Arthritis Intervention Trial. *Arthritis Rheum* 2008; 58(10): 3183–3191.

41 Sawitzke AD, Shi H, Finco MF, *et al.* Clinical efficacy and safety of glucosamine, chondroitin sulphate, their combination, celecoxib or placebo taken to treat osteoarthritis of the knee: 2-year results from GAIT. *Ann Rheum Dis* 2010; 69(8): 1459–1464.

42 Scholtissen S, Bruyere O, Neuprez A, *et al.* Glucosamine sulphate in the treatment of knee osteoarthritis: cost-effectiveness comparison with paracetamol. *Int J Clin Pract* 2010; 64(6): 756–762.

43 Towheed TE, Maxwell L, Anastassiades TP, *et al.* Glucosamine therapy for treating osteoarthritis. *Cochrane Database Syst Rev* 2005; 18(2): CD002946.

44 Vlad SC, LaValley MP, McAlindon TE, *et al.* Glucosamine for pain in osteoarthritis: why do trial results differ? *Arthritis Rheum* 2007; 56(7): 2267–2277.

45 Wandel S, Juni P, Tendal B, *et al.* Effects of glucosamine, chondroitin, or placebo in patients with osteoarthritis of hip or knee: network meta-analysis. *BMJ* 2010; 341(16): c4675.

46 Wangroongsub Y, Tanavalee A, Wilairatana V, *et al.* Comparable clinical outcomes between glucosamine sulfate–potassium chloride and glucosamine sulfate–sodium chloride in patients with mild and moderate knee osteoarthritis: a randomized, double-blind study. *J Med Assoc Thai* 2010; 93(7): 805–811.

47 Wilkens P, Scheel IB, Grundnes O, *et al.* Effect of glucosamine on pain-related disability in patients with chronic low back pain and degenerative lumbar osteoarthritis: a randomized controlled trial. *JAMA* 2010; 304(1): 45–52.

48 Yoshimura M, Sakamoto K, Tsuruta A, *et al.* Evaluation of the effect of glucosamine administration on biomarkers for cartilage and bone metabolism in soccer players. *Int J Mol Med* 2009; 24(4): 487–494.

49 Balkan B, Dunning BE. Glucosamine inhibits glucokinase in vitro and produces a glucose-specific impairment of in vivo insulin secretion in rats. *Diabetes* 1994; 43: 1173–1179.

50 Shankar R, Zhu R, Baron JS, A.D. Glucosamine infusion in mice mimics the beta-cell dysfunction of non-insulin dependent diabetes mellitus. *Metab Clin Exp* 1998; 47: 573–577.

51 Han DH, Chen MM, Holloszy JO. Glucosamine and glucose induce insulin resistance by different mechanisms in rat skeletal muscle. *Am J Physiol Endocrinol Metab* 2003; 285(6): E1267–E1272.

52 Wallis MG, Smith ME, Kolka CM, *et al.* Acute glucosamine-induced insulin resistance in muscle in vivo is associated with impaired capillary recruitment. *Diabetologia* 2005; 48(10): 2131–2139.

53 Bailey CJ, Turner SL. Glucosamine-induced insulin resistance in L6 muscle cells. *Diabetes Obes Metab* 2004; 6(4): 293–298.

54 Yu JG, Boies SM, Olefsky JM. The effect of oral glucosamine sulfate on insulin sensitivity in human subjects. *Diabetes Care* 2003; 26(6): 1941–1942.

55 Muniyappa R, Karne RJ, Hall G, et al. Oral glucosamine for 6 weeks at standard doses does not cause or worsen insulin resistance or endothelial dysfunction in lean or obese subjects. *Diabetes* 2006; 55(11): 3142–3150.

56 Scroggie DA, Albright A, Harris MD. The effect of glucosamine-chondroitin supplementation on glycosylated hemoglobin levels in patients with type 2 diabetes mellitus: a placebo-controlled, double-blinded, randomized controlled trial. *Arch Intern Med* 2003; 163: 1587–1590.

57 Tannis AJ, Barban J, Conquer JA. Effect of glucosamine supplementation on fasting and non-fasting plasma glucose and serum insulin concentrations in healthy individuals. *Osteoarthritis Cartilage* 2004; 12: 506–511.

58 Biggee BA, Blinn CM, Nuite M, et al. Effects of oral glucosamine sulphate on serum glucose and insulin during an oral glucose tolerance test of subjects with osteoarthritis. *Ann Rheum Dis* 2007; 66(2): 260–262.

59 Anderson JW, Nicolosi RJ, Borzelleca JF. Glucosamine effects in humans: a review of effects on glucose metabolism, side effects, safety considerations and efficacy. *Food Chem Toxicol* 2005; 43(2): 187–201.

60 Stumpf JL, Lin SW. Effect of glucosamine on glucose control. *Ann Pharmacother* 2006; 40(4): 694–698.

61 Albert SG, Fishman Oiknine R, Parseghian S, et al. The effect of glucosamine on serum HDL cholesterol and apolipoprotein A1 levels in people with diabetes. *Diabetes Care* 2007; 30(11): 2800–2803.

62 Dostrovsky NR, Towheed TE, Hudson RW, et al. The effect of glucosamine on glucose metabolism in humans: a systematic review of the literature. *Osteoarthritis Cartilage* 2011; 2011: 18.

63 Hathcock JN, Shao A. Risk assessment for coenzyme Q_{10} (ubiquinone). *Regul Toxicol Pharmacol* 2006; 45(3): 282–288.

64 Medicines Healthcare products Regulatory Agency. Glucosamine adverse reactions and interactions. *Curr Probl Pharmacovigilance* 2006; 31: 8.

65 Knudsen JF, Sokol GH. Potential glucosamine–warfarin interaction resulting in increased international normalized ratio: case report and review of the literature and MedWatch database. *Pharmacotherapy* 2008; 28(4): 540–548.

Glutathione

Description

Glutathione (N-(N-L-gamma-glutamyl-L-cysteinyl)glycine) is an endogenous tripeptide made up of gamma-glutamic acid, cysteine and glycine. It is also known as GSH and is synthesised in the liver. It has antioxidant and other metabolic functions.

Action

Glutathione is a primary participant in cellular antioxidant systems.[1] It is abundant in cytoplasm, nuclei and mitochondria. Glutathione contains a sulphydryl group, which can accommodate the loss of an electron and also partially ionise at cellular pH to produce more reactive anions. Such anions are extremely reactive and participate in oxidation and reduction (redox) reactions. Glutathione is also a component part of the enzymes glutathione peroxidase and glutathione reductase, which act as mediators in the oxidation and reduction of glutathione. One of the primary antioxidant roles of glutathione is protection of protein sulphydryl groups. These reactive amino acids must be kept in a reduced state to function in their various unique roles inside the cells.[2]

The concentration of cellular glutathione has a major effect on its antioxidant function because it acts as a trap for various oxidants produced by oxidative stress. Its concentration varies considerably as a result of nutrient limitation, exercise, ageing and oxidative stress. Under oxidative stress, the concentration of glutathione can be reduced significantly. The rate of glutathione synthesis may be compromised during ageing, leading to a decrease in the total pool of this antioxidant. An imbalance in glutathione and associated enzymes has been implicated in a variety of conditions such as cancer, neurodegenerative diseases, cystic fibrosis and human immunodeficiency virus (HIV) infection.[3]

As part of its antioxidant and metabolic roles, glutathione is involved in DNA synthesis and repair, protein and prostaglandin synthesis, amino acid transport, metabolism of toxins and carcinogens, immune system function, prevention of oxidative cell damage and enzyme activation.[1]

Possible uses

Orally, glutathione has been used to increase levels of glutathione in people who have low levels of this peptide. Suggested benefits of increased levels of glutathione include reduction in fatigue, depression, obesity, anxiety, vertigo, allergies, periodontal gum disease and arthritis, and an improved immune system. Orally, glutathione has also been used for treating cataracts, asthma, cardiovascular disease, cancer, Alzheimer's disease, Parkinson's disease and HIV infection. There is insufficient reliable information on the effects of oral glutathione.

Intravenously, glutathione has been used to prevent the adverse effects of antineoplastic therapy with some evidence of benefit.[4,5] It has also been used by inhalation in lung disorders, including cystic fibrosis, but the evidence of benefit is unclear.

Precautions/contraindications

Not adequately studied.

Pregnancy and breast-feeding

Insufficient data; avoid in pregnancy and breast-feeding.

Adverse effects

Oral administration is insufficiently studied.

Interactions

Insufficiently studied.

Dose

Typical doses in supplements vary between 50 and 500 mg daily, with a typical daily dose of 250 mg. However, the bioavailability of oral glutathione is not adequately studied.

> **Conclusion**
> Glutathione has been used in many conditions, but given orally there is insufficient evidence of benefit.

References

1 Lomaestro BM, Malone M. Glutathione in health and disease: pharmacotherapeutic issues. *Ann Pharmacother* 1995; 29: 1263–1273.
2 Thomas J. Oxidant defense and nitrosative stress. In Shils, M, Shike, M, Ross, AC, Caballero, B, Cousins, RJ, eds. *Modern Nujtrition in Health and Disease*, 10th edn. Philadelphia, PA: Lippincott, Williams & Wilkins; 2006: 685–695.
3 Townsend DM, Tew KD, Tapiero H. The importance of glutathione in human disease. *Biomed Pharmacother* 2003; 57: 145–155.
4 Cascinu S, Catalano V, Cordella L, *et al.* Neuroprotective effect of reduced glutathione on oxaliplatin-based chemotherapy in advanced colorectal cancer: a randomized, double-blind, placebo-controlled trial. *J Clin Oncol* 2002; 20: 3478–3483.
5 Cascinu S, Cordella L, Del Ferro E, Fronzoni M, Catalano G. Neuroprotective effect of reduced glutathione on cisplatin-based chemotherapy in advanced gastric cancer: a randomized double-blind placebo-controlled trial. *J Clin Oncol* 1995; 13: 26–32.

Grape seed extract

Description

Grape seed extract is an extract from the tiny seeds of red grapes.

Constituents

Grape seed extract is a source of oligomeric proanthocyanidin complexes (OPCs), sometimes known as proanthocyanidins, which are one of the categories of flavonoids (see Flavonoids). Proanthocyanidins are polyphenol oligomers derived from flavan-3-ols and flavan-3,4-diols. Grape seed extract contains OPCs made up of dimers or trimers of catechin and epicatechin. Additional active ingredients in grape seed extract include essential fatty acids and tocopherols.

Action

Grape seed is a potent antioxidant,[1] which:

- neutralises free radicals, including hydroxyl groups and lipid peroxides, blocking lipid peroxidation and stabilising cell membranes;[2]
- produces an endothelium-dependent relaxation of blood vessels[3]
- inhibits the destruction of collagen by stabilising the activity of 1-antitrypsin, which inhibits the activity of destructive enzymes such as elastase and hyaluronidase (this is thought to prevent fluid exudation by allowing red blood cells to cross the capillaries);
- inhibits the release of inflammatory mediators, such as histamine and prostaglandins and inhibits tumour necrosis factor-alpha-mediated inflammatory status,[4] which protects the heart from inflammation during the consumption of a high-fat diet;[5]
- inhibits platelet aggregation;[6]
- protects against endothelial injury by enhancing endothelial nitric oxide synthase expression and nitric oxide production;[7] and
- may protect the human lens from oxidative stress linked with cataract.[8]

In addition, grape seed extract is thought to have antibacterial, antiviral and anticarcinogenic[9,10] actions.

Possible uses

Grape seed extract is promoted as an antioxidant to prevent coronary heart disease and stroke, and to strengthen fragile capillaries and improve circulation to the extremities. It is promoted for the treatment of conditions associated with poor vascular function such as diabetes mellitus, varicose veins, impotence and tingling in the arms and legs. Anecdotally it has been reported to be useful for treating inflammatory conditions and cancer. It has also been suggested to be useful for helping to prevent macular degeneration and cataracts.

Cardiovascular disease

Oral administration of proanthocyanidins from grape seed extract reduced serum cholesterol in a high-cholesterol animal feed model.[11] Specifically, it prevented the increase of total and LDL cholesterol.

In a double-blind study, 71 patients with peripheral venous insufficiency received 300 mg daily OPCs from grape seed. A reduction in functional symptoms was observed in 75% of the treated patients compared with 41% of the patients given a placebo.[12]

In a double-blind clinical trial, a group of elderly patients with either spontaneous or drug-induced poor capillary resistance were treated with 100–150 mg OPCs from grape extract daily, or placebo. There was a significant improvement in capillary resistance in the treated group after approximately 2 weeks.[13]

A further trial evaluated the effect of a standardised formulation of a polyphenolic extract of grapes on LDL susceptibility to oxidation in a group of heavy smokers. This was a randomised, double-blind, crossover study involving 24 healthy male heavy smokers aged 50 years or over. Subjects were given two capsules (containing 75 mg of a grape procyanidin extract) twice daily for 4 weeks. This was followed by a washout period of 3 weeks and placebo for 4 weeks. Subjects did not show significant modification of total cholesterol, triglycerides, HDL or LDL cholesterol during grape seed extract treatment. However, among oxidative indices, the concentration of thiobarbituric acid-reactive substances was significantly reduced in subjects taking grape seed extract compared with placebo and basal values. The authors concluded that the antioxidant potential of grape seed extract polyphenols may prove effective as a model of oxidative stress (smoking). However, more investigational data are needed before use in wider clinical settings can be recommended.[14]

Grape seed extract has been found to lower blood pressure in people with metabolic syndrome. In this trial, subjects were randomized into three groups: placebo, 150 mg grape seed extract per day, and 300 mg grape seed extract per day. Patients were treated for 4 weeks, and serum lipids, blood glucose and ambulatory blood pressure were measured at the beginning of the study and at the end. Both systolic and diastolic blood pressure was lowered after treatment with grape seed extract compared with placebo. There were no significant changes in serum lipids or blood glucose values.[15]

Miscellaneous

Grape seed extract is increasingly being investigated for other conditions. A double-blind RCT investigated the effect of grape seed extract in the treatment of seasonal allergic rhinitis. Patients with seasonal allergic rhinitis and skin prick test sensitivity to ragweed were randomised to 8 weeks' treatment with grape seed extract 100 mg twice daily or placebo, which was begun before the ragweed pollen season. Over the period of the study, no significant differences were observed between active and placebo groups in rhinitis quality of life assessments, symptom diary scores or requirements for rescue antihistamine. No significant laboratory abnormalities were detected. Overall, this study showed no trends towards supporting the efficacy of grape seed extract in the treatment of seasonal allergic rhinitis.[16]

Grape seed extract has been shown to stimulate lipolysis *in vitro* and reduce food intake in rats. Leading on from these findings, a study has assessed the efficacy of grape seed extract with respect to energy intake and satiety. In a randomised, placebo-controlled, double-blind crossover study, 51 subjects (age 18–65 years; body mass index 22–30) were given a grape seed supplement for 3 days, 30–60 min prior to *ad libitum* lunch and dinner in a university restaurant. In the total study population, no difference in 24-h energy intake was found between grape seed extract and placebo. However, in a subgroup of 23 subjects with an energy requirement ≥7.5 MJ/day, energy intake was reduced by 4% after grape seed compared with placebo. There were no significant differences in macronutrient composition, attitude towards eating, satiety, mood or tolerance. The authors concluded that these findings suggest that grape seed could be effective in reducing 24-h energy intake

in normal to overweight dietary unrestrained subjects and could, therefore, play a role in body weight management.[17]

Grapeseed extract has also been shown to improve liver function in people with non-alcoholic fatty liver change.[18]

> ### Conclusion
> Preliminary evidence suggests that grape seed extract might lower lipid levels, improve symptoms of venous insufficiency and capillary resistance, reduce oxidative stress and play a role in body weight management. However, there are no well-controlled studies, and evidence for efficacy is promising but not yet robust.

Precautions/contraindications

No known contraindications, but based on the potential pharmacological activity of OPCs (i.e. that they may inhibit platelet aggregation), grape seed extract should be used with caution in patients with a history of bleeding or haemostatic disorders. It is probably wise to discontinue use 14 days before any surgery, including dental surgery.

Pregnancy and breast-feeding

No problems have been reported, but there have not been sufficient studies to guarantee the safety of grape seed extract in pregnancy and breast-feeding.

Adverse effects

None reported. However, there are no long-term studies assessing the safety of grape seed extract.

Interactions

Drugs

None reported, but in theory bleeding tendency may be increased with anticoagulants, aspirin and anti-platelet drugs.

Dose

Grape seed extract is available in the form of tablets and capsules. Supplements should be standardised (and labelled) to contain 92–95% proanthocyanidins or OPCs.

The dose is not established, but doses of 100–300 mg daily have been used in studies.

References

1 Bagchi D, Sen CK, Ray SD, *et al.* Molecular mechanisms of cardioprotection by a novel grape seed proanthocyanidin extract. *Mutat Res* 2003; 523524: 87–97.

2 Murray M, Pizzorono J. Procyanidolic oligomers. In: Murray M, Pizzorono J, eds. *The Textbook of Natural Medicine*, 2nd edn. London: Churchill Livingstone, 1999: 899–902.

3 Edirisinghe I, Burton-Freeman B, Tissa Kappagoda C. Mechanism of the endothelium-dependent relaxation evoked by a grape seed extract. *Clin Sci (Lond)* 2008; 114(4): 331–337.

4 Chao CL, Chang NC, Weng CS, *et al.* Grape seed extract ameliorates tumor necrosis factor-alpha-induced inflammatory status of human umbilical vein endothelial cells. *Eur J Nutr* 2010; 2010: 28.

5 Charradi K, Sebai H, Elkahoui S, *et al.* Grape seed extract alleviates high-fat diet-induced obesity and heart dysfunction by preventing cardiac siderosis. *Cardiovasc Toxicol* 2011; 2011: 14.

6 Shenoy SF, Keen CL, Kalgaonkar S, *et al.* Effects of grape seed extract consumption on platelet function in postmenopausal women. *Thromb Res* 2007; 121 (3): 431–432.

7 Feng Z, Wei RB, Hong Q, *et al.* Grape seed extract enhances eNOS expression and NO production through regulating calcium-mediated AKT phosphorylation in H_2O_2-treated endothelium. *Cell Biol Int* 2010; 34(10): 1055–1061.

8 Jia Z, Song Z, Zhao Y, *et al.* Grape seed proanthocyanidin extract protects human lens epithelial cells from oxidative stress via reducing NF-κB and MAPK protein expression. *Mol Vis* 2011; 17: 210–217.

9 Kaur M, Agarwal C, Agarwal R. Anticancer and cancer chemopreventive potential of grape seed extract and other grape-based products. *J Nutr* 2009; 139(9): 1806S–1812S.

10 Park SY, Lee YH, Choi KC, *et al.* Grape seed extract regulates androgen receptor-mediated transcription in prostate cancer cells through potent anti-histone acetyltransferase activity. *J Med Food* 2011; 14(12): 9–16.

11 Tebib K, Bessanicon P, Roaunet J. Dietary grape seed tannins affect lipoproteins, lipoprotein lipases and tissue lipids in rats fed hypercholesterolemic diets. *J Nutr* 1994; 124: 2451–2457.

12 Thebaut JF, Thebaut P, Vin F. Study of Endotolon in functional manifestations of peripheral venous insufficiency. *Gaz Med France* 1985; 92: 96–100.

13 Dartenuc JY, Marache P, Choussat H. Capillary resistance in geriatry. A study of a microangioprotector – Endotolon. *Bord Med* 1980; 13: 903–907.

14 Vigna GB, Costantini F, Aldini G, *et al.* Effect of standardized grape seed extract on low-density lipoprotein susceptibility to oxidation in heavy smokers. *Metabolism* 2003; 52: 1250–1257.

15 Sivaprakasapillai B, Edirisinghe I, Randolph J, *et al.* Effect of grape seed extract on blood pressure in subjects with the metabolic syndrome. *Metabolism* 2009; 58(12): 1743–1746.

16 Bernstein DI, Bernstein CK, Deng C, *et al.* Evaluation of the clinical efficacy and safety of grapeseed extract in the treatment of fall seasonal allergic rhinitis: a pilot study. *Ann Allergy Asthma Immunol* 2002; 88: 272–278.

17 Vogels N, Nijs IM, Westerterp-Plantenga MS. The effect of grape-seed extract on 24 h energy intake in humans. *Eur J Clin Nutr* 2004; 58: 667–673.

18 Khoshbaten M, Aliasgarzadeh A, Masnadi K, *et al.* Grape seed extract to improve liver function in patients with nonalcoholic fatty liver change. *Saudi J Gastroenterol* 2010; 16(3): 194–197.

Grapefruit seed extract

Description

Grapefruit seed extract is a substance extracted from grapefruit seeds. It is available as a liquid concentrate, tablets and capsules.

Action

Grapefruit seeds contain numerous constituents, including naringin, nomilin, deacetyl-nomilin, nomilinic-acid-17-O-beta-D-glucoside, deacetylnomilinic-acid-17-O-beta-D-glucoside, limonol, deoxy-limonol, 7-obacunol, obacunone, epi-iso-obacunoic-acid-17-O-beta-D-glucoside, iso-oba-cunoic-acid-17-O-beta-D-glucoside and *trans*-obacunoic-acid-17-O-beta-D-glucoside.

Grapefruit seed extract has antibacterial[1–6] and antifungal[4,7] activity. It may also have a hypolipidaemic action.[8]

Possible uses

Human research using grapefruit seed extract is very limited. In one study, 25 people with symptoms associated with irritable bowel syndrome such as intermittent diarrhoea, constipation, flatulence, bloating and abdominal discomfort were treated with either 2 drops of a 0.5% oral solution of grapefruit seed extract twice daily or 150 mg of encapsulated grapefruit seed extract three times daily.[9] After 1 month, symptoms had improved in 20% of people taking the liquid, while all of the patients taking the capsules noted a definite improvement of constipation, flatulence, abdominal discomfort and night rest. However, this study is now more than 20 years old and its findings have not been confirmed in double-blind trials.

In a study in rats, grapefruit seed extract was found to reduce the extent of pancreatitis.[10] In another rat study, oral treatment of diabetic rats with 100–600 mg/kg/day grapefruit juice for 30 days resulted in significant reductions in fasting plasma glucose, triglyceride, total cholesterol, low-density lipoprotein (LDL) cholesterol and very-low-density lipoprotein (VLDL) cholesterol, effects that were comparable to those of metformin.[8] The researchers concluded that the results of this study lend support to the traditional use of grapefruit seeds in the management of people with type 1 diabetes and may suggest a role in orthodox management of this disease. Further research is required to confirm these findings.

Conclusion
Grapefruit seed extract has antimicrobial properties. However, human research using this ingredient is very limited. One trial showed that it improved symptoms of irritable bowel syndrome.

Precautions/contraindications

Insufficient reliable information.

Pregnancy and breast-feeding

Insufficient data.

Adverse effects

None reported.

Interactions

In a case study involving one man and one woman on lifelong treatment with warfarin, grapefruit seed extract appeared to result in an interaction.[11] After taking grapefruit seed extract for 3 days, the woman experienced a minor subcutaneous haematoma and her international normalised ratio (INR) value was 7.9. This was reported to the Swedish Medical Products Agency (MPA) as a spontaneous post-marketing report concerning adverse drug reactions/interactions and was found to be due to the presence of the synthetic preservative benzethonium chloride (BTC) in the grapefruit seed products. Furthermore, BTC was found to be a potent inhibitor of CYP3A4 and CYP2C9 activity *in vitro*.

Whether grapefruit seed extract interacts with the drugs associated with the grapefruit juice interaction such as anti-arrhythmics, ciclosporin, sirolimus and tacrolimus, atorvastatin and simvastatin is not clear.

Dose

The typical recommendation for the liquid concentrate is 10–12 drops in water one to three times daily. For capsules and tablets containing dried grapefruit seed extract, the usual recommendation is 100–200 mg one to three times daily.

References

1 Von Woedtke T, Schluter B, Pflegel P, Lindequist U, Julich WD. Aspects of the antimicrobial efficacy of

grapefruit seed extract and its relation to preservative substances contained. *Pharmazie* 1999; 54: 452–456.

2 Heggers JP, Cottingham J, Gusman J, *et al*. The effectiveness of processed grapefruit-seed extract as an antibacterial agent: II. Mechanism of action and in vitro toxicity. *J Altern Complement Med* 2002; 8: 333–340.

3 Reagor L, Gusman J, McCoy L, Carino E, Heggers JP. The effectiveness of processed grapefruit-seed extract as an antibacterial agent: I. An in vitro agar assay. *J Altern Complement Med* 2002; 8: 325–332.

4 Cvetnic Z, Vladimir-Knezevic S. Antimicrobial activity of grapefruit seed and pulp ethanolic extract. *Acta Pharm* 2004; 54: 243–250.

5 Brorson Ø, Brorson SH. Grapefruit seed extract is a powerful in vitro agent against motile and cystic forms of *Borrelia burgdorferi sensu lato*. *Infection* 2007; 35: 206–208.

6 Alonso D, Gimeno M, Sepulveda-Sanchez JD, Shirai K. Chitosan-based microcapsules containing grapefruit seed extract grafted onto cellulose fibers by a non-toxic procedure. *Carbohydr Res* 2010; 345: 854–859.

7 Krajewska-Kulak E, Lukaszuk C, Niczyporuk W. [Effects of 33% grapefruit extract on the growth of the yeast-like fungi, dermatopytes and moulds]. *Wiad Parazytol* 2001; 47: 845–849.

8 Adeneye AA. Hypoglycemic and hypolipidemic effects of methanol seed extract of *Citrus paradisi Macfad* (Rutaceae) in alloxan-induced diabetic Wistar rats. *Nig Q J Hosp Med* 2008; 18: 211–215.

9 Ionescu G, Kiehl R, Wichmann-Kunz F, *et al*. Oral citrus seed extract in atopic eczema: in vitro and in vivo studies on intestinal microflora. *J Orthomol Med* 1990; 5: 155–158.

10 Dembinski A, Warzecha Z, Konturek SJ, *et al*. Extract of grapefruit-seed reduces acute pancreatitis induced by ischemia/reperfusion in rats: possible implication of tissue antioxidants. *J Physiol Pharmacol* 2004; 55: 811–821.

11 Brandin H, Myrberg O, Rundlof T, Arvidsson AK, Brenning G. Adverse effects by artificial grapefruit seed extract products in patients on warfarin therapy. *Eur J Clin Pharmacol* 2007; 63: 565–570.

Green-lipped mussel

Description

Green-lipped mussel extract comes from *Perna canaliculata*, a salt-water shellfish indigenous to New Zealand.

Constituents

Green-lipped mussel extract contains amino acids, fats, carbohydrates and minerals. The lipid fraction consists of n-3 polyunsaturated fatty acids (PUFA), phospholipids and sterols.[1–4] It has the capacity to inhibit cyclo-oxygenase (COX) 1 and 2[5] and modulate inflammatory cytokines[6–8] and prostaglandins[9] which are likely to be functions of its n-3 PUFA content.

Possible uses

Arthritis

Green-lipped mussel extract is claimed to be effective in the treatment of rheumatoid arthritis and osteoarthritis. The small number of human studies published have generally shown that green-lipped mussel is not effective in arthritis,[10–12] but two studies have shown positive effects.[13,14] A more recent study has indicated that green-lipped mussel, added to a complete dry diet, can help alleviate symptoms of arthritis in dogs.[15]

A systematic review of studies using freeze-dried green-lipped mussel found mixed outcomes and was not conclusive. Of five RCTs, only two attested benefits for rheumatoid and osteoarthritic patients. Similarly, animal studies have yielded mixed findings. In both cases, according to the authors, this could be due to lack of stabilisation of the omega-3 fatty acids in the product.[16]

A Cochrane systematic review evaluated green-lipped mussel for osteoarthritis: four RCTs, three placebo-controlled and the fourth a comparative trial of green-lipped mussel extract vs stabilised powder extract, were included. No RCTs comparing green-lipped mussel with conventional treatment were identified. All four studies assessed green-lipped mussel as an adjunctive treatment to conventional medication for a clinically relevant time in mild to moderate osteoarthritis. All trials reported clinical benefits in the green-lipped mussel treatment group, but the findings from two studies were not included because of possible unblinding and inappropriate statistical analysis. The data from the two more rigorous trials, in conjunction with a re-analysis of the authors' original data, indicated that green-lipped mussel may be superior to placebo for the treatment of mild to moderate osteoarthritis.[17]

Asthma

Experimental studies have shown that lipid extract of green-lipped mussel is effective at inhibiting 5′-lipoxygenase and cyclo-oxygenase pathways responsible for production of eicosanoids, including leukotrienes and prostaglandins, and it has been suggested that this compound could help patients with asthma. An RCT assessed the effect of green-lipped mussel on asthma symptoms, peak expiratory flow and hydrogen peroxide as a marker of airway inflammation in patients in expired breath condensate as a marker of airway inflammation. Forty-six patients with atopic asthma received two capsules of a lipid extract of green-lipped mussel or placebo three times a day for 8 weeks. Each capsule of extract contained 50 mg omega-3 polyunsaturated fatty acids and 100 mg olive oil, while the placebo contained only 100 mg olive oil. There was a significant decrease in daytime wheeze, the concentration of exhaled hydrogen peroxide and an increase in morning peak expiratory flow rate. The authors concluded that lipid extract of New Zealand green-lipped mussel may have some beneficial effect in patients with atopic asthma.[18]

Conclusion

Green-lipped mussel is claimed to be effective in arthritis. Trial data are somewhat inconsistent and methodology is poor in some cases. However, this preparation may be superior to placebo. As a credible biological mechanism exists for this treatment, further rigorous investigations are required to assess efficacy and optimal dosage.

Adverse effects

Green-lipped mussel is relatively non-toxic, but allergic reactions (e.g. gastrointestinal discomfort, nausea and flatulence) have been reported occasionally. Hepatic toxicity was noted in two patients in a trial evaluating green-lipped mussel in prostate and breast cancer.[19]

Interactions

None reported.

Dose

Green-lipped mussel extract is available in the form of capsules.

The dose is not established; dietary supplements provide approximately 1 g per daily dose.

References

1 Murphy KJ, Mann NJ, Sinclair AJ. Fatty acid and sterol composition of frozen and freeze-dried New Zealand green lipped mussel (*Perna canaliculus*) from three sites in New Zealand. *Asia Pac J Clin Nutr* 2003; 12(1): 50–60.
2 Murphy KJ, Mooney BD, Mann NJ, *et al.* Lipid, FA, and sterol composition of New Zealand green lipped mussel (*Perna canaliculus*) and Tasmanian blue mussel (*Mytilus edulis*). *Lipids* 2002; 37(6): 587–595.
3 Treschow AP, Hodges LD, Wright PF, *et al.* Novel anti-inflammatory omega-3 PUFAs from the New Zealand green-lipped mussel, *Perna canaliculus*. *Comp Biochem Physiol B Biochem Mol Biol* 2007; 147(4): 645–656.
4 Singh M, Hodges LD, Wright PF, *et al.* The CO_2-SFE crude lipid extract and the free fatty acid extract from *Perna canaliculus* have anti-inflammatory effects on adjuvant-induced arthritis in rats. *Comp Biochem Physiol B Biochem Mol Biol* 2008; 149(2): 251–258.
5 McPhee S, Hodges LD, Wright PF, *et al.* Anti-cyclo-oxygenase effects of lipid extracts from the New Zealand green-lipped mussel, *Perna canaliculus*. *Comp Biochem Physiol B Biochem Mol Biol* 2007; 146(3): 346–356.
6 Mani S, Lawson JW. In vitro modulation of inflammatory cytokine and IgG levels by extracts of *Perna canaliculus*. *BMC Complement Altern Med* 2006; 6 (1): 1.
7 Lee CH, Butt YK, Wong MS, *et al.* A lipid extract of *Perna canaliculus* affects the expression of pro-inflammatory cytokines in a rat adjuvant-induced arthritis model. *Eur Ann Allergy Clin Immunol* 2008; 40(4): 148–153.

8 Lee CH, Lum JH, Ng CK, *et al.* Pain controlling and cytokine-regulating effects of lyprinol, a lipid extract of *Perna canaliculus*, in a rat adjuvant-induced arthritis model. *Evid Based Complement Alternat Med* 2009; 6(2): 239–245.

9 Halpern GM. Anti-inflammatory effects of a stabilized lipid extract of *Perna canaliculus* (Lyprinol). *Allerg Immunol (Paris)* 2000; 32(7): 272–278.

10 Caughey DE, Grigor RR, Caughey EB. *Perna canaliculus* in the treatment of rheumatoid arthritis. *Eur J Rheumatol Inflamm* 1983; 6: 197–200.

11 Huskisson EC, Scott J, Bryans R. Seatone is ineffective in rheumatoid arthritis. *Br Med J (Clin Res Ed)* 1981; 282(6273): 1358–1359.

12 Larkin JG, Capell HA, Sturrock RD. Seatone in rheumatoid arthritis: a six-month placebo-controlled study. *Ann Rheum Dis* 1985; 44(3): 199–201.

13 Gibson RG, Gibson SL. Seatone in arthritis. *Br Med J* 1981; 282: 1795.

14 Gibson RG, Gibson SL, Conway V, *et al.* *Perna canaliculus* in the treatment of arthritis. *Practitioner* 1980; 224(1347): 955–960.

15 Bui LM, Bierer TL. Influence of green lipped mussels (*Perna canaliculus*) in alleviating signs of arthritis in dogs. *Vet Ther* 2003; 4(4): 397–407.

16 Cobb CS, Ernst E. Systematic review of a marine nutriceutical supplement in clinical trials for arthritis: the effectiveness of the New Zealand green-lipped mussel *Perna canaliculus*. *Clin Rheumatol* 2006; 25(3): 275–284.

17 Brien S, Prescott P, Coghlan B, *et al.* Systematic review of the nutritional supplement *Perna canaliculus* (green-lipped mussel) in the treatment of osteoarthritis. *Q J Med* 2008; 101(3): 167–179.

18 Emelyanov A, Fedoseev G, Krasnoschekova O, *et al.* Treatment of asthma with lipid extract of New Zealand green-lipped mussel: a randomised clinical trial. *Eur Respir J* 2002; 20(3): 596–600.

19 Sukumaran S, Pittman KB, Patterson WK, *et al.* A phase I study to determine the safety, tolerability and maximum tolerated dose of green-lipped mussel (*Perna canaliculus*) lipid extract, in patients with advanced prostate and breast cancer. *Ann Oncol* 2010; 21(5): 1089–1093.

Green tea extract

Description

Green tea is prepared from the steamed and dried leaves of *Camellia sinensis*. It is different from black tea in that black tea is produced from leaves that have been withered, rolled, fermented and dried. The lack of fermentation gives green tea its unique flavour and also preserves the naturally present flavonoids, which are antioxidants.

Constituents

Green tea contains flavonoids, a large group of polyphenolic compounds with antioxidant properties. Of the flavonoids found in green tea, catechins make up 30–50% of the dry tea leaf weight. These include epigallocatechin gallate, epicatechin and epicatechin gallate. Green tea also contains flavonols, tannins, minerals, free amino acids and methylxanthines (caffeine, theophylline and theobromine).

Action

Green tea appears to have the following effects:

- An antioxidant effect. Green tea may protect against oxidative damage to cells and tissues.[1,2]
- A chemoprotective effect. This is attributed to the catechins, compounds that are thought to inhibit cell proliferation. *In vitro* studies have shown that green tea polyphenols induce programmed cell death (apoptosis) in human cancer cells[3,4] and block tumour growth by inhibition of tumour necrosis factor-α as well as a variety of other potential anti-cancer effects.[5–9] Animal studies have also shown the inhibitory effect of green tea against carcinogens.[10–12]
- Antibacterial and antiviral activity. *In vitro* studies have demonstrated that green tea polyphenols block the growth of micro-organisms that cause diarrhoea[13] and influenza.[14]
- Reduction of serum cholesterol.

- Reduction in LDL cholesterol oxidation. Two *in vitro* studies[15,16] showed that green tea can inhibit oxidation of LDL.
- Inhibition of platelet aggregation.

Possible uses

Green tea has been investigated mainly for supposed protective effects in cancer and cardiovascular disease (CVD).

Cancer

A review of 31 epidemiological studies of green tea consumption and cancer risk found no overall consistent effect.[8] Of the total studies reviewed, 17 showed reduced cancer risk, seven increased risk, three no association and five an increased risk. Of the 10 studies on stomach cancer, six suggested a reduced risk and three an increased risk. Of the nine studies investigating colorectal cancer, four suggested a reduced risk and three an increased risk. Both studies on bladder cancer showed a reduced risk, and two out of the three studies on pancreatic cancer showed reduced risk. Studies examining oesophageal cancer showed mixed results, but very hot or scalding tea was associated with increased risk.

In the Ohsaki National Health Insurance Cohort Study, a prospective cohort study initiated in 40 530 Japanese middle-aged adults without history of stroke, coronary heart disease or cancer at baseline, green tea consumption was not associated with reduced mortality due to cancer. However, green tea consumption was associated with reduced mortality due to all causes and with reduced mortality due to CVD.[17]

In a study of 472 Japanese patients with stage I, II and III breast cancer,[18] the level of green tea consumption before clinical diagnosis of cancer was evaluated. Increased consumption of green tea was significantly associated with decreased numbers of axillary lymph node metastases among pre-menopausal patients with stage I and II breast cancer and increased expression of progesterone receptor and oestrogen receptor in postmenopausal patients. In a follow-up study, increased consumption of green tea was correlated with reduced recurrence of stage I and II breast cancer; the recurrence rate was 16.7% among those consuming five or more cups daily or 24.3% in those consuming four or more cups daily. However, no improvement was seen in those with stage III breast cancer.

In a case–control study in South East China (1009 cases of breast cancer in patients aged 20–87 years, 1009 age-matched controls), green tea consumption (after adjusting for established and potential confounders) was associated with reduced risk of breast cancer. The odds ratios were 0.87 (95% confidence interval (CI), 0.73 to 1.04) in women consuming 1–249 g dried green tea leaves per annum, 0.68 (95% CI, 0.54 to 0.86) for 250–499 g per annum, 0.59 (95% CI, 0.45 to 0.77) for 500–749 g per annum and 0.61 (95% CI, 0.48 to 0.78) for >750 g per annum. The authors concluded that regular consumption of green tea can protect against breast cancer.[19]

Green tea may block the frequency of sister chromatid exchange (SCE), a biomarker of mutagenesis. A study in 52 Korean smokers[20] showed that SCE rates were significantly higher in smokers than non-smokers. However, the frequency of SCE in smokers who consumed green tea was comparable to that of non-smokers.

A systematic review and meta-analysis of observational studies linking green tea with breast cancer found that the pooled relative risk of developing breast cancer for the highest levels of green tea consumption in cohort studies was 0.89 (95% CI, 0.71 to 1.1; $P = 0.28$), and in case–control studies, the odds ratio was 0.44 (95% CI, 0.14 to 1.31; $P = 0.14$). The pooled relative risk of cohort studies for breast cancer recurrence in all stages was 0.75 (95% CI, 0.47 to 1.19; $P = 0.22$). The authors' conclusion was that, to date, the epidemiological data indicate that consumption of five or more cups of green tea a day shows a non-statistically significant trend towards the prevention of breast cancer. There is some evidence that green tea consumption may help to prevent breast cancer recurrence in early stage (I and II) cancers.[21]

Genetic factors may play a role in the influence of green tea on breast cancer. A case–control study involving 297 incident breast cancer cases and 665 control subjects in Singapore found no association of green tea consumption and breast cancer among all women or those with low activity of angiotensin-converting enzyme genotype. However, among women with a genotype giving high enzyme activity, frequency of intake for green tea was associated with a significantly decreased risk of breast cancer.[22]

Green tea has also been associated with reduced risk of prostate cancer. In a prospective study based in Japan, 49 920 men aged 40–69 years were asked about their green tea consumption. The study began in 1990 with follow up to the end of 2004. During this time, 404 men were newly diagnosed with prostate cancer, of whom 114 had advanced cancer, 271 were localised and 19 were of an undetermined stage. Green tea was not associated with localised prostate cancer. However, consumption was associated with a dose-dependent decrease in the risk of advanced prostate cancer. The multivariate relative risk was 0.52 (95% CI, 0.28 to 0.96) for men drinking more than five cups of green tea daily compared with fewer than one cup daily (P(trend) = 0.01). The authors concluded that green tea may be associated with decreased risk of advanced prostate cancer.[23]

A further prospective study, this time in 69 710 Chinese women aged 40–70 years, evaluated the effect of green consumption on colorectal cancer. The relative risk of colorectal cancer was 0.63 (95% CI, 0.45 to 0.88) for women who reported drinking green tea regularly. A significant dose–response relationship was found for both the amount of tea consumed and the duration in years of lifetime tea consumption. The reduction in risk was most evident among those who consistently reported drinking tea regularly at baseline and follow up (over 2–3 years). The inverse association was observed for both colon and rectal cancers.[24]

Overall the evidence relating green tea consumption to cancer risk is unclear. Three meta-analyses looking specifically at the link between green tea and risk of breast cancer,[25] stomach cancer[26] and lung cancer[27] have concluded that green tea has limited or no effect on risk of these cancers, while a Cochrane review of 51 studies (>1.6 million participants) concluded that there is insufficient and conflicting evidence to make firm recommendations about green tea consumption and cancer risk.[28] This is mainly because most of the studies are conducted in Asian countries where a large proportion of the tea consumed is green tea.

Cardiovascular disease

A cross-sectional study of the effects of drinking green tea on cardiovascular and liver disease[29] in 1371 Japanese men aged over 40 showed that increased consumption of green tea was associated with reduced serum concentrations of total cholesterol and triglyceride and an increased proportion of HDL cholesterol, with a decreased proportion of low and very LDL cholesterol. In addition, increased consumption of green tea was associated with reduced concentrations of hepatic markers in serum (aspartate aminotransferase, alanine transferase and ferritin).

However, another cross-sectional study in 371 individuals from five districts of Japan[30] showed that green tea was not associated with serum concentrations of total cholesterol, triglycerides or HDL cholesterol.

Another study examined the relation between green tea consumption and arteriographically determined coronary atherosclerosis.[31] The subjects were 512 patients (302 men and 210 women) aged 30 years or older, who had undergone coronary arteriography for the first time between September 1996 and August 1997. Green tea consumption tended to be inversely associated with coronary atherosclerosis in men but not in women.

A further study investigated the impact of theaflavin-enriched green tea extract on the lipids and lipoproteins of subjects with mild to moderate hypercholesterolaemia. A total of 240 men and women aged 18 or over on a low-fat diet with mild to moderate hypercholesterolaemia were randomly assigned to receive a daily capsule containing theaflavin-enriched green tea extract (375 mg) or placebo for 12 weeks. In the green tea group, mean total cholesterol fell by 11.3% and mean LDL cholesterol by 16.4%, both statistically significant changes compared with baseline. There were no significant changes in the placebo group. The authors concluded that the green tea extract studied is an effective adjunct to a low-saturated fat diet to reduce LDL cholesterol in hypercholesterolaemic adults and is well tolerated.[32] Green tea has also been shown to improve overall antioxidant status and to protect against oxidative damage in humans,[2] and to attenuate the increase in plasma triacylglycerol (triglyceride) levels following a fat load.[33]

In a Portugese study involving 29 subjects, 1 L of green tea daily for 4 weeks was associated with significant improvement in lipid profiles. A decrease in total cholesterol, LDL cholesterol, apolipoprotein B, and ratio of total cholesterol to HDL cholesterol, but an increase in HDL cholesterol and apolipoprotein A1 was observed. No significant differences were observed for triacylglycerol and lipoprotein(a).[34]

Short-term administration of green tea (8 g daily) for 2 weeks has been associated with improved endothelial function in smokers, suggesting that consumption of green tea could reduce cardiovascular risk in smokers.[35] In a study involving 42 subjects with coronary artery disease, dietary supplementation with epigallocatechin 3-gallate (EGCG) (300 mg daily) significantly improved endothelial function.[36] Cardiovascular risk markers did not change in a group of healthy men consuming green tea polyphenols for 3 weeks.[37] A recent meta-analysis supported only a tentative association between green tea consumption and a reduced risk of coronary artery disease.[38]

Body weight

Green tea is being increasingly investigated for its potential influence on body weight. One study found that weight maintenance after 7.5% body weight loss was not affected by green tea treatment.[39] In another study, a green tea/caffeine mixture improved weight maintenance, partly through thermogenesis and fat oxidation, but only in habitual low-caffeine consumers.[40] Further evidence for a thermogenic effect of green tea was found in another study where there was an increase in 24-h energy expenditure with mixtures of caffeine and EGCG, a catechin in green tea.[41] However, green tea had no significant effect on body weight in Chinese obese women with polycystic ovary syndrome.[27]

A 12-week double-blind parallel, multicentre trial evaluated the effect of green tea ingestion (583 mg catechins) versus control (96 mg catechins) on body fat in 240 subjects. Reductions in body weight, body mass index, body fat ratio, body fat mass, waist circumference, hip circumference, visceral fat and subcutaneous fat were found to be greater in the catechin group than the control group. A greater decrease in systolic blood pressure was also found in the catechin group compared with the control group in

those subjects with a systolic blood pressure ≥ 130 mmHg. LDL cholesterol was also decreased to a greater extent in the catechin group. No adverse effects were found. The authors concluded that green tea high in catechins is associated with a decrease in obesity and cardiovascular disease risk.[42]

A further 12-week RCT involved 78 obese women aged 16–60 years receiving green tea extract (400 mg three times a day) or placebo for 12 weeks. Body weight, body mass index and waist circumference were measured at the beginning and end of the study but there were no statistical differences between green tea extract and placebo.[43]

A meta-analysis of 11 studies found that green tea catechins significantly decreased body weight and significantly maintained body weight after a period of weight loss. Habitual caffeine intake had a small inhibitory influence on this effect as did ethinicity in that there was a smaller effect in Caucasians than in Asian people.[44]

Miscellaneous

Green tea has been studied for its effect on insulin resistance, blood glucose level, HbA1c level and markers of inflammation, but without any clear effects in an initial study.[45] However, a further trial produced more positive results. This was a crossover trial in 60 subjects (aged 32–73 years) with borderline diabetes which evaluated the effect of green tea extract powder (containing 544 mg polyphenols) daily for 2 months on glucose abnormalities. A significant reduction in haemoglobin A1c and a borderline significant reduction in diastolic blood pressure were associated with the intervention. The intervention resulted in no significant changes in weight, body mass index, body fat, systolic blood pressure, fasting serum glucose, serum lipid level or C-reactive protein.[46] A more recent trial in 12 healthy men undertaking a moderate cycling programme found that green tea extract could improve fat oxidation, insulin sensitivity and glucose tolerance.[47] Another trial in athletes undertaking endurance cycling showed no influence of green tea extract supplementation on energy metabolism or any measure of performance.[48]

Green tea polyphenols have been postulated to protect human skin from photoageing, but clinically significant changes were not detected in one study.[49]

A further study found that green tea extracts can be a potential therapy for patients with human papilloma virus (HPV) infected cervical lesions.[50] This study evaluated the influence of green tea extracts delivered in the form of an ointment or capsules in 51 patients with HPV-infected cervical lesions. Overall, a 69% response rate was noted for treatment with green tea extracts compared with a 10% response rate from untreated controls.

A recent Japanese cross-sectional study has evaluated the effect of green tea on cognitive function. The frequency of green tea consumption was examined in 1003 Japanese subjects aged 70 or over. Higher consumption of green tea was associated with lower levels of cognitive impairment.[51]

Conclusion

Green tea has been investigated for protective effects in CVD and cancer, in which it shows some promise, but there is insufficient and conflicting evidence on which to base firm recommendations for either consumption of green tea as a drink or a food supplement. There is also some evidence that it helps to maintain body weight after weight loss. However, there is still a dearth of good-quality controlled trials and firm conclusions must await results from such trials.

Precautions/contraindications

No known contraindications, but based on the potential pharmacological activity of polyphenols (i.e. that they may inhibit platelet aggregation), green tea extract should be used with caution in patients with a history of bleeding or haemostatic disorders. It is probably wise to discontinue use 14 days before any surgery, including dental surgery.

Pregnancy and breast-feeding

No problems have been reported, but there have been insufficient studies to guarantee the safety of green tea supplements in pregnancy and breast-feeding.

Adverse effects

There is a lack of tolerance and safety data on supplements of this substance. However, green tea has been consumed safely in China for more than 4000 years. Recently there have been case reports of green tea extracts (not the beverage) being associated with liver toxicity. As with any plant-containing substance, this may be due to the presence of contaminants.

Interactions

Drugs

None are known, but in theory bleeding tendency may be increased with anticoagulants, aspirin and antiplatelet drugs.

Dose

Green tea is available in the form of capsules as well as tea for drinking.

The dose is not established, but doses of 250–300 mg daily have been used. Supplements should be standardised (and labelled) to contain 50–97% polyphenols, containing per dose at least 50% (–)-EGCG. Four to six cups of freshly brewed green tea should provide similar levels of polyphenols.

References

1 Coimbra S, Castroa E, Rocha-Pereirab P, *et al.* The effect of green tea in oxidative stress. *Clin Nutr* 2006; 25(5): 790–796.
2 Erba D, Riso P, Bordoni A, *et al.* Effectiveness of moderate green tea consumption on antioxidative status and plasma lipid profile in humans. *J Nutr Biochem* 2005; 16: 144–149.
3 Ahmad N, Feyes DK, Niemenen Al, *et al.* Green tea constituent epigallocatechin-3-gallate and induction of apoptosis and cell cycle arrest in human carcinoma cells. *J Natl Cancer Inst* 1997; 89: 1881–1886.
4 Hibasami H, Komiya T, Achiwa Y, *et al.* Induction of apoptosis in human stomach cancer cells by green tea catechins. *Oncol Rep* 1998; 5: 527–529.
5 Kuroda Y, Hara Y. Antimutagenic and anticarcinogenic activity of tea polyphenols. *Mutat Res* 1999; 436: 69–97.
6 Leanderson P, Faresjo AO, Tagesson C. Green tea polyphenols inhibit oxidant-induced DNA strand breakage in cultured lung cells. *Free Rad Biol Med* 1997; 23: 235–242.

7   Fujiki H, Suganuma M, Okabe S, *et al.* Mechanistic findings of green tea as cancer preventive for humans. *Proc Soc Exp Biol Med* 1999; 220: 225–228.

8   Bushman JL. Green tea and cancer in humans: a review of the literature. *Nutr Cancer* 1998; 31: 151–159.

9   Nihal A, Hasan M. Green tea polyphenols and cancer: biological mechanisms and practical implications. *Nutr Rev* 1999; 57: 78–83.

10 Yang CS, Yang GY, Landau JM, *et al.* Tea and tea polyphenols inhibit cell proliferation, lung tumorigenesis and tumour progression. *Exp Lung Res* 1998; 24: 629–639.

11 Wang ZY, Huang MT, Ferraro T, *et al.* Inhibitory effect of green tea in the drinking water on tumorigenesis by ultraviolet light and 12-O-tetradecanoyl-phorbol-13-acetate in the skin of SKH-1 mice. *Cancer Res* 1992; 52: 1162–1170.

12 Paschka GA, Butler R, Young CY. Induction of apoptosis in prostate cancer lines by the green tea component (−)epigallocatechin-3-gallate. *Cancer Lett* 1998; 130: 1–7.

13 Shetty M, Subbannaya K, Shivananda PG. Antibacterial activity of tea (*Camellia sinensis*) and coffee (*Coffee arabica*) with special reference to *Salmonella typhimurium*. *J Commun Dis* 1994; 26: 147–150.

14 Nakayama M, Suzuki K, Toda M, *et al.* Inhibition of the infectivity of influenza virus by tea polyphenols. *Antiviral Res* 1993; 21: 289–299.

15 vanhet Kof KH, deBoer HS, Wiseman SA, *et al.* Consumption of green or black tea does not increase resistance of low-density lipoprotein to oxidation in humans. *Am J Clin Nutr* 1997; 66: 1125–1132.

16 Yokozawa T, Dong E. Influence of green tea and its three major components upon low density lipoprotein oxidation. *Exp Toxicol Pathol* 1997; 49: 329–335.

17 Kuriyama S, Shimazu T, Ohmori K, *et al.* Green tea consumption and mortality due to cardiovascular disease, cancer, and all causes in Japan: the Ohsaki study. *JAMA* 2006; 296: 1255–1265.

18 Nakachi K, Suemasu K, Suga K, *et al.* Influence of drinking green tea on breast cancer malignancy among Japanese patients. *Jpn J Cancer Res* 1998; 89: 254–261.

19 Zhang M, Holman CD, Huang JP, Xie X. Green tea and the prevention of breast cancer: a case-control study in southeast China. *Carcinogenesis* 2007; 28: 1074–1078.

20 Lee IP, Kim JH, Kang MH, *et al.* Chemoprotective effect of green tea (*Camellia sinensis*) against cigarette smoke-induced mutations (SCE) in humans. *J Cell Biochem Suppl* 1997; 27: 68–75.

21 Seely D, Mills EJ, Wu P, *et al.* The effects of green tea consumption on incidence of breast cancer and recurrence of breast cancer: a systematic review and meta-analysis. *Integr Cancer Ther* 2005; 4: 144–155.

22 Yuan J-M, Koh W-P, Sun C-L, *et al.* Green tea intake, ACE gene polymorphism and breast cancer risk among Chinese women in Singapore. *Carcinogenesis* 2005; 26: 1389–1394.

23 Kurahashi N, Sasazuki S, Iwasaki M, *et al.* Green tea consumption and prostate cancer risk in Japanese men: a prospective study. *Am J Epidemiol* 2008; 167: 71–77.

24 Yang G, Shu X-O, Li H, *et al.* Prospective cohort study of green tea consumption and colorectal cancer risk in women. *Cancer Epidemiol Biomarkers Prev* 2007; 16: 1219–1223.

25 Ogunleye AA, Xue F, Michels KB. Green tea consumption and breast cancer risk or recurrence: a meta-analysis. *Breast Cancer Res Treat* 2009; 119 (2): 477–484.

26 Myung SK, Bae WK, Oh SM, *et al.* Green tea consumption and risk of stomach cancer: a meta-analysis of epidemiologic studies. *Int J Cancer* 2009; 124(3): 670–677.

27 Chan CC, Koo MW, Ng EH, *et al.* Effects of Chinese green tea on weight, and hormonal and biochemical profiles in obese patients with polycystic ovary syndrome: a randomized placebo-controlled trial. *J Soc Gynecol Invest* 2006; 13(1): 63–68.

28 Boehm K, Borrelli F, Ernst E, *et al.* Green tea (*Camellia sinensis*) for the prevention of cancer. *Cochrane Database Syst Rev* 2009; 8(3): CD005004.

29 Imai K, Nakachi K. Cross sectional study of effects of drinking green tea on cardiovascular and liver disease. *BMJ* 1995; 310: 693–696.

30 Tsubono Y, Tsugane S. Green tea intake in relation to serum lipid levels in middle-aged Japanese men and women. *Ann Epidemiol* 1997; 7: 280–284.

31 Sasazuki S, Kodama H, Yoshimasu K, *et al.* Relation between green tea consumption and the severity of coronary atherosclerosis among Japanese men and women. *Ann Epidemiol* 2000; 10: 401–408.

32 Maron DJ, Lu GP, Cai NS, *et al.* Cholesterol lowering effect of a theaflavin-enriched green tea extract: a randomized controlled trial. *Arch Intern Med* 2003; 163: 1448–1453.

33 Unno T, Tago M, Suzuki Y, *et al.* Effect of tea catechins on postprandial plasma lipid responses in human subjects. *Br J Nutr* 2005; 93: 543–547.

34 Coimbra S, Santos-Silva A, Rocha-Pereira P, *et al.* Green tea consumption improves plasma lipid profiles in adults. *Nutrition Res* 2006; 26: 604–607.

35 KimW Jeong MH, Cho SH, *et al.* Effect of green tea consumption on endothelial function and circulating endothelial progenitor cells in chronic smokers. *Circ J* 2006; 70: 1052–1057.

36 Widlansky ME, Hamburg NM, Anter E, *et al.* Acute EGCG supplementation reverses endothelial dysfunction in patients with coronary artery disease. *J Am Coll Nutr* 2007; 26: 95–102.

37 Frank J, George TW, Lodge JK, *et al.* Daily consumption of an aqueous green tea extract supplement does not impair liver function or alter cardiovascular disease risk biomarkers in healthy men. *J Nutr* 2009; 139(1): 58–62.

38 Wang ZM, Zhou B, Wang YS, *et al.* Black and green tea consumption and the risk of coronary artery disease: a meta-analysis. *Am J Clin Nutr* 2011; 93(3): 506–515.

39 Kovacs EM, Lejeune MP, Nijs I, Westerterp-Plantenga MS. Effects of green tea on weight maintenance after body-weight loss. *Br J Nutr* 2004; 91: 431–437.

40 Westerterp-Plantenga MS, Lejeune MP, Kovacs EM. Body weight loss and weight maintenance in relation to habitual caffeine intake and green tea supplementation. *Obes Res* 2005; 13: 1195–1204.

41 Berube-Parent S, Pelletier C, Dore J, Tremblay A. Effects of encapsulated green tea and guarana extracts containing a mixture of epigallocatechin-3-gallate and caffeine on 24 h expenditure and fat oxidation in men. *Br J Nutr* 2005; 94: 432–436.

42 Nagao T, Hase T, Tokimitsu I. A green tea extract high in catechins reduces body fat and cardiovascular risks in humans. *Obesity (Silver Spring)* 2007; 15: 1473–1483.

43 Hsu CH, Tsai TH, Kao YH, *et al.* Effect of green tea extract on obese women: a randomized, double-blind, placebo-controlled clinical trial. *Clin Nutr* 2008; 27(3): 363–370.

44 Hursel R, Viechtbauer W, Westerterp-Plantenga MS. The effects of green tea on weight loss and weight maintenance: a meta-analysis. *Int J Obes (Lond)* 2009; 33(9): 956–961.

45 Fukino Y, Shimbo M, Aoki N, *et al.* Randomized controlled trial for an effect of green tea consumption on insulin resistance and inflammation markers. *J Nutr Sci Vitaminol (Tokyo)* 2005; 51: 335–342.

46 Fukino Y, Ikeda A, Maruyama K, *et al.* Randomized controlled trial for an effect of green tea-extract powder supplementation on glucose abnormalities. *Eur J Clin Nutr* 2007.

47 Venables MC, Hulston CJ, Cox HR, *et al.* Green tea extract ingestion, fat oxidation, and glucose tolerance in healthy humans. *Am J Clin Nutr* 2008; 87 (3): 778–784.

48 Eichenberger P, Mettler S, Arnold M, *et al.* No effects of three-week consumption of a green tea extract on time trial performance in endurance-trained men. *Int J Vitam Nutr Res* 2011; 80(1): 54–64.

49 Chiu AE, Chan JL, Kern DG, *et al.* Double-blind, placebo-controlled trial of green tea extracts in the clinical and histology appearance of photoaging skin. *Dermatol Surg* 2005; 31(7Pt2): 855–860.

50 Ahn WS, Yoo J, Huh SW, *et al.* Protective effects of green tea extracts (polyphenon E and EGCG) on human cervical lesions. *Eur J Cancer Prev* 2003; 12: 383–390.

51 Kuriyama S, Hozawa A, Ohmori K, *et al.* Green tea consumption and cognitive function: a cross sectional study from the Tsurugaya Project. *Am J Clin Nutr* 2006; 83: 355–361.

Guarana

Description

Guarana is produced from the dried and powdered seeds of a South American shrub, *Paullinia cupana*.

Constituents

Guarana contains a substance called guaranine (a synonym for caffeine). It also contains theobromine, theophylline and tannins.

Action

Guarana acts as a CNS stimulant, increases heart rate and contractility, increases blood pressure, inhibits platelet aggregation, stimulates gastric acid secretion, causes diuresis, relaxes bronchial smooth muscle and stimulates the release of catecholamines.

Possible uses

Guarana is claimed to:

- improve mental alertness, endurance, vitality, immunity, stamina in athletes and sexual drive;
- retard ageing;
- alleviate migraine, diarrhoea, constipation and tension; and
- act as an appetite suppressant to aid slimming.

The effects of guarana on mental alertness have often been assumed to reflect its caffeine content. However, recent trial evidence indicates that this might not be correct. A double-blind placebo-controlled trial evaluating guarana, ginseng and their combination in 28 healthy young participants showed that all three treatments resulted in improved task performance throughout the day compared with placebo. In the case of guarana, improvements were seen across 'attention' tasks (but with some evidence of reduced accuracy), and on a sentence verification task. While also increasing the speed of attention task performance, both ginseng and the ginseng/guarana combination also enhanced the speed of memory task performance, with little evidence of modulated accuracy. Guarana and the combination, and to a lesser extent ginseng, also led to significant improvements in serial subtraction task performance.[1] This trial employed guarana with a low caffeine content (9 mg) so these effects are unlikely to be caused by caffeine. A further placebo-controlled trial by the same research group looked at the effect of a guarana/vitamin/mineral supplement on cognitive performance and found that the supplement improved task performance in terms of speed and accuracy in a visual processing task. Increase in mental fatigue associated with performance of an extended task was attenuated by the supplement.[2]

A dose–response trial evaluating the behavioural effects of guarana also found that the effects of guarana cannot be attributed to caffeine alone. This double-blind, counterbalanced, placebo-controlled study of 26 subjects assessed the acute mood and cognitive effects throughout the day of four different doses (37.5, 75, 150 and 300 mg) of a standardised guarana extract (PC-102). Guarana improved secondary memory performance and increased alert and content mood ratings. The two lower doses produced more positive cognitive effects than the higher doses.[3]

A trial in patients with breast cancer undergoing radiation therapy failed to show any effect of guarana 75 mg daily on fatigue and depressive sysmptoms.[4]

Conclusion

Guarana has been shown to have psychoactive properties, improving alertness, mood and task performance and reducing fatigue. Such results have been found at low doses, suggesting that they may not be entirely attributable to caffeine.

Precautions/contraindications

Guarana should be avoided by people with heart conditions, peptic ulcer, anxiety disorders, and renal impairment. It should also not be taken within 2 h of bedtime.

Pregnancy and breast-feeding

Guarana should be avoided during pregnancy and breast-feeding.

Adverse effects

High doses of guarana may cause insomnia, nervousness, irritability, palpitations, gastric irritation, flushing and elevated blood pressure.

Interactions

None have been reported.

Dose

Guarana is available in the form of tablets and capsules, either in isolation or with vitamins and minerals in other dietary supplements.

The dose is not established. Guarana should not be recommended. Dietary supplements provide 50–200 mg.

References

1 Kennedy DO, Haskell CF, Wesnes KA, *et al*. Improved cognitive performance in human volunteers following administration of guarana (*Paullinia cupana*) extract: comparison and interaction with *Panax* ginseng. *Pharmacol Biochem Behav* 2004; 79(3): 401–411.

2 Kennedy DO, Haskell CF, Robertson B, *et al*. Improved cognitive performance and mental fatigue following a multi-vitamin and mineral supplement with added guarana (*Paullinia cupana*). *Appetite* 2008; 50(2-3): 506–513.

3 Haskell CF, Kennedy DO, Wesnes KA, *et al*. A double-blind, placebo-controlled, multi-dose evaluation of the acute behavioural effects of guarana in humans. *J Psychopharmacol* 2007; 21(1): 65–70.

4 da Costa Miranda V, Trufelli DC, Santos J, *et al*. Effectiveness of guarana (*Paullinia cupana*) for postradiation fatigue and depression: results of a pilot double-blind randomized study. *J Altern Complement Med* 2009; 15(4): 431–433.

Hyaluronic acid

Description

Hyaluronic acid (also known as hyaluronan, hyaluronate) is a disaccharide glycosaminoglycan polymer composed of D-glucuronic acid and N-acetyl-D-glucosamine, linked together via alternating β-1,4 and β-1,3 glycosidic bonds. Polymers of hyaluronic acid can have up to 25 000 disaccharide repeating structures and range in size from 5000 to 20 000 000 Daltons *in vivo*.[1]

Hyaluronic acid is distributed widely throughout connective, epithelial and neural tissues, principally in the cartilage, synovial fluid and aqueous humour. It is one of the chief components of the extracellular matrix, where it contributes significantly to cell proliferation and migration. An average 70 kg man has approximately 15 g of hyaluronic acid in his body, one-third of which is turned over every day.[2,3]

Action

Hyaluronic acid has a key role in articular cartilage, where it surrounds each chondrocyte, and exists together with proteoglycans in the form of macromolecular aggregates, the stability of which is enhanced by link protein. These large aggregates absorb water and contribute to the structure and resilience of cartilage.[4] The size of these aggregans decreases with age, which seems to be related to a modification in the chain length of hyaluronic acid.[4]

Hyaluronic acid is also a major component of skin, where it is involved in tissue repair. On excessive exposure to UVB rays, the skin becomes inflamed and hyaluronic acid synthesis in the dermal cells is reduced.[5] Degradation products of hyaluronic acid accumulate in the skin following UVB exposure.[6]

Hyaluronic acid also contributes to cellular movement and proliferation and may be involved in the progression of some malignant tumours. The principal receptor for hyaluronic acid is CD44 and up-regulation of CD44 is considered to be a marker of cell activation in lymphocytes. CD44 also participates in cell adhesion interactions required by tumour cells. The interaction of hyaluronic acid with CD44 may explain its contribution to tumour growth. Hyaluronic acid degradation products are potent activators of dendritic cells and appear to induce maturation of dendritic cells via Toll-like receptor 2 (TLR2), TLR4 or both TLR2 and TLR4.[7,8] TLR and hyaluronic acid play a role in innate immunity.

Possible uses

Medicinal use

Hyaluronic acid is used by injection as an adjunct in ophthalmic surgery (e.g. cataract, corneal transplant, glaucoma, retinal detachment) and in osteoarthritis.[2] A meta-analysis found that intra-articular injection of hyaluronic acid can decrease symptoms of osteoarthritis of the knee with significant improvements in pain and functional outcomes and few adverse events. However, there was significant between-study heterogeneity in the estimates of the efficacy of hyaluronic acid, indicating the need for further well-controlled trials.[9] A further systematic review and meta-analysis found no consistent evidence that hyaluronic acid is clinically effective in the treatment of osteoarthritis of the knee and that it may be associated with a greater risk of adverse events.[10] A Cochrane analysis concluded that hyaluronic derivatives, given by injection, are an effective treatment for osteoarthritis of the knee with beneficial effects on pain, function and patient global assessment, and at different post-injection periods (but especially at the 5- to 13-week post-injection period). It is of note that the magnitude of the clinical effect is different for different products, comparisons, timepoints, variables and trial designs.[11]

Hyaluronic acid is involved in wound healing[12] and when used topically may be of value in the prevention and treatment of various inflammatory skin diseases (e.g. venous leg ulcers, diabetic foot lesions).[13]

Dietary supplement

Oral preparations of hyaluronic acid are promoted on the Internet for relief of joint pain, lubrication of joints, younger, softer-looking skin, clear eyes and to delay ageing. There is no robust scientific evidence to back up these claims.

> **Conclusion**
> There is no scientific evidence of benefit for oral supplements containing hyaluronic acid.

Precautions/contraindications

Hyaluronic acid should not be recommended as a dietary supplement.

Adverse effcts

Hyaluronic acid contributes to cell proliferation and may contribute to progression of malignant tumours. Levels of hyaluronic acid may be high in patients with cancer and may fall with treatment. The clinical relevance of these findings in relation to administration of hyaluronic acid is unclear.

Interactions

None reported.

Dose

Hyaluronic acid should be avoided as an oral supplement and should not be used by injection without medical supervision. Oral supplements are available on the Internet.

References

1 Percival SP. Sodium hyaluronate in perspective: experiences from a four-year clinical trial. *Trans Ophthalmol Soc UK* 1985; 104 (Pt 6): 616–620.
2 Goa KL, Benfield P. Hyaluronic acid. A review of its pharmacology and use as a surgical aid in ophthalmology, and its therapeutic potential in joint disease and wound healing. *Drugs* 1994; 47: 536–566.
3 Stern R. Hyaluronan catabolism: a new metabolic pathway. *Eur J Cell Biol* 2004; 83: 317–325.
4 Holmes MW, Bayliss MT, Muir H. Hyaluronic acid in human articular cartilage. Age-related changes in content and size. *Biochem J* 1988; 250: 435–441.
5 Averbeck M, Gebhardt CA, Voigt S, *et al.* Differential regulation of hyaluronan metabolism in the epidermal and dermal compartments of human skin by UVB irradiation. *J Invest Dermatol* 2007; 127: 687–697.
6 Dai G, Freudenberger T, Zipper P, *et al.* Chronic ultraviolet B irradiation causes loss of hyaluronic acid from mouse dermis because of down-regulation of hyaluronic acid synthases. *Am J Pathol* 2007; 171: 1451–1461.
7 Termeer C, Benedix F, Sleeman J, *et al.* Oligosaccharides of Hyaluronan activate dendritic cells via Toll-like receptor 4. *J Exp Med* 2002; 195: 99–111.
8 Robertson SM, Davey RT, Voell J, *et al.* Effect of *Ginkgo biloba* extract on lopinavir, midazolam and fexofenadine pharmacokinetics in healthy subjects. *Curr Med Res Opin* 2008; 24: 591–599.
9 Wang CT, Lin J, Chang CJ, *et al.* Therapeutic effects of hyaluronic acid on osteoarthritis of the knee. A meta-analysis of randomized controlled trials. *J Bone Joint Surg Am* 2004; 86-A(3): 538–545.
10 Arrich J, Piribauer F, Mad P, *et al.* Intra-articular hyaluronic acid for the treatment of osteoarthritis of the knee: systematic review and meta-analysis. *CMAJ* 2005; 172: 1039–1043.
11 Bellamy N, Campbell J, Welch V, *et al.* Viscosupplementation for the treatment of osteoarthritis of the knee. *Cochrane Database Syst Rev* 2006; (2): CD005321.
12 Chen WY, Abatangelo G. Functions of hyaluronan in wound repair. *Wound Repair Regen* 1999; 7: 79–89.
13 Weindl G, Schaller M, Schafer-Korting M, Korting HC. Hyaluronic acid in the treatment and prevention of skin diseases: molecular biological, pharmaceutical and clinical aspects. *Skin Pharmacol Physiol* 2004; 17: 207–213.

Hydroxycitric acid

Description

Hydroxycitric acid (HCA) is derived from the small fruit of the plant *Garcinia cambogia* found in South-East Asia.

Action

HCA is a potent inhibitor of the enzyme ATP-citrate-lyase. This enzyme converts citric acid, a carbohydrate product of the Krebs cycle into acetyl coenzyme A. Acetyl coenzyme A is a substrate for fatty acid and cholesterol synthesis. Inhibition of ATP-citrate-lyase has the capacity to prevent carbohydrate conversion to fat. This is thought to induce the body to oxidise the excess carbohydrates, resulting in increased glycogen storage which could, in turn, contribute to suppression of appetite. Inhibition of conversion of carbohydrate to fat may also inhibit adipose tissue synthesis.

Possible uses

In vitro and animal studies have suggested that HCA suppresses appetite and reduces food intake, with body weight loss in rats. However, clinical trials in humans do not support the use of HCA as a weight loss supplement.

A 12-week randomised, double-blind, controlled trial in 135 overweight men and women given 1500 mg HCA daily found that patients in both the intervention and the control groups lost a significant amount of weight over 12 weeks with no significant differences between the groups. There were no significant differences in estimated percentage of body fat mass loss between groups and the fraction of weight loss as fat was not influenced by treatment group.[1]

A double-blind RCT in 10 overweight men studied the effect of 3-day HCA supplementation (3 g daily) or placebo on metabolic parameters that could influence body weight regulation, with or without moderately intense exercise.

However, neither respiratory quotient, energy expenditure nor the blood parameters measured (glucose, insulin, lactate, beta-hydroxybutyrate) were significantly different between the groups with or without exercise. HCA appeared to have no effect on the rate of fat oxidation.[2]

Similar findings were derived from two further studies. One trial in 10 exercise-trained cyclists found that HCA supplementation even in large quantities had no significant effect on oxidation of carbohydrate and fat. Plasma glucose, glycerol and fatty acids did not differ.[3] Two weeks of supplementation with HCA or HCA plus medium chain triglycerides (MCT) in 11 overweight men did not increase fat oxidation. Compared with placebo in this study there was also no increased satiety, fat oxidation, 24-hour energy expenditure or body weight loss in those taking HCA. (Both groups lost weight.)[4]

However, two 5-day trials involving the use of 250 mg HCA or placebo (one in trained cyclists,[5] one in untrained women[6]) and a further 5-day trial with 500 mg HCA or placebo in untrained men[7] found increased fat oxidation and increased endurance.

A further 2-week trial, this time in normal to moderately obese subjects (seven men and 14 women) found that HCA (500 mg daily) and HCA combined with MCT did not result in increased satiety of decreased energy intake compared with placebo. There was significant weight loss in both intervention groups and placebo.[8]

A placebo-controlled, single-blind crossover trial in 12 overweight men and 12 overweight women found that 24-hour energy intake was decreased by 15–30% with 300 mg HCA compared with placebo, with sustained satiety. However, body weight tended to decrease ($P = 0.1$).[9]

A double-blind, placebo-controlled, randomised and crossover design trial in 10 sedentary, lean men evaluated the effect of HCA in limiting the capacity for *de novo* fat synthesis during overfeeding and, hence, the possibility that HCA could promote weight maintenance in this situation. The trial involved 10 days of overfeeding (3-day high fat and 7-day high carbohydrate). During overfeeding the men ingested 3 × 500 mg HCA daily or placebo. *De novo* fat synthesis was reduced in the HCA group ($P <$ 0.01) and activity-induced energy expenditure was higher ($P < 0.5$), indicating that treatment with HCA during overfeeding may reduce *de novo* fat synthesis, which could help to ensure that body weight does not increase.[10]

Trials employing a HCA preparation of increased biovailability have yielded better results. A novel, water-soluble calcium-potassium salt of HCA in a dose equivalent to 2800 mg of HCA daily resulted in reduced body weight, improved lipid profiles, suppression of appetite and increased fat oxidation in comparison with placebo.[11,12]

> ### Conclusion
> Preclinical trials have suggested that HCA reduces appetite and body weight. However, RCTs in humans have been largely disappointing. There is insufficient justification to recommend HCA for weight loss. However, the use of a preparation of increased biovailability has shown more positive results. Further controlled clinical trials are required to build on already existing data.

Precautions/contraindications

No long-term studies have assessed the safety of HCA.

Pregnancy and breast-feeding

There are no data in pregnant and breast-feeding women. HCA is best avoided during pregnancy and lactation.

Adverse effects

No serious side-effects have been noted. There were no reports of side-effects during supplementation of HCA 1500 mg daily for 12 weeks in overweight subjects.[1,13] In a recent safety assessment of HCA, doses of up to 2800 mg daily have been suggested to be safe for human consumption.[14]

Interactions

None have been reported.

Dose

HCA is available in the form of tablets, capsules and powders. Extract of *Garcinia cambogia* is also available. The dose is not established. Manufacturers recommend taking 250–1500 mg daily of HCA.

References

1 Heymsfield SB, Allison DB, Vasselli JR, *et al.* *Garcinia cambogia* (hydroxycitric acid) as a potential antiobesity agent: a randomized controlled trial. *JAMA* 1998; 280: 1596–1600.

2 Kriketos AD, Thompson HR, Greene H, Hill JO. (−)-Hydroxycitric acid does not affect energy expenditure and substrate oxidation in adult males in a post-absorptive state. *Int J Obes Relat Metab Disord* 1999; 23: 867–873.

3 van Loon LJ, van Rooijen JJ, Niesen B, *et al.* Effects of acute (−)-hydroxycitrate supplementation on substrate metabolism at rest and during exercise in humans. *Am J Clin Nutr* 2000; 72: 1445–1450.

4 Kovacs EM, Westerterp-Plantenga MS, de Vries M, *et al.* Effects of 2-week ingestion of (−)-hydroxycitrate and (−)-hydroxycitrate combined with medium-chain triglycerides on satiety and food intake. *Physiol Behav* 2001; 74: 543–549.

5 Lim K, Ryu S, Ohishi Y, *et al.* Short-term (−)-hydroxycitrate ingestion increases fat oxidation during exercise in athletes. *J Nutr Sci Vitaminol (Tokyo)* 2002; 48: 128–133.

6 Lim K, Ryu S, Nho HS, *et al.* (−)-Hydroxycitric acid ingestion increases fat utilization during exercise in untrained women. *J Nutr Sci Vitaminol (Tokyo)* 2003; 49: 163–167.

7 Tomita K, Okuhara Y, Shigematsu N, *et al.* (−)-Hydroxycitrate ingestion increases fat oxidation during moderate intensity exercise in untrained men. *Biosci Biotechnol Biochem* 2003; 67: 1999–2001.

8 Kovacs EM, Westerterp-Plantenga MS, Saris WH. The effects of 2-week ingestion of (−)-hydroxycitrate and (−)-hydroxycitrate combined with medium-chain triglycerides on satiety, fat oxidation, energy expenditure and body weight. *Int J Obes Relat Metab Disord* 2001; 25: 1087–1094.

9 Westerterp-Plantenga MS, Kovacs EM. The effect of (−)-hydroxycitrate on energy intake and satiety

in overweight humans. *Int J Obes Relat Metab Disord* 2002; 26: 870–872.

10   Kovacs EM, Westerterp-Plantenga MS. Effects of (−)-hydroxycitrate on net fat synthesis as de novo lipogenesis. *Physiol Behav* 2006; 88: 371–381.

11   Preuss HG, Bagchi D, Bagchi M, *et al*. Effects of a natural extract of (−)-hydroxycitricacid (HCA-SX) and a combination of HCA-SX plus niacin-bound chromiumand *Gymnema sylvestre* extract on weight loss. *Diabetes Obes Metab* 2004; 6: 171–180.

12   Preuss HG, Garis RI, Bramble JD, *et al*. Efficacy of a novel calcium/potassium salt of (−)-hydroxycitric acid in weight control. *Int J Clin Pharmacol Res* 2005; 25: 133–144.

13   Mattes RD, Bormann L. Effects of (−)-hydroxycitric acid on appetitive variables. *Physiol Behav* 2000; 71: 87–94.

14   Soni MG, Burdock GA, Preuss HG, *et al*. Safety assessment of (−)-hydroxycitric acid and Super CitriMax, a novel calcium/potassium salt. *Food Chem Toxicol* 2004; 42: 1513–1529.

5-Hydroxytryptophan (5-HTP)

Description

5-Hydroxytryptophan (5-HTP) is an amino acid synthesised endogenously from tryptophan, which is then converted to serotonin. 5-HTP is available in the form of supplements and marketed for conditions related to low serotonin levels. Supplements were banned in 1990 as a result of the association of 5-HTP with eosinophilic myalgia syndrome (EMS) and several fatalities. However, following the suggestion that this could be caused by contaminants in 5-HTP supplements rather than 5-HTP itself, supplements have been available since 2001.

Action

5-HTP may help to raise serotonin (5-HT) levels in the brain, which may have beneficial effects on disorders associated with low serotonin levels (e.g. depression, anxiety, sleep, aggression, pain and sexual behaviour).[1]

Dietary sources

5-HTP is not commonly found in food but the amino acid tryptophan, from which the body makes 5-HTP, can be found in turkey, chicken, milk, potatoes, pumpkin, sunflower seeds, turnip and collard greens, and seaweed.

Bioavailability

The amount of 5-HTP reaching the central nervous system (CNS) is affected by the extent to which 5-HTP is converted to serotonin in the periphery. This conversion is controlled by the enzyme amino acid decarboxylase. 5-HTP is well absorbed from an oral dose, with about 70% ending up in the bloodstream. It easily crosses the blood–brain barrier and effectively increases CNS synthesis of serotonin.[1] Oral availability of 5-HTP has been found to be 47–84% (mean value 69.2%).[2]

Possible uses

5-HTP has been studied for a wide variety of mood disorders (particularly depression) and poor sleep.

Depression and anxiety

Low levels of 5-HT in the brain can contribute to thedevelopment of depression and negative mood.[3] Many antidepressant drugs (e.g. selectiveserotonin re-uptake inhibitors; SSRIs) increase 5-HT levels. Some studies indicate that 5-HTP may be effective in mild to moderate depression.[4,5] Many of these studies were conducted during the 1970s and 1980s and the methodology is not robust.

A Cochrane review of 5-HTP in depression concluded that of the many studies evaluating 5-HTP in depression and insomnia, only two trials involving a total of 64 patients were of sufficient quality to meet inclusion criteria for the review. As a consequence the review stated that evidence is of insufficient quality to be conclusive.[6] Evidence suggests that 5-HTP may be synergistic with SSRIs in the treatment of depression,[7] in that SSRIs prevent re-uptake of serotonin, while 5-HTP improves its synthesis.

Preliminary evidence suggests that 5-HTP could be beneficial in anxiety.[8]

Sleep

Some evidence from small older studies indicates that 5-HTP can help to induce sleep.[9,10] 5-HTP crosses the blood–brain barrier more effectively than L-tryptophan. A dose of 100 mg daily has been associated with improvement in slow-wave sleep in human subjects.[9]

Fibromyalgia

Fibromyalgia syndrome is a musculoskeletal pain and fatigue disorder characterised by diffuse myalgia, localised areas of tenderness, fatigue, lowered pain thresholds, and non-restorative sleep. Evidence indicates that reduced 5-HT flux could be a factor in this condition and supplementation with 5-HTP and L-tryptophan has been shown to improve symptoms.[11–13]

Headache

5-HT plays a crucial role in mediating the descending pain inhibitory systems and in the pathophysiology of migraine. Small studies have shown beneficial effects of 5-HTP in migraine[14] and other chronic primary headaches.[15]

Body weight

Low 5-HT levels may contribute to excess fat and carbohydrate intake (which can result in weight gain). In overweight individuals with diabetes, supplementation with 5-HTP has been shown to decrease fat and carbohydrate intake by promoting a feeling of satiety (fullness).[16] Other similar studies of obese men and women without diabetes found that supplementation with 5-HTP resulted in decreased food intake and weight loss.[17]

> ### Conclusion
> 5-HTP supplements may help to increase serotonin levels in the brain, and as a consequence 5-HTP has been evaluated for benefits on mood, depression, sleep, headache and appetite. Small trials have shown positive effects, but large, well-controlled trials remain to be conducted.

Precautions/contraindications

There is a great deal of controversy about the safety of 5-HTP. Use of L-tryptophan has been associated with eosinophilic myalgia syndrome (EMS), a potentially fatal muscle disorder diagnosed in at least 1500 individuals and responsible for at least 38 deaths. Analysis of several different 5-HTP products led to the identification of the same contaminant as the one in L-tryptophan. The contaminant can be identified by gas chromatography and named 'peak X'.18–20 EMS has been reported in 10 people taking 5-HTP. Such reports prompted the FDA to ban the sale of all tryptophan supplements in 1989 and the UK followed suit in 1990. So far, evidence is insufficient to show whether EMS is caused by 5-HTP or contaminants.

Pregnancy and breast-feeding

Avoid during pregnancy and breast-feeding.

Adverse effects

5-HTP may cause mild gastrointestinal disturbances including nausea, heartburn, flatulence and satiety. See also precautions related to EMS (above). High doses (>100 mg) can cause serotonin syndrome (excessive 5-HT). Signs include: euphoria, drowsiness, sustained rapid eye movement, reflex hyperreactivity, rapid muscle contraction and relaxation in the ankle causing abnormal movements of the foot, clumsiness, restlessness, feeling drunk and dizzy, muscle contraction and relaxation in the jaw, sweating, intoxication, muscle twitching, rigidity, high body temperature. Drugs which increase 5-HT (see Interactions) can also cause serotonin syndrome if taken with 5-HTP.

Interactions

Drugs

Antidepressants
Selective serotonin inhibitors (SSRIs), mono-amine oxidaseinhibitors (MAOIs), trazodone and venlafaxine interfere with 5-HT uptake. 5-HTP may increase serotonin levels with these drugs and should be avoided.

Carbidopa
5-HTP has been associated with scleroderma (hard, thick inflamed skin) in patients taking carbidopa.

Sumatriptan
May increase 5-HT levels with 5-HTP.

Tramodol
May increase 5-HT levels with 5-HTP.

Zolpidem
Theoretically could cause hallucinations with 5-HTP.

Dose

5-HTP is best avoided until there is clear evidence of its safety.

References

1 Birdsall TC. 5-Hydroxytryptophan: a clinically-effective serotonin precursor. *Altern Med Rev* 1998; 3: 271–280.

2 Magnussen I, Nielsen-Kudsk F. Bioavailability and related pharmacokinetics in man of orally administered L-5-hydroxytryptophan in steady state. *Acta Pharmacol Toxicol (Copenh)* 1980; 46: 257–262.

3 Dayan P, Huys QJ. Serotonin, inhibition, and negative mood. *PLoS Comput Biol* 2008; 4: e4.

4 Byerley WF, Judd LL, Reimherr FW, Grosser BI. 5-Hydroxytryptophan: a review of its antidepressant efficacy and adverse effects. *J Clin Psychopharmacol* 1987; 7: 127–137.

5 Turner EH, Loftis JM, Blackwell AD. Serotonin a la carte: supplementation with the serotonin precursor 5-hydroxytryptophan. *Pharmacol Ther* 2006; 109: 325–338.

6 Shaw K, Turner J, Del. Mar C. Tryptophan and 5-hydroxytryptophan for depression. *Cochrane Database Syst Rev* 2002; CD003198.

7 Turner EH, Blackwell AD. 5-Hydroxytryptophan plus SSRIs for interferon-induced depression: synergistic mechanisms for normalizing synaptic serotonin. *Med Hypotheses* 2005; 65: 138–144.

8 Kahn RS, Westenberg HG. L-5-Hydroxytryptophan in the treatment of anxiety disorders. *J Affect Disord* 1985; 8: 197–200.

9 Soulairac A, Lambinet H. [Effect of 5-hydroxytryptophan, a serotonin precursor, on sleep disorders]. *Ann Med Psychol (Paris)* 1977; 1: 792–798.

10 Wyatt RJ, Zarcone V, Engelman K, *et al*. Effects of 5-hydroxytryptophan on the sleep of normal human subjects. *Electroencephalogr Clin Neurophysiol* 1971; 30: 505–509.

11 Juhl JH. Fibromyalgia and the serotonin pathway. *Altern Med Rev* 1998; 3: 367–375.

12 Sarzi Puttini P, Caruso I. Primary fibromyalgia syndrome and 5-hydroxy-L-tryptophan: a 90-day open study. *J Int Med Res* 1992; 20: 182–189.

13 Caruso I, Sarzi Puttini,P, Cazzola M, Azzolini V. Double-blind study of 5-hydroxytryptophan versus placebo in the treatment of primary fibromyalgia syndrome. *J Int Med Res* 1990; 18: 201–209.

14 De Benedittis,G, Massei R. Serotonin precursors in chronic primary headache. A double-blind crossover study with L-5-hydroxytryptophan vs. placebo. *J Neurosurg Sci* 1985; 29: 239–248.

15 Ribeiro CA. L-5-Hydroxytryptophan in the prophylaxis of chronic tension-type headache: a double-blind, randomized, placebo-controlled study. For the Portuguese Head Society. *Headache* 2000; 40: 451–456.

16 Cangiano C, Laviano A, Del BenM, *et al*. Effects of oral 5-hydroxy-tryptophan on energy intake and macronutrient selection in non-insulin dependent diabetic patients. *Int J Obes Relat Metab Disord* 1998; 22: 648–654.

17 Cangiano C, Ceci F, Cascino A, *et al*. Eating behavior and adherence to dietary prescriptions in obese adult subjects treated with 5-hydroxytryptophan. *Am J Clin Nutr* 1992; 56: 863–867.

18 Food and Drug Administration. FDA Talk Paper. Impurities confirmed in dietary supplement 5-hydroxytryptophan. 1998. Available at: http://vm.cfsan.fda.gov/~lrd/tp5htp.html (accessed 29 February 2008).

19 Food and Drug Administration. Information paper on L-tryptophan and 5-hydroxy-L-tryptophan. Office of Nutritional Products, Labeling, Dietary Supplements. Center for Food Safety and Applied Nutrition. February 2001.

20 Johnson KL, Klarskov K, Benson LM, *et al*. Presence of peak X and related compounds: the reported contaminant in case related 5-hydroxy-L-tryptophan associated with eosinophilia-myalgia syndrome. *J Rheumatol* 1999; 26: 2714–2717.

Iodine

Description

Iodine is an essential trace element.

Human requirements

See Table 1 for Dietary Reference Values for iodine.

Dietary intake

In the UK, the average adult diet provides: for men, 220 µg daily; for women, 159 µg.

Action

Iodine is an essential part of the thyroid hormones thyroxine (T$_4$) and triiodothyronine (T$_3$).

Dietary sources

See Table 2 for dietary sources of iodine.

Metabolism

Absorption
Inorganic iodine is rapidly and efficiently absorbed. Organically bound iodine is less well absorbed.

Distribution
Iodine is transported to the thyroid gland (for the synthesis of thyroid hormones), and to a lesser extent to the salivary and gastric glands.

Elimination
Excretion of inorganic iodine is mainly via the urine. Some organic iodine is eliminated in the faeces. Iodine is excreted in the breast milk.

Deficiency

Iodine deficiency leads to goitre and hypothyroidism.

Possible uses

Supplements containing iodine may be required by vegans (strict vegetarians who consume no dairy products). In a study in Greater London that included 38 vegans,[1] intakes of iodine in the vegan individuals were below the DRVs. The authors of the study concluded that the impact of these low iodine intakes should be studied further and that vegans should use appropriate dietary supplements. Further studies have confirmed a markedly reduced iodine intake with a lactovegetarian diet compared with an ordinary diet,[2] and a higher prevalence of iodine deficiency in vegans and vegetarians.[3]

Precautions/contraindications

None reported.

Pregnancy and breast-feeding

Doses exceeding the RDA should not be used (they may result in abnormal thyroid function in the infant).

Adverse effects

High iodine intake may induce hyperthyroidism (particularly in those over the age of 40 years) and toxic modular goitre or hypothyroidism in autoimmune thyroid disease. There is a risk of hyperkalaemia with prolonged use of high doses. Toxicity is rare with intakes below 5000 µg daily and extremely rare at intakes below 1000 µg daily.

Hypersensitivity reactions including headache, rashes, symptoms of head cold, swelling of lips, throat and tongue, and arthralgia (joint pain) have been reported.

Table 1 Dietary Reference Values for iodine (µg/day)

	UK			USA		WHO/FAO RNI
						EU RDA = 150 µg
Age	LRNI	RNI	EVM	RDA	TUL	
0–3 months	40	50		110[1]	–	90
4–6 months	40	60		110[1]	–	90
7–12 months	40	60		130	–	90
1–3 years	40	70		90	200	90
4–6 years	50	100		–	–	
4–8 years	–	–		90	300	
7–10 years	55	110		–	–	120[3]
9–13 years	–	–		120	600	–
14–18 years	–	–		150	900	150[4]
Males and females						
11–14 years	65	130		–	–	–
15–18 years	70	140		–	–	–
19–50+	70	140	500[1]	150	1100	150
Pregnancy	*	*		220	1100[2]	200
Lactation	*	*		290	1100[2]	200

* No increment.
[1] Adequate Intakes (AIs).   [2] < 18 years, 90 µg.   [3] 6–12 years.   [4] 13–18 years.
EVM = Likely upper safe daily intake from supplements alone.
LRNI = Lowest Reference Nutrient Intake.
RNI = Reference Nutrient Intake.
TUL = Tolerable Upper Intake Level.

Interactions

Drugs
Antithyroid drugs: iodine may interfere with thyroid control.

Dose

Iodine is available mostly as an ingredient in multivitamin and mineral products.

Dietary supplements usually provide 50–100% of the RDA.

Upper safety levels

The UK Expert Group on Vitamins and Minerals (EVM) has identified a likely safe total intake of iodine for adults from supplements alone of 500 µg daily.

Table 2 Dietary sources of iodine

Food portion	Iodine content (µg)
Milk and dairy products	
Milk, whole, semi-skimmed or skimmed (284 ml; ¹/₂ pint)	*45*
1 pot yoghurt (150 g)	90
Cheese (50 g)	*25*
Fish	
Cod, cooked (150 g)	150
Haddock, cooked (150 g)	300
Mackerel, cooked (150 g)	200
Plaice, cooked (150 g)	*50*

Excellent sources (**bold**); good sources (*italics*).
Note: Iodised salt contains 150 µg/5 g.

References

1 Draper A, Lewis J, Malhotra N, Wheeler E. The energy and nutrient intakes of different types of vegetarian: a case for supplements? *Br J Nutr* 1993; 69: 3–19.

2 Remer T, Neubert A, Manz F. Increased risk of iodine deficiency with vegetarian nutrition. *Br J Nutr* 1999; 81: 45–49.

3 Krajovicova-Kuldlackova M, Buckova K, Klimes I, Sebokova E. Iodine deficiency in vegetarians and vegans. *Ann Nutr Metab* 2003; 47: 183–185.

Iron

Description

Iron is an essential trace mineral.

Human requirements

See Table 1 for Dietary Reference Values of iron.

Dietary intake

In the UK, the average adult diet provides: for men 13.2 mg daily; for women, 10.0 mg. Dietary iron consists of haem and non-haem iron; in animal foods, about 40% of the iron is haem iron and 60% is non-haem iron; all the iron in vegetable products is non-haem iron.

Action

Iron is a component of haemoglobin, myoglobin and many enzymes that are involved in a variety of metabolic functions, including transport and storage of oxygen, the electron transport chain, DNA synthesis and catecholamine metabolism.[1]

Dietary sources

See Table 2 for dietary sources of iron.

Metabolism

Absorption

Absorption of iron occurs principally in the duodenum and proximal jejunum. Absorption of food iron varies between 5% and 15%.[1] Haem iron is more efficiently absorbed than non-haem iron. Body iron content is regulated mainly through changes in absorption.

Distribution

Iron is transported in the blood bound to the protein transferrin, and is stored in the liver, spleen and bone marrow as ferritin and haemosiderin.

Elimination

The body has a limited capacity to eliminate iron, and it can accumulate in the body to toxic amounts. Small amounts are excreted in the faeces, urine, skin, sweat, hair, nails and menstrual blood.

Bioavailability

The absorption of non-haem iron is enhanced by concurrent ingestion of meat, poultry and fish, and by various organic acids, especially ascorbic acid; it is inhibited by phytates (found in bran and high-fibre cereals), tannins (found in tea and coffee), egg yolk and by some drugs and nutrients (see Interactions). Ferrous salts are more efficiently absorbed than ferric salts.

Deficiency

Iron deficiency leads to microcytic, hypochromic anaemia. Symptoms include fatigue, weakness, pallor, dyspnoea on exertion and palpitations. Non-haematological effects include impairment in work capacity, intellectual performance, neurological function and immune function and, in children, behavioural disturbances.[1] Gastrointestinal symptoms are also fairly common and the fingernails may become lustreless, brittle, flattened and spoon-shaped. *Helicobacter pylori* infection is also associated with iron deficiency.[2]

Table 1 Dietary Reference Values for iron (mg/day)

Age	UK				USA		EU RDA $=$ 14 mg
	LRNI	EAR	RNI	EVM	RDA	TUL	FAO/WHO RNI[1]
0–3 months	0.9	1.3	1.7		0.27[2]	40	–
4–6 months	2.3	3.3	4.3		0.27[2]	40	–
7–12 months	4.2	6.0	7.8		11	40	6.2–18.6
1–3 years	3.7	5.3	6.9		7	40	3.9–11.6
4–6 years	3.3	4.7	6.1		–	–	4.2–12.6
4–8 years	–	–	–		10	40	–
7–10 years	4.7	6.7	8.7		10	–	5.9–17.8[3]
9–13 years	–	–	–		8	40	–
Males							
11–14 years	6.1	8.7	11.3		–	–	9.7–29.2[4]
15–18 years	6.1	8.7	11.3		–	–	12.5–37.6
14–18 years	–	–	–		11	45	–
19–50+ years	4.7	6.7	8.7	17	8	45	9.2–27.4
Females							
11–14 years	8.0	11.4	14.8[5]		–	–	9.3–28.0[4,6]/21.8–65.4[4,7]
14–18 years	–	–	–		15	45	–
15–50+ years	8.0	11.4	14.8[1]	17	–	–	–
19–50 years	–	–	–		18	45	19.6–58.8
50+ years	4.7	6.7	8.7		8	45	9.1–27.4
Pregnancy	*	*	*		27	45	NS
Lactation	*	*	*		9[8]	45	10.0–30.0
Post-menopause						8	
Pre-menopause					18		

*No increment.
[1]Requirement depends on iron bioavailability of the diet.   [2]Adequate Intakes (AIs).   [3]7–9 years.   [4]10–14 years.
[5]Insufficient level for women who have high menstrual losses who may need iron supplements.   [6]Pre-menarche.
[7]Post-menarche.   [8]Aged <18 years, 10 mg daily.
EAR, Estimated Average Requirement; EVM, likely safe daily intake from supplements alone; LRNI, Lowest Reference Nutrient Intake; RNI, Reference Nutrient Intake; TUL, Tolerable Upper Intake Level from diet and supplements.

Possible uses

Requirements may be increased and/or supplements needed in:

- infants and children from the age of 6 months to 4 years;
- early adolescence;
- the female reproductive period;
- pregnancy; and
- vegetarians.

Mental health

There is some evidence that iron supplementation improves cognition in children and adults. A blinded, placebo-controlled, stratified intervention study among women aged 18–35 years of

Table 2 Dietary sources of iron

Food portion	Iron content (mg)	Food portion	Iron content (mg)
Breakfast cereals		Liver, lambs, cooked (90 g)	9
1 bowl **All-Bran** (45 g)	5	Kidney, lambs, cooked (75 g)	9
1 bowl **Bran Flakes** (45 g)	9	**Fish**	
1 bowl *Corn Flakes* (30 g)	2	**Cockles** (80 g)	21
1 bowl **muesli** (95 g)	5	**Mussels** (80 g)	6
2 pieces *Shredded Wheat*	2	*Pilchards, canned* (105 g)	2.8
1 bowl *Special K* (35 g)	4	*Sardines, canned* (70 g)	3
1 bowl **Start** (30 g)	5	**Vegetables**	
1 bowl **Sultana Bran** (35 g)	5	*Green vegetables, average, boiled* (100 g)	1.5
2 *Weetabix*	3	*Potatoes, boiled* (150 g)	0.5
Cereal products		*1 small can baked beans* (200 g)	3
Bread, brown, 2 slices	1.5	*Lentils, kidney beans or other pulses* (105 g)	2
white,[1] *2 slices*	1	**Dahl, chickpea** (155 g)	5
wholemeal, 2 slices	2	*lentil* (155 g)	2.5
1 chapati	1.5	*Soya beans, cooked* (100 g)	3
1 naan bread	3.5	**Fruit**	
Pasta, brown, boiled (150 g)	2.0	*8 dried apricots*	2
white, boiled (150 g)	1.0	*4 figs*	2.5
Rice, brown, boiled (165 g)	0.7	*$^1/_2$ avocado pear*	1.5
white, boiled (165 g)	0.3	Blackberries (100 g)	1
Dairy products		Blackcurrants (100 g)	1
1 egg, size 2 (60 g)	1	**Nuts**	
Meat		20 almonds	1
Red meat, roast (85 g)	2.5	10 Brazil nuts	1
1 beef steak (155 g)	5.4	1 small bag peanuts (25 g)	0.5
Minced beef, lean, stewed (100 g)	3	*Milk chocolate* (100 g)	1.6
1 chicken leg (190 g)	1	*Plain chocolate* (100 g)	2.4

[1]White bread is supplemented with additional iron in the UK.
Excellent sources (**bold**); good sources (*italics*).

varied iron status found that iron-sufficient women ($n = 42$) performed better on cognitive tasks and completed them faster than did the women with iron-deficiency anaemia ($n = 34$). Factors representing performance accuracy and the time needed to complete the tasks by iron-deficient but non-anaemic women ($n = 73$) were intermediate between the two extremes of iron status. After treatment with iron, a significant improvement in serum ferritin was associated with a five- to seven-fold improvement in cognitive performance, whereas a significant improvement in haemoglobin was related to improved speed in completing the cognitive tasks.[3]

In an Australian placebo-controlled study, the influence of iron supplementation during pregnancy on child behaviour during the early years was studied. Mean behaviour and temperament scores and the proportion of parent-rated and teacher-rated abnormal total difficulties scores did not differ between the iron and placebo groups. However, the incidence of children with an abnormal score on the teacher-rated peer problems subscale was higher in the iron group (11 of 112 subjects; 8%) than in the placebo group (3 of 113 subjects; 2%); the relative risk was 3.70 (95% confidence interval (CI), 1.06 to 12.91; $P = 0.026$). Overall, prenatal iron supplementation had no consistent effect on child behaviour at early school age in this study population.[4] Further studies by this same research group found no influence of iron supplementation during pregnancy on child IQ and behaviour at early school age[5] or on iron status of children at 6 months and 4 years.[6]

A meta-analysis of 14 randomised controlled trials among children over 6 years, adolescents and adult women found that iron supplementation in anaemic (but not non-anaemic) individuals improved attention, concentration and IQ.[7] However, many of the included trials were small and methodologically weak and these findings require confirmation with well powered, blinded trials.

Iron deficiency has been suggested as a possible contributing cause of attention-deficit hyperactivity disorder (ADHD) in children. A trial in 23 non-anaemic children (aged 5–8 years) with serum ferritin levels <30 ng/mL who met DSM-IV criteria for ADHD were randomized (3 : 1 ratio) to either oral iron (ferrous sulphate, 80 mg daily; $n = 18$) or placebo ($n = 5$) for 12 weeks. There was a progressive significant decrease in the ADHD Rating Scale after 12 weeks with iron but not placebo. Improvement of the study children with iron-supplementation therapy on parent and teacher rating scales failed to reach significance. Iron therapy was well tolerated and its effectiveness was found to be comparable to stimulants.[8]

Iron status has been shown to be diminished among female soldiers during combat training, and iron supplementation may prove to be beneficial for mood and physical performance during the training period.[9]

Miscellaneous

Anaemia as a consequence of surgery is often treated with iron therapy, but the evidence base for this practice is limited. In a prospective, randomised controlled trial among 300 patients who had undergone hip fracture with a haemoglobin level of <11.0 g/dL, a 28-day course of ferrous sulphate had no clinically relevant benefit compared with placebo.[10]

Frequent blood donations may lead to a negative iron balance and iron depletion may be prevented by iron supplementation after whole blood donations. A Norwegian study examined the short time changes in iron status after donation in two groups randomised to iron supplementation or no additional iron. Iron supplementation had a significant positive impact on the restoration of iron status 1 week after donation.[11]

Iron supplementation has been associated with an influence on physical growth in children. However, a systematic review of 25 trials did not document a statistically significant positive effect of iron supplementation on any anthropometric variable (weight for age, weight for height, height for age, mid upper-arm circumference, skinfold thickness or head circumference).[12]

Precautions/contraindications

Iron supplements should be avoided in conditions associated with iron overload (e.g. haemochromatosis, haemosiderosis, thalassaemia); gastrointestinal disease, particularly inflammatory bowel disease, intestinal stricture, diverticulitis and peptic ulcer.

Pregnancy and breast-feeding

The Reference Nutrient Intake for iron during pregnancy is no greater than for other adult women. Requirements during pregnancy are partly offset by lack of menstruation and partly by increased efficiency of absorption. A Cochrane review concluded that women who receive daily antenatal iron supplementation are less likely to have iron deficiency and iron-deficiency anaemia at term, as defined by current cut-off values. Side-effects and haemoconcentration (haemoglobin > 13.0 g/dL) are more common in women who receive daily iron supplementation. No differences were evident between daily and weekly supplementation with regard to gestational anaemia; haemoconcentration during pregnancy appeared less frequent with the weekly regimen.[13] Routine iron supplementation is not required in pregnancy, but iron status should be monitored.

Adverse effects

Iron supplements may cause gastrointestinal irritation, nausea and constipation, which may lead to faecal impaction, particularly in the elderly. Patients with inflammatory bowel disease may suffer exacerbation of diarrhoea. Any reduced incidence of side-effects associated with modified-release preparations may be due to the fact that only small amounts of iron are released in the intestine. Liquid iron preparations may stain the teeth. Iron supplementation in women with low iron stores has been associated with lipid peroxidation.[14]

Interactions

Drugs

Antacids: reduced absorption of iron; give 2 h apart.

Bisphosphonates: reduced absorption of bisphosphonates; give 2 h apart.

Co-careldopa: reduced plasma levels of carbidopa and levodopa.

Levodopa: absorption of levodopa may be reduced.

Methyldopa: reduced absorption of methyldopa.

Penicillamine: reduced absorption of penicillamine.

4-Quinolones: absorption of ciprofloxacin, norfloxacin and ofloxacin reduced by oral iron; give 2 h apart.

Tetracyclines: reduced absorption of iron and vice versa; give 2 h apart.

Trientine: reduced absorption of iron; give 2 h apart.

Nutrients

Calcium: calcium carbonate or calcium phosphate may reduce absorption of iron; give 2 h apart (absorption of iron in multiple formulations containing iron and calcium is not significantly altered).

Copper: large doses of iron may reduce copper status and vice versa.

Manganese: reduced absorption of manganese.

Vitamin E: large doses of iron may increase requirement for vitamin E; vitamin E may impair haematological response to iron in patients with iron-deficiency anaemia.

Zinc: reduced absorption of iron and vice versa. However, a recent trial in pregnant women found that iron supplementation did not prejudice zinc metabolism.[15]

Dose

Iron is best taken on an empty stomach, but food reduces the possibility of stomach upsets; oral

Table 3 Iron content of commonly used iron supplements

Iron salt	Iron (mg/g)	Iron (%)
Ferrous fumarate	330	33
Ferrous gluconate	120	12
Ferrous glycine sulphate	180	18
Ferrous orotate	150	15
Ferrous succinate	350	35
Ferrous sulphate	200	20
Ferrous sulphate, dried	300	30
Iron amino acid chelate	100	10

liquid preparations should be well diluted with water or fruit juice and drunk through a straw.

As a dietary supplement, 10–17 mg daily.

Upper safety levels

The UK Expert Group on Vitamins and Minerals (EVM) has identified a likely safe total intake of iron for adults from supplements alone of 17 mg daily.

Note: Doses are given in terms of elemental iron; patients should be advised that iron supplements are not identical and provide different amounts of elemental iron; iron content of various iron salts commonly used in supplements is shown in Table 3.

References

1 MacPhail P. Iron. In: Mann J, Truswell AS, eds. *Essentials of Human Nutrition*, 3rd edn. Oxford: Oxford University Press, 2007: 125–137.

2 Cardenas VM, Mulla ZD, Ortiz M, *et al.* Iron deficiency and *Helicobacter pylori* infection in the United States. *Am J Epidemiol* 2006; 163(2): 127–134.

3 Murray-Kolb LE, Beard JL. Iron treatment normalizes cognitive functioning in young women. *Am J Clin Nutr* 2007; 85(3): 778–787.

4 Parsons AG, Zhou SJ, Spurrier NJ, *et al.* Effect of iron supplementation during pregnancy on the behaviour of children at early school age: long-term follow-up of a randomised controlled trial. *Br J Nutr* 2008; 99(5): 1133–1139.

5   Zhou SJ, Gibson RA, Crowther CA, *et al.* Effect of iron supplementation during pregnancy on the intelligence quotient and behavior of children at 4 y of age: long-term follow-up of a randomized controlled trial. *Am J Clin Nutr* 2006; 83(5): 1112–1117.

6   Zhou SJ, Gibson RA, Makrides M. Routine iron supplementation in pregnancy has no effect on iron status of children at six months and four years of age. *J Pediatr* 2007; 151(4): 438–440.

7   Falkingham M, Abdelhamid A, Curtis P, *et al.* The effects of oral iron supplementation on cognition in older children and adults: a systematic review and meta-analysis. *Nutr J* 2010; 9(4): 4.

8   Konofal E, Lecendreux M, Deron J, *et al.* Effects of iron supplementation on attention deficit hyperactivity disorder in children. *Pediatr Neurol* 2008; 38(1): 20–26.

9   McClung JP, Karl JP, Cable SJ, *et al.* Randomized, double-blind, placebo-controlled trial of iron supplementation in female soldiers during military training: effects on iron status, physical performance, and mood. *Am J Clin Nutr* 2009; 90(1): 124–131.

10 Parker MJ. Iron supplementation for anemia after hip fracture surgery: a randomized trial of 300 patients. *J Bone Joint Surg Am* 2010; 92(2): 265–269.

11 Rosvik AS, Hervig T, Wentzel-Larsen T, *et al.* Effect of iron supplementation on iron status during the first week after blood donation. *Vox Sang* 2009; 98(3 Pt1): e249–256.

12 Sachdev H, Gera T, Nestel P. Effect of iron supplementation on physical growth in children: systematic review of randomised controlled trials. *Public Health Nutr* 2006; 9(7): 904–920.

13 Pena-Rosas JP, Viteri FE. Effects of routine oral iron supplementation with or without folic acid for women during pregnancy. *Cochrane Database Syst Rev* 2006; (3): CD004736.

14 King SM, Donangelo CM, Knutson MD, *et al.* Daily supplementation with iron increases lipid peroxidation in young women with low iron stores. *Exp Biol Med* 2008; 233(6): 701–707.

15 Harvey LJ, Dainty JR, Hollands WJ, *et al.* Effect of high-dose iron supplements on fractional zinc absorption and status in pregnant women. *Am J Clin Nutr* 2007; 85(1): 131–136.

Isoflavones

Description

Isoflavones belong to the class of compounds known as flavonoids, and they are found principally in soya beans and products made from them, including soya flour, soya milk, tempeh and tofu. They are present in varying amounts depending on the type of soya product and how it is processed. Isoflavones are also found in dietary supplements.

Constituents

The principal isoflavones in the soya bean are genistein, daidzein and glycetin, which are present mainly as glycosides. After ingestion, the glycosides are hydrolysed in the large intestine by the action of bacteria to release genistein, daidzein and glycetin. Daidzein can be metabolised by the bacteria in the large intestine to form either equol, which is oestrogenic, or O-des-methylangolensin, which is non-oestrogenic, while genistein is metabolised to the non-oestrogenic *p*-ethyl phenol. Variation in the ability to metabolise daidzein could therefore have an influence on the health effects of isoflavones.

Action

Isoflavones are naturally-occurring weak oestrogens, also known as phytoestrogens, which are capable of binding to oestrogen receptors where, depending on the hormonal status of the individual, they may seem to exert either oestrogenic or anti-oestrogenic effects. Premenopausally, isoflavones may therefore be anti-oestrogenic, while postmenopausally they could act oestrogenically, although further research is required to confirm this concept.

There are two types of oestrogen receptors – alpha and beta – and different tissues appear to have different ratios of each type. Thus, alpha-receptors appear to predominate in breast, uterus and ovary, while beta-receptors appear to predominate in prostate, bone and vascular tissue. Phytoestrogens, although less potent than endogenous or synthetic oestrogens, have been shown to bind to beta-oestrogen receptors, raising the possibility that phytoestrogens could produce beneficial effects on, for example, bone and vascular tissue, without causing adverse effects on the breast and ovary.

In addition to these hormonal effects, animal and *in vitro* evidence indicates that isoflavones arrest growth of cancer cells through inhibition of DNA replication, interference of signal transduction pathways and reduction in the activity of various enzymes. Isoflavones also exhibit antioxidant effects, suppress angiogenesis and inhibit the actions of various growth factors and cytokines.[1]

Possible uses

Isoflavones have been investigated for a potential role in cardiovascular disease (CVD), cancer, osteoporosis and menopausal symptoms. A significant majority of trials have been conducted in menopausal and postmenopausal women (see Table 1).

Cardiovascular disease

Soya protein
Products containing soya protein have been shown to reduce both total and LDL cholesterol in some – but not all – studies in animals and humans with raised cholesterol levels. The mechanisms by which soya foods could reduce cholesterol are being investigated, but may include enhancement of bile acid secretion and reduced cholesterol metabolism. Other mechanisms, independent of cholesterol lowering, by which soya could be cardioprotective, include reduction of platelet aggregation and clot formation, and inhibition of atherosclerosis by an antioxidant effect and by inhibiting cell adhesion and proliferation in the arteries.[76] However, further studies are required to confirm these possibilities.

In addition, the question of which constituents of soya are actually responsible for lipid lowering is under discussion, and it is not certain that isoflavones are the components responsible for any beneficial effect. Animal studies specifically comparing the effects of isoflavone-rich soya with isoflavone-free soya on a range of blood lipids have produced conflicting results.

A meta-analysis of 38 controlled clinical trials looking at the effects of soya protein on serum lipid levels in humans showed that there was a statistically significant association between soya protein intake and improvement in serum lipid levels.[77] Of the 38 trials, 34 reported a reduction in serum cholesterol, and overall there was a 9.3% decrease in total cholesterol, a 12.9% decrease in LDL cholesterol and a 10.5% decrease in triacylglycerols. HDL cholesterol increased, but this change was not significant.

A double-blind, randomised 6-month trial involving 66 postmenopausal women with hypercholesterolaemia found that compared to control, soya protein providing either 56 or 90 mg isoflavones significantly reduced non-HDL cholesterol and raised HDL cholesterol, with no change in total cholesterol.[78] The effects of consuming a soya protein beverage powder compared with a casein supplement were evaluated in 20 male subjects randomly allocated to the two groups.[79] There were no significant differences in plasma total and HDL cholesterol or in platelet aggregation between the groups, possibly because the men were normocholesterolaemic at entry into the study.

In a further study, soya protein was found to enhance the effect of a low-fat, low-cholesterol diet by reducing serum LDL cholesterol and increasing the ratio of LDL cholesterol to HDL cholesterol in men with both normal and high serum lipid levels.[80]

In a double-blind, placebo-controlled trial involving 156 healthy men and women, soya protein providing 62 mg isoflavones was associated with a significant reduction in total and LDL cholesterol compared with isoflavone-free soya protein (the placebo).[81] Moreover, soya protein providing 37 mg isoflavones was also associated with a decrease in total and LDL cholesterol, but the reduction was significant only in those subjects with a baseline LDL exceeding 4.24 mmol/L. There was no effect on HDL levels or triacylglycerols. Soya protein providing a lower dose of isoflavones (27 mg daily) had no effect on any of the measured indices. In subjects with baseline LDL levels between 3.62 and 4.24 mmol/L there was no significant effect of any dose of isoflavones.

Table 1 Clinical trials and systematic reviews evaluating isoflavones in menopausal and postmenopausal women

Reference	Duration and type of trial	Dose of soy/ isoflavone	Study group	Outcome measures	Observed effects
Albertazzi et al. (1998)[2]	12-week double-blind, parallel, multicentre, randomised placebo-controlled study	40 g isolated soya protein	104 postmenopausal women.	Number of moderate to severe hot flushes (including night sweats)	Soya was significantly superior to placebo ($P < 0.01$) in reducing the mean number of hot flushes per 24 h after 4, 8 and 12 weeks of treatment
Albertazzi et al. (2005)[3]	6-week crossover, placebo-controlled study	90 mg genistein	100 postmenopausal women	Hot flushes	In women with significant hot flushes (score (intensity × number) ≥ 9, genistein reduced symptoms by 30% compared with baseline and the difference compared with placebo was statistically significant
Alekel et al. (2000)[4]	24-week randomised, double-blind, placebo-controlled trial	Soya protein isolate with isoflavones (80.4 mg/day)	48 perimenopausal women	Lumbar spine BMD, BMC	Soya isoflavones attenuated bone loss from the lumbar spine
Alekel et al. (2009)[5]	3 year randomised, double-blind, placebo-controlled trial	224 healthy postmenopausal women (aged 45.8–65.0 years)	Placebo vs 2 soya isoflavone groups (80 compared with 120 mg/day); + 500 mg calcium and 600 IU vitamin D₃ 474 white women (45–70 years) with low BMD	Lumbar spine, total proximal femur, femoral neck, and whole-body BMD	No bone-sparing effect of soya isoflavones except for a small effect at the femoral neck
Alexandersen et al. (2001)[6]	4 year RCT	Ipriflavone 200 mg three times a day vs placebo		Bone metabolism	No effect of ipriflavone on bone loss or none metabolism
Atkinson et al. (2004)[7]	1 year a double-blind, randomised, placebo-controlled trial	A red clover-derived isoflavone tablet (26 mg biochanin A, 16 mg formononetin, 1 mg genistein and 0.5 mg daidzein)	205 women (49–65 years)	Breast density, oestradiol, gonadotrophins, menopausal symptoms	No effects on any measures

(Continued)

Table 1 (continued)

Reference	Duration and type of trial	Dose of soy/ isoflavone	Study group	Outcome measures	Observed effects
Aubertin-Leheudre et al. (2008)[8]	6-month randomised double-blind placebo-controlled trial	Isoflavone supplement (70 mg)	Obese postmenopausal women	CVD risk factors	Isoflavones did not favourably affect risk factors predisposing to CVD (biochemical or body composition)
Basaria et al. (2009)[9]	12-week double-blind, randomised, placebo-controlled trial	20 g of soya protein containing 160 mg of total isoflavones vs taste-matched placebo (20 g whole milk protein)	93 healthy, ambulatory, postmenopausal women (mean age 56 years)	Self-reported QOL, cognition, lipoproteins and androgen status	Significant improvement in all 4 QOL subscales (vasomotor, psychosexual, physical and sexual); no significant changes in cognition, serum androgens or plasma lipids were seen with isoflavone or placebo
Baum et al. (1998)[10]	6-month parallel-group, double-blind trial with 3 interventions.	Healthy diet vs healthy diet + soya protein vs healthy diet + soya protein + isoflavones	66 hypercholesterolemic, free-living, postmenopausal women	Blood lipids	Non-HDL cholesterol reduced and HDL cholesterol increased in both soya groups; total cholesterol unchanged
Blakesmith et al. (2003)[11]	A double-blind, randomised, parallel study for 4 menstrual cycles	Isoflavone supplement (86 mg/ day, derived from red clover)	25 healthy premenopausal women	Blood lipids, glucose, insulin	No significant effects on total, LDL or HDLcholesterol; HDL subfractions; triacylglycerol; lipoprotein(a); glucose; insulin
Bolanos et al. (2010)[12]	Meta-analysis	Soya (dietary, extract, or concentrate) vs placebo	19 RCTs of at least 12 weeks in duration	Vasomotor symptoms	A significant tendency in favour of soya, but high heterogeneity in studies
Burke et al. (2003)[13]	A double-masked, randomised, controlled, clinical trial	25 g soya protein placebo vs soya protein + 42 mg isoflavones vs soya protein + 58 mg isoflavones	241 community-dwelling women reporting vasomotor symptoms at baseline	Change in reported vasomotor symptoms	No significant differences in the number and severity of vasomotor symptoms observed among the 3 groups.
Casini et al. (2006)[14]	6 month randomised, double-blind, crossover, placebo-controlled trial	60 mg/day isoflavones	78 postmenopausal women	Cognitive performance and mood	Cognitive performance and mood improved with isoflavones

Study	Design	Intervention	Participants	Outcomes measured	Results
Charles et al. (2009)[15]	12-week RCT	160 mg total isoflavones (64 mg genistein, 63 mg daidzein, 34 mg glycitein) or 20 g soya protein placebo	75 healthy postmenopausal women	Inflammatory and metabolic markers (adipokines, cytokines)	No improvement in metabolic parameters
Chedraui et al. (2008)[16]	90-day RCT	Trifolium pratense-derived isoflavone supplement (80 mg red clover isoflavones)	60 postmenopausal women aged >40 years,	Blood lipids	Significant decrease in total cholesterol, LDL cholesterol and lipoprotein A levels
Chen et al. (2004)[17]	RCT	Three treatment groups: 67 in placebo group (daily dose 0 mg isoflavones + 500 mg calcium), 68 in mid-isoflavone group (40 mg isoflavones + 500 mg calcium), 68 in high-isoflavone group (80 mg isoflavones + 500 mg calcium)	203 Chinese postmenopausal women (48–62 years)	Bone mineral content	Significant favourable effect of isoflavone supplementation on rates of change in BMC at the total hip and trochanter among later postmenopausal women (> 4 years), women with lower body weight (≤ median of 55.5 kg), and women with lower calcium intake (≤ median of 1095 mg/day)
Cheng et al. (2004)[18]	6-month randomised, double-blind, active placebo-controlled clinical trial	100 mg isoflavone soft capsules, 300 mg calcium, and a blank vitamin capsule per day; oestrogen active control group received 0.625 mg conjugated oestrogen, 300 mg calcium, and blank isoflavone soft capsules per day	30 postmenopausal Taiwanese women	Fasting blood glucose, insulin	Soya isoflavones and conjugated oestrogen equally lower fasting blood glucose and insulin levels
Colacurci et al. (2005)[19]	6-month RCT	Isoflavone vs placebo tablets	60 postmenopausal women	Endothelial function	Improvement in endothelium-dependent vasodilatation and a reduction in plasma adhesion molecule levels
Crisafulli et al. (2004)[20]	1-year RCT	Genistein 54 mg/day vs HRT	90 healthy, postmenopausal women (47–57 years)	Hot flushes and endometrial thickness	Positive effects on hot flushes without a negative impact on endometrial thickness
Crisafulli et al. (2005)[21]	6-month double-blind, placebo-controlled, randomised study	Genistein 54 mg/day vs placebo	60 healthy postmenopausal women (52–60 years)	Fasting glucose, fasting insulin, insulin resistance, fibrinogen, SHBG	Isoflavones reduced cardiometabolic markers and increased SHBG
D'Anna et al. (2005)[22]	6-month RCT	Genistein 54 mg/day vs HRT vs placebo	90 healthy postmenopausal women (50–60 years)	Homocysteine, CRP	Isoflavone did not modify homocysteine or CRP

(Continued)

Table 1 (continued)

Reference	Duration and type of trial	Dose of soy/isoflavone	Study group	Outcome measures	Observed effects
De-Fu Maa et al. (2008)[23]	Meta-analysis of RCTs	Soya isoflavones	10 studies	BMD or BMC	Isoflavone intervention significantly attenuated bone loss in spines of menopausal women
Engelman et al. (2005)[24]	A double-blind 6-week study	4 treatments with soya protein (40 g/day) isolate: low phytate/low isoflavone, normal phytate/low isoflavone, low phytate/normal isoflavone or normal phytate/normal isoflavone	55 postmenopausal women	Blood lipids and measures of oxidative stress	Isoflavones did not have significant effect on reducing oxidative damage or improving blood lipids
Ferrari (2009)[25]	12-week prospective, randomised, double-blind, placebo-controlled multicentre trial	80 mg isoflavones vs placebo	180 women (40–65 years) with a minimum of 5 moderate-to-severe hot flushes in the last 7 days at baseline and absence of menstruation for at least 6 months	Hot flushes	Number of hot flushes reduced significantly with isoflavones
Gambacciani et al. (1997)[26]	2 year longitudinal comparative study	Calcium (500 mg/day); high-dose ipriflavone (600 mg/day) + the same calcium dose; low-dose conjugated oestrogens (0.3 mg/day) + calcium; or low-dose ipriflavone (400 mg/day) + low-dose conjugated oestrogens (0.3 mg/day) plus calcium	Postmenopausal women	Bone turnover, BMD	High dose iipriflavone or low-dose ipriflavone + low-dose conjugated oestrogens can prevent the increase in bone turnover and the decrease in BMD that follow ovarian failure
Hall et al. (2005)[27]	24-week randomised, double-blind, placebo-controlled, crossover dietary intervention trial	Isoflavone-enriched (genistein-to-daidzein ratio, 2 : 1; 50 mg/day) or placebo	117 healthy European postmenopausal women	Inflammatory biomarkers for CVD risk	Isoflavones improved CRP but not other inflammatory biomarkers

Reference	Study type	Intervention	Subjects	Outcome measures	Results
Hall et al. (2008)[28]	Acute study	80 mg isoflavones in a test meal vs placebo	22 healthy postmenopausal women	Endothelium-dependent vasodilatation	Increased endothelium-dependent vasodilatation with isoflavones
Hidalgo et al. (2005)[29]	90-day RCT	80 mg isoflavones (red clover) vs placebo	60 postmenopausal women (>40 years)	Menopausal symptoms, vaginal cytology, blood lipids	Compared with placebo, isoflavone supplementation significantly decreased menopausal symptoms and had a positive effect on vaginal cytology and triglyceride levels
Hooper et al. (2009)[30]	Meta-analysis	Soya or isoflavones for > 4 weeks	47 studies (pre- and postmenopausal women)	Circulating hormones	Isoflavone-rich soya products decrease FSH and LH in pre-menopausal women and may increase oestradiol in postmenopausal women
Howes et al. (2000)[31]	Three-period (4-weeks each) randomised, double blind, ascending dose study	Red clover tablet containing approx. biochanin A 26 mg, formononetin 16 mg, daidzein 0.5 mg, genistein 1 mg; dosage 1–2 tablets per day vs placebo	66 postmenopausal women with plasma cholesterol levels 5.0–9.0 mmol/L	Blood lipids	Isoflavones did not significantly alter total plasma cholesterol, LDL cholesterol, HDL cholesterol or plasma triglyceride levels
Howes et al. (2003)[32]	4-week randomised double-blind crossover trial	Red clover (approx. 50 mg/day) vs placebo	16 postmenopausal type 2 diabetics treated with diet or oral hypoglycaemic therapy	Blood pressure and forearm vascular endothelial function	Isoflavones improved blood pressure and endothelial function
Howes et al. (2004)[33]	6 month RCT	Red clover (tablet containing formononetin 25 mg, biochanin 2.5 mg, < 1 mg daidzein and genistein)	30 postmenopausal women (> 60 years)	Cognitive function	No improvement
Huntley & Ernst (2004)[34]	Systematic review	Soya preparations	13 RCTs	Menopausal symptoms	Results not conclusive; four RCTs were positive, suggesting soya preparations are beneficial for peri-menopausal symptoms; six were negative; with one of the six showing a positive trend
Hutchins et al. (2005)[35]	Placebo-controlled crossover trial	500 mg vitamin C; 5 mg/kg body weight isoflavones; 500 mg vitamin C + 5 mg/kg body weight isoflavones; placebo	10 healthy postmenopausal women	Total lipid peroxides, plasma vitamin C, blood pressure	Isoflavones reduced lipid peroxides, increased blood pressure; no synergistic antioxidant effect with vitamin C

(Continued)

Table 1 (continued)

Reference	Duration and type of trial	Dose of soy/isoflavone	Study group	Outcome measures	Observed effects
Imhof et al. (2008)[36]	2-week controlled stdy	200 mg isoflavones or with 2 mg 17β-estradiol per day, or combination of both	Postmenopausal women	Proliferation of breast cancer cells	In women with normal oestradiol levels, isoflavones were antiproliferative, but they were proliferative in women with low oestrdiol levels
Jou et al. (2008)[37]	6-month RCT; women divided into equol and non-equol producers	135 mg/day isoflavones	96 healthy postmenopausal women	Menopausal symptoms	Isoflavone improved menopausal symptoms only in women with the ability to produce equol
Katase et al. (2001)[38]	24 month RCT	Ipriflavone 600 mg/day vs placebo	89 pre-menopausal ovariectomised women (early-stage group) and postmenopausal women (late-stage group)	BMD	Overall, ipriflavone suppressed bone loss compared with placebo, but did not prevent acute bone loss in the early-stage group
Kok et al. (2005)[39]	12-month double-blind randomised trial	Soya protein containing 99 mg isoflavones/day (aglycone weights) vs milk protein (placebo)	202 postmenopausal women (60–75 years)	Body composition, physical performance	No change
Kok et al. (2005)[40]	1-year double-blind randomised placebo-controlled trial	Soya protein, containing 52 mg genistein, 41 mg daidzein, and 6 mg glycitein (aglycone weights), or milk protein (placebo) daily	202 postmenopausal women (60–75 years)	QOL (health status, life satisfaction and depression)	No improvement in QOL measures with isoflavones
Krebs et al. (2004)[41]	Systematic review	Phytoestrogen vs control >4 weeks in duration	25 trials involving 2348 participants	Menopausal symptoms	Phytoestrogens available as soya foods, soya extracts, and red clover extracts do not improve hot flushes or other menopausal symptoms
Kreijkamp-Kaspers et al. (2005)[42]	12-month double-blind randomised trial	Soya protein containing 99 mg/day isoflavones (aglycone weights) vs milk protein (placebo)	202 postmenopausal women (60–75 years)	Blood pressure and endothelial function	Increase in blood pressure with soya isoflavones; no change in endothelial function

Study	Study design	Intervention	Participants	Outcome measure	Findings
Kwak et al. (2009)[43]	Randomised, double-blind, placebo-controlled study over 3 menstrual cycles	Soya isoflavones	53 pre-menopausal women divided into groups according to excretion of equol	Bone turnover	An anti-oestrgenic effect of isoflavones on bone turnover was observed in pre-menopausal equol producers
Lipovac et al. (2009)[44]	90-day RCT	80 mg red clover isoflavones vs placebo	109 postmenopausal women (>40 years)	Anxiety and depression	Red clover isoflavones effective in reducing depressive and anxiety symptoms
Lissin et al. (2004)[45]	6-week RCT	90 mg/day isoflavones versus placebo	40 postmenopausal, hypercholesterolaemic women not on HRT	Vascular reactivity, lipid levels, markers of inflammation	Improved vascular reactivity but no change in lipids with isoflavones
Liu et al. (2009)[46]	6-month double-blind randomised placebo-controlled trial	15 g soya protein + 100 mg isoflavones; 15 g milk protein + 100 mg isoflavones; 15 g milk protein (placebo group)	180 postmenopausal Chinese women with mild hyperglycaemia	Body weight, body fat	Soya protein + isoflavones had mild favourable effect on body composition and body weight
Liu et al. (2010)[47]	6-month double-blind, randomised, placebo-controlled trial	5 g soya protein + 100 mg isoflavones; 15 g milk protein + 100 mg isoflavones; 15 g milk protein daily	180 postmenopausal Chinese women with prediabetes or untreated early diabetes	Glycaemic control	No effects of isoflavones on glycaemic control
Llaneza et al. (2010)[48]	24-month RCT	40 mg soya isoflavones vs placebo (+ Mediterranean diet)	116 postmenopausal women with insulin resistance	Changes in insulin resistance	Daily intake of 40 mg soya isoflavones + Mediterranean diet and exercise reduced insulin resistance in postmenopausal women who had resistance in the first place
Marini et al. (2007)[49]	24-month RCT	Genistein 54 mg/day or placebo	389 postmenopausal women with low BMD	BMD	Positive effects of isoflavones on BMD
Maskarinec et al. (2009)[50]	2-year multisite, randomised, double-blinded, placebo-controlled trial	80 or 120mg/day isoflavones each or a placebo	406 postmenopausal women	Mammographic density (marker for breast cancer risk)	Isoflavone supplements did not modify breast density
McMichael-Phillips et al. (1998)[51]	14-day placebo-controlled trial	60 g soya supplement (containing 45 mg isoflavones)	48 women with benign or malignant breast disease	Breast cell proliferation	Isoflavones increased breast cell proliferation
Merz-Demlow et al. (2000)[52]	3 × 3 menstrual cycles; randomised, crossover-controlled trial	Three soya isoflavone intakes provided as soya protein isolate: control (10.0 ± 1.1 mg/day), low (64.7 ± 9.4 mg/day); high (128.7 ± 15.7 mg/day)	13 healthy, free-living, pre-menopausal women with normal cholesterol	Blood lipids	Isoflavones significantly improved the lipid profile

(Continued)

Table 1 (continued)

Reference	Duration and type of trial	Dose of soy/isoflavone	Study group	Outcome measures	Observed effects
Messina & Hughes (2003)[53]	Systematic review	Soya isoflavones	13 trials	Hot flushes	A statistically significant relationship ($P = 0.01$) between initial hot flush frequency and treatment efficacy
Moraes et al. (2009)[54]	24-week controlled trial	Topical oestrogen vs topical isoflavone	36 postmenopausal women	Skin morphollology	Topical oestrogen had better effect on skin morphology than topical isoflavones
Murkies et al. (1995)[55]	12-week double-blind RCT	Soya vs wheat flour	58 postmenopausal women (mean age 54 years; range 30–70) with at least 14 hot flushes per week	Menopausal symptoms	Hot flushes decreased in both groups
Ohta et al. (1999)[56]	Prospective 1 year study	600 mg/day ipriflavone or 0.8 g/day calcium lactate	60 postmenopausal women with osteopaenia or osteoporosis	BMD	Bone resorption was lower with ipriflavone
Potter et al. (1998)[57]	6-month, parallel-group, double-blind trial with 3 interventions	Low-fat diet with 40 g/day protein: protein obtained from (a) casein and non-fat dry milk (control), (b) isolated soya protein containing 1.39 mg isoflavones/g protein (ISP56), (c) isolated soya protein containing 2.25 mg isoflavones/g protein (ISP90)	66 free-living, hypercholesterolaemic, postmenopausal women	BMC, BMD, blood lipids	Significant increases occurred in both BMC and BMD in the lumbar spine but not elsewhere for the ISP90 group compared with the control group ($P < 0.05$); HDL cholesterol increased in both ISP56 and ISP90 groups ($P < 0.05$)
Powles et al. (2008)[58]	3 year pilot RCT	40 mg isoflavones daily	401 healthy women (35–70 years)	Breast density, endometrial thickness, serum cholesterol, plasma FSH, BMD	No changes with isoflavones
Ricci et al. (2010)[59]	Meta-analysis of 10 RCTs	Soya isoflavone supplementation	794 non-Asian peri- and postmenopausal women not taking HRT	Glucose metabolism	Soya isoflavones did not affect fasting blood glucose significantly

Reference	Study design	Intervention	Subjects	Outcome measured	Results
Rios et al. (2008)[60]	6-month, double-blind, placebo-controlled study	40 mg isoflavone (n = 25) or 40 mg casein placebo (n = 22)	47 postmenopausal women (47–66 years)	Lipid and endogenous hormone levels	In both placebo and isoflavone groups total and LDL cholesterol decreased, HDL and VLDL cholesterol increased and triacylglycerol increased
Rios et al. (2008)[61]	6-month, double-blinded, placebo-controlled study	40 mg isoflavone (n = 25) or 40 mg casein placebo (n = 22).	47 postmenopausal women (47–66 years)	Effects on coagulation and fibrinolytic factors	Haemostatic variables did not change significantly throughout the study in the isoflavone group
Samman et al. (1999)[62]	4-month randomised crossover trial	86 mg isoflavones daily for the duration of 2 menstrual cycles followed by placebo for an equivalent period, or vice versa	14 healthy pre-menopausal women	Plasma lipids and oxidisability of LDL	No change in LDL oxidisability, total cholesterol or triacylglycerol
Samman et al. (2009)[63]	4-month double-blind, randomised, parallel study	Placebo or purified red clover (Trifolium pratense) isoflavone (86 mg/day) tablets	23 pre-menopausal women	Serum homocysteine (CVD risk marker)	No effect on serum homocysteine or folic acid
Schult et al. (2004)[64]	A 12-week randomised, double-blind, placebo-controlled trial	Promensil (82 mg total isoflavones), Rimostil (57.2 mg total isoflavones), or placebo	252 menopausal women (45–60 years) experiencing ≥ 35 hot flashes per week	Lipids and bone turnover markers	Compared with placebo, both of the supplements decreased levels of triglycerides; no differences in markers of bone turnover
Simons et al. (2000)[65]	8-week double-blind, placebo-controlled, randomised crossover trial	Soya bean phytoestrogen tablet (80 mg/day isoflavones)	20 healthy, postmenopausal women (50–70 years), with evidence of endothelial dysfunction	Plasma lipids and endothelial function	No effects on lipid and lipoprotein levels or on endothelial function
Spence et al. (2005)[66]	3-month randomised, crossover design	Soya protein isolate enriched with isoflavones; soya protein isolate devoid of isoflavones; or casein-whey protein isolate (control)	15 postmenopausal women	Calcium metabolism	Soya isoflavones did not significantly affect calcium metabolism
Terzic et al. (2009)[67]	12-month RCT	Red clover vs placebo	40 healthy postmenopausal women (average age 56 years)	Total blood cholesterol, cholesterol fractions, triacylglycerol	Isoflavones reduced total and LDL cholesterol, and triacylglycerol; HDL cholesterol increased

(Continued)

Table 1 (continued)

Reference	Duration and type of trial	Dose of soy/ isoflavone	Study group	Outcome measures	Observed effects
Tice et al. (2003)[68]	12-week randomised, double-blind, placebo-controlled trial	Promensil (82 mg/day total isoflavones), Rimostil (57 mg/ day total isoflavones), or an identical placebo	Menopausal women (45–60 years) who were experiencing at least 35 hot flushes per week	Change in hot flushes and QOL	Reductions in hot flush count at 12 weeks were similar for the Promensil, Rimostil and placebo groups; in comparison with the placebo group, participants in the Promensil group, but not in the Rimostil group, reduced hot flushes more rapidly; QOL improvements and adverse events were comparable in the three groups
Uesugi et al. (2003)[69]	3-month RCT	Isoflavone extract (61.8 mg) vs placebo	22 postmenopausal women	Bone metabolism, vaginal cytology	Isoflavones produced maturational changes of vaginal epithelia without affecting serum FSH levels and decreased urinary pyridinoline excretion (marker of reduced bone turnover)
Uesugi et al. (2004)[70]	8-week double-blind, placebo-controlled crossover study	40 mg/day isoflavones	58 Japanese menopausal women	Urinary deoxypyridinoline, (marker of bone resorption); plasma osteocalcin, BMD, hot flushes	Compared with placebo, isoflavone produced significantly reduced urinary deoxypyridinoline, (this tendency was remarkable among equol producers); plasma osteocalcin and BMD did not change by week 4; hot flushes decreased significantly; systolic and diastolic blood pressure of hypertensive participants decreased significantly after isoflavone treatment

Reference	Study design	Intervention	Subjects	Outcomes measured	Results
Verheus et al. (2008)[71]	1 year double-blind, randomised, controlled trial	Soya protein intake with 99 mg isoflavones daily or milk protein (placebo)	202 Dutch postmenopausal women (60–75 years)	Mammographic density	No difference between groups in mammographic density; no influence of equol production
Verhoeven et al. (2005)[72]	12-week randomised, placebo-controlled, double-blind study	Soya isoflavones and Actaea racemosa L.	124 women experiencing at least five vasomotor symptoms every 24 h	Hot flushes, QOL	No significant effect on menopausal symptoms
Verhoeven et al. (2007)[73]	12-week randomised, placebo-controlled, double-blind study	Soya isoflavones and Actaea racemosa L.	124 menopausal women	Fasting dimethylarginine, lipids, CRP	No influence of supplement on any measured parameter
Williamson-Hughes et al. (2006)[74]	Systematic review	Well-characterised isoflavone supplements	11 studies using similar doses of isoflavones	Hot flushes related to isoflavone content of study products	Only study products with >15 mg genistein: caused a significant reduction in hot flushes (5 trials)
Wu et al. (2006)[75]	12-month RCT	4 groups: (a) placebo, (b) walking (45 min/day, 3 days/week) with placebo, (c) isoflavone intake (75 mg/day isoflavone conjugates), (d) combination of isoflavone plus walking	136 postmenopausal women at <5 years after the onset of menopause	BMD, fat mass, serum lipid,	Combined intervention of 75 mg/day isoflavone intake and walking exercise for 1 year showed a trend for a greater effect on BMD at total hip and Ward's triangle regions than either alone; intervention with isoflavone in postmenopausal Japanese women showed a modest effect on BMD compared with those in Westerners

BMC, bone mineral content; BMD, bone mineral density; CRP, C-reactive protein; CVD, cardiovascular disease; FSH, follicle-stimulating hormone; HRT, hormone replacement therapy; LH, luteinising hormone; QOL, quality of life; SHBG, sex hormone-binding globulin.

A further study, involving 81 men with moderate hypercholesterolaemia (total serum cholesterol 5.7–7.7 mmol/L) found that soya protein (20 g daily, providing 37.5 mg isoflavones) reduced non-HDL cholesterol by 2.6% and total cholesterol by 1.8% after 6 weeks.[82] Another trial involving healthy young men compared the effects of milk protein isolate, low isoflavone soya protein isolate (1.64 ± 0.19 mg aglycone isoflavones daily) and high isoflavone soya protein isolate (61.7 ± 7.4 mg aglycone isoflavones daily) on lipid levels. The differences produced by the three treatments were not significant, but the ratios of total to HDL cholesterol, LDL to HDL cholesterol and apolipoprotein (apo) B to A1 were significantly lower with both the soya protein treatments than with the milk protein isolate.[83]

A study in 13 pre-menopausal women with normal serum cholesterol levels found that total cholesterol, HDL cholesterol and LDL cholesterol levels changed significantly across menstrual cycle phases. During specific phases of the cycle, soya protein providing 128.7 mg isoflavones significantly lowered LDL cholesterol by 7.6–10.0%, the ratio of total to HDL cholesterol by 10.2% and the ratio of LDL to HDL cholesterol by 13.8%. Despite the high intake of isoflavones, the changes in lipid concentrations were small, but the authors concluded that over a lifetime the small effects observed could slow the development of atherosclerosis and reduce the risk of coronary heart disease (CHD) in women with normal cholesterol levels.[84]

A preliminary study in six subjects investigated the effect of soya (providing genistein 12 mg and daidzein 7 mg) daily for 2 weeks on resistance of LDL to oxidation, because it appears that LDL has to be oxidised before it can damage the arteries. The results from this small study indicated that isoflavones could offer protection against LDL oxidation.[85]

A randomised crossover study in 24 subjects compared soya-enriched diets that were providing 1.9 or 66 mg of isoflavones daily. The aim was to investigate the effects of the diets on biomarkers of lipid peroxidation and resistance of LDL to oxidation, because oxidative damage to lipids may be involved in the aetiology of atherosclerosis and CVD. The diet high in isoflavones reduced lipid peroxidation and increased the resistance of LDL to oxidation.[86]

Isoflavone supplements

Studies giving isoflavones in tablet form have yielded less positive results than those using soya protein. A group of 46 men and 13 postmenopausal women not taking HRT, all with average serum cholesterol levels, participated in an 8-week randomised, double-blind, placebo-controlled trial of two-way parallel design. One tablet containing 55 mg isoflavones (predominantly in the form of genistein) or placebo was taken daily. Post-intervention, there were no significant differences in total, LDL and HDL cholesterol and lipoprotein(a).[87]

Another trial, this time in 14 pre-menopausal women, found that a supplement providing 86 mg daily for 2 months produced no change compared with placebo in plasma concentrations of total cholesterol and triacylglycerol, nor in the oxidisability of LDL.[88] A further study in 20 healthy postmenopausal women (50–70 years old) with evidence of endothelial dysfunction, found that a soya bean tablet providing 80 mg of isoflavones daily for 8 weeks produced no significant effects on plasma lipids compared with placebo.[89]

The effects of dietary isoflavone supplementation using a purified red clover supplement (containing approximately biochanin A 26 mg, formononetin 16 mg, daidzein 0.5 mg and genistein 1 mg per tablet) at doses of one to two tablets daily were compared with placebo in a three-period, randomised, double-blind, ascending-dose study in 66 postmenopausal women with moderately elevated plasma cholesterol levels (5.0–9.0 mmol/L).[90] Each of the three treatment periods lasted for 4 weeks. The dietary supplement did not significantly alter plasma total cholesterol, LDL or HDL cholesterol, or plasma triglycerides. Further trials with red clover have also shown that this preparation has no effect on blood lipids.[11,91] However, at least one trial has shown that red clover may favourably influence blood pressure and endothelial function in postmenopausal women with type 2 diabetes.[92]

Recent trials have looked at other cardiovascular risk factors besides lipids that soya isoflavones might influence. Results to date have not been promising. Isoflavones were found to have no significant effect on reducing oxidative damage.[93,94] Studies looking at effects of isoflavones on vascular function have been conflicting, some showing improved function,[95,96] while others showed no effect.[97] One trial in healthy postmenopausal women suggested a positive influence of soya isoflavones on endothelial function, as evidenced by improvement in endothelium-dependent vasodilatation and a reduction in plasma adhesion molecule levels.[98] Another trial in postmenopausal women suggested that isoflavones could have beneficial effects on C-reactive protein concentrations, but not on other inflammatory markers of cardiovascular risk in postmenopausal women. This study also assessed whether there were any differences in response according to equol production, but there were not.[49] A study looking at the effect of a specific isoflavone – genistein – suggested that genistein may have a favourable effect on some cardiovascular markers, including fasting glucose, fasting insulin, insulin resistance and fibrinogen.[99] However, a further trial involving genistein found that after 6 months' treatment, genistein did not modify circulating homocysteine levels or C-reactive protein.[100] Isoflavones have been studied in healthy young men and found to reduce plasma homocysteine and to have antioxidant activity.[101] Daily intake of soya isoflavones (80 mg) in high-risk, middle-aged men has been found to reduce blood pressure, total cholesterol and non-HDL cholesterol, while raising HDL cholesterol.[102] A 12-week study of 29 healthy postmenopausal women evaluated the effect of soya isoflavones (100 mg daily) on platelet thromboxane A2 receptor density (a marker of platelet function) as well as lipoprotein status. Platelet thromboxane A2 receptor density declined significantly in the intervention group, remaining mostly unchanged in the experimental group. The change in plasma thromboxane A2 receptors was inversely correlated with serum isoflavones. The authors concluded that the beneficial effects of isoflavones could be more related to platelet function than to improving classical risk factors.[103] More recent trials have continued to show inconsistent effects. A 90-day controlled trial in 60 postmenopausal women with the isoflavone supplement *Trifolium pratense* showed a reduction in total and LDL cholesterol.[16] Two trials in women by Rios *et al.*[60,61] demonstrated improved lipid profiles but no change in haemostatic factors with isoflavone supplements, while another trial in 60 obese postmenopausal women showed no effect of isoflavone supplementation.[58]

Meta-analyses and systematic reviews

Several systematic reviews and meta-analyses evaluating the effect of soya/isoflavones on lipids and cardiovascular risk factors have now been conducted. A 2003 meta-analysis of 10 studies, which included 21 treatments in total, found that soya-associated isoflavones were not related to changes in LDL or HDL cholesterol.[104]

A 2004 meta-analysis of eight RCTs found that under conditions of identical soya protein intake, high isoflavone intake led to significantly greater decreases in serum LDL cholesterol than low isoflavone intake, demonstrating that isoflavones have LDL cholesterol-lowering effects independent of soya protein.[105]

A 2005 meta-analysis of 23 RCTs published from 1995 to 2002 found that soya protein with isoflavones intact was associated with significant decreases in serum total cholesterol, LDL cholesterol and triacylglycerols and significant increases in serum HDL cholesterol. The reductions in total and LDL cholesterol were larger in men than in women. Initial total cholesterol concentrations had a powerful effect on changes in total and HDL cholesterol, especially in subjects with hypercholesterolaemia. The strongest lowering effects on total cholesterol, LDL cholesterol and triacylglycerol occurred within the short initial period of intervention, while increases in HDL cholesterol were only observed in studies lasting longer than 12 weeks. However, tablets containing extracted soya isoflavones did not have a significant effect on total cholesterol reduction.[106]

The American Heart Association Science Advisory assessed the more recent work on soya protein and isoflavones. In the majority of 22 randomised trials, isolated soya protein with isoflavones (as compared with other proteins) decreased LDL cholesterol concentrations, but the reduction of approximately 3% was very small relative to the large amount of soya protein consumed (averaging 50 g, about half the usual total daily protein intake). No significant effects on HDL cholesterol, triglycerides or blood pressure were evident. Among 19 studies of soya isoflavones, the average effect on LDL cholesterol and other lipid risk factors was nil.[107] A further critical analysis of investigations into the effect of soya protein and isoflavones on plasma lipoproteins concluded that the data are not quantitatively impressive and raise substantial questions about the clinical importance of the hypocholesterolaemic effects observed.[108]

A more recent US meta-analysis of 41 RCTs in which isolated protein supplementation was the only intervention found that supplementation was associated with a significant (albeit small) reduction in serum total cholesterol, LDL cholesterol and triglycerides and a significant increase in HDL cholesterol. There was a dose–response relation between soya protein and isoflavone supplementation and net changes in serum lipids, and serum lipids were reduced among adults with or without hypercholesterolaemia.[109]

Another meta-analysis including 11 studies found that soya isoflavones decreased total cholesterol by 0.10 mmol/L (1.77%) and LDL cholesterol by 0.13 mmol/L (3.58%). No significant changes in HDL cholesterol or triacylyglycerol were found. Isoflavone-depleted soya protein significantly decreased LDL cholesterol by 0.18 mmol/L (4.98%) and significantly increased HDL cholesterol by 0.04 mmol/L (3%). The reductions in LDL cholesterol were larger in those with raised cholesterol than in those with normal values.[110]

Cancer

Epidemiological studies have shown that populations with high intakes of soya foods – such as in China, Japan and other Asian countries – usually have a lower risk of cancers of the breast, uterus, prostate and colon.[111,112] Epidemiological evidence from the USA suggests that dietary phytoestrogens (of which isoflavones are one type) are associated with a decreased risk of lung cancer.[113] Experimental evidence from in vitro and animal studies on the effects of isoflavones on cancerous cells[114–116] has led to the suggestion that isoflavones could reduce the risk of cancer in humans.

Substantial reduction in risk of breast cancer has been reported among women with high intakes of phytoestrogens (as evidenced from urinary excretion).[117] Lower urinary daidzein and genistein concentrations were found in postmenopausal women with recently diagnosed breast cancer compared with controls.[118] Isoflavones appear to protect against cancer by influences on growth factor, malignant cell proliferation and cell differentiation. A more recent study found no evidence that isoflavone treatment reduces colorectal epithelial cell proliferation or the average height of proliferating cells in the caecum, sigmoid colon or rectum, and that it increases cell-proliferating measures in the sigmoid colon.[119]

Another study found no evidence that isoflavones alter the concentration of serum prostate-specific antigen.[120] Increasing plasma isoflavones failed to produce a corresponding modulation of serum steroid hormone levels in men with localised prostate cancer.[121] A pilot study of high-dose isoflavones in men undergoing androgen deprivation for prostate cancer showed no significant improvement in cognition, vasomotor symptoms or any other aspect of quality of life measures compared with placebo.[122] However, soy isoflavones taken in conjunction with radiation therapy were associated with a reduction in the urinary, intestinal and sexual adverse effects in patients with prostate cancer.[123]

The American Heart Association Science Advisory has concluded that the efficacy and safety of soya isoflavones for preventing or treating cancer of the breast, endometrium and prostate are not established.[107] A recent systematic review concluded that isoflavone intake does not alter breast density in postmenopausal women, but may increase it in pre-menopausal women.[124]

Osteoporosis

There is some evidence from animal studies that soya isoflavones preserve bone mineral density (BMD).[125,126] A preliminary study in 66 hypercholesterolaemic, postmenopausal women supplemented with soya protein (providing either 1.39 or 2.2 mg isoflavones/g protein) or placebo for 6 months showed that the higher dose of isoflavones was associated with a significant increase in BMD at the lumbar spine site.[127] The lower dose was not associated with any change in BMD. HDL cholesterol (the beneficial type) increased significantly with both soya treatments.

A later study examined the effects of 24-week consumption of soya protein isolate with isoflavones (80.4 mg daily) on bone loss in perimenopausal women.[128] The randomised double-blind study showed that soya isoflavones attenuated the reduction in lumbar spine BMD and bone mineral content, both of which occurred in the control group.

More recent studies evaluating the effect of isoflavones on bone have continued to show mixed results. One 3-month trial in 22 postmenopausal women found that isoflavones (61.8 mg daily) could slow down bone turnover as judged by decreased urinary pyridinoline excretion.[129] A further trial in 58 menopausal Japanese women found that isoflavones (40 mg daily) for 8 weeks produced a significant decrease in urinary deoxypyridoline and may therefore have a beneficial effect on bone resorption.[130] Another trial involving 136 Japanese women, who were < 5 years after the onset of the menopause, found that a combined intervention of isoflavone conjugates (75 mg daily) with walking 45 min a day on 3 days a week for 1 year produced a trend for an increased effect on BMD at total hip compared with placebo and either intervention alone.[75] A trial in 203 Chinese women aged 48–62 years found that isoflavones have a mild, but significant, effect on maintenance of hip bone mineral content. This effect was more marked in women in later menopause or those with lower body weight or lower calcium intake.[131,132] A 1-year supplementation study in postmenopausal Taiwanese women found that isoflavones 100 mg daily were associated with a protective effect on oestrogen-related bone loss, and the BMD of lumbar vertebrae 1–3 was increased.[133]

Other trials have shown no significant effect of isoflavones on bone turnover markers,[134] bone sparing,[5] BMD[135,136] or calcium retention,[137] while other trials have shown that isoflavones do not appear to have oestrogenic effects on markers of bone resorption.[43,138]

A meta-analysis including nine studies with a total of 432 subjects found that isoflavone supplementation significantly inhibits bone resorption and stimulates bone formation. These effects occurred even with doses of isoflavones < 90 mg daily or in interventions lasting 12 weeks.[139] A further meta-analysis of 10 studies concluded that isoflavone intervention significantly attenuates bone loss of the spine in menopausal women. Spine bone mineral content and spine bone mineral density increased significantly.[23]

Studies conducted with ipriflavone, a synthetic isoflavone available as a dietary supplement, have found that ipriflavone reduced bone loss in postmenopausal women.[140–143] However, a large multicentre RCT in 472 postmenopausal women aged 45–75 years found that ipriflavone does not prevent bone loss or affect biochemical markers of bone metabolism. In addition, in this study, ipriflavone was found to induce lymphocytopaenia in a significant number of women.[144]

Menopausal symptoms

Reduction of oestrogen production in middle-aged women is associated with symptoms of the menopause, such as hot flushes, vaginal dryness and atrophic vaginitis, and is also thought to contribute to the increased risk of CHD and osteoporosis. The main symptoms of the menopause were thought to occur universally, but women in some countries, such as Japan, appear to experience symptoms such as hot flushes less frequently than women in Western countries,[145] yet far fewer Japanese women use HRT postmenopausally.[146]

Several preliminary studies on the effects of administration of soya isoflavones on menopausal symptoms indicated possible benefit. One study involved 58 postmenopausal women with at least 14 hot flushes a week.[147] They received either 45 g soya flour or wheat flour each day as a supplement to their regular diet over 12 weeks in a randomised double-blind design. Hot flushes decreased in both groups (45% in the soya group and 25% in the controls), with a rapid response in the soya group at 6 weeks. Menopausal symptoms also decreased significantly in both groups. The authors concluded that the lack of difference between the two groups could be due either to a strong placebo effect or a decline in symptoms with time.

Another study provides more persuasive evidence. One hundred and forty-five postmenopausal women were randomised to receive either three servings of soya foods daily or control for 12 weeks.[148] Menopausal symptom scores, hot flushes and vaginal dryness decreased by 50, 54 and 60%, respectively, in women on the soya diet. These three parameters also fell in the control group, but only the reduction in menopausal symptom score was significant.

More recently, a double-blind placebo-controlled study involved 104 postmenopausal women who were randomised to receive 60 g soya protein isolate containing 76 mg isoflavones, or a control.[149] In comparison with placebo, subjects on the soya supplement reported a statistically lower mean number of flushes per 24 h after 4, 8 and 12 weeks. By week 3, the treated group experienced a 26% reduction in the mean number of hot flushes, a 33% reduction by week 4, and by week 12 a 45% reduction, compared with 30% in the control group.

A study in 241 women reporting vasomotor symptoms suggested that soya protein containing 42 or 58 mg of isoflavones is no more effective than isoflavone-extracted soya protein for improving the number and severity of vasomotor symptoms in peri- and postmenopausal women.[150] In another study, which evaluated the effects of a supplement containing both soya isoflavones and black cohosh, there was no statistically significant effect on climacteric effects compared with placebo in perimenopausal women experiencing at least five vasomotor symptoms per day.[72] A 6-month study in 79 postmenopausal women comparing a soya extract providing 120 mg isoflavones with 0.625 mg conjugated equine oestrogens and placebo found that there was a decrease in symptoms in both treatment groups and that the effects of soya with isoflavones were similar to those of oestrogen. However, soya isoflavone had no effect on endometrium and vaginal mucosa during the treatment.[151]

Red clover (another source of isoflavones) has also been investigated for an effect on menopausal symptoms. An RCT in 252 women aged 45–60 years compared two red clover supplements (Promensil and Rimostil, providing 82 and 57 mg isoflavones, respectively) with placebo. The reductions in mean hot flush count at 12 weeks were similar for Promensil (5.1), Rimostil (5.4) and placebo (5.0). In comparison with the placebo group, participants in the Promensil group, but not in the Rimostil group, reduced hot flushes more rapidly. Quality of life improvements and adverse events were comparable in the three groups. The authors concluded that neither supplement had a clinically important effect on hot flushes or other symptoms of menopause.[68] Another trial in 60 postmenopausal women found that a red clover supplement (80 mg isoflavones) significantly decreased menopausal symptoms and had a positive effect on vaginal cytology and triglyceride levels.[152]

Studies evaluating the effect of genistein have found that this compound can have a beneficial effect on menopausal hot flushes.[153,154]

Systematic reviews have considered the effects of soya and red clover isoflavones on menopausal symptoms. A UK systematic review including 10 RCTs that investigated the value of soya preparations for perimenopausal symptoms found that the results were not conclusive. Four of the trials were positive, but six were negative, with one of these six showing a positive trend. The conclusions were that there is some evidence of benefit for soya preparations in perimenopausal symptoms, but the heterogeneity of the studies performed to date means it is difficult to make a definitive statement.[155] A US systematic review identified 25 trials involving 2348 participants; the researchers concluded that the available evidence suggests that phytoestrogens available as soya foods, soya extracts and red clover extracts do not improve hot flushes or other menopausal symptoms.[156] Evidence from a further systematic review and meta-analysis suggests that frequency of hot flushes is not reduced by red clover isoflavone extracts and results were mixed for soya isoflavone extracts.[157] An Australian meta-analysis evaluating the effect of isoflavone therapy in reducing the number of daily menopausal flushes found, despite heterogeneity in the studies, that isoflavones were associated with a significant, slight to moderate reduction in flushes. The percentage reduction in flushes was significantly related to the number of baseline flushes a day and the dose of isoflavone studied. The benefit was more apparent in women experiencing a high number of hot flushes a day.[158] In another trial, relief of hot flushes was related to time since the menopause, with a greater than 12 month gap being related to better hot flush relief.[25]

Cognitive function

Isoflavones have been evaluated for effects on cognitivefunction. Results to date have been inconsistent. In a6-month, double-blind RCT involving 53 women aged 55–74 years, women taking the isoflavone supplement(110 mg) did consistently better compared with their ownbaseline scores and placebo responses at 6 months. Isoflavone supplementation had a favourable effect on cognitive function, particularly veral memory, in these postmenopausal women.[159] In a further 6-month trial in 30 women aged over 60, a red clover isoflavone supplement did not appear to have major cognitive effects.[160] A Dutch trial in 202 healthy postmenopausal women aged 60–65 years found that cognitive function and also BMD and plasma lipids did not differ significantly between the isoflavone and placebo groups after a year.[161]

Miscellaneous

Other symptoms and conditions have been a recent focus of trials involving isoflavones. Isoflavones have been found to have no effect on quality of life (health status, life satisfaction, depression) in elderly postmenopausal women,[161] while another study found benefit among women who have become menopausal recently.[9]

Another study suggested that isoflavones do not have beneficial effects on body composition and physical performance in postmenopausal women.[39] A further trial found that soya isoflavones (100 mg) and 0.625 mg conjugated oestrogen equally lower fasting glucose and insulin levels in postmenopausal women,[162] while another trial found that isoflavones did not result in favourable changes in fasting glucose and insulin.[47] A meta-analysis of 10 RCTs showed that isoflavone supplementation was not associated with glycaemic control.[59]

Another study showed that soya isoflavones may have thepotential to reduce specific premenstrual symptoms (e.g. headache,breast tenderness, cramps, swelling).[163] A pilot study in 12 women with polycysticovary syndrome found that genistein 36 mg/day for 6 months was associated with improved lipid profile but no change in hormone status.[164]

Conclusion
The effects of isoflavones have been studied in many clinical trials. The scientific literature is conflicting because of inconsistencies in populations studied, lack of appropriate controlgroups, selection of end points and types of study. There is asuggestion, but no conclusive evidence, that isoflavones have a beneficial effect on bone health. The consumption of whole soya bean foods and soya bean protein isolates has some beneficial effects on lipid markers of cardiovascular risk. The consumption of isolated isoflavones does not affect blood lipid levels or blood pressure, although it may improve endothelial function. For menopausal symptoms, there is currently limited evidence that soya bean protein isolates, soya bean foods or red clover (*Trifolium pratense* L.) extract are effective, but soya bean isoflavone extracts may be effective in reducing hot flushes. There are too few RCT studies to reach conclusions on the effects of isoflavones on breast cancer, colon cancer, diabetes or cognitive function. The health benefits of soya bean phytoestrogens in healthy postmenopausal women are subtle, and even some well-designed studies do not show protective effects. Future studies should focus on high-risk postmenopausal women, especially in the areas of diabetes, CVD, breast cancer and bone health.

There are some data to suggest that isoflavones have beneficialphysiological effects, but the clinical implications of these effectsare unclear. The consumption of whole soya bean foods and soya bean protein isolates has beneficial effects on lipid markers of cardiovascular risk. The consumption of isolated isoflavones does not appear to have a significant effect on blood lipids or blood pressure, although it may improve endothelial function. For menopausal symptoms there is some evidence that soya bean protein isolates, soya foods or red clover extracts are effective, but soya bean isoflavone extracts may be effective in reducing hot flushes. There is a suggestion, but no conclusive evidence, that isoflavones may have a beneficial effect on bone health. There are too few RCTs to reach conclusions on the effects of isoflavones on breast cancer, colon cancer, diabetes or cognitive function.[165]

Precautions/contraindications

Use with caution in individuals at risk of hormone-dependent cancers. The efficacy and safety of soya isoflavones for preventing or treating cancer of the breast, endometrium and prostate are not established.[107]

Pregnancy and breast-feeding

No problems have been reported, but there have not been sufficient studies to guarantee the safety of isoflavones in pregnancy and breast-feeding. Because of their hormonal effects, isoflavones are probably best avoided.

Adverse effects

Soya foods have been consumed in Asian cultures for centuries.However, studies are needed to assess the long-term safety ofsupplemental soya protein isolates or isoflavonesupplements. In addition, isoflavones are oestrogenic – albeit weakly so– and there is some evidence that they may stimulate cancer cell proliferation in women with breast cancer.[166] However, in studies in healthy women, soya isoflavones do not appear to increase mammographic breast density.[50,166,167] A 3-year study found that red clover isoflavones were safe and well tolerated in healthy women with a first-degree relative with breast cancer.[58] A dose of 80 mg daily of isoflavones over 12 weeks produced no evidence of toxicity in men with early stage prostate cancer.[121] Nevertheless, until more is known about these compounds, women with breast cancer and men with prostate cancer should consult their doctors before taking isoflavones.

Interactions

None reported.

Dose

Supplements
Isoflavones are available in the form of tablets and capsules.

The dose is not established. Dietary supplements containing mixed isoflavones provide 50–100 mg in a dose.

Health claims
In 2002, the UK Joint Health Claims Initiative (JHCI: http://www.jhci.org.uk) proposed a generic health claim for soya protein that may be included on the labels of appropriate foods as follows: 'The inclusion of at least 25 g soya protein per day as part of a diet low in saturated fat can help reduce blood cholesterol.'

In 1999, the US Food and Drug Administration (FDA: http://www.fda.gov) approved a similar claim: 'Diets low in saturated fat and cholesterol that include 25 g of soya protein a day may reduce the risk of heart disease. One serving of [name of food] provides _____ grams of soya protein.'

References

1 Potter JD, Steinmetz K. Vegetables, fruit and phyto-estrogens as preventive agents. In: Stewart BW, McGregor D, Kleihues P, eds. *Principles of Chemoprevention*. Lyon, France: International Agency for Research on Cancer, 1996: 61–90.

2 Albertazzi P, Pansini F, Bonaccorsi G, *et al*. The effect of dietary soy supplementation on hot flushes. *Obstet Gynecol* 1998; 91(1): 6–11.

3 Albertazzi P, Steel SA, Bottazzi M. Effect of pure genistein on bone markers and hot flushes. *Climacteric* 2005; 8(4): 371–379.

4 Alekel DL, Germain AS, Peterson CT, *et al*. Isoflavone-rich soy protein isolate attenuates bone loss in the lumbar spine of perimenopausal women. *Am J Clin Nutr* 2000; 72(3): 844–852.

5 Alekel DL, VanLoan MD, Koehler KJ, *et al*. The soy isoflavones for reducing bone loss (SIRBL) study: a 3-y randomized controlled trial in postmenopausal women. *Am J Clin Nutr* 2009; 91(1): 218–230.

6 Alexandersen P, Toussaint A, Christiansen C, *et al*. Ipriflavone in the treatment of postmenopausal osteoporosis: a randomized controlled trial. *JAMA* 2001; 285(11): 1482–1488 .

7 Atkinson C, Warren RM, Sala E, *et al*. Red-clover-derived isoflavones and mammographic breast density: a double-blind, randomized, placebo-controlled trial [ISRCTN42940165]. *Breast Cancer Res* 2004; 6(3): R170–R179.

8 Aubertin-Leheudre M, Lord C, Khalil A, *et al*. Isoflavones and clinical cardiovascular risk factors in obese postmenopausal women: a randomized double-blind placebo-controlled trial. *J Womens Health (Larchmt)* 2008; 17(8): 1363–1369.

9 Basaria S, Wisniewski A, Dupree K, *et al*. Effect of high-dose isoflavones on cognition, quality of life, androgens, and lipoprotein in post-menopausal women. *J Endocrinol Invest* 2009; 32(2): 150–155.

10 Baum JA, Teng H, Erdman JWJr, *et al*. Long-term intake of soy protein improves blood lipid profiles and increases mononuclear cell low-density-lipoprotein receptor messenger RNA in hypercholesterolemic, postmenopausal women. *Am J Clin Nutr* 1998; 68(3): 545–551.

11 Blakesmith SJ, Lyons-Wall PM, George C, *et al*. Effects of supplememtation with purified red clover

(*Trifolium pratense*) isoflavones on plasma lipids and insulin resistance in healthy premenopausal women. *Br J Nutr* 2003; 89: 467–474.

12 Bolanos R, DelCastillo A, Francia J. Soy isoflavones versus placebo in the treatment of climacteric vasomotor symptoms: systematic review and meta-analysis. *Menopause* 2010; 17(3): 660–666.

13 Burke GL, Legault C, Anthony M, *et al.* Soy protein and isoflavone effects on vasomotor symptoms in peri- and postmenopausal women: the Soy Estrogen Alternative Study. *Menopause* 2003; 10(2): 147–153.

14 Casini ML, Marelli G, Papaleo E, *et al.* Psychological assessment of the effects of treatment with phytoestrogens on postmenopausal women: a randomized, double-blind, crossover, placebo-controlled study. *Fertil Steril* 2006; 85(4): 972–978.

15 Charles C, Yuskavage J, Carlson O, *et al.* Effects of high-dose isoflavones on metabolic and inflammatory markers in healthy postmenopausal women. *Menopause* 2009; 16(2): 395–400.

16 Chedraui P, San Miguel G, Hidalgo L, *et al.* Effect of *Trifolium pratense*-derived isoflavones on the lipid profile of postmenopausal women with increased body mass index. *Gynecol Endocrinol* 2008; 24(11): 620–624.

17 Chen YM, Ho SC, Lam SS, *et al.* Beneficial effect of soy isoflavones on bone mineral content was modified by years since menopause, body weight, and calcium intake: a double-blind, randomized, controlled trial. *Menopause* 2004; 11(3): 246–254.

18 Cheng SY, Shaw NS, Tsai KS, *et al.* The hypoglycemic effects of soy isoflavones on postmenopausal women. *J Womens Health (Larchmt)* 2004; 13(10): 1080–1086.

19 Colacurci N, Chiantera A, Fornaro F, *et al.* Effects of soy isoflavones on endothelial function in healthy postmenopausal women. *Menopause* 2005; 12(3): 299–307.

20 Crisafulli A, Marini H, Bitto A, *et al.* Effects of genistein on hot flushes in early postmenopausal women: a randomized, double-blind EPT- and placebo-controlled study. *Menopause* 2004; 11(4): 400–404.

21 Crisafulli A, Altavilla D, Marini H, *et al.* Effects of the phytoestrogen genistein on cardiovascular risk factors in postmenopausal women. *Menopause* 2005; 12(2): 186–192.

22 D'Anna R, Baviera G, Corrado F, *et al.* The effect of the phytoestrogen genistein and hormone replacement therapy on homocysteine and C-reactive protein level in postmenopausal women. *Acta Obstet Gynecol Scand* 2005; 84(5): 474–477.

23 Maa DF, Qinc LQ, Wanga PY, *et al.* Soya isoflavone intake increases bone mineral density in the spine of menopausal women: meta-analysis of randomized controlled trials. *Clin Nutr* 2008; 27(?): 57–64.

24 Engelman HM, Alekel DL, Hanson LN, *et al.* Blood lipid and oxidative stress responses to soy protein with isoflavones and phytic acid in postmenopausal women. *Am J Clin Nutr* 2005; 81(3): 590–596.

25 Ferrari A. Soy extract phytoestrogens with high dose of isoflavones for menopausal symptoms. *J Obstet Gynaecol Res* 2009; 35(6): 1083–1090.

26 Gambacciani M, Ciaponi M, Cappagli B, *et al.* Effects of combined low dose of the isoflavone derivative ipriflavone and estrogen replacement on bone mineral density and metabolism in postmenopausal women. *Maturitas* 1997; 28(1): 75–81.

27 Hall WL, Vafeiadou K, Hallund J, *et al.* Soy-isoflavone-enriched foods and inflammatory biomarkers of cardiovascular disease risk in postmenopausal women: interactions with genotype and equol production. *Am J Clin Nutr* 2005; 82(6): 1260–1268 quiz 13651366.

28 Hall WL, Formanuik NL, Harnpanich D, *et al.* A meal enriched with soy isoflavones increases nitric oxide-mediated vasodilation in healthy postmenopausal women. *J Nutr* 2008; 138(7): 1288–1292.

29 Hidalgo LA, Chedraui PA, Morocho N, *et al.* The effect of red clover isoflavones on menopausal symptoms, lipids and vaginal cytology in menopausal women: a randomized, double-blind, placebo-controlled study. *Gynecol Endocrinol* 2005; 21(5): 257–264.

30 Hooper L, Ryder JJ, Kurzer MS, *et al.* Effects of soy protein and isoflavones on circulating hormone concentrations in pre- and post-menopausal women: a systematic review and meta-analysis. *Hum Reprod Update* 2009; 15(4): 423–440.

31 Howes JB, Sullivan D, Lai N, *et al.* The effects of dietary supplementation with isoflavones from red clover on the lipoprotein profiles of post menopausal women with mild to moderate hypercholesterolaemia. *Atherosclerosis* 2000; 152(1): 143–147.

32 Howes JB, Tran D, Brillante D, *et al.* Effects of dietary supplementation with isoflavones from red clover on ambulatory blood pressure and endothelial function in postmenopausal type 2 diabetes. *Diabetes Obes Metab* 2003; 5(5): 325–332.

33 Howes JB, Bray K, Lorenz L, *et al.* The effects of dietary supplementation with isoflavones from red clover on cognitive function in postmenopausal women. *Climacteric* 2004; 7(1): 70–77.

34 Huntley AL, Ernst E. Soy for the treatment of perimenopausal symptoms: a systematic review. *Maturitas* 2004; 47(1): 1–9.

35 Hutchins AM, McIver IE, Johnston CS. Soy isoflavone and ascorbic acid supplementation alone or in combination minimally affect plasma lipid peroxides in healthy postmenopausal women. *J Am Diet Assoc* 2005; 105(7): 1134–1137.

36 Imhof M, Molzer S, Imhof M. Effects of soy isoflavones on 17β-estradiol-induced proliferation of MCF-7 breast cancer cells. *Toxicol In Vitro* 2008; 22(6): 1452–1460.

37 Jou HJ, Wu SC, Chang FW, *et al.* Effect of intestinal production of equol on menopausal symptoms in

women treated with soy isoflavones. *Int J Gynaecol Obstet* 2008; 102(1): 44–49.

38 Katase K, Kato T, Hirai Y, *et al.* Effects of ipriflavone on bone loss following a bilateral ovariectomy and menopause: a randomized placebo-controlled study. *Calcif Tissue Int* 2001; 69(2): 73–77.

39 Kok L, Kreijkamp-Kaspers S, Grobbee DE, *et al.* Soy isoflavones, body composition, and physical performance. *Maturitas* 2005; 52(2): 102–110.

40 Kok L, Kreijkamp-Kaspers S, Grobbee DE, *et al.* A randomized, placebo-controlled trial on the effects of soy protein containing isoflavones on quality of life in postmenopausal women. *Menopause* 2005; 12(1): 56–62.

41 Krebs EE, Ensrud KE, MacDonald R, *et al.* Phytoestrogens for treatment of menopausal symptoms: a systematic review. *Obstet Gynecol* 2004; 104(4): 824–836.

42 Kreijkamp-Kaspers S, Kok L, Bots ML, *et al.* Randomized controlled trial of the effects of soy protein containing isoflavones on vascular function in postmenopausal women. *Am J Clin Nutr* 2005; 81(1): 189–195.

43 Kwak HS, Park SY, Kim MG, *et al.* Marked individual variation in isoflavone metabolism after a soy challenge can modulate the skeletal effect of isoflavones in premenopausal women. *J Korean Med Sci* 2009; 24(5): 867–873.

44 Lipovac M, Chedraui P, Gruenhut C, *et al.* Improvement of postmenopausal depressive and anxiety symptoms after treatment with isoflavones derived from red clover extracts. *Maturitas* 2009; 65(3): 258–261.

45 Lissin LW, Oka R, Lakshmi S, *et al.* Isoflavones improve vascular reactivity in post-menopausal women with hypercholesterolemia. *Vasc Med* 2004; 9(1): 26–30.

46 Liu ZM, Ho SC, Chen YM, *et al.* A mild favorable effect of soy protein with isoflavones on body composition: a 6-month double-blind randomized placebo-controlled trial among Chinese postmenopausal women. *Int J Obes (Lond)* 2009; 34(2): 309–138.

47 Liu ZM, Chen YM, Ho SC, *et al.* Effects of soy protein and isoflavones on glycemic control and insulin sensitivity: a 6-mo double-blind, randomized, placebo-controlled trial in postmenopausal Chinese women with prediabetes or untreated early diabetes. *Am J Clin Nutr* 2010; 91(5): 1394–1401.

48 Llaneza P, Gonzalez C, Fernandez-Inarrea J, *et al.* Soy isoflavones, Mediterranean diet, and physical exercise in postmenopausal women with insulin resistance. *Menopause* 2010; 17(2): 372–378.

49 Marini H, Minutoli L, Polito F, *et al.* Effects of the phytoestrogen genistein on bone metabolism in osteopenic postmenopausal women: a randomized trial. *Ann Intern Med* 2007; 146(12): 839–847.

50 Maskarinec G, Verheus M, Steinberg FM, *et al.* Various doses of soy isoflavones do not modify mammographic density in postmenopausal women. *J Nutr* 2009; 139(5): 981–986.

51 McMichael-Phillips DF, Harding C, Morton M, *et al.* Effects of soy-protein supplementation on epithelial proliferation in the histologically normal human breast. *Am J Clin Nutr* 1998; 68(6Suppl): 1431S–1435S.

52 Merz-Demlow BE, Duncan AM, Wangen KE, *et al.* Soy isoflavones improve plasma lipids in normocholesterolemic, premenopausal women. *Am J Clin Nutr* 2000; 71(6): 1462–1469.

53 Messina M, Hughes C. Efficacy of soyfoods and soybean isoflavone supplements for alleviating menopausal symptoms is positively related to initial hot flush frequency. *J Med Food* 2003; 6(1): 1–11.

54 Moraes AB, Haidar MA, Soares Junior JM, *et al.* The effects of topical isoflavones on postmenopausal skin: double-blind and randomized clinical trial of efficacy. *Eur J Obstet Gynecol Reprod Biol* 2009; 146(2): 188–192.

55 Murkies AL, Lombard C, Strauss BJ, *et al.* Dietary flour supplementation decreases post-menopausal hot flushes: effect of soy and wheat. *Maturitas* 1995; 21(3): 189–195.

56 Ohta H, Komukai S, Makita K, *et al.* Effects of 1-year ipriflavone treatment on lumbar bone mineral density and bone metabolic markers in postmenopausal women with low bone mass. *Horm Res* 1999; 51(4): 178–183.

57 Potter SM, Baum JA, Teng H, *et al.* Soy protein and isoflavones: their effects on blood lipids and bone density in postmenopausal women. *Am J Clin Nutr* 1998; 68(6Suppl): 1375S–1379S.

58 Powles TJ, Howell A, Evans DG, *et al.* Red clover isoflavones are safe and well tolerated in women with a family history of breast cancer. *Menopause Int* 2008; 14(1): 6–12.

59 Ricci E, Cipriani S, Chiaffarino F, *et al.* Effects of soy isoflavones and genistein on glucose metabolism in perimenopausal and postmenopausal non-Asian women: a meta-analysis of randomized controlled trials. *Menopause* 2010; 17(5): 1080–1086.

60 Rios DR, Rodrigues ET, Cardoso AP, *et al.* Lack of effects of isoflavones on the lipid profile of Brazilian postmenopausal women. *Nutrition* 2008; 24(11-12): 1153–1158.

61 Rios DR, Rodrigues ET, Cardoso AP, *et al.* Effects of isoflavones on the coagulation and fibrinolytic system of postmenopausal women. *Nutrition* 2008; 24(2): 120–126.

62 Samman S, Lyons Wall PM, Chan GS, *et al.* The effect of supplementation with isoflavones on plasma lipids and oxidisability of low density lipoprotein in premenopausal women. *Atherosclerosis* 1999; 147(2): 277–283.

63 Samman S, Koh HS, Flood VM, *et al.* Red clover (*Trifolium pratense*) isoflavones and serum homocysteine in premenopausal women: a pilot study. *J Womens Health (Larchmt)* 2009; 18(11): 1813–1816.

64 Schult TM, Ensrud KE, Blackwell T, *et al.* Effect of isoflavones on lipids and bone turnover markers in menopausal women. *Maturitas* 2004; 48(3): 209–218.

65 Simons LA, von Konigsmark M, Simons J, *et al.* Phytoestrogens do not influence lipoprotein levels or endothelial function in healthy, postmenopausal women. *Am J Cardiol* 2000; 85(11): 1297–1301.

66 Spence LA, Lipscomb ER, Cadogan J, *et al.* The effect of soy protein and soy isoflavones on calcium metabolism in postmenopausal women: a randomized crossover study. *Am J Clin Nutr* 2005; 81(4): 916–922.

67 Terzic MM, Dotlic J, Maricic S, *et al.* Influence of red clover-derived isoflavones on serum lipid profile in postmenopausal women. *J Obstet Gynaecol Res* 2009; 35(6): 1091–1095.

68 Tice JA, Ettinger B, Ensrud K, *et al.* Phytoestrogen supplements for the treatment of hot flashes: the Isoflavone Clover Extract (ICE) Study: a randomized controlled trial. *JAMA* 2003; 290(2): 207–214.

69 Uesugi T, Toda T, Okuhira T, *et al.* Evidence of estrogenic effect by the three-month-intervention of isoflavone on vaginal maturation and bone metabolism in early postmenopausal women. *Endocr J* 2003; 50(5): 613–619.

70 Uesugi S, Watanabe S, Ishiwata N, *et al.* Effects of isoflavone supplements on bone metabolic markers and climacteric symptoms in Japanese women. *Biofactors* 2004; 22(14): 221–228.

71 Verheus M, vanGils CH, Kreijkamp-Kaspers S, *et al.* Soy protein containing isoflavones and mammographic density in a randomized controlled trial in postmenopausal women. *Cancer Epidemiol Biomarkers Prev* 2008; 17(10): 2632–2638.

72 Verhoeven MO, van der Mooren MJ, van de Weijer PH, *et al.* Effect of a combination of isoflavones and *Actaea racemosa* Linnaeus on climacteric symptoms in healthy symptomatic perimenopausal women: a 12-week randomized, placebo-controlled, double-blind study. *Menopause* 2005; 12 (4): 412–420.

73 Verhoeven MO, Teerlink T, Kenemans P, *et al.* Effects of a supplement containing isoflavones and *Actaea racemosa* L. on asymmetric dimethylarginine, lipids, and C-reactive protein in menopausal women. *Fertil Steril* 2007; 87(4): 849–857.

74 Williamson-Hughes PS, Flickinger BD, Messina MJ, *et al.* Isoflavone supplements containing predominantly genistein reduce hot flash symptoms: a critical review of published studies. *Menopause* 2006; 13(5): 831–839.

75 Wu J, Oka J, Tabata I, *et al.* Effects of isoflavone and exercise on BMD and fat mass in postmenopausal Japanese women: a 1-year randomized placebo-controlled trial. *J Bone Miner Res* 2006; 21 (5): 780–789.

76 Setchell KDR. Phytoestrogens: the biochemistry, physiology, and implications for human health of soy isoflavones. *Am J Clin Nutr* 1998; 68: 1333S–1346S.

77 Anderson JW, Johnstone BW, Cook-Newell ME. Meta-analysis of the effects of soy protein intake on serum lipids. *New Engl J Med* 1995; 333: 276–282.

78 Baum JA, Teng H, Erdman Jr JEA. Long-term intake of soya protein improves blood lipid profiles and increases mononuclear cell low-density-lipoprotein receptor messenger RNA in hypercholesterolemic, postmenopausal women. *Am J Clin Nutr* 1998; 68: 545–551.

79 Gooderham MH, Adlercreutz H, Ojala ST, *et al.* A soy protein isolate rich in genistein and daidzein and its effects on plasma isoflavone concentration, platelet aggregation, blood lipids and fatty acid composition of plasma phospholipid in normal men. *J Nutr* 1996; 126: 2000–2006.

80 Wong W, O'Brian Smith E, Stuff JE, *et al.* Cholesterol-lowering effect of soy protein in normocholesterolemic and hypercholesterolemic men. *Am J Clin Nutr* 1998; 68: 1385S–1389S.

81 Crouse JR 3rd, Morgan T, Terry JG, *et al.* Soy protein containing isoflavones reduces plasma concentrations of lipids. *Arch Int Med* 1999; 159: 2070–2076.

82 Teixera SR, Potter SM, Weigel R, *et al.* Effects of feeding 4 levels of soy protein for 3 and 6 wk on blood lipids and apolipoproteins in moderately hypercholesterolemic men. *Am J Clin Nutr* 2000; 71: 1077–1084.

83 McVeigh BL, Dillingham BL, Lampe JW, *et al.* Effect of soy protein varying in isoflavone content on serum lipids in healthy young men. *Am J Clin Nutr* 2006; 83: 244–251.

84 Merz-Demlow BE, Duncan AM, Wangen KE, *et al.* Soy isoflavones improve plasma lipids in normocholesterolemic, premenopausal women. *Am J Clin Nutr* 2000; 71: 1462–1469.

85 Tikkanen MJ, Wahala K, Ojala S, *et al.* Effect of soybean phytoestrogen intake on low density lipoprotein oxidation resistance. *Proc Natl Acad Sci USA* 1998; 95: 3106–3110.

86 Wiseman H, O'Reilly JD, Adlercreutz H, *et al.* Isoflavone phytoestrogens consumed in soy decrease F2-isoprostane concentrations and increase resistance of low-density lipoprotein to oxidation in humans. *Am J Clin Nutr* 2000; 72: 395–400.

87 Hodgson JM, Puddey IB, Beilin LJ, *et al.* Supplementation with isoflavonoid phytoestrogens does not alter serum lipid concentrations: a randomized controlled trial in humans. *J Nutr* 1998; 128: 728–732.

88 Samman S, Lyons Wall PM, Chan GS, *et al.* The effect of supplementation with isoflavones on plasma lipids and oxidisability of low density lipoprotein in premenopausal women. *Atherosclerosis* 1999; 147: 277–283.

89 Simons LA, von Koningsmark M, Simons J, *et al.* Phytoestrogens do not influence lipoprotein levels or endothelial function in healthy, postmenopausal women. *Am J Cardiol* 2000; 85: 1297–1301.

90 Howes JB, Sullivan D, Lai N, *et al.* The effects of dietary supplementation with isoflavones from red clover on the lipoprotein profiles of postmenopausal women with mild to moderate hypercholesterolaemia. *Atherosclerosis* 2000; 152: 143–147.

91 Atkinson C, Oosthuizen W, Scollen S, *et al.* Modest protective effects of isoflavones from a red clover-derived dietary supplement on cardiovascular risk factors in perimenopausal woman, and evidence of an interaction with ApoE genotype in 49–65 year old women. *J Nutr* 2004; 134: 1759–1764.

92 Howes JB, Tran D, Brilliante D, *et al.* Effects of dietary supplementation with isoflavones from red clover on ambulatory blood pressure and endothelial function in postmenopausal type 2 diabetes. *Diabetes Obes Metab* 2003; 5: 325–332.

93 Engelman HM, Alekel DL, Hanson LN, *et al.* Blood lipid and oxidative stress responses to soy protein with isoflavones and phytic acid in postmenopausal women. *Am J Clin Nutr* 2005; 81: 590–596.

94 Hutchins AM, McIver JE, Johnston CS. Soy isoflavones and ascorbibd acid supplementation alone or in combination minimally affect plasma lipid peroxides in healthy postmenopausal women. *J Am Diet Assoc* 2005; 105: 1134–1137.

95 Kreijkamp-Kaspers S, Kok L, Bots ML, *et al.* Randomized controlled trial of the effects of soy protein containing isoflavones on vascular function in postmenopausal women. *Am J Clin Nutr* 2005; 81: 5189–5189.

96 Lissin LW, Okra R, Lakshmi S, *et al.* Isoflavones improve vascular reactivity in post-menopausal women with hypercholesesterolaemia. *Vasc Med* 2004; 9: 26–30.

97 Hermansen K, Hansen B, al JRe. Effects of soy supplementation on blood lipids and arterial function in hypercholesterolaemic subjects. *Eur J Clin Nutr* 2005; 59: 843–850.

98 Colacurci N, Chiantera A, Fornaro F, *et al.* Effects of soy isoflavones on endothelial function in healthy postmenopausal women. *Menopause* 2005; 12: 299–307.

99 Crisafulli A, Altavilla D, Marini H, *et al.* Effects of the phytoestrogen genistein on cardiovascular risk factors in postmenopausal women. *Menopause* 2005; 12: 186–192.

100 D'Anna R, Baviera G, Corrado F, *et al.* The effect of the phytoestrogen genistein and hormone replacement therapy on homocysteine and C-reactive protein level in postmenopausal women. *Acta Obstet Gynecol Scand* 2005; 84: 474–477.

101 Chen CY, Bakhiet RM, Hart V, *et al.* Isoflavones improve plasma homocysteine status and antioxidant defense system in healthy young men at rest but do not ameliorate oxidative stress induced by 80% VO_2pk exercise. *Ann Nutr Metab* 2005; 49: 33–41.

102 Sagara M, Kanda T, Jelekera M, *et al.* Effects of dietary intake of soy protein and isoflavones on cardiovascular risk factors in high-risk, middle-aged men in Scotland. *J Am Coll Nutr* 2004; 23: 85–91.

103 Garrido A, De laMaza MP, Hirsch S, *et al.* Soy isoflavones affect platelet thromboxane A2 receptor density but not plasma lipids in menopausal women. *Maturitas* 2006; 54(3): 270–276.

104 Weggermans RM, Trautwein EA. Relation between soya-associated isoflavones and LDL and HDL cholesterol concentrations in humans: a meta-analysis. *Eur J Clin Nutr* 2003; 57: 940–946.

105 Zhuo XG, Melby MK, Watanabe S. Soy isoflavone intake lowers serum LDL cholesterol: a meta-analysis of 8 randomized controlled trials in humans. *J Nutr* 2004; 134: 2395–2400.

106 Zhan S, Ho SC. Meta-analysis of the effects of soy protein containing isoflavones on the lipid profile. *Am J Clin Nutr* 2005; 81: 397–408.

107 Sacks FM, Lichtenstein A, VanHorn L, *et al.* Soy protein, isoflavones, and cardiovascular health: an American Heart Association Science Advisory for professionals from the Nutrition Committee. *Circulation* 2006; 113(7): 1034–1044.

108 Dewell A, Hollenbeck PL, Hollenbeck CB. Clinical review: a critical evaluation of the role of soy protein and isoflavone supplementation in the control of plasma cholesterol concentrations. *J Clin Endocrinol Metab* 2006; 91(3): 772–780.

109 Reynolds K, Chin A, Lees KA, *et al.* A meta-analysis of the effect of soy protein supplementation on serum lipids. *Am J Cardiol* 2006; 98: 633–640.

110 Taku K, Umegaki K, Sato Y, *et al.* Soy isoflavones lower serum total and LDL cholesterol in humans: a meta-analysis of 11 randomized controlled trials. *Am J Clin Nutr* 2007; 85(4): 1148–1156.

111 Messina MJ, Persky V, Setchell KD, *et al.* Soy intake and cancer risk: a review of the in vitro and in vivo data. *Nutr Cancer* 1994; 21: 113–131.

112 Goodman MT, Wilkens LR, Hankin JH, *et al.* Association of soy and fiber consumption with the risk of endometrial cancer. *Am J Epidemiol* 1997; 146: 294–306.

113 Schabath MB, Hernandez LM, Wu X, *et al.* Dietary phytoestrogens and lung cancer risk. *JAMA* 2005; 294: 1493–1504.

114 Barnes S. Effect of genistein on in vitro and in vivo models of cancer. *J Nutr* 1995; 125: 777S– 1995; 783S.

115 Hawrylewicz EJ, Zapata JJ, Blair WH. Soy and experimental cancer. *J Nutr* 1995; 125: 698S–708S.

116 Kennedy AR. The evidence for soybean products as cancer preventive agents. *J Nutr* 1995; 125: 733S–743S.

117 Ingram D, Sanders K, Kolybaba M, *et al.* Case-control study of phyto-estrogens and breast cancer. *Lancet* 1997; 350: 990–994.

118 Murkies A, Dalais FS, Briganti EM, *et al.* Phytoestrogens and breast cancer in postmenopausal women: a case control study. *Menopause* 2000; 7: 289–296.

119 Adams KF, Lampe PD, Newton KM, *et al.* Soy protein containing isoflavones does not decrease colorectal epithelial cell proliferation in a randomized controlled trial. *Am J Clin Nutr* 2005; 82: 620–626.

120 Adams KF, Chen C, Newton KM, *et al.* Soy isoflavones do not modulate prostate-specific antigen concentrations in older men in a randomized controlled trial. *Cancer Epidemiol Biomarkers Prev* 2004; 13: 644–648.

121 Kumar NB, Krischer JP, Allen K, *et al.* Safety of purified isoflavones in men with clinically localized prostate cancer. *Nutr Cancer* 2007; 59(2): 169–175.

122 Sharma P, Wisniewski A, Braga-Basaria M, *et al.* Lack of an effect of high dose isoflavones in men with prostate cancer undergoing androgen deprivation therapy. *J Urol* 2009; 182(5): 2265–2272.

123 Ahmad IU, Forman JD, Sarkar FH, *et al.* Soy isoflavones in conjunction with radiation therapy in patients with prostate cancer. *Nutr Cancer* 2010; 62(7): 996–1000.

124 Hooper L, Madhavan G, Tice JA, *et al.* Effects of isoflavones on breast density in pre- and postmenopausal women: a systematic review and meta-analysis of randomized controlled trials. *Hum Reprod Update* 2010; 16(6): 745–760.

125 Arjmandi BH, Alekel L, Hollis BW, *et al.* Dietary soybean protein prevents bone loss in an ovariectomized rat model of osteoporosis. *J Nutr* 1996; 126: 161–167.

126 Anderson JJ, Ambrose WW, Garner SC. Biphasic effects of genistein on bone tissue in the ovariectomized, lactating rat model. *Proc Soc Exp Biol Med* 1998; 217: 345–350.

127 Potter SM, Baum JA, Teng H, *et al.* Soy protein and isoflavones: their effects on blood lipids and bone mineral density in postmenopausal women. *Am J Clin Nutr* 1998; 68: 1375S– 1998; 1379S.

128 Alekel DL, St Germain A, Peterson CT, *et al.* Isoflavone-rich soy protein isolate attenuates bone loss in the lumbar spine of perimenopausal women. *Am J Clin Nutr* 2000; 72: 844–852.

129 Uesugi T, Toda T, Okuhira T, *et al.* Evidence of estrogenic effect by the three-month-intervention of isoflavone on vaginal maturation and bone metabolism in early postmenopausal women. *Endocr J* 2003; 50: 613–619.

130 Useugi S, Watanabe S, Ishiwata N, *et al.* Effects of isoflavone supplements on bone metabolic markers and climacteric symptoms in Japanese women. *Biofactors* 2004; 22: 221–228.

131 Chen YM, Ho SC, Lam SS, *et al.* Beneficial effect of soy isoflavones on bone mineral content was modified by years since menopause, body weight and calcium intake: a double-blind, randomized, controlled trial. *Menopause* 2004; 11: 246–254.

132 Chen YM, Ho SC, Lam SS, *et al.* Soy isoflavones have a favourable effect on bone mass in Chinese postmenopausal women with lower bone mass: a double-blind, randomized, controlled trial. *J Clin Endocrinol Metab* 2003; 88: 4740–4747.

133 Hui-Ying H, Hsiao-Ping Y, Hui-Ting Y, *et al.* One-year isoflavone supplementation prevents early postmenopausal bone loss but without a dose-dependent effect. *J Nutr Biochem* 2006; 17: 509–517.

134 Schult TM, Ensrud KE, Blackwell T, *et al.* Effects of isoflavones on lipids and bone turnover markers in menopausal women. *Maturitas* 2004; 48: 209–218.

135 Kenny AM, Mangano KM, Abourizk RH, *et al.* Soy proteins and isoflavones affect bone mineral density in older women: a randomized controlled trial. *Am J Clin Nutr* 2009; 90(1): 234–242.

136 Liu J, Ho SC, Su YX, *et al.* Effect of long-term intervention of soy isoflavones on bone mineral density in women: a meta-analysis of randomized controlled trials. *Bone* 2009; 44(5): 948–953.

137 Spence LA, Lipscomb ER, Cadogan J, *et al.* The effect of soy protein and soy isoflavones on calcium metabolism in postmenopausal women: a randomized crossover study. *Am J Clin Nutr* 2005; 81: 916–922.

138 Dalais FS, Ebeling PR, Kotsopoulos D, *et al.* The effects of soy protein containing isoflavones on lipids and indices of bone resorption in postmenopausal women. *Clin Endocrinol* 2003; 58: 704–709.

139 Ma DF, Qin LQ, Wang PY, *et al.* Soy isoflavone intake inhibits bone resorption and stimulates bone formation in menopausal women: meta-analysis of randomized controlled trials. *Eur J Clin Nutr* 2007;.

140 Agnusdei D, Crepaldi G, Isaia G, *et al.* A double-blind, placebo-controlled diet of ipriflavone for prevention of postmenopausal spinal bone loss. *Calcif Tissue Int* 1997; 61: 142–147.

141 Gambacciani M, Ciaponi M, Cappagli B, *et al.* Effects of combined low dose of the isoflavone derivative ipriflavone and estrogen replacement on bone mineral density and metabolism in postmenopausal women. *Maturitas* 1997; 28: 75–81.

142 Ohta H, Komukai S, Makita K, *et al.* Effects of 1-year ipriflavone treatment on bone mineral density and bone metabolic markers in postmenopausal women with low bone mass. *Horm Res* 1999; 51: 178–183.

143 Katase K, Kato T, Hirai Y, *et al.* Effects of ipriflavone on bone loss following a bilateral ovariectomy and menopause: a randomized placebo-controlled study. *Calcif Tissue Int* 2001; 69: 73–77.

144 Alexandersen P, Toussaint A, Chistiansen C, *et al.* Ipriflavone in the treatment of postmenopausal osteoporosis: a randomized controlled trial. *JAMA* 2001; 285: 1482–1488.

145 Lock M. Contested meanings of the menopause. *Lancet* 1991; 337: 1270–1272.

146 Kurzer MS, Xu X. Dietary phytoestrogens. *Ann Rev Nutr* 1997; 17: 353–381.

147 Murkies AL, Lombard C, Strauss BJG, *et al.* Dietary flour supplementation decreases post-menopausal hot flushes: effect of soy and wheat. *Maturitas* 1995; 21: 189–195.

148 Brzezinski A, Aldercreutz H, Shaoul R, *et al.* Short-term effects of phytoestrogen-rich diet on postmenopausal women. *J North Am Menopause Soc* 1997; 4: 89–94.

149 Albertazzi P, Pansini F, Bonaccorsi G, *et al.* The effect of dietary soy supplementation on hot flushes. *Obstet Gynecol* 1998; 91: 6–11.

150 Burke GL, Legault C, Anthony M, *et al.* Soy protein and isoflavone effects on vasomotor symptoms in peri-and postmenopausal women: the Soy Estrogen Alternative Study. *Menopause* 2003; 10: 147–143.

151 Kaari C, Haidar MA, Junior JM, *et al.* Randomized clinical trial comparing conjugated equine estrogens and isoflavones in postmenopausal women: a pilot study. *Maturitas* 2006; 53: 49–58.

152 Hidalgo LA, Chedraui PA, Morocho N, *et al.* The effect of red clover isoflavones on menopausal symptoms, lipids and vaginal cytology in menopausal women: a randomized, double-blind, placebo-controlled study. *Gynecol Endocrinol* 2005; 21: 257–264.

153 Crisafulli A, Marini H, Bitto A, *et al.* Effects of genistein on hot flushes in early postmenopausal women: a randomized, double-blind EPT- and placebo-controlled study. *Menopause* 2004; 11: 400–404.

154 Albertazzi P, Steel SA, Bottazzi M. Effect of genistein on bone markers and hot flushes. *Climcateric* 2005; 8: 371–379.

155 Huntley AL, Ernst E. soyafor the treatment of perimenopausal symptoms – a systematic review. *Maturitas* 2004; 47: 1–9.

156 Krebs EE, Ensrud KE, MacDonald R, *et al.* Phytoestrogens for treatment of menopausal symptoms: a systematic review. *Obstet Gynecol* 2004; 104: 824–836.

157 Nelson HD, Vesco KK, Haney E, *et al.* Nonhormonal therapies for menopausal hot flashes. *JAMA* 2006; 295: 2057–2071.

158 Howes LG, Howes JB, Knight DC. Isoflavone therapy for menopausal flushes: a systematic review and meta-analysis. *Maturitas* 2006; 55(3): 203–211.

159 Kritz-SilversteinD Von Muhlen D, Barrett-Connor E, *et al.* Isoflavones and cognitive function in older women: the soya and Postmenopausal Health in Ageing (SOPHIA) Study. *Menopause* 2003; 10: 196–202.

160 Howes JB, Bray K, Lorenz L, *et al.* The effects of dietary supplementation with isoflavones from red clover on cognitive function in postmenopausal women. *Climacteric* 2004; 7: 70–77.

161 Kreijkamp-Jaspers S, Kok L, Grobbee DL, *et al.* Effect of soya protein containing isoflavones on cognitive function, bone mineral density, and plasma lipids in postmenopausal women: a randomized controlled trial. *JAMA* 2004; 292: 65–74.

162 Cheng SY, Shaw NS, Tsai KS, *et al.* The hypoglycemic effects of soya isoflavones on postmenopausal women. *J Womens Health (Larchmt)* 2004; 13: 1080–1086.

163 Bryant M, Cassidy A, Hill C, *et al.* Effect of consumption of soya isoflavones on behavioural, somatic and affective symptoms in women with premenstrual symptoms. *Br J Nutr* 2005; 93: 731–739.

164 Romualdi D, Costantini B, Campagna G, *et al.* Is there a role for soya isoflavones in the therapeutic approach to polycystic ovary syndrome? Results from a pilot study *Fertil Steril* 2008; 90(5): 1826–1833.

165 Cassidy A, Albertazzi A, Lise Nielsen I, *et al.* Critical review of health effects of soybean phyto-oestrogens in post-menopausal women. *Proc Nutr Soc* 2006; 65: 76–92.

166 McMichael-Phillips DF, Harding C, Morton M, *et al.* Effects of soy-protein supplementation on epithelial proliferation in the histologically normal human breast. *Am J Clin Nutr* 1998; 68: 1431S–1416S.

167 Atkinson C, Warren RM, Sala E, *et al.* Red-clover derived isoflavones and mammographic breast density: a double-blind, randomized, placebo-controlled trial (ISRCTN42940165). *Breast Cancer Res* 2004; 6: R170–R179.

Kelp

Description

Kelp is a long-stemmed seaweed, derived from various species (e.g. *Fucus*, *Laminaria*) of brown algae, known as a preparation of dried seaweed of various species.

Constituents

Kelp is a source of several minerals and trace elements, especially iodine.

Possible uses

Kelp is claimed to be a slimming aid (some herbal products containing kelp are licensed in the UK for this purpose). Its main use is as a source of iodine.

Precautions/contraindications

Kelp should be avoided in patients with thyroid disease, unless recommended by a doctor. It may be contaminated with toxic trace elements (e.g. antimony, arsenic, lead, strontium).

Pregnancy and breast-feeding

Avoid (because of contaminants – see Precautions).

Adverse effects

A few case reports have linked hyperthyroidism to kelp ingestion.[1–7] Hypothyroidism may also be more prevalent in people who consume excess amounts of iodine in the form of kelp.[8] A US guideline on detection of thyroid dysfunction notes that patients who ingest iodine compounds (e.g. kelp) are at increased risk of developing thyroid dysfunction.[9] Nausea and diarrhoea have been reported occasionally. Kelp supplements have also been linked with arsenic toxicosis,[10] although this has been questioned.[11,12]

Interactions

See Iodine monograph.

Dose

Kelp is available in the form of capsules, tablets, powder and liquid.

The dose is not established. Dietary supplements contain 200–500 mg kelp. The iodine content is variable and not always quoted on the label.

References

1 Shilo S, Hirsch HJ. Iodine-induced hyperthyroidism in a patient with a normal thyroid gland. *Postgrad Med J* 1986; 62: 661–662.
2 Ishizuki Y, Yamauchi K, Miura Y. Transient thyrotoxicosis induced by Japanese kombu. *Nippon Naibunpi Gakkai Zasshi* 1989; 65: 91–98.
3 deSmet PA, Stricker BH, Wilderink F, Wiersinga WM. Hyperthyroidism during treatment with kelp tablets. *Ned Tijdschr Geneeskd* 1990; 134: 1058–1059.
4 Hartmann AA. Hyperthyroidism during administration of kelp tablets. *Ned Tijdschr Geneeskd* 1990; 134: 1373.
5 Eliason BC. Transient hyperthyroidism in a patient taking dietary supplements containing kelp. *J Am Board Fam Pract* 1998; 11: 478–480.
6 Clark CD, Bassett B, Burge MR. Effects of kelp supplementation on thyroid function in euthyroid subjects. *Endocr Pract* 2003; 9(5): 363–369.
7 Arum SM, He X, Braverman LE. Excess iodine from an unexpected source. *N Engl J Med* 2009; 360(4): 424–426.
8 Konno N, Iizuka N, Kawasaki K, *et al*. Screening for thyroid dysfunction in adults residing in Hokkaido, Japan: in relation to urinary iodide

concentration and thyroid autoantibodies. *Hokkaido Igaku Zasshi* 1994; 69: 614–626.

9 Landenson PW, Singer PA, Ain KB, *et al.* American Thyroid Association guidelines for detection of thyroid dysfunction. *Arch Intern Med* 2000; 160: 1573–1575.

10 Amster E, Tiwary A, Schenker MB. Case report: potential arsenic toxicosis secondary to herbal kelp supplement. *Environ Health Perspect* 2007; 115(4): 606–608.

11 Lewis AS. Organic versus inorganic arsenic in herbal kelp supplements. *Environ Health Perspect* 2007; 115(12): A575 author reply A576A577.

12 McGuffin M, Dentali S. Safe use of herbal kelp supplements. *Environ Health Perspect* 2007; 115 (12): A575–A576; author reply A576A577.

Lactase

Description

Lactase (beta-galactosidase) is the enzyme responsible for the breakdown of lactose. Lactase is found in the brush border cells of the intestine. These cells regenerate continually and have a half-life of 2–3 days. In the absence of a challenge from lactose, production of lactase decreases ad eventually ceases altogether. Lactase is available in the form of a food supplement.

Action

Lactase breaks down lactose into the monosaccharides, galactoseand glucose. Deficiency of lactase can occur to varying degrees leading to impaired ability to digest lactose. (The sole sources of lactose in the diet are cows' milk and human milk.) Lactose remaining in the intestine can cause osmotic diarrhoea and is also fermented by colonic bacteria, resulting in symptoms such as watery diarrhoea, which is often acidic in nature and may cause perianal dermatitis. Lactase deficiency may be:

- *Congenital*. A severe and rare condition, this is characterised by complete absence of lactase which requires total and permanent lactose exclusion. Symptoms of profuse watery diarrhoea appear soon after birth. Breastfeeding is contraindicated and the use of lactose-free infant formulas is essential. Dietetic expertise is required to ensure the diet remains lactose free and nutritionally adequate from weaning onwards.
- *Primary (ethnic)*. This is an autosomal recessive disorder wherelactase may disappear slowly between infancy and adulthood if thereis no demand for it. Lactose maldigestion is low in children under 4 years of age and plateaus from the age of 13 years. Primary lactasedeficiency is common in people whose genetic origins lie in countries where milk consumption after infancy is traditionally rare (i.e. South East Asia, India, the

Middle East and parts of Africa). Prevalence may exceed 50% in South America, Africa and Asia, reaching 100% in some Asian countries. In Europe, prevalence ranges from 2% in Scandinavia to 70% in Sicily, and in the USA from 15% in white people to 80% in black people. Symptoms are similar to those in congenital lactase deficiency but are dose related and become marked only at high levels of intake (e.g. 50 g loads; cows' milk contains 50 g lactose per litre). Many people with primary lactase deficiency can therefore tolerate moderate intakes of milk and milk products, and complete lactose avoidance is unnecessary. Individual tolerance varies but most people with low lactase levels can consume 12–15 g of lactose per day (equivalent to 250 mL or half a pint of milk) without discomfort. Symptoms may be less likely if lactose is consumed with food. Lactose may be better tolerated in the form of fermented milk products such as yogurt.
- *Secondary lactase deficiency*. This is a temporary deficiency of lactase due to damage to the intestinal brush border as a result of severe gastroenteritis, intestinal surgery, untreated coeliac disease or cows' milk protein intolerance. It is characterised by diarrhoea, which persists until after the primary disorder has been treated.

Lactase deficiency can cause osteoporosis, possibly due to poorcalcium intake.[1,2]

Possible uses

Lactase (as a food supplement) is used for preventing the symptoms of lactose intolerance. Small preliminary studies have shown that lactase may reduce symptoms of lactose intolerance. An acute challenge test in 24 subjects compared lactase tablets (9900 IU) with placebo in a randomised, double-blind crossover manner. The subjects also consumed 224 ml (8 oz) whole milk to which was added 37.5 g lactose (total lactose intake, 50 g). In 21 of the subjects, the area under the hydrogen concentration–time curve (AUC) was lower after lactase than after placebo. There were no significant differences in plasma glucose levels. Subjective ratings of the severity of abdominal cramping, belching, flatulence, and diarrhoea were lower during the first 8 h after challenge in lactase-treated subjects; ratings for bloating were lower during the next 8 h.[3] A study in 52 lactose malabsorbers found that lactase 2000 IU added to 500 mL milk also reduced breath hydrogen and symptoms of lactose malabsorption,[4] while another study in eight lactose malabsorbers also found that lactase combined with milk resulted in a reduction in symptoms of lactose intolerance and an increase in blood glucose concentrations, indicating that lactose was being digested.[5] A more recent trial in 11 men and 19 women (all lactose malabsorbers) evaluated the effect of lactase (3000 IU 10 hours before milk consumption) and lactase 6000 IU 5 min before milk consumption. Breath hydrogen and clinical symptom score fell significantly in both cases compared with placebo.[6]

Lactase has been studied in children. A study in 18 older children (mean age 11.4 years) found that lactase tablets reduced breath hydrogen excretion and clinical symptoms of lactose intolerance.[7]

Trials have evaluated specific lactase preparations. One trial compared three beta-galactosidase enzyme preparations – Lactogest (soft gel capsule), Lactaid (caplet), and DairyEase (chewable tablet) with placebo – in lactose maldigesters who were fed with 20 g or 50 g of lactose. All three enzyme preparations reduced both the peak and total breath hydrogen production when fed with milk containing 20 g of lactose. Four capsules of Lactogest, two caplets of Lactaid, or two tablets of DairyEase (each treatment containing approx 6000 IU) reduced total hydrogen production significantly ($P < 0.05$) below that observed with two capsules of Lactogest (containing approximately 3000 IU) in a stoichiometric manner. Symptoms were significantly ($P < 0.05$) less severe with all the beta-galactosidase products. In contrast, with 50 g of lactose in water, peak and total hydrogen production was modestly, but not significantly, reduced by the enzyme treatment. Furthermore, symptom scores for bloating, cramping, nausea, pain, diarrhoea,

and flatus were not different between treatments and the control. The 50 g lactose dose appeared to overwhelm the ability of either 3000 or 6000 IU of beta-galactosidase to assist significantly with lactose digestion.[8] A further trial that evaluated three oral lactase preparations (Lactrase, Lactaid and DairyEase) in 10 lactose intolerant subjects found that the three products differed in their abilities to influence symptoms and breath hydrogen excretion following an 18 g lactose challenge (in ice cream). Only Lactaid reduced the breath hydrogen excretion with lactose (mean peak, area under the curve and cumulative breath hydrogen excretion; ($P < 0.05$). Lactrase and DairyEase influenced symptoms: Lactrase reduced pain, bloating and total symptomatic scores ($P < 0.05$), whereas DairyEase only reduced pain ($P < 0.05$). Lactaid administration did not reduce symptoms.[9]

Conclusion

In small controlled trials, lactase supplements have been shown to reduce symptoms of lactose malabsorption and to reduce breath hydrogen excretion. However, many patients with lactase deficiency can tolerate significant amounts of lactose without developing gastrointestinal symptoms.

Precautions/contraindications

None reported. However, lactase supplements should not be recommended in cases of congenital lactase deficiency as this condition should be managed by use of a lactose-free diet.

Pregnancy and breastfeeding

Insufficient data; avoid in pregnancy and breast feeding.

Adverse effects

None reported. Doses up to 9000 IU have been used without adverse effects.[3,8,9]

Interactions

None reported.

Dose

The typical dose of lactase is 6000–9000 IU tablets chewed and swallowed at the start of a lactose-containing meal or 2000 IU of the solution added to 500 mL of milk immediately before consumption.[4]

References

1 Horowitz M, Wishart J, Mundy L, Nordin BE. Lactose and calcium absorption in postmenopausal osteoporosis. *Arch Intern Med* 1987; 147(3): 534–536.
2 Newcomer AD, Hodgson SF, McGill DB, Thomas PJ. Lactase deficiency: prevalence in osteoporosis. *Ann Intern Med* 1978; 89(2): 218–220.
3 Sanders SW, Tolman KG, Reitberg DP. Effect of a single dose of lactase on symptoms and expired hydrogen after lactose challenge in lactose-intolerant subjects. *Clin Pharm* 1992; 11(6): 533–538.
4 Lami F, Callegari C, Tatali M, *et al.* Efficacy of addition of exogenous lactase to milk in adult lactase deficiency. *Am J Gastroenterol* 1988; 83 (10): 1145–1149.
5 Xenos K, Kyroudis S, Anagnostidis A, Papastathopoulos P. Treatment of lactose intolerance with exogenous beta-D-galactosidase in pellet form. *Eur J Drug Metab Pharmacokinet* 1998; 23 (2): 350–355.
6 Montalto M, Nucera G, Santoro L, *et al.* Effect of exogenous beta-galactosidase in patients with lactose malabsorption and intolerance: a crossover double-blind placebo-controlled study. *Eur J Clin Nutr* 2005; 59(4): 489–493.
7 Medow MS, Thek KD, Newman LJ, *et al.* Beta-galactosidase tablets in the treatment of lactose intolerance in pediatrics. *Am J Dis Child* 1990; 144(11): 1261–1264.
8 Lin MY, Dipalma JA, Martini MC, Gross CJ, Harlander SK, Savaiano DA, *et al.* Comparative effects of exogenous lactase (beta-galactosidase) preparations on in vivo lactose digestion. *Dig Dis Sci* 1993; 38(11): 2022–2027.
9 Ramirez FC, Lee K, Graham DY. All lactase preparations are not the same: results of a prospective, randomized, placebo-controlled trial. *Am J Gastroenterol* 1994; 89(4): 566–570.

Lecithin

Description

Lecithin is a phospholipid and is known as phosphatidylcholine.

Constituents

Lecithin is composed of phosphatidyl esters, mainly phosphatidylcholine, phosphatidylethanolamine, phosphatidylserine and phosphatidylinositol. It also contains varying amounts of other substances such as fatty acids, triglycerides and carbohydrates. One teaspoon (3.5 g) lecithin granules provides on average: energy 117 kJ (28 kcal), phosphatidyl choline 750 mg, phosphatidyl inositol 500 mg, choline 100 mg, inositol 100 mg, phosphorus 110 mg.

Human requirements

Lecithin is not an essential component of the diet. It is synthesised from choline.

Action

Lecithin is a source of choline (see Choline) and inositol. It is an essential component of cell membranes and a precursor to acetylcholine.

Dietary sources

Soya beans, peanuts, liver, meat, eggs.

Metabolism

About 50% of ingested lecithin enters the thoracic duct intact. The rest is degraded to glycerophosphorylcholine in the intestine, and then to choline in the liver. Plasma choline levels reflect lecithin intake.

Deficiency

Not established.

Possible uses

Lecithin is claimed to be beneficial in the treatment of disease related to impaired cholinergic function (see Choline). It has also been claimed to be of benefit in lowering serum cholesterol levels and improving memory. It is sometimes taken for dementia and Alzheimer's disease.

Cholesterol

An open clinical trial in the 1970s showed that oral lecithin in large doses (20–30 g daily) led to a significant reduction in cholesterol concentration in one out of the three healthy subjects studied and three out of the seven people with hypercholesterolaemia.[1]

However, in a double-blind study, 20 hyperlipidaemic men were randomised to receive frozen yoghurt, frozen yoghurt with 20 g soya bean lecithin or frozen yoghurt with 17 g sunflower oil. Sunflower oil was used to control for the increased intake in energy and linoleic acid from the lecithin. Lecithin treatment had no independent effect on serum lipoprotein or plasma fibrinogen levels in this group of men.[2]

A review of 24 papers examining the effect of consuming lecithin on serum cholesterol raised concern about the small size and lack of control groups in many of the studies. The authors concluded that there was no evidence for a specific effect of lecithin on serum cholesterol independent of its linoleic acid content or secondary changes in food intake. The observed lecithin-induced hypocholesterolaemic effects in the studies were artefacts caused by the manner and design of the data analysis, were mediated by dietary changes or were due to the linoleic acid present in lecithin.[3]

Alzheimer's disease

A double-blind, placebo-controlled crossover study in 11 outpatients with Alzheimer's disease found that lecithin 10 g three times a day for 3 months was associated with an improvement in tests of learning ability, but there was no improvement in any of the psychological tests used.[4]

Two further double-blind studies (one in patients with Alzheimer's disease,[5] one in normal adults[6]) showed no effect of lecithin on memory.

Another double-blind RCT in 53 subjects with probable Alzheimer's disease involved the use of lecithin and tacrine or lecithin and placebo for 36 weeks. No clinically relevant improvement was found in any of the groups over 36 weeks.[7]

A Cochrane review investigating the efficacy of lecithin in the treatment of dementia or cognitive impairment found 12 RCTs involving patients with Alzheimer's disease (265 patients), Parkinsonian dementia (21 patients) and subjective memory problems (90 patients). No trials reported any clear benefit of Alzheimer's disease or Parkinsonian dementia. A dramatic result in favour of lecithin was obtained in a trial of subjects with subjective memory problems. The authors concluded that evidence from randomised trials does not support the use of lecithin in the treatment of dementia. A moderate effect could not be ruled out, but they concluded that results from the small trials to date do not indicate priority for a large randomised trial.[8]

Conclusion

Controlled clinical trials have provided no evidence that lecithin lowers cholesterol or helps to improve memory in patients with Alzheimer's disease. Claims for the value of lecithin in lowering blood pressure and also in hepatitis, gallstones, psoriasis and eczema are unsubstantiated. Further trials are needed to assess the role of lecithin.

Precautions/contraindications

None known.

Pregnancy and breast-feeding

No problems have been reported, but there have not been sufficient studies to guarantee the safety of lecithin (in amounts greater than those found in foods) in pregnancy and breast-feeding.

Adverse effects

None reported.

Interactions

None reported.

Dose

Lecithin is available in the form of tablets, capsules and powder. Lecithin supplements provide between 20 and 90% phosphatidylcholine (depending on the product).

The dose is not established. On current evidence, lecithin is unlikely to be useful. Product manufacturers recommend 1200–2400 mg daily.

References

1 Simons LA, Hickie JB, Ruys J. Treatment of hypercholesterolaemia with oral lecithin. *Aust NZ J Med* 1977; 7: 262–266.

2 Oosthuizen W, Vorster HH, Vermaak WJ, *et al.* Lecithin has no effect on serum lipoprotein, plasma fibrinogen and macromolecular protein complex levels in hyperlipidaemic men in a double-blind controlled study. *Eur J Clin Nutr* 1998; 52: 419–424.

3 Knuiman JT, Beynen AC, Katan MB. Lecithin intake and serum cholesterol. *Am J Clin Nutr* 1989; 49: 266–268.

4 Etienne P, Dastoor D, Gauthier S, *et al.* Alzheimer disease: lack of effect of lecithin treatment for 3 months. *Neurology* 1981; 31: 1552–1554.

5 Brinkman SD, Smith RC, Meyer JS, *et al.* Lecithin and memory training in suspected Alzheimer's disease. *J Gerontol* 1982; 37: 4–9.

6 Harris CM, Dysken MW, Fovall P, Davis JM. Effect of lecithin on memory in normal adults. *Am J Psychiatry* 1983; 140: 1010–1012.

7 Maltby N, Broe GA, Creasey H, *et al.* Efficacy of tacrine and lecithin in mild to moderate Alzheimer's disease: double-blind trial. *BMJ* 1994; 308: 879–883.

8 Higgins JPT, Flicker L. Lecithin for dementia and cognitive impairment. *Cochrane Database. Syst Rev* 2000; (4): CD001015.

Magnesium

Description

Magnesium is an essential mineral. It is the second most abundant intracellular cation in the body.

Human requirements

See Table 1 for Dietary Reference Values for magnesium.

Dietary intake

In the UK, the average diet provides: for males, 336 mg daily; for females, 250 mg daily.

Action

Magnesium is an essential cofactor for enzymes requiring ATP (these are involved in glycolysis, fatty acid oxidation and amino acid metabolism). It is also required for the synthesis of RNA and replication of DNA; neuromuscular transmission; and calcium metabolism.

Dietary sources

See Table 2 for dietary sources of magnesium.

Metabolism

Absorption
Absorption of magnesium occurs principally in the jejunum and ileum by active carrier-mediated processes (partly dependent on vitamin D and parathyroid hormone) and by diffusion.

Distribution
Magnesium is widely distributed in the soft tissues and skeleton.

Elimination

Excretion is largely via the urine (magnesium homeostasis is controlled mainly by the kidneys), with unabsorbed and endogenously secreted magnesium in the faeces. Small amounts are excreted in saliva and breast milk.

Bioavailability

Bioavailability appears to be enhanced by vitamin D, but is decreased by phytates and non-starch polysaccharides (dietary fibre).

Deficiency

Signs and symptoms include hypocalcaemia and hypokalaemia; muscle spasm, tremor and tetany; personality changes, lethargy and apathy; convulsions, delirium and coma; anorexia, nausea, vomiting, abdominal pain and paralytic ileus; cardiac arrhythmias, tachycardia and sudden cardiac death.

Possible uses

Magnesium has been investigated for a role in cardiovascular disease (CVD) (including hypertension), diabetes mellitus, migraine, osteoporosis and premenstrual syndrome (PMS).

Cardiovascular disease

Low dietary and serum magnesium has been associated with CVD,[1,2] particularly in men.[3] This association has not been found in women.[4] However, dietary magnesium intake in women has been inversely associated with some markers of systemic inflammation and endothelial dysfunction[5] and heart rhythm changes.[6] Some epidemiological data have suggested a reduced mortality from coronary artery disease in populations living in hard water areas with high concentrations of magnesium in drinking water[7,8]

Table 1 Dietary Reference Values for magnesium (mg/day)

	UK				USA		WHO
						EU RDA = 14 mg	
Age	LRNI	EAR	RNI	EVM	RDA	TUL	RNI
0–3 months	30	40	55		30	–	26–36
4–6 months	40	50	60		30	–	26–36
7–9 months	45	60	75		75	–	54
10–12 months	45	60	80		75	–	54
1–3 years	50	65	85		80	65	60
4–6 years	70	90	120		–	–	76
4–8 years	–	–	–		130	110	–
7–10 years	115	150	200		170	–	100[1]
9–13 years	–	–	–	–	240	350	–
Males							
11–14 years	180	230	280		–	–	230[2]
14–18 years	–	–	–		410	350	230
15–18 years	190	250	280		–	–	–
19–50+ years	190	250	300	300	–	–	260[3]
19–30 years	–	–	–		400	350	–
31–70+ years	–	–	–		420	350	–
Females							
11–14 years	180	230	280		–	–	220[2]
14–18 years	–	–	–		360	350	220
15–18 years	190	250	300		310	–	–
19–50 years	190	250	300	300	280	–	260[4]
50+ years	150	200	270	300	280	–	–
19–30 years	–	–	–		310	350	–
31–70+ years	–	–	–		320	350	–
Pregnancy	*	*	*	360–400	350	220	–
Lactation			+50		320–360	350	270

* No increment.
[1] 7–9 years;   [2] 10–14 years;   [3] > 65 years = 224 mg;   [4] > 65 years = 190 mg.
EAR = Estimated Average Requirement.
EVM = Likely safe daily intake from supplements alone.
LRNI = Lowest Reference Nutrient Intake.
RNI = Reference Nutrient Intake.
TUL = Tolerable Upper Intake Level.

Other data, however, have indicated no such association,[9] and a large cohort study in which 2512 older men were followed for 10 years also provided no evidence of a protective role for magnesium in CVD.

Marginal magnesium status has been implicated in myocardial infarction, but reduced serum magnesium levels found in some patients with myocardial infarct patients may be a result of the infarction rather than the cause of it. However, one double-blind placebo-controlled study in patients with acute myocardial infarction showed reduced serum triglyceride concentrations and tendencies towards increased HDL

Table 2 Dietary sources of magnesium

Food portion	Magnesium content (mg)
Breakfast cereals	
1 bowl *All-Bran* (45 g)	90
1 bowl *Bran Flakes* (45 g)	50
1 bowl Corn Flakes (30 g)	5
1 bowl *muesli* (95 g)	90
2 pieces *Shredded Wheat*	50
2 *Weetabix*	50
Cereal products	
Bread, brown, 2 slices	40
white, 2 slices	15
wholemeal, 2 slices	60
1 chapati	30
Pasta, brown, boiled (150 g)	60
white, boiled (150 g)	25
Rice, brown, boiled (165 g)	60
white, boiled (165 g)	15
Milk and dairy products	
Milk, whole, semi-skimmed or	35
skimmed (284 ml; $^1/_2$ pint)	
1 pot yoghurt (150 g)	30
Cheese (50 g)	12
1 egg, size 2 (60 g)	10
Meat and fish	
Meat, cooked (100 g)	25
Liver, lambs, cooked (90 g)	20
Kidney, lambs, cooked (75 g)	20
White fish, cooked (150 g)	30
Pilchards, canned (105 g)	40
Sardines, canned (70 g)	35
Shrimps (80 g)	49
Tuna, canned (95 g)	30
Vegetables	
Green vegetables, average, boiled (100 g)	20
Potatoes, boiled (150 g)	20
1 small can *baked beans* (200 g)	60
Lentils, kidney beans or other pulses (105 g)	50
Fruit	
1 banana	35
1 orange	20
Nuts	
20 *almonds*	50
10 *Brazil nuts*	80
30 *hazelnuts*	50
30 *peanuts*	70

Note: Hard drinking water may contribute significantly to intake. Excellent sources (**bold**); good sources (*italics*).

cholesterol concentrations after oral magnesium supplementation.[10]

Oral magnesium supplementation therapy has been associated in placebo-controlled trials with inhibition of platelet-dependent thrombosis,[11,12] improved endothelial function[13,14] in patients with coronary artery disease, reduced levels of C-reactive protein (a biomarker of inflammation),[15] improved heart rate variability in patients with heart failure,[16] and improved post-meal hyperlipidaemia in healthy people.[17] In people with low dietary magnesium intake (<50% of the RDA), individuals taking magnesium supplements were 22% less likely to have elevated C-reactive protein (a marker of inflammation).[18]

A trial in 187 people found that oral magnesium 365 mg daily for 6 months increased exercise duration time compared with placebo, and decreased exercise-induced chest pain. Quality of life parameters significantly improved in the magnesium group. The authors concluded that these findings suggest that oral magnesium supplementation for 6 months in patients with coronary artery disease results in a significant improvement in exercise tolerance, exercise-induced chest pain and quality of life, suggesting a mechanism whereby magnesium could beneficially alter outcomes in patients with coronary artery disease.[19]

A more recent trial in 53 men with stable coronary artery disease found that magnesium therapy (15 mmol; 375 mg daily) for 6 months improved exercise tolerance (as judged by increase in maximal oxygen uptake) and left ventricular function.[20]

Some controlled studies have suggested that intravenous magnesium given early after suspected myocardial infarction could reduce the frequency of serious arrhythmias and mortality. However, magnesium has been given as a prescription medicine in these cases and not as a dietary supplement.

Blood pressure

There is some evidence that magnesium reduces blood pressure.[21] A 20 mmol increase in daily magnesium intake resulted in a diastolic blood pressure fall of 3.4 mmHg in a trial in Dutch women.[22] A reduction in blood pressure occurred with a low-sodium, high-potassium, high-magnesium salt in older patients with mild to moderate hypertension and suggested that the increased magnesium intake could have contributed to the fall in blood pressure.[23]

However, another study[24] showed that magnesium supplementation did not have an additive hypotensive effect in mild hypertensive subjects on a reduced sodium intake. Another group,[25] using a double-blind randomised crossover design, detected no fall in blood pressure with magnesium supplementation, despite a significant increase in plasma magnesium concentration.

More recent double-blind placebo-controlled trials[26,27] have shown no effect of magnesium supplementation (300–360 mg) on blood pressure in healthy subjects and those with mild to moderate hypertension.[28]

A meta-analysis of 20 randomised trials involving 1220 subjects found that magnesium supplementation produced a modest dose-dependent blood pressure lowering effect.[29] For each 250 mg daily increase in magnesium intake, systolic blood pressure fell by a further 4.3 mmHg and diastolic blood pressure by 2.3 mmHg.

In a Cochrane review of 12 RCTs (total of 545 subjects and inclusion of trials with 8–26 weeks follow-up), magnesium supplementation did not significantly reduce systolic blood pressure (mean difference −1.3 mmHg, 95% confidence interval (CI), −4.0 to 1.5) but did significantly reduce diastolic blood pressure (mean difference: −2.2 mmHg, 95% CI, −3.4 to −0.9). However, the reviewers concluded that trials were of poor quality and therefore likely to have overestimated effects, making the evidence in favour of a causal association between magnesium supplementation and blood pressure reduction weak.[30]

Further studies conducted since this meta-analysis have continued to be inconsistent in their findings. A 12-week study in which 24 mildly hypertensive patients were assigned to 600 mg magnesium daily or lifestyle advice found that magnesium reduced blood pressure to a small but consistent extent.[31] Results from a trial in 155 overweight, non-diabetic adults with normal plasma magnesium suggested that magnesium supplementation (300 mg daily) does not reduce blood pressure and enhance insulin sensitivity in normo-magnesaemic non-diabetic overweight people. However, in a subgroup analysis, magnesium supplementation lowered blood pressure in healthy adults with higher blood pressure.[32]

Lack of effect of magnesium on blood pressure was also found in a trial of 17 patients with mild to moderate essential hypertension and whose average blood pressure after two months of observation with no treatment was 154/100 mmHg. They were entered into a double-blind randomised crossover study of 1 month's treatment with magnesium aspartate (15 mmol magnesium daily) and treatment with placebo for a further month. This preparation of magnesium was well tolerated and did not cause diarrhoea. Despite a significant increase in plasma magnesium concentration and a significant increase in urinary excretion of magnesium while taking magnesium aspartate, there was no fall in blood pressure compared with either treatment with placebo or values before treatment.[33]

Diabetes mellitus

Magnesium modulates glucose transport across cell membranes, and is a cofactor in various pathways involving enzymatic oxidation. Individuals with diabetes, especially those with glycosuria and ketoacidosis, may have excessive urinary losses of magnesium.[34,35] Hypomagnesaemia is common in these patients and can potentially cause insulin resistance.[36] Magnesium intake was not related to diabetes risk in the European Prospective Investigation Into Cancer cohort study,[37] but a meta-analysis published as part of the same paper showed a significant inverse association (relative risk of extreme categories of magnesium intake, 0.77; 95% CI, 0.72 to 0.84).[37]

In a cohort study involving 1223 men and 1485 women without diabetes, magnesium intake was inversely associated with fasting insulin, post-glucose challenge plasma insulin and insulin resistance. No significant association was found between magnesium intake and fasting glucose or 2-hour post-challenge glucose.[38]

One study has shown that insulin secretory capacity improved with dietary magnesium supplementation for 4 weeks.[39] The effect of diabetes on tissue content of magnesium is variable and cannot always be predicted from serum magnesium measurements. Epidemiologically, magnesium deficiency has been associated with diabetic neuropathy,[40] and although there is no evidence to indicate that magnesium supplementation can alter this complication, the magnesium status of patients at risk of magnesium depletion (e.g. those on thiazides) should be assessed. However, monitoring is difficult and a dose for patients with diabetes mellitus has not been established.

In an open trial, 11 patients with type 1 diabetes and persistently low erythrocyte magnesium levels were given 450 mg magnesium following an intravenous loading dose of magnesium. During intravenous loading, plasma magnesium decreased and erythrocyte magnesium increased. Supplementation did not normalise magnesium status, and there were no significant changes in glycated haemoglobin or serum lipid levels. The authors concluded that chronic magnesium depletion may occur in type 1 diabetes and that it is difficult to replete and maintain body stores.[41]

In a double-blind, placebo-controlled trial, 128 Brazilian patients with type 2 diabetes were randomised to receive 497 mg magnesium, 994 mg magnesium or placebo. At the start of the study, 47.7% of the patients had low plasma magnesium and 31.1% had low intramononuclear magnesium levels. Intracellular magnesium was significantly lower than in the normal population and was lower in those with peripheral neuropathy than those without. However, there was no correlation between plasma and intracellular magnesium and glycaemic control. In the groups on placebo and lower-dose magnesium, neither a change in plasma nor intracellular magnesium occurred and there was no change in glycaemic control. The higher dose of magnesium was associated with an increase in plasma and intracellular magnesium and a significant fall in fructosamine.[42]

In a placebo-controlled (not blinded) study, involving 50 patients with type 2 diabetes, supplementation with 360 mg magnesium daily over 3 months increased plasma magnesium and urinary magnesium excretion, but had no effect on glycaemic control or lipid concentration.[43]

More recent trials have shown that oral magnesium supplementation improves insulin sensitivity and metabolic control in type 2 diabetic patients with decreased serum magnesium levels,[44] and also improves insulin sensitivity in non-diabetic subjects with decreased magnesium levels.[45]

Premenstrual syndrome

Reduced magnesium levels have been reported in women affected by PMS. An Italian double-blind randomised study[46] in 32 women showed that a supplement of 360 mg magnesium daily improved premenstrual symptoms related to mood changes. More recently, a randomised, double-blind, placebo-controlled study[47] in 38 women showed no effect of magnesium supplementation (200 mg daily) in the first month, but symptoms including weight gain, swelling of extremities, breast tenderness and abdominal bloating, improved during the second month. A further study[48] in 44 women lasting 1 month showed that magnesium 200 mg daily plus vitamin B_6 50 mg daily produced a modest effect on anxiety-related premenstrual symptoms.

Migraine

There is some evidence that magnesium supplementation is effective in migraine, but results from studies are equivocal. Thus, oral magnesium was effective in reducing the frequency of migraine in a 12-week, placebo-controlled, double-blind study.[49] There was also a reduction in the average duration of pain and need for acute medication, although these changes were not significant. However, in another similar study, magnesium had no effect.[50] A further trial compared a placebo containing riboflavin 25 mg with a treatment containing riboflavin 400 mg, magnesium 300 mg and feverfew 100 mg. The placebo response in this trial was high and there was no difference between placebo and treatment.[51] The possibility that magnesium supplementation has differing effects depending on type of migraine was investigated in a study looking at 30 patients who suffered migraine without aura. The dose of magnesium was 600 mg daily, which significantly reduced the frequency and severity of attacks and was associated with changes in cortical blood flow compared with placebo.[52]

Osteoporosis

Magnesium is a constituent of bone, and supplementation has been shown to increase bone density in individuals with osteoporosis. Increased magnesium intake is associated with a lower decline in BMD after the menopause.[53] Supplements have been shown to decrease markers of bone turnover in young men,[54] but not young women.[55] Bone density increased in adolescent girls,[56] patients with gluten-sensitive enteropathy and associated osteoporosis,[57] and also in menopausal women[58] who were given oral magnesium. Oral magnesium has also been shown to suppress bone turnover in post-menopausal women.[59]

Gallstones

Magnesium has recently been evaluated for a role in gallstone disease. Since magnesium deficiency can cause dyslipidaemia and insulin hypersecretion, this may facilitate gallstone formation. In a US cohort study involving 42 705 men, the multivariate relative risk (RR) of total magnesium intake was 0.72 (CI, 0.61 to 0.86; P (trend) $= 0.006$) and for dietary magnesium it was 0.68 (CI, 0.57 to 0.82; P(trend) $= 0.0006$), indicating a protective role of magnesium consumption in the prevention of symptomatic gallstones among men.[60]

Athletes

Magnesium supplementation has been suggested to improve athletic performance. In one double-blind, placebo-controlled study,[61] magnesium (507 mg versus 246 mg daily) improved muscular strength, and in another similar study,[62] swimming, running and cycling performance was improved. However, in a 2-week study,[63] athletes taking magnesium 500 mg daily did not demonstrate improved performance or reduced muscle tiredness.

Cancer

Epidemiological studies have shown an association between magnesium and colon cancer in women. A prospective cohort study among 61 433 Swedish women aged 40–75 years found an inverse association of magnesium intake with colorectal cancer.[64] Another prospective cohort study among 35 196 Iowa women aged 55–69 years found an inverse association between magnesium intake and colon cancer, but this association was largely lacking for rectal cancer.[65]

Pregnancy

Many women, particularly those from disadvantaged backgrounds, have intakes of magnesium below recommended levels. Magnesium supplementation has been investigated for possible benefit in reducing foetal growth retardation and pre-eclampsia, and increasing birth weight. A Cochrane review found seven trials involving 2689 women. Six of these trials randomly allocated women to either oral magnesium or control, while the largest trial with 985 women had a cluster design where randomisation was according to a study centre. The analysis was conducted with and without this trial. When all seven trials were included, oral magnesium from the 25th week of pregnancy was associated with lower frequency of pre-term birth, a lower frequency of low birth weight, fewer small for gestational age infants and fewer cases of antepartum haemorrhage compared with placebo. In the analysis excluding the cluster trial the effects were no different between treatment and placebo. Only one of the trials was judged to be of high quality, with the others likely to have resulted in a bias favouring magnesium supplementation. The review concluded that there is not enough high-quality evidence to show that dietary magnesium supplementation during pregnancy is beneficial.[66] A further review concluded that magnesium, used after threatened pre-term labour, does not reduce pre-term birth or improve the outcome for the infant.[67]

Miscellaneous

In preliminary trials, magnesium supplementation has been shown to exert antioxidant activity in children with asthma,[68] to improve symptoms of depression in elderly patients with diabetes,[69] prevent reduction of thyroid hormone activity in sports people[70] and to lead to changes in gene expression and proteomic profiling consistent with improved metabolic outcomes in overweight individuals.[71]

Conclusion

Epidemiological studies show an association between marginal magnesium status and CVD and hypertension. However, the effect of supplementation is equivocal and any effect appears to be small. Patients with diabetes often have poor magnesium status, but supplementation does not appear to have an effect on glucose control, possibly because it is difficult to replete and maintain adequate magnesium levels. Preliminary evidence suggests that magnesium could reduce the frequency and pain of migraine and may help the symptoms of PMS. There is no good evidence that magnesium improves performance in athletes.

Precautions/contraindications

Doses exceeding the RDA are best avoided in renal impairment.

Pregnancy and breast-feeding

No problems reported with normal intakes.

Adverse effects

Toxicity from oral ingestion is unlikely in individuals with normal renal function. Doses of 3–5 g have a cathartic effect. High blood levels of magnesium related to laxative abuse and high antacid use has been associated with reduced survival probability.[72]

Interactions

Drugs

Alcohol: excessive alcohol intake increases renal excretion of magnesium.
Loop diuretics: increased excretion of magnesium.
4-quinolones: may reduce absorption of 4-quinolones; give 2 h apart.
Tetracyclines: may reduce absorption of tetracyclines; give 2 h apart.
Thiazide diuretics: increased excretion of magnesium.

Dose

Magnesium is available in the form of tablets and capsules. It is available in isolation, in combination with calcium (and sometimes with vitamin D) and in multivitamin and mineral preparations.

The dose is not established. Dietary supplements provide 100–500 mg per dose.

References

1 Liao F, Folsom AR, Brancati FL. Is low magnesium concentration a risk factor for coronary heart disease? The Atherosclerosis Risk in Communities (ARIC) Study. *Am Heart J* 1998; 136: 480–490.

2 Abbott RD, Ando F, Masaki KH, *et al.* Dietary magnesium intake and the future risk of coronary heart disease (the Honolulu Heart Program). *Am J Cardiol* 2003; 92: 665–669.

3 Al-Delaimy WK, Rimm EB, Willett WC, *et al.* Magnesium intake and risk of coronary heart disease among men. *J Am Coll Nutr* 2004; 23: 63–70.

4 Song Y, Manson JE, Cook NR, *et al.* Dietary magnesium intake and risk of cardiovascular disease among women. *Am J Cardiol* 2005; 96: 1135–1141.

5 Song Y, Li TY, vanDam RM, *et al.* Magnesium intake and plasma concentrations of markers of systemic inflammation and endothelial dysfunction in women. *Am J Clin Nutr* 2007; 85: 1068–1074.

6 Nielsen FH, Milne DB, Klevay LM, *et al.* Dietary magnesium deficiency induces heart rhythm changes, impairs glucose tolerance, and decreases serum cholesterol in post menopausal women. *J Am Coll Nutr* 2007; 26: 121–132.

7 The Caerphilly and Speedwell Collaborative Group Caerphilly and Speedwell collaborative heart disease studies. *J Epidemiol Community Health* 1984; 38: 259–262.

8 Rubenowitz E, Molin I, Axelsson G, Rylander R. Magnesium in drinking water in relation to morbidity and mortality from acute myocardial infarction. *Epidemiology* 2000; 11: 416–421.

9 Rosenlund M, Berglind N, Hallqvist J, *et al.* Daily intake of magnesium and calcium from drinking water in relation to myocardial infarction. *Epidemiology* 2005; 16: 570–576.

10 Rasmussen HS, Aurup P, Goldstein K, *et al.* Influence of magnesium substitution therapy on blood lipid composition in patients with ischaemic heart disease. A double-blind, placebo controlled study. *Arch Intern Med* 1989; 149: 1050–1053.

11 Shechter M, Merz CN, Paul-Labrador M, *et al.* Oral magnesium supplementation inhibits platelet dependent thrombosis in patients with coronary artery disease. *Am J Cardiol* 1999; 84: 152–156.

12 Shechter M, Merz CN, Paul-Labrador M, *et al.* Beneficial antithrombotic effects of the association of pharmacological oral magnesium therapy with aspirin in coronary heart disease patients. *Magnes Res* 2000; 13: 275–284.

13 Shechter M, Sharir M, Labrador MJ, *et al.* Oral magnesium therapy improves endothelial function in patients with coronary artery disease. *Circulation* 2000; 102: 2353–2358.

14 Fuentes JC, Salmon AA, Silver MA. Acute and chronic oral magnesium supplementation: effects on endothelial function, exercise capacity, and quality of life in patients with symptomatic heart failure. *Congest Heart Fail* 2006; 12: 9–13.

15 Almoznino-Sarafian D, Berman S, Mor A, *et al.* Magnesium and C-reactive protein in heart failure: an anti-inflammatory effect of magnesium administration? *Eur J Nutr* 2010; 46: 230–237.

16 Almoznino-Sarafian D, Sarafian G, Berman S, *et al.* Magnesium administration may improve heart rate variability in patients with heart failure. *Nutr Metab Cardiovasc Dis* 2010; 19: 641–645.

17 Kishimoto T, Tani M, Uto-Kondo H, *et al.* Effects of magnesium on postprandial serum lipid responses in healthy human subjects. *Br J Nutr* 2010; 103: 469–472.

18 King DE, Mainous AG,III Geesey ME, *et al.* Magnesium supplement intake and C-reactive protein levels in adults. *Nutrition Res* 2006; 26: 193–196.

19 Shechter M, Bairey Merz CN, Stuchlinger HG, *et al.* Effects of oral magnesium therapy on exercise tolerance, exercise-induced chest pain, and quality of life in patients with coronary artery disease. *Am J Cardiol* 2003; 91: 517–521.

20 Pokan R, Hofmann P, von Duvillard SP, *et al.* Oral magnesium therapy, exercise heart rate, exercise tolerance, and myocardial function in coronary artery disease patients. *Br J Sports Med* 2006; 40: 773–778.

21 Widman L, Webster PO, Stegmayr BK, Wirell M. The dose-dependent reduction in blood pressure through administration of magnesium. *Am J Hypertension* 1993; 6: 41–45.

22 Witteman JCM, Grobbee DE, Derkx FHM, *et al.* Reduction of blood pressure with oral magnesium supplementation in women with mild to moderate hypertension. *Am J Clin Nutr* 1994; 60: 129–135.

23 Geleijnse JM, Witteman JCM, Bak AAA, *et al.* Reduction in blood pressure with a low sodium, high potassium, high magnesium salt in older subjects with mild to moderate hypertension. *BMJ* 1994; 309: 436–440.

24 Nowson CA, Morgan TO. Magnesium supplementation in mild hypertensive patients on a moderately low sodium diet. *Clin Exp Pharmacol Physiol* 1989; 16: 299–302.

25 Cappuccio FP, Markandu ND, Beynon GW, *et al.* Lack of effect of oral magnesium on high blood pressure: a double-blind study. *BMJ* 1985; 291: 235–238.

26 Sacks FM, Willet WC, Smith A, *et al.* Effect on blood pressure of potassium, calcium and magnesium in women with low habitual intake. *Hypertension* 1998; 31: 131–138.

27 Yamamoto ME, Applegate WB, Klag MJ, *et al.* Lack of blood pressure effect with calcium and magnesium supplementation in adults with high-normal blood pressure. Reports from phase I of the Trials of Hypertension Prevention (TOHP). Trials of Hypertension Prevention (TOHP) Collaborative Research Group. *Ann Epidemiol* 1995; 5: 96–107.

28 Ferrara LA, Iannuzzi R, Castaldo A, *et al.* Long-term magnesium supplementation in essential hypertension. *Cardiology* 1992; 81: 25–33.

29 Jee SH, Miller ER, Gullar E, *et al.* The effect of magnesium supplementation on blood pressure: a metaanalysis of randomized controlled trials. *Am J Hypertens* 2002; 15: 691–696.

30 Dickinson HO, Nicolson DJ, Campbell F, *et al.* Magnesium supplementation for the management of essential hypertension in adults. *Cochrane Database Syst Rev* 2006; (3): CD004640.

31 Hatzistavri LS, P.A. S, Georgianos P.I., *et al.* Oral magnesium supplementation reduces ambulatory blood pressure in patients with mild hypertension. *Am J Hypertens* 2009; 22: 1070–1075.

32 Lee S, Park HK, Son SP, *et al.* Effects of oral magnesium supplementation on insulin sensitivity and blood pressure in normo-magnesemic nondiabetic overweight Korean adults. *Nutr Metab Cardiovasc Dis* 2009; 19: 781–788.

33 Cappuccio FP, Markandu ND, Beynon GW, *et al.* Lack of effect of oralmagnesium on high blood pressure: a double blindstudy. *BMJ* 1985; 291: 235–238.

34 Fujii S, Takemura T, Wada M, *et al.* Magnesium levels in plasma, erythrocyte and urine in patients with diabetes mellitus. *Horm Metab Res* 1982; 14: 161–162.

35 McNair P, Christensen MS, Christiansen C, *et al.* Renal hypomagnesaemia in human diabetes mellitus: its relation to glucose homeostasis. *Eur J Clin Invest* 1982; 12: 81–85.

36 Jain AP, Gupta NN, Kumar A. Some metabolic effects of magnesium in diabetes mellitus. *J Assoc Physicians India* 1976; 24: 827–831.

37 Schulze MB, Schulz M, Heidemann C, *et al.* Fiber and magnesium intake and incidence of type 2 diabetes: a prospective study and meta-analysis. *Arch Intern Med* 2007; 167: 956–965.

38 Rumawas ME, McKeown NM, Rogers G, *et al.* Magnesium intake is related to improved insulin homeostasis in the Framingham offspring cohort. *J Am Coll Nutr* 2006; 25: 486–492.

39 Paolisso G, Passariello N, Pizza G, *et al.* Dietary magnesium supplements improve cell response to glucose and arginine in elderly non-insulin dependent diabetic subjects. *Acta Endocrinol* 1989; 121: 16–20.

40 McNair P, Christiansen C, Madsbad S, *et al.* Hypomagnesaemia, a risk factor in diabetic nephropathy. *Diabetes* 1978; 27: 1075–1077.

41 De Leeuw I, Engelen W, Vertommen J, *et al.* Effect of intensive IV + oral magnesium supplementation on circulating ion levels, lipid parameters, and metabolic control in Mg-depleted insulin-dependent diabetic patients (IDDM). *Magnes Res* 1997; 10: 135–141.

42 Lima Mde L, Cruz T, Pousada JC, *et al.* The effect of magnesium supplementation in increasing doses on the control of type 2 diabetes. *Diabetes Care* 1998; 21: 682–686.

43 de Valk HW, Verkaaik R, van Rijn HJ, *et al.* Oral magnesium supplementation in insulin-requiring type 2 diabetic patients. *Diabet Med* 1998; 15: 503–507.

44 Rodriguez-Moran M, Guerrero-Romero F. Oral magnesium supplementation improves insulin sensitivity and metabolic control in type 2 diabetic subjects: a randomized double-blind controlled trial. *Diabetes Care* 2003; 26: 1147–1152.

45 Guerrero-Romero F, Tamez-Perez HE, Gonzalez-Gonzalez G, *et al.* Oral magnesium supplementation improves insulin sensitivity in non-diabetic subjects with insulin resistance. A double-blind placebo controlled randomized trial. *Diabetes Metab* 2004; 30: 253–258.

46 Facchinetti F, Borella P, Sances G, *et al.* Oral magnesium successfully relieves premenstrual mood changes. *Obstet Gynecol* 1991; 78: 177–181.

47 Walker AF, DeSouza MC, Vickers MF, *et al.* Magnesium supplementation alleviates premenstrual symptoms of fluid retention. *J Womens Health* 1998; 7: 1157–1165.

48 De Souza MC, Walker AF, Robinson PA, Bolland K. A synergistic effect of a daily supplement for 1 month of 200 mg magnesium plus 50 mg vitamin B6 for the relief of anxiety related premenstrual symptoms: a randomized, double-blind, crossover study. *J Women's Health Gend Based Med* 2000; 9: 131–139.

49 Peikert A, Wilimzig C, Kohne-Volland R. Prophylaxis of migraine with oral magnesium: results from a progressive multi-center, placebo-controlled and double blind randomized study. *Cephalagia* 1996; 16: 257–263.

50 Pfaffenrath V, Wessely P, Meyer C. Magnesium in the prophylaxis of migraine: a double blind, placebo-controlled study. *Cephalagia* 1996; 16: 436–440.

51 Maizels M, Blumenfeld A, Burchette R. A combination of riboflavin, magnesium, and feverfew for migraine prophylaxis: a randomized trial. *Headache* 2004; 44: 885–890.

52 Koseoglu E, Talaslioglu A, Gonul AS, *et al.* The effects of magnesium prophylaxis in migraine without aura. *Magnes Res* 2008; 21: 101–108.

53 Tucker AK, Hannan MT, Chen H. Potassium, magnesium, and fruit and vegetable intakes are associated with greater bone mineral density in elderly men and women. *Am J Clin Nutr* 1999; 69: 727–736.

54 Dimai HP, Porta S, Wirnsberger G. Daily oral magnesium supplementation suppresses bone turnover in young adult males. *J Clin Endocrinol Metab* 1998; 83: 2742–2748.

55 Doyle L, Flynn A, Cashman K. The effect of magnesium supplementation on biochemical markers of bone metabolism or blood pressure in healthy young adult females. *Eur J Clin Nutr* 1999; 53: 255–261.

56 Carpenter TO, DeLucia MC, Zhang JH, *et al.* A randomized controlled study of effects of dietary magnesium oxide supplementation on bone mineral content in healthy girls. *J Clin Endocrinol Metab* 2006; 91: 4866–4872.

57 Rude RK, Olerich M. Magnesium deficiency: possible role in osteoporosis associated with gluten-sensitive enteropathy. *Osteoporosis Int* 1996; 6: 453–461.

58 Stendig-Limberg G, Tepper R, Leichter R. Trabecular bone density in a two year controlled trial of peroral magnesium in osteoporosis. *Magnes Res* 1993; 6: 155–163.

59 Aydin H, Deyneli O, Yavuz D, *et al.* Short-term oral magnesium supplementation suppresses bone turnover in postmenopausal osteoporotic women. *Biol Trace Elem Res* 2010; 133: 136–139.

60 Tsai CJ, Leitzmann MF, Willett WC, Giovannucci EL. Long-term effect of magnesium consumption on the risk of symptomatic gallstone disease among men. *Am J Gastroenterol* 2008; 103: 375–382.

61 Brilla LR, Haley TF. Effect of magnesium supplementation on strength training in humans. *J Am Coll Nutr* 1992; 11: 326–329.

62 Golf SW, Bender S, Gruttner J. On the significance of magnesium in extreme physical stress. *Cardiovasc Drugs Ther* 1998; 12(Suppl 2): 197–202.

63 Weller E, Backert P, Meinck HM. Lack of effect of oral Mg-supplementation on magnesium in serum, blood cells, and calf muscle. *Med Sci Sport Exerc* 1998; 30: 1584–1591.

64 Larsson SC, Bergkvist L, Wolk A. Magnesium intake in relation to risk of colorectal cancer in women. *JAMA* 2005; 293: 87–89.

65 Folsom AR, Hong Ching-Ping. Magnesium intake and reduced risk of colon cancer in a prospective study of women. *Am J Epidemiol* 2006; 163: 232–235.

66 Makrides M, Crowther CA. Magnesium supplementation in pregnancy. *Cochrane Database Syst Rev* 2001; (4): CD000937.

67 Crowther CA, Moore V. Magnesium maintenance therapy for preventing preterm birth after threatended preterm labour. *The Cochrane Database of Systematic Reviews* 1998;(1): CD000940.

68 Bede O, Nagy D, Suranyi A, *et al.* Effects of magnesium supplementation on the glutathione redox system in atopic asthmatic children. *Inflamm Res* 2010; 57: 279–286.

69 Barragan-Rodriguez M, Rodriguez-Moran M, Guerrero-Romero F. Efficacy and safety of oral magnesium supplementation in the treatment of depression in the elderly with type 2 diabetes: a randomized, equivalent trial. *Magnes Res* 2010; 21: 218–223.

70 Cinar V. The effects of magnesium supplementation on thyroid hormones of sedentars and Tae-Kwon-Do sportsperson at resting and exhaustion. *Neuroendocrinol Lett* 2010; 28: 708–712.

71 Chacko SA, Sul J, Song Y, *et al.* Magnesium supplementation, metabolic and inflammatory markers, and global genomic and proteomic profiling: a randomized, double-blind, controlled, crossover trial in overweight individuals. *Am J Clin Nutr* 2011; 93(2): 463–473.

72 Corbi G, Ancafora D, Iannuzzi GL, *et al.* Hypermagnesemia predicts mortality in elderly withcongestive heart disease: relationship with laxative and antacid use. *Rejuvenation Res* 2008; 11: 129–138.

Manganese

Description

Manganese is an essential trace mineral.

Human requirements

No Reference Nutrient Intake or Estimated Average Requirement has been set for manganese in the UK, but a safe and adequate intake is: for adults, 1.4 mg daily; infants, 10 μg daily. The UK safe upper intake from supplements alone is 5 mg daily for adults.

In the USA, the daily adequate intakes (AIs) are: for infants 0–6 months, 0.003 mg, 7–12 months, 0.6 mg; children, 1–3 years, 1.2 mg, 4–8 years, 1.5 mg; males, 9–13 years, 1.9 mg, 14–18 years, 2.2 mg, 19–70+ years, 2.3 mg; females 9–18 years, 1.6 mg, 19–70+ years, 1.8 mg, pregnancy 2.0 mg, breast-feeding 2.6 mg.

The daily Tolerable Upper Intake Level from food, water and supplements is: for children 1–3 years, 2 mg, 4–8 years, 3 mg; 9–13 years, 6 mg, 14–18 years, 9 mg, 19–70+ years, 11 mg, pregnancy, 9 mg, breast-feeding 11 mg.

Dietary intake

In the UK, the average adult diet provides 4.6–5.4 mg daily.

Action

Manganese activates several enzymes, including hydroxylases, kinases, decarboxylases and transferases. It is also a constituent of several metalloenzymes, such as arginase, pyruvate carboxylase, and also superoxide dismutase, which protects cells from free radical attack. It may have a role in the regulation of glucose homeostasis and in calcium mobilisation.

Dietary sources

See Table 1 for dietary sources of manganese.

Table 1 Dietary sources of manganese

Food portion	Manganese content (mg)
Cereal products	
Bread, brown, 2 slices	**1**
white, 2 slices	0.3
wholemeal, 2 slices	**1.5**
Milk and dairy products	
Milk and cheese	Traces
Meat and fish	
Meat and fish	Traces
Liver, lambs, cooked (90 g)	0.4
Vegetables	
1 small can baked beans (200 g)	0.6
Lentils, kidney beans or other pulses (105 g)	**1–1.5**
Green vegetables, average, boiled (100 g)	0.2
Fruit	
1 banana	0.5
Blackberries, stewed (100 g)	**1.5**
Pineapple, canned (150 g)	**1.5**
Nuts	
20 almonds	0.3
10 Brazil nuts	0.4
30 hazelnuts	**1.0**
30 peanuts	0.7
Tea, 1 cup	0.3

Note: Some other foods (e.g. breakfast cereals) contain significant quantities, but there is no reliable information on the amount.
Excellent sources (>1 mg/portion) (**bold**).

Metabolism

Absorption

Absorption of manganese occurs throughout the length of the small intestine, probably via a saturable carrier mechanism, but absorptive efficiency is believed to be poor.

Distribution

Manganese is transported in the blood bound to plasma proteins. Organs with the highest concentrations include the liver, kidney and pancreas, but 25% of the body pool is found within the skeleton. Homeostasis is maintained by hepatobiliary and intestinal secretion.

Elimination

Manganese is eliminated primarily in the faeces.

Bioavailability

Bioavailability of manganese appears to be enhanced by vitamin C and meat-containing diets, but is decreased by iron and non-starch polysaccharides (dietary fibre). Although tea contains large amounts of manganese, it is essentially unavailable to humans.

Deficiency

Manganese deficiency in individuals consuming mixed diets is very rare. Symptoms thought to be associated with deficiency (which have occurred only on semi-purified diets) include weight loss, dermatitis, hypocholesterolaemia, depressed growth of hair and nails and reddening of black hair.

Possible uses

Diabetes

Manganese has been claimed to be useful in diabetes mellitus. A relationship between dietary manganese and carbohydrate metabolism in humans has been suggested.[1] This paper described the case of a diabetic patient resistant to insulin therapy who responded to oral manganese with a consistent drop in blood glucose levels. However, there is insufficient evidence to warrant recommendation of manganese supplements to patients with diabetes.

Miscellaneous

Manganese supplements have also been used to treat inflammatory conditions such as rheumatoid arthritis, on the basis that manganese

supplementation has been shown to raise levels of superoxide dismutase, which may protect against oxidative damage.[2]

Precautions/contraindications

No problems reported.

Pregnancy and breast-feeding

No problems reported at normal doses.

Adverse effects

Manganese is essentially non-toxic when administered orally. Toxic reactions in humans occur only as the result of the chronic inhalation of large amounts of manganese found in mines and some industrial plants. Signs include severe psychiatric abnormalities and neurological disorders similar to Parkinson's disease.

Interactions

None reported.

Dose

Manganese is available in the form of tablets and capsules.

The dose is not established. Dietary supplements provide 5–50 mg per dose.

Upper safety levels

The UK Expert Group on Vitamins and Minerals (EVM) has identified a likely safe total intake of manganese for adults from supplements alone of 4 mg daily.

References

1   Rubenstein AH, Levin NW, Elliot GA. Manganese-induced hypoglycaemia. *Lancet* 1962; 2: 1348–1351.
2   Pasquier C. Manganese containing superoxide dismutase deficiency in polymorphonuclear lymphocytes in rheumatoid arthritis. *Inflammation* 1984; 8: 27–32.

Melatonin

Description

Melatonin is a hormone synthesised by the pineal gland. It is synthesised from tryptophan, which is converted to serotonin and this in turn is converted to melatonin. Melatonin is secreted in a 24-h circadian rhythm, regulating the normal sleep–wake periods. Secretion starts as soon as darkness falls, normally peaking between 02:00 and 04:00, and synthesis is inhibited by exposure to light. Daily output is greatest in young adults and production declines after the age of 20 years.

Action

Melatonin has a role in the regulation of sleep, and as a supplement it can reset the sleep–wake cycle and help to promote sleep. In addition, it regulates the secretion of growth hormone and gonadotrophic hormones, and it has antioxidant activity. It may also have anti-cancer properties.

Possible uses

Melatonin has been investigated for jet lag, sleeping difficulties and cancer prevention.

Jet lag

A small double-blind, placebo-controlled trial evaluated 17 volunteers who flew from London to San Francisco, where they stayed for 2 weeks before returning. For 3 days before returning to London, subjects were given 5 mg melatonin or placebo at 18:00 local time. Following their return to Britain, the dose was continued for 4 more days between 14:00 and 16:00. On day 7, the volunteers were asked to rate their jet lag, and those taking melatonin reported significantly less severe jet lag than those taking placebo.[1]

In a similar study, 20 subjects flew east from Auckland, New Zealand, to London and returned after 3 weeks. Subjects took either melatonin 5 mg or placebo for the first journey and vice versa for the return journey. Less jet lag was experienced in the volunteers taking melatonin.[2]

In a further double-blind placebo-controlled trial, 52 flight crew were randomly assigned to three groups: early melatonin (5 mg melatonin for 3 days before arrival, continuing for 5 days after returning home), late melatonin (placebo for 3 days, followed by melatonin 5 mg for 5 days) and placebo. The flight was from Los Angeles to New Zealand and all subjects began taking capsules at 07:00 to 08:00 Los Angeles time (corresponding to 02:00 to 03:00 New Zealand time) 2 days before departure and continued for 5 days after arrival in New Zealand. Subjects in the late melatonin group reported less jet lag and sleep disturbance than the placebo group, while those in the early melatonin group reported a worse recovery than the placebo group. The authors concluded that the timing of melatonin appeared to influence the subjective symptoms of jet lag.[3]

In another double-blind placebo-controlled study, 257 subjects on a flight from New York to Oslo were randomised to receive either 5 mg melatonin or placebo at bedtime, 0.5 mg melatonin at bedtime or 0.5 mg melatonin taken on a shifting schedule. In this study, melatonin showed no difference from placebo. However, the authors acknowledged that the study had various limitations, including the fact that the subjects stayed only 4 days at their destination before flying back and may not have had enough time to adapt to the new time. In addition, time of sleep onset at night, awakening in the morning and daytime sleepiness were assessed rather than night-time sleep disturbance, and it is night-time disturbance that is most associated with jet lag. Moreover, subjects knew that they had three out of four chances of receiving melatonin, and the placebo effect may have been quite large, diluting the influence of melatonin.[4]

In a study in baboons (which have similar sleep patterns to humans), various doses of melatonin were given at various times of day to see if melatonin shifted circadian rhythms. Activity patterns of the baboons were constantly monitored in a darkened room. Melatonin did not shift circadian rhythms, but it did induce sleep when given at night. However, the same dose given during the day did not cause sleep.[5] The authors concluded that melatonin does not shift circadian phase in baboons using doses similar to those prescribed for treating human circadian system disorders, suggesting that melatonin may not help to overcome the effects of jet lag.

Melatonin has been compared with zolpidem and also used in combination with zolpidem for jet lag in relation to eastwards travel. In a study involving 137 people, zolpidem was rated as producing the best sleep quality during the night flight and as the most effective jet lag medication. However, all active treatments led to a decrease in jet lag. Zolpidem and the combination of zolpidem and melatonin were less well tolerated than melatonin alone. Adverse reports included nausea, vomiting, amnesia and somnambulia to the point of incapacitation. Confusion, morning sleepiness and nausea were highest in the combination group.[6]

Another trial measured the effects of slow-release caffeine and melatonin on sleep and daytime sleepiness after a seven time zone eastbound flight. Three groups of nine subjects were given either caffeine (300 mg) at 08:00 on recovery days 1 to 5, or melatonin 5 mg on the pre-flight day (at 17:00), the flight day (at 16:00) and from days 1 to 3 after the flight (at 23:00) or placebo at the same times. Compared with baseline there was a significant rebound of slow-wave sleep on nights 1 to 2 with placebo and melatonin and a significant decrease in rapid eye movement (REM) sleep on night 1 with placebo and on nights 1 to 3 with melatonin. Caffeine reduced sleepiness but also tended to affect sleep quality until the last drug day. The authors concluded that both caffeine and melatonin have positive effects on some jet lag symptoms after an eastbound flight, caffeine on daytime sleepiness and melatonin on sleep.[7]

A Cochrane review involving 10 trials found that in eight of these trials melatonin, when taken close to the target bedtime at the destination (22:00 to midnight), decreased jet lag from flights crossing five or more time zones. Daily doses of 0.5–5 mg were effective except that people fell asleep faster and slept better after 5 mg than 0.5 mg. Doses above 5 mg appear to be more effective. The relative ineffectiveness of 2 mg slow-release melatonin suggests that a short-lived higher peak concentration of melatonin works better. The reviewers said that timing of the melatonin dose is crucial. If taken early in the day, it can cause sleepiness and delay adaptation to local time. The authors concluded that melatonin is effective in preventing or reducing jet lag, and occasional short-term use appears to be safe. They also recommended it should be offered to travellers crossing five or more time zones, particularly in an easterly direction, and especially if they have experienced jet lag on previous journeys.[8]

Sleep disorders

In a study of six healthy young men, doses of 0.3 mg and 1 mg melatonin given at night produced acute hypnotic effects. There were no residual hypnotic effects the next morning, as shown from the results on mood and performance tests carried out by the volunteers.[9]

In a double-blind, placebo-controlled, crossover study, 12 elderly patients were randomised to receive 2 mg controlled-release melatonin daily for 3 weeks. There were no differences in sleep time, but there was a reduction in time to onset of sleep, and an increase in sleep quality, as measured by wrist actigraphy.[10]

In a further double-blind, placebo-controlled, crossover study, 14 patients with insomnia (55–80 years) received 0.5 mg melatonin either as an immediate-release dose 30 min before bedtime, a controlled-release dose 30 min before bedtime, an immediate-release dose 4 h after bedtime, or placebo. Each trial lasted for 2 weeks with 2-week washout periods. All melatonin doses resulted in significant reductions in time to sleep onset, but no improvement in sleep quality and no increase in sleep time.[11]

A 2001 systematic review of melatonin in older people with insomnia included six crossover RCTs. Five of the RCTs reported some positive effects, with decreased sleep latency in four studies, an increase in sleep efficiency in three studies and a decrease in wake time during sleep in two studies. Subjective sleep quality was not improved in the two studies that assessed this. There were no adverse effects with melatonin. The authors concluded that further research is required before widespread use of melatonin in geriatric populations can be advocated. They also consider it worthwhile investigating whether melatonin could be used to reduce the amount of benzodiazepines used by older people.[12]

A later RCT involving older people with age-related sleep maintenance problems found that 5 mg melatonin taken at bedtime did not improve sleep quality.[13] In 10 patients (aged 30–75 years) with primary insomnia, there were no differences in sleep electroencephalographic (EEG) records, the amount or subjective quality of sleep or side-effects between a placebo, 0.3 mg melatonin or 1 mg melatonin.[14] In a further study in patients (mean age 50 years) with reduced REM sleep duration, melatonin 3 mg administered between 22:00 and 23:00 for 4 weeks significantly increased percentage of REM sleep compared with placebo.[15] Melatonin has also been found to restore sleep efficiency in individuals with mental retardation and insomnia.[16]

A 2004 systematic review of melatonin in sleep disorders concluded that melatonin is not effective in treating most primary sleep disorders with short-term use, although there is some evidence to suggest that melatonin is effective in treating delayed sleep phase syndrome with short-term use. The review also stated that evidence suggests that melatonin is not effective in treating most secondary sleep disorders with short-term use and no evidence suggests that melatonin is effective in alleviating the sleep disturbance aspect of jet lag and shift work disorder. Evidence also suggests that melatonin is safe with short-term use.[17]

A meta-analysis published in 2005 by the same group as the 2004 systematic review also suggested that melatonin is not effective in treating most primary sleep disorders with short-term use (4 weeks or less), but there is some evidence that melatonin is effective in treating delayed sleep phase syndrome with short-term use.[18] A further 2005 meta-analysis of 15 studies found that melatonin significantly reduced sleep latency by 4 min, increased sleep efficiency by 3.1% and increased sleep duration by 13.7 min.[19]

A meta-analysis published in 2006 (by the same group as the 2004 systematic review[17] and the 2005 meta-analysis[18]) included six RCTs, which showed no evidence that melatonin had an effect on sleep latency in people with secondary disorders. Analysis of nine RCTs found no evidence that melatonin had an effect on sleep latency in people with sleep disorders accompanying sleep restriction (e.g. jet lag, shift work). Analysis of 17 RCTs showed no evidence of adverse events of melatonin in short-term use (3 months or less).[20]

More recently, studies have begun to evaluate prolonged release melatonin (PRM) in sleep disorders as PRM is licensed in Europe and other countries for the short-term treatment of primary insomnia in patients aged 55 years and over. However, a clear definition of the target patient population and well-controlled studies of long-term efficacy and safety are lacking. Two recent placebo-controlled trials involving 40 patients[21] and 791 patients[22] demonstrated short and longer-term efficacy and safety of melatonin in elderly patients.

Transdermal melatonin has been shown to improve sleep maintenance during daytime and may have advantages over oral melatonin which has a short half life and, therefore, is of limited use in night shift workers and people with jet lag. One small study found that transdermal melatonin can improve sleep maintenance during attempts to sleep out of phase with circadian rhythm.[23]

Melatonin has also been evaluated in children with insomnia and mental disorders. It has been found to advance the sleep–wake rhythm in children with idiopathic chronic sleep-onset insomnia.[24] In young patients with epilepsy, melatonin has been shown to reduce wake–sleep disorders[25] and to be of potential use as an adjunct to anti-epileptic therapy in reducing oxidant stress.[26–28] In a systematic review of melatonin treatment in children with neurodevelopmental disabilities and sleep impairment, melatonin was found to significantly reduce time to sleep onset, but there was no significant effect on the other outcome measures of total sleep time, night-time awakenings and parental opinions on their children's sleep.[29]

Studies have also evaluated melatonin for potential benefit for sleep disorders in patients with dementia. Three studies have shown no evidence that melatonin is effective in improving sleep in patients with dementia.[30-32] A Cochrane review found some – albeit insufficient – evidence to support the use of melatonin in managing cognitive disturbances in people with dementia. However, there was some evidence of benefit on some behavioural symptoms.[33]

A meta-analysis of nine studies involving 183 people with intellectual disabilities showed that melatonin reduced time to fall asleep by a mean of 34 min and increased total sleep time by a mean of 50 min while significantly decreasing the number of waking episodes each night.[34]

A prospective open-label study has evaluated the potential for melatonin to improve tinnitus, particularly in those with sleep disturbance caused by tinnitus. A total of 24 patients took 3 mg melatonin per day for 4 weeks, followed by 4 weeks of observation. Melatonin use was associated with improvement in tinnitus and sleep. There was an association between the amount of improvement in sleep and tinnitus. The impact of melatonin on sleep was greatest in those with the worst sleep quality, but its impact on tinnitus was not associated with the severity of tinnitus. The authors concluded that melatonin may be a safe treatment for patients with idiopathic tinnitus, especially those with sleep disturbance due to tinnitus.[35]

Cancer

A group of 80 patients with advanced solid tumours, all of whom refused chemotherapy or who did not respond to previous chemotherapy, were randomised to receive either interleukin 2 (IL-2) or IL-2 and melatonin (40 mg) starting 1 week before IL-2. Melatonin increased the anti-tumour activity of IL-2, resulting in accelerated tumour regression rate, increased progression-free survival and longer overall survival in these patients.[36]

In a small preliminary study involving 14 women with metastatic breast cancer, melatonin was shown to increase the effects of tamoxifen.[37]

In a controlled study, 50 patients with brain metastases caused by solid neoplasms were randomised to receive supportive care alone (steroids and anticonvulsants) or supportive care plus melatonin 20 mg daily. Survival at 1 year, free from brain progression, and mean survival

time were significantly higher in the melatonin group.[38]

Another study randomised 80 patients with metastatic tumours to receive chemotherapy or chemotherapy plus melatonin (20 mg daily). Melatonin was associated with a significant reduction in frequency of thrombocytopaenia, malaise and asthenia, and a non-significant trend towards less stomatitis and neuropathy compared with controls. However, melatonin had no effect on alopecia and vomiting.[39]

A systematic review of 10 RCTs of melatonin in the treatment of cancer found that melatonin reduced the risk of death at 1 year (relative risk, 0.66; 95% confidence interval, 0.59 to 0.73). Effects were consistent across melatonin dose and type of cancer. No adverse events were reported. The authors concluded that the reduction in risk of death and lack of adverse events suggest potential for melatonin in cancer management, but these effects must be confirmed by further good-quality RCTs.[40]

Blood pressure

The biological clock has been shown to be involved in autonomic cardiovascular regulation. Recent research has investigated the effect of enhancing the functioning of the biological clock by melatonin in blood pressure. A double-blind, crossover RCT in 16 men with untreated essential hypertension evaluated the influence of oral melatonin 2.5 mg daily, 1 h before sleep, on 24-h ambulatory blood pressure and actigraphic estimates of sleep quality. Repeated melatonin intake over 3 weeks (but not an acute single dose) reduced systolic and diastolic blood pressure during sleep by 6 and 4 mmHg, respectively. The treatment did not affect heart rate. The day–night amplitudes of the rhythms in systolic and diastolic blood pressures were increased by 15% and 25%, respectively. Repeated (but not acute) melatonin also improved sleep. The authors concluded that support of circadian pacemaker function may provide a new strategy in the treatment of essential hypertension.[41]

A further trial has found a similar effect in women. In a double-blind RCT 18 women (aged 47–63 years) with normal blood pressure ($n = 9$) or treated essential hypertension ($n = 9$)

received a 3-week course of slow-release melatonin (3 mg) 1 h before going to bed. They were then crossed over for 3 weeks. In comparison with placebo, melatonin administration did not influence diurnal blood pressure but did significantly decrease nocturnal systolic (-3.77 ± 1.7 mmHg; $P = 0.04$) and diastolic (-3.63 ± 1.3 mmHg; $P = 0.013$) pressure without modifying heart rate. The effect was inversely related to the day–night difference in blood pressure, suggesting that prolonged administration may improve the day–night rhythm of blood pressure, particularly in women with a blunted nocturnal decline.[42]

Another RCT in young patients with type 1 diabetes also found that melatonin (5 mg daily) amplifies the nocturnal decline in blood pressure and suggested that melatonin should be considered in trials of prevention of hypertension in type 1 diabetes.[43]

However, consideration should be given before giving melatonin to patients with cardiovascular disease and abnormal circadian pattern of blood pressure. In a trial of 60 patients (40–80 years) with coronary artery disease, melatonin (5 mg daily) caused not only a nocturnal decrease in blood pressure but also a daytime increase.[44] Melatonin should not, therefore, be recommended in patients with 'high normal' values of blood pressure because of the danger of induction of arterial hypertension.

Cognitive impairment

A number of studies suggest a relationship between decline of melatonin function and the symptoms of dementia. A Cochrane review of three RCTs designed to evaluate melatonin for sleep disorders associated with dementia found no evidence of efficacy for cognitive function, with evidence from a single small trial that there may be some benefit for behavioural problems.[33]

An RCT evaluated the change in cognitive and non-cognitive symptoms in 189 residents of 12 care facilities in The Netherlands in response to melatonin and bright light (the two major synchronizers of the circadian timing system). Light attenuated cognitive deterioration, the increase in functional limitations and depression. Melatonin shortened sleep onset and increased sleep duration, but had adverse effects on mood, which were not seen if melatonin was given in combination with bright light. Combined treatment also attenuated aggressive behaviour and improved night restlessness.[45] Melatonin treatment alone has been associated with reduced depression in patients with circadian rhythm sleep disorders and associated comorbid depression,[46] and may be beneficial in treating major depressive disorder associated with sleep disorder.[47]

Miscellaneous

Melatonin has been evaluated in other disorders. Studies have shown insufficient evidence of benefit for melatonin in chronic fatigue syndrome[48] migraine[49] and in tardive dyskinesia.[50] However, supplemental melatonin has been associated with significant reduction in nocturia in men with benign prostatic enlargement.[51] In relation to the gastrointestinal tract, melatonin supplementation has produced attenuation of abdominal pain, reduced rectal pain sensitivity,[52,53] prolonged colonic transit time[53] in patients with irritable bowel syndrome and reduced oxidative damage in the stomach of individuals with dyspepsia.[54] Results from a preliminary study suggest that melatonin either alone or in combination with omeprazole could help in the management of gastro-oesophageal reflux disease (GORD).[55] Animal models suggest that melatonin could be a candidate neuroprotective agent for human stroke.[56] Melatonin has also been evaluated as an anxiolytic and analgesic during various types of surgery with positive results in cataract surgery[57] but not in laparoscopic cholecystectomy[58] or general surgery[59]

Conclusion

Melatonin has been promoted widely for the prevention and treatment of jet lag and sleep disorders. For jet lag, melatonin appears promising, but results from studies on supplements and sleep have been conflicting. Use of melatonin supplementation is associated with improved sleep quality and latency in elderly people with sleep disorder, but people with disturbed sleep should seek advice from their doctor. Reduced secretion has also been associated with cancer, and preliminary research suggests that melatonin may reduce adverse effects associated with chemotherapy and increase survival time. Reduced secretion has also been linked with CVD, epilepsy and depression, but its role as a potential supplement in these conditions is unclear.

Precautions/contraindications

Caution in taking melatonin (as any other sleep therapy) for prolonged periods without medical assessment of the patient. Melatonin should be avoided in women wishing to conceive (large doses may inhibit ovulation); in children and in patients with mental illness, including depression.

Pregnancy and breast-feeding

Melatonin should be avoided in pregnancy.

Adverse effects

No known toxicity or serious side-effects, but the effects of long-term supplementation are unknown. However, there have been reports of headaches, abdominal cramp, inhibition of fertility and libido, gynaecomastia, exacerbation of symptoms of fibromyalgia and also sleep disturbance. In addition, there have been reports of increased seizures in children suffering from neurological disorders. Inhibition of ovulation has been observed with high doses, but melatonin should not be used as a contraceptive.

Interactions

No data are available, but in theory melatonin may be additive with medication that causes CNS depression. In addition, beta-blockers inhibit melatonin release, and this may be the mechanism by which beta-blockers cause sleep disturbance. Other drugs, including fluoxetine, ibuprofen and indomethacin, may also reduce nocturnal melatonin secretion. Melatonin may influence the effects of warfarin.

Dose

Not established. Manufacturers recommend 3–5 mg.

References

1 Arendt J, Aldhous M, Marks V. Alleviation of jet lag by melatonin: preliminary results of controlled double blind trial. *Br Med J* 1986; 292: 1170.
2 Petrie K, Conaglen JV, Thompson L, *et al*. Effect of melatonin on jet lag after long haul flights. *BMJ* 1989; 298(6675): 705–707.
3 Petrie K, Dawson AG, Thompson L, *et al*. A double-blind trial of melatonin as a treatment for jet lag in international cabin crew. *Biol Psychiatry* 1993; 33 (7): 526–530.
4 Spitzer RL, Terman M, Williams JB, *et al*. Jet lag: clinical features, validation of a new syndrome-specific scale, and lack of response to melatonin in a randomized, double-blind trial. *Am J Psychiatry* 1999; 156(9): 1392–1396.
5 Hao H, Rivkees S. Melatonin does not shift circadian phase in baboons. *J Clin Endocrinol Metab* 2000; 85(10): 3618–3622.
6 Suhner A, Schlagenhauf P, Hofer I, *et al*. Effectiveness and tolerability of melatonin and zolpidem for the alleviation of jet lag. *Aviat Space Environ Med* 2001; 72(7): 638–646.
7 Beaumont M, Batejat D, Pierard C, *et al*. Caffeine or melatonin effects on sleep and sleepiness after rapid eastward transmeridian travel. *J Appl Physiol* 2004; 96(1): 50–58.
8 Herxheimer A, Petrie KJ, *et al*. Melatonin for preventing and treating jet lag. *Cochrane Database Syst Rev* 2001;(1): CD001520.
9 Zhdanova IV, Wurtman RJ, Lynch HJ, *et al*. Sleep-inducing effects of low doses of melatonin ingested in the evening. *Clin Pharmacol Ther* 1995; 57(5): 552–558.
10 Garfinkel D, Laudon M, Nof D, *et al*. Improvement of sleep quality in elderly people by controlled-release melatonin. *Lancet* 1995; 346(8974): 541–544.
11 Hughes RJ, Sack RL, Lewy AJ. The role of melatonin and circadian phase in age-related sleep-maintenance insomnia: assessment in a clinical trial of melatonin replacement. *Sleep* 1998; 21(1): 52–68.
12 Olde Rikkert M, Rigaud AS. Melatonin in elderly patients with insomnia: a systematic review. *Z Gerontol Geriatr* 2001; 34: 491–497.
13 Baskett JJ, Broad JB, Wood PC, *et al*. Does melatonin improve sleep in older people? A randomised crossover trial *Age Ageing* 2003; 32(2): 164–170.
14 Almeida Montes LG, Ontiveros Uribe MP, Cortes Sotres J, *et al*. Treatment of primary insomnia with melatonin: a double-blind, placebo-controlled, crossover study. *J Psychiatr Neurosci* 2003; 28: 191–196.
15 Kunz D, Mahlberg R, Muller C, *et al*. Melatonin in patients with reduced REM sleep duration: two randomized controlled trials. *J Clin Endocrinol Metab* 2004; 89(1): 128–134.
16 Niederhofer H, Staffen W, Mair A, *et al*. Brief report: melatonin facilitates sleep in individuals with mental retardation and insomnia. *J Autism Dev Disord* 2003; 33: 469–472.

17 Buscemi N, Vandermeer B, Pandya R, *et al.* Melatonin for treatment of sleep disorders. *Evid Rep Technol Assess (Summ)* 2004(108): 1–7.

18 Buscemi N, Vandermeer B, Hooton N, *et al.* The efficacy and safety of exogenous melatonin for primary sleep disorders. A meta-analysis. *J Gen Intern Med* 2005; 20(12): 1151–1158.

19 Brzezinski A, Vangel MG, Wurtman RJ, *et al.* Effects of exogenous melatonin on sleep: a meta-analysis. *Sleep Med Rev* 2005; 9(1): 41–50.

20 Buscemi N, Vandermeer B, Hooton N, *et al.* Efficacy and safety of exogenous melatonin for secondary sleep disorders and sleep disorders accompanying sleep restriction: meta-analysis. *BMJ* 2006; 332(7538): 385–393.

21 Luthringer R, Muzet M, Zisapel N, *et al.* The effect of prolonged-release melatonin on sleep measures and psychomotor performance in elderly patients with insomnia. *Int Clin Psychopharmacol* 2009; 24(5): 239–249.

22 Wade AG, Ford I, Crawford G, *et al.* Nightly treatment of primary insomnia with prolonged release melatonin for 6 months: a randomized placebo controlled trial on age and endogenous melatonin as predictors of efficacy and safety. *BMC Med* 2010; 8: 51.

23 Aeschbach D, Lockyer BJ, Dijk DJ, *et al.* Use of transdermal melatonin delivery to improve sleep maintenance during daytime. *Clin Pharmacol Ther* 2009; 86(4): 378–382.

24 Smits MG, van Stel HF, van der Heijden K, *et al.* Melatonin improves health status and sleep in children with idiopathic chronic sleep-onset insomnia: a randomized placebo-controlled trial. *J Am Acad Child Adolesc Psychiatry* 2003; 42(11): 1286–1293.

25 Coppola G, Iervolino G, Mastrosimone M, *et al.* Melatonin in wake-sleep disorders in children, adolescents and young adults with mental retardation with or without epilepsy: a double-blind, cross-over, placebo-controlled trial. *Brain Dev* 2004; 26 (6): 373–376.

26 Gupta M, Aneja S, Kohli K. Add-on melatonin improves quality of life in epileptic children on valproate monotherapy: a randomized, double-blind, placebo-controlled trial. *Epilepsy Behav* 2004; 5(3): 316–321.

27 Gupta M, Gupta YK, Agarwal S, *et al.* A randomized, double-blind, placebo controlled trial of melatonin add-on therapy in epileptic children on valproate monotherapy: effect on glutathione peroxidase and glutathione reductase enzymes. *Br J Clin Pharmacol* 2004; 58(5): 542–547.

28 Gupta M, Gupta YK, Agarwal S, *et al.* Effects of add-on melatonin administration on antioxidant enzymes in children with epilepsy taking carbamazepine monotherapy: a randomized, double-blind, placebo-controlled trial. *Epilepsia* 2004; 45(12): 1636–1639.

29 Phillips L, Appleton RE. Systematic review of melatonin treatment in children with neurodevelopmental disabilities and sleep impairment. *Dev Med Child Neurol* 2004; 46: 771–775.

30 Serfaty M, Kennell-Webb S, Warner J, *et al.* Double blind randomised placebo controlled trial of low dose melatonin for sleep disorders in dementia. *Int J Geriatr Psychiatry* 2002; 17(12): 1120–1127.

31 Singer C, Tractenberg RE, Kaye J, *et al.* A multicenter, placebo-controlled trial of melatonin for sleep disturbance in Alzheimer's disease. *Sleep* 2003; 26(7): 893–901.

32 Gehrman PR, Connor DJ, Martin JL, *et al.* Melatonin fails to improve sleep or agitation in double-blind randomized placebo-controlled trial of institutionalized patients with Alzheimer disease. *Am J Geriatr Psychiatry* 2009; 17(2): 166–169.

33 Jansen SL, Forbes DA, Duncan V, *et al.* Melatonin forcognitive impairment. *Cochrane Database Syst Rev* 2006;(1): CD003802.

34 Braam W, Smits MG, Didden R, *et al.* Exogenous melatonin for sleep problems in individuals with intellectual disability: a meta-analysis. *Dev Med Child Neurol* 2009; 51(5): 340–349.

35 Megwalu U, Finnell JE, Piccirillo JF. The effects of melatonin on tinnitus and sleep. *Otolaryngol Head Neck Surg* 2006; 134: 210–213.

36 Lissoni P, Barni S, Tancini G, *et al.* A randomised study with subcutaneous low-dose interleukin 2 alone vs interleukin 2 plus the pineal neurohormone melatonin in advanced solid neoplasms other than renal cancer and melanoma. *Br J Cancer* 1994; 69 (1): 196–199.

37 Lissoni P, Barni S, Meregalli S, *et al.* Modulation of cancer endocrine therapy by melatonin: a phase II study of tamoxifen plus melatonin in metastatic breast cancer patients progressing under tamoxifen alone. *Br J Cancer* 1995; 71(4): 854–856.

38 Lissoni P, Barni S, Ardizzoia A, *et al.* A randomized study with the pineal hormone melatonin versus supportive care alone in patients with brain metastases due to solid neoplasms. *Cancer* 1994; 73(3): 699–701.

39 Lissoni P, Tancini G, Barni S, *et al.* Treatment of cancer chemotherapy-induced toxicity with the pineal hormone melatonin. *Support Care Cancer* 1997; 5(2): 126–129.

40 Mills E, Wu P, Seely D, *et al.* Melatonin in the treatment of cancer: a systematic review of randomized controlled trials and meta-analysis. *J Pineal Res* 2005; 39: 360–366.

41 Scheer FA, Van Montfrans GA, van Someren EJ, *et al.* Daily nighttime melatonin reduces blood pressure in male patients with essential hypertension. *Hypertension* 2004; 43(2): 192–197.

42 Cagnacci A, Cannoletta M, Renzi A, *et al.* Prolonged melatonin administration decreases nocturnal blood pressure in women. *Am J Hypertens* 2005; 18(Pt1): 1614–1618.

43 Cavallo A, Daniels SR, Dolan LM, *et al.* Blood pressure response to melatonin in type 1 diabetes. *Pediatr Diabetes* 2004; 5(1): 26–31.

44 Rechcinski T, Trzos E, Wierzbowska-Drabik K, *et al.* Melatonin for nondippers with coronary artery disease: assessment of blood pressure profile and heart rate variability. *Hypertens Res* 2009; 33 (1): 56–61.

45 Riemersma-van der Lek RF, Swaab DF, Twisk J, *et al.* Effect of bright light and melatonin on cognitive and noncognitive function in elderly residents of group care facilities: a randomized controlled trial. *JAMA* 2008; 299(22): 2642–2655.

46 Rahman SA, Kayumov L, Shapiro CM. Antidepressant action of melatonin in the treatment of delayed sleep phase syndrome. *Sleep Med* 2009; 11(2): 131–136.

47 Serfaty MA, Osborne D, Buszewicz MJ, *et al.* A randomized double-blind placebo-controlled trial of treatment as usual plus exogenous slow-release melatonin (6 mg) or placebo for sleep disturbance and depressed mood. *Int Clin Psychopharmacol* 2010; 25(3): 132–142.

48 Williams G, Waterhouse J, Mugarza J, *et al.* Therapy of circadian rhythm disorders in chronic fatigue syndrome: no symptomatic improvement with melatonin or phototherapy. *Eur J Clin Invest* 2002; 32(11): 831–837.

49 Alstadhaug KB, Odeh F, Salvesen R, *et al.* Prophylaxis of migraine with melatonin: a randomized controlled trial. *Neurology* 2010; 75(17): 1527–1532.

50 Nelson LA, McGuire JM, Hausafus SN. Melatonin for the treatment of tardive dyskinesia. *Ann Pharmacother* 2003; 37(7-8): 1128–1131.

51 Drake MJ, Mills IW, Noble JG. Melatonin pharmacotherapy for nocturia in men with benign prostatic enlargement. *J Urol* 2004; 171(3): 1199–1202.

52 Song GH, Leng PH, Gwee KA, *et al.* Melatonin improves abdominal pain in irritable bowel syndrome patients who have sleep disturbances: a randomised, double blind, placebo controlled study. *Gut* 2005; 54(10): 1402–1407.

53 Lu WZ, Song GH, Gwee KA, *et al.* The effects of melatonin on colonic transit time in normal controls and IBS patients. *Dig Dis Sci* 2009; 54(5): 1087–1093.

54 Klupinska G, Poplawski T, Smigielski J, *et al.* The effect of melatonin on oxidative DNA damage in gastric mucosa cells of patients with functional dyspepsia. *Pol Merkur Lekarski* 2009; 26(155): 366–369.

55 Kandil TS, Mousa AA, El-Gendy AA, *et al.* The potential therapeutic effect of melatonin in gastro-esophageal reflux disease. *BMC Gastroenterol* 2010; 10(7): 7.

56 Macleod MR, O'Collins T, Horky LL, *et al.* Systematic review and meta-analysis of the efficacy of melatonin in experimental stroke. *J Pineal Res* 2005; 38(1): 35–41.

57 Ismail SA, Mowafi HA. Melatonin provides anxiolysis, enhances analgesia, decreases intraocular pressure, and promotes better operating conditions during cataract surgery under topical anesthesia. *Anesth Analg* 2009; 108(4): 1146–1151.

58 Gogenur I, Kucukakin B, Bisgaard T, *et al.* The effect of melatonin on sleep quality after laparoscopic cholecystectomy: a randomized, placebo-controlled trial. *Anesth Analg* 2009; 108(4): 1152–1156.

59 Capuzzo M, Zanardi B, Schiffino E, *et al.* Melatonin does not reduce anxiety more than placebo in the elderly undergoing surgery. *Anesth Analg* 2006; 103(1): 121–123.

Methylsulfonylmethane

Description

Methylsulfonylmethane (MSM) is an organic sulphur-containing compound. It is an oxidation product of the organic solvent, dimethyl sulfoxide (DMSO). DMSO has been used (although is of unproven efficacy) in the treatment of arthritis and connective tissue injuries.

Action

MSM is claimed by manufacturers to be an organic source of sulphur for synthetic processes. However, there is no evidence to support the need for this in humans. There are many other dietary sources of sulphur, including the sulphur-containing amino acids cysteine and methionine, which are found in dietary protein.

Because cartilage has a high content of sulphur, and sulphur is needed for the formation of connective tissue, it has been suggested that MSM as a source of sulphur could be useful in the management of conditions such as osteoarthritis and joint injuries where there is degeneration or destruction of cartilage. Because MSM is a metabolite of DMSO, it has been suggested that some of the supposed benefits of DMSO (see above) could be attributed to MSM.

There is some very preliminary evidence that MSM reduces homocysteine levels and that it might reduce lipid peroxidation.[1]

Dietary sources

MSM is found naturally in a variety of fruits, vegetables, milk, meat, fish, coffee, tea and chocolate.

Possible uses

Extravagant claims for MSM have been made since the 1980s. Many of these claims have been made by manufacturers and marketers of supplements, and one website was warned by the US Food and Drug Administration (FDA) about making illegal claims. Claims and a rationale for taking MSM can be found on a website that describes two unpublished studies showing benefits of MSM on firstly arthritis, muscle and joint pain and, secondly, on muscle strain and other athletic injuries.[2]

There is some evidence from two small controlled trials that MSM, either in combination with glucosamine or alone, could improve symptoms of pain in arthritis. In one double-blind RCT, 188 patients with mild to moderate osteoarthritis were randomised to glucosamine 500 mg three times daily, MSM 500 mg three times daily or glucosamine 500 mg plus MSM 500 mg three times daily for 12 weeks. All three treatments produced an analgesic and anti-inflammatory effect. Compared with the individual agents, the combination of glucosamine and MSM produced more rapid onset of analgesia and was associated with better anti-inflammatory effect, better efficacy in reducing pain and swelling and better improvement in the functional ability of joints.[3]

A pilot clinical trial randomised 50 men and women with knee osteoarthritis pain to MSM 3 g twice daily or placebo twice daily for 12 weeks. MSM improved symptoms of pain and physical function, but did not reduce stiffness or a total aggregate of osteoarthritis symptom scores. The authors cautioned that the benefits and safety of MSM in managing osteoarthritis and long-term use cannot be confirmed with this pilot trial.[1]

A systematic review of six studies evaluated a total of 681 patients with osteoarthritis of the knee taking DMSO (297 taking the active treatment) or MSM (52 taking the active treatment). Two of the four DMSO trials and both MSM trials reported significant improvement in pain outcomes in the treatment group compared with comparator treatments; however, methodological issues and concerns over optimal dosage and treatment period were highlighted. The review found that no definitive conclusion can currently be drawn for either supplement. The findings from all the DMSO studies need to be viewed with caution because of poor methodology including possible unblinding and questionable treatment duration and dose. The data from the more rigorous MSM trials provide positive but not definitive evidence that MSM is superior to placebo in the treatment of mild to moderate osteoarthritis of the knee. The authors concluded that further studies are now required to identify both the optimum dosage and the longer-term safety of MSM and DMSO, and for definitive efficacy trials.[4]

Preliminary evidence from an open trial found that MSM 2600 mg daily for 30 days could relieve respiratory symptoms in seasonal allergic rhinitis with no adverse events. No significant changes were observed in plasma IgE or histamine levels. The authors concluded that the results merited further investigation in a larger controlled trial.[5]

MSM has also been used for snoring, scleroderma, fibromyalgia, systemic lupus erythromatosus, repetitive stress injuries, HIV/AIDS, depression, breast and colon cancer, eye inflammation, insect bites and Alzheimer's disease. However there are no data from clinical trials in humans to support these uses.

Conclusion

MSM has been studied as a source of sulphur for the management of arthritic conditions. The findings of a systematic review of six trials suggest that MSM could reduce pain and improve physical function in patients with osteoarthritis, but longer term, larger trials are needed. Many extravagant claims have been made for the value of MSM in other conditions, but evidence is lacking and further trials are needed to confirm suggested benefits.

Precautions/contraindications

None reported.

Pregnancy and breast-feeding

No problems have been reported, but there have not been sufficient studies to guarantee the safety of MSM in pregnancy and breast-feeding.

Adverse effects

MSM is a component of foods and has not been reported to be toxic. No adverse effects were reported when rats were given 1–5 g/kg body weight for 3 months.[6] A 30-day study in humans revealed no side-effects with a 2600 mg daily dosage.[5]

Interactions

None reported.

Dose

The dose is not established. Supplements typically provide 1500–3000 mg in a daily dose.

References

1 Kim LS, Axelrod LJ, Howard P, *et al.* Efficacy of methylsulfonylmethane (MSM) in osteoarthritis pain of the knee: a pilot clinical trial. *Osteoarthritis Cartilage* 2006; 14: 286–294.
2 Fine Nutraceuticals Inc. http://www.msm.com (accessed 8 November 2006).
3 Usha PR, Naidu MUR. Randomised, double-blind, parallel, placebo-controlled study of oral glucosamine, methylsulfonylmethane and their combination in osteoarthritis. *Clin Drug Invest* 2004; 24: 353–363.
4 Brien S, Prescott P, Bashir N, *et al.* Systematic review of the nutritional supplements dimethyl sulfoxide (DMSO) and methylsulfonylmethane (MSM) in the treatment of osteoarthritis. *Osteoarthritis Cartilage* 2008; 16(11): 1277–1288.
5 Barrager E, Veltmann JR,Jr Schauss AG, Schiller RN. A multicentered, open-label trial on the safety and efficacy of methylsulfonylmethane in the treatment of seasonal allergic rhinitis. *J Altern Complement Med* 2002; 8: 167–173.
6 Horvath K, Noker PE, Somfai-Relle S, *et al.* Toxicity of methylsulfonylmethane in rats. *Food Chem Toxicol* 2002; 40: 1459–1462.

Molybdenum

Description

Molybdenum is an essential ultratrace mineral.

Human requirements

No Reference Nutrient Intake or Estimated Average Requirement has been set for molybdenum in the UK but a safe and adequate daily intake is: for adults, 50–400 µg; infants, children and adolescents, 0.5–1.5 µg/kg. The UK Food Standards Agency has not set a safe upper level.

In the USA, daily adequate intakes (AIs) are: for infants, 0–6 months, 2 µg, 7–12 months, 3 µg. RDAs are: for children, 1–3 years, 17 µg, 4–8 years, 22 µg; for males and females, 9–13 years, 34 µg, 14–18 years, 43 µg, 19–70+ years, 45 µg; pregnancy and breast-feeding, 50 µg. The daily Tolerable Upper Intake Level from food, water and supplements is: for children 1–3 years, 300 µg, 4–8 years, 600 µg; 9–13 years, 1100 µg, 14–18 years, 1700 µg, 19–70+ years, 2000 µg, pregnancy, 1700 µg, breast-feeding 2000 µg.

Dietary intake

Average adult intakes of molybdenum are 120–140 µg daily (US figures).

Action

Molybdenum functions as an essential cofactor for several enzymes, including aldehyde oxidase (oxidises and detoxifies various pyrimidines, purines and related compounds involved in DNA metabolism); xanthine oxidase/dehydrogenase (catalyses the formation of uric acid); sulphite oxidase (involved in sulphite metabolism).

Dietary sources

The richest sources of molybdenum include milk and milk products, dried beans and peas, wholegrain cereals and liver and kidney.

Metabolism

Absorption
Molybdenum is readily absorbed, but the mechanism of absorption is uncertain.

Distribution
Molybdenum is transported in the blood, loosely attached to erythrocytes, and binds specifically β_2-macroglobulin. The highest concentrations are found in the liver and kidney.

Elimination
Excretion of molybdenum is mainly via the kidneys, but significant amounts are eliminated in the bile.

Deficiency

A precise description of molybdenum deficiency in humans has not been clearly documented.

Evidence so far has been limited to a single patient on long-term total parenteral nutrition, who developed hypermethioninaemia, decreased urinary excretion of sulphate and uric acid, and increased urinary excretion of sulphite and xanthine. In addition, the patient suffered irritability and mental disturbances that progressed into coma. Supplementation with molybdenum improved the clinical condition and normalised uric acid production.

Possible uses

None established.

Adverse effects

Molybdenum is a relatively non-toxic element. High dietary intakes (10–15 mg daily) have been associated with elevated uric acid concentrations in blood and an increased incidence of gout, and may also result in impaired bioavailability of copper and altered metabolism of nucleotides.

Interactions

None reported.

Dose

Molybdenum is available mainly in multivitamin and mineral supplements.

There is no established dose.

Multivitamins

Description

Many supplements contain more than one vitamin and mineral. The majority of these products are classed as so-called 'multivitamins', which contain a wide variety of essential vitamins, and often minerals and trace elements too. A significant proportion of multivitamins sold on the UK high street contain amounts of vitamins and minerals around the Recommended Daily Amount (RDA). (The European Union (EU) RDA, rather than the UK Dietary Reference Values, is the reference figure used to compare amounts of vitamins and minerals on the labels of food supplements in the UK and throughout the EU.) Other multivitamins contain vitamins and minerals in higher doses than the RDA and are often labelled 'high potency', 'megavitamins' or 'maximum strength'. Still other products contain a combination of fewer vitamins and/or minerals, marketed for specific purposes or specific stages of life (e.g. women's health, men's health, sports, menopause, pregnancy).

Action

The potential action of multivitamins depends on the vitamins and minerals they contain. However, both vitamins and minerals are important for good health: normal growth and development; overall health and well-being; release of energy from food; healthy teeth and bones; healing and repair of body tissue; healthy eyes; normal healthy structure of skin, hair and nails; and the health of muscles, the nervous system and the circulatory system.

Possible uses

Recent UK national diet and nutrition surveys[1-5] have shown that some population groups are at risk from marginal intakes of vitamins and minerals. Thus, a 'moderate' one-a-day multivitamin/mineral containing the RDA of a wide range of vitamins and minerals recognised as essential for health may be beneficial. Although supplements are not a substitute for a poor diet, evidence shows they can help to reduce nutritional gaps.

Groups of people at particular risk from inadequate intake or poor absorption of a range of vitamins and minerals (rather than isolated nutrients) include elderly people, strict vegetarians (vegans) or alcohol-dependent individuals.[6] Those on restricted diets for cultural or medical reasons (e.g. allergies and intolerances) or those on poorly managed weight-reduction diets may also have inadequate intakes of vitamins and minerals.

However, it is well recognised that people who take supplements may be the ones who least need them. Intakes of fruit and vegetables[7] and micronutrients from food[8-10] have been found to be higher in supplement users, although one study found no difference.[11] In a Canadian study, calcium and vitamin D intakes from food were actually lower in supplement users than in non-supplement users,[12] possibly because of lower dairy consumption in those taking supplements.

An epidemiological study in 4384 US adults evaluated the influence of supplement use on the overall intake of nutrients and the possibility that supplements could compensate for dietary deficits. Of the total, 1777 took supplements daily, 428 were infrequent users and 2179 did not take supplements. Attitude about the importance of following a healthful diet was a consistent predictor of supplement use for both men and women.[13]

A significantly smaller proportion of supplement users than non-users had intakes from food alone that were below the estimated average requirement (EAR) for vitamins A, B_6 and C, and for folate, zinc and magnesium. However, fewer than 50% of both users and non-users met the EAR for folate, vitamin E and magnesium from food sources alone, indicating that a large proportion of older US adults do not achieve the EAR for several nutrients from food alone. Overall, supplements improved the nutrient intake of older adults. After accounting for the contribution of supplements, 80% or more of users met the EAR for vitamins A, B_6, B_{12}, C, E, folate, iron and zinc, but not magnesium, showing that supplements compensate to some extent. However, some supplement users, particularly men, exceeded Tolerable Upper Intake Levels (ULs) for iron and zinc, and a small percentage of women exceeded the UL for vitamin A.[13]

Benefits observed in those who consumed multivitamins may result from their concerns about health and attempts to live healthier lifestyles.[14-16] The general association between multivitamin supplement use and healthy lifestyle makes it difficult to interpret the potential influence of multivitamins on health outcomes.

Improvement in nutritional intake

Studies in adults have shown that supplement use can make a significant contribution to vitamin and mineral intake. The National Diet and Nutrition Survey (NDNS) in British adults found that supplement users had higher intakes of vitamins and minerals and were less likely to have intakes below the Reference Nutrient Intake (RNI) than non-supplement users.[2] Similar findings have been shown in Ireland,[8] Germany,[17,18] the USA[19] and Canada.[12] Food supplements have also been shown to make a substantial contribution to the intakes of vitamins and minerals in toddlers[11,20] and teen-agers.[9,10,21,22] In addition, several studies[23–25] have shown that supplementation with vitamins and minerals can improve plasma levels of micronutrients and reduce the prevalence of suboptimal plasma concentrations.

Chronic disease

Use of multivitamins has also been associated with reduced risk of chronic disease in some epidemiological studies, but not all. However, there have been few well-controlled RCTs from which to draw solid evidence-based conclusions about the effect of multivitamins on chronic disease risk.[14,16]

Cancer

In the Cancer Prevention Study II cohort, past multivitamin use (> 10 years before enrolment) but not recent (< 10 years before enrolment) was associated with modestly reduced risk of colorectal cancer,[26] but a small increase in prostate cancer.[27] A recent prospective study of > 295 000 men enrolled in the US National Institutes of Health Diet and Health Study found that regular multivitamin use was not associated with the risk of early or localised prostate cancer.[28]

In the Health Professionals' Follow-up Study, men who reported folate consumption from multivitamins for >10 years had a 25% reduction in colon cancer risk.[29] Also, in the Nurses' Health Study, women who reported multivitamin use (with folate) for ≥15 years had a 75% reduction in colorectal cancer risk.[30] However, in a pooled analysis of eight prospective studies, use of multivitamins and specific vitamin supplements was not significantly associated with lung cancer risk.[31]

Infection

Several studies have evaluated the influence of multivitamin use on immune function and infection. However, evidence for the benefit of multivitamins in the prevention of infection is weak and conflicting, as confirmed by two systematic reviews/meta-analyses, one in elderly people[32] and one in adults of all ages.[33] A more recent observational study among 83 165 women in the Nurses' Health Study II found that higher intake of vitamins from diet and supplements

was not likely to reduce pneumonia risk in well-nourished women.[34]

A double-blind RCT in Tanzania among 1078 pregnant women with HIV infection found that multivitamin supplementation delayed the progress of HIV and delayed the initiation of anti-retroviral therapy.[35] In the same trial, the risk of hypertension was also reduced in these HIV-infected pregnant women.[36]

Cardiovascular disease

Evidence from observational studies suggests a reduced risk of cardiovascular disease in users of multivitamins in some studies[37,38] but not others.[39]

Evidence from an RCT in 69 patients with type 2 diabetes suggested that a combination of vitamins could reduce blood pressure[40] and improve lipid profiles by increasing HDL cholesterol and apolipoprotein A-1.[41]

Cognitive function

A recent RCT involving 910 men and women aged >65 years living in the community evaluated the effect of daily supplementation with 11 vitamins and five minerals on cognitive function. There was no evidence of overall benefit on cognitive function, but there was weak evidence for a beneficial effect in those aged >75 years and in those at increased risk of micronutrient deficiency.[42]

Behaviour in youngsters

A double-blind RCT in 231 young adult prisoners found that antisocial behaviour in prisons, including violence, was reduced by vitamins and minerals and essential fatty acids.[43] Reduced violence and antisocial behaviour was also observed in a group of children aged 6–12 years given multivitamin supplements compared with those given placebo.[44]

Eye health

Multivitamin use has been associated with reduced risk of cataract in two observational studies.[45,46] In another observational study, use of vitamins combined with zinc had no influence on the risk of early age-related macular degeneration (ARMD).[47]

The Age Related Eye Disease Study (AREDS), a large randomised controlled intervention study, evaluated the effect of anti-oxidant vitamins combined with zinc (80 mg daily) and copper (2 mg daily) on ARMD. Both zinc alone and antioxidants plus zinc significantly reduced the odds of developing advanced ARMD in the higher risk group, but showed no benefits at other stages of the disease.[48] However, supplementation had no significant effect on cataract development.

Conclusions

Multivitamin supplements are not a substitute for poor diet. However, a daily multivitamin/mineral containing RDA doses of a wide range of micronutrients could potentially benefit population groups at risk of poor intakes. In observational studies, use of multivitamins and antioxidants, particularly in the long term, has been linked with reduced risk of cardiovascular disease, cancer and cataract. Evidence for benefit of multivitamins in reducing infection is weak and conflicting. Results of intervention trials with multivitamin supplements have been somewhat disappointing, although multivitamins have been associated with reduced risk of certain stages of ARMD, and of antisocial and violent behaviour in children and youngsters in prison.

Precautions/contraindications

Care should be taken not to exceed safe upper levels of any vitamin and mineral, particularly if taken long term. Caution should be exercised if a multivitamin is taken with one or several other dietary supplements.

Adverse effects

Multivitamin products containing the RDA of vitamins and minerals are generally thought to be safe.

Interactions

Multivitamins may affect warfarin anticoagulation in susceptible patients.[49,50]

See also the monographs on individual vitamins and minerals.

References

1 Office of Population Censuses and Surveys Social Survey Division and Department of Health. *The National Diet and Nutrition Survey: Children Aged 1½ to 4½ Years*. London: HMSO, 1995.

2 Henderson L, Irving K, Gregory J *et al*. *The National Diet and Nutrition Survey: Adults Aged 19 to 64 Years*. Vol. 3: *Vitamin and Mineral Intake and Urinary Analysis*. London: The Stationery Office, 2003.

3 Office for National Statistics Social Survey Division. *National Diet and Nutrition Survey: Young People Aged 4 to 18 Years*. London: The Stationery Office, 2000.

4 Ministry of Agriculture, Fisheries and Food. *National Diet and Nutrition Survey: People Aged 65 Years and Over. Report of the Diet and Nutrition Survey*. London: The Stationery Office, 1998.

5 Bates B, Lennox A, Swan G. National Diet and Nutrition Survey. Headline Results from Year, of the Rolling Programme (2008/2009). A Survey Carried out on Behalf of the Food Standards Agency and the Department of Health. London: The Stationary Office, 2010.

6 Fairfield KM, Fletcher RH. Vitamins for chronic disease prevention in adults: scientific review. *JAMA* 2002; 287: 3116–3126.

7 Harrison RA, Holt D, Pattison DJ, Elton PJ. Are those in need taking dietary supplements? A survey of 21 923 adults. *Br J Nutr* 2004; 91: 617–623.

8 Kiely M, Flynn A, Harrington KE, *et al*. The efficacy and safety of nutritional supplement use in a representative sample of adults in the North/South Ireland Food Consumption Survey. *Public Health Nutr* 2001; 4: 1089–1097.

9 Dwyer JT, Garcea AO, Evans M, *et al*. Do adolescent vitamin-mineral supplement users have better nutrient intakes than nonusers? Observations from the CATCH tracking study *J Am Diet Assoc* 2001; 101: 1340–1346.

10 Stang J, Story MT, Harnack L, Neumark-Sztainer D. Relationships between vitamin and mineral supplement use, dietary intake, and dietary adequacy among adolescents. *J Am Diet Assoc* 2000; 100: 905–910.

11 Briefel R, Hanson C, Fox MK, *et al*. Feeding Infants and Toddlers Study: do vitamin and mineral supplements contribute to nutrient adequacy or excess among US infants and toddlers? *J Am Diet Assoc* 2006; 106(Suppl1): S52–S65.

12 Troppmann L, Gray-Donald K, Johns T. Supplement use: is there any nutritional benefit? *J Am Diet Assoc* 2002; 102: 818–825.

13 Sebastian RS, Cleveland LE, Goldman JD, Moshfegh AJ. Older adults who use vitamin/mineral supplements differ from nonusers in nutrient intake adequacy and dietary attitudes. *J Am Diet Assoc* 2007; 107: 1322–1332.

14 NIH State-of-the-Science Panel. NIH State-of-the-Science Conference: multivitamin/mineral supplements and chronic disease prevention, May 15–17, 2006, Bethesda, Maryland, USA. *Am J Clin Nutr* 2007; 85: 251S–327S.

15 NIH State-of-the-Science Panel. NIH State-of-the-Science Conference statement on multivitamin/mineral supplements and chronic disease prevention. *NIH Consens State Sci Statements* 2006; 23: 1–30.

16 NIH State-of-the-Science Panel. NIH State-of-the-Science Conference statement on multivitamin/mineral supplements and chronic disease prevention. *Ann Intern Med* 2006; 145: 364–371.

17 Beitz R, Mensink GB, Fischer B, Thamm M. Vitamins: dietary intake and intake from dietary supplements in Germany. *Eur J Clin Nutr* 2002; 56: 539–545.

18 Schwarzpaul S, Strassburg A, Luhrmann PM, Neuhauser-Berthold M. Intake of vitamin and mineral supplements in an elderly German population. *Ann Nutr Metab* 2006; 50: 155–162.

19 Archer SL, Stamler J, Moag-Stahlberg A, *et al.* Association of dietary supplement use with specific micronutrient intakes among middle-aged American men and women: the INTERMAP Study. *J Am Diet Assoc* 2005; 105: 1106–1114.

20 Fox MK, Reidy K, Novak T, Ziegler P. Sources of energy and nutrients in the diets of infants and toddlers. *J Am Diet Assoc* 2006; 106(Suppl 1): S28–S42.

21 Kim SH, Han JH, Keen CL. Vitamin and mineral supplement use by healthy teenagers in Korea: motivating factors and dietary consequences. *Nutrition* 2001; 17: 373–380.

22 Sichert-Hellert W, Wenz G, Kersting M. Vitamin intakes from supplements and fortified food in German children and adolescents: results from the DONALD study. *J Nutr* 2006; 136: 1329–1333.

23 Girodon F, Blache D, Monget AL, *et al.* Effect of a two-year supplementation with low doses of antioxidant vitamins and/or minerals in elderly subjects on levels of nutrients and antioxidant defense parameters. *J Am Coll Nutr* 1997; 16: 357–365.

24 Navarro M, Wood RJ. Plasma changes in micronutrients following a multivitamin and mineral supplement in healthy adults. *J Am Coll Nutr* 2003; 22: 124–132.

25 Wolters M, Hermann S, Hahn A. Effects of 6-month multivitamin supplementation on serum concentrations of alpha-tocopherol, beta-carotene, and vitamin C in healthy elderly women. *Int J Vitam Nutr Res* 2004; 74: 161–168.

26 Jacobs EJ, Connell CJ, Chao A, *et al.* Multivitamin use and colorectal cancer incidence in a US cohort: does timing matter? *Am J Epidemiol* 2003; 158: 621–628.

27 Stevens VL, McCullough ML, Diver WR, *et al.* Use of multivitamins and prostate cancer mortality in a large cohort of US men. *Cancer Causes Control* 2005; 16: 643–650.

28 Lawson KA, Wright ME, Subar A, *et al.* Multivitamin use and risk of prostate cancer in the National Institutes of Health-AARP Diet and Health Study. *J Natl Cancer Inst* 2007; 99: 754–764.

29 Giovannucci E, Rimm EB, Ascherio A, *et al.* Alcohol, low methionine, low folate diets and risk of colon cancer in men. *J Natl Cancer Inst* 1995; 87: 265–273.

30 Giovannucci E, Stampfer MJ, Colditz GA, *et al.* Multivitamin use, folate and colon cancer in women in the Nurses' Health Study. *Ann Intern Med* 1998; 129: 517–524.

31 Cho E, Hunter DJ, Spiegelman D, *et al.* Intakes of vitamins A, C and E and folate and multivitamins and lung cancer: a pooled analysis of 8 prospective studies. *Int J Cancer* 2006; 118: 970–978.

32 El-Kadiki A, Sutton AJ. Role of multivitamins and mineral supplements in preventing infections in elderly people: systematic review and meta-analysis of randomised controlled trials. *BMJ* 2005; 330: 871.

33 Stephen AI, Avenell A. A systematic review of multivitamin and multimineral supplementation for infection. *J Hum Nutr Diet* 2006; 19: 179–190.

34 Neuman MI, Willett WC, Curhan GC. Vitamin and micronutrient intake and the risk of community-acquired pneumonia in US women. *Am J Med* 2007; 120: 330–336.

35 Fawzi WW, Msamanga GI, Spiegelman D, *et al.* A randomized trial of multivitamin supplements and HIV disease progression and mortality. *N Engl J Med* 2004; 351: 23–32.

36 Merchant AT, Msamanga G, Villamor E, *et al.* Multivitamin supplementation of HIV-positive women during pregnancy reduces hypertension. *J Nutr* 2005; 135: 1776–1781.

37 Rimm EB, Willett WC, Hu FB, *et al.* Folate and vitamin B_6 from diet and supplements in relation to risk of coronary heart disease among women. *JAMA* 1998; 279: 359–364.

38 Holmquist C, Larsson S, Wolk A, deFaire U. Multivitamin supplements are inversely associated with risk of myocardial infarction in men and women: Stockholm Heart Epidemiology Program (SHEEP). *J Nutr* 2003; 133: 2650–2654.

39 Muntwyler J, Hennekens CH, Manson JE, *et al.* Vitamin supplement use in a low-risk population of US male physicians and subsequent cardiovascular mortality. *Arch Intern Med* 2002; 162: 1472–1476.

40 Farvid MS, Jalali M, Siassi F, *et al.* The impact of vitamins and/or mineral supplementation on blood pressure in type 2 diabetes. *J Am Coll Nutr* 2004; 23: 272–279.

41 Farvid MS, Siassi F, Jalali M, *et al.* The impact of vitamin and/or mineral supplementation on lipid profiles in type 2 diabetes. *Diabetes Res Clin Pract* 2004; 65: 21–28.

42 McNeill G, Avenell A, Campbell MK, *et al.* Effect of multivitamin and multimineral supplementation on cognitive function in men and women aged 65

years and over: a randomised controlled trial. *Nutr J* 2007; 6: 10.

43 Gesch CB, Hammond SM, Hampson SE, *et al.* Influence of supplementary vitamins, minerals and essential fatty acids on the antisocial behaviour of young adult prisoners. Randomised, placebo-controlled trial. *Br J Psych* 2002; 181: 22–28.

44 Schoenthaler SJ, Bier ID. The effect of vitamin-mineral supplementation on juvenile delinquency among American schoolchildren: a randomized, double-blind placebo-controlled trial. *J Altern Complement Med* 2000; 6: 7–17.

45 Kuzniarz M, Mitchell P, Cumming RG, Flood VM. Use of vitamin supplements and cataract: the Blue Mountains Eye Study. *Am J Ophthalmol* 2001; 132: 19–26.

46 Leske MC, Chylack LT, Jr. He Q, *et al.* Antioxidant vitamins and nuclear opacities: the longitudinal study of cataract. *Ophthalmology* 1998; 105: 831–836.

47 Kuzniarz M, Mitchell P, Flood VM, Wang JJ. Use of vitamin and zinc supplements and age-related maculopathy: the Blue Mountains Eye Study. *Ophthalmic Epidemiol* 2002; 9: 283–295.

48 Age-Related Eye Disease Study Research Group. A randomized, placebo-controlled, clinical trial of high-dose supplementation with vitamins C and E and beta-carotene for age-related cataract and vision loss: AREDS report no. 9. *Arch Ophthalmol* 2001; 119: 1439–1452.

49 Kurnik D, Lubetsky A, Loebstein R, *et al.* Multivitamin supplements may affect warfarin anticoagulation in susceptible patients. *Ann Pharmacother* 2003; 37: 1603–1606.

50 Kurnik D, Loebstein R, Rabinovitz H, *et al.* Over-the-counter vitamin K_1-containing multivitamin supplements disrupt warfarin anticoagulation in vitamin K_1-depleted patients. A prospective, controlled trial. *Thromb Haemost* 2004; 92: 1018–1024.

N-Acetyl cysteine

Description

N-Acetyl cysteine (NAC) is a derivative of the dietary amino acid L-cysteine. It is a source of sulphydryl groups and, as such, can stimulate the synthesis of reduced glutathione (GSH), an endogenous antioxidant. It has been in clinical use for more than 30 years as a mucolytic agent for a variety of respiratory conditions, but is now available as a dietary supplement.

Action

By stimulating the production of glutathione, NAC acts as an antioxidant. It also helps to protect the liver from various toxicants and is used at high doses for the treatment of paracetamol-induced toxicity. NAC also chelates heavy metals such as cadmium, lead and mercury, and may be useful for the treatment of heavy metal toxicity.

Possible uses

NAC is promoted for influenza, bronchitis and the management of symptoms related to HIV and cancer.

Respiratory conditions

Oral NAC has been used since the 1960s for the treatment of bronchitis and it has also been advocated as a prophylactic in patients with chronic bronchitis. Various trials have also reported that supplementation may reduce the duration of bronchitic exacerbations.

In a study in nine patients for 4 weeks,[1] regular use of NAC 200 mg three times a day resulted in no significant differences in lung function, mucociliary clearance curves or sputum viscosity compared with placebo. In another study involving 181 patients randomised to receive either NAC 200 mg three times a day or placebo for 5 months in a double-blind manner, the number of exacerbations of bronchitis and the total number of days taking an antibiotic was reduced in the NAC group compared with placebo, but the differences were not significant.[2]

A further study in 526 patients suffering from chronic bronchitis found no significant differences between NAC and placebo in the number of exacerbations, but there was a significant reduction with NAC in the number of days patients were incapacitated.[3] Yet another double-blind, randomised, placebo-controlled trial found that NAC tablets 300 mg three times a day were associated with a significant reduction in the number of sick leave days after 4 months of treatment during the winter. After 6 months, the number of sick leave days and exacerbations of bronchitis remained lower in the NAC group, but the differences were not significant.[4]

An open randomised study involving 169 patients with chronic obstructive pulmonary disease (COPD) found that NAC 600 mg daily plus standard treatment compared with placebo plus standard treatment was associated with a reduction in the number of sick leave days and exacerbations.[5]

A meta-analysis of nine double-blind, placebo-controlled trials of oral NAC in chronic bronchopulmonary disease concluded that a prolonged course of NAC prevents acute exacerbations of chronic bronchitis, thus possibly reducing morbidity and healthcare costs.[6]

A quantitative systematic review of 11 trials published between 1976 and 1994 found that oral NAC reduces the risk of exacerbations and improves symptoms in patients with chronic bronchitis compared with placebo, without increasing the risk of adverse effects. However, the question of whether this benefit is sufficient to justify the routine use of NAC in all patients with bronchitis should be addressed with further studies, the authors concluded.[7]

More recent trials have not demonstrated positive results. An NAC/vitamin C combination had no clinical benefit in chronic bronchitis.[8] In one RCT involving 523 patients in 50 centres, oral NAC 600 mg daily and placebo produced similar clinical outcomes (fall in vital capacity, number of exacerbations). However, amongst patients not taking inhaled corticosteroids, those on NAC had significantly fewer exacerbations.[9] Two further trials have found that NAC reduced the oxidative burden (as shown by reduced exhaled hydrogen peroxide) in airways of stable COPD patients.[10,11]

A multinational study in 155 patients with idiopathic pulmonary fibrosis found that mortality was no different between groups treated with NAC and placebo. However, the NAC group had 9% better vital capacity and improved carbon monoxide diffusing capacity. There was also a slightly lower rate of myelotoxicity in the NAC group.[12] An Italian trial evaluated the impact of oxygen treatment on oxidation free radicals and the effect of NAC in that process. Forty-five stable COPD patients were given oxygen along with placebo or NAC (1200 or 1800 mg daily). Oxygen therapy increased free radical production and disturbed redox balance, but this was prevented by NAC.[13]

Influenza

In a randomised, double-blind study, 262 subjects, 62% of whom had chronic but non-respiratory degenerative disease (e.g. cardiovascular disease, diabetes, arthritis) received NAC 1200 mg daily or placebo for 6 months. In the NAC group, there was a significant reduction in influenza-like episodes, severity of illness and length of time confined to bed as compared with the placebo group.[14] However, NAC did not prevent subclinical influenza infection (as assessed by antibody response to A/H_1N_1 virus), but the authors concluded that it reduced the incidence of clinically apparent disease.

Human immunodeficiency virus

In general, HIV-positive individuals have low levels of cysteine and GSH, and it has been suggested that NAC may benefit these patients by raising GSH levels,[15,16] but evidence for the value of NAC supplementation is equivocal.

In a double-blind, placebo-controlled trial, 45 HIV-positive patients on antiretroviral therapy were randomised to receive 800 mg NAC or placebo for 4 months. In the NAC group, cysteine levels increased from their low pretreatment levels, and tumour necrosis factor-alpha levels fell. In addition, the decline in CD4 lymphocyte count found at the start of the study was less severe in the NAC group compared with placebo.[17] Another trial found that NAC was capable of raising the CD cell count faster than a placebo.[18]

NAC has also been investigated in combination with trimethoprim–sulfamethoxazole in the prophylaxis of *Pneumocystis jiroveci* (was *carinii*) in HIV-positive patients.[19,20] It has been suggested that adverse reactions to the antibiotics are due to low GSH levels in these patients, which may be improved by NAC supplementation. However, NAC did not reduce the risk of adverse reactions to trimethoprim–sulfamethoxazole in either study.

A further 180-day RCT found that there were no measurable benefits of supplementing antiretroviral therapy with NAC in terms of viral load, tumour necrosis factor-alpha and lymphocyte apoptosis. Baseline levels of GSH were not recovered.[21]

Cancer

Preliminary *in vitro* studies have indicated that NAC could have a role in the prevention and management of some forms of cancer. In a large randomised trial, 2592 patients (60% with head and neck cancer and 40% with lung cancer), most of whom were previous or current smokers, received vitamin A (300 000 units daily for 1 year, followed by 150 000 units daily during the second year), NAC (600 mg daily for 2 years), both compounds or placebo.[22] However, there was no benefit in terms of survival, event-free survival or second primary tumours with either vitamin A or NAC. A further small trial in smokers found that NAC has the potential to modulate certain cancer-associated biomarkers in specific organs, and could therefore impact upon tobacco smoke carcinogenicity in humans.[23]

Infertility

NAC is being evaluated in an obstetric setting (not as a dietary supplement in the community) for a possible role in augmenting ovulation (in combination with clomiphene citrate) in the management of unexplained infertility or infertility caused by polycystic ovary syndrome. Results from trials have been inconsistent, with some trials showing improved ovulation rate[24,25] or reduced pregnancy loss[26] while others have not.[27–29] One trial has shown that supplemental selenium with NAC improves semen quality in infertile men.[30]

Miscellaneous

NAC has been evaluated for a range of other conditions. Preliminary trials have suggested that NAC may improve depressive symptoms in bipolar disorder,[31] improve glutathione regulation in schizophrenia,[32] manipulate the glutamate system to reduce reward-seeking addictive behaviours such as gambling,[33] protect people with identifiable genotypes against noise-induced loss of hearing,[34] and, in combination with mesalazine, improve the clinical picture in ulcerative colitis compared with mesalazine alone.[35]

> ### Conclusion
> NAC may be useful as prophylaxis in patients with chronic bronchitis and COPD. There is preliminary evidence from one study that it may also reduce symptoms of influenza in older people. Preliminary studies in HIV-positive patients suggest that NAC may improve the clinical picture in such patients, although further research is required. *In vitro* work has indicated that NAC could reduce the risk of cancer, although one large study has shown no significant benefits.

Precautions/contraindications

None reported.

Pregnancy and breast-feeding

No problems have been reported, but there have not been sufficient studies to guarantee the safety of NAC in pregnancy and breast-feeding.

Adverse effects

None reported, but there are no long-term studies assessing the safety of NAC. It has been used since the 1970s with few side-effects (e.g. mild gastrointestinal side-effects and skin rash). Such adverse effects that have been noted have occurred mainly with large oral doses of NAC given for paracetamol poisoning.

Interactions

None reported.

Dose

NAC is available in the form of tablets.

The dose is not established (for use as a supplement). Clinical trials have used 600–1200 mg daily.

References

1   Millar AB, Pavia D, Agnew JE, *et al.* Effect of oral *N*-acetylcysteine on mucus clearance. *Br J Dis Chest* 1985; 79: 262–266.
2   British Thoracic Society Research Committee. Oral *N*-acetylcysteine and exacerbation rates in patients with chronic bronchitis and severe airways obstruction. *Thorax* 1985; 40: 832–835.
3   Parr GD, Huitson A, Oral Fabrol (oral *N*-acetyl cysteine) in chronic bronchitis. *Br J Dis Chest* 1987; 81: 341–348.
4   Rasmussen JB, Glennow C. Reduction in days of illness after long-term treatment with *N*-acetyl-cysteine controlled-release tablets in patients with chronic bronchitis. *Eur Respir J* 1988; 1: 341–345.
5   Pela R, Calcagni AM, Subiaco S, *et al.* *N*-Acetyl-cysteine reduces the exacerbation rate in patients with moderate to severe COPD. *Respiration* 1999; 66: 495–500.
6   Grandjean EM, Berthet P, Ruffmann R, Leuenberger P. Efficacy of oral long-term *N*-acetylcysteine in chronic bronchopulmonary disease: a meta-analysis of published double-blind, placebo-controlled clinical trials. *Clin Ther* 2000; 22: 209–221.
7   Stey C, Steurer J, Bachmann S, *et al.* The effect of *N*-acetylcysteine in chronic bronchitis: a quantitative systematic review. *Eur Respir J* 2000; 16: 253–262.
8   Lukas R, Scharling B, Schultze-Werninghaus G, Gillissen A. Antioxidant treatment with *N*-acetyl-cysteine and vitamin C in patients with chronic bronchitis. *Deutsch Med Wochenschr* 2005; 130: 563–567.
9   Decramer M, Rutten-van Molken M, Dekhuijzen PN, *et al.* Effects of *N*-acetylcysteine on outcomes in chronic obstructive pulmonary disease (Bronchitis Randomized NAC Cost-Utility Study, BRONCUS): a randomized placebo-controlled study. *Lancet* 2005; 365: 1552–1560.
10 DeBenedetto F, Aceto A, Dragani B, *et al.* Long-term oral *N*-acetylcysteine reduces exhaled

hydrogen peroxide in stable COPD. *Pulm Pharmacol Ther* 2005; 18: 41–47.

11 Kasielski M, Nowak D. Long-term administration of N-acetylcysteine decreases hydrogen peroxide exhalation in subjects with chronic obstructive airways disease. *Respir Med* 2001; 95: 448–456.

12 Demedts M, Behr J, Buhl R, *et al.* High dose acetylcysteine in idiopathic pulmonary fibrosis. *N Engl J Med* 2005; 353: 2229–2242.

13 Foschino Barbaro MP, Serviddio G, Resta O, *et al.* Oxygen therapy at low flow causes oxidative stress in chronic obstructive pulmonary disease. Prevention by N-acetylcysteine. *Free Radic Res* 2005; 39: 1111–1118.

14 De Flora S, Grassi C, Carati L. Attenuation of influenza-like symptomatology and improvement of cell-mediated immunity with long-term N-acetyl cysteine treatment. *Eur Respir J* 1997; 10: 1535–1541.

15 Herzenbeg LA, De Rosa SC, Dubs JG, *et al.* Glutathione deficiency is associated with impaired survival in HIV disease. *Proc Natl Acad Sci USA* 1997; 94: 1967–1972.

16 De Rosa SC, Zaretsky MD, Dubs JG, *et al.* N-Acetylcysteine replenishes glutathione in HIV infection. *Eur J Clin Invest* 2000; 30: 915–929.

17 Akerlund B, Jarstrand C, Lindeke B, *et al.* Effect of N-acetylcysteine (NAC) treatment on HIV-1 infection: a double-blind placebo-controlled trial. *Eur J Clin Pharmacol* 1996; 50: 457–461.

18 Spada C, Treitlinger A, Reis M, *et al.* The effect of N-acetylcysteine supplementation upon viral load, CD4, CD8 total lymphocyte count and haematocrit in individuals undergoing antiretroviral treatment. *Clin Chem Lab Med* 2002; 40: 452–455.

19 Akerlund B, Tynell E, Bratt G, *et al.* N-Acetylcysteine treatment and the risk of toxic reactions to trimethoprim-sulphamethoxazole in primary *Pneumocystis carinii* prophylaxis in HIV-infected patients. *J Infect* 1997; 35: 143–147.

20 Walmsley SL, Khorasheh S, Singer J, *et al.* A randomised trial of N-acetylcysteine for prevention of trimethoprim-sulphamethoxazole hypersensitivity reactions in *Pneumocystis carinii* pneumonia prophylaxis (CTN 057). Canadian HIV Trials Network 057 Study Group. *J Acquir Immune Defic Syndr Hum Retrovir* 1998; 19: 498–505.

21 Treitinger A, Spada C, Masokawa IY, *et al.* Effect of N-acetyl-L-cysteine on lymphocyte apoptosis, lymphocyte viability, TNF-alpha and IL-8 in HIV infected patients undergoing antiretroviral treatment. *Br J Infect Dis* 2004; 8: 363–371.

22 Van Zandwijk N, Dalesio O, Pastorino U, *et al.* EUROSCAN, a randomized trial of vitamin A and N-acetylcysteine in patients with head and neck cancer or lung cancer. For the European Organization for Research and Treatment of Cancer Head and Neck and Lung Cancer Cooperative Groups. *J Natl Cancer Inst* 2000; 92: 977–986.

23 Van Schooten FJ, Besaratinia A, De Flora S, *et al.* Effects of oral administration of N-acetyl-L-cysteine: a multi-biomarker study in smokers. *Cancer Epidemiol Biomarkers Prev* 2002; 11: 167–175.

24 Badawy A, State O, Abdelgawad S. N-Acetyl cysteine and clomiphene citrate for induction of ovulation in polycystic ovary syndrome: a cross-over trial. *Acta Obstet Gynecol Scand* 2007; 86(2): 218–222.

25 Nasr A. Effect of N-acetyl-cysteine after ovarian drilling in clomiphene citrate-resistant PCOS women: a pilot study. *Reprod Biomed Online* 2009; 20(3): 403–409.

26 Amin AF, Shaaban OM, Bediawy MA. N-acetyl cysteine for treatment of recurrent unexplained pregnancy loss. *Reprod Biomed Online* 2008; 17 (5): 722–726.

27 Badawy A, Baker El Nashar A, El Totongy M. Clomiphene citrate plus N-acetyl cysteine versus clomiphene citrate for augmenting ovulation in the management of unexplained infertility: a randomized double-blind controlled trial. *Fertil Steril* 2006; 86(3): 647–650.

28 Elnashar A, Fahmy M, Mansour A, *et al.* N-Acetyl cysteine vs. metformin in treatment of clomiphene citrate-resistant polycystic ovary syndrome: a prospective randomized controlled study. *Fertil Steril* 2007; 88(2): 406–409.

29 Abu Hashim H, Anwar K, El-Fatah RA. N-Acetyl cysteine plus clomiphene citrate versus metformin and clomiphene citrate in treatment of clomiphene-resistant polycystic ovary syndrome: a randomized controlled trial. *J Womens Health (Larchmt)* 2010; 19(11): 2043–2048.

30 Safarinejad MR, Safarinejad S. Efficacy of selenium and/or N-acetyl-cysteine for improving semen parameters in infertile men: a double-blind, placebo controlled, randomized study. *J Urol* 2009; 181(2): 741–751.

31 Berk M, Copolov D, Dean O, *et al.* N-Acetyl cysteine as a glutathione precursor for schizophrenia— a double-blind, randomized, placebo-controlled trial. *Biol Psychiatry* 2008; 64(5): 361–368.

32 Lavoie S, Murray MM, Deppen P, *et al.* Glutathione precursor, N-acetyl-cysteine, improves mismatch negativity in schizophrenia patients. *Neuropsychopharmacology* 2008; 33(9): 2187–2199.

33 Grant JE, Kim SW, Odlaug BL. N-Acetyl cysteine, a glutamate-modulating agent, in the treatment of pathological gambling: a pilot study. *Biol Psychiatry* 2007; 62(6): 652–657.

34 Lin CY, Wu JL, Shih TS, *et al.* N-Acetyl-cysteine against noise-induced temporary threshold shift in male workers. *Hear Res* 2010; 269(12): 42–47.

35 Guijarro LG, Mate J, Gisbert JP, *et al.* N-Acetyl-L-cysteine combined with mesalamine in the treatment of ulcerative colitis: randomized, placebo-controlled pilot study. *World J Gastroenterol* 2008; 14(18): 2851–2857.

Niacin

Description

Niacin is a water-soluble vitamin of the vitamin B complex.

Nomenclature

Niacin is a generic term used to describe the compounds that exhibit the biological properties of nicotinamide. It occurs in food as nicotinamide and nicotinic acid. It is sometimes known as niacinamide.

Units

Requirements and food values for niacin are the sum of the amounts of nicotinic acid and nicotinamide. Niacin is also obtained in the body from the amino acid tryptophan. On average, 60 mg tryptophan is equivalent to 1 mg niacin.

Niacin (mg equivalents) = nicotinic acid (mg)

+ nicotinamide (mg)

+ tryptophan (mg)/60

Human requirements

Niacin requirements depend on energy intake; values are therefore given as mg/1000 kcal and also as total values based on estimated average energy requirements for the majority of people in the UK (Table 1).

Dietary intake

In the UK, the average adult diet provides (niacin equivalents): for men, 44.7 mg daily; for women, 30.9 mg.

Action

Nutritional

As a vitamin, niacin functions as a component of two coenzymes, nicotinamide adenine dinucleotide (NAD) and nicotinamide adenine dinucleotide diphosphate (NADP). These coenzymes participate in many metabolic processes including glycolysis, tissue respiration, lipid, amino acid and purine metabolism.

Pharmacological

In doses in excess of nutritional requirements, nicotinic acid (but not nicotinamide) reduces serum cholesterol and triglycerides by inhibiting the synthesis of VLDLs, which are the precursors of LDLs. Nicotinic acid also causes direct peripheral vasodilatation.

Dietary sources

See Table 2 for dietary sources of niacin.

Metabolism

Absorption

Both nicotinamide and nicotinic acid are absorbed in the duodenum by facilitated diffusion (at low concentrations) and by passive diffusion (at high concentrations).

Distribution

Conversion of niacin to its coenzymes occurs in most tissues.

Elimination

Elimination occurs mainly via the urine. Niacin appears in breast milk.

Bioavailability

Niacin is remarkably stable and can withstand reasonable periods of heating, cooking and storage with little loss. Bioavailability of niacin from cereals may be low, but much of the niacin in breakfast cereals comes from fully available synthetic niacin added to fortify such products.

Table 1 Dietary Reference Values for niacin (nicotinic acid equivalent) (mg/day)

Age	UK					USA		EU RDA = 18 mg
								FAO/WHO
	LRNI[1]	EAR[1]	RNI[1]	RNI[2]	EVM	RDA[2]	TUL[2]	RNI[2]
0–6 months	4.4	5.5	6.6	3		2	–	2
7–12 months	4.4	5.5	6.6	5		3	–	4
1–3 years	4.4	5.5	6.6	8		6	10	6
4–6 years	4.4	5.5	6.6	11		–	–	9
4–8 years	–	–	–	–		8	15	–
7–10 years	4.4	5.5	6.6	12		–	–	12[a]
9–13 years	–	–	–	–		12	20	–
Males								
11–14 years	4.4	5.5	6.6	15		–	–	16[b]
15–18 years	4.4	5.5	6.6	18		–	–	16
14–18 years	–	–	–	–		16	30	–
19–50 years	4.4	5.5	6.6	17	17[3]	16	35	16
51–65+ years	–	–	–	–		–	–	16
51–70+ years	–	–	–	–		16	35	–
Females								
11–14 years	4.4	5.5	6.6	12		–	–	14[b]
15–18 years	4.4	5.5	6.6	14		–	–	14
14–18 years	–	–	–	–		14	30	–
19–50 years	4.4	5.5	6.6	13	17[3]	14	35	14
51–65+ years	–	–	–	–		–	–	14
51–70+ years	–	–	–	–		14	35	–
Pregnancy	*	*	*	–		18	35[4]	18
Lactation	*	*	+2.3	+2		17	35[4]	17

[a] 7–9 years. [b] 10–14 years. [1] mg/1000 kcal. [2] mg/day.
[3] Likely safe daily intake of nicotinamide from supplements alone is 500 mg daily. [4] Women < 18 years = 30 mg daily.
EAR = Estimated Average Requirement.
EVM = Likely safe daily intake of nicotinic acid from supplements alone.
LRNI = Lowest Reference Nutrient Intake.
RNI = Reference Nutrient Intake.
TUL = Tolerable Upper Intake Level.

Deficiency

Niacin deficiency (rare in the UK) may lead to pellagra. Early signs of deficiency are vague and non-specific and may include reduced appetite, weight loss, gastrointestinal discomfort, weakness, irritability and inability to concentrate. Signs of more advanced deficiency include sore mouth, glossitis and stomatitis. The severe deficiency state of pellagra is characterised by dermatitis (predominantly in the areas of skin exposed to sunlight), dementia (associated with confusion, disorientation, seizures and hallucinations) and diarrhoea.

Possible uses

Despite claims made for niacin, it is of unproven value in arthritis, alcohol dependence,

Table 2 Dietary sources of niacin

Food portion	Niacin content[1] (mg)
Breakfast cereals	
1 bowl All-Bran (45 g)	*6.5*
1 bowl Bran Flakes (45 g)	*7.5*
1 bowl Corn Flakes (30 g)	*5.0*
1 bowl muesli (95 g)	**8.0**
1 bowl Start (40 g)	**10.0**
2 pieces Shredded Wheat	*3.0*
2 Weetabix	*6.0*
Cereal products	
Bread, brown, 2 slices	*3.0*
white, 2 slices	*2.5*
wholemeal, 2 slices	*4.0*
1 chapati	*2.5*
1 naan bread	*5.0*
1 white pitta bread	*2.5*
Pasta, brown, boiled (150 g)	*3.5*
white, boiled (150 g)	*2.0*
Rice, brown, boiled (160 g)	*3.0*
white, boiled (160 g)	*2.0*
2 heaped tablespoons wheatgerm	*1.5*
Milk and dairy products	
Milk, whole, semi-skimmed, or skimmed (284 ml; ¹/₂ pint)	*2.5*
Soya milk (284 ml; ¹/₂ pint)	*1.5*
1 pot yoghurt (150 g)	*1.5*
Cheese (50 g)	*1.5*
1 egg, size 2 (60 g)	*2.5*
Meat and fish	
Beef, roast (85 g)	**10.0**
Lamb, roast (85 g)	**10.0**
Pork, roast (85 g)	**10.0**
1 chicken leg portion	**16.0**
Liver, lambs, cooked (90 g)	**18.0**
Kidney, lambs, cooked (75g)	**11.5**
Fish, cooked (150 g)	**10–15**
Vegetables	
Peas, boiled (100 g)	*2.5*
Potatoes, boiled (150 g)	*1.5*
1 small can baked beans (200 g)	*2.6*
Chickpeas, cooked (105 g)	*2.0*
Red kidney beans (105 g)	*2.0*
Dahl, lentil (150 g)	*1.5*
Nuts	
30 peanuts	*6.5*
Yeast	
Brewer's yeast (10 g)	*1.5*
Marmite, spread on 1 slice bread	*3.5*

Niacin equivalents (includes both preformed niacin and niacin obtained from tryptophan).
Excellent sources (**bold**); good sources (*italics*).

schizophrenia and other mental disorders unrelated to niacin deficiency. Nicotinic acid is prescribable on the NHS for hyperlipidaemia, but should not be sold as a supplement for this purpose.

Niacin (nicotinamide) is being evaluated in studies either alone or with cholesterol-lowering drugs for effect in cholesterol lowering and other cardiovascular risk factors. Some studies,[1–5] a meta-analysis[6] and a review[6] have demonstrated efficacy in cholesterol lowering while others have demonstrated efficacy of niacin in endothelial dysfunction.[7–9] However, doses used are high (500–1000 mg daily) and exceed the UK safe upper level, which makes this use unsuitable for dietary supplementation. In any case, further studies are required to confirm these findings.

In combination with coenzyme Q and riboflavin, niacin has been shown in patients with breast cancer to reduce cytokine levels[10] and serum tumour marker levels,[11] and to increase DNA repair enzyme and disappearance of DNA methylation.[12]

Oral nicotinamide (500 mg or 1500 mg daily) may inhibit the suppression of skin immunity induced by ultraviolet light.[13] (Cutaneous immunity is a significant defence against skin cancer.) In an epidemiological study, high intake of niacin was associated with reduced DNA damage in airline pilots exposed to ionising radiation.[14]

Precautions/contraindications

Large doses of niacin are best avoided in gout (may increase uric acid levels); peptic ulcer (large doses may activate an ulcer); and liver disease (large doses cause deterioration). Large doses should also be used with caution in diabetes mellitus owing to possible effects on glycaemic control.[6] However, studies suggest that lipid-modifying doses can safely be used in patients with diabetes.[15] Supplements containing nicotinic acid should not be used as a cholesterol-lowering agent without medical advice.

Pregnancy and breast-feeding

No problems reported.

Adverse effects

Both nicotinamide and nicotinic acid can be toxic in excessive amounts, but the effects are somewhat different.

Nicotinamide

In normal doses, nicotinamide is not toxic, but chronic administration at doses of 3 g daily for periods of more than 3 months may cause nausea, headaches, heartburn, fatigue, sore throat, dry hair, dry skin and blurred vision.

Nicotinic acid

Acute flushing (at doses of 100–200 mg, but reduced risk with sustained-release preparations), pounding headache, dizziness, nausea, vomiting, pruritis; occasionally decreased glucose tolerance and increased uric acid levels; rarely hepatic impairment (risk may be increased with sustained-release preparations) and hypertension.

Oral niacin has been associated with an increase in intraocular pressure in a patient with glaucoma. The intraocular pressure of a 73-year-old man with a history of primary open-angle glaucoma had been approximately 21 and 17 mmHg in the right and left eyes, respectively, while taking latanoprost 0.005% and dorzolamide hydrochloride 2%. When taking 500 mg oral niacin, his intraocular pressure increased to 37 and 27 mmHg in the right and left eyes, respectively, on one occasion. On re-examination, the intraocular pressure had increased to 28 and 23 mmHg in the right and left eyes, respectively. Each time the niacin was stopped, the intraocular pressure decreased to the original levels.[16]

Interactions

Drugs

Lipid-lowering drugs: increased risk of rhabdomyolysis and myopathy (combined therapy should include careful monitoring).

Nutrients

Adequate amounts of all B vitamins are required for optimal functioning; deficiency or excess of one B vitamin may lead to abnormalities in the metabolism of another.

Dose

Nicotinamide is available in the form of tablets, but is found mainly in multivitamin and mineral products.

Dietary supplements generally provide 30–50 mg daily.

References

1   Whitney EJ, Krasuski RA, Personius BE, *et al.* A randomized trial of a strategy for increasing high-density lipoprotein cholesterol levels: effects on progression of coronary heart disease and clinical events. *Ann Intern Med* 2005; 142(2): 95–104.
2   Taylor AJ, Sullenberger LE, Lee HJ, *et al.* Arterial Biology for the Investigation of the Treatment Effects of Reducing Cholesterol (ARBITER) 2: a double-blind, placebo-controlled study of extended-release niacin on atherosclerosis progression in secondary prevention patients treated with statins. *Circulation* 2004; 110(23): 3512–3517.
3   McKenney JM, McCormick LS, Schaefer EJ, *et al.* Effect of niacin and atorvastatin on lipoprotein subclasses in patients with atherogenic dyslipidemia. *Am J Cardiol* 2001; 88(3): 270–274.
4   Maccubbin D, Bays HE, Olsson AG, *et al.* Lipid-modifying efficacy and tolerability of extended-release niacin/laropiprant in patients with primary hypercholesterolaemia or mixed dyslipidaemia. *Int J Clin Pract* 2008; 62(12): 1959–1970.
5   Karas RH, Kashyap ML, Knopp RH, *et al.* Long-term safety and efficacy of a combination of niacin extended release and simvastatin in patients with dyslipidemia: the OCEANS study. *Am J Cardiovasc Drugs* 2008; 8(2): 69–81.
6   Goldberg RB, Jacobson TA. Effects of niacin on glucose control in patients with dyslipidemia. *Mayo Clin Proc* 2008; 83(4): 470–478.
7   Taylor AJ, Lee HJ, Sullenberger LE. The effect of 24 months of combination statin and extended-release niacin on carotid intima-media thickness: ARBITER 3. *Curr Med Res Opin* 2006; 22(11): 2243–2250.
8   Taylor AJ, Villines TC, Stanek EJ, *et al.* Extended-release niacin or ezetimibe and carotid intima-media thickness. *N Engl J Med* 2009; 361(22): 2113–2122.
9   Warnholtz A, Wild P, Ostad MA, *et al.* Effects of oral niacin on endothelial dysfunction in patients with coronary artery disease: results of the randomized, double-blind, placebo-controlled INEF study. *Atherosclerosis* 2009; 204(1): 216–221.
10 Premkumar VG, Yuvaraj S, Vijayasarathy K, *et al.* Serum cytokine levels of interleukin-1beta, -6, -8, tumour necrosis factor-alpha and vascular endothelial growth factor in breast cancer patients treated

with tamoxifen and supplemented with co-enzyme Q(10), riboflavin and niacin. *Basic Clin Pharmacol Toxicol* 2007; 100(6): 387–391.

11 Premkumar VG, Yuvaraj S, Vijayasarathy K, *et al.* Effect of coenzyme Q10, riboflavin and niacin on serum CEA and CA 15-3 levels in breast cancer patients undergoing tamoxifen therapy. *Biol Pharm Bull* 2007; 30(2): 367–370.

12 Premkumar VG, Yuvaraj S, Shanthi P, *et al.* Co-enzyme Q10, riboflavin and niacin supplementation on alteration of DNA repair enzyme and DNA methylation in breast cancer patients undergoing tamoxifen therapy. *Br J Nutr* 2008; 100(6): 1179–1182.

13 Yiasemides E, Sivapirabu G, Halliday GM, *et al.* Oral nicotinamide protects against ultraviolet

radiation-induced immunosuppression in humans. *Carcinogenesis* 2009; 30(1): 101–105.

14 Yong LC, Petersen MR. High dietary niacin intake is associated with decreased chromosome translocation frequency in airline pilots. *Br J Nutr* 2010; 105(4): 496–505.

15 Elam MB, Hunninghake DB, Davis KB, *et al.* Effect of niacin on lipid and lipoprotein levels and glycemic control in patients with diabetes and peripheral arterial disease: the ADMIT study: A randomized trial. Arterial Disease Multiple Intervention Trial. *JAMA* 2000; 284(10): 1263–1270.

16 Tittler EH, deBarros DS, Navarro JB, *et al.* Oral niacin can increase intraocular pressure. *Ophthalmic Surg Lasers Imaging* 2008; 39(4): 341–342.

Nickel

Description

Nickel is a trace element. It can exist in oxidation states –I, 0, +I, +II, +III and +IV. State II is the most important in biological systems.[1] Nickel has not been shown to be essential in humans, but it is present in a few multivitamin/multimineral supplements in the UK.

Human requirements

Human requirements for nickel have not been established. There are no Dietary Reference Values. The Food Standards Agency Expert Vitamins and Minerals (EVM) group stated that UK dietary intake of nickel would not be expected to have any harmful effects but did not set a safe upper level or guidance level for adults for supplemental nickel intake.[2] The US Food and Nutrition Board set a Tolerable Upper Intake Level of 1 mg daily for adolescents and all adults.

Intake

Mean intake of dietary nickel in the UK is 130 µg daily, with an estimated maximum intake of 260 µg daily.[2]

Action

Nickel is an essential component in the enzymes of many plants, bacteria, algae and fungi. In humans, nickel influences iron absorption and metabolism and may be essential in red blood cell metabolism.[2]

Dietary sources

Nickel is present in a variety of foods, particularly pulses, grains (especially oats) and nuts. It is also present in drinking water.

Metabolism

Absorption

Dietary nickel is poorly absorbed. Absorption takes place in the small intestine via a carrier-mediated mechanism, but passive diffusion may also occur.

Distribution

The majority of nickel in human serum is bound to albumin, with some bound to nickeloplasmin, an α-macroglobulin, and some to amino acids, such as histidine, cysteine and aspartic acid.[1] It is distributed widely throughout the tissues with the highest concentrations in bone, lung, liver, kidney and endocrine glands. Nickel is also found in hair, nails, saliva and breast milk.

Elimination

Absorbed nickel is excreted predominantly in the urine, but some is also lost through sweat.

Bioavailability

Reported values of nickel absorption are $< 1\%$ when consumed with food, ascorbic acid, milk, tea, coffee and orange juice.[1] In a fasting state, 20–25% of nickel (from a nickel salt) may be absorbed.[2] Absorption is increased under conditions of low nickel and iron bioavailability.

Deficiency

Nickel deficiency has not been observed in humans. In animals, deficiency is associated with delayed sexual maturity, perinatal mortality, reduced growth and reduced haematopoiesis.

Possible uses

There are no known beneficial human health effects from consuming dietary nickel.

Precautions/contraindications

None reported.

Pregnancy and breast-feeding

There are no data in humans, but in animal studies, nickel toxicity is associated with perinatal mortality.

Adverse effects

Acute nickel exposure is associated with gastro-intestinal disturbances, visual disturbance, headache, cough, wheezing and giddiness. Approximately 7–10% of the population (predominantly women) is affected by nickel-allergic dermatitis. Ingestion of nickel may exacerbate eczema due to nickel sensitivity. Iron deficiency may increase the risk of nickel sensitisation.[2]

Interactions

None reported.

Dose

The dose is not established. Supplements in the UK contain up to 5 µg in a daily dose.

References

1 Eckert C. Other trace elements. In: Shils ME, Shike M, Ross AC, *et al. Modern Nutrition in Health and Disease*, 10th edn. London: Lippincott, Williams and Wilkins, 2006; 338–350.
2 Food Standards Agency. Risk assessment: nickel. http://www.eatwell.gov.uk/healthydiet/nutritionessentials/vitaminsandminerals/nickel (accessed 9 July 2006).

Octacosanol

Description

Octacosanol is the main component of poli-cosanol, which is isolated from sugar cane wax. Octacosanol has also been isolated from *Eupolyphaga sinensis*, some *Euphorbia* species, *Acacia modeseta*, *Serenoa repens* and other plants, including whole grains, fruit and vege-tables. It is a 28-carbon long-chain alcohol.

Action

Octacosanol appears to have a lipid-lowering effect, and there is some evidence (albeit limited) that octacosanol may improve muscle endur-ance. However, almost all of the studies con-ducted to date have emanated from a few research groups in Cuba and use one source of policosanol from Cuban cane sugar. The results from these groups have not been consistently replicated elsewhere.

Possible uses

It has been claimed that octacosanol is protect-ive against CVD, can improve endurance in athletes, and is beneficial in patients with Parkinson's disease.

Cardiovascular disease

Animal studies have shown that policosanol reduces serum lipids,[1–3] platelet aggregation[4] and atherosclerosis,[5,6] and that it may help to protect against cerebral ischaemia.[7]

Platelet aggregation

In a double-blind, placebo-controlled study, 37 healthy volunteers were randomised to receive either placebo or policosanol 10 mg daily for 7 days, 20 mg daily for the next 7 days, then 40 mg daily for the next 7 days. Platelet aggre-gation (induced by ADP and epinephrine)

reduced as the dose of policosanol increased, with significant effects observed after the second and third but not the first dose level. Coagulation time remained unchanged during the trial.[8]

In a further randomised, placebo-controlled, double-blind study involving healthy volun-teers, policosanol (5, 10, 25 and 50 mg), admin-istered orally, inhibited platelet aggregation (induced by ADP and epinephrine), and at a dose of 20 mg daily for 7 days the inhibition was significant. A modest effect on collagen-induced platelet aggregation was observed only at the highest dose (50 mg daily) while the low-est dose (5 mg daily) was ineffective. Policosanol did not affect coagulation time.[9] Further studies in healthy volunteers[10] and those with type II hypercholesterolaemia[11] have shown similar effects on platelet aggregation.

A randomised, double-blind, placebo-con-trolled study was carried out in 43 healthy volunteers to compare the effects of policosanol (20 mg daily), aspirin (100 mg daily) and com-bination therapy (policosanol 20 mg daily plus aspirin 100 mg daily) on platelet aggregation. With policosanol, platelet aggregation induced by ADP, epinephrine and collagen was signifi-cantly reduced. Aspirin reduced platelet aggre-gation induced by collagen and epinephrine but not by ADP. Combined therapy significantly inhibited platelet aggregation by all agonists. Coagulation time did not change during the trial. The authors concluded that policosanol (20 mg daily) was as effective as aspirin (100 mg daily), and that combination therapy showed some advantages over the respective monotherapies.[12]

A further double-blind RCT compared the antiplatelet effects of two doses of policosanol (20 and 40 mg daily) with placebo. Both doses significantly reduced platelet aggregation, com-pared with placebo, but no differences were observed in the effects produced by the two doses. Effects on platelet aggregation were similar in normal and hypercholesterolaemic patients. In addition, after 30 days, both 20 mg and 40 mg policosanol reduced LDL and total cholesterol and raised HDL cholesterol.[13]

Lipid lowering

A pilot single-blind, randomised, placebo-controlled trial was conducted in 23 middle-aged outpatients with well-documented chronic CHD and primary or marginal hyperlipidaemia. Twelve patients received 1 mg policosanol twice a day and 11 patients received placebo. The treated group showed a significant reduction in total (14.8%) and LDL (15.6%) cholesterol. The authors stated there was also a clinical tendency in five out of 12 of the treated patients towards improvement of CHD.[14]

In a 2-year, double-blind, randomised, placebo-controlled trial involving 69 patients with total and LDL cholesterol poorly controlled by diet, octacosanol 5 mg twice a day was associated with a 25% reduction in LDL cholesterol and an 18% reduction in total cholesterol. Ratios of LDL to HDL cholesterol were also reduced. All changes were significant and were maintained throughout the 2 years of the study.[15]

Another double-blind, placebo-controlled trial in 29 patients with non-insulin-dependent diabetes mellitus (NIDDM) and hypercholesterolaemia found that 10 mg policosanol daily significantly reduced total cholesterol by 17.5% and LDL cholesterol by 21.8%, non-significantly reduced triglycerides by 6.6%, and non-significantly raised HDL cholesterol by 11.3%. Glycaemic control was unaffected and no adverse effects were attributable to policosanol. The authors concluded that policosanol is safe and effective in patients with NIDDM and hypercholesterolaemia.[16]

A further double-blind, randomised study comparing the effect of policosanol (10 mg daily; 55 patients) with the two HMG-CoA reductase inhibitors, lovastatin (20 mg daily; 26 patients) or simvastatin (10 mg daily; 25 patients), showed that LDL cholesterol was reduced by 24% with policosanol, 22% with lovastatin and 15% with simvastatin. HDL cholesterol was increased in the policosanol group but not in the two groups using the HMG-CoA reductase inhibitors.[17]

A similar study comparing policosanol (10 mg daily) with acipimox (750 mg daily), involving 63 patients, showed that policosanol reduced total cholesterol and LDL cholesterol by 15.8% and 21%, respectively, and lowered the ratio of LDL to HDL cholesterol by 15.8%. Acipimox reduced both total cholesterol and LDL cholesterol by 7.5%.[18]

A further study comparing policosanol (10 mg daily) and pravastatin (10 mg daily) showed reductions in total and LDL cholesterol with policosanol of 13.9% and 19.3%, respectively, and lowered the LDL:HDL cholesterol ratio by 28.3%. Pravastatin lowered total cholesterol by 11.8% and LDL cholesterol by 15.6%. Policosanol reduced platelet aggregation to a greater extent than pravastatin. The authors concluded that policosanol (10 mg daily) produces more favourable effects on serum lipids and platelet aggregation than pravastatin (10 mg daily).[19] A further study comparing policosanol (10 mg daily) with lovastatin (20 mg daily) in 53 patients showed similar effects on serum lipid levels.[20] A further study comparing policosanol 10 mg daily with lovastatin 20 mg daily found that policosanol was slightly more effective than lovastatin in reducing the LDL/HDL and total cholesterol:HDL ratios, in increasing HDL levels and preventing LDL oxidation.[21] A Russian study found that policosanol 10 mg daily was superior than to bezafibrate 400 mg daily in lowering cholesterol.[22] In a study comparing policosanol 10 mg daily with atorvastatin 10 mg daily, policosanol was less effective than atorvastatin in reducing serum LDL and triglyceride levels in elderly patients with hypercholesterolaemia. Policosanol, but not atorvastatin, significantly increased serum HDL, while both reduced serum triglycerides and other measures of atherogenesis.[23]

Further studies have shown that policosanol reduced serum total and LDL cholesterol and raised HDL cholesterol in a study involving 437 individuals with type II hypercholesterolaemia and additional coronary risk factors,[24] and in a study involving 69 healthy subjects, policosanol decreased the susceptibility of LDL cholesterol to oxidation *in vitro*.[25] Similar influences on cholesterol with policosanol have been shown in a trial involving 244 post-menopausal women with hypercholesterolaemia.[26]

Newer studies have found that policosanol is effective, safe and well tolerated in older patients with hypercholesterolaemia and high coronary risk,[27] in post-menopausal women with hypercholesterolaemia,[28] and in older patients with hypertension and hypercholesterolaemia.[29] A dose of 40 mg policosanol was not found to offer any lipid-lowering advantage over a dose of 20 mg daily.[30] In a study comparing policosanol with mixtures of higher aliphatic primary alcohols, policosanol was found to reduce LDL cholesterol while the other mixtures did not.[31] A study evaluating the effect of policosanol with omega-3 fatty acids found that the combination lowered LDL and total cholesterol and triglycerides, and raised HDL cholesterol.[32] Another study found that policosanol could provide additional benefits in lowering blood pressure in people taking beta-blockers.[33]

However, a Dutch study investigating policosanol from wheatgerm found that a dose of 20 mg daily had no beneficial effect on blood lipids.[34]

A recent meta-analysis[35] compared the effect of policosanol with plant sterols and stanols and found that policosanol is more effective for LDL cholesterol reduction and more favourably alters the lipid profile. A Bandolier review[36] concluded that policosanol from Cuban sugar cane reduces total and LDL cholesterol by an amount equivalent to statins and has fewer, less serious, adverse events. However, all the Cuban trials show exactly the same 10–15% reduction in total cholesterol regardless of patient characteristics, duration of study (although most were longer than 6 weeks) or dose of policosanol. The inter-subject variation in cholesterol lowering with statins is much greater, making the policosanol results appear quite strange.

A recent South African RCT investigated the effect of a policosanol supplement (20 mg daily) for 12 weeks on 19 subjects with hypercholesterolaemia (some of whom had familial hypercholesterolaemia). However, the supplement had no significant effect on total or LDL cholesterol compared with placebo.[37] A further trial has evaluated policosanol derived from Cuban sugar cane in lipid outpatient clinics and general practices in Germany. A total of 143 patients with hypercholesterolaemia or combined hyperlipidaemia were randomised to receive policosanol 10, 20, 40 or 80 mg daily or placebo. No statistically significant difference between policosanol and placebo was observed in lipid lowering.[38]

Intermittent claudication

The Cuban researchers have also investigated the effect of policosanol in patients with intermittent claudication. A 2-year study found that policosanol 10 mg twice daily was more effective in improving walking distance than placebo.[39] A further study comparing policosanol (10 mg daily) with lovastatin (20 mg daily) found that policosanol (not lovastatin) was effective in improving walking distance,[40] while another study found policosanol (10 mg twice a day) to be as effective as ticlopidine (now discontinued in the UK) (250 mg three times a day).[41]

Parkinson's disease

Octacosanol has been evaluated in patients with mild to moderate Parkinson's disease. In a double-blind crossover trial, 10 patients received either 5 mg octacosanol or placebo (both three times a day) for 6 weeks. Only three patients improved significantly at the study's end. Some responded slightly or had no disease progression during the study. Activities of daily living and mood improved, but physical endurance and parkinsonian symptoms did not. One patient experienced dizziness and another experienced exacerbation of dyskinesias. The authors concluded that octacosanol might be beneficial for patients with mild Parkinson's disease, but that the benefit is likely to be small and less than that exerted by existing treatments.[42]

Amyotrophic lateral sclerosis

Anecdotally, octacosanol has been claimed to improve symptoms of amyotrophic lateral sclerosis (AMS), but a placebo-controlled, double-blind, crossover trial in which patients received either 40 mg octacosanol or placebo for 3 months and were then crossed over showed no difference between octacosanol and placebo.[43]

Athletes

Octacosanol is now being widely advertised for enhancing performance in athletes, particularly in the USA and Australia. However, there are almost no supporting data.

One study in 33 male student athletes (20 controls, 13 supplemented) showed that supplementation with a pack containing 29 supplements including 2000 µg octacosanol was associated with a decrease in body fat and increase in muscle girth measurement, indicating the formation of lean body mass. However, the study was not blinded, the diet not controlled and the pack contained a variety of supplements in addition to octacosanol.[44]

Another study in 16 subjects (students and lecturers in physical education) measured grip strength, chest strength, and reaction time to both auditory and visual stimuli. Following supplementation with 1000 µg octacosanol for 8 weeks, only grip strength and reaction time to visual stimuli were improved.[45]

Conclusion

A number of human studies have now been conducted with policosanol and have shown benefits in lipid lowering and platelet aggregation compared with placebo. They have also shown similar effects to various lipid-lowering drugs. However, nearly all of the studies have been conducted by one research group in Havana, Cuba, and with policosanol from Cuban sugar cane. They have not been replicated outside Cuba or using policosanol from other sources. There is very little evidence that octacosanol is useful for athletes.

Precautions/contraindications

None reported.

Pregnancy and breast-feeding

No problems have been reported, but there have not been sufficient studies to guarantee the safety of octacosanol in pregnancy and breast-feeding. The effects are unknown, and octacosanol is best avoided.

Adverse effects

None reported, but there are no long-term studies assessing the safety of octacosanol. In a trial investigating the effects of placebo and policosanol, 5 mg, 10 mg and 20 mg daily, policosanol was said by the authors to be well tolerated with

no disturbances of blood or clinical biochemistry. Adverse effects were found to be mild and transient with no differences between the groups.[46]

Interactions

None reported. A study in rats investigated the effect of adding policosanol to warfarin. Policosanol did not enhance the prolongation of bleeding time induced by warfarin alone.[47]

Dose

Octacosanol is available in the form of tablets and capsules.

The dose is not established. Doses used in studies have varied from 1 to 20 mg policosanol daily.

References

1   Arruzazabala ML, Carbajal D, Mas R, *et al.* Cholesterol-lowering effect of policosanol in rabbits. *Biol Res* 1994; 27: 205–208.

2   Menendez R, Amor AM, Gonzalez RM, *et al.* Effect of policosanol on the hepatic cholesterol biosynthesis of normocholesterolemic rats. *Biol Res* 1996; 29: 253–257.

3   Menendez R, Arruzazabala L, Mas R, *et al.* Cholesterol-lowering effect of policosanol on rabbits with hypercholesterolaemia induced by a wheat starch-casein diet. *Br J Nutr* 1997; 77: 923–932.

4   Arruzazabala ML, Carbajal D, Mas R, *et al.* Effects of policosanol on platelet aggregation in rats. *Thromb Res* 1993; 69: 321–327.

5   Noa M, Mas R, de la Rosa MC, *et al.* Effect of policosanol on lipofundin-induced atherosclerotic lesions in rats. *J Pharm Pharmacol* 1995; 47: 289–291.

6   Arruzazabala ML, Noa M, Menendez R, *et al.* Protective effect of policosanol on atherosclerotic lesions in rabbits with exogenous hypercholesterolaemia. *Braz J Med Biol Res* 2000; 33: 835–840.

7   Molina V, Arruzazabala D, Carbajal D, *et al.* Effect of policosanol on cerebral ischemia in Mongolian gerbils. *Braz J Med Biol Res* 1999; 32: 1269–1276.

8   Arruzazabala ML, Valdes S, Mas R, *et al.* Effect of policosanol successive dose increases on platelet aggregation in healthy volunteers. *Phamacol Res* 1996; 34: 181–185.

9   Valdes S, Arruzazabala ML, Fernandez L, *et al.* Effect of policosanol on platelet aggregation in

healthy volunteers. *Int J Clin Pharmacol Res* 1996; 16: 67–72.

10 Carbajal D, Arruzazabala ML, Valdes S, *et al.* Effect of policosanol on platelet aggregation and serum levels of arachidonic acid metabolites in healthy volunteers. *Prostaglandins Leukot Essent Fatty Acids* 1998; 58: 61–64.

11 Arruzazabala ML, Mas R, Molina V, *et al.* Effect of policosanol on platelet aggregation in type II hypercholesterolemic patients. *Int J Tissue React* 1998; 20: 119–124.

12 Arruzazabala ML, Valdes S, Mas R, *et al.* Comparative study of policosanol, aspirin and the combination therapy policosanol-aspirin on platelet aggregation in healthy volunteers. *Pharmacol Res* 1997; 36: 293–297.

13 Arruzazabala ML, Molina V, Mas R, *et al.* Antiplatelet effects of policosanol (20 and 40mg/day) in healthy volunteers and dyslipidaemic patients. *Clin Exp Pharmacol Physiol* 2002; 29: 891–897.

14 Batista J, Stusser R, Saez F, *et al.* Effect of policosanol on hyperlipidemia and coronary heart disease in middle-aged patients. A 14-month pilot study. *Int J Clin Phamacol Ther* 1996; 34: 134–137.

15 Canetti M, Moreira M, Mas R, *et al.* A two-year study on the efficacy and tolerability of policosanol in patients with type II hyperlipoproteinaemia. *Int J Clin Pharmacol Res* 1995; 15: 159–165.

16 Torres O, Agramonte AJ, Illnait J, *et al.* Treatment of hypercholesterolemia in NIDDM with policosanol. *Diabetes Care* 1995; 18: 393–397.

17 Prat H, Roman O, Pino E. Comparative effects of policosanol and two HMG-CoA reductase inhibitors on type II hypercholesterolemia. *Rec Med Chil* 1999; 127: 286–294.

18 Alcocer L, Fernandez L, Campos E, *et al.* A comparative study of policosanol versus acipimox in patients with type II hypercholesterolemia. *Int J Tissue React* 1999; 21: 85–92.

19 Castano G, Mas R, Arruzazabala ML, *et al.* Effect of policosanol and pravastatin on lipid profile, platelet aggregation and endothelemia in older hypercholesterolemic patients. *Int J Clin Pharmacol Res* 1999; 19: 105–116.

20 Crespo N, Illnait J, Mas R, *et al.* Comparative study of the efficacy and tolerability of policosanol and lovastatin in patients with hypercholesterolemia and noninsulin dependent diabetes mellitus. *Int J Clin Pharmacol Res* 1999; 19: 117–127.

21 Castano G, Menendez R, Mas R, *et al.* Effects of policosanol and lovastatin on lipid profile and lipid peroxidation in patients with dyslipidaemia associated with type 2 diabetes mellitus. *Int J Clin Pharmacol Res* 2002; 22: 89–99.

22 Nitkin IuP, Slepchenko NV, Gratsianskii NA, *et al.* Results of the multicenter controlled study of the hypolipidemic drug polycosanol in Russia. *Ter Arkh* 2000; 72: 7–10.

23 Castano G, Mas R, Fernandez L, *et al.* Comparison of the efficacy and tolerability of policosanol with atorvastatin in elderly patients with type II hypercholesterolaemia. *Drugs Aging* 2003; 20: 153–163.

24 Mas R, Castano G, Illnait J, *et al.* Effects of policosanol in patients with type II hypercholesterolemia and additional risk factors. *Clin Pharmacol Ther* 1999; 65: 439–447.

25 Menendez R, Mas R, Amor AM, *et al.* Effects of policosanol treatment on the susceptibility of low density lipoprotein (LDL) isolated from healthy volunteers to oxidative modification *in vitro*. *Br J Clin Pharmacol* 2000; 50: 255–262.

26 Castano G, Mas R, Fernandez L, *et al.* Effects of policosanol on postmenopausal women with type II hypercholesterolemia. *Gynecol Endocrinol* 2000; 14: 187–195.

27 Castano G, Mas R, Fernandez JC, *et al.* Effects of policosanol in older patients with type II hypercholesterolemia and high coronary risk. *J Gerontol A Biol Sci Med Sci* 2001; 56: M186–M192.

28 Mirkin A, Mas R, Martino M, *et al.* Efficacy and tolerability of policosanol in hypercholesterolaemic, postmenopausal women. *Int J Pharmacol Res* 2001; 21: 31–41.

29 Castano G, Mas R, Fernandez JC, *et al.* Effects of policosanol on older patients with hypertension and type II hypercholesterolaemia. *Drugs R D* 2002; 3: 159–172.

30 Castano G, Mas R, Fernandez L, *et al.* Effects of policosanol 20 versus 40 mg/day in the treatment of patients with type II hypercholesterolemia: a 6-month double-blind study. *Int J Clin Pharmacol Res* 2001; 21: 43–57.

31 Castano G, Fernandez L, Mas R, *et al.* Comparison of the efficacy, safety and tolerability of original policosanol versus other mixtures of higher aliphatic primary alcohols in patients with type II hypercholesterolemia. *Int J Pharmacol Res* 2002; 22: 55–66.

32 Castano G, Fernandez L, Mas R, *et al.* Effects of addition of policosanol to omega-3 fatty acids therapy on the lipid profile of patients with type II hypercholesterolaemia. *Drugs R D* 2005; 6: 207–219.

33 Castano G, Mas R, Gamez R, *et al.* Concomitant use of policosanol and beta-blockers in older patients. *Int J Clin Pharmacol Res* 2004; 24: 65–77.

34 Lin Y, Rudrum M, van der Wielen RP, *et al.* Wheat germ policosanol failed to lower plasma cholesterol in subjects with normal to mildly elevated cholesterol concentrations. *Metabolism* 2004; 53: 1309–1314.

35 Chen JT, Wesley R, Shanburek RD, *et al.* Meta-analysis of natural therapies for hyperlipidemia: plant sterols and stanols versus policosanol. *Pharmacotherapy* 2005; 25: 171–183.

36 Anonymous. Policosanol for lipid-lowering. *Bandolier* January 2005 (available from http://www.jr2.ox.ac.uk/bandolier/Extraforbando/Policosanol.pdf).

37 Greyling A, De Witt C, Oosthuizen W, Jerling JC. Effects of a policosanol supplement on serum lipid concentrations in hypercholesterolaemic and heterozygous familial hypercholesterolaemic subjects. *Br J Nutr* 2006; 95: 968–975.

38 Berthold HK, Unverdorben S, Degenhardt R, *et al*. Effect of policosanol on lipid levels among patients with hypercholesterolaemia or combined hyperlipidaemia. *JAMA* 2006; 295: 2262–2269.

39 Castano G, Mas Ferreiro R, Fernandez L, *et al*. A long-term study of policosanol in the treatment of intermittent claudication. *Angiology* 2001; 52: 115–125.

40 Castano G, Mas R, Fernandez L, *et al*. Effects of policosanol and lovastatin in patients with intermittent claudication: a double-blind comparative pilot study. *Angiology* 2003; 54: 25–38.

41 Castano G, Mas R, Gamez R, *et al*. Effects of policosanol and ticlodipidine in patients with

intermittent claudication: a double-blinded pilot comparative study. *Angiology* 2004; 55: 361–371.

42 Snider SR. Octacosanol in Parkinsonism. *Ann Neurol* 1984; 16: 273 (letter).

43 Norris FH, Denys EH, Fallat RJ. Trial of octacosanol on amyotrophic lateral sclerosis. *Neurology* 1986; 36: 1263–1264.

44 Cockerill DL, Bucci LR. Increases in muscle girth and decreases in body fat associated with a nutritional supplement program. *Chiro Sports Med* 1987; 1: 73–76.

45 Saint-John M, McNaughton L. Octacosanol ingestion and its effects on metabolic responses to submaximal cycle ergometry, reaction time, and chest and grip strength. *Int Clin Nutr Rev* 1986; 6: 81–87.

46 Pons P, Rodriguez M, Robaina C, *et al*. Effects of successive dose increases of policosanol on the lipid profile of patients with type II hypercholesterolaemia and tolerability to treatment. *Int J Clin Pharmacol Res* 1994; 14: 27–33.

47 Carbajal D, Arruzazabala ML, Valdes S, *et al*. Interaction of policosanol-warfarin on bleeding time and thrombosis in rats. *Pharmacol Res* 1998; 38: 89–91.

Olive leaf

Description

Olive leaf is the leaf of the olive tree (*Olea europaea*). The medicinal use of the olive leaf can be traced back thousands of years to treat a variety of medical conditions. However, contemporary interest in olive leaf has increased on the basis of the role of olives and olive oil in the Mediterranean diet. Olive oil (extracted from the olive fruit) is associated with cardioprotective effects, which probably result from not only its content of oleic acid (a fatty acid) but also, in the case of extra virgin olive oil, from the presence of the antioxidant polyphenols such as oleuropein and hydroxytyrosol.[1] Unprocessed olive leaf also contains oleuropein and hydroxytyrosol, as well as several other polyphenols and flavonoids, including oleocanthal. Extracts of olive leaf have, therefore, been evaluated in

recent research studies for potential health benefit.

Action

The polyphenols contained in olive leaf and extra virgin olive oil have antioxidant activity, which is potentially beneficial against the oxidation of low-density lipoprotein (LDL).[2,3] However, there is an opinion that a clinically meaningful intake of the antioxidant polyphenols may be difficult to achieve.[4] Evidence suggests that olive polyphenols are 55–65% bioavailable in humans.[3]

A recent review of the evidence on the antioxidant activity of olive polyphenols suggests that olive polyphenols decrease the levels of oxidized LDL in plasma and positively affect several biomarkers of oxidative damage.[5] An intake of about 10 mg per day of olive polyphenols is suggested to be required to achieve an antioxidant effect.

Possible uses

Traditionally, olive leaf taken orally has been used for the treatment of viral, bacterial and protozoal infections, including influenza, pneumonia, the common cold, meningitis, encephalitis, tuberculosis, malaria, gonorrhoea, herpes, shingles, human immunodeficiency virus (HIV), chronic fatigue and hepatitis B, as well as non-infective conditions such as hypertension, diabetes and allergic rhinitis, to improve renal and digestive function, and as a diuretic and antipyretic.

Olive leaf extract could potentially be of benefit in cardiovascular disease and metabolic syndrome. Evidence from a recent trial in rats suggests that olive leaf extract containing polyphenols such as oleuropein and hydroxytyrosol reverses (in this rat model) the chronic inflammation and oxidative stress that induces the cardiovascular, hepatic and metabolic symptoms of diet-induced obesity and diabetes, but with no change in blood pressure.[1]

However, human studies are now needed to clarify the effect of olive polyphenols on markers of oxidative stress, particularly DNA damage and plasma isoprostane levels, as well as their potential to reduce metabolic symptoms in obesity, diabetes and cardiovascular disease.

Precautions/contraindications

None reported; insufficient reliable information.

Pregnancy and breast-feeding

Insufficient data.

Adverse effects

Possible respiratory allergy.

Interactions

None reported.

Dose

No typical dose.

Conclusion

Traditionally, olive leaf has been taken orally for the treatment of a variety of infective and non-infective conditions. It is the subject of recent interest based on the beneficial properties of the polyphenols, which it contains in common with the olive fruit and olive oil. The overall evidence from *in vitro* assays and animal and human studies support the antioxidant effect of olive polyphenols. However, further larger-scale human studies are needed to clarify the effect of olive polyphenols on markers of oxidative stress.

References

1 Poudyal H, Campbell F, Brown L. Olive leaf extract attenuates cardiac, hepatic, and metabolic changes in high carbohydrate-, high fat-fed rats. *J Nutr* 2010; 140: 946–953.

2 Masella R, Giovannini C, Vari R, *et al.* Effects of dietary virgin olive oil phenols on low density lipoprotein oxidation in hyperlipidemic patients. *Lipids* 2001; 36: 1195–1202.

3 Vissers MN, PL. Roodenburg AJC, Leenen R, Katan MB. Olive oil phenols are absorbed in humans. *J Nutr* 2002; 132: 409–417.

4 Vissers MN, Zock PL, Katan MB. Bioavailability and antioxidant effects of olive oil phenols in humans: a review. *Eur J Clin Nutr* 2004; 58: 955–965.

5 Raederstorff D. Antioxidant activity of olive polyphenols in humans: a review. *Int J Vitam Nutr Res* 2009; 79: 152–165.

Pangamic acid

Description and nomenclature

An alternative name for pangamic acid is vitamin B_{15}, but it is not an officially recognised vitamin. Pangamic acid is the name given to a product originally claimed to contain D-gluconodimethyl aminoacetic acid, which was obtained from apricot kernels and later from rice bran.

Constituents

The composition of supplements is undefined, but they may contain one or more of the following substances: calcium gluconate, glycine, *N,N*-dimethylglycine and *N,N*-diisopropylamine dichloroacetate (*N,N*-diisopropylamine dichloroacetate has pharmacological activity).

Dietary sources

Apricot kernels, brewer's yeast, liver, wheatgerm, bran and wholegrains.

Possible uses

Research by Soviet sports scientists focused attention on pangamic acid, but very little research has been done in other countries. Pangamic acid is claimed to enhance athletic performance and to be beneficial in CVD, asthma and diabetes mellitus. Scientific studies show no evidence of therapeutic efficacy for pangamic acid.

Precautions/contraindications

Pangamic acid should not be taken at all, by anyone.

Adverse effects

Pangamic acid may be mutagenic and thus potentially able to cause cancer. It may cause occasional transient flushing of the skin.

Interactions

None reported.

Dose

Pangamic acid should be avoided. Dietary supplements are rarely available in UK high-street outlets, but may be available on the Internet.

Pantothenic acid

Description

Pantothenic acid is a water-soluble B complex vitamin.

Human requirements

See Table 1 for Dietary Reference Values for pantothenic acid.

Dietary intake

In the UK, the average adult diet provides 5.1 mg daily.

Action

Pantothenic acid functions mainly as a component of coenzyme A and acyl carrier protein.

Table 1 Dietary Reference Values for pantothenic acid (mg/day)

| Age | UK | | USA | | EU RDA = 6 mg |
	Safe intake	EVM	AI	TUL	FAO/WHO RNI
0–6 months	1.7		1.7	–	1.7
7–12 months	1.7		1.8	–	1.8
1–3 years	1.7		2.0	–	2.0
4–10 years	3–7		–	–	3.0[1]4.0[2]
4–8 years				3.0	
9–13 years			4.0	–	
Males and females					
11–50+ years	3–7	200	–	5.0	
14–70+ years			5.0	–	–
Pregnancy	–		6.0	–	6.0
Lactation	–		7.0	–	7.0

[1] 4–6 years.   [2] 7–9 years.
EVM = Likely safe daily intake from supplements alone.
TUL = Tolerable Upper Intake Level (not determined for pantothenic acid).

Coenzyme A has a central role as a cofactor for enzymes involved in the metabolism of lipids, carbohydrates and proteins; it is also required for the synthesis of cholesterol, steroid hormones, acetylcholine and porphyrins. As a component of acyl carrier protein, pantothenic acid is involved in various transfer reactions and in the assembly of acetate units into longer-chain fatty acids.

Dietary sources

See Table 2 for dietary sources of pantothenic acid.

Metabolism

Absorption
Absorption occurs in the small intestine.

Distribution
Pantothenic acid is widely distributed in body tissues (particularly in the liver, adrenal glands, heart and kidneys), mainly as coenzyme A.

Elimination
About 70% is excreted unchanged via the urine and 30% in the faeces.

Bioavailability

Bioavailability may be reduced by some drugs (see Interactions) and a high fat intake, and increased by a diet high in protein.

Deficiency

Deficiency has not been clearly identified in humans consuming a mixed diet.

Possible uses

Pantothenic acid has been used for a wide range of disorders such as acne, alopecia, allergies, burning feet, asthma, grey hair, dandruff, cholesterol lowering, improving exercise performance, depression, osteoarthritis, rheumatoid arthritis, multiple sclerosis, stress, shingles, ageing and Parkinson's disease. It has been investigated in clinical trials for arthritis, cholesterol lowering and exercise performance.

Table 2 Dietary sources of pantothenic acid

Food portion	Pantothenic acid content (mg)
Breakfast cereals	
1 bowl All-Bran (45 g)	0.7
1 bowl Bran Flakes (45 g)	0.7
1 bowl Corn Flakes (30 g)	0.1
1 bowl muesli (95 g)	**1.1**
2 pieces Shredded Wheat	0.4
2 Weetabix	0.3
Cereal products	
Bread, brown, 2 slices	0.2
white, 2 slices	0.2
wholemeal, 2 slices	0.4
1 chapati	0.1
Milk and dairy products	
Milk, whole, semi-skimmed or	0.8
skimmed (284 ml; $^1/_2$ pint)	
1 pot yoghurt (150 g)	0.6
Cheese (50 g)	0.2
1 egg, size 2 (60 g)	**1.0**
Meat and fish	
Beef, roast (85 g)	0.5
Lamb, roast (85 g)	0.5
Pork, roast (85 g)	0.8
1 chicken leg portion	**1.5**
Liver, lambs, cooked (90 g)	**7.0**
Kidney, lambs,	**4.0**
cooked (75 g)	
Fish, cooked (150 g)	0.5
Vegetables	
1 small can baked	0.4
beans (200 g)	
Chickpeas, cooked (105 g)	0.3
Red kidney beans (105 g)	0.2
Peas, boiled (100 g)	0.1
Potatoes, boiled (150 g)	0.6
Green vegetables, average,	0.2
boiled (100 g)	
Fruit	
1 banana	0.5
1 orange	0.6
Nuts	
30 peanuts	0.7
Yeast	
Brewer's yeast (10 g)	**1.0**

Excellent sources (> 1 mg/portion) (**bold**).

Arthritis

In an uncontrolled trial, patients treated with pantothenate 12.5 mg twice a day showed a limited, variable improvement within 1–2 weeks of therapy, which ended upon discontinuation of therapy.[1] In a double-blind, placebo-controlled trial,[2] 94 patients with arthritis (of whom 27 had rheumatoid arthritis) were randomised to receive large doses of calcium pantothenate (titrated up from 500 mg daily to 2000 mg daily) or a placebo for 8 weeks. There was no significant reduction in either group in the duration of morning stiffness or disability, but both groups experienced significant relief from pain. When the subjects with rheumatoid arthritis were analysed separately, the group receiving pantothenate showed statistically significant reduction in morning stiffness, disability and pain compared with placebo.

Cholesterol lowering

A double-blind, placebo-controlled, crossover study in 29 patients with various types of dyslipidaemia found that 900 mg pantothenic acid daily reduced total and LDL cholesterol in type IIb hyperlipidaemia, with varying effects in type IV patients.[3]

Exercise performance

Two double-blind, placebo-controlled studies with pantothenic acid in runners[4] and cyclists[5] showed that pantothenic acid had no effect on exercise performance.

> **Conclusion**
> Research is too limited to be able to make recommendations for pantothenic acid.

Precautions/contraindications

None reported.

Pregnancy and breast-feeding

No problems reported.

Adverse effects

No adverse effects, except for occasional diarrhoea, have been reported in humans. High intake of pantothenic acid (and biotin and riboflavin) with low intake of calcium, folate, nicotinic acid, vitamin E, retinol and beta-carotene, has been associated with increased genome instability.[6]

Interactions

Drugs

Alcohol: excessive alcohol intake may increase requirement for pantothenic acid.

Oral contraceptives: may increase requirement for pantothenic acid.

Nutrients

Adequate amounts of all B vitamins are required for optimal functioning; deficiency or excess of one B vitamin may lead to abnormalities in the metabolism of another.

Dose

Pantothenic acid and calcium pantothenate are available in the form of tablets and capsules, but they are found mainly in multivitamin and mineral preparations.

The dose is not established. Dietary supplements contain up to 100 mg daily.

References

1 Annand J. Pantothenic acid and OA. *Lancet* 1963; 41: 1168.
2 General Practitioner Research Group. Calcium pantothenate in arthritic conditions. A report from the General Practitioner Research Group. *Practitioner* 1980; 224: 208–211.
3 Gaddi A, Descovich GC, Noseda G, *et al.* Controlled evaluation of pantethine, a natural hypolipemic compound, in patients with hyperlipidaemia. *Atherosclerosis* 1984; 50: 73–83.
4 Nice C, Reeves AG, Brinck-Johnsen T, *et al.* The effects of pantothenic acid on human exercise capacity. *J Sports Med Phys Fitness* 1984; 24: 26–29.
5 Webster MJ. Physiological and performance responses to supplementation with thiamin and pantothenic acid derivatives. *Eur J Appl Physiol* 1998; 77: 486–491.
6 Fenech M, Baghurst P, Luderer W, *et al.* Low intake of folate, nicotinic acid, vitamin E, retinol, beta-carotene, and high intake of pantothenic acid, biotin and riboflavin are significantly associated with increased genome instability – result from a dietary intake and micronutrients intake survey in South Australia. *Carcinogenesis* 2005; 26: 991–999.

Para-amino benzoic acid

Description and nomenclature

Para-amino benzoic acid (PABA) is a member of the vitamin B complex, but is not an officially recognised vitamin.

Dietary sources

Brewer's yeast, liver, wheatgerm, bran and wholegrains.

Possible uses

PABA is claimed to prevent greying hair and to be useful as an anti-ageing supplement. It has been used in digestive disorders, arthritis, insomnia and depression. There is no convincing scientific evidence available.

A derivative of PABA is used topically as a sunscreen agent; this is effective in the prevention of sunburn.

Adverse effects

Toxicity is low, but high doses (>30 mg) may cause anorexia, nausea, vomiting, liver toxicity, fever, itching and skin rash.

Interactions

Sulphonamides: kill bacteria by mimicking PABA; supplements containing PABA should be avoided while taking these drugs.

Dose

PABA is available in the form of tablets and capsules.

There is no established dose. Supplements are not justified. Dietary supplements provide 100–500 mg per dose.

Phosphatidylserine

Description

Phosphatidylserine belongs to a class of fat-soluble compounds called phospholipids. Phospholipids are essential components of cell membranes, with high concentrations found in the brain. Phosphatidylserine is the most abundant phospholipid in the brain.

Action

Phosphatidylserine helps to ensure fluidity, flexibility and permeability in cell membranes. It stimulates the release of various transmitters, such as acetylcholine and dopamine, enhances ion transport and increases the number of neurotransmitter receptor sites in the brain.

Possible uses

Phosphatidyl serine is claimed to be useful in enhancing memory, treating depression and preventing age-related neurotransmitter defects.

Age-related cognitive decline

A double-blind, randomised, controlled study was conducted in 42 hospitalised demented patients, in which half the patients received 300 mg phosphatidylserine and the other half placebo. The trial lasted for 6 weeks. Two distinct rating scales were used: the Crighton Scale and the Peri Scale. Results showed a trend towards improvement in the treated patients and analysis of covariance showed a significant treatment effect on the Peri Scale. The results at the end of treatment were compared with results obtained 3 weeks later and there was still a significant difference on the Peri Scale, indicating (according to the authors) a drug-related effect.[1]

The effects of phosphatidylserine on cognitive, affective and behavioural symptoms were studied in a group of elderly women with depressive disorders. The treatment was not blinded or randomised. Patients were treated with placebo for 15 days followed by phosphatidylserine (300 mg daily) for 30 days. Changes in depression, memory and general behaviour were measured according to four different scales before and after placebo, and after treatment. Depressive symptoms were marked before placebo, did not change after placebo, and were significantly reduced by phosphatidylserine treatment. There was also improvement in memory (recall, long-term retrieval), but there were no changes in plasma levels of various neurochemicals.[2]

In a double-blind, placebo-controlled study, 149 patients with age-associated memory impairment were treated with phosphatidylserine 300 mg or placebo for 12 weeks. The supplemented subjects improved relative to placebo on performance tests related to learning and memory tasks of daily life. Analysis of subgroups showed that subjects who performed at a relatively low level before treatment were most likely to respond to phosphatidylserine. The authors concluded that phosphatidylserine may be a promising candidate for treating memory loss in later life.[3]

In a double-blind, placebo-controlled study, 51 patients with probable Alzheimer's disease were treated with phosphatidylserine (300 mg daily) or placebo for 12 weeks. Two rating scales were used to assess the patients, and after 12 weeks, the treated group improved on three of the 12 variables on one scale and five of the 25 variables on the other scale. Family members rated significant improvements with phosphatidylserine after 6 and 9 weeks but not at 12 weeks. The authors stressed that phosphatidylserine could be helpful in patients with early-stage disease, but might have no effect in middle and later stages.[4]

In a double-blind, placebo-controlled, crossover study, 33 patients with mild primary degenerative dementia received either phosphatidylserine 300 mg daily or placebo for 8 weeks. Clinical global rating scales showed significantly more patients improving with phosphatidylserine than placebo. However, there were no significant improvements in dementia rating scale or psychometric tests.[5]

In a double-blind, placebo-controlled study 494 elderly patients (aged 65–93 years) with moderate to severe cognitive decline were randomised to receive either phosphatidylserine 300 mg daily or placebo for 6 months. Sixty-nine patients dropped out of the trial. Patients were examined before the study, and 3 and 6 months after. Statistically significant improvements in the treated group compared with placebo were observed in terms of both behavioural and cognitive parameters.[6]

More recent trials have demonstrated similar findings. In a 6-month trial in 78 elderly Japanese people with mild cognitive impairment (50–69 years), phosphatidylserine (100 mg, 300 mg/day) improved memory compared with baseline and placebo in those with the lowest memory scores at the start of the trial. Memory improvements in the phosphatidylserine-treated groups were mostly attributed to the increase in delayed verbal recall, a memory ability attenuated in the earliest stage of dementia.[7] Further trials have shown that phosphatidylserine combined with omega-3 fatty acids[8] and ginkgo biloba[9] may also improve cognitive function.

Physical stress

In a double-blind trial, eight healthy men underwent three experiments with a bicycle ergometer. Before the exercise, each subject received intravenously 50 or 75 mg of phosphatidylserine or placebo. Blood samples were collected before and after the exercise and analysed for epinephrine, norepinephrine, dopamine, adrenocorticotrophic hormone (ACTH), cortisol, growth hormone, prolactin and glucose. Physical stress induced a clear-cut increase in plasma epinephrine, norepinephrine, ACTH, cortisol, growth hormone and prolactin, whereas no significant change was found in plasma dopamine and glucose. Pretreatment with both 50 mg and 75 mg phosphatidylserine significantly blunted the ACTH and cortisol responses to physical stress.[10]

In a study using the same exercise protocol in the same research centre, nine healthy men were treated for three 10-day periods with placebo, 400 mg and 800 mg phosphatidylserine daily. Oral phosphatidylserine rather than the intravenous formulation was used. Phosphatidylserine 800 mg significantly blunted the ACTH and cortisol responses to physical exercise. The authors concluded that chronic oral administration of phosphatidylserine might counteract stress-induced activation of the hypothalamic–pituitary–adrenal axis in men.[11]

A further study in 10 healthy men assigned to either phosphatidylserine 600 mg daily or placebo and a cycle test showed that phosphatidylserine reduced cortisol concentrations and was effective in reducing physical stress and physical deterioration associated with acute exercise.[12]

More recent trials have shown less promising effects. A randomised controlled trial in 16 soccer players found that supplementation with phosphatidylserine was not effective in attenuating the cortisol response, perceived soreness and markers of muscle damage and lipid peroxidation following exhaustive running. However, supplementation tended to increase running time to exhaustion, suggesting that phosphatidylserine might have an ergogenic effect.[13] A further RCT by the same research group in eight active men found that supplementation with 750 mg daily of phosphatidylserine for 10 days did not afford additional protection against delayed onset of muscle soreness and markers of muscle damage, inflammation and oxidative stress that follow prolonged downhill running.[14]

Psychological stress

Recent research has investigated the effects of phosphatidylserine on psychological stress. A study assigned four groups of 20 subjects to 400 mg, 600 mg or 800 mg phosphatidylserine complex (PAS) or placebo for 3 weeks, then exposed them to the Trier Social Stress Test. Treatment with 400 mg PAS resulted in a pronounced blunting of both serum ACTH and cortisol, but did not affect heart rate. The effect was not seen with the larger doses of PAS. After the test, the placebo group showed the expected increased distress while the 400 mg PAS group showed reduced distress. The authors concluded that this study provides initial evidence of a selective stress dampening effect of PAS on the pituitary–adrenal axis, suggesting the potential for PAS in the treatment of stress-related disorders.[15]

Similar findings emerged from a trial in 16 healthy subjects in whom stress was induced followed by phosphatidylserine supplementation or placebo. Supplementation with phosphatidylserine was associated with a more relaxed state compared with placebo.[16]

Conclusion

There is evidence from controlled trials that phosphatidylserine improves memory and other symptoms of cognitive decline in elderly patients. There is also some limited evidence that phosphatidylserine attenuates the cortisol response to exercise. However, this response is a natural phenomenon and interfering with it could delay recovery in athletes. Further research is required to ascertain whether phosphatidylserine is beneficial in athletes or not.

Precautions/contraindications

None reported.

Pregnancy and breast-feeding

No problems have been reported, but there have not been sufficient studies to guarantee the safety of phosphatidylserine in pregnancy and breast-feeding.

Adverse effects

No known toxicity or side-effects, but there are no long-term studies assessing the safety of phosphatidylserine. There have been concerns about phosphatidylserine supplements derived from bovine brain tissue, because of concerns about diseases such as bovine spongiform encephalopathy, and supplements based on soya have been developed. The two supplements are slightly different and there has been discussion about whether they have the same level of efficacy. Most research to date has been conducted with bovine-based supplements. Preliminary research in animals suggests that the effects are similar, but further work needs to be done in this area.

Interactions

None reported.

Dose

Phosphatidylserine is available in the form of tablets, capsules and powder.

The dose is not established. Doses used in studies have been 300 mg daily in investigations on cognitive function, and up to 800 mg daily in studies on physical stress. Supplements provide 100–800 mg daily.

References

1   Delwaide PJ, Gyselynck-Mambourg AM, Hurlet A, *et al.* Double-blind randomized controlled study of phosphatidyserine in senile demented patients. *Acta Neurol Scand* 1986; 73: 136–140.
2   Maggioni M, Picotti GB, Bondiolotti GP, *et al.* Effects of phosphatidylserine in geriatric patients with depressive disorders. *Acta Psychiatr Scand* 1990; 81: 265–270.
3   Crook TH, Tinklenberg Yesavage J, *et al.* Effects of phosphatidylserine in age-associated memory impairment. *Neurology* 1991; 41: 644–649.
4   Crook T, Petrie W, Wells C, *et al.* Effects of phosphatidylserine in Alzheimer's disease. *Psychopharmacol Bull* 1992; 28: 61–66.
5   Cenacchi T, Bertoldin T, Farina C, *et al.* Cognitive decline in the elderly: a double-blind, placebo-controlled multicenter study on efficacy of phosphatidylserine administration. *Aging (Milano)* 1993; 5: 123–133.
6   Engel RR, Satzger W, Gunther W, *et al.* Double-blind, crossover study of phosphatidylserine versus placebo in patients with early dementia of the Alzheimer's type. *Eur Neuropsychopharmacol* 1992; 2: 149–155.
7   Kato-Kataoka A, Sakai M, Ebina R, *et al.* Soybean-derived phosphatidylserine improves memory function of the elderly Japanese subjects with memory complaints. *J Clin Biochem Nutr* 2010; 47(3): 246–255.
8   Vakhapova V, Cohen T, Richter Y, *et al.* Phosphatidylserine containing omega-3 fatty acids may improve memory abilities in non-demented elderly with memory complaints: a double-blind placebo-controlled trial. *Dement Geriatr Cogn Disord* 2010; 29(5): 467–474.
9   Kennedy DO, Haskell CF, Mauri PL, *et al.* Acute cognitive effects of standardised *Ginkgo biloba* extract complexed with phosphatidylserine. *Hum Psychopharmacol* 2007; 22(4): 199–210.
10 Monteleone P, Beinat L, Tanzillo C, *et al.* Effects of phosphatidylserine on the neuroendocrine response to physical stress in humans. *Neuroendocrinology* 1990; 52: 243–248.

11 Monteleone P, Maj M, Beinat L, *et al.* Blunting by chronic phosphatidylserine administration of the stress-induced activation of the hypothalamic-pituitary-adrenal axis in healthy men. *Eur J Clin Pharmacol* 1992; 42: 385–388.

12 Starks MA, Starks SL, Kingsley M, *et al.* The effects of phosphatidylserine on endocrine response to moderate intensity exercise. *J Int Soc Sports Nutr* 2008; 5(11): 11.

13 Kingsley MI, Wadsworth D, Kilduff LP, *et al.* Effects of phosphatidylserine on oxidative stress following intermittent running. *Med Sci Sports Exerc* 2005; 37(8): 1300–1306.

14 Kingsley MI, Kilduff LP, McEneny J, *et al.* Phosphatidylserine supplementation and recovery following downhill running. *Med Sci Sports Exerc* 2006; 38(9): 1617–1625.

15 Hellhammer J, Fries E, Buss C, *et al.* Effects of soy lecithin phosphatidic acid and phosphatidylserine complex (PAS) on the endocrine and psychological responses to mental stress. *Stress* 2004; 7: 119–126.

16 Baumeister J, Barthel T, Geiss KR, *et al.* Influence of phosphatidylserine on cognitive performance and cortical activity after induced stress. *Nutr Neurosci* 2008; 11(3): 103–110.

Phytosterols

Description

Phytosterols are plant compounds found naturally in the diet, with a similar chemical structure to cholesterol. They are also added to foods such as spreads, cream cheese, yoghurt, salad dressings, bread and drinks. A small, but increasing, number of food supplements in the form of tablets and capsules also contain them. Most phytosterols, like cholesterol, have a double bond in the steroid nucleus, but they contain an extra methyl or ethyl group in a side chain. Their role in plants is to stabilise the phospholipid bilayers in plant cell membranes, as cholesterol does in animal cell membranes.

Constituents

There are more than 100 different phytosterols, but the most abundant are the unsaturated compounds sitosterol, campesterol and stigmasterol, and the saturated compounds sitosterol and campestanol. Clinical studies generally focus on free phytosterols and phytosterol esters.[1] *Note*: the term phytosterol is used here to include both the saturated (stanols) and the unsaturated plant sterols.

Dietary intake

The daily dietary intake varies between 100 and 400 mg.[1,2] However, plant sterol intake would have been considerably higher 5–7 million years ago, up to 1 g per day (because the intake of fruit, vegetables and other plant foods was much higher than it is today).

Absorption

Absorption efficiency for plant sterols in humans is low, around 2–5%, which is considerably less than that of cholesterol, which is about 60%.[2] The saturated stanols are less well absorbed than the unsaturated sterols. Percentage absorption of beta-sitostanol is <1% while that of beta-sitosterol is around 5%. However, the stanols are as effective as the unsaturated sterols in lowering serum cholesterol, but because absorption of the former is lower, there is less chance of adverse consequences.

Dietary sources

Phytosterols exist in all plant foods and are mainly associated with the cell wall as structural components. Vegetarians, therefore, consume more phytosterols than do omnivores. Plant foods with a high fat and/or fibre content (e.g. oils, nuts, seeds and grains) are the most concentrated dietary sources.[1] A US analysis of the phytosterol content of nuts and seeds found that sesame seeds and wheatgerm had the highest concentration (>400 mg/100 g), followed by pistachio nuts (279 mg/100 g), sunflower seeds (270 mg/100 g), with English walnuts and Brazil nuts having a lower content (113 mg/100 g and 95 mg/100 g, respectively). Peanut butter (smooth) contains 135 mg/100 g.[3]

Action

The cholesterol lowering effect of phytosterols is well documented.[1,2,4–10] At intakes of 2–2.5 g daily, products enriched with phytosterol esters lower plasma LDL cholesterol levels by 10–14%.[9] The phytosterol component of typical diets is generally considered to be too small to influence cholesterol absorption.

Phytosterols reduce blood levels of total cholesterol and LDL cholesterol through reduction of cholesterol absorption,[9] although they may also influence cellular cholesterol metabolism within intestinal enterocytes.[9] The reduction of cholesterol absorption by phytosterols leads to increased synthesis of hepatic cholesterol. However, a reduction in LDL cholesterol occurs because of up-regulation of LDL receptor synthesis. Generally, phytosterols have no effect on HDL cholesterol or triglycerides.[11]

Plant stanol esters have been suggested to be more effective in lowering cholesterol than sterol esters. However, evidence for a significant difference in efficacy between stanols and sterols when they are esterified is limited.[1] One trial did find that the cholesterol-lowering effect of plant sterol esters was attenuated between 1 and 2 months, while plant stanol esters maintained their cholesterol-lowering efficacy.[12] In this same study, the effect of plant sterol esters after 2 months was not significantly different from baseline. This was accompanied by an increase in plasma plant sterols and a reduction in bile acid synthesis, which results in attenuation of cholesterol-lowering efficacy.[13] One placebo-controlled trial in 10 subjects with normal lipid levels found that unesterified sitostanol was more effective in reducing LDL cholesterol than was esterified sitostanol.[14]

Possible uses

Cholesterol reduction

Cholesterol reduction with free phytosterols and phytosterol esters has been studied in more than 60 human trials that have investigated subjects with normal lipid levels, hypercholesterolaemia, familial hypercholesterolaemia and diabetes mellitus. The mean reduction of LDL cholesterol with an average dose of 2.4 g daily is 9.9%.[1] A meta-analysis in familial hypercholesterolaemic subjects found that fat spreads enriched with 2.3 ± 0.5 g phytosterols daily reduced total cholesterol by 7–11% and LDL cholesterol by 10–15% in 6.5 ± 1.9 weeks compared with control treatment.[10]

Phytosterols seem to be effective against a background of both low- and high-fat diets.[15] However, one study has found that they are more effective when cholesterol intake is high,[16] while another found the plant stanol effect in lowering plasma cholesterol and LDL cholesterol was independent of and additive to the effect from dietary fat reduction.[17] Individual response also varies in that phytosterols decrease cholesterol absorption to a different extent in different people,[18] with emerging evidence that response varies according to genetic makeup,[19] for example apolipoprotein E genotype.[20] Preliminary evidence also indicates that the cholesterol lowering response does not depend on baseline serum plant sterol concentrations.[21]

Most studies have investigated the effect of phytosterols administered in a fat-spread vehicle. A trial in an outpatient setting found that routine prescription of 25 g daily of a spread containing 2 g phytosterols is effective for management of hypercholesterolaemia in this setting.[22] Customary use of phytosterol-/stanol-enriched spreads in free-living conditions (as opposed to controlled trial conditions) has also been found to produce benefit – with a stabilising effect on serum cholesterol levels compared with no use of such spreads, which produced an increase in serum cholesterol.[23]

The source of plant sterols within the fortified spread seems to have no effect on the capacity to reduce serum cholesterol. A 6-week trial found that plant sterols from soya bean oil, tall oil and a mixture of tall oil with rapeseed oil were equally effective in lowering LDL cholesterol, with the absolute decrease in LDL dependent on baseline concentrations.[24] A 4-week trial in 59 hypercholesterolaemic subjects showed that plant sterols from tall and rapeseed oils reduced atherogenic lipids and lipoproteins similarly.[25]

Giving phytosterols in other vehicles such as low-fat milk,[26–28] fermented milk,[29,30] soya drink,[31,32] yoghurt,[27,33–35] low-fat cheese,[34,36] orange juice,[37,38] and in a lemon-flavoured drink or egg white has also been shown to reduce serum cholesterol.[39] However, other studies have suggested that phytosterols added to non-fat and low-fat beverages are not effective in modifying lipid levels.

Phytosterols present naturally in foods can also lower cholesterol. A recent trial involved 106 subjects at high risk for cardiovascular disease (CVD) who were assigned to two Mediterranean diets supplemented with virgin olive oil (VOO) or nuts, which are phytosterol-rich foods, or to advice on a low-fat diet. The average phytosterol intake increased by 76, 158 and 15 mg daily in participants assigned VOO, nuts and low-fat diets, respectively. Compared with participants in the low-fat diet group, changes in outcome variables were observed only in those in the Mediterranean diet with nuts group, with increases in intake of fibre, polyunsaturated fatty acids and phytosterols (all $P < 0.020$) and significant reductions of LDL cholesterol (0.27 mmol/L (8.3%); $P < 0.05$) and the ratio of LDL to HDL cholesterol (0.29 mmol/l (11.5%); $P < 0.05$). Variations in saturated fat, cholesterol or fibre intake were unrelated to LDL cholesterol changes.[40]

Trials with pharmaceutical formulations

Trials have investigated the effect on LDL cholesterol of phytosterols in tablet form. A rapidly disintegrating stanol lecithin tablet (1.26 g stanols daily) produced a decrease in LDL cholesterol of 10.4% and a reduction in the ratio of LDL to HDL cholesterol of 11.4% in a trial involving 52 subjects. By comparison, slowly disintegrating tablets had no effect on any lipid paramenter.[41]

Another trial in 26 patients following the American Heart Association Heart Healthy Diet and on long-term statin therapy found that 1.8 g daily of dispersible soya stanols in tablet form reduced LDL cholesterol by a further 9.1% (beyond statins alone), providing evidence that stanol tablets could offer potential adjunctive therapy for patients who have not reached their target LDL cholesterol goal during statin therapy.[42]

Softgel and capsule formulations have also been investigated. A placebo-controlled trial randomised 30 hypercholesterolaemic subjects to either phytostanol ester (2.7 g stanol esters) in a softgel formulation or placebo for 28 days. Phytostanol supplementation resulted in a significant decrease in total cholesterol (8%) and LDL cholesterol (9%). There were no alterations in concentrations of HDL-cholesterol or triglycerides. Neither LDL cholesterol/HDL cholesterol ratios nor total cholesterol/HDL cholesterol ratios altered significantly.[43]

A double-blind, placebo-controlled trial with a 4-week treatment phase tested the efficacy of plant sterol esters (1.3 g plant stanol esters daily) in 16 free-living hypercholesterolaemic subjects. In comparison with placebo, LDL cholesterol was significantly reduced by 7% and 4% ($P < 0.05$) at week 3 and week 4. HDL cholesterol at week 4 was significantly increased by 9% but not at week 4 (4%). Total cholesterol was not significantly different from placebo throughout the study period. Total cholesterol/HDL cholesterol and LDL cholesterol/HDL cholesterol were significantly reduced by 8% and 6%, respectively, at week 3 and by 8% and 10%, respectively, at week 4. C-reactive protein and triglycerides did not differ throughout the study.[44]

A further trial in 17 patients after colectomy who were administered plant stanol esters in a pastille for 1 week showed that serum levels of total and LDL cholesterol decreased by 9% and 14%, respectively, and absorption of esterified and free cholesterol reduced by over 40%. Faecal elimination of cholesterol was increased by about 35%, and 60% of plant stanol esters were hydrolysed in the gastrointestinal tract. Hydrolysis of plant stanol esters was more pronounced in a normal than a low fat diet.[45]

A randomised, double-blind, two-group parallel, placebo-controlled study to test the cholesterol-lowering properties of stearate-enriched plant sterol esters in 32 normo- and hypercholesterolaemic adults randomised participants to consume 3 g daily of either plant sterol esters (1 g three times per day with meals) or placebo delivered in capsules. Serum LDL cholesterol concentration significantly decreased by 0.42 mmol/L (11%) and the ratio of LDL to HDL cholesterol decreased 10% with plant sterol ester supplementation, whereas LDL particle size and lipoprotein subclass particle concentrations (as measured by NMR) were not affected. The percentage change in LDL cholesterol was positively correlated with baseline lathosterol concentration, indicating an association between the magnitude of LDL change and the rate of whole-body cholesterol synthesis. Serum campesterol (but not sitosterol) concentration significantly increased in the plant sterol ester group. Serum tocopherol, retinol and beta-carotene concentrations were not affected by plant sterol ester supplementation.[46]

Although phytosterols favourably influence total cholesterol and LDL cholesterol levels, their effects on other indicators of risk for CVD have not been so intensively studied. One trial showed that phytosterols could attenuate exercise-induced beneficial increase in HDL cholesterol,[47] another concluded that these compounds have no effect on coronary heart disease risk,[48] while yet another found no influence on endothelial function in type 1 diabetes.[49]

Miscellaneous

Phytosterols have been studied *in vitro* and in animals for other activity, including anti-athero-genic activity, anti-cancer activity, antioxidant activity and anti-inflammatory activity. Results are promising but require confirmation in controlled clinical trials in humans.

Conclusion

The cholesterol-reducing effect of phytosterols is well documented. Intakes of 2–2.5 g daily of products enriched with phytosterol esters lower plasma LDL cholesterol levels by 10–14%. The mean reduction in LDL cholesterol with an average dose of 2.4 g daily is 9.9%. Despite the cholesterol-lowering effect, the benefit of phytosterols in reducing cardiovascular risk remains to be proven. Whether stanol esters or sterol esters are the most beneficial is debatable and more evidence is required. Most studies have investigated the effect of phytosterols given in fat spreads. However, there is evidence that these compounds can also lower cholesterol if given in the form of milks, yoghurts, orange juice and low-fat cheese. Preliminary evidence from trials incorporating phytosterols in tablets have also demonstrated efficacy in cholesterol reduction, but the formulation must be well dispersible. There is preliminary evidence that phytosterols may have activity against cancer.

Precautions/contraindications

There are a few people with rare genetic defects such as phytosterolaemia, who are susceptible to high phytosterol intakes.[2] The impact of phytosterols in these people is unknown, but there is increased absorption of phytosterols, which may lead to increased atherosclerosis, as excess cholesterol does, and also to cell fragility. In addition, the larger number of people who are heterozygous for such conditions may also have some increased susceptibility to high phytosterol intakes.

There are no data in children under 5 years with normocholesterolaemia. It would seem prudent, pending such data, to caution against the use of phytosterols in children because of the potential risk of reduced absorption of fat-soluble nutrients. Phytosterols have the same cholesterol-reducing effect in hypercholesterolaemic children as in hypercholesterolaemic adults.

Pregnancy and breast-feeding

There are no long-term data in pregnancy and breast-feeding.

Adverse effects

Within the range of intake that causes desirable reduction in blood levels of cholesterol and LDL cholesterol, phytosterols are thought to be clinically safe.[2] However, because phytosterols reduce the absorption of cholesterol it has been suggested that they might reduce the absorption of other lipid-soluble substances such as carotenoids (e.g. beta-carotene and lycopene) and vitamin E. The clinical evidence is controversial, with some studies showing that plant sterols do reduce blood levels of carotenoids and vitamin E, while other studies show no effect.[2] Macular pigment optical density could change as a result of any reduction in serum carotenoids but a recent study has refuted this suggestion.[50] A study involving 15-weeks of consumption of natural non-esterified plant sterol-enriched food indicated no serious adverse effects during this period. However, serum alpha-tocopherol levels were somewhat reduced in the sterol group, suggesting that long-term effects of plant sterols on serum fat-soluble vitamin concentrations should be further explored, especially in relation to very-low-fat diets.[51] It would, therefore, seem prudent to advise patients to include sources of fat-soluble vitamins in their diets.

Interactions

Drugs

Statins: in theory, combination treatment of statins and phytosterols could have an additive effect on reduction of LDL cholesterol, because phytosterols and statins have different mechanisms of action. A review including five trials of combination therapy found that the addition of phytosterols reduced LDL cholesterol by a further 4.5% per gram of phytosterols.[1] Consumption of spread that provided 5.1 g daily of plant stanol esters effectively reduced elevated total and LDL cholesterol levels in participants on a stable regimen of a statin.[52] In another study, the addition of stanol ester margarine to statin therapy produced LDL cholesterol reduction equivalent to doubling the dose of statin.[53] A further trial in patients optimally treated with statins found that intensive dietary treatment with plant stanol spreads and lipid-lowering diet resulted in a significant reduction of LDL cholesterol (15.6%) compared with a reduction of 7.7% in the control group (who were optimally treated with statins).[54] In another study, a tablet containing stanols further reduced LDL cholesterol by 9.1% in patients taking statins.[42]

However, in a Dutch study, plant stanol or sterol consumption for 16 weeks had no effect on markers of oxidative stress, antioxidant status, endothelial dysfunction and low-grade inflammation in patients on stable statin treatment, despite a significant reduction in LDL cholesterol.[55] A study of 90 weeks' duration by this same Dutch group among patients well stabilised on statins found that consumption of both plant sterol and stanol esters effectively lowered LDL cholesterol in these long-term statin users.[56] Moreover, this study also indicated that consumption of 2.5 g plant stanols or sterols daily in people taking statins does not affect neurocognitive function or mood.[57]

A recent meta-analysis of eight controlled trials evaluating the influence of plant stanols/sterols in patients with hypercholesterolaemia who were taking statins found that this combination significantly lowered total cholesterol and LDL cholesterol but not HDL cholesterol or triglycerides.[58]

Nutrients

Lipid-soluble nutrients: in theory, phytosterols could reduce the absorption of lipid-soluble substances such as carotenoids and vitamin E, but evidence for this is conflicting.

Dose

Doses of phytosterols used in clinical studies have varied between 1 and 3 g daily (free sterol/stanol equivalent). The mean reduction of LDL cholesterol with an average dose of 2.4 g daily is 9.9%.[1] There is some evidence to suggest that to obtain optimal cholesterol-reducing impact, plant sterols should be consumed as smaller doses given more often, rather than one large daily dose.[59]

Few studies have looked at higher doses, but there is concern that higher doses might increase systemic availability of these substances. However, a 10-week controlled trial involving an 8.8 g daily dose of plant stanols showed that serum plant stanol levels remained at comparable low levels as in studies with daily intake of 2–3 g, and were normalized in 4 weeks, while effectively reducing serum cholesterol levels.[60] Nevertheless, further research is needed to identify the optimal dose of phytosterols, the relative efficacy of phytosterols in different populations and the efficacy of these compounds when incorporated into different foods (other than fat spread) and tablet formulations. On current evidence, patients should be advised not to exceed a 2–3 g daily dose.

References

1 Normen L, Holmes D, Frohlich J. Plant sterols and their role in combined use with statins for lipid lowering. *Curr Opin Invest Drugs* 2005; 6(3): 307–316.

2 Berger A, Jones PJ, Abumweis SS. Plant sterols: factors affecting their efficacy and safety as functional food ingredients. *Lipids Health Dis* 2004; 3: 5.

3 Phillips KM, Ruggio DM, Ashraf-Khorassani M. Phytosterol composition of nuts and seeds commonly consumed in the United States. *J Agric Food Chem* 2005; 53(24): 9436–9445.

4 Ling WH, Jones PJ. Dietary phytosterols: a review of metabolism, benefits and side effects. *Life Sci* 1995; 57(3): 195–206.

5 Jones PJ, MacDougall DE, Ntanios F, *et al.* Dietary phytosterols as cholesterol-lowering agents in humans. *Can J Physiol Pharmacol* 1997; 75(3): 217–227.

6 Moghadasian MH, Frohlich JJ. Effects of dietary phytosterols on cholesterol metabolism and atherosclerosis: clinical and experimental evidence. *Am J Med* 1999; 107(6): 588–594.

7 Law M. Plant sterol and stanol margarines and health. *BMJ* 2000; 320(7238): 861–864.

8 Katan MB, Grundy SM, Jones P, *et al.* Efficacy and safety of plant stanols and sterols in the management of blood cholesterol levels. *Mayo Clin Proc* 2003; 78(8): 965–978.

9 Plat J, Mensink RP. Plant stanol and sterol esters in the control of blood cholesterol levels: mechanism and safety aspects. *Am J Cardiol* 2005; 96 (Suppl 1A): 15D–22D.

10 Moruisi KG, Oosthuizen W, Opperman AM. Phytosterols/stanols lower cholesterol concentrations in familial hypercholesterolemic subjects: a systematic review with meta-analysis. *J Am Coll Nutr* 2006; 25(1): 41–48.

11 Plat J, Mensink RP. Effects of plant stanol esters on LDL receptor protein expression and on LDL receptor and HMG-CoA reductase mRNA expression in mononuclear blood cells of healthy men and women. *FASEB J* 2002; 16(2): 258–260.

12 O'Neill FH, Brynes A, Mandeno R, *et al.* Comparison of the effects of dietary plant sterol and stanol esters on lipid metabolism. *Nutr Metab Cardiovasc Dis* 2004; 14(3): 133–142.

13 O'Neill FH, Sanders TA, Thompson GR. Comparison of efficacy of plant stanol ester and sterol ester: short-term and longer-term studies. *Am J Cardiol* 2005; 96(Suppl 1A): 29D–36D.

14 Sudhop T, Lutjohann D, Agna M, *et al.* Comparison of the effects of sitostanol, sitostanol-lacetate, and sitostanol oleate on the inhibition of cholesterolabsorption in normolipemic healthy male volunteers. A placebo controlled randomized cross-over study. *Arzneimittelforschung* 2003; 53 (10): 708–713.

15 Hernandez-Mijares A, Banuls C, Rocha M, *et al.* Effects of phytosterol ester-enriched low-fat milk on serum lipoprotein profile in mildly hypercholesterolaemic patients are not related to dietary cholesterol or saturated fat intake. *Br J Nutr* 2010; 104 (7): 1018–1025.

16 Mussner MJ, Parhofer KG, von Bergmann K, *et al.* Effects of phytosterol ester-enriched margarine on plasma lipoproteins in mild to moderate hypercholesterolemia are related to basal cholesterol and fat intake. *Metabolism* 2002; 51(2): 189–194.

17 Chen SC, Judd JT, Kramer M, *et al.* Phytosterol intake and dietary fat reduction are independent and additive in their ability to reduce plasma LDL cholesterol. *Lipids* 2009; 44(3): 273–281.

18 Rudkowska I, AbuMweis SS, Nicolle C, *et al.* Association between non-responsiveness to plant sterol intervention and polymorphisms in cholesterol metabolism genes: a case-control study. *Appl Physiol Nutr Metab* 2008; 33(4): 728–734.

19 Gylling H, Hallikainen M, Raitakari OT, *et al.* Long-term consumption of plant stanol and sterol esters, vascular function and genetic regulation. *Br J Nutr* 2009; 101(11): 1688–1695.

20 Sanchez-Muniz FJ, Maki KC, Schaefer EJ, *et al.* Serum lipid and antioxidant responses in hypercholesterolemic men and women receiving plant sterol esters vary by apolipoprotein E genotype. *J Nutr* 2009; 139(1): 13–19.

21 Houweling AH, Vanstone CA, Trautwein EA, *et al.* Baseline plasma plant sterol concentrations do not predict changes in serum lipids. C-reactive protein (CRP) and plasma plant sterols following intake of a plant sterol-enriched food. *Eur J Clin Nutr* 2009; 63(4): 543–551.

22 Patch CS, Tapsell LC, Williams PG. Plant sterol/stanol prescription is an effective treatment strategy for managing hypercholesterolemia in outpatient clinical practice. *J Am Diet Assoc* 2005; 105(1): 46–52.

23 Wolfs M, de Jong N, Ocke MC, *et al.* Effectiveness of customary use of phytosterol/-stanol enriched margarines on blood cholesterol lowering. *Food Chem Toxicol* 2006; 44(10): 1682–1688.

24 Clifton PM, Mano M, Duchateau GS, *et al.* Dose-response effects of different plant sterol sources in fat spreads on serum lipids and C-reactive protein and on the kinetic behavior of serum plant sterols. *Eur J Clin Nutr* 2008; 62(8): 968–977.

25 Heggen E, Granlund L, Pedersen JI, *et al.* Plant sterols from rapeseed and tall oils: effects on lipids, fat-soluble vitamins and plant sterol concentrations. *Nutr Metab Cardiovasc Dis* 2009; 20(4): 258–265.

26 Clifton PM, Noakes M, Sullivan D, *et al.* Cholesterol-lowering effects of plant sterol esters differ in milk, yoghurt, bread and cereal. *Eur J Clin Nutr* 2004; 58(3): 503–509.

27 Noakes M, Clifton PM, Doornbos AM, *et al.* Plant sterol ester-enriched milk and yoghurt effectively reduce serum cholesterol in modestly hypercholesterolemic subjects. *Eur J Nutr* 2005; 44(4): 214–222.

28 Thomsen AB, Hansen HB, Christiansen C, *et al.* Effect of free plant sterols in low-fat milk on serum lipid profile in hypercholesterolemic subjects. *Eur J Clin Nutr* 2004; 58(6): 860–870.

29 Plana N, Nicolle C, Ferre R, *et al.* Plant sterol-enriched fermented milk enhances the attainment of LDL-cholesterol goal in hypercholesterolemic subjects. *Eur J Nutr* 2008; 47: 32–39.

30 Mannarino E, Pirro M, Cortese C, *et al.* Effects of a phytosterol-enriched dairy product on lipids, sterols and 8-isoprostane in hypercholesterolemic patients: a multicenter Italian study. *Nutr Metab Cardiovasc Dis* 2009; 19(2): 84–90.

31 Weidner C, Krempf M, Bard JM, *et al.* Cholesterol lowering effect of a soy drink enriched with plant sterols in a French population with moderate hypercholesterolemia. *Lipids Health Dis* 2008; 7: 35.

32 Rideout TC, Chan YM, Harding SV, *et al.* Low and moderate-fat plant sterol fortified soymilk in modulation of plasma lipids and cholesterol kinetics in subjects with normal to high cholesterol concentrations: report on two randomized crossover studies. *Lipids Health Dis* 2009; 8: 45.

33 Mensink RP, Ebbing S, Lindhout M, *et al.* Effects of plant stanol esters supplied in low-fat yoghurt on serum lipids and lipoproteins, non-cholesterol sterols and fat soluble antioxidant concentrations. *Atherosclerosis* 2002; 160(1): 205–213.

34 Korpela R, Tuomilehto J, Hogstrom P, *et al.* Safety aspects and cholesterol-lowering efficacy of low fat dairy products containing plant sterols. *Eur J Clin Nutr* 2006; 60(5): 633–642.

35 Niittynen LH, Jauhiainen TA, Poussa TA, *et al.* Effects of yoghurt enriched with free plant sterols on the levels of serum lipids and plant sterols in moderately hypercholesterolaemic subjects on a high-fat diet. *Int J Food Sci Nutr* 2008; 59(5): 357–367.

36 Jauhiainen T, Salo P, Niittynen L, *et al.* Effects of low-fat hard cheese enriched with plant stanol esters on serum lipids and apolipoprotein B in mildly hypercholesterolaemic subjects. *Eur J Clin Nutr* 2006; 60: 1253–1257.

37 Devaraj S, Jialal I, Vega-Lopez S. Plant sterol-fortified orange juice effectively lowers cholesterol levels in mildly hypercholesterolemic healthy individuals. *Arterioscler Thromb Vasc Biol* 2004; 24 (3): e25–e28.

38 Devaraj S, Autret BC, Jialal I. Reduced-calorie orange juice beverage with plant sterols lowers C-reactive protein concentrations and improves the lipid profile in human volunteers. *Am J Clin Nutr* 2006; 84(4): 756–761.

39 Spilburg CA, Goldberg AC, McGill JB, *et al.* Fat-free foods supplemented with soy stanol–lecithin powder reduce cholesterol absorption and LDL cholesterol. *J Am Diet Assoc* 2003; 103(5): 577–581.

40 Escurriol V, Cofan M, Serra M, *et al.* Serum sterol responses to increasing plant sterol intake from natural foods in the Mediterranean diet. *Eur J Nutr* 2009; 48(6): 373–382.

41 McPherson TB, Ostlund RE, Goldberg AC, *et al.* Phytostanol tablets reduce human LDL-cholesterol. *J Pharm Pharmacol* 2005; 57(7): 889–896.

42 Goldberg AC, Ostlund RE,Jr Bateman JH, *et al.* Effect of plant stanol tablets on low-density lipoprotein cholesterol lowering in patients on statin drugs. *Am J Cardiol* 2006; 97(3): 376–379.

43 Woodgate D, Chan CH, Conquer JA. Cholesterol-lowering ability of a phytostanol softgel supplement in adults with mild to moderate hypercholesterolemia. *Lipids* 2006; 41(2): 127–132.

44 Acuff RV, Cai DJ, Dong ZP, *et al.* The lipid lowering effect of plant sterol ester capsules in hypercholesterolemic subjects. *Lipids Health Dis* 2007; 611:.

45 Nissinen MJ, Gylling H, Miettinen TA. Effects of plant stanol esters supplied in a fat free milieu by pastilles on cholesterol metabolism in colectomized human subjects. *Nutr Metab Cardiovasc Dis* 2006; 16(6): 426–435.

46 Carr TP, Krogstrand KL, Schlegel VL, *et al.* Stearate-enriched plant sterol esters lower serum LDL cholesterol concentration in normo- and hypercholesterolemic adults. *J Nutr* 2009; 139(8): 1445–1450.

47 Alhassan S, Reese KA, Mahurin J, *et al.* Blood lipid responses to plant stanol ester supplementation and aerobic exercise training. *Metabolism* 2006; 55(4): 541–549.

48 Varady KA, St-Pierre AC, Lamarche B, *et al.* Effect of plant sterols and endurance training on LDL particle size and distribution in previously sedentary hypercholesterolemic adults. *Eur J Clin Nutr* 2005; 59(4): 518–525.

49 Hallikainen M, Lyyra-Laitinen T, Laitinen T, *et al.* Effects of plant stanol esters on serum cholesterol concentrations, relative markers of cholesterol metabolism and endothelial function in type 1 diabetes. *Atherosclerosis* 2008; 199(2): 432–439.

50 Berendschot TT, Plat J, de Jong A, *et al.* Long-term plant stanol and sterol ester-enriched functional food consumption, serum lutein/zeaxanthin concentration and macular pigment optical density. *Br J Nutr* 2009; 101(11): 1607–1610.

51 Tuomilehto J, Tikkanen MJ, Hogstrom P, *et al.* Safety assessment of common foods enriched with natural nonesterified plant sterols. *Eur J Clin Nutr* 2009; 63(5): 684–691.

52 Blair SN, Capuzzi DM, Gottlieb SO, *et al.* Incremental reduction of serum total cholesterol and low-density lipoprotein cholesterol with the addition of plant stanol ester-containing spread to statin therapy. *Am J Cardiol* 2000; 86(1): 46–52.

53 Simons LA. Additive effect of plant sterol-ester margarine and cerivastatin in lowering low-density lipoprotein cholesterol in primary hypercholesterolemia. *Am J Cardiol* 2002; 90(7): 737–740.

54 Castro Cabezas M, de Vries JH, Van Oostrom AJ, *et al.* Effects of a stanol-enriched diet on plasma cholesterol and triglycerides in patients treated with statins. *J Am Diet Assoc* 2006; 106(10): 1564–1569.

55 de Jong A, Plat J, Bast A, *et al.* Effects of plant sterol and stanol ester consumption on lipid metabolism, antioxidant status and markers of oxidative stress, endothelial function and low-grade inflammation in patients on current statin treatment. *Eur J Clin Nutr* 2008; 62(2): 263–273.

56 de Jong A, Plat J, Lutjohann D, *et al.* Effects of long-term plant sterol or stanol ester consumption on lipid and lipoprotein metabolism in subjects on statin treatment. *Br J Nutr* 2008; 100(5): 937–941.

57 Schiepers OJ, de Groot RH, van Boxtel MP, *et al.* Consuming functional foods enriched with plant

sterol or stanol esters for 85 weeks does not affect neurocognitive functioning or mood in statin-treated hypercholesterolemic individuals. *J Nutr* 2009; 139(7): 1368–1373.

58 Scholle JM, Baker WL, Talati R, *et al.* The effect of adding plant sterols or stanols to statin therapy in hypercholesterolemic patients: systematic review and meta-analysis. *J Am Coll Nutr* 2009; 28(5): 517–524.

59 AbuMweis SS, Vanstone CA, Lichtenstein AH, *et al.* Plant sterol consumption frequency affects plasma lipid levels and cholesterol kinetics in humans. *Eur J Clin Nutr* 2009; 63(6): 747–755.

60 Gylling H, Hallikainen M, Nissinen MJ, *et al.* Very high plant stanol intake and serum plant stanols and non-cholesterol sterols. *Eur J Nutr* 2009; 49(2): 111–117.

Pomegranate

Description

Pomegranate is a fruit-bearing deciduous shrub cultivated throughout the Mediterranean region, India, South East Asia, California and Arizona. Parts of the pomegranate that have been studied for human use include the fruit, fruit juice, seed, seed oil, bark, rind, root, stem, leaf and flower.

The constituent compounds are mainly anti-oxidant polyphenols with some vitamins, minerals, amino acids and fatty acids (Table 1). Some dietary supplement manufacturers use the juice for their products, while others use polyphenolic extracts derived from the juice, but extracts from all parts of the fruit, bark, roots and leaves of the tree have been used historically for therapeutic effects.

The most therapeutically active pomegranate constituent appears to be ellagic acid, with activity also found in ellagitannins (including punicalagins), punicic acid, flavonoids, anthocyanidins, anthocyanins, flavones and flavonols. Ellagic acid has powerful anticarcinogenic[2] and antioxidant[3] properties, which have helped to propel pomegranate into the research limelight, but the other active constituents should not be ignored. Increased plasma and urinary polyphenolic concentrations[4–6] and *in vivo* antioxidant effects have been demonstrated following ingestion of pomegranate.

Action

Pomegranate has several properties, including antioxidant, anticarcinogenic and anti-inflammatory properties. Studies in animals have shown that pomegranate extracts reduce oxidative stress and lipid peroxidation in animals[7] and increase plasma antioxidant capacity in humans.[8,9] Pomegranate has been shown to have activity against prostate cancer,[10–12] colon cancer and breast cancer[11] cells *in vitro*. *In vitro* studies have also provided evidence that pomegranate has anti-inflammatory activity.[13,14]

Possible uses

Pomegranate extract and juice have been studied in a few human trials for several conditions, particularly cancers and cardiovascular disease.

Cancer

A preliminary trial in men with rising prostate-specific antigen (PSA) following treatment for prostate cancer found that pomegranate juice had positive effects on measures of PSA turnover, cell proliferation and oxidative stress.[15]

Cardiovascular disease

The effects of pomegranate juice consumption on lipid peroxidation in plasma and high-density lipoprotein (HDL) and low-density lipoprotein (LDL) cholesterol was examined in a double-armed human trial. In the first study, 13 healthy, non-smoking men (aged 20–35 years) were given 50 ml of pomegranate juice daily for 2 weeks. In the second study (duration ≤10 weeks), three healthy men (aged 20–35 years) were given increasing doses of pomegranate juice, ranging from 20 ml to 80 ml daily. No significant effect was shown in either study on plasma lipid profile or lipoprotein patterns.

Table 1 Pomegranate constituents[1]

Pomegranate plant component	Constituents
Juice	Anthocyanins, caffeic acid, catechin, ellagic acid, gallic acid, epigallocatechin gallate (EGCG), quercetin, rutin, glucose, ascorbic acid, minerals (particularly iron), amino acids
Seed oil	95% punicic acid, ellagic acid, fatty acid, sterols
Pericarp (peel, rind)	Phenolic punicalagins, gallic acid, catechin, EGCG, quercetin, rutin, other flavonols, flavones, flavonones, anthocyanidins, fatty acids
Leaves	Tannins (punicalin and punicafolin), flavone glycosides, including luteolin and apigenin
Flower	Gallic acid, ursolic acid, triterpenoids, including maslinic and asiatic acid
Roots and bark	Ellagitannins, including punicalin and punicalagin, piperidine alkaloids

However, pomegranate juice had an inhibitory effect on lipid peroxidation in plasma and in lipoproteins, with the 50 ml dose being most effective, yielding a 32% decrease in plasma lipid peroxidation. Pomegranate also demonstrated up to 90% inhibition of collagen-induced platelet aggregation in human platelets *ex vivo*.[16]

A placebo-controlled trial involving 10 patients with carotid artery stenosis found that pomegranate juice over 1–3 years reduced carotid intima media thickness (CIMT) and blood pressure and improved plasma antioxidant status. For all studied parameters, maximal effects were observed after 1 year of pomegranate juice consumption.[16] A further trial in men and women found that in people with moderate coronary heart disease risk, pomegranate juice consumption had no significant effect on overall CIMT progression rate, but it may have slowed CIMT progression in people with increased oxidative stress and disturbances in the triglyceride-rich lipoprotein/HDL axis.[17]

Pomegranate juice has also been found to increase the association between HDL cholesterol and the enzyme paraoxanase 1 in people with diabetes mellitus,[18,19] leading the researchers to suggest that pomegranate might inhibit atherosclerosis in these patients. A pilot study involving 22 people with type 2 diabetes given 40 g of pomegranate juice for 8 weeks found statistically significant reductions in total cholesterol, LDL cholesterol, total/HDL cholesterol ratio and LDL/HDL cholesterol ratio.[20]

A small clinical trial showed that pomegranate juice inhibits serum angiotensin-converting enzyme (ACE) and reduces systolic blood pressure in people with hypertension. Seven out of 10 people in the trial experienced a 36% average decrease in serum ACE activity and a small but significant (5%) decrease in systolic blood pressure.[21]

In a double-blind randomised placebo-controlled trial involving 39 people with coronary heart disease, 240 ml of pomegranate juice daily for 3 months resulted in a reduction in myocardial ischaemia and improved myocardial perfusion. Angina episodes reduced by 50% in the pomegranate juice group and increased by 38% in the placebo group.[22]

Conclusion

Pomegranate is a potent antioxidant with anticarcinogenic and anti-inflammatory properties. However, the possibility that it could have a beneficial effect on diseases such as cancer and cardiovascular disease in humans requires more clinical research. Currently, several clinical trials are in progress exploring the therapeutic potential of pomegranate.

Precautions/contraindications

Insufficient reliable information.

Pregnancy and breast-feeding

Insufficient data.

Adverse effects

Allergic reactions have been reported.

Interactions

In theory, pomegranate could increase the effects of anti-hypertensive medication and ACE inhibitors because of its potential activity. In animal studies, pomegranate has been shown to inhibit various cytochrome P450 enzymes[23] and has increased tolbutamide[24] and carbamazepine[25] bioavailability in rats. Evidence from a single case study suggests that pomegranate juice consumption could reduce the bioavailability of warfarin.[26]

Dose

None established. Studies have used 50–240 ml of pomegranate juice daily or 40 g concentrated pomegranate juice daily. Some commercially available pomegranate extracts are being standardised to contain 40% or more ellagic acid.

References

1 Jurenka J. Therapeutic applications of pomegranate (*Punica granatum* L.): a review. *Alt Med Rev* 2008; 13: 128–144.

2 Falsaperla M, Morgia G, Tartarone A, Ardito R, Romano G. Support ellagic acid therapy in patients with hormone refractory prostate cancer (HRPC) on standard chemotherapy using vinorelbine and estramustine phosphate. *Eur Urol* 2005; 47: 449–454 discussion 454455.

3 Hassoun EA, Vodhanel J, Abushaban A. The modulatory effects of ellagic acid and vitamin E succinate on TCDD-induced oxidative stress in different brain regions of rats after subchronic exposure. *J Biochem Mol Toxicol* 2004; 18: 196–203.

4 Seeram NP, Henning SM, Zhang Y, *et al.* Pomegranate juice ellagitannin metabolites are present in human plasma and some persist in urine for up to 48 hours. *J Nutr* 2006; 136: 2481–2485.

5 Seeram NP, Lee R, Heber D. Bioavailability of ellagic acid in human plasma after consumption of ellagitannins from pomegranate (*Punica granatum* L.) juice. *Clin Chim Acta* 2004; 348: 63–68.

6 Seeram NP, Zhang Y, McKeever R, *et al.* Pomegranate juice and extracts provide similar levels of plasma and urinary ellagitannin metabolites in human subjects. *J Med Food* 2008; 11: 390–394.

7 Rosenblat M, Volkova N, Coleman R, Aviram M. Pomegranate byproduct administration to apolipoprotein E-deficient mice attenuates atherosclerosis development as a result of decreased macrophage oxidative stress and reduced cellular uptake of oxidized low-density lipoprotein. *J Agric Food Chem* 2006; 54: 1928–1935.

8 Rosenblat M, Hayek T, Aviram M. Anti-oxidative effects of pomegranate juice (PJ) consumption by diabetic patients on serum and on macrophages. *Atherosclerosis* 2006; 187: 363–371.

9 Guo C, Wei J, Yang J, Xu J, Pang W, Jiang Y. Pomegranate juice is potentially better than apple juice in improving antioxidant function in elderly subjects. *Nutr Res* 2008; 28: 72–77.

10 Seeram NP, Aronson WJ, Zhang Y, *et al.* Pomegranate ellagitannin-derived metabolites inhibit prostate cancer growth and localize to the mouse prostate gland. *J Agric Food Chem* 2007; 55: 7732–7737.

11 Adams LS, Zhang Y, Seeram NP, Heber D, Chen S. Pomegranate ellagitannin-derived compounds exhibit antiproliferative and antiaromatase activity in breast cancer cells in vitro. *Cancer Prev Res (Phila)*; 3: 108–113.

12 Sartippour MR, Seeram NP, Rao JY, *et al.* Ellagitannin-rich pomegranate extract inhibits angiogenesis in prostate cancer in vitro and in vivo. *Int J Oncol* 2008; 32: 475–480.

13 Schubert SY, Lansky EP, Neeman I. Antioxidant and eicosanoid enzyme inhibition properties of pomegranate seed oil and fermented juice flavonoids. *J Ethnopharmacol* 1999; 66: 11–17.

14 Larrosa M, Gonzalez-Sarrias A, Yanez-Gascon MJ, *et al.* Anti-inflammatory properties of a pomegranate extract and its metabolite urolithin-A in a colitis rat model and the effect of colon inflammation on phenolic metabolism. *J Nutr Biochem* 2009; 21: 717–725.

15 Pantuck AJ, Leppert JT, Zomorodian N, *et al.* Phase II study of pomegranate juice for men with rising prostate-specific antigen following surgery or radiation for prostate cancer. *Clin Cancer Res* 2006; 12: 4018–4026.

16 Aviram M, Dornfeld L, Rosenblat M, *et al.* Pomegranate juice consumption reduces oxidative stress, atherogenic modifications to LDL, and platelet aggregation: studies in humans and in atherosclerotic apolipoprotein E-deficient mice. *Am J Clin Nutr* 2000; 71: 1062–1076.

17 Davidson MH, Maki KC, Dicklin MR, *et al.* Effects of consumption of pomegranate juice on carotid intima-media thickness in men and women at moderate risk for coronary heart disease. *Am J Cardiol* 2009; 104: 936–942.

18 Rock W, Rosenblat M, Miller-Lotan R, *et al.* Consumption of Wonderful variety pomegranate juice and extract by diabetic patients increases paraoxonase 1 association with high-density lipoprotein and stimulates its catalytic activities. *J Agric Food Chem* 2008; 56: 8704–8713.

19 Fuhrman B, Volkova N, Aviram M. Pomegranate juice polyphenols increase recombinant paraoxonase-1 binding to high-density lipoprotein: studies in vitro and in diabetic patients. *Nutrition* 2009; 26: 359–366.

20 Esmaillzadeh A, Tahbaz F, Gaieni I, Alavi-Majd H, Azadbakht L. Cholesterol-lowering effect of concentrated pomegranate juice consumption in type II diabetic patients with hyperlipidemia. *Int J Vitam Nutr Res* 2006; 76: 147–151.

21 Aviram M, Dornfeld L. Pomegranate juice consumption inhibits serum angiotensin converting enzyme activity and reduces systolic blood pressure. *Atherosclerosis* 2001; 158: 195–198.

22 Sumner MD, Elliott-Eller M, Weidner G, *et al.* Effects of pomegranate juice consumption on myocardial perfusion in patients with coronary heart disease. *Am J Cardiol* 2005; 96: 810–814.

23 Faria A, Monteiro R, Azevedo I, Calhau C. Pomegranate juice effects on cytochrome P450S expression: in vivo studies. *J Med Food* 2007; 10: 643–649.

24 Nagata M, Hidaka M, Sekiya H, *et al.* Effects of pomegranate juice on human cytochrome P450 2C9 and tolbutamide pharmacokinetics in rats. *Drug Metab Dispos* 2007; 35: 302–305.

25 Hidaka M, Okumura M, Fujita K, *et al.* Effects of pomegranate juice on human cytochrome p450 3A (CYP3A) and carbamazepine pharmacokinetics in rats. *Drug Metab Dispos* 2005; 33: 644–648.

26 Komperda KE. Potential interaction between pomegranate juice and warfarin. *Pharmacotherapy* 2009; 29: 1002–1006.

Potassium

Description

Potassium is an essential mineral.

Human requirements

See Table 1 for Dietary Reference Values for potassium.

Dietary intake

In the UK, the average adult diet provides: for men, 3279 mg daily; for women, 2562 mg.

Action

Potassium is the principal intracellular cation, and is fundamental to the regulation of acid–base and water balance. It contributes to transmission of nerve impulses, control of skeletal muscle contractility and maintenance of blood pressure.

Dietary sources

See Table 2 for dietary sources of potassium.

Metabolism

Absorption

Absorption occurs principally in the small intestine.

Table 1 Dietary Reference Values for potassium (mg/day)

Age	UK		US minimum requirement[1]
	LRNI	RNI	EU RDA = none
0–3 months	400	800	500
4–6 months	400	850	500
7–9 months	400	700	700
10–12 months	450	700	700
1–3 years	450	800	1000
4–6 years	600	1100	1400
7–10 years	950	2200	1600
11–14 years	1600	3100	2000
15–50+ years	2000	3500	2000
Pregnancy	*	*	*
Lactation	*	*	*

*No increment.
[1]Desirable intakes may exceed these values.
LRNI = Lowest Reference Nutrient Intake.
RNI = Reference Nutrient Intake.
Note: No EAR has been derived for potassium.

Table 2 Dietary sources of potassium

Food portion	Potassium content (mg)	Food portion	Potassium content (mg)
Breakfast cereals		*Vegetables*	
1 bowl All-Bran (45 g)	450	Green vegetables, average, boiled (100 g)	100–200
1 bowl Bran Flakes (45 g)	250		
1 bowl Corn Flakes (30 g)	30	Potatoes, boiled (150 g)	450
1 bowl muesli (95 g)	500	baked (150 g)	950
		1 small can baked beans (200 g)	600
2 pieces Shredded Wheat	150		
2 Weetabix	150	Lentils, kidney beans or other pulses, cooked (105 g)	300
		Soya beans, cooked (100 g)	500
Cereal products		*Mixed vegetable curry (300 g)*	1250
Bread, brown, 2 slices	100	*Fruit*	
white, 2 slices	70	1 apple	100
wholemeal, 2 slices	160	8 *dried apricots*	600
1 chapati	110	1 banana	350
Pasta, brown, boiled (150 g)	200	$^1/_2$ *cantaloupe melon*	750
white, boiled (150 g)	40	10 dates	300
Rice, brown, boiled (165 g)	150	4 *figs*	600
white, boiled (165 g)	80	1 orange	300
Milk and dairy products		1 handful raisins	350
Milk, whole, semi-skimmed or skimmed (284 ml; $^1/_2$ pint)	400	*Nuts*	
		20 almonds	150
1 pot yoghurt (150 g)	370	10 Brazil nuts	200
Cheese (50 g)	50	30 hazelnuts	250
1 egg, size 2 (60 g)	50	30 peanuts	200
Meat and fish		*Beverages*	
Meat, cooked (100 g)	200–300	1 mug hot chocolate	350
Liver, lambs, cooked (90 g)	300	1 mug *Build-Up*	700
Kidney, lambs, cooked (75 g)	250	1 mug *Complan (sweet)*	600
White fish, cooked (150 g)	400–500	1 mug *Horlicks*	600
Herring or mackerel (110 g)	460	1 large glass grapefruit juice	200
Pilchards, canned (105 g)	450	1 large glass orange juice	300
Sardines, canned (70 g)	300	1 large glass tomato juice	460

Good sources (*italics*).

Elimination

Excretion is mainly via the urine (the capacity of the kidneys to conserve potassium is poor); unabsorbed and intestinally-secreted potassium is eliminated in the faeces; some is lost in saliva and sweat.

Deficiency

Potassium deficiency leads to hypokalaemia, symptoms of which include anorexia, nausea, abdominal distension, paralytic ileus; muscle weakness, reduced or absent reflexes, paralysis; listlessness, apprehension, drowsiness, irrational behaviour; respiratory failure; polydypsia, polyuria; and cardiac arrhythmias.

Possible uses

Hypertension

Potassium may lower blood pressure,[1,2] but there is evidence for a stronger relationship of the sodium/potassium ratio to blood pressure than potassium alone.[3,4] However, a case–cohort analysis of the Rotterdam study showed no consistent association of urinary sodium, potassium or sodium/potassium ratio with cardiovascular disease (CVD) and all-cause mortality over the range of intakes observed in this population. Dietary potassium estimated by a food frequency questionnaire, however, was associated with a lower risk of all-cause mortality in subjects initially free of CVD and hypertension. A significant positive association between urinary sodium/potassium ratio and all-cause mortality was observed but only in overweight subjects who were initially free of CVD and hypertension.[5]

Several other minerals (see Calcium and Magnesium) may affect blood pressure, and dietary measures to reduce blood pressure might be more effective if the intake of several minerals is changed simultaneously.

There is some evidence from double-blind, placebo-controlled trials that potassium supplementation (1500–3000 mg daily) can lower blood pressure in normotensive[6–8] and hypertensive[8,9] individuals, but two other trials have failed to show any benefit.[10,11]

Precautions/contraindications

Excessive doses are best avoided in patients with chronic renal failure (particularly in the elderly), gastrointestinal obstruction or ulceration, peptic ulcer, Addison's disease, heart block, severe burns or acute dehydration.

Pregnancy and breast-feeding

No data are available on potassium supplements in pregnancy. They should be avoided.

Adverse effects

Nausea, vomiting, diarrhoea and abdominal cramps may occur, particularly if potassium is taken on an empty stomach. Modified-release preparations may cause gastrointestinal ulceration. Hyperkalaemia is almost unknown with oral administration provided renal function is normal. Intakes exceeding 17 g daily (unlikely from oral supplements) would be required to cause toxicity.

Interactions

Drugs

Angiotensin-converting enzyme inhibitors: increased risk of hyperkalaemia.
Carbenoxolone: reduced serum potassium levels.
Corticosteroids: increased excretion of potassium.
Cyclosporin: increased risk of hyperkalaemia.
Laxatives: chronic use reduces absorption of potassium.
Loop diuretics: increased risk of hypokalaemia (but potassium supplements seldom necessary with small dose of diuretic).
Non-steroidal inflammatory drugs: increased risk of hyperkalaemia.
Potassium-sparing diuretics: increased risk of hyperkalaemia.
Thiazide diuretics: increased risk of hypokalaemia (but potassium supplements seldom necessary with small dose of diuretic).

Dose

Mild deficiency, oral, 1500–4000 mg daily, with plenty of fluid (liquid preparations should be diluted well).

As a dietary supplement, no dose has been established.

References

1 Khaw KT, Thom S. Randomized double-blind crossover trial of potassium on blood pressure in normal subjects. *Lancet* 1982; 2: 1127–1129.
2 Cappuccio FP, MacGregor DA. Does potassium supplementation lower blood pressure? A meta-analysis of published trials *J Hypertension* 1991; 9: 465–473.
3 Grobbee DE, Hofman A, Roelandt JT, *et al.* Sodium restriction and potassium supplementation in young people with mildly elevated blood pressure. *J Hypertension* 1987; 5: 115–119.
4 Geleijnse JM, Kok FJ, Grobbee DE. Blood pressure response to changes in sodium and potassium intake: a metaregression analysis of randomised trials. *J Hum Hypertens* 2003; 17(7): 471–480.
5 Geleijnse JM, Witteman JC, Stijnen T, *et al.* Sodium and potassium intake and risk of cardiovascular events and all-cause mortality: the Rotterdam Study. *Eur J Epidemiol* 2007; 22(11): 763–770.
6 Brancati FL, Appel LJ, Seidler AJ, *et al.* Effect of potassium supplementation on blood pressure in African Americans on a low-potassium diet. A

randomized, double-blind, placebo-controlled trial. *Arch Intern Med* 1996; 156(1): 61–67.

7 Sacks FM, Willett WC, Smith A, *et al.* Effect on blood pressure of potassium, calcium, and magnesium in women with low habitual intake. *Hypertension* 1998; 31(1): 131–138.

8 Braschi A, Naismith DJ. The effect of a dietary supplement of potassium chloride or potassium citrate on blood pressure in predominantly normotensive volunteers. *Br J Nutr* 2008; 99(6): 1284–1292.

9 Fotherby MD, Potter JF. Potassium supplementation reduces clinic and ambulatory blood pressure

in elderly hypertensive patients. *J Hypertension* 1992; 10: 1403–1408.

10 Sacks FM, Willett WC, Smith A, *et al.* Effect on blood pressure of potassium, calcium and magnesium in women with low habitual intake. *Hypertension* 1995; 26: 950–956.

11 Berry SE, Mulla UZ, Chowienczyk PJ, *et al.* Increased potassium intake from fruit and vegetables or supplements does not lower blood pressure or improve vascular function in UK men and women with early hypertension: a randomised controlled trial. *Br J Nutr* 2010; 104(12): 1839–1847.

Probiotics and prebiotics

Description

A probiotic is a live microbial food supplement that beneficially affects the host animal by improving its intestinal microbial balance.[1,2] For human adult use, this includes fermented milk products and over-the-counter products, such as powders, tablets and capsules that contain lyophilised bacteria. The micro-organisms involved are usually producers of lactic acid, such as lactobacilli and bifidobacteria, which are widely used in yoghurt and dairy products. However, yeasts have also been used (Table 1).[3,4] These microbes are non-pathogenic and survive passage through the stomach and small bowel.

A prebiotic is a non-digestible food ingredient, which beneficially affects the host by selectively stimulating the growth, activity, or both, of one or a limited number of bacterial species already resident in the colon.[5] Prebiotics are not digested by intestinal enzymes, instead passing through the upper gastrointestinal tract to the colon where they are selectively used as fuel by beneficial bacteria.

Although any food residue entering the colon is a potential prebiotic candidate, it is the influence of the food residue on certain specific microbes that is important. Lactulose was used more than 40 years ago as a prebiotic infant formula food supplement to increase numbers of lactobacilli in the infant intestine,[6] but the specificity of this substrate for enhancing these micro-organisms has not been effectively proven

scientifically. In humans, consumption of fructo-oligosaccharides increases the proportion of bifidobacteria in faeces.[7] Similar effects have been observed in rats fed with galacto-oligosaccharides and colonised with human faecal flora.[8]

Possible uses

The possible benefits to health of probiotics and prebiotics are to:

- prevent and treat diarrhoea, including acute diarrhoea, travellers' diarrhoea and antibiotic-associated diarrhoea);
- alleviate lactose intolerance;
- treat inflammatory bowel conditions (e.g. irritable bowel syndrome (IBS), ulcerative colitis and Crohn's disease);
- contribute to the management of *Helicobacter pylori* infection and the side-effects of therapy;
- enhance the immune system;
- treat allergic conditions, such as atopic ezcema;
- prevent and treat vaginal infections;
- lower serum cholesterol; and
- prevent cancer and tumour growth.

Acute diarrhoea

There is a relatively large volume of literature supporting the use of probiotics in diarrhoeal conditions, but it is only recently that the scientific

Table 1 Examples of commonly used probiotics and prebiotics[45]

Probiotics	Prebiotics
Lactobacilli	Fructo-oligosaccharides
Lactobacillus	Galacto-
acidophilus	oligosaccharides
L. casei	Inulin
L. delbrueckii subsp.	Lactulose
bulgaricus	Lactitol
L. reuteri	
L. brevis	
L. cellobiosus	
L. curvatus	
L. fermentium	
L.plantarum	
L. gasseri	
L. rhamnosus	
Gram-positive cocci	
Lactococcus lactis subsp.	
cremoris	
Streptococcus salivarius	
subsp. thermophilus	
Enterococcus faecium	
Streptococcus	
diacetylactis	
Streptococcus	
intermedius	
Bifidobacteria	
Bifidobacterium bifidum	
B. adolescentis	
B. animalis	
B. infantis	
B. longum	
B. thermophilum	
Yeasts	
Saccharomyces	
boulardii	
Saccharomyces	
cerevisiae	

basis for this has started to become established, with the publication of a number of respectable clinical studies. Probiotics have been examined for their effectiveness in the prevention and treatment of several types of diarrhoea, including antibiotic-associated diarrhoea, bacterial and viral diarrhoea (including travellers' diarrhoea), as well as that caused by lactose intolerance. The effects of probiotics, particularly with some bacterial strains and in some types of diarrhoea, appear promising, but the effects of prebiotics on diarrhoea are currently unknown.

Various mechanisms by which probiotics could be of benefit in diarrhoea have been proposed and summarised in two reviews.[9,10] These include reduction in gastrointestinal pH through stimulation of lactic acid-producing bacteria; a direct antagonistic action on gastrointestinal pathogens; competition with pathogens for binding and receptor sites; improved immune function and competition for limited nutrients.

A detailed review in the mid-1990s[11] of all placebo-controlled human studies supplementing *Lactobacillus acidophilus*, *Bifidobacterium longum*, *L. casei* GG and other selected microorganisms from 1966 to 1995 concluded that: 'these studies have shown that biotherapeutic agents have been used successfully to prevent antibiotic-associated diarrhoea, to prevent acute infantile diarrhoea, to treat recurrent *Clostridium difficile* disease, and to treat various other diarrhoeal illnesses'. The authors also noted that many of the studies included small numbers of subjects.

A more recent systematic review concluded that available evidence does not support the administration of probiotics with antibiotics to prevent the development of *C. difficile* disease and is inadequate to justify its introduction as a treatment for *C. difficile* antibiotic-associated disease (at the McGill University Health Centre, where the study was conducted).[12] A meta-analysis of six RCTs found that the probiotic, *Saccharomyces boulardii*, significantly reduced the risk of *C. difficile* disease, but was the only probiotic that was effective.[13]

Evidence for a beneficial effect of probiotics in diarrhoea appears to be strongest for that caused by rotavirus. Rotavirus infection causes gastroenteritis, which is characterised by acute diarrhoea and vomiting. Gastroenteritis is a leading cause of morbidity and mortality among children worldwide. A review of studies that used *Lactobacillus*, *Bifidobacterium* and *Enterococcus* concluded that *Lactobacillus* GG (a *Lactobacillus* strain isolated from human intestine) consistently shortened the diarrhoeal phase of rotavirus by 1 day,[14] but that evidence was less strong for a role of *Lactobacillus* GG and other probiotics in the prevention of diarrhoea due to bacterial or other viral infections.

A systematic review of 10 RCTs (treatment) and three RCTs (prevention) concluded that probiotics significantly reduced the duration of acute infectious diarrhoea in infants and children, especially diarrhoea caused by rotavirus. No conclusions could be reached about the use of probiotics in the prevention of diarrhoea, because of clinical and statistical heterogeneity among the studies.[15] A meta-analysis of 18 RCTs confirmed the efficacy of probiotic supplements in reducing duration of symptoms among children up to 5 years of age with acute, non-bacterial diarrhoea. Probiotics, particularly lactobacilli, reduced the duration of an acute diarrhoeal episode in an infant or child by approximately 1 day.[16] A further meta-analysis involving nine trials that had used *Lactobacillus* in children with acute infectious diarrhoea found a reduction in diarrhoea duration of 0.7 days and a reduction in diarrhoea frequency of 1.6 stools on day 2 of treatment in participants receiving lactobacilli.[17]

The role of probiotic bacteria in the prevention and treatment of paediatric diarrhoea is increasingly well established, but their role in adults has been less well investigated. However, an RCT involving 541 young men found a non-significant trend for reduction in the incidence of diarrhoea with yoghurt containing *L. casei* compared with placebo.[18]

A Cochrane review involving 23 studies found that probiotics reduced the risk of diarrhoea (in adults and children) at 3 days (relative risk (RR), 0.66; 95% confidence interval (CI), 0.55 to 0.77; 15 studies) and the mean duration of diarrhoea by 30.48 h (95% CI, 18.51 to 42.46; 12 studies). The authors concluded that probiotics appear to be a useful adjunct to rehydration therapy in treating acute infectious diarrhoea in adults and children, and that more research is needed to identify the use of particular probiotic regimens in specific patient groups.[19] Two further meta-analyses have added further weight to the evidence that probiotics reduce the duration and severity of acute diarrhoea.[20,21]

Further trials have continued to show encouraging results. *L. rhamnosus* 19070-2 and *L. reuteri* DSM 12246 ameliorated acute diarrhoea in hospitalised children[22] and in children from daycare centres[23] and reduced the period of rotavirus excretion. The beneficial effects were most prominent in children treated early in the diarrhoeal phase. *B. lactis* strain Bb12[24] or *B. breve* C50

with *S. thermophilus* 065[25] or *L. reuteri* with *B. lactis*,[26] added to an infant formula, appear to have some protective effect against acute diarrhoea in healthy children. *S. boulardii* significantly reduced the duration of acute diarrhoea and the duration of hospital stay in children with acute diarrhoea.[27] The feeding of a cereal containing *S. thermophilus*, *B. lactis*, *L. acidophilus* and zinc reduced the severity and duration of acute gastroenteritis in young children, but whether the combination is better than either probiotics or zinc alone is unknown.[28] Administration of *L. rhamnosus* strains shortened the duration of rotaviral diarrhoea in children but not of diarrhoea of any aetiology.[29]

Travellers' diarrhoea

The prevention of travellers' diarrhoea by lactobacilli, bifidobacteria, enterococci and streptococci has been investigated in several studies, but results have been inconsistent. In a double-blind, placebo-controlled trial, 820 Finnish travellers to two holiday resorts in Turkey were randomised to receive either *Lactobacillus* GG or placebo.[30] The overall incidence of diarrhoea was 43.8%. Of the 331 sufferers, 178 (46.5%) were in the placebo group and 153 (41%) were in the *Lactobacillus* group, but the difference was not significant. However, in one of the resorts, the treatment significantly reduced the incidence of diarrhoea from 39.5% (30 out of 76) in the placebo group to 23.9% (17 out of 71) in the treatment group. In another study involving 245 travellers to developing countries, the risk of diarrhoea on any one day in travellers who took *Lactobacillus* GG was 3.9% compared with 7.4% in the control group.[31]

In another study, the incidence of diarrhoea was reduced from 71% to 43% in travellers to Egypt who were given capsules of *S. thermophilus*, *L. bulgaricus*, *L. acidophilus* and *B. bifidum*.[32] However, neither *L. acidophilus* nor *Enterococcus faecium* had any beneficial effects on diarrhoea in groups of Austrian tourists.[33] In addition, no effect of *L. acidophilus* or *L. fermentum* was observed in soldiers who were sent to Belize in Central America.[34] No effect of *L. acidophilus* on the prevention of travellers' diarrhoea was seen in a study where half of the travellers went to West Africa,[35] and it seems that the effect of probiotics on travellers' diarrhoea depends on the bacterial strain used and the destination of the traveller.[14] A meta-analysis concluded that some probiotics (notably *S. boulardii* and a mixture of *L. acidophilus* and *B. bifidum*) had significant efficacy.[36]

Antibiotic-associated diarrhoea

Diarrhoea caused by the growth of pathogenic bacteria is the most common side-effect of antibiotic use, and *in vitro* studies have shown that some bacterial strains can inhibit this growth. *Lactobacillus* GG (in yoghurt) reduced the incidence and duration of diarrhoea in healthy men receiving erythromycin for 7 days,[37] and successfully eradicated *C. difficile* in five patients with relapsing colitis.[38] A meta-analysis of six trials evaluating the efficacy of *Lactobacillus* GG found that four of the trials were associated with a significant reduction in the risk of antibiotic-associated diarrhoea, one of the trials reduced the number of days of antibiotic-associated diarrhoea, while the sixth trial found no benefit with *Lactobacillus* GG.[39] *Lactobacillus* F19 had a limited effect on the emergence of resistant isolates during treatment with penicillin and quinolones.[40] *S. boulardii* has been shown to reduce the risk of antibiotic-associated diarrhoea in children.[41]

Enterococcus SF68 reduced the incidence of diarrhoea caused by antibiotics,[42] whereas studies with *L. acidophilus*[43,44] have provided no conclusive evidence of benefit with this strain in prevention of diarrhoea caused by antibiotics. A daily dose of *B. lactis* and *S. thermophilus* has been shown to prevent antibiotic-associated diarrhoea.[45]

A meta-analysis of nine RCTs suggested that probiotics can be used to prevent antibiotic-associated diarrhoea, and that both *S. boulardii* and lactobacilli have the potential for benefit in this situation. However, the meta-analysis also concluded that the efficacy of probiotics in treating antibiotic-associated diarrhoea remains unproven.[46] Another meta-analysis that included seven RCTs also suggested that probiotic supplements were associated with a significant decrease in the incidence of antibiotic-associated diarrhoea, while concluding that evidence of benefit is not conclusive, partly because of poor study design.[47] A further meta-analysis of five RCTs found that *S. boulardii* is moderately effective in preventing antibiotic-associated diarrhoea in children and adults treated with antibiotics for any reason (mainly respiratory tract infections). In this meta-analysis, for every 10 patients receiving daily *S. boulardii* with antibiotics, one fewer would develop antibiotic-associated diarrhoea.[48] A more recent meta-analysis including 25 RCTs found that probiotics significantly reduced the relative risk of antibiotic-associated diarrhoea (RR, 0.43; 95% CI, 0.31 to 0.58; $P < 0.001$). Three types of probiotic were associated with this benefit: *S. boulardii*, *L. rhamnosus* GG and probiotic mixtures.[13] A further meta-analysis evaluating the use of probiotics for prevention of antibiotic-associated diarrhoea in children concluded that intention to treat analysis showed non-significant effects overall. The per-protocol analysis for 9 out of the 10 included trials reporting on the incidence of diarrhoea showed statistically significant benefit of probiotics over controls. The authors concluded that the data were promising but that further research into probiotic strains, and the effect of age (infant versus older children) and antibiotic duration should be conducted.[49]

A randomised double-blind placebo-controlled trial post-dating these meta-analyses found that consumption of 100 g of a probiotic drink (Actimel) twice a day containing *L. casei*, *L. bulgaricus* and *S. thermophilus* could reduce incidence of antibiotic-associated diarrhoea and *C. difficile* associated diarrhoea when taken during a course of antibiotics and for 1 week after.[50] A trial conducted in Poland among 78 children treated with antibiotics for various infections showed that a food supplement containing *B. longum*, *L. rhamnosus* and *L. plantarum* did not reduce the incidence of diarrhoea but reduced stool frequency.[51] A recent Swedish trial among adults treated with antibiotics demonstrated that *L. plantarum* was able to prevent the milder gastrointestinal symptoms associated with antibiotic treatment.[52]

Lactose intolerance

Lactose intolerance is a problem for a large proportion of the world's population for whom lactose acts like an osmotic non-digestible carbohydrate because they have a low amount of intestinal lactase. During fermentation of yoghurt and acidophilus milk, lactobacilli produce lactase that hydrolyses lactose to glucose and galactose. This pre-digestion of lactose could potentially reduce the symptoms associated with lactose intolerance in susceptible individuals, and probiotics have been shown to improve lactose digestion and intolerance in some studies[53,54] but not others.[55] A systematic review assessing the efficacy of oral probiotics in adults with lactose intolerance found that probiotics did not alleviate the signs and symptoms of this condition, but that specific strains, concentrations and preparations may be effective.[56] Further trials of specific strains and concentrations are necessary to clarify this potentially beneficial effect.

Irritable bowel syndrome

Recent research has investigated the potential benefit of probiotics in irritable bowel syndrome (IBS). A double-blind RCT in 40 patients found that *L. plantarum* 299V was associated with resolution of abdominal pain and a trend towards normalisation of stool frequency in constipated patients.[57] In another study, however, the same probiotic had no apparent benefit in patients with IBS and no influence on colonic fermentation.[58] In a further study, short-term therapy with *L. plantarum* LP01 and *B. breve* BR03 or *L. plantarum* LP01 and *L. acidophilus* LA02 reduced the pain score and severity of characteristic IBS symptoms.[59] *B. infantis* 35624 was associated with a significant reduction in abdominal pain and/or discomfort, bloating and/or distension and bowel movement difficulty. This response was associated with normalisation of the ratio of an anti-inflammatory to a pro-inflammatory cytokine, suggesting an immune-modulating role for this organism in IBS.[60]*Lactobacillus* GG has been associated with a lower incidence of perceived abdominal distension (but no other symptomatic differences)[61] and a probiotic combination (VSL#3) with reduced flatulence and slower colonic transit in patients with IBS and bloating.[62] Live combined *Bifidobacterium, Lactobacillus* and *Enterococcus* capsules administered over 4 weeks improved symptoms of IBS, which may have been related to observed alterations in the gastrointestinal flora.[63] However, *L. reuteri* was not associated with significant improvement in IBS symptoms compared with placebo.[64] Two further controlled trials using probiotic mixtures[65,66] demonstrated reduction in IBS symptoms. Oral administration of

Lactobacillus strains has been shown to induce opioid and cannabinoid receptors in intestinal epithelial cells, mediating analgesia in the gut, suggesting a mechanism whereby probiotics could help to manage the symptoms of IBS.[67]

In a UK study, *B. infantis* in a dose of 1×10^8 cfu was found to be significantly superior to both placebo and other doses of bifidobacteria for abdominal pain, bloating, bowel dysfunction, incomplete evacuation, straining and the passage of gas[68] while a French study among 371 adults employing *B. lactis* in a fermented milk demonstated improved digestive comfort.[69] However, a further French study employing four strains of lactobacilli among 100 patients with IBS found that the probiotic combination was not significantly superior to placebo in relieving symptoms of IBS.[70]

The large number of trials conducted with probiotics in IBS has allowed for meta-analysis and systematic review. Recent reviews have concluded that probiotics reduce some symptoms of IBS, but the magnitude of benefit and the most effective species and strain are uncertain.[71–75]

Ulcerative colitis

The evidence base for probiotics in ulcerative colitis is broader than that for Crohn's disease and generally more encouraging. Placebo-controlled RCTs showed significant clinical improvement,[76–78] while other studies reported that probiotics (or prebiotics) were at least as effective as conventional treatment in reducing symptoms, obtaining remission and preventing relapse.[79–84] When given as adjunct to conventional drug treatment, various probiotics including VSL 3,[85,86] *S. boulardii*,[87] bifidobacteria,[77,83,88] and lactobacilli[89,90] have significantly improved inflammation, prevented relapse or prolonged relapse-free time.

Pouchitis

Ileoanal pouchitis is the inflammation of an internal pouch created surgically for the storage of stool in patients who have had part of their colon removed to treat ulcerative colitis or familial adenomatous polyposis. Pouchitis can cause symptoms similar to ulcerative colitis, such as diarrhoea, crampy abdominal pain, increased frequency of stool, bleeding, fever, dehydration and joint pain. About one-third of patients with an ileoanal pouch have had at least one episode of pouchitis and the likelihood increases with the length of time since the pouch was created.

Several trials have evaluated probiotics in the management of pouchitis. A nine-month trial of VSL#3 in 40 patients with chronic relapsing pouchitis in remission showed a significantly lower rate of relapse (3/20 patients) compared with placebo (20/20 patients).[91] A trial in 40 patients randomised for 1 year after creation of an ileal pouch for ulcerative colitis found that 2 out of 20 patients taking VSL#3 had an episode of acute pouchitis compared with 8 out of 20 taking placebo. Mean stool frequency was also significantly lower in the VSL#3 group and improvements in quality of life scores were observed in the VSL#3 group but not the placebo group.[92] A trial in 36 patients with recurrent pouchitis (in whom remission was induced by combined metronidazole and ciprofloxacin) found that remission was maintained at 1 year in 17 out of 20 patients on VSL#3, but in only one patient on VSL#3.[93] Three controlled trials with a fermented milk product (Cultura) containing live lactobacilli and bifidobacteria have found beneficial effects on symptoms and inflammation but no changes in histology.[78,94,95] A 3 year Dutch RCT among 117 patients with surgical creation of a pouch showed *L. rhamnosus* reduced the frequency of first episodes of pouchitis.[96]

Crohn's disease

Human trial evidence for probiotics in Crohn's disease is generally not positive so far. Among five controlled trials to date,[97–101] only one has shown potentially positive effects of *S. boulardii* in the maintenance treatment of Crohn's disease.[97] A meta-analysis of eight RCTs failed to demonstrate the efficacy of probiotics in maintaining remission and preventing clinical and endoscopic recurrence in Crohn's disease.[102]

Helicobacter pylori infection

Probiotics are being investigated for potential benefit in reducing *H. pylori* colonisation and also in reducing the side-effects associated with *H. pylori* treatment. Ingestion of a product containing *Lactobacillus* La1,[103,104] *L. johnsonii*[105] and yoghurt containing *Lactobacillus* and *Bifidobacterium*,[106,107] inhibited *H. pylori*

colonisation. Supplementation with *L. casei*[108] and *S. boulardii*[109] conferred an enhanced therapeutic benefit on *H. pylori* eradication in subjects on triple therapy. In a further study evaluating *S. boulardii*, the effectiveness of this probiotic appeared to lie in its ability to reduce side effects of triple therapy and hence improve compliance.[110] A 4-week pretreatment with a yoghurt containing *Lactobacillus* and *Bifidobacterium* reduced *H. pylori* load, improving eradication rate with quadruple therapy after triple therapy had failed.[111] A 3-week RCT in 14 *H. pylori*-infected patients showed that the probiotic product Yakult slowed growth of the bacterium.[112] A yogurt containing lactobacilli, *B. longum* and *S. thermophilus* successfully helped to reduce eradication rates alongside triple therapy but not the incidence of side-effects.[113] No improvement in eradication rates was observed in a 14-day RCT with *Bifidobacterium* DN-173[114]

B. clausii reduced the incidence of the most common side effects related to *H. pylori* antibiotic therapy.[115] *L. casei* supplementation has also been shown to reduce the side-effects of 10-day quadruple therapy and result in a slight improvement in eradicating *H. pylori*.[116] *Lactobacillus* GG has been shown to have a beneficial impact on *H. pylori* related side-effects,[117] while in another study a range of probiotics (*Lactobacillus* GG, *S. boulardii*, a combination of *Lactobacillus* spp. and bifidobacteria) were found to be superior to placebo for side-effect prevention.[118] A further study also showed that a probiotic supplement improved tolerance to the eradication regimen.[119]

Two systematic reviews have concluded that intake of lactobacilli or lactobacilli combined with bifidobacteria may increase eradication rates of *H. pylori* colonisation and/or reduce some side-effects associated with conventional therapy.[120,121]

Immunity

The colonic microflora affects systemic and mucosal immunity in the host. Probiotics are claimed to stimulate the immune system and preliminary evidence suggests that these substances could increase the immune response.[122–126] An RCT involving 136 university students under examination stress (which has been associated with a suppressed immune response) were given milk fermented with yoghurt cultures plus *L. casei* or a placebo of semi-skimmed milk for 3 weeks prior to and during the 3-week examination period. The fermented milk modulated the number of lymphocytes and CD56 cells, indicating an effect on the immune system.[127] In another human trial, a fermented product containing two probiotic strains (*L. gasser* CECT 5714, *L. coryniformis* CECT 5711) increased the proportion of phagocytic cells (monocytes and neutrophils) as well as their phagocytic activity, and increased the proportion of natural killer cells and IgA concentrations. The fermented product enhanced immunity to a greater extent than a standard yoghurt.[128] *L. casei* has been associated with positive effects on immune competence in middle-aged people.[129,130] Oral *L. rhamnosus GG* has been shown in infants to enhance generation of interleukin-10 and hence anti-inflammatory status.[131]

Allergic conditions

Recent research interest has focused on the potential role of probiotics in various conditions known to have an allergic component. There is evidence that *Lactobacillus* GG[123,132–135] and *Bifidobacterium* Bb-12[136] could improve symptoms in infants with atopic eczema. A combination of *L. rhamnosus* 19070–2 and *L. reuteri* DSM 122460,[137] *L. rhamnosus* and *B. lactis*,[138] *B. bifidium, B. lactis* and *L. acidophilus*,[139] and supplementation with the probiotic *L. fermentum* VRI-033 PCC[140] have also been found to be effective in the management of atopic dermatitis or in reducing the risk of its development. The benefits associated with *Lactobacillus* GG in atopic eczema and/or dermatitis have been observed to a greater extent in infants who are sensitised to immunoglobulin-E (IgE) than those who are non-IgE-sensitised.[141–143] Impairment of the intestinal mucosal barrier appears to be involved in the pathogenesis of atopic dermatitis and there is evidence that probiotic supplementation can stabilise the intestinal barrier function.[144] However, a more recent trial with *L. rhamnosus* found no clinical effect on atopic dermatitis.[145]

Clinical studies also suggest that probiotics could be effective in the primary prevention of atopic disease. In infants at high risk of atopic disease, administration of probiotics to their mothers prenatally[139,142,146–148] and during breast-feeding[149] has been shown to prevent atopic disease, particularly eczema.

Three meta-analyses have come to somewhat different conclusions about the effect of probiotics in atopic eczema, with two[150,151] suggesting that symptoms can be improved in some cases, particularly in those with moderate to severe disease,[151] although findings are inconsistent;[150] the third concluded that probiotic administration did not reduce the severity of eczema.[152]

There is also preliminary evidence that fermented milk containing *L. paracasei* LP-33 can improve the quality of life of patients with allergic rhinitis and may serve as an alternative treatment.[153,154] In a further preliminary trial, *L. gasseri* was shown to improve symptoms of asthma and allergic rihinitis in schoolchildren.[155]

Vaginal infections

One of the claims frequently made for probiotics, specifically for *L. acidophilus*, is that they can prevent vaginal infections. The conclusions of a review were that there was evidence (albeit limited) for *L. acidophilus* in the prevention of candidal vaginitis.[156]

In a double-blind, controlled, crossover trial of 46 women with a history of vaginal infections, participants were randomised to receive either *L. acidophilus* yoghurt (150 mL daily) containing live organisms or pasteurised yoghurt (150 mL daily) for 2 months each with a 2-month washout period between interventions.[157] However, only seven subjects completed the whole study, and the reason for the high dropout rate was not explained. The yoghurt containing live organisms was associated with a significant reduction in episodes of bacterial vaginosis. Both yoghurts were associated with a decrease in candidal vaginitis, but there was no significant difference between the treatments.[157]

A more recent RCT investigated the effect of *Lactobacillus* preparations taken orally or vaginally, or both, on vulvovaginitis following antibiotic treatment for a non-gynaecological infection. The study involved 235 Australian women aged 18–50 years. Overall 55/235 women developed post-antibiotic vulvovaginitis, but neither oral nor vaginal *Lactobacillus* treatment influenced the incidence of this condition compared with placebo.[158]

Two more recent trials have demonstrated positive results of probiotics in bacterial vaginosis. The first involved 49 women who were treated with metronidazole for 7 days or the same schedule, then a once-weekly vaginal application of 40 mg of *L. rhamnosus* for 6 months. During the first 6 months of follow-up, a constant percentage (96%) of patients in the probiotic group had a balanced vaginal ecosystem. Follow-up over 12 months showed no statistically significant difference among vaginal ecosystems in patients in the probiotic group, whereas in the other group there was a significant increase in the number of women with abnormal flora over time ($P = 0.01$).[159] In the second trial, which involved 40 women with bacterial vaginosis, administration of vaginal tablets containing *L. rhamnosus* for a period of 24 months was found to be effective and safe both for restoring the physiological vaginal pH and controlling symptoms of bacterial vaginosis.[160]

Cardiovascular disease

Probiotics have been evaluated for a potential effect on serum cholesterol and other cardiovascular risk factors. The influence of probiotics on serum cholesterol levels is the subject of controversy. Studies in the 1970s and 1980s frequently reported significant reductions in serum cholesterol with daily consumption of fermented milk, but these studies have been criticised on methodological grounds, including the fact that in most of the studies showing positive results, large volumes of yoghurt (0.5–8.4 L) were consumed.[161] Two controlled trials have shown that yoghurt (200 mL daily) containing live cultures of *L. acidophilus*[162] or yoghurt (375 mL daily) fermented with *L. acidophilus* with added fructo-oligosaccharides[163] (prebiotic) reduced serum cholesterol by 2.9% and 4.4%, respectively. Another study indicated that inulin (a prebiotic) may also lower cholesterol.[164] A further study found that the probiotic *B. longum* resulted in a significant reduction in serum total cholesterol in subjects with moderate hypercholesterolaemia,[165] while a yoghurt enriched with *L. acidophilus* and *B. longum*, and oligofructose (a synbiotic) increased serum HDL cholesterol and led to an improvement in the LDL cholesterol/HDL cholesterol ratio.[166]

However, a trial in postmenopausal women found that probiotic capsules containing bacteria *L. acidophilus* and *B. longum* had no effect on cholesterol either independently or in addition to soya.[167] A further trial in 80 volunteers with raised cholesterol found no effect of capsules containing freeze-dried *L. acidophilus* for 6 weeks on serum lipids.[168]

Probiotics have also been associated with a reduction in blood pressure[169,170] and other cardiovascular risk factors (e.g. fibrinogen, monocyte adhesion and pro-inflammatory markers).[169]

Osteoporosis

There is some evidence that prebiotics (inulin and oligofructose) can improve calcium absorption,[171–173] and this effect could enhance bone mineral density with a consequent reduction in the risk of osteoporosis. However, there are no human studies with prebiotics assessing the risk of osteoporosis.

Respiratory tract infections

Regular intake of probiotics may reduce nasal colonisation with pathogenic bacteria.[174] There is also evidence that intake of probiotic bacteria over at least 3 months shortens common cold episodes.[175] Probiotic therapy may reduce respiratory infections in infants,[176] and in elderly adults, the incidence of influenza[177] and the risk of catching a cold.[178]

Miscellaneous

Probiotics are being evaluated in a number of other conditions, including constipation,[179,180] necrotising enterocolitis in preterm infants,[181] infantile colic,[182] pulmonary exacerbations in cystic fibrosis,[183] intensive care patients,[184,185] oral thrush,[186] acute otitis media,[187] stress-induced gastrointestinal symptoms,[188] prevention of colorectal cancer,[189] rheumatoid arthritis and other disorders of the immune system. Probiotics may also reduce the number of *Escherichia coli* colonies in the faeces, which could help to prevent urinary tract infections.[190] Results from research are promising but await confirmation from controlled clinical trials.

Summary of uses

Table 2 summarises the studies and systematic reviews evaluating probiotics for the uses outlined above.

Table 2 Clinical trials and systematic reviews evaluating the effect of probiotics on gastrointestinal disease and eczema

Reference	Duration and type of trial	Type of probiotic	Study group	Outcome measures	Observed effects
Acute diarrhoea					
Szajewska & Mrukowicz (2001)[15]	Systematic review	Various	RCTs in infants and children	Treatment and prevention of acute infectious diarrhoea in infants and children	Probiotics significantly reduced the duration of acute infectious diarrhoea
Rosenfeldt et al. (2002)[22]	5-day randomised controlled trial (Denmark)	Lactobacillus rhamnosus 19070-2 and Lactobacillus reuteri DSM12246 10[10] cfu of each strain or placebo twice daily	Hospitalised children with diarrhoea	Acute diarrhoea	Probiotics reduced acute diarrhoea, reduced hospital stay and period of rotavirus excretion
Rosenfeldt et al. (2002)[23]	5-day randomised controlled trial (Denmark)	L. rhamnosus 19070-2 and L. reuteri DSM 12246 10[10] cfu of each strain or placebo twice daily	Children in day centres with diarrhoea	Acute diarrhoea	Probiotics reduced the duration of diarrhoea
Huang et al. (2002)[16]	Meta-analysis	Probiotics with rehydration therapy	18 trials (in children)	Duration of diarrhoea	Probiotics reduced duration of acute diarrhoea by 1 day
Van Niel et al. (2002)[17]	Meta-analysis	Various Lactobacillus	9 RCTs in children	Outcomes in acute infectious diarrhoea	Reduction in diarrhoea and diarrhoea frequency
Allen et al. (2004)[19]	Meta-analysis	Probiotics with rehydration therapy	23 studies (1917 participants)	Severity and duration of acute infectious diarrhoea	Probiotics reduced the risk of diarrhoea and duration of diarrhoea by 30 h
Salazar-Lindo et al. (2004)[195]	120 hour randomised controlled trial (Peru)	A milk formula containing 1 × 10[9] cfu/mL of Lactobacillus casei strain GG	179 male infants with acute watery diarrhoea (3–36 months)	Acute diarrhoea	No positive benefit of Lactobacillus GG on watery diarrhoea
Thibault et al. (2004)[25]	5-month randomised controlled trial	Fermented infant formula (fermentation with Bifidobacterium breve C50 and Streptococcus thermophilus O65) or a standard infant formula of the same nutritional composition	971 infants (4–6 months)	Acute diarrhoea	Reduced severity of acute diarrhoea with fermented milk formula
Chouraqui et al. (2004)[24]	Randomised controlled trial (France)	A milk formula supplemented with viable Bifidobacterium lactis strain Bb 12	99 infants (<8 months)	Prevention of acute diarrhoea	Reduced risk of diarrhoea; insignificant trend for shorter episodes of diarrhoea

Study	Design	Intervention	Subjects	Indication	Findings
Kurugol & Koturoglu (2005)[27]	5 day randomised controlled trial (Turkey)	S. boulardii (250 mg daily)	200 children with diarrhoea	Acute diarrhoea	Probiotic reduced duration of acute diarrhoea and hospital stay
Dendukuri et al. (2005)[12]	Systematic review	Varied	4 trials	Prevention and treatment of CDAD	Insufficient evidence for the routine clinical use of probiotics to prevent or treat CDAD
Pereg et al. (2005)[18]	Randomised controlled trial (Israel)	Yoghurt with L. casei	541 young male military recruits	Prevention of acute diarrhoea	A non-significant trend for reduction of the incidence of diarrhoea
Weizman et al. (2005)[26]	12-week randomised controlled trial (Israel)	Formula supplemented with B. lactis (BB-12), L. reuteri (ATCC 55730), or no probiotics	201 infants (4–10 months)	Prevention of diarrhoea and other infections	Fewer and shorter episodes of diarrhoea
Shamir et al. (2005)[28]	Double-blind, prospective study	Daily 6×10^9 cfu S. thermophilus, 2×10^9 cfu B. lactis, 2×10^9 cfu Lactobacillus acidophilus + 10 mg zinc + 0.3 g fructo-oligosaccharides or placebo	65 infants (6–12 months)	Acute gastroenteritis	Reduction in severity and duration of acute gastroenteritis
Billoo et al. (2006)[196]	5-day randomised controlled trial with 2 month follow-up (Pakistan)	S. boulardii (250 mg twice a day)	100 children	Acute diarrhoea	S. boulardii significantly reduced frequency and duration of acute diarrhoea
Szymanski et al. (2006)[29]	5-day randomised controlled trial (Poland)	Lakcid L at a dose 1.2×10^{10} cfu or placebo, twice daily	87 children (2 months-6 years)	Duration of diarrhoea	Reduced duration of rotavirus diarrhoea
Sazawal et al. (2006)[197]	Meta-analysis	Various	34 trials	Acute diarrhoea	Some evidence of effect, but dependent on the age of the host and genera of strain used
McFarland et al. (2006)[13]	Systematic review	Various	6 randomised controlled trials	CDAD	S. boulardii was effective
Allen at al (2010)[20]	Meta-analysis	Various	63 studies (8014 participants)	Acute infectious diarrhoea	Probiotics shorten duration and stool frequency in acute infectious diarrhoea
Bernaola Aponte et al. (2010)[21]	Meta-analysis	Various	4 trials (464 subjects)	Persistent diarrhoea	Probiotics reduced duration of persistent diarrhoea

(continued)

Table 2 (continued)

Reference	Duration and type of trial	Type of probiotic	Study group	Outcome measures	Observed effects
Travellers' diarrhoea					
Oksanen et al. (1990)[30]	Randomised controlled trial	Lactobacillus GG	820 adults on holiday in Turkey	TD	Lactobacillus GG reduced TD
Briand et al. (2006)[35]	Randomised controlled trial	L. acidophilus	174 travellers (West Africa)	TD	No benefit of L. acidophilus
McFarland et al. (2007)[36]	Meta-analysis	Various	12 randomised controlled trials	TD	Several probiotics (S. boulardii and a mixture of L. acidophilus and Bifidobacteria lactis) had significant efficacy
Antibiotic associated diarrhoea					
Wunderlich et al. (1989)[42]	Double-blind placebo-controlled trial (Switzerland)	One capsule twice daily of either Enterococcus SF68 or placebo	123 patients	AAD	Probiotic effective in reducing AAD
Siitonen et al. (1990)[37]	1 week randomised controlled trial (Finland)	125 mL of either Lactobacillus GG fermented yoghurt or pasteurised regular yoghurt	16 volunteers taking erythromycin 400 mg three times a day	AAD	Reduced diarrhoea with probiotics
D'Souza et al. (2002)[46]	Meta-analysis	Various	9 randomised controlled trials	AAD	S. boulardii and lactobacilli have potential to prevent AAD
Correa et al. (2005)[45]	15-day randomised controlled trial (Brazil)	Commercial formula containing 10 viable cells of B. lactis and 10 viable cells of S. thermophilus at the initiation of antibiotics	80 infants (6–36 months)	AAD	Reduction in AAD with probiotic
Kotowska et al. (2005)[41]	Randomised controlled trial (Poland)	S. boulardii (250 mg twice daily for duration of antibiotic treatment)	?>269 children with otitis media and/or respiratory tract infections (6 months to 14 years)	AAD	S. boulardii effectively reduces the risk of AAD in children
Hawrelak et al. (2005)[39]	Meta-analysis	Various	6 trials	AAD	4/6 trials found a significant reduction in the risk of AAD with co-administration of Lactobacillus GG; 1 trial found a reduced number of days with AAD with Lactobacillus GG administration, while the sixth trial found no benefit of Lactobacillus GG supplementation

Reference	Study type	Intervention	Participants	Condition	Findings
Cremonini et al. (2005)[47]	Meta-analysis	Various	7 studies	AAD	Strong preventive effect of probiotics
Szajewska & Mrukowicz (2005)[48]	Meta-analysis	S. boulardii	5 randomised controlled trials (1076 participants)	AAD	S. boulardii is moderately effective in preventing AAD in children and adults
Johnston et al. (2006)[198]	Meta-analysis	Various	6 randomised controlled trials (707 patients)	AAD	Lactobacillus GG, Lactobacillus sporogens or S. boulardii showed strong evidence for the preventative effects of probiotics for AAD
Szajewska et al. (2006)[199]	Meta-analysis	Various	6 randomised controlled trials	AAD	Reduced AAD in children with probiotics
McFarland et al. (2006)[13]	Systematic review	Various	25 randomised controlled trials	AAD	Three types of probiotics (S. boulardii, L. rhamnosus GG, and probiotic mixtures) significantly reduced the development of AAD
Hickson et al. (2007)[50]	Randomised controlled trial (UK)	100 g (97 mL) drink containing L. casei, Lactobacillus bulgaricus and S. thermophilus twice a day during a course of antibiotics and for 1 week after the course finished	135 hospital patients taking antibiotics	AAD	Reduced incidence of AAD and CDAD with specific probiotics
Johnston et al. (2007)[49]	Meta-analysis	Lactobacilli spp., Bifidobacterium spp., Streptococcus spp. or S. boulardii alone or in combination (5×10^9 to 40×10^9 cfu day)	10 studies	AAD	Evidence for benefit is promising
Safdar et al. (2008)[200]	Randomised controlled trial (US)	Probiotic (Florajen)	40 patients	AAD	Reduction in AAD
Szymanski et al. (2008)[51]	Randomised controlled trial (Poland)	A food supplement containing 10^8 cfu Bifidobacterium longum, L. rhamnosus and Lactobacillus plantarum (n = 40) or a placebo (n = 38) orally twice daily for the duration of antibiotic treatment	78 children with otitis media, and/or respiratory tract infections, and/or urinary tract infections treated with antibiotics (5 months to 16 years)	AAD	Probiotics did not reduce rate of diarrhoea but reduced stool frequency

(continued)

Table 2 (continued)

Reference	Duration and type of trial	Type of probiotic	Study group	Outcome measures	Observed effects
Kale-Pradhan et al. (2010)[201]	Meta-analysis	Lactobacillus spp.	10 studies (862 patients)	AAD	Lactobacilllus reduced risk of AAD in adults but not children
Lonnermark et al. (2010)[52]	Randomised controlled trial (Sweden)	L. plantarum 299V (10^{10} cfu) or a placebo drink daily, until a week after termination of antibiotic treatment	Subjects treated with antibiotics	AAD	L. plantarum had a preventive effect on milder gastrointestinal symptoms during treatment with antibiotics
Irritable bowel syndrome					
O'Sullivan &O'Morain (2000)[202]	Randomised controlled trial (Ireland)	Lactobacillus GG	25 with IBS	IBS outcomes	No significant improvement of symptoms
Niedzielin et al. (2001)[57]	4-week randomised controlled trial (Poland)	L. plantarum 299V	40 patients	IBS outcomes	Resolution of abdominal painand trend towards reduced stool frequency
Sen et al. (2002)[58]	4-week randomised controlled trial (UK)	L. plantarum 299V	12 untreated patients with IBS	IBS outcomes	No improvement in colonic fermentation or IBS symptoms
Saggioro et al. (2004)[59]	4-week randomised controlled trial (Italy)	L. plantarum LP01 and B. breve BR 03 or L. plantarum LP01 and L. acidophilus LA 02, all strains at concentrations of 5×10^9 cfu/g powder containing starch	70 with IBS (25–64 years)	IBS symptoms	Severity of symptoms reduced with both probiotic formulations
Bausserman & Michail (2005)[61]	6-week randomised controlled trial (US)	Lactobacillus GG	50 children with IBS	IBS outcomes	Lactobacillus GG was not superior to placebo in the treatment of abdominal pain in children with IBS but may help to relieve such symptoms as perceived abdominal distension
Bittner et al. (2005)[65]	2-week randomised controlled trial (US)	Prescript-Assist (proprietary probiotic–prebiotic); one 500 mg capsule twice a day	25 with IBS	IBS outcomes	Significant improvement in some IBS symptoms

(continued)

Study	Trial	Intervention	Participants	Outcome	Results
Kajander et al. (2005)[66]	6-month randomised controlled trial (Finland)	Probiotic capsule	103 with IBS	IBS symptoms (abdominal pain, distension, flatulence, borborygmi)	The probiotic mixture produced a significant, though slight, beneficial effect on symptoms of IBS
Kim et al. (2005)[62]	4 to 8-week randomised controlled trial	VSL# 3 twice daily	48 with IBS	IBS symptoms	Reduced flatulence and colonic transit
Niv et al. (2005)[64]	6-month randomised controlled trial (Israel)	L. reuteri (ATCC 55730) 1×10^8 cfu/tablet twice a day	54 with IBS	IBS symptoms	No improvement in IBS symptoms
O'Mahony et al. (2005)[60]	8-week randomised controlled trial (Ireland)	Lactobacillus salivarius UCC4331 or Bifidobacterium infantis 35624, each in a dose of 1×10^{10} live bacterial cells in a malted milk drink	77 with IBS	IBS symptoms	B. infantis 35624 alleviated symptoms in IBS
Fan et al. (2006)[63]	4-week randomised controlled trial (China)	Capsules of live combined Bifidobacterium, Lactobacillus and Enterococcus spp. 1260 mg day in three spearate doses	85 with IBS	IBS symptoms	Combined probiotic improved IBS symptoms
Kim et al. (2006)[203]	4-week randomised controlled trial (Korea)	Medilac DS (Bacillus subtilis, Streptococcus faecium)	40 with IBS	IBS symptoms	Pain and frequency of pain decreased, but not bloating, flatulence, stool consistency
Whorwell et al. (2006)[68]	4-week randomised controlled trial (UK)	Bacteria B. infantis 35624 at a dose of 1×10^6, 1×10^8 or 1×10^{10} cfu/mL	326 with IBS	IBS symptoms	B. infantis 35624 at a dose of 1×10^8 cfu was significantly superior to placebo and all other Bifidobacterium doses for the primary efficacy variable of abdominal pain as well as the composite score and scores for bloating, bowel dysfunction, incomplete evacuation, straining, and the passage of gas at the end of the 4-week study
Drouault-Holowacz et al. (2008)[70]	4-week randomised controlled trial (France)	4 strains of lactobacilli	100 with IBS	IBS outcomes	The probiotic combination was not significantly superior to the placebo in relieving symptoms of IBS
McFarland & Dublin (2008)[71]	Meta-analysis	Various	20 trials (1404 patients)	IBS outcomes	Reduced symptoms; less abdominal pain with probiotics

Table 2 *(continued)*

Reference	Duration and type of trial	Type of probiotic	Study group	Outcome measures	Observed effects
Moayyedi et al. (2008)[72]	Systematic review	Various	19 randomised controlled trials (1650 patients)	IBS outcomes	Probiotics appear to be efficacious in IBS, but the magnitude of benefit and the most effective species and strain are uncertain
Nikfar et al. (2009)[73]	Meta-analysis	Various	8 randomised controlled trials	IBS outcomes	Improvement in symptoms of IBS
Brenner et al. (2009)[74]	Meta-analysis	Various	16 randomised controlled trials	IBS symptoms	*B. infantis* 35624 has shown efficacy for improvement of IBS symptoms
Guyonnet et al. (2009)[69]	A randomised, open-label, controlled, pilot study (France)	Fermented milk containing *B. lactis* DN-173010	371 adults reporting digestive discomfort	Abdominal symptoms	Improved digestive comfort with probiotics
Hoveyda et al. (2009)[75]	Meta-analysis	Various	14 randomised controlled trials	IBS outcomes	Improvement in some symptoms of IBS
Ulcerative colitis					
Kruis et al. (1997)[79]	12-week, double-blind, double-dummy study (Germany)	Oral preparation of viable *Escherichia. coli* Nissle (serotype 06:K5:H1) vs mesalazine 500 mg three times a day	120 with inactive UC	Relapse of UC	Relapse rates and time were similar between probiotic and standard treatment
Rembacken et al. (1999)[84]	12-month single-centre, randomised, double-dummy study (UK)	Non-pathogenic *E. coli* vs mesalazine	116 with active UC	UC relapse	Non-pathogenic *E.coli* had an equivalent effect to mesalazine in maintaining remission of UC
Venturi et al. (1999)[85]	12 month intervention (Italy)	VSL#3 containing 5×10^{11} cells/g of 3 strains of bifidobacteria, 4 strains of lactobacilli and 1 strain of *Streptococcus salivarius* ssp. *thermophilus* (3 g each day for 12 months)	20 with UC in remission	UC relapse	15/20 treated patients remained in remission during the study; 1 patient was lost to follow up, while the remaining 4 relapsed

Study	Trial type	Intervention	Sample	Outcome measure	Results
Guslandi et al. (2003)[87]	4-week open, pilot trial (Italy)	S. boulardii 250 mg three times a day (as additional treatment to mesalazine)	25 with UC on maintenance treatment with mesalazine	UC relapse	17/24 patients remained in remission
Ishikawa et al. (2003)[83]	12-month randomised controlled trial (Japan)	Bifidobacteria-fermented milk supplement as a dietary adjunct	21 with UC	UC relapse	Significant reduction in exacerbations in intervention group
Cui et al. (2004)[88]	8-week randomised controlled trial (China)	Bifid triple viable capsule (BIFICO) (1.26 g/day), or an identical placebo (starch)	30 with UC treated with sulfasalazine + glucocorticoid	Intestinal mucosae; relapse of UC	Probiotic effective in preventing flare-ups in UC
Kato et al. (2004)[77]	12-week randomised controlled trial (Japan)	100 mL/day Bifidobacteria-fermented milk + conventional treatment	20 with mild to moderate, active UC	UC clinical activity	Clinical activity index significantly lower in the probiotic treatment
Kruis et al. (2004)[80]	A double-blind, double-dummy trial (Germany)	E. coli Nissle 1917 (200 mg three times a day) or mesalazine	327 with UC	Maintenance of remission of UC	Probiotic was as efficient as mesalazine in maintaining remission
Tursi et al. (2004)[81]	8-week randomised controlled trial (Italy)	Low-dose balsalazide (2.25 g/day) plus 3 g/day VSL#3 (group A) with medium-dose balsalazide alone (group B) and with mesalazine (group C)	90 with mild to moderate UC	Relapse of UC	Balsalazide/VSL#3 may was more effective than balsalazide alone or mesalazine
Bibiloni et al. (2005)[86]	6 week open label trial (Canada)	VSL#3, 3.6×10^{12} bacteria daily in two divided doses	34 with active UC	Relapse of UC	Treatment with VSL#3 resulted in a combined induction of remission/response rate of 77% with no adverse events
Furrie et al. (2005)[76]	1 month randomised controlled trial (UK)	B. longum with a prebiotic	18 with active UC	Clinical status	Improvement in clinical status with synbiotic
Zocco et al. (2006)[89]	12 month randomised controlled trial (Italy)	Lactobacillus GG 18×10^9 viable bacteria/day (n = 65), mesalazine 2400 mg/day (n = 60) or Lactobacillus GG + mesalazine (n = 62)	187 with quiescent UC	Relapse of UC	Lactobacillus GG was more effective than mesalazine in prolonging relapse-free time; no differences between the 3 groups in relapse rate
Zigra et al. (2007)[204]	Systematic review	Various	9 studies	Comparison of probiotics with anti-inflammatory drugs or placebo in the remission of UC	Existing studies suggest similar safety and efficacy of probiotics in comparison with anti-inflammatory drugs

(continued)

Table 2 *(continued)*

Reference	Duration and type of trial	Type of probiotic	Study group	Outcome measures	Observed effects
Hegazy & El-Bedewy (2010)[90]	8-week randomised controlled trial (Egypt)	Probiotic (*Lactobacillus delbruekii* and *Lactobacillus fermentum*) vs sulfasalazine vs sulfasalazine + probiotic vs control	30 with mild to moderate UC	Effect on pro-inflammatory cytokines and NF-κB activation	Probiotic significantly ameliorated the inflammation by decreasing inflammatory cytokines compared with sulfasalazine group and the control group
Sang *et al.* (2010)[205]	Meta-analysis	Various	13 randomised controlled trials	Remission in UC	Probiotic treatment was more effective than placebo in maintaining remission in UC
Pouchitis					
Gionchetti *et al.* (2003)[92]	1 year randomised controlled trial (Italy)	VSL#3	40 with IPAA for UC	Prevention of pouchitis	Treatment with VSL#3 is effective in the prevention of the onset of acute pouchitis and improves quality of life of patients with IPAA
Laake *et al.* (2003)[94]	4-week open label study (Norway)	A fermented milk product (Cultura; 500 mL) containing live lactobacilli (LA-5) and bifidobacteria (Bb-12)	10 with IPAA for UC	Ileal pouch inflammation and perfusion in the pouch	Change in gross appearance of mucosa at endoscopy but no change in histological picture (after 4 weeks)
Gosselink *et al.* (2004)[96]	3 year randomised controlled trial (Netherlands)	*L. rhamnosus* GG	117 with IPAA for UC	Pouchitis	First episodes of pouchitis were observed less frequently
Laake *et al.* (2004)[95]	4-week randomised controlled trial (Norway)	A fermented milk product (Cultura), containing live lactobacilli (LA-5) and bifidobacteria (Bb-12)	51 with IPAA for UC	Mucosal histology, inflammation	No change in histology; reduction in disease activity index
Laake *et al.* (2005)[78]	A 4-week randomised controlled trial (Norway)	A fermented milk product (Cultura) containing live lactobacilli (LA-5) and bifidobacteria (Bb-12)	61 with IPAA for UC; 6 after surgery for ileorectal anastomosis	Mucosal histology, inflammation	Beneficial effect on symptoms and endoscopic inflammation in patients with UC and IPAA

Crohn's disease

Gupta et al. (2000)[206]	6 month open-label study (US)	Lactobacillus GG (10^{10} cfu) in enterocoated tablets twice a day	4 children with mildly to moderately active Crohn's disease	Clinical activity	Significant improvement in clinical activity 1 week after starting Lactobacillus GG
Guslandi et al. (2000)[97]	6-month randomised controlled trial (Italy)	Mesalamine 1 g three times a day or mesalamine 1 g two times a day plus a preparation of S. boulardii 1 g daily	32 with Crohn's disease in clinical remission	Maintenance of remission	Fewer clinical relapses with mesalamine plus probiotic than mesalamine alone
Guandalini et al. (2002)[207]	Open-label, preliminary study (US)	Lactobacillus GG	4 children with active Crohn's disease (mean age 14.5 years; range 10–18)	Crohn's disease outcomes	Significant improvement
Prantera et al. (2002)[98]	1 year controlled trial (Italy)	12×10^9 cfu Lactobacillus or identical placebo	45 with Crohn's disease who had all diseased gut removed	Recurrence of Crohn's disease	Lactobacillus GG did not prevent endoscopic recurrence at 1 year nor reduce the severity of recurrent lesions
Schultz et al. (2004)[99]	6 month randomised controlled trial (Germany)	Lactobacillus GG (2×10^9 cfu/day) or placebo	11 with moderate to active Crohn's disease	Induction or maintenance of medically induced remission of Crohn's disease	No benefit of Lactobacillus GG in inducing or maintaining medically induced remission in Crohn's disease
Bousvaros et al. (2005)[100]	2-year randomised controlled trial	L. rhamnosus strain GG	75 children with Crohn's disease on standard medication	Relapse in Crohn's disease	Lactobacillus GG did not prolong time to relapse
Marteau et al. (2006)[101]	6-month randomised controlled trial (France)	Two packets per day of lyophilised Lactobacillus johnsonii LA-1 (2×10^9 cfu) or placebo	98 with surgical resection for Crohn's disease	Recurrence of Crohn's disease	L. johnsonii LA-1 (4×10^9 cfu/day) did not have a sufficient effect, if any, to prevent endoscopic recurrence of Crohn's disease
Rahimi et al. (2008)[102]	Meta-analysis	Various	8 randomised controlled trials	Remission in Crohn's disease	Failed to demonstrate the efficacy of probiotics in maintaining remission and preventing clinical and endoscopic recurrence in Crohn's disease

(continued)

Table 2 (continued)

Helicobacter pylori infection

Reference	Duration and type of trial	Type of probiotic	Study group	Outcome measures	Observed effects
Canducci et al. (2000)[208]	7 day randomised controlled trial (Italy)	Triple therapy or triple therapy + L. acidophilus	120 H. pylori-positive patients	Effect on H. pylori	Increase in eradication rate with probiotic
Armuzzi et al. (2001)[117]	14-day randomised controlled trial (Italy)	Triple therapy + placebo or triple therapy + Lactobacillus GG	60 H. pylori-positive patients	Effect on H. pylori treatment side-effects	Lactobacillus GG supplementation showed a positive impact on H. pylori therapy-related side-effects and on overall treatment tolerability
Felley et al. (2001)[104]	3-week randomised controlled trial (Switzerland)	L. johnsonii LA-1-acidified milk (LC-1) or placebo + clarithromycin	53 H. pylori-infected volunteers	Effect on H. pylori	Reduced H. pylori density and gastric inflammation
Cremonini et al. (2002)[118]	2-week randomised controlled trial (Italy)	Lactobacillus GG vs S. boulardii vs a combination, vs placebo + triple therapy for 1 week	85 H. pylori-infected subjects	Effect on H. pylori treatment side-effects	All probiotics superior to placebo for side-effects but not for compliance with triple therapy
Sheu et al. (2002)[107]	5-week randomised controlled trial (Taiwan)	Lactobacillus- and Bifidobacterium-containing yogurt with triple therapy or triple therapy alone; 1-week triple therapy + 4 additional weeks for probiotic group	160 H. pylori-infected subjects	Effect on H. pylori eradication	Probiotics improved the intention-to-treat eradication rates of H. pylori, and restored the depletion of Bifidobacterium in stools after triple therapy
Cats et al. (2003)[112]	3-week randomised controlled trial (Netherlands)	Yakult	14 H. pylori-infected subjects	H. pylori growth	Some reduction in H. pylori growth with Yakult
Cruchet et al. (2003)[103]	4-week randomised controlled trial (Chile)	4 groups: live or heat-killed L. johnsonii LA-1 or Lactobacillus paracasei ST11	326 H. pylori-infected children	H. pylori colonisation	Moderate reduction in H. pylori with L. johnsonii
Pantoflickova et al. (2003)[105]	16-week randomised controlled trial (Switzerland)	L. johnsonii vs placebo	50 H. pylori-positive adults	H. pylori-associated gastritis	Favourable effect of probiotic on H. pylori gastritis
Nista et al. (2004)[115]	14-day randomised controlled trial (Italy)	Bacillus clausii + triple therapy or placebo + triple therapy	120 H. pylori-positive patients	Antibiotic-associated side-effects in H. pylori therapy	Reduced incidence of side-effects with probiotic

Tursi et al. (2004)	5-week randomised controlled trial	10-day triple therapy with 16 × 10⁹ bacteria L. casei ssp. casei DG or triple therapy with placebo	70 H. pylori-positive patients	Side-effects of H. pylori treatment	Probiotic reduced side-effects; slight improvement in H. pylori eradication rate
Wang et al. (2004)[106]	8-week controlled trial (China)	Lactobacillus and Bifidobacterium-containing yogurt	59 H. pylori-positive adults	H. pylori infection	Probiotic effectively suppressed H. pylori infection
Myllyluoma et al. (2005)[119]	4-week randomised controlled trial (Finland)	L. rhamnosus GG, L. rhamnosus LC705, B. breve Bb99 and Propionibacterium freudenreichii ssp. shermanii JS, or a placebo + standard drug treatment	47 H. pylori-infected adults	Symptoms of H. pylori treatment	No influence of probiotic onnew or aggravated symptoms during H. pylori treatment, buttotal symptom severity was reduced
Sykora et al. (2005)[108]	14-day randomised controlled trial (Czech Republic)	L. casei DN-114 001 + triple therapy or triple therapy alone	86 symptomatic H. pylori-positive children	H. pylori eradication rates	Probiotic conferred an enhanced therapeutic effect in H. pylori gastritis
Gotteland et al. (2006)[120]	Systematic review	Lactobacillus and Bifidobacterium spp.		H. pylori colonisation and side-effects of treatment	Probiotics do not eradicate H. pylori but maintain lower levels of this pathogen in the stomach; in combination with antibiotics; probiotics may increase eradication rate and/or decrease adverse effects
Sheu et al. (2006)[111]	1-week therapy with or without 4 weeks of pretreatment with probiotic yogurt (randomised controlled trial, Taiwan)	Lactobacillus and Bifidobacterium-containing yogurt + standard quadruple therapy or standard quadruple therapy alone	138 for whom triple therapy had failed (antimicrobial resistance)	H. pylori load	A 4-week pretreatment with probioitic yogurt could decrease H. pylori loads despite antimicrobial resistance, thus improving the efficacy of quadruple therapy in eradicating residual H. pylori
Kim et al. (2008)[113]	3-week randomised controlled trial (Korea)	Triple therapy + yogurt (L. acidophilus HY2177, L. casei HY2743, B. longum HY8001, and S. thermophilus B-1) or triple therapy alone	347 H. pylori-infected patients	Side-effects of H. pylori treatment and eradication rates	Probiotic reduced eradication rates but not side-effects of therapy

(continued)

Table 2 (continued)

Reference	Duration and type of trial	Type of probiotic	Study group	Outcome measures	Observed effects
Zou et al. (2009)[121]	Meta-analysis	Lactobacilli	8 randomised controlled trials (1372 participants)	H. pylori eradication and side-effects of treatment	Lactobacilli improved H. pylori eradication therapy and improved some side-effects of therapy (diarrhoea, bloating, taste disturbance)
Song et al. (2010)[205]	4-week randomised controlled trial (Korea)	Proton pump inhibitor-based triple therapy for 7 days plus S. boulardii for 4 weeks, plus S. boulardii and mucoprotective agent for 4 weeks, or with no addition	991 H. pylori-infected patients	H. pylori eradication rates and side-effects of therapy	No significant effects on H. pylori eradication rates; S. boulardii possibly effective for improving eradication rates by reducing side-effects and improving completion of therapy
Yasar et al. (2010)[114]	14-day randomised controlled trial	Triple therapy + 125 mL of probiotic-containing yogurt (Bifidobacterium DN-173 10^{10} cfu/g) before breakfast or triple therapy alone	76 patients with H. pylori infection	H. pylori eradication rates; prevention of side-effects related to eradication therapy	No improvement in eradication rates with probiotic; improvement in constipation and stomatitis
Eczema					
Isolauri et al. (2000)[136]	Randomised controlled trial (Finland)	Extensively hydrolysed whey formula ± B. lactis Bb-12 or Lactobacillus GG (ATCC 53103)	27 infants who manifested atopic eczema during breast feeding (4–6 months)	Extent and severity of atopic eczema	Improvement in eczema and inflammatory cytokines
Pessi et al. (2000)[131]	8 week randomised controlled trial	Oral L. rhamnosus GG	9 infants with atopic dermatitis	Effects on immune mediators	Enhanced interleukin-10 generation and anti-inflammatory state
Kalliomaki et al. (2001)[146]	Randomised controlled trial (Finland)	Lactobacillus GG prenatally and postnatally to infants	Mothers who had at least one first-degree relative (or partner) with atopic eczema, allergic rhinitis or asthma	Chronic recurring atopic eczema and other allergic disease	Lactobacillus GG was effective in prevention of early atopic disease (eczema, asthma, allergic rhinitis) in children at high risk

Kirjavainen et al. (2002)[209]	Randomised controlled trial (Finland)	Extensively hydrolysed whey formula with or without B. lactis Bb-12	21 infants with early onset atopic eczema	Gut microflora and allergic sensitisation	Probiotic modified the gut microflora in a manner that may alleviate allergic inflammation
Rautava et al. (2002)[149]	Randomised controlled trial (Finland)	Probiotics given to mother	62 mother–infant pairs	Immunoprotective quality of breast milk	Probiotics promoted the immunoprotective potential of breast milk and potentially provides protection against atopic eczema during the first 2 years of life
Kalliomaki et al. (2003)[132]	4-year follow-up of randomised controlled trial	L. rhamnosus strain GG (ATCC 53103)	107 children	Development of atopic disease	Preventive effect of Lactobacillus GG is prolonged beyond infancy
Kirjavainen et al. (2003)[133]	Randomised controlled trial (Finland)	Lactobacillus GG in extensively hyrolysed whey formula or formula alone	35 infants with atopic eczema and allergy to cow's milk	Symptoms of atopic eczema	Improvement in atopic eczema with viable Lactobacillus GG
Rosenfeldt et al. (2003)[137]	6 week randomised controlled trial (Finland)	2 probiotic strains (lyophilised L. rhamnosus 19070-2 and L. reuteri DSM 122460)	Children with atopic dermatitis (1–13 years)	Severity of eczema	Extent of eczema decreased with probiotic
Pohjavuori et al. (2004)[134]	4-week randomised controlled trial (Finland)	L. rhamnosus GG and a mixture of 4 bacterial species + elimination diet and skin treatment	Infants with suspected cows' milk allergy	Modulation of immune response	Improved immune response with probiotic
Rosenfeldt et al. (2004)[144]	6 week randomised controlled trial (Finland)	L. rhamnosus 19070-2 and L. reuteri DSM 12246	41 children with atopic dermatitis	Gastrointestinal symptoms	Gastrointestinal symptoms reduced with probiotic
Viljanen et al. (2005)[135]	4-week randomised controlled trial (Finland)	Lactobacillus GG, a mixture of four probiotic strains	230 infants with atopic eczema	Markers of intestinal inflammation	Improvement in inflammation with probiotic
Viljanen et al. (2005)[210]	4-week randomised controlled trial (Finland)	Lactobacillus GG, a mixture of four probiotic strains	230 infants with atopic eczema and suspected cows' milk allergy	Inflammatory markers	Probiotics induced systemically detectable low-grade inflammation
Viljanen et al. (2005)[141]	4-week randomised controlled trial (Finland)	Lactobacillus GG, a mixture of four probiotic strains	120 infants with suspected cows' milk allergy	Effect on atopic eczema	Treatment with Lactobacillus GG may alleviate symptoms of atopic eczema/dermatitis in IgE-sensitized infants but not in non-IgE-sensitized infants

(continued)

Table 2 *(continued)*

Reference	Duration and type of trial	Type of probiotic	Study group	Outcome measures	Observed effects
Weston et al. (2005)[140]	8-week randomised controlled trial (Australia)	1 × 10^9 Lactobacillus fermentum VRI-033 PCC) or an equivalent volume of placebo, twice daily	56 children with atopic dermatitis (6–18 months)	Severity and extent of atopic dermatitis	Improved atopic dermatitis with probiotic
Brouwer et al. (2006)[211]	3 month randomised controlled trial (Netherlands)	L. rhamnosus (n = 17), Lactobacillus GG (n = 16) or placebo (n = 17)	Infants with atopic dermatitis	Clinical and immunological effects	No clinical or immunological effect of probiotics
Sistek et al. (2006)[138]	Randomised controlled trial (New Zealand)	L. rhamnosus and Bifidobacteria lactis	59 infants with atopic dermatitis	Improvements in atopic dermatitis	Improved atopic dermatitis only in food-sensitised infants
Abrahamsson et al. (2007)[142]	Randomised controlled trial (Sweden)	L. reuteri from gestational week 36 until delivery	232 families with allergic disease	Allergic disease	Treated infants had less IgE-associated eczema at 2 years of age
Osborn & Sinn (2007)[150]	Meta-analysis	Various	12 studies	Allergic disease	Reduction in clinical eczema but findings not consistent
Boyle et al. (2008)[212]	Meta-analysis	Various	12 randomised controlled trials (781 patients)	Eczema	No significant difference in eczema severity
Michail et al. (2008)[151]	Meta-analysis	Various	10 studies (n = 678)	Severity of atopic dermatitis	Improved symptoms particularly in those with moderate to severe disease
Wickens et al. (2008)[147]	Randomised controlled trial (New Zealand)	L. rhamnosus HN001, Bifidobacterium animalis ssp. lactis strain HN019 or placebo daily from 35 weeks of gestation until 6 months if breastfeeding; their infants randomised to receive the same treatment from birth to 2 years (n = 474)	Infants (pregnant women) at risk of allergic disease	Development of eczema and atopy at 2 years	Supplementation with L. rhamnosus, but not B. animalis ssp. lactis, substantially reduced the cumulative prevalence of eczema, but not atopy, by 2 years

Reference	Study type	Intervention	Population	Outcome measured	Result
Kim et al. (2009)[139]	Randomised controlled trial (Korea)	Bifidobacteria lactis BGN4, B. lactis AD011, and L. acidophilus AD031, or placebo, starting at 4–8 weeks before delivery and continuing until 6 months after delivery	112 pregnant women with a family history of allergic diseases	Development of eczema or atopic dermatitis	Reduced risk of eczema during first year of life in the offspring
Kuitunen et al. (2009)[213]	Randomised controlled trial (Finland)	A probiotic mixture (2 lactobacilli, bifidobacteria, and propionibacteria) or placebo during the last month of pregnancy and to the infants from birth until age 6 months	1223 mothers with infants at high risk for allergy	Cumulative incidence of allergic diseases (eczema, food allergy, allergic rhinitis, and asthma) and IgE sensitisation at 5 years	No allergy-preventive effect that extended to age 5 years was achieved with perinatal supplementation of probiotic bacteria to high-risk mothers and children; it conferred protection only to caesarean-delivered children
West et al. (2009)[214]	Randomised controlled trial (Sweden)	Cereals with (n = 89) or without Lactobacillus F19 (n = 90) from 4 to 13 months of age	179 infants	Cumulative incidence of eczema at 13 months of age	Reduced risk of eczema with probiotic
Dotterud et al. (2010)[148]	Randomised controlled trial (Norway)	L. rhamnosus GG, L. acidophilus LA-5 and B. animalis subsp. lactis Bb-12 from 36 weeks of gestation to 3 months postnatally during breastfeeding	415 pregnant women	Prevention of atopic sensitisation or allergic diseases during the child's first 2 years	Probiotic reduced the cumulative incidence of atopic dermatitis, but had no effect on atopic sensitization
Rose et al. (2010)[145]	6 month randomised controlled trial (Germany)	L. rhamnosus (LGG, 10^{10} cfu) or placebo	131 children with at least two wheezing episodes and a first-degree family history of atopic disease (6–24 months)	Impact on allergic sensitisation	Oral Lactobacillus GG had no clinical effect on atopic dermatitis or asthma-related events, and only mild effects on allergic sensitisation

AAD, antibiotic-associated diarrhoea; ATCC, American Type Culture Collection; CDAD, Clostridium difficile acute diarrhoea; cfu, colony-forming units; IBS, irritable bowel syndrome; IPAA, ileal pouch-anal anastomosis; TD, travellers' diarrhoea; UC, ulcerative colitis.

Conclusion

The colonic microflora is important to health, and modification of the bacterial species inhabiting the large bowel – using probiotics and prebiotics – has been suggested to produce potential health benefits. There are a growing number of published papers on the use of both probiotics and prebiotics, and although they show ability to alter the colonic microflora, evidence that they can reduce the risk of diseases is more limited. This may in part be because of differences in methodology, particularly the large number of different strains that have been used. The evidence for an effect of probiotics in acute diarrhoea appears to be greatest for rotavirus infection. Study results in travellers' diarrhoea have been inconsistent. Evidence has increased considerably in recent years that probiotics can reduce the risk of atopic eczema and be effective in its management. Probiotics can be effective in preventing antibiotic-associated diarrhoea. There is also some evidence that probiotics can improve lactose intolerance, boost immunity, prevent vaginal infections and lower serum cholesterol, but further research is required. Moreover there is, as yet, no conclusive evidence that either prebiotics or probiotics can prevent cancer in humans.

Precautions/contraindications

None reported.

Pregnancy and breast-feeding

No known problems.

Adverse effects

Probiotics have a long history of apparently safe use.[215–217] However, they can exert potentially powerful immune effects so caution is required until more data are available. This may be relevant for probiotics added to infant formula or given to seriously immunocompromised patients, in whom there have been isolated cases of opportunistic infections from probiotic species.[215,216,218]

Interactions

None reported.

Dose

Probiotics are available in the form of tablets and capsules of *L. acidophilus*, often with other bacteria. They are also available in the form of yoghurts and various fermented milks. Many probiotics require refrigeration to maintain viability and like any other product should be used before the expiry date. Commercial products have not always been found to contain the bacterial strain listed on the label, and in some cases, the bacteria may not be viable.[44]

Prebiotics are available in the form of tablets, capsules and powders of fructo-oligosaccharides and inulin.

There is no established dose for any of these products. Specific probiotics have been used in studies evaluating different conditions. The species and strain of probiotic for different indications is likely to be important.

References

1   Fuller R. *Probiotics. The Scientific Basis*. London: Chapman & Hall, 1992.
2   Fuller R. A review: probiotics in man and animals. *J Appl Bacteriol* 1989; 66: 365–378.
3   Sadler MJ, Saltmarsh M. *Functional Foods*. Cambridge: Royal Society of Chemistry, 1998: 4–5.
4   Macfarlane GT, Cummings JH. Probiotics and prebiotics: can regulating the activities of intestinal bacteria benefit health? *BMJ* 1999; 318: 999 L 1003.
5   Gibson GR, Roberfroid MB. Dietary modulation of the human colonic microbiota: introducing the concept of prebiotics. *J Nutr* 1995; 125: 1401–1412.
6   MacGillivray PC, Finlay HVL, Binns TB. Use of lactulose to create a preponderance of lactobacilli in the intestine of bottle-fed infants. *Scott Med J* 1959; 4: 182–189.
7   Gibson GR, Beatty EB, Wang X, Cummings JH. Selective stimulation of bifidobacteria in the human colon by oligofructose and inulin. *Gastroenterology* 1995; 108: 975–982.
8   Rowland IR, Tanaka R. The effects of transgalactosylated oligosaccharides on gut flora metabolism in rats associated with human faecal microflora. *J Appl Bacteriol* 1993; 74: 667–674.
9   Collins MD, Gibson GR. Probiotics, prebiotics, and synbiotics: approaches for modulating the microbial ecology of the gut. *Am J Clin Nutr* 1999; 69: 1052S–1057S.

10 Rolfe RD. The role of probiotic cultures in the control of gastrointestinal health. *J Nutr* 2000; 130: S396–S402.

11 Elmer GW Surawicz CM, MacFarland LV. Biotherapeutic agents. A neglected modality for the treatment and prevention of selected intestinal and vaginal infections. *JAMA* 1996; 275: 870–876.

12 Dendukuri N, Costa V, McGregor M, *et al*. Probiotic therapy for the prevention and treatment of *Clostridium difficile*-associated diarrhea: a systematic review. *Cmaj* 2005; 173(2): 167–170.

13 McFarland LV. Meta-analysis of probiotics for the prevention of antibiotic associated diarrhoea and the treatment of *Clostridium difficile* disease. *Am J Gastroenterol* 2006; 101: 812–822.

14 de Roos NM, Katan MB. Effects of probiotic bacteria on diarrhea, lipid metabolism, and carcinogenesis: a review of papers published between 1988 and 1998. *Am J Clin Nutr* 2000; 71: 405–411.

15 Szajewska H, Mrukowicz JZ. Probiotics in the treatment and prevention of acute infectious diarrhoea in infants and children: a systematic review of published, randomized, double-blind, placebo-controlled trials. *J Pediatr Gastroenterol Nutr* 2001; 33: S17–S25.

16 Huang JS, Bousvaros A, Lee JW, *et al*. Efficacy of probiotic use in acute diarrhoea in children: a metaanalysis. *Dig Dis Sci* 2002; 47: 2625–2634.

17 Van Niel CW, Feudtner C, Garrison MM, Christakis DA. *Lactobacillus* therapy for acute infectious diarrhea in children: a meta-analysis. *Pediatrics* 2002; 109: 678–684.

18 Pereg D, Kimhi O, Tirosh A, *et al*. The effect of fermented yogurt on the prevention of diarrhea in a healthy adult population. *Am J Infect Control* 2005; 33: 122–125.

19 Allen SJ, Okoko B, Martinez E, *et al*. Probiotics for treating infectious diarrhoea. *Cochrane Database Syst Rev* 2004; (2): CD003048.

20 Allen SJ, Martinez EG, Gregorio GV, *et al*. Probiotics for treating acute infectious diarrhoea. *Cochrane Database Syst Rev* 2010; 10(11): CD003048.

21 Bernaola Aponte G, Bada Mancilla CA, Carreazo Pariasca NY, *et al*. Probiotics for treating persistent diarrhoea in children. *Cochrane Database Syst Rev* 2010; 10(11): CD007401.

22 Rosenfeldt V, Michaelsen KF, Jakobsen M, *et al*. Effect of probiotic *Lactobacillus* strains in young children hospitalized with acute diarrhoea. *Pediatr Infect Dis J* 2002; 21: 411–416.

23 Rosenfeldt V, Michaelsen KF, Jakobsen M, *et al*. Effect of probiotic *Lactobacillus* strains on acute diarrhea in a cohort of nonhospitalized children in day-care centers. *Pediatr Infect Dis J* 2002; 21: 417–419.

24 Chouraqui JP, Van Egroo LD, Fichot MC. Acidified milk formula supplemented with *Bifidobacterium lactis*: impact on infant diarrhea in residential care settings. *J Pediatr Gastroenterol Nutr* 2004; 38: 288–292.

25 Thibault H, Aubert-Jacquin C, Goulet O. Effects of long-term consumption of a fermented infant formula (with *Bifidobacterium breve* c50 and *Streptococcus thermophilus* 065) on acute diarrhea in healthy infants. *J Pediatr Gastroenterol Nutr* 2004; 39: 147–152.

26 Weizman Z, Asli G, Alsheikh A. Effect of a probiotic infant formula on infections in child care centers: comparison of two probiotic agents. *Pediatrics* 2005; 115: 5–9.

27 Kurugol Z, Koturoglu G. Effects of *Saccharomyces boulardii* in children with acute diarrhoea. *Acta Paediatr* 2005; 94: 44–47.

28 Shamir R, Makhoul IR, Etzioni A, Shehadeh N. Evaluation of a diet containing probiotics and zinc for the treatment of mild diarrheal illness in children younger than one year of age. *J Am Coll Nutr* 2005; 24: 370–375.

29 Szymanski H, Pejcz J, Jawien M, *et al*. Treatment of acute infectious diarrhoea in infants and children with a mixture of three *Lactobacillus rhamnosus* strains – a randomized, double-blind, placebo-controlled trial. *Aliment Pharmacol Ther* 2006; 23: 247–253.

30 Oksanen PJ, Salminen S, Saxelin M, *et al*. Prevention of travellers' diarrhoea by *Lactobacillus* GG. *Ann Med* 1990; 22: 53–56.

31 Hilton E, Kolakowski P, Singer C, Smith M. Efficacy of *Lactobacillus* GG as a diarrheal preventive in travellers. *J Travel Med* 1997; 4: 41–43.

32 Black FT, Andersen PL, Orskov J, *et al*. Prophylactic efficacy of lactobacilli on travellers' diarrhoea. In: Steffen R (ed.). *Travel Medicine. Conference on International Travel Medicine 1, Zurich, Switzerland*. Berlin: Springer, 1989: 333–335.

33 Kollaritsch H, Wiedermann G. Travellers' diarrhoea among Austrian tourists: epidemiology, clinical features and attempts at non-antibiotic drug prophylaxis. In: Pasini W (ed.). *Proceedings of the Second International Conference on Tourist Health*. Rimini: World Health Organization, 1990: 74–82.

34 Katelaris PH, Salam I, Farthing MJG. Lactobacilli to prevent travellers' diarrhea? *NEngl J Med* 1995; 333: 1360–1361.

35 Briand V, Buffet P, Genty S, *et al*. Absence of efficacy of nonviable *Lactobacillus acidophilus* for the prevention of traveler's diarrhea: a randomized, double-blind, controlled study. *Clin Infect Dis* 2006; 43: 1170–1175.

36 McFarland LV. Meta-analysis of probiotics for the prevention of traveler's diarrhea. *Travel Med Infect Dis* 2007; 5: 97–105.

37 Siitonen S, Vapaatalo H, Salminen S, *et al*. Effect of *Lactobacillus* GG yoghurt in prevention of antibiotic associated diarrhoea. *Ann Med* 1990; 22: 57–59.

38 Gorbach SL, Chang TW, Goldin B. Successful treatment of relapsing *Clostridium difficile* colitis with *Lactobacillus* GG. *Lancet* 1987; 2: 1519. (letter).

39 Hawrelak JA, Whiten DL, Myers SP. Is *Lactobacillus rhamnosus* GG effective in preventing the onset of antibiotic-associated diarrhoea: a systematic review. *Digestion* 2005; 72: 51–56.

40 Sullivan A, Johansson A, Svenungsson B, Nord CE. Effect of *Lactobacillus* F19 on the emergence of antibiotic-resistant microorganisms in the intestinal microflora. *J Antimicrob Chemother* 2004; 54: 791–797.

41 Kotowska M, Albrecht P, Szajewska H. *Saccharomyces boulardii* in the prevention of antibiotic associated diarrhoea in children: a randomized double-blind placebo-controlled trial. *Aliment Pharmacol Ther* 2005; 21: 583–590.

42 Wunderlich PF, Braun L, Fumagalli I, *et al.* Doubleblind report on the efficacy of lactic acid producing *Enterococcus* SF68 in the prevention of antibiotic associated diarrhoea in the treatment of acute diarrhoea. *J Int Med Res* 1989; 17: 333–338.

43 Tankanow RM, Ross MB, Ertel IJ, *et al.* A double blind, placebo-controlled study of the efficacy of Lactinex in the prophylaxis of amoxicillin-induced diarrhoea. *Ann Pharmacol* 1990; 24: 382–384.

44 Black F, Einarsson K, Lidbeck A, *et al.* Effect of lactic acid producing bacteria on the human intestinal microflora during ampicillin treatment. *Scand J Infect Dis* 1991; 23: 247–254.

45 Correa NB, Perret Filho LA, Penna FJ, *et al.* A randomized formula controlled trial of *Bifidobacterium lactis* and *Streptococcus thermophilus* for prevention of antibiotic-associated diarrhea in infants. *J Clin Gastroenterol* 2005; 39: 385–389.

46 D'Souza AL, Rajkumar C, Cooke J, Bulpitt CJ. Probiotics in prevention of antibiotic-associated diarrhoea: meta-analysis. *BMJ* 2002; 324: 1361–1364.

47 Cremonini F, Di Caro S, Nista EC, *et al.* A meta-analysis: the effect of probiotic administration on antibiotic-associated diarrhoea. *Aliment Pharmacol Ther* 2002; 16: 1461–1467.

48 Szajeska H, Mrukowicz J. Meta-analysis: non-pathogenic yeast *Saccharomyces boulardii* in the prevention of antibiotic-associated diarrhoea. *Aliment Pharmacol Ther* 2005; 22: 365–372.

49 Johnston BC, Supina AL, Ospina M, Vohra S. Probiotics for the prevention of pediatric antibiotic associated diarrhea. *Cochrane Database Syst Rev* 2007; (2): CD004827 .

50 Hickson M, D'Souza AL, Muthu N, *et al.* Use of probiotic *Lactobacillus* preparation to prevent diarrhoea associated with antibiotics: randomised double blind placebo controlled trial. *BMJ* 2007; 335: 80.

51 Szymanski H, Armanska M, Kowalska-Duplaga K, *et al.* *Bifidobacterium longum* PL03, *Lactobacillus rhamnosus* KL53A, and *Lactobacillus plantarum* PL02 in the prevention

52 Lonnermark E, Friman V, Lappas G, *et al.* Intake of *Lactobacillus plantarum* reduces certain gastro-intestinal symptoms during treatment with antibiotics. *J Clin Gastroenterol* 2010; 44(2): 106–112.

53 Sanders ME. Summary of the conclusions from a consensus panel of experts on health attributes of lactic cultures: significance to fluid milk products containing cultures. *J Dairy Sci* 1993; 76: 1819–1828.

54 Mustapha A, Jiang T, Savaino DA. Improvement of lactose digestion by humans following ingestion of unfermented acidophilus milk: influence of bile sensitivity, lactose transport, and acid tolerance of *Lactobacilllus acidophilus*. *J Dairy Sci* 1997; 80: 1537–1545.

55 Saltzman JR, Russell RM, Golner B, *et al.* A randomized trial of *Lactobacillus acidophilus* BG2F04 to treat lactose intolerance. *Am J Clin Nutr* 1999; 69: 140–146.

56 Levri KM, Ketvertis K, Deramo M, *et al.* Do probiotics reduce adult lactose intolerance? A systematic review *J Fam Pract* 2005; 54: 613–620.

57 Niedzielin K, Kordecki H, Birkenfeld B. A controlled, double-blind, randomized study on the efficacy of *Lactobacillus plantarum* 299V in patients with irritable bowel syndrome. *Eur J Gastroenterol Hepatol* 2001; 13: 1143–1147.

58 Sen S, MullanMM Parker TJ, *et al.* Effect of *Lactobacillus plantarum* 299V on colonic fermentation and symptoms of irritable bowel syndrome. *Dig Dis Sci* 2002; 47: 2615–2620.

59 Saggioro A. Probiotics in the treatment of irritable bowel syndrome. *J Clin Gastroenterol* 2004; 38: S104–S106.

60 O'Mahony L, McCarthy J, Kelly P, *et al.* *Lactobacillus* and *Bifidobacterium* in irritable bowel syndrome: symptom responses and relationship to cytokine profiles. *Gastroenterology* 2005; 128: 541–551.

61 Bausserman M, Michail S. The use of *Lactobacillus* GG in irritable bowel syndrome in children: a double-blind randomized control trial. *J Pediatr* 2005; 147: 197–201.

62 Kim HJ, Vazquez-Roque MI, Camilleri M, *et al.* A randomized controlled trial of a probiotic combination VSL#3 and placebo in irritable bowel syndrome with bloating. *Neurogastroenterol Motil* 2005; 17: 687–696.

63 Fan YJ, Chen SJ, Yu YC, *et al.* A probiotic treatment containing *Lactobacillus*, *Bifidobacterium* and *Enterococcus* improves IBS symptoms in an open label trial. *J Zhejiang Univ Sci B* 2006; 7: 987–991.

64 Niv E, Naftali T, Hallak R, Vaisman N. The efficacy of *Lactobacillus reuteri* ATCC 55730 in the treatment of patients with irritable bowel

syndrome – a double blind, placebo-controlled, randomized study. *Clin Nutr* 2005; 24: 925–931.

65 Bittner AC, Croffut RM, Stranahan MC. Prescript-Assist probiotic-prebiotic treatment for irritable bowel syndrome: a methodologically oriented, 2-week, randomized, placebo-controlled, doubleblind clinical study. *Clin Ther* 2005; 27: 75–61.

66 Kajander K, Hatakka K, Poussa T, *et al.* A probiotic mixture alleviates symptoms in irritable bowel syndrome patients: a controlled 6-month intervention. *Aliment Pharmacol Ther* 2005; 22: 387–394.

67 Rousseaux C, Thuru X, Gelot A, *et al.* *Lactobacillus acidophilus* modulates intestinal pain and induces opioid and cannabinoid receptors. *Nat Med* 2007; 13: 35–37.

68 Whorwell PJ, Altringer L, Morel J, *et al.* Efficacy of an encapsulated probiotic *Bifidobacterium infantis* 35624 in women with irritable bowel syndrome. *Am J Gastroenterol* 2006; 101(7): 1581–1590.

69 Guyonnet D, Woodcock A, Stefani B, *et al.* Fermented milk containing *Bifidobacterium lactis* DN-173 010 improved self-reported digestive comfort amongst a general population of adults. A randomized, open-label, controlled, pilot study. *J Dig Dis* 2009; 10(1): 61–70.

70 Drouault-Holowacz S, Bieuvelet S, Burckel A, *et al.* A double blind randomized controlled trial of a probiotic combination in 100 patients with irritable bowel syndrome. *Gastroenterol Clin Biol* 2008; 32(2): 147–152.

71 McFarland LV, Dublin S. Meta-analysis of probiotics for the treatment of irritable bowel syndrome. *World J Gastroenterol* 2008; 14(17): 2650–2661.

72 Moayyedi P, Ford AC, Talley NJ, *et al.* The efficacy of probiotics in the treatment of irritable bowel syndrome: a systematic review. *Gut* 2008; 59(3): 325–332.

73 Nikfar S, Rahimi R, Rahimi F, *et al.* Efficacy of probiotics in irritable bowel syndrome: a meta-analysis of randomized, controlled trials. *Dis Colon Rectum* 2008; 51(12): 1775–1780.

74 Brenner DM, Moeller MJ, Chey WD, *et al.* The utility of probiotics in the treatment of irritable bowel syndrome: a systematic review. *Am J Gastroenterol* 2 009; 104(4): 1033–1049; quiz 1050.

75 Hoveyda N, Heneghan C, Mahtani KR, *et al.* A systematic review and meta-analysis: probiotics in the treatment of irritable bowel syndrome. *BMC Gastroenterol* 2009; 9(15): 15.

76 Furrie E, Macfarlane S, Kennedy A, *et al.* Synbiotic therapy (*Bifidobacterium longum/*Synergy 1) initiates resolution of inflammation in patients with active ulcerative colitis: a randomised controlled pilot trial. *Gut* 2005; 54: 242–249.

77 Kato K, Misumo S, Umesaki Y, *et al.* Randomized placebo-controlled trial assessing the effect of bifidobacteria-fermented milk on active ulcerative colitis. *Aliment Pharmacol Ther* 2004; 20: 11333–11341.

78 Laake KO, Bjorneklett A, Aamodt G, *et al.* Outcome of four weeks' intervention with probiotics on symptoms and endoscopic appearance after surgical reconstruction with a J-configured ilealpouch-anal anastomosis in ulcerative colitis. *Scand J Gastroenterol* 2005; 40: 43–51.

79 Kruis W, Schutz E, Fric P, *et al.* Double-blind comparison of an oral *Escherichia coli* preparation and mesalazine in maintaining remission of ulcerative colitis. *Aliment Pharmacol Ther* 1997; 11: 853–858.

80 Kruis W, Fric P, Pokrotnieks J, *et al.* Maintaining remission of ulcerative colitis with the probiotic *Escherichia coli* Nissle 1917 is as effective as standard mesalazine. *Gut* 2004; 53: 1617–1623.

81 Tursi A, Brandimarte G, Giorgetti GM, *et al.* Low dose balsalazide plus a high-potency probiotic preparation is more effective than balsalazide alone or mesalazine in the treatment of acute mild to moderate ulcerative colitis. *Med Sci Monit* 2004; 10: 1126–1131.

82 Hanai H, Kanauchi O, Mitsuyama K, *et al.* Germinated barley foodstuff prolongs remission in patients with ulcerative colitis. *Int J Mol Med* 2004; 13: 643–647.

83 Ishikawa H, Akedo I, Umesaki Y, *et al.* Randomized controlled trial of the effect of bifidobacteria fermented milk on ulcerative colitis. *J Am Coll Nutr* 2003; 22: 53–63.

84 Rembacken BJ, Snellin Am Hawkey PM, *et al.* Non-pathogenic *Escherichia coli* versus mesalazine for the treatment of ulcerative colitis: a randomised trial. *Lancet* 1999; 354: 635–639.

85 Venturi A, Gionchetti P, Rizzello F, *et al.* Impact on the composition of the faecal flora by a new probiotic preparation: preliminary data on maintenance treatment of patients with ulcerative colitis. *Aliment Pharmacol Ther* 1999; 13(8): 1103–1108.

86 Bibiloni R, Fedorak RN, Tannock GW, *et al.* VSL3 probiotic-mixture induces remission in patients with active ulcerative colitis. *Am J Gastroenterol* 2005; 100(7): 1539–1546.

87 Guslandi M, Giollo P, Testoni PA. A pilot trial of *Saccharomyces boulardii* in ulcerative colitis. *Eur J Gastroenterol Hepatol* 2003; 15(6): 697–698.

88 Cui HH, Chen CL, Wang JD, *et al.* Effects of probiotic on intestinal mucosa of patients with ulcerative colitis. *World J Gastroenterol* 2004; 10(10): 1521–1525.

89 Zocco MA, dal Verme LZ, Cremonini F, *et al.* Efficacy of *Lactobacillus* GG in maintaining remission of ulcerative colitis. *Aliment Pharmacol Ther* 2006; 23(11): 1567–1574.

90 Hegazy SK, El-Bedewy MM. Effect of probiotics on pro-inflammatory cytokines and NF-κB activation in ulcerative colitis. *World J Gastroenterol* 2010; 16(33): 4145–4151.

91 Gionchetti P, Rizzello F, Venturi A, *et al.* Oral bacteriotherapy as maintenance treatment in

patients with chronic pouchitis: a double-blind, placebo-controlled trial. *Gastroenterology* 2000; 119(2): 305–309.

92 Gionchetti P, Rizzello F, Helwig U, *et al.* Prophylaxis of pouchitis onset with probiotic therapy: a double-blind, placebo-controlled trial. *Gastroenterology* 2003; 124(5): 1202–1209.

93 Mimura T, Rizzello F, Helwig U, *et al.* Once daily high dose probiotic therapy (VSL3) for maintaining remission in recurrent or refractory pouchitis. *Gut* 2004; 53(1): 108–114.

94 Laake KO, Line PD, Aabakken L, *et al.* Assessment of mucosal inflammation and circulation in response to probiotics in patients operated with ileal pouch anal anastomosis for ulcerative colitis. *Scand J Gastroenterol* 2003; 38(4): 409–414.

95 Laake KO, Line PD, Grzyb K, *et al.* Assessment of mucosal inflammation and blood flow in response to four weeks' intervention with probiotics in patients operated with a J-configurated ileal-pouch-anal-anastomosis (IPAA). *Scand J Gastroenterol* 2004; 39(12): 1228–1235.

96 Gosselink MP, Schouten WR, van Lieshout LM, *et al.* Delay of the first onset of pouchitis by oral intake of the probiotic strain *Lactobacillus rhamnosus* GG. *Dis Colon Rectum* 2004; 47(6): 876–884.

97 Guslandi M, Mezzi G, Sorghi M, Testoni PA. *Saccharomyces boulardii* in maintenance treatment of Crohn's disease. *Dig Dis Sci* 2000; 45: 1462–1464.

98 Prantera C, Scribano ML, Flasco G, Andreoli A, Luzi C. Ineffectiveness of probiotics in preventing recurrence after curative resection for Crohn's disease: a randomised controlled trial with *Lactobacillus* GG. *Gut* 2002; 51: 405–409.

99 Schultz M, Timmer A, Herfarth HH, *et al.* *Lactobacillus* GG in inducing and maintaining remission of Crohn's disease. *BMC Gastroenterol* 2004; 4: 5.

100 Bousvaros A, Guandalini S, Baldassano RN, *et al.* A randomized, double-blind trial of *Lactobacillus* GG versus placebo in addition to standard maintenance therapy for children with Crohn's disease. *Inflamm Bowel Dis* 2005; 11: 833–839.

101 Marteau P, Lemann M, Seksik P, *et al.* Ineffectiveness of *Lactobacillus johnsonii* LA1 for prophylaxis of postoperative recurrence in Crohn's disease: a randomised, double-blind, placebo controlled GETAID trial. *Gut* 2006; 55(6): 842–847 .

102 Rahimi R, Nikfar S, Rahimi F, *et al.* A meta-analysis on the efficacy of probiotics for maintenance of remission and prevention of clinical and endoscopic relapse in Crohn's disease. *Dig Dis Sci* 2008; 53(9): 2524–2531.

103 Cruchet S, Obregon MC, Salazar G, *et al.* Effect of ingestion of a dietary product containing *Lactobacillus johnsonii* La1 on *Helicobacter*

pylori colonization in children. *Nutrition* 2003; 19: 716–721.

104 Felley CP, Corthesy-Theulaz I, Rivero JL, *et al.* Favourable effect of an acidified milk (LC-1) on *Helicobacter pylori* gastritis in man. *Eur J Gastroenterol Hepatol* 2001; 13(1): 25–29.

105 Pantoflickova D, Corthesy-Theulaz I, Dorta G, *et al.* Favourable effect of regular intake of fermented milk containing *Lactobacillus johnsonii* on *Helicobacter pylori* associated gastritis. *Aliment Pharmacol Ther* 2003; 18(8): 805–813.

106 Wang KY, Li SN, Liu CS, *et al.* Effects of ingesting *Lactobacillus*- and *Bifidobacterium*-containing yogurt in subjects with colonized *Helicobacter pylori*. *Am J Clin Nutr* 2004; 80: 737–741.

107 Sheu BS, Wu JJ, Lo CY, *et al.* Impact of supplement with *Lactobacillus*- and *Bifidobacterium*-containing yogurt on triple therapy for *Helicobacter pylori* eradication. *Aliment Pharmacol Ther* 2002; 16(9): 1669–1675.

108 Sykora J, Valeckova K, Amlerova J, *et al.* Effects of a specially designed fermented milk product containing probiotic *Lactobacillus casei* DN-114001 and the eradication of *H. pylori* in children: a prospective double-blind study. *J Clin Gastroenterol* 2005; 39: 692–698.

109 Gotteland M, Poliak L, Cruchet S, Brunser O. Effect of regular ingestion of *Saccharomyces boulardii* plus inulin or *Lactobacillus acidophilus* LB in children colonized by *Helicobacter pylori*. *Acta Paediatr* 2005; 94: 1747–1751.

110 Song MJ, Park DI, Park JH, *et al.* The effect of probiotics and mucoprotective agents on PPI-based triple therapy for eradication of *Helicobacter pylori*. *Helicobacter* 2010; 15(3): 206–213.

111 Sheu B-S, Cheng H-C, Kao A-W, *et al.* Pretreatment with *Lactobacillus* and *Bifidobacterium*-containing yogurt can improve the efficacy of quadruple therapy in eradicating residual *Helicobacter pylori* infection after failed triple therapy. *Am J Clin Nutr* 2006; 83: 864–869.

112 Cats A, Kuipers EJ, Bosschaert MA, *et al.* Effect of frequent consumption of a *Lactobacillus casei*-containing milk drink in *Helicobacter pylori*-colonized subjects. *Aliment Pharmacol Ther* 2003; 17(3): 429–435.

113 Kim MN, Kim N, Lee SH, *et al.* The effects of probiotics on PPI-triple therapy for *Helicobacter pylori* eradication. *Helicobacter* 2008; 13(4): 261–268.

114 Yasar B, Abut E, Kayadibi H, *et al.* Efficacy of probiotics in *Helicobacter pylori* eradication therapy. *Turk J Gastroenterol* 2010; 21(3): 212–217.

115 Nista EC, Candelli M, Cremonini GF, *et al.* *Bacillus clausii* therapy to reduce side effects of anti-*Helicobacter pylori* treatment: randomized, double-blind, placebo-controlled trial. *Aliment Pharmacol Ther* 2004; 20: 1181–1188.

116 Tursi A, Barndimarte G, Giogetti GM, Modeo ME. Effect of *Lactobacillus casei* supplementation on the effectiveness and tolerability of a new

secondline 10-day quadruple therapy after failure of a first attempt to cure *Helicobacter pylori* infection. *Med Sci Monit* 2004; 10: CR662–CR666.

117 Armuzzi A, Cremonini F, Bartolozzi F, *et al.* The effect of oral administration of *Lactobacillus* GG on antibiotic-associated gastrointestinal side-effects during *Helicobacter pylori* eradication therapy. *Aliment Pharmacol Ther* 2001; 15(2): 163–169.

118 Cremonini F, Di Caro S, Covino M, *et al.* Effect of different probiotic preparations on anti-*Helicobacter pylori* therapy-related side effects: a parallel group, triple blind, placebo-controlled strudy. *Am J Gastroenterol* 2002; 97: 2744–2749.

119 Myllyloma E, Veijola L, Ahlroos T, *et al.* Probiotic supplementation improves tolerance to *Helicobacter pylori* eradication therapy – a placebocontrolled, double-blind randomized pilot study. *Aliment Pharmacol Ther* 2005; 21: 1263–1272.

120 Gotteland M, Brunser O, Cruchet S. Systematic review: are probiotics useful in controlling gastric colonization by *Helicobacter pylori*? *Aliment Pharmacol Ther* 2006; 23: 1077–1086.

121 Zou J, Dong J, Yu X. Meta-analysis. *Lactobacillus* containing quadruple therapy versus standard triple first-line therapy for *Helicobacter pylori* eradication. *Helicobacter* 2009; 14(5): 97–107.

122 Schiffrin EJ, Rochat F, Link-Amster H, *et al.* Immunomodulation of human blood cells following the ingestion of lactic acid bacteria. *J Dairy Sci* 1995; 78: 491–497.

123 Majaama M, Isolauri E. Probiotics. a novel approach in the management of food allergy. *J Allergy Clin Immunol* 1997; 99: 179–185.

124 Galdeano CM, Perdigon G. The probiotic bacterium *Lactobacillus casei* induces activation of the gut mucosal immune system through innate immunity. *Clin Vaccine Immunol* 2006; 13: 219–226.

125 Kim YG, Ohta T, Takahashi T, *et al.* Probiotic *Lactobacillus casei* activates innate immunity via NFkappaB and p38 MAP kinase signalling pathways. *J Microbes Infect* 2006; 8: 994–1004.

126 Berman SH, Eichelsdoerfer P, Yim D, *et al.* Daily ingestion of a nutritional probiotic supplement enhances innate immune function in healthy adults. *Nutrition Research* 2006; 9: 454–459.

127 Marcos A, Warnberg J, Nova E, *et al.* The effect of milk fermented by yogurt cultures plus *Lactobacillus casei* DN-11401 on the immune response of subjects under academic examination stress. *Eur J Nutr* 2004; 43: 381–389.

128 Olivares M, Diaz-Ropero MP, Gomez N, *et al.* The consumption of two new probiotic strains, *Lactobacillus gasseri* CECT 5714 and *Lactobacillus coryniformis* CECT 5711 boosts the immune system of healthy humans. *Int Microbiol* 2006; 9: 47–52.

129 Parra MD, Martinez de Morentin BE, Cobo JM, *et al.* Daily ingestion of fermented milk containing *Lactobacillus casei* DN114001 improves innate defense capacity in healthy middle-aged people. *J Physiol Biochem* 2004; 60: 85–91.

130 Parra D, Morentin BM, Cobo JM, *et al.* Monocyte function in healthy middle-aged people receiving fermented milk containing *Lactobacillus casei*. *J Nutr Health Aging* 2004; 8: 208–211.

131 Pessi T, Sutas Y, Hurme M, *et al.* Interleukin-10 generation in atopic children following oral *Lactobacillus rhamnosus* GG. *Clin Exp Allergy* 2000; 30(12): 1804–1808.

132 Kalliomaki M, Salminen S, Poussa T, *et al.* Probiotics and prevention of atopic disease: 4-year follow-up of a randomised placebo-controlled trial. *Lancet* 2003; 361(9372): 1869–1871.

133 Kirjavainen PV, Salminen SJ, Isolauri E. Probiotic bacteria in the management of atopic disease: underscoring the importance of viability. *J Pediatr Gastroenterol Nutr* 2003; 36(2): 223–227.

134 Pohjavuori E, Viljanen M, Korpela R, *et al.* *Lactobacillus* GG effect in increasing IFN-gamma production in infants with cow's milk allergy. *J Allergy Clin Immunol* 2004; 114(1): 131–136.

135 Viljanen M, Kuitunen M, Haahtela T, *et al.* Probiotic effects on faecal inflammatory markers and on faecal IgA in food allergic atopic eczema/ dermatitis syndrome infants. *Pediatr Allergy Immunol* 2005; 16(1): 65–71.

136 Isolauri E, Arvola T, Sutas Y, *et al.* Probiotics in the management of atopic eczema. *Clin Exp Allergy* 2000; 30: 1604–1610.

137 Rosenfeldt V, Benfeldt E, Nielsen SD, *et al.* Effect of probiotic *Lactobacillus* strains in children with atopic dermatitis. *J Allergy Clin Immunol* 2003; 111: 389–395.

138 Sistek D, Kelly R, Wickens K, *et al.* Is the effect of probiotics on atopic dermatitis confined to food sensitized children? *Clin Exp Allergy* 2006; 36(5): 629–633.

139 Kim JY, Kwon JH, Ahn SH, *et al.* Effect of probiotic mix (*Bifidobacterium bifidum*, *Bifidobacterium lactis*, *Lactobacillus acidophilus*) in the primary prevention of eczema: a double-blind, randomized, placebo-controlled trial. *Pediatr Allergy Immunol* 2009; 21(2): e386–e393.

140 Weston S, Halbert A, Richmond P, Prescott SL. Effects of probiotics on atopic dermatitis: a randomized controlled trial. *Arch Dis Child* 2005; 892–897.

141 Viljanen M, Savilahti E, Haahtela T, *et al.* Probiotics in the treatment of atopic eczema/dermatitis syndrome in infants: a double-blind placebo controlled trial. *Allergy* 2005; 60: 494–500.

142 Abrahamsson TR, Jakobsson T, Böttcher MF, *et al.* Probiotics in prevention of IgE-associated eczema: a double-blind, randomized, placebo-controlled trial. *J Allergy Clin Immunol* 2007; 119: 1174–1180.

143 Kukkonen K, Savilahti E, Haahtela T, *et al.* Probiotics and prebiotic galacto-oligosaccharides

in the prevention of allergic diseases: a random-ized, double-blind, placebo-controlled trial. *J Allergy Clin Immunol* 2007; 119: 192–198.

144 Rosenfeldt V, Benfeldt E, Valerius NH, *et al.* Effect of probiotics on gastrointestinal symp-toms and small intestinal permeability in chil-dren with atopic dermatitis. *J Pediatr* 2004; 145: 612–616.

145 Rose MA, Stieglitz F, Koksal A, *et al.* Efficacy of probiotic *Lactobacillus* GG on allergic sensitiza-tion and asthma in infants at risk. *Clin Exp Allergy* 2010; 40(9): 1398–1405.

146 Kalliomaki M, Salkminen S, Arvilommi H, *et al.* Probiotics in primary prevention of atopic disease: a randomized placebo-controlled trial. *Lancet* 2001; 357: 1076–1079.

147 Wickens K, Black PN, Stanley TV, *et al.* A differ-ential effect of 2 probiotics in the prevention of eczema and atopy: a double-blind, randomized, placebo-controlled trial. *J Allergy Clin Immunol* 2008; 122(4): 788–794.

148 Dotterud CK, Storro O, Johnsen R, *et al.* Probiotics in pregnant women to prevent allergic disease: a randomized, double-blind trial. *Br J Dermatol* 2010; 163(3): 616–623.

149 Rautava S, Kalliomaki M, Isolauri E. Probiotics during pregnancy and breast-feeding might confer immunomodulatory protection against atopic dis-ease in the infant. *J Allergy Clin Immunol* 2002; 109: 119–121.

150 Osborn DA, Sinn JK. Probiotics in infants for pre-vention of allergic disease and food hypersensitivity. *Cochrane Database Syst Rev* 2007; (4): CD006475.

151 Michail SK, Stolfi A, Johnson T, *et al.* Efficacy of probiotics in the treatment of pediatric atopic der-matitis: a meta-analysis of randomized controlled trials. *Ann Allergy Asthma Immunol* 2008; 101 (5): 508–516.

152 Boyle RJ, Bath-Hextall FJ, Leonardi-Bee J, *et al.* Probiotics for the treatment of eczema: a systematic review. *Clin Exp Allergy* 2009; 39(8): 1117–1127.

153 Wang MF, Lin HC, Wang YY, Hus CH. Treatment of perennial allergic rhinitis with lactic acid bacteria. *Pediatr Allergy Immunol* 2004; 15: 152–158.

154 Peng GC, Hsu CH. The efficacy and safety of heat-killed *Lactobacillus paracasei* for treatment of perennial allergic rhinitis induced by house-dust mite. *Pediatr Allergy Immunol* 2005; 16: 433–438.

155 Chen YS, Jan RL, Lin YL, *et al.* Randomized placebo-controlled trial of *Lactobacillus* on asth-matic children with allergic rhinitis. *Pediatr Pulmonol* 2010; 45(11): 1111–1120.

156 Shalev E, Battino S, Weiner E, *et al.* Ingestion of yogurt containing *Lactobacillus acidophilus* com-pared with pasteurized yoghurt as prophylaxis for recurrent candidal vaginitis and bacterial vagino-sis. *Arch Fam Med* 1996; 5: 593–596.

157 De Simone C, Ciardi A, Grassi A, *et al.* Effect of *Bifidobacterium bifidum* and *Lactobacillus*

acidophilus on gut mucosa and peripheral blood B lymphocytes. *Immunopharmacol Immunotoxi-col* 1992; 14: 331–340.

158 Pirotta M, Gunn J, Chondros P, *et al.* Effect of *Lactobacillus* in preventing post-antibiotic vulvo-vaginal candidiasis: a randomised controlled trial. *BMJ* 2004; 329: 548.

159 Marcone V, Rocca G, Lichtner M, *et al.* Long-term vaginal administration of *Lactobacillus rhamnosus* as a complementary approach to man-agement of bacterial vaginosis. *Int J Gynaecol Obstet* 2010; 110(3): 223–226.

160 Rossi A, Rossi T, Bertini M, *et al.* The use of *Lactobacillus rhamnosus* in the therapy of bacter-ial vaginosis. Evaluation of clinical efficacy in a population of 40 women treated for 24 months. *Arch Gynecol Obstet* 2010; 281(6): 1065–1069.

161 Anderson JW, Gillialand SE. Effect of fermented milk (yogurt) containing *Lactobacillus acidophil-us* L1 on serum cholesterol by hypercholesterol-emic humans. *J Am Coll Nutr* 1999; 18: 43–50.

162 Schaafsma G, Meuling WJ, van Dokkum W, Bouley C. Effects of a milk product, fermented by *Lactobacillus acidophilus* and with fructo-oligosaccharides added, on blood lipids in male volunteers. *Eur J Clin Nutr* 1998; 52: 436–440.

163 Davidson MH, Maki KC, Synecki C. Evaluation of the influence of dietary inulin on serum lipids in adults with hypercholesterolemia. *Nutrition* 1998; 18: 503–517.

164 Mital BK, Garg SK. Anticarcinogenic, hypochol-esterolemic and antagonistic activities of *Lactobacillus acidophilus*. *Crit Rev Microbiol* 1995; 21: 175–214.

165 Xiao JZ, Kondo S, Takahashi N, *et al.* Effects of milk products fermented by *Bifidobacterium longum* on blood lipids in rats and healthy adult male volunteers. *J Dairy Sci* 2003; 86: 2452–2461.

166 Kiessling G, Schneider J, Jahreis G. Long-term consumption of fermented dairy products over 6 months increases HDL cholesterol. *Eur J Clin Nutr* 2002; 56: 843–849.

167 Greany KA, Nettleton JA, Wangen KE, *et al.* Probiotic consumption does not enhance the chol-esterol lowering effect of soy in postmenopausal women. *J Nutr* 2004; 134: 3277–3283.

168 Lewis SJ, Burmeister S. A double-blind placebo-controlled study of the effects of *Lactobacillus acidophilus* on plasma lipids. *Eur J Clin Nutr* 2005; 59: 776–780.

169 Naruszewicz M, Johansson ML, Zapolska-Downar D, Bukowska H. Effect of *Lactobacillus plantarum* 299v on cardiovascular disease risk factors in smokers. *Am J Clin Nutr* 2002; 76: 1249–1255.

170 Aihara K, Kajimoto O, Hirata H, *et al.* Effect of powdered fermented milk with *Lactobacillus helveticus* on subjects with high-normal blood pressure or mild hypertension. *J Am Coll Nutr* 2005; 24: 257–265.

171 Coudray C, Bellanger J, Catiglia-Delavaud C, *et al.* Effect of soluble and partly soluble dietary fibres supplementation on absorption and balance of calcium, magnesium, iron and zinc in healthy young men. *Eur J Clin Nutr* 1997; 51: 375–380.

172 van den Heuvel EGHM, Muys T, van Dokkum W, Schaafsma G. Oligofructose stimulates calcium absorption in adolescents. *Am J Clin Nutr* 1999; 69: 544–548.

173 Abrams SA, Griffin IJ, Hawthorne KM, *et al.* A combination of prebiotic short- and long-chain inulin-type fructans enhances calcium absorption and bone mineralization in young adolescents. *Am J Clin Nutr* 2005; 82: 471–476.

174 Gluck U, Gebbers JO. Ingested probiotics reduce nasal colonization with pathogenic bacteria (*Staphylococcus aureus, Streptococcus pneumoniae* and beta-hemolytic streptococci). *Am J Clin Nutr* 2003; 77: 517–520.

175 de Vrese M, Winkler P, Rautenberg P, *et al.* Effect of *Lactobacillus gasseri* PA 16/8, *Bifidobacterium longum* SP07/3, *B. bifidum* MF 20/5 on common cold episodes: a double-blind, randomized, controlled trial. *Clin Nutr* 2005; 24: 481–491.

176 Taipale T, Pienihakkinen K, Isolauri E, *et al.* *Bifidobacterium animalis* subsp. *lactis* BB-12 in reducing the risk of infections in infancy. *Br J Nutr* 2011; 105(3): 409–416.

177 Namba K, Hatano M, Yaeshima T, *et al.* Effects of *Bifidobacterium longum* BB536 administration on influenza infection, influenza vaccine antibody titer, and cell-mediated immunity in the elderly. *Biosci Biotechnol Biochem* 2010; 74(5): 939–945.

178 Makino S, Ikegami S, Kume A, *et al.* Reducing the risk of infection in the elderly by dietary intake of yoghurt fermented with *Lactobacillus delbrueckii* ssp. *bulgaricus* OLL1073R-1. *Br J Nutr* 2010; 104 (7): 998–1006.

179 Bekkali NL, Bongers ME, Van den Berg MM, *et al.* The role of a probiotics mixture in the treatment of childhood constipation: a pilot study. *Nutr J* 2007; 6: 17.

180 Tabbers MM, Chmielewska A, Roseboom MG, *et al.* Effect of the consumption of a fermented dairy product containing *Bifidobacterium lactis* DN-173 010 on constipation in childhood: a multicentre randomised controlled trial (NTRTC. 1571). *BMC Pediatr* 2009; 9(22): 22.

181 Deshpande G, Rao S, Patole S. Probiotics for prevention of necrotising enterocolitis in preterm neonates with very low birthweight: a systematic review of randomised controlled trials. *Lancet* 2007; 369: 1614–1620.

182 Savino F, Pelle E, Palumeri E, *et al.* *Lactobacillus reuteri* (American Type Culture Collection Strain 55 730) versus simethicone in the treatment of infantile colic: a prospective randomized study. *Pediatrics* 2007; 119: e124–130.

183 Bruzzese E, Raia V, Spagnuolo MI, *et al.* Effect of *Lactobacillus* GG supplementation on pulmonary exacerbations in patients with cystic fibrosis: a pilot study. *Clin Nutr* 2007; 26: 322–328.

184 Watkinson PJ, Barber VS, Dark P, Young JD. The use of pre- pro- and synbiotics in adult intensive care unit patients: systematic review. *Clin Nutr* 2007; 26: 182–192.

185 Alberda C, Gramlich L, Meddings J, *et al.* Effects of probiotic therapy in critically ill patients: a randomized, double-blind, placebo-controlled trial. *Am J Clin Nutr* 2007; 85: 816–823.

186 Hatakka K, Ahola AJ, Yli-Knuuttila H, *et al.* Probiotics reduce the prevalence of oral candida in the elderly–a randomized controlled trial. *J Dent Res* 2007; 86: 125–130.

187 Hatakka K, Blomgren K, Pohjavuori S, *et al.* Treatment of acute otitis media with probiotics in otitis prone children: a double-blind, placebo-controlled randomised study. *Clin Nutr* 2007; 26: 314–321.

188 Diopa L, Guilloub S, Durandc H. Probiotic food supplement reduces stress-induced gastrointestinal symptoms in volunteers: a double-blind, placebo controlled, randomized trial. *Nutr Res* 2008; 28: 1–5.

189 Rafter J, Bennett M, Caderni G, *et al.* Dietary synbiotics reduce cancer risk factors in polypecto-mized and colon cancer patients. *Am J Clin Nutr* 2007; 85: 488–496.

190 Akil I, Yilmaz O, Kurutepe S, *et al.* Influence of oral intake of *Saccharomyces boulardii* on *Escherichia coli* in enteric flora. *Pediatr Nephrol* 2006; 21: 807–810.

191 Ezendam J, van Loveren H. Probiotics: immunomodulation and evaluation of safety and efficacy. *Nutr Rev* 2006; 64(1): 1–14.

192 Senok AC, Ismaeel AY, Botta GA. Probiotics: facts and myths. *Clin Microbiol Infect* 2005; 11 (12): 958–966.

193 Hammerman C, Bin-Nun A, Kaplan M. Safety of probiotics: comparison of two popular strains. *BMJ* 2006; 333(7576): 1006–1008.

194 Boyle RJ, Robins-Browne RM, Tang ML. Probiotic use in clinical practice: what are the risks? *Am J Clin Nutr* 2006; 83(6): 1256–1264 quiz 1446–1447.

195 Salazar-Lindo E, Miranda-Langschwager P, Campos-Sanchez M, *et al.* *Lactobacillus casei* strain GG in the treatment of infants with acute watery diarrhea: a randomized, double-blind, placebo controlled clinical trial [ISRCTN67363048]. *BMC Pediatr* 2004; 4: 18.

196 Billoo AG, Memon MA, Khaskheli SA, *et al.* Role of a probiotic (*Saccharomyces boulardii*) in management and prevention of diarrhoea. *World J Gastroenterol* 2006; 12(28): 4557–4560.

197 Sazawal S, Hiremath G, Dhingra U, *et al.* Efficacy of probiotics in prevention of acute diarrhoea: a meta-analysis of masked, randomised, placebo-controlled trials. *Lancet Infect Dis* 2006; 6(6): 374–382.

198 Johnston BC, Supina AL, Vohra S. Probiotics for pediatric antibiotic-associated diarrhea: a meta-

analysis of randomized placebo-controlled trials. *CMAJ* 2006; 175(4): 377–383.

199 Szajewska H, Ruszczynski M, Radzikowski A. Probiotics in the prevention of antibiotic-associated diarrhea in children: a meta-analysis of randomized controlled trials. *J Pediatr* 2006; 149(3): 367–372.

200 Safdar N, Barigala R, Said A, *et al.* Feasibility and tolerability of probiotics for prevention of antibiotic-associated diarrhoea in hospitalized US military veterans. *J Clin Pharm Ther* 2008; 33(6): 663–668.

201 Kale-Pradhan PB, Jassal HK, Wilhelm SM. Role of *Lactobacillus* in the prevention of antibiotic-associated diarrhea: a meta-analysis. *Pharmacotherapy* 2010; 30(2): 119–26.

202 O'Sullivan MA, O'Morain CA. Bacterial supplementation in the irritable bowel syndrome. A randomised double-blind placebo-controlled crossover study. *Dig Liver Dis* 2000; 32(4): 294–301.

203 Kim YG, Moon JT, Lee KM, *et al.* [The effects of probiotics on symptoms of irritable bowel syndrome]. *Korean J Gastroenterol* 2006; 47(6): 413–419.

204 Zigra PI, Maipa VE, Alamanos YP. Probiotics and remission of ulcerative colitis: a systematic review. *Neth J Med* 2007; 65(11): 411–418.

205 Sang LX, Chang B, Zhang WL, *et al.* Remission induction and maintenance effect of probiotics on ulcerative colitis: a meta-analysis. *World J Gastroenterol* 2010; 16(15): 1908–1915.

206 Gupta P, Andrew H, Kirschner BS, *et al.* Is *Lactobacillus* GG helpful in children with Crohn's disease? Results of a preliminary, open-label study *J Pediatr Gastroenterol Nutr* 2000; 31(4): 453–457.

207 Guandalini S. Use of *Lactobacillus*-GG in paediatric Crohn's disease. *Dig Liver Dis* 2002; 34 (Suppl 20): S63–S65.

208 Canducci F, Armuzzi A, Cremonini F, *et al.* A lyophilized and inactivated culture of

Lactobacillus acidophilus increases *Helicobacter pylori* eradication rates. *Aliment Pharmacol Ther* 2000; 14: 1625–1629.

209 Kirjavainen PV, Arvola T, Salminen SJ, *et al.* Aberrant composition of gut microbiota of allergic infants: a target of bifidobacterial therapy at weaning? *Gut* 2002; 51(1): 51–55.

210 Viljanen M, Pohjavuori E, Haahtela T, *et al.* Induction of inflammation as a possible mechanism of probiotic effect in atopic eczema-dermatitis syndrome. *J Allergy Clin Immunol* 2005; 115(6): 1254–1259.

211 Brouwer ML, Wolt-Plompen SA, Dubois AE, *et al.* No effects of probiotics on atopic dermatitis in infancy: a randomized placebo-controlled trial. *Clin Exp Allergy* 2006; 36(7): 899–906.

212 Boyle RJ, Bath-Hextall FJ, Leonardi-Bee J, *et al.* Probiotics for treating eczema. *Cochrane Database Syst Rev* 2008; 8(4): CD006135.

213 Kuitunen M, Kukkonen K, Juntunen-Backman K, *et al.* Probiotics prevent IgE-associated allergy until age 5 years in cesarean-delivered children but not in the total cohort. *J Allergy Clin Immunol* 2009; 123(2): 335–341.

214 West CE, Hammarstrom ML, Hernell O. Probiotics during weaning reduce the incidence of eczema. *Pediatr Allergy Immunol* 2009; 20(5): 430–437.

215 Ezendam J, van Loveren H. Probiotics: immunomodulation and evaluation of safety and efficacy. *Nutr Rev* 2006; 64: 1–14.

216 Senok AC, Ismaeel AY, Botta GA. Probiotics: facts and myths. *Clin Microbiol Infect* 2005; 11: 958–966.

217 Hammerman C, Bin-Nun A, Kaplan M. Safety of probiotics: comparison of two popular strains. *BMJ* 2006; 333: 1006–1008.

218 Boyle RJ, Robins-Browne RM, Tang ML. Probiotic use in clinical practice: what are the risks? *Am J Clin Nutr* 2006; 83: 1256–1264; quiz 1446–1447.

Psyllium

Description

Psyllium (ispaghula) is the mucilage obtained from the seed coat (husk or hull) of *Plantago ovata*. It is a rich source of dietary fibre.

Constituents

The main active ingredient in psyllium is a water-soluble, gel-forming polysaccharide, which appears chemically to be a highly branched arabinoxylan, with the main chain of 1,4-linked xylopyranose residues densely substituted with either single xylose units or trisaccharides. The arabinoxylan has been found to contain 74.1% xylose, 22.4% arabinose, 1.8% galactose and trace amounts of glucose, rhamnose and uronic acid.[1]

Action

The water-soluble polysaccharide in psyllium forms a viscous gel in the intestine. As a result of this gel formation, psyllium has several effects, acting to:

- stimulate peristalsis, reduce gastrointestinal transit time, increase stool weight and function as a bulk laxative;[2,3]
- lubricate the stools, so facilitating defecation;[4]
- increase the water-absorbing capacity and viscosity of the faeces, delaying gastric emptying time and improving the consistency of the faeces in both diarrhoea and constipation;[2,5]
- reduce the production of gastric acid;
- prolong gastrointestinal transit time in cases of diarrhoea, possibly by delaying the production of gaseous fermentation products;[5]
- reduce serum cholesterol by elimination of cholesterol in bile acids[6] and reducing absorption of dietary fats;[7,8]
- delay the rate of absorption of carbohydrates, which can reduce post-meal blood glucose levels in patients with diabetes mellitus;[9,10] and
- decrease glucose, insulin, ghrelin, and peptide YY (PYY) responses after a meal.[11]

Psyllium, like other soluble fibres, appears to be partially fermented by the bacteria in the colon to produce short-chain fatty acids (e.g. butyrate).[5,12]

Possible uses

Psyllium has a long history of use as a dietary fibre supplement to promote the regulation of large bowel function and, more recently, has been shown to lower blood cholesterol levels.

Constipation
Psyllium is effective as a bulk laxative in the management of constipation,[2,4,13,14] and several commercial preparations of ispaghula husk are licensed and prescribable as bulk laxatives in the UK.

Diarrhoea
Psyllium has been shown to improve faecal consistency in patients with diarrhoea.[4,5] Studies in tube-fed patients have also shown an improvement in diarrhoea with psyllium.

Hypercholesterolaemia
Psyllium is effective in reducing serum cholesterol in people with hypercholesterolaemia.

Psyllium 5.1 g twice a day for 8 weeks produced a modest but significant improvement in total cholesterol and LDL cholesterol in men and women on either high- or low-fat diets.[15] In a further study, psyllium 3.4 g three times a day for 8 weeks reduced total and LDL cholesterol in men.[16] Another study with psyllium 6.7 g daily for 2 weeks and a low-fat diet reduced total, LDL, HDL cholesterol and the LDL/HDL ratio with no effect on triglycerides.[8] Further studies have indicated that psyllium supplementation is effective in lowering LDL cholesterol, but has no or limited effect on HDL cholesterol and triglycerides.[17,18] Studies of 6 months' duration have demonstrated the potential for long-term benefit of psyllium in lowering LDL cholesterol.[19,20]

There appear to be some advantages in combining psyllium with other agents: with mono-unsaturated fat to further reduce the LDL/HDL cholesterol ratio,[21] with phytosterols to improve not only overall lipid profile but also lipoprotein particles sizes,[22,23] and with guar to improve lipoprotein profiles and reduce blood pressure.[24]

Trials of psyllium in children have also shown potential benefits in cholesterol lowering.[25,26] Meta-analyses have confirmed the cholesterol-lowering effect of psyllium in adults as an adjunct to a low-fat diet.[27,28] However, a recent meta-analysis of 21 studies that included psyllium with any type of dietary background showed that, compared with placebo, psyllium consumption lowered serum total cholesterol by 0.375 mmol/L (95% confidence interval (CI), 0.257 to 0.494) and LDL cholesterol by 0.278 mmol/L (95% CI, 0.213 to 0.312) in a manner that was both time and dose dependent.[29]

Psyllium supplementation in patients taking 10 mg simvastatin seems to be as effective in lowering cholesterol as 20 mg simvastatin alone.[30] A combination of psyllium and colestipol at half the usual doses lowered cholesterol as effectively as either psyllium or colestipol alone.[31] Addition of psyllium to colestyramine produced further reduction in total and LDL cholesterol levels and also helped to improve compliance by reducing the gastrointestinal side-effects of colestyramine.[32]

Psylliujm has also been shown to reduce exposure to triacylglycerols in the post-meal phase[33] but had no effect on C-reactive protein and fibrinogen.[34]

Diabetes

Preliminary evidence has indicated that psyllium has some influence on post-prandial blood glucose, glycated haemoglobin, insulin, total cholesterol, LDL cholesterol and triacylglycerol in patients with type 2 diabetes and hypercholesterolaemia.[9,10,35–40] However, studies are not totally consistent.

Irritable bowel syndrome

Studies evaluating the effect of psyllium in irritable bowel syndrome (IBS) have produced inconsistent results, with some showing no benefit[41] and others showing benefit.[42–44]

Ulcerative colitis

There is some evidence of benefit of psyllium in ulcerative colitis. It has been shown to be helpful in maintaining remission[45] and to be as effective as mesalazine in maintaining remission.[46] However, a trial of psyllium in juvenile ulcerative colitis patients found no influence on faecal bile acid excretion.[47]

Side-effects of orlistat

In one trial, psyllium has been shown to relieve the side-effects of orlistat (e.g. flatulence, diarrhoea, abdominal cramps, oily discharge).[48]

Conclusion

Psyllium has been well studied for its effect on bowel function, with studies generally showing an increase in stool weight and reduced gastrointestinal transit time in patients with constipation. Faecal consistency is also generally improved in patients with diarrhoea. Psyllium produces a modest reduction in total and LDL cholesterol in patients with hypercholesterolaemia and is effective as an adjunct to dietary management and possibly to drug management. It does not appear to influence HDL cholesterol or triglycerides. In patients with diabetes, psyllium has produced modest reductions in post-prandial blood glucose, glycated haemoglobin and insulin, but further research is needed to confirm these effects. There is conflicting evidence for the value of psyllium in IBS and ulcerative colitis.

Precautions/contraindications

Psyllium is contraindicated in people with conditions causing gastrointestinal obstruction, hypersensitivity to psyllium and swallowing disorders.

Psyllium may cause reduction in blood glucose levels. People with diabetes should be monitored.

Some psyllium preparations are sweetened with aspartame. These products should be avoided in people with phenylketonuria.

Pregnancy and breast-feeding

Psyllium is considered to be safe in pregnancy and breast-feeding, although studies in humans have not been conducted.

Adverse effects

Psyllium can cause flatulence, abdominal pain, bloating, diarrhoea, constipation and nausea. Starting with a dose and building up gradually can help to minimise gastrointestinal effects. Psyllium can also cause gastrointestinal obstruction, especially in patients with dysphagia and other swallowing disorders, but it can occur in anyone, unless it is consumed with plenty of water.

Allergic reactions (e.g. rhinitis, sneezing, headache, conjunctivitis, urticaria, itching, dyspnoea and flushing) can occur. Severe allergic reactions include wheezing, angio-oedema, asthma, cough, diarrhoea and anaphylactic shock.

Interactions

Drugs

Anti-diabetic drugs: psyllium may lower blood glucose and have an additive effect with anti-diabetic drugs.

Aspirin: absorption may be reduced.

Carbamazepine: absorption may be reduced.

Digoxin: absorption may be reduced.

Lithium: absorption may be reduced.

Statins: psyllium may have an additive effect in reducing blood cholesterol.

Warfarin: theoretical risk of reduced absorption, but clinical studies have not demonstrated an effect.

Nutrients

Minerals and vitamins: psyllium may reduce the absorption of all nutrients (in particular minerals such as calcium, iron, zinc and magnesium).

Dose

Wide ranges of doses have been used in studies, but are not clearly established.

- In constipation, 7–40 g daily in two to three divided doses has been used.
- In cholesterol lowering, the most commonly used doses in adults have ranged from 10 to 20 g psyllium daily and in children 5–10 g daily, in two or three divided doses.
- In type 2 diabetes, up to 45 g daily has been given to lower blood glucose.
- For IBS, 6–30 g daily has been used.

For commercial licensed and prescribable preparations of ispaghula, doses can be found in the *British National Formulary*.

Psyllium should always be taken with plenty of fluid and doses avoided just before bedtime (to prevent gastrointestinal obstruction).

References

1   Fischer M, Nanxiong Y, Gray G, *et al.* The gel-forming polysaccharide of psyllium husk. *Carbohydr Res* 2004; 339: 2009–2017.

2   Ashraf W, Park F, Lof J, Quigley EM. Effects of psyllium therapy on stool characteristics, colon transit and anorectal function in chronic idiopathic constipation. *Aliment Pharmacol Ther* 1995; 9: 639–647.

3   Marteau P, Flourie B, Cherbut C, *et al.* Digestibility and bulking effect of ispaghula husks in healthy humans. *Gut* 1994; 35: 1747–1752.

4   Marlett JA, Kajs TM, Fischer MH. An unfermented gel component of psyllium seed husk promotes laxation as a lubricant in humans. *Am J Clin Nutr* 2000; 72: 784–789.

5   Washington N, Harris M, Mussellwhite A, Spiller RC. Moderation of lactulose-induced diarrhea by psyllium: effects on motility and fermentation. *Am J Clin Nutr* 1998; 67: 317–321.

6   Chaplin MF, Chaudhury S, Dettmar PW, *et al.* Effect of ispaghula husk on the faecal output of bile acids in healthy volunteers. *J Steroid Biochem Mol Biol* 2000; 72: 283–292.

7   Ganji V, Kies CV. Psyllium husk fibre supplementation to soybean and coconut oil diets of humans: effect on fat digestibility and faecal fatty acid excretion. *Eur J Clin Nutr* 1994; 48: 595–597.

8   Wolever TM, Jenkins DJ, Mueller S, *et al.* Psyllium reduces blood lipids in men and women with hyperlipidemia. *Am J Med Sci* 1994; 307: 269–273.

9   Anderson JW, Allgood LD, Turner J, *et al.* Effects of psyllium on glucose and serum lipid responses in men with type 2 diabetes and hypercholesterolemia. *Am J Clin Nutr* 1999; 70: 466–473.

10 Wolever TM, Vuksan V, Eshuis H, *et al.* Effect of method of administration of psyllium on glycemic response and carbohydrate digestibility. *J Am Coll Nutr* 1991; 10: 364–371.

11 Karhunen LJ, Juvonen KR, Flander SM, *et al.* A psyllium fiber-enriched meal strongly attenuates postprandial gastrointestinal peptide release in healthy young adults. *J Nutr* 2010; 140(4): 737–744.

12 Wolever TM, Robb PA. Effect of guar, pectin, psyllium, soy polysaccharide, and cellulose on breath hydrogen and methane in healthy subjects. *Am J Gastroenterol* 1992; 87: 305–10.

13 Ashraf W, Pfeiffer RF, Park F, *et al.* Constipation in Parkinson's disease: objective assessment and response to psyllium. *Mov Disord* 1997; 12: 946–951.

14 Marlett JA, Li BU, Patrow CJ, Bass P. Comparative laxation of psyllium with and without senna in an ambulatory constipated population. *Am J Gastroenterol* 1987; 82: 333–337.

15 Sprecher DL, Harris BV, Goldberg AC, *et al.* Efficacy of psyllium in reducing serum cholesterol levels in hypercholesterolemic patients on high- or low-fat diets. *Ann Intern Med* 1993; 119(7Pt1): 545–554.

16 Anderson JW, Zettwoch N, Feldman T, *et al.* Cholesterol-lowering effects of psyllium hydrophilic mucilloid for hypercholesterolemic men. *Arch Intern Med* 1988; 148: 292–296.

17 Anderson JW, Riddell-Mason S, Gustafson NJ, *et al.* Cholesterol-lowering effects of psyllium-enriched cereal as an adjunct to a prudent diet in the treatment of mild to moderate hypercholesterolemia. *Am J Clin Nutr* 1992; 56: 93–98.

18 Roberts DC, Truswell AS, Bencke A, *et al.* The cholesterol-lowering effect of a breakfast cereal containing psyllium fibre. *Med J Aust* 1994; 161: 660–664.

19 Davidson MH, Maki KC, Kong JC, *et al.* Long-term effects of consuming foods containing psyllium seed husk on serum lipids in subjects with hypercholesterolemia. *Am J Clin Nutr* 1998; 67: 367–376.

20 Anderson JW, Davidson MH, Blonde L, *et al.* Long-term cholesterol-lowering effects of psyllium as an adjunct to diet therapy in the treatment of hypercholesterolemia. *Am J Clin Nutr* 2000; 71: 1433–1438.

21 Jenkins DJ, Wolever TM, Vidgen E, *et al.* Effect of psyllium in hypercholesterolemia at two mono-unsaturated fatty acid intakes. *Am J Clin Nutr* 1997; 65: 1524–1533.

22 Shrestha S, Freake HC, McGrane MM, *et al.* A combination of psyllium and plant sterols alters lipoprotein metabolism in hypercholesterolemic subjects by modifying the intravascular processing of lipoproteins and increasing LDL uptake. *J Nutr* 2007; 137(5): 1165–1170.

23 Shrestha S, Volek JS, Udani J, *et al.* A combination therapy including psyllium and plant sterols lowers LDL cholesterol by modifying lipoprotein metabolism in hypercholesterolemic individuals. *J Nutr* 2006; 136(10): 2492–2497.

24 Cicero AF, Derosa G, Manca M, *et al.* Different effect of psyllium and guar dietary supplementation on blood pressure control in hypertensive overweight patients: a six-month, randomized clinical trial. *Clin Exp Hypertens* 2007; 29(6): 383–394.

25 Dennison BA, Levine DM. Randomized, double-blind, placebo-controlled, two-period crossover clinical trial of psyllium fiber in children with hypercholesterolemia. *J Pediatr* 1993; 123: 24–29.

26 Davidson MH, Dugan LD, Burns JH, *et al.* A psyllium-enriched cereal for the treatment of hypercholesterolemia in children: a controlled, double-blind, crossover study. *Am J Clin Nutr* 1996; 63: 96–102.

27 Olson BH, Anderson SM, Becker MP, *et al.* Psyllium-enriched cereals lower blood total cholesterol and LDL cholesterol, but not HDL cholesterol, in hypercholesterolemic adults: results of a meta-analysis. *J Nutr* 1997; 127: 1973–1980.

28 Anderson JW, Allgood LD, Lawrence A, *et al.* Cholesterol-lowering effects of psyllium intake adjunctive to diet therapy in men and women with hypercholesterolemia: meta-analysis of 8 controlled trials. *Am J Clin Nutr* 2000; 71: 472–479.

29 Wei ZH, Wang H, Chen XY, *et al.* Time- and dose-dependent effect of psyllium on serum lipids in mild-to-moderate hypercholesterolemia: a meta-analysis of controlled clinical trials. *Eur J Clin Nutr* 2009; 63(7): 821–827.

30 Moreyra AE, Wilson AC, Koraym A. Effect of combining psyllium fiber with simvastatin in lowering cholesterol. *Arch Intern Med* 2005; 165: 1161–1166.

31 Spence JD, Huff MW, Heidenheim P, *et al.* Combination therapy with colestipol and psyllium mucilloid in patients with hyperlipidemia. *Ann Intern Med* 1995; 123: 493–499.

32 Maciejko JJ, Brazg R, Shah A, *et al.* Psyllium for the reduction of cholestyramine-associated gastrointestinal symptoms in the treatment of primary hypercholesterolemia. *Arch Fam Med* 1994; 3: 955–960.

33 Khossousi A, Binns CW, Dhaliwal SS, *et al.* The acute effects of psyllium on postprandial lipaemia and thermogenesis in overweight and obese men. *Br J Nutr* 2008; 99(5): 1068–1075.

34 King DE, Mainous AG3rd, Egan BM, *et al.* Effect of psyllium fiber supplementation on C-reactive protein: the trial to reduce inflammatory markers (TRIM). *Ann Fam Med* 2008; 6(2): 100–106.

35 Pastors JG, Blaisdell PW, Balm TK, *et al.* Psyllium fiber reduces rise in postprandial glucose and insulin concentrations in patients with non-insulin-dependent diabetes. *Am J Clin Nutr* 1991; 53: 1431–1435.

36 Frati Munari AC, Benitez Pinto W, Raul Ariza Andraca C, Casarrubias M. Lowering glycemic index of food by acarbose and *Plantago psyllium* mucilage. *Arch Med Res* 1998; 29: 137–41.

37 Rodriguez-Moran M, Guerrero-Romero F, Lazcano-Burciaga G. Lipid- and glucose-lowering efficacy of *Plantago psyllium* in type II diabetes. *J Diabetes Complications* 1998; 12: 273–278.

38 Ziai SA, Larijani B, Akhoondzadeh S, *et al.* Psyllium decreased serum glucose and glycosylated hemoglobin significantly in diabetic outpatients. *J Ethnopharmacol* 2005; 102: 202–207.

39 Sierra M, Garcia JJ, Fernandez N, *et al.* Therapeutic effects of psyllium in type 2 diabetic patients. *Eur J Clin Nutr* 2002; 56: 830–842.

40 Sartore G, Reitano R, Barison A, *et al.* The effects of psyllium on lipoproteins in type II diabetic patients. *Eur J Clin Nutr* 2009; 63(10): 1269–1271.

41 Longstreth GF, Fox DD, Youkeles L, *et al.* Psyllium therapy in the irritable bowel syndrome. A double-blind trial. *Ann Intern Med* 1981; 95: 53–56.

42 Prior A, Whorwell PJ. Double blind study of ispaghula in irritable bowel syndrome. *Gut* 1987; 28: 1510–1513.

43 Jalihal A, Kurian G. Ispaghula therapy in irritable bowel syndrome: improvement in overall well-being is related to reduction in bowel dissatisfaction. *J Gastroenterol Hepatol* 1990; 5: 507–513.

44 Misra SP, Thorat VK, Sachdev GK, Anand BS. Long-term treatment of irritable bowel syndrome: results of a randomized controlled trial. *Q J Med* 1989; 73: 931–939.

45 Hallert C, Kaldma M, Petersson BG. Ispaghula husk may relieve gastrointestinal symptoms in ulcerative colitis in remission. *Scand J Gastroenterol* 1991; 26: 747–750.

46 Fernandez-Banares F, Hinojosa J, Sanchez-Lombrana JL, *et al.* Randomized clinical trial of *Plantago ovata* seeds (dietary fiber) as compared with mesalamine in maintaining remission in ulcerative colitis. Spanish Group for the Study of Crohn's Disease and Ulcerative Colitis (GETECCU). *Am J Gastroenterol* 1999; 94: 427–433.

47 Ejderhamn J, Hedenborg G, Strandvik B. Long-term double-blind study on the influence of dietary fibres on faecal bile acid excretion in juvenile ulcerative colitis. *Scand J Clin Lab Invest* 1992; 52: 697–706.

48 Cavaliere H, Floriano I, Medeiros-Neto G. Gastrointestinal side effects of orlistat may be prevented by concomitant prescription of natural fibers (psyllium mucilloid). *Int J Obes Relat Metab Disord* 2001; 25: 1095–1099.

Pumpkin seed

Description

Pumpkin seed is the seed of *Curcubita pepo*.

Constituents

Pumpkin seeds contain 30–50% oil.[1–4] The main fatty acids are linoleic (n-6 polyunsaturated fatty acid), oleic (n-9 monounsaturated fatty acid) and the saturated fatty acids palmitic and stearic acids, which collectively make up 98% of the total fatty acids.[1,3,4] Pumpkin seeds also contain a small amount of linolenic acid (n-3 polyunsaturated fatty acid) and phytosterols. Pumpkin seed oil is rich in vitamin E,[2,4] especially gamma-tocopherol, of which it contains 5–10 times as much as alpha-tocopherol. It also contains a range of other vitamins and minerals (e.g. vitamin A, B vitamins, magnesium, iron, zinc and copper). Another constituent is cucurbitin, which is associated with anthelmintic effects. Pumpkin seed also contains acyl coenzyme A oxidase, which catalyses fatty acid oxidation.[5] Concentration of constituents varies significantly according to growth.

Action

Pumpkin seed is associated with diuretic, anthelmintic, antihypertensive, antidiabetic, anti-inflammatory, antioxidant, antitumour, hypocholesterolaemic and immunomodulatory activity.[6] Pumpkin seed extract has also been shown to have ACE inhibitory and alpha-glucosidase activity, further suggesting that pumpkin seed could reduce the risk of complications linked to hypertension and hyperglycaemia.[7] A rat study found that pumpkin seed had antioxidative effects and was effective in alleviating the peroxidative effects associated with protein energy malnutrition and carbon tetrachloride-induced liver injury.[8]

Possible uses

Pumpkin seed is claimed to have several benefits, predominantly on the reproductive and urinary systems. It is claimed to be beneficial in benign prostatic hyperplasia (BPH), kidney stones, cholesterol lowering, arthritis and diabetes. It is also claimed to be beneficial for skin care.

German Commission E Monographs include pumpkin seed, stating that it is used for irritable bladder condition, micturition problems of BPH (stages 1 and 2).

Several preclinical studies in animals have evaluated the effects of pumpkin seeds on the urinary system. In rabbits, pumpkin seed oil was associated with lower bladder pressure, increased bladder compliance and reduced urethral pressure.[9] In rats, pumpkin seed oil-inhibited, testosterone-induced prostatic hyperplasia[10] and prostate growth induced by testosterone/prazosin.[11]

Clinical trials in humans have also suggested beneficial effects of pumpkin seed on the urinary system. A trial in 20 boys (aged 2–7 years) evaluated the effect of pumpkin seed on crystalluria in an endemic area of Thailand and found that pumpkin seed lowered calcium-oxalate crystal occurrence.[12] A further trial in Thailand involving adolescents found that pumpkin seed improved inhibition of crystal formation or aggregation compared with placebo, suggesting that pumpkin seed could reduce the risk of urinary stone disease in this group of Thai adolescents.[13]

A 3-month randomised, double-blind trial in 53 men with prostatic hyperplasia found that curbicin (a preparation obtained from pumpkin seeds and dwarf palm plants) improved urinary flow, micturition time, residual urine, frequency of micturition and subjective symptom assessment compared with placebo.[14]

> **Conclusion**
> Pumpkin seed is used traditionally for problems of micturition in BPH and bladder irritation. Preclinical trials in animals suggest benefit, but good quality RCTs in humans are needed to confirm these benefits. There is no convincing evidence to make positive recommendations for pumpkin seed.

Precautions/contraindications

None known.

Pregnancy and breast-feeding

No harmful effects of pumpkin seed or pumpkin seed oil are known. No long-term data exist on pumpkin seed supplements.

Adverse effects

Adverse effects seem to be limited to allergic reactions. However, there is one case report involving a herbal blend containing pumpkin seeds, and also saw palmetto and nettle root extract with bioflavonoid and beta-carotene, in which ejaculatory volume was reduced.[15]

Interactions

None reported.

Dose

The dose is not established. Pumpkin seeds can be taken orally in the form of whole seeds, ground seeds, seed oil or in the form of capsules containing pumpkin seed oil. Supplements generally contain 300–600 mg of pumpkin seed oil. For BPH, pumpkin seed oil, 480 mg in three divided doses has been used.[14]

References

1 Murkovic M, Hillebrand A, Winkler J, *et al.* Variability of fatty acid content in pumpkin seeds (*Cucurbita pepo* L.). *Z Lebensm Unters Forsch* 1996; 203: 216–219.

2 Murkovic M, Hillebrand A, Winkler J, Pfannhauser W. Variability of vitamin E content in pumpkin seeds (*Cucurbita pepo* L.). *Z Lebensm Unters Forsch* 1996; 202: 275–278.

3 Younis YM, Ghirmay S, al-Shihry SS. African *Cucurbita pepo* L.: properties of seed and variability in fatty acid composition of seed oil. *Phytochemistry* 2000; 54: 71–75.

4 Stevenson DG, Eller FJ, Wang L, *et al.* Oil and tocopherol content and composition of pumpkin seed oil in 12 cultivars. *J Agric Food Chem* 2007; 55: 4005–4013.

5 De Bellis L, Gonzali S, Alpi A, *et al.* Purification and characterization of a novel pumpkin short-chain acyl-coenzyme A oxidase with structural similarity to acyl-coenzyme A dehydrogenases. *Plant Physiol* 2000; 123: 327–334.

6 Caili F, Huan S, Quanhong L. A review on pharmacological activities and utilization technologies of pumpkin. *Plant Foods Hum Nutr* 2006; 61: 73–80.

7 Kwon YI, Apostolidis E, Kim YC, Shetty K. Health benefits of traditional corn, beans, and pumpkin: in vitro studies for hyperglycemia and hypertension management. *J Med Food* 2007; 10: 266–275.

8 Nkosi CZ, Opoku AR, Terblanche SE. Antioxidative effects of pumpkin seed (*Cucurbita pepo*) protein isolate in CCl$_4$-induced liver injury in low-protein fed rats. *Phytother Res* 2006; 20: 935–940.

9 Zhang X, Ouyang JZ, Zhang YS, *et al.* Effect of the extracts of pumpkin seeds on the urodynamics of rabbits: an experimental study. *J Tongji Med Univ* 1994; 14: 235–238.

10 Gossell-Williams M, Davis A, O'Connor N. Inhibition of testosterone-induced hyperplasia of the prostate of Sprague-Dawley rats by pumpkin seed oil. *J Med Food* 2006; 9: 284–286.

11 Tsai YS, Tong YC, Cheng JT, *et al.* Pumpkin seed oil and phytosterol-F can block testosterone/prazosin-induced prostate growth in rats. *Urol Int* 2006; 77: 269–274.

12 Suphakarn VS, Yarnnon C, Ngunboonsri P. The effect of pumpkin seeds on oxalcrystalluria and urinary compositions of children in hyperendemic area. *Am J Clin Nutr* 1987; 45: 115–121.

13 Suphiphat V, Morjaroen N, Pukboonme I *et al.* The effect of pumpkin seeds snack on inhibitors and promoters of urolithiasis in Thai adolescents. *J Med Assoc Thai* 1993; 76: 487–493.

14 Carbin BE, Larsson B, Lindahl O. Treatment of benign prostatic hyperplasia with phytosterols. *Br J Urol* 1990; 66: 639–641.

15 Marks LS, Partin AW, Epstein JI, *et al.* Effects of a saw palmetto herbal blend in men with symptomatic benign prostatic hyperplasia. *J Urol* 2000; 163: 1451–1456.

Pycnogenol

Description

Pycnogenol is a registered trade name for a specific standardised extract of procyanidins (a category of flavonoids) from the bark of the French maritime pine (*Pinus pinaster* ssp. *atlantica*), which is grown in the Bay of Biscay in southwest France. The term pycnogenol was originally intended to serve as a scientific name for this category of flavonoids and was therefore applied to any preparation consisting of procyanidins.

Constituents

Pycnogenol is a mixture of monomeric and polymeric procyanidins. Catechin is the main monomeric procyanidin, while epicatechin is present in trace amounts. Catechin and epicatechin units are linked together to form bipolymers and larger procyanidin units. Other constituents of pycnogenol include another flavonoid, taxifolin, and a range of phenolic acids such as *p*-hydroxybenzoic acid, protocatechic acid, vanillic acid, gallic acid, caffeic acid, ferulic acid and *p*-coumaric acid. Calcium, copper, iron, manganese, potassium and zinc are also present.[1,2]

Action

Pycnogenol stimulates production of nitric oxide *in vitro* and *in vivo* from the natural substrate L-arginine.[1] Nitric oxide prevents platelet aggregation and causes the release of cyclic guanosine monophosphate in smooth muscle cells, leading to vasodilatation. By virtue of these effects, pycnogenol has a range of pharmacological activities on the vascular system including:

- inhibition of platelet aggregation and vasodilation; pycnogenol also appears to improve the efficacy of acetylsalicylic acid in inhibition of platelet function;[3]

- inhibition of angiotensin-converting enzyme (ACE) with reduction in blood pressure;[1,4]
- improved endothelial function;[5]
- improved lipid profiles;[6]
- enhanced capillary integrity and stabilisation of cell membranes;[7]
- improved erectile function.[8]

Other effects that have been demonstrated *in vitro* and in animals include:

- antioxidant and free radical activity;[2,6,7]
- inhibition of nuclear factor-κB, various interleukins and other factors centrally involved in inflammatory processes;[9]
- inhibition of histamine realease;[1]
- stimulation of the immune system (e.g. enhanced phagocytosis and natural killer cell activity);[10]
- lowering of blood glucose;[11]
- inhibiting alpha-glucosidase (which may help to explain the blood glucose lowering effect)[12]
- inhibition of cyclo-oxygenase 1 and 2 activity.[13]

Possible uses

A variety of claims have been made for pycnogenol and there is enormous research interest in this substance. Traditionally, pycnogenol was used in the treatment of scurvy and wound healing. Today it is marketed mainly for its supposed effects on the circulation, and its antioxidant, free radical and anti-inflammatory activity.

Cardiovascular function

Pycnogenol supplementation of 60 patients with cardiovascular disease (CVD) has been shown to increase vasodilatation and reduce the incidence of cardiovascular events,[1] while a preliminary study in 16 subjects found that pycnogenol improved endothelium dependent vasodilatation.[14] Inhibition of platelet aggregation has been demonstrated in smokers and in cardiovascular patients.[1] A double-blind crossover study in 11 patients with mild hypertension found that supplementation with 200 mg pycnogenol normalised blood pressure and lowered thromboxane levels.[1] A further double-blind placebo-controlled trial involved 58 patients on the calcium channel blocker nifedipine. Supplementation with 100 mg pycnogenol allowed a reduction in the dosage of nifedipine used in the management of hypertension with a reduction in plasma concentration of endothelin-1 and increase in prostacyclin.[5]

In another study involving 25 subjects, pycnogenol 150 mg daily significantly reduced LDL cholesterol levels and raised HDL cholesterol.[6] Two further small studies also found that supplementation with pycnogenol significantly lowered total cholesterol and LDL.[8,15]

Pycnogenol has been associated with significant reduction in symptoms of chronic venous insufficiency (CVI).[1] A prospective trial in 86 patients with chronic CVI, ankle swelling and previous history of venous ulceration compared pycnogenol 150 mg or 300 mg daily for 8 weeks with a combination of diosmin and hersperidin (Daflon) 1000 mg daily. Clinical improvement in the pycnogenol group was significantly greater than in the Daflon group.[16] Pycnogenol has been demonstrated to be more efficacious in CVI than a commercial horse chestnut extract (a remedy for CVI).[15]

Pycnogenol has also been shown to prevent deep vein thrombosis after long-haul flights,[17] to help to prevent oedema in patients treated with anti-hypertensive drugs,[18] and in combination with coenzyme Q_{10} to improve management of heart failure with reduced blood pressure, heart rate and oedema.[19]

Analgesic activity
Clinical trials have examined the effect of pycnogenol in pain. A study in 47 patients with menstrual pain found that pycnogenol 30 mg twice a day through three menstrual cycles was associated with significant abdominal and back pain relief during the second and third cycles.[20] A further study found that pycnogenol prevents cramps, muscular pain at rest and pain after/during exercise in healthy subjects, athletes prone to cramps, patients with venous disease, patients with intermittent claudication and patients with diabetic microangiopathy.[21] Pycnogenol has also been found to reduce levels of C-reactive protein and fibrinogen (both makerts of inflammation) in osteoarthritis,[22] and to reduce symptoms of

pain and gastrointestinal symptoms associated with drug treatment and use of medication and, therefore, treatment costs associated with osteoarthritis.[23,24]

Diabetes
Two clinical trials have provided evidence that pycnogenol could be beneficial in type 2 diabetes. An open, controlled trial in 18 men and 12 women found that pycnogenol lowered postprandial glucose, HBA_{1c} and endothelin 1.[11] This finding was confirmed in a double-blind, placebo-controlled study in 77 patients.[25] A placebo-controlled trial in 48 patients with type 2 diabetes and treated with ACE inhibitors found that, compared with controls, pycnogenol resulted in improved diabetes control, lowered CVD risk factors and reduced antihypertensive medicine use.[26] A further RCT among diabetic patients taking ramipril combined with pycnogenol found that the addition of pycnogenol improved kidney function and lowering serum creatinine and urinary albumin.[27,28] Combined local and systemic treatment with pycnogenol has been associated with reduced area of diabsetic ulceration and increased speed of ulcer healing.[29,30] Pycnogenol taken at the early stage of diabetic retinopathy may enhance retinal blood circulation accompanied by regression of oedema, which favourably improves vision of patients.[31]

Sexual function
Supplementation with pycnogenol has been found to improve erectile function.[8,32] Pycnogenol has also been associated with improvement in sperm quality and function.[33]

Attention deficit hyperactivity disorder
There have been anecdotal reports of benefit of pycnogenol in attention deficit hyperactivity disorder (ADHD). A randomised, placebo-controlled, double-blind trial involving 61 children (mostly boys) supplemented with 1 mg/kg pycnogenol daily or placebo over 4 weeks found improvements in some ADHD scores in the treatment compared with placebo group, but not all aspects of the condition improved. Scores measured a month after stopping treatment returned to baseline. Based on these results, the authors suggested that pycnogenol has some activity in relieving ADHD symptoms

in children.[34] Two further studies have come to a similar conclusion and indicated that there might be a link between improvement in symptoms of ADHD and reduced oxidative damage to DNA with pycnogel treatment[35] or reduced catecholamine concentrations.[36]

Miscellaneous

Pycnogenol has been found to improve lung function in asthma,[37] minimise gingival bleeding and plaque accumulation,[38] reduce inflammation in systemic lupus erthyromatosus,[39] improve menopausal symptoms,[40] improve cognitive performance in older people,[41] relieve tinnitus by improving cochlear blood flow,[42] reduce bleeding from haemorrhoids[43] and improve allergic rhinitis symptoms when supplementation was started at least 5 weeks before the onset of the allergy season.[44]

Conclusion

Trials have shown pycnogenol to have beneficial effects in cardiovascular conditions, pain, diabetes, sexual function, ADHD, asthma, gingivitis, systemic lupus erthyromatosus, menopausal symptoms, cognitive performance, tinnitus, haemorrhoids and allergic rhinitis. However, these trials should be treated with circumspection as some have been open-label, and those that have been placebo-controlled have been small, short-term studies. However, the benefits observed justify further larger controlled trials.

Precautions/contraindications

None reported.

Pregnancy and breast-feeding

No teratogenic effects have been observed, but pycnogenol should be avoided as a general precaution.

Adverse effects

No serious side-effects reported. Mild side-effects such as gastrointestinal problems, nausea, headache, dizziness and skin sensitisation are rare and transient in most cases.

Interactions

None reported.

Dose

The dose is not established. Clinical trials have used 40–100 mg pycnogenol daily or 1 mg/kg body weight daily.

References

1 Rohdewald P. A review of the French maritime pine bark extract (Pycnogenol), a herbal medication with a diverse clinical pharmacology. *Int J Clin Pharmacol Ther* 2002; 40: 158–168.
2 Packer L, Rimbach G, Virgili F. Antioxidant activity and biologic properties of a procyanidin-rich extract from pine (*Pinus maritima*) bark, pycnogenol. *Free Radic Biol Med* 1999; 27: 704–724.
3 Golanski J, Muchova J, Golanski R, *et al.* Does pycnogenol intensify the efficacy of acetylsalicylic acid in the inhibition of platelet function? In vitro experience *Postepy Hig Med Dosw (Online)* 2006; 60: 316–321.
4 Hosseini S, Lee J, Sepulveda RT, *et al.* A randomized, double-blind, placebo-controlled, prospective 16 week crossover study to determine the role of Pycnogenol in modifying blood pressure in mildly hypertensive patients. *Nutr Res* 2001; 21: 1251–1260.
5 Liu X, Wei J, Tan F, Zhou S, *et al.* Pycnogenol, French maritime pine bark extract, improves endothelial function of hypertensive patients. *Life Sci* 2004; 74: 855–862.
6 Devaraj S, Vega-Lopez S, Kaul N, *et al.* Supplementation with a pine bark extract rich in polyphenols increases plasma antioxidant capacity and alters the plasma lipoprotein profile. *Lipids* 2002; 37: 931–934.
7 Grimm T, Schafer A, Hogger P. Antioxidant activity and inhibition of matrix metalloproteinases by metabolites of maritime pine bark extract (pycnogenol). *Free Radic Biol Med* 2004; 36: 811–822.
8 Durackova Z, Trebaticky B, Novotny V, *et al.* Lipid metabolism and erectile function improvement by Pycnogenol R extract from the bark of *Pinus pinaster* in patients suffering from erectile dysfunction – a pilot study. *Nutr Res* 2003; 23: 1189–1198.
9 Grimm T, Chovanova Z, Muchova J, *et al.* Inhibition of NF-kappaB activation and MMP-9 secretion by plasma of human volunteers after ingestion of maritime pine bark extract (Pycnogenol). *J Inflamm (Lond)* 2006; 3: 1.
10 Kim HC, Healey JM. Effects of pine bark extract administered to immunosuppressed adult mice infected with *Cryptosporidium parvum*. *Am J Chin Med* 2001; 29: 469–475.

11 Liu X, Zhou HJ, Rohdewald P. French maritime pine bark extract Pycnogenol dose-dependently lowers glucose in type 2 diabetic patients. *Diabetes Care* 2004; 27: 839.

12 Schafer A, Hogger P. Oligomeric procyanidins of French maritime pine bark extract (Pycnogenol(R)) effectively inhibit alpha-glucosidase. *Diabetes Res Clin Pract* 2007; 77(1): 41–46.

13 Schafer A, Chovanova Z, Muchova J, *et al.* Inhibition of COX-1 and COX-2 activity by plasma of human volunteers after ingestion of French maritime pine bark extract (Pycnogenol). *Biomed Pharmacother* 2006; 60: 5–9.

14 Nishioka K, Hidaka T, Nakamura S, *et al.* Pycnogenol, French maritime pine bark extract, augments endothelium-dependent vasodilation in humans. *Hypertens Res* 2007; 30(9): 775–780.

15 Koch R. Comparative study of venostatin and pycnogenol in chronic venous insufficiency. *Phytother Res* 2002; Suppl1: S1–S5.

16 Cesarone MR, Belcaro G, Rohdewald P, *et al.* Comparison of Pycnogenol and Daflon in treating chronic venous insufficiency: a prospective, controlled study. *Clin Appl Thromb Hemost* 2006; 12: 205–212.

17 Belcaro G, Cesarone MR, Rohdewald P, *et al.* Prevention of venous thrombosis and thrombophlebitis in long-haul flights with pycnogenol. *Clin Appl Thromb Hemost* 2004; 10: 373–377.

18 Belcaro G, Cesarone MR, Ricci A, *et al.* Control of edema in hypertensive subjects treated with calcium antagonist (nifedipine) or angiotensin-converting enzyme inhibitors with pycnogenol. *Clin App Thromb Hemost* 2006; 12(4): 440–444.

19 Belcaro G, Cesarone MR, Dugall M, *et al.* Investigation of pycnogenol(R) in combination with coenzyme Q_{10} in heart failure patients (NYHA II/III). *Panminerva Med* 2010; 52 (Suppl 1): 21–25.

20 Kohama T, Suzuki N, Ohno S. Inoue M. Analgesic efficacy of French maritime pine bark extract in dysmenorrhea: an open clinical trial. *J Reprod Med* 2004; 49: 828–832.

21 Vinciguerra G, Belcaro G, Cesarone MR, *et al.* Cramps and muscular pain: prevention with pycnogenol in normal subjects, venous patients, athletes, claudicants and in diabetic microangiopathy. *Angiology* 2006; 57: 331–339.

22 Belcaro G, Cesarone MR, Errichi S, *et al.* Variations in C-reactive protein, plasma free radicals and fibrinogen values in patients with osteoarthritis treated with pycnogenol. *Redox Rep* 2008; 13(6): 271–276.

23 Belcaro G, Cesarone MR, Errichi S, *et al.* Treatment of osteoarthritis with pycnogenol. The SVOS (San Valentino Osteo-arthrosis Study). Evaluation of signs, symptoms, physical performance and vascular aspects. *Phytother Res* 2008; 22(4): 518–523.

24 Cisar P, Jany R, Waczulikova I, *et al.* Effect of pine bark extract (pycnogenol) on symptoms of knee osteoarthritis. *Phytother Res* 2008; 22(8): 1087–1092.

25 Liu X, Wei J, Tan F, *et al.* Antidiabetic effect of pycnogenol French maritime pine bark extract in patients with diabetes type II. *Life Sci* 2004; 75: 2505–2513.

26 Zibadi S, Rohdewald PJ, Park D, *et al.* Reduction of cardiovascular risk factors in subjects with type 2 diabetes by pycnogenol supplementation. *Nutr Res* 2008; 28(5): 315–320.

27 Stuard S, Belcaro G, Cesarone MR, *et al.* Kidney function in metabolic syndrome may be improved with pycnogenol(R). *Panminerva Med* 2010; 52 (Suppl 1): 27–32.

28 Cesarone MR, Belcaro G, Stuard S, *et al.* Kidney flow and function in hypertension: protective effects of pycnogenol in hypertensive participants: a controlled study. *J Cardiovasc Pharmacol Ther* 2010; 15(1): 41–46.

29 Belcaro G, Cesarone MR, Errichi BM, *et al.* Diabetic ulcers: microcirculatory improvement and faster healing with pycnogenol. *Clin Appl Thromb Hemost* 2006; 12(3): 318–323.

30 Cesarone MR, Belcaro G, Rohdewald P, *et al.* Rapid relief of signs/symptoms in chronic venous microangiopathy with pycnogenol: a prospective, controlled study. *Angiology* 2006; 57(5): 569–576.

31 Steigerwalt R, Belcaro G, Cesarone MR, *et al.* Pycnogenol improves microcirculation, retinal edema, and visual acuity in early diabetic retinopathy. *J Ocul Pharmacol Ther* 2009; 25(6): 537–540.

32 Stanislavov R, Nikolova V. Treatment of erectile dysfunction with pycnogenol and L-arginine. *J Sexual Marital Ther* 2003; 29: 207–213.

33 Roseff SJ. Improvement in sperm quality and function with French maritime pine tree bark extract. *J Reprod Med* 2002; 47: 821–824.

34 Trebaticka J, Kopasova S, Hradecna Z, *et al.* Treatment of ADHD with French maritime pine bark extract, pycnogenol(R). *Eur Child Adolesc Psychiatry* 2006; 15: 329–335.

35 Chovanova Z, Muchova J, Sivonova M, *et al.* Effect of polyphenolic extract, pycnogenol, on the level of 8-oxoguanine in children suffering from attention deficit/hyperactivity disorder. *Free Radic Res* 2006; 40(9): 1003–1010.

36 Dvorakova M, Jezova D, Blazicek P, *et al.* Urinary catecholamines in children with attention deficit hyperactivity disorder (ADHD): modulation by a polyphenolic extract from pine bark (pycnogenol). *Nutr Neurosci* 2007; 10(34): 151–157.

37 Lau BH, Riesen SK, Truong KP, *et al.* Pycnogenol as an adjunct in the management of childhood asthma. *J Asthma* 2004; 41: 825–832.

38 Kimbrough C, Chun M, de la Roca G, Lau BH. PYCNOGENOL chewing gum minimizes gingival bleeding and plaque formation. *Phytomedicine* 2002; 9: 410–413.

39 Stefanescu M, Matache C, Onu A, *et al.* Pycnogenol efficacy in the treatment of systemic lupus

erythematosus patients. *Phytother Res* 2001; 15: 698–704.

40 Yang HM, Liao MF, Zhu SY, *et al.* A randomised, double-blind, placebo-controlled trial on the effect of pycnogenol on the climacteric syndrome in peri-menopausal women. *Acta Obstet Gynecol Scand* 2007; 86(8): 978–985.

41 Ryan J, Croft K, Mori T, *et al.* An examination of the effects of the antioxidant pycnogenol on cognitive performance, serum lipid profile, endocrinological and oxidative stress biomarkers in an elderly population. *J Psychopharmacol* 2008; 22(5): 553–562.

42 Grossi MG, Belcaro G, Cesarone MR, *et al.* Improvement in cochlear flow with pycnogenol(R) in patients with tinnitus: a pilot evaluation. *Panminerva Med* 2010; 52(Suppl 1): 63–67.

43 Belcaro G, Cesarone MR, Errichi B, *et al.* Pycnogenol treatment of acute hemorrhoidal episodes. *Phytother Res* 2010; 24(3): 438–444.

44 Wilson D, Evans M, Guthrie N, *et al.* A randomized, double-blind, placebo-controlled exploratory study to evaluate the potential of pycnogenol for improving allergic rhinitis symptoms. *Phytother Res* 2010; 24(8): 1115–1119.

Quercetin

Description

Quercetin (3,3',4',5,7-pentahydroxyflavone)[1] is a flavonoid that forms the chemical backbone for other flavonoids such as hesperidin, naringin, rutin and tangeritin. Rutin is the most common flavonoid containing the quercetin backbone, in which quercetin is attached to a glucose-rhamnose moiety. Quercetin is also found bound to one or two glucose molecules (monoglycoside and diglycoside forms).[2]

Dietary sources

Quercetin is one of the most abundant dietary flavonoids. It is found in apples; black, green and buckwheat tea; onions (particularly the outer rings); raspberries; red wine; red grapes; cherries; citrus fruits; broccoli and other green leafy vegetables.[3] Preliminary work by the University of Queensland, Australia, suggests that quercetin is also found in varieties of honey such as that derived from eucalyptus and tea tree. Quercetin is also found in ginkgo biloba and St John's wort.

Dietary intake

Estimated dietary intake is 25–50 mg daily.[4]

Action

Quercetin has a range of activities. It has been shown *in vitro* to:

- act as an antioxidant;[5]
- inhibit LDL oxidation;[4,6,7]
- inhibit the nitric oxide synthase pathway;[8,9]
- have anti-inflammatory activity, possibly due to an influence on the production of eicosanoids, including leukotrienes and prostaglandins,[4] and also cytokines;[10]
- have potential as an anti-cancer agent through interaction with type II oestrogen-binding sites,[11] inhibition of tyrosine kinase,[12] up-

regulation of tumour suppressor genes,[13,14] induction of apoptosis,[15,16] and inhibition of tumour necrosis factor-alpha[17] (however, no effects on gene expression were demonstrated in a placebo-controlled trial[18]);
- have antihistamine activity.[19]

However, in a clinical trial, daily supplementation of healthy humans with graded concentrations of quercetin for 2 weeks did not affect antioxidant status, oxidised LDL, inflammation or metabolism.[20] A further clinical study shows that quercetin increases antioxidant capacity *in vivo* in a dose-dependent manner and displays anti-inflammatory effects *in vitro*, but not *in vivo* or *ex vivo*, in the blood of healthy volunteers.[21] A lack of effect of quercetin (500 or 100 mg daily) on oxidative stress and antioxidant capacity was confirmed in a larger study among 1002 subjects aged 18–85 years,[22] but this trial did demonstrate a reduction in upper respiratory tract infection duration and severity in the middle-aged and older subjects consuming 1000 mg quercetin daily.[23] No effects of quercetin (500 or 1000 mg daily) on immune function or inflammation were observed in a placebo-controlled trial among 120 women,[24] and no effects of quercetin 1000 mg daily for 7 days on oxygen uptake (VO_{2max}) were found in a study among 11 sedentary men and women.[25]

Possible uses

Quercetin offers several potential therapeutic uses in the prevention of cardiovascular disease (CVD), cancer, cataract, schizophrenia and prostatitis. However, there are few clinical trials in humans to date.

Cardiovascular disease

Quercetin may have a role in the prevention of CVD. An epidemiological study suggested that high intakes of dietary flavonoids, particularly quercetin, are associated with a reduced risk of CVD in older men.[26] This protective effect is thought to be due to a variety of quercetin's activities, such as its antioxidant capacity,[4] including inhibition of LDL oxidation,[6] nitric oxide synthase inhibition,[8] improved endothelial function,[27] inhibition of tissue factor (the cellular receptor that initiates blood coagulation),[28] platelet aggregation,[29] and a range of anti-inflammatory activities. However, quercetin supplementation does not appear to reduce total and LDL cholesterol or to increase HDL cholesterol.[29,30]

Evidence is emerging that quercetin could reduce blood pressure. A placebo-controlled crossover clinical trial in 19 men and women with prehypertension and 22 with stage 1 hypertension showed that quercetin 730 mg daily for 28 days reduced blood pressure compared with placebo, but only in those with stage 1 hypertension.[31] A further 6-week controlled trial conducted by the same research group among 93 overweight or obese subjects with traits of metabolic syndrome (and, therefore, at risk of CVD) showed that quercetin 150 mg daily reduced systolic blood pressure and plasma oxidized LDL concentrations.[32] These effects varied by apolipoprotein genotype in that quercetin exhibited blood pressure-lowering effects in overweight-obese carriers of the apo ε3/ε3 genotype but not in carriers of the ε4 allele. Furthermore, quercetin supplementation resulted in a reduction in HDL cholesterol and apoA1 in apo ε4 carriers.[33]

Cancer

In vitro studies have shown quercetin to have various properties that could give it anti-cancer activity (e.g. cell cycle regulation, interaction with type II oestrogen-binding sites, inhibition of tyrosine kinase and reduction in the number of aberrant crypt foci,[34] inhibition of tyrosine kinase,[12] inhibition of tumour necrosis factor-alpha[17] and inhibition of tumour angiogenesis.[1]

Quercetin has been shown *in vitro* to inhibit growth of colorectal cancer cells,[14,35,36] possibly by up-regulation in the expression of tumour suppressor genes[14] and modulation of cell-cycle related and apoptosis genes.[36]

It has also been shown to have potential activity against prostate cancer. It can attenuate the function of the androgen receptor (AR), inhibiting AR-mediated expression of prostate-specific antigen,[37] up-regulating tumour suppressor genes while down-regulating oncogenes

and cell cycle genes,[13] and inhibit other receptors involved in growth and metastasis of prostate cancer.[38]

Quercetin has also been shown *in vitro* to have activity against leukaemia cells[15,16] and pancreatic tumour cells.[39] Other preliminary studies suggest that quercetin could have inhibitory effects on other cancer types, including breast, ovary, endometrial, non-small-cell lung, gastric and squamous cell.[40]

Athletics

Quercetin has been evaluated for an influence on muscle metabolism during exercise, but findings to date have not been promising.[41] A placebo-controlled trial in 40 trained male cyclists showed that quercetin 1 g daily over a 24-day period diminished postexercise expression of mRNA for leukocyte interleukin (IL)-8 and IL-10, indicating that elevated plasma quercetin levels exerted some effects within the blood compartment. Quercetin did not, however, influence any of the muscle measures, including NF-κB content, cytokine mRNA, or cyclo-oxygenase 2 mRNA expression across a 3-day intensified exercise period.[42] Within this same trial, quercetin versus placebo ingestion did not alter exercise-induced changes in several measures of immune function, but it significantly reduced upper respiratory tract infection incidence in cyclists during the 2-week period after intensified exercise.[43] No effects were seen on exercise performance in this[44] and another trial[45] in military cadets.

In a further trial among 63 athletes by the same research group, quercetin ingestion (1 g daily) for 3 weeks before a competitive 160-km race significantly increased plasma quercetin levels but failed to attenuate muscle damage, inflammation, increases in plasma cytokine and hormone levels, and alterations in leukocyte cytokine mRNA expression[46] or plasma lipid, antioxidant capacity or oxidative damage;[47] it also had no effect on markers of immune function or upper respiratory tract infection rates.[48] Lack of effect of quercetin on exercise-induced oxidative stress and inflammation was observed in another trial in 40 athletes,[49] and no effects were found on perceived exertion.[50] However, a more recent trial among 26 untrained adult men by the same group demonstrated a slight improvement in 12-min treadmill time performance with quercetin 1000 mg daily compared with placebo,[51] while a trial among 12 untrained volunteers found that quercetin 100 mg daily for 7 days can increase endurance.[52]

Cataract

One study in rats has shown that quercetin could have a possible role in reducing the incidence of cataracts, by inhibiting oxidative damage in the lens. Quercetin was converted to its metabolite 3-O-methyl quercetin by catechol-O-methyltransferase (COMT) in the rat lens, and both compounds were found to inhibit hydrogen peroxide-induced opacification.[53]

Autoimmune disease

Quercetin was found in one study to ameliorate experimental allergic encephalomyelitis by blocking IL-12 signalling and Th1 differentiation, suggesting that it may be effective in treating multiple sclerosis and other Th1-cell-mediated autoimmune diseases.[54]

Schizophrenia

Evidence from one study suggests that quercetin (in combination with other antioxidants) might benefit patients with schizophrenia.[55]

Miscellaneous

Preliminary evidence suggests that quercetin may be of benefit in allergic rhinitis and against various viruses, including herpes simplex and respiratory syncytial viruses.[4]

Conclusion

Quercetin is the subject of intense research on the basis of its antioxidant, anti-inflammatory and anti-cancer activities. *In vitro* studies have demonstrated that quercetin offers potential in preventing CVD and cancer, and possibly cataract. Evidence is emerging that quercetin could reduce blood pressure in those with hypertension, but a number of recent trials evaluating quercetin for exercise performance have found almost no benefits. Further controlled clinical trials in humans are needed before any conclusions can be drawn about the value of quercetin supplementation.

Precautions/contraindications

None reported.

Pregnancy and breast-feeding

No problems have been reported, but there have not been sufficient studies to guarantee the safety of quercetin in pregnancy and breast-feeding.

Adverse effects

Orally, quercetin may cause headache and tingling of the extremities.

Interactions

Quercetin is a bioflavonoid that inhibits P-glycoprotein and has been investigated for potential interactions with various drugs. One study showed no influence of quercetin on plasma saquinivir,[56] while another showed that short-term use of quercetin elevated plasma concentrations of fexofenadine.[57]

Dose

The dose is not established. Typical oral doses range from 400 to 500 mg three times daily. Doses of 500–1000 mg daily have been shown to cause highly variable increases in plasma quercetin concentrations.[58]

Quercetin is administered by injection (but this is not a dietary supplement use).

References

1 Igura K, Ohta T, Kuroda Y, *et al.* Resveratrol and quercetin inhibit angiogenesis in vitro. *Cancer Lett* 2001; 171(1): 11–16.

2 Erlund I, Kosonen T, Alfthan G, *et al.* Pharmacokinetics of quercetin from quercetin aglycone and rutin in healthy volunteers. *Eur J Clin Pharmacol* 2000; 56(8): 545–553.

3 Hertog MG, Hollman PC. Potential health effects of the dietary flavonol quercetin. *Eur J Clin Nutr* 1996; 50(2): 63–71.

4 Formica JV, Regelson W. Review of the biology of quercetin and related bioflavonoids. *Food Chem Toxicol* 1995; 33(12): 1061–1080.

5 Filipe P, Haigle J, Silva JN, *et al.* Anti- and pro-oxidant effects of quercetin in copper-induced low

density lipoprotein oxidation. Quercetin as an effective antioxidant against pro-oxidant effects of urate. *Eur J Biochem* 2004; 271(10): 1991–1999.

6   Janisch KM, Williamson G, Needs P, *et al.* Properties of quercetin conjugates: modulation of LDL oxidation and binding to human serum albumin. *Free Radic Res* 2004; 38(8): 877–884.

7   Yamamoto N, Moon JH, Tsushida T, *et al.* Inhibitory effect of quercetin metabolites and their related derivatives on copper ion-induced lipid peroxidation in human low-density lipoprotein. *Arch Biochem Biophys* 1999; 372(2): 347–354.

8   Chan MM, Mattiacci JA, Hwang HS, *et al.* Synergy between ethanol and grape polyphenols, quercetin, and resveratrol, in the inhibition of the inducible nitric oxide synthase pathway. *Biochem Pharmacol* 2000; 60(10): 1539–1548.

9   Mu MM, Chakravortty D, Sugiyama T, *et al.* The inhibitory action of quercetin on lipopolysaccharide-induced nitric oxide production in RAW 264.7 macrophage cells. *J Endotoxin Res* 2001; 7(6): 431–438.

10 Wadsworth TL, Koop DR. Effects of the wine polyphenolics quercetin and resveratrol on pro-inflammatory cytokine expression in RAW 264.7 macrophages. *Biochem Pharmacol* 1999; 57(8): 941–949.

11 Shenouda NS, Zhou C, Browning JD, *et al.* Phytoestrogens in common herbs regulate prostate cancer cell growth in vitro. *Nutr Cancer* 2004; 49(2): 200–208.

12 Huang YT, Hwang JJ, Lee PP, *et al.* Effects of luteolin and quercetin, inhibitors of tyrosine kinase, on cell growth and metastasis-associated properties in A431 cells overexpressing epidermal growth factor receptor. *Br J Pharmacol* 1999; 128(5): 999–1010.

13 Nair HK, Rao KV, Aalinkeel R, *et al.* Inhibition of prostate cancer cell colony formation by the flavonoid quercetin correlates with modulation of specific regulatory genes. *Clin Diagn Lab Immunol* 2004; 11(1): 63–69.

14 van Erk MJ, Roepman P, van der Lende TR, *et al.* Integrated assessment by multiple gene expression analysis of quercetin bioactivity on anticancer-related mechanisms in colon cancer cells in vitro. *Eur J Nutr* 2005; 44(3): 143–156.

15 Mertens-Talcott SU, Talcott ST, Percival SS. Low concentrations of quercetin and ellagic acid synergistically influence proliferation, cytotoxicity and apoptosis in MOLT-4 human leukemia cells. *J Nutr* 2003; 133(8): 2669–7264.

16 Mertens-Talcott SU, Percival SS. Ellagic acid and quercetin interact synergistically with resveratrol in the induction of apoptosis and cause transient cell cycle arrest in human leukemia cells. *Cancer Lett* 2005; 218(2): 141–151.

17 Wadsworth TL, McDonald TL, Koop DR. Effects of *Ginkgo biloba* extract (EGb 761) and quercetin on lipopolysaccharide-induced signaling pathways involved in the release of tumor necrosis factor alpha. *Biochem Pharmacol* 2001; 62(7): 963–974.

18 Boomgaarden I, Egert S, Rimbach G, *et al.* Quercetin supplementation and its effect on human monocyte gene expression profiles in vivo. *Br J Nutr* 2010; 104(3): 336–345.

19 Marozzi FJ, Jr, Kocialski AB, Malone MH. Studies on the antihistaminic effects of thymoquinone, thymohydroquinone and quercetin. *Arzneimittelforschung* 1970; 20(10): 1574–1577.

20 Egert S, Wolffram S, Bosy-Westphal A, *et al.* Daily quercetin supplementation dose-dependently increases plasma quercetin concentrations in healthy humans. *J Nutr* 2008; 138(9): 1615–1621.

21 Boots AW, Wilms LC, Swennen EL, *et al.* In vitro and ex vivo anti-inflammatory activity of quercetin in healthy volunteers. *Nutrition* 2008; 24(78): 703–710.

22 Shanely RA, Knab AM, Nieman DC, *et al.* Quercetin supplementation does not alter antioxidant status in humans. *Free Radic Res* 2010; 44(2): 224–231.

23 Heinz SA, Henson DA, Austin MD, *et al.* Quercetin supplementation and upper respiratory tract infection: a randomized community clinical trial. *Pharmacol Res* 2010; 62(3): 237–242.

24 Heinz SA, Henson DA, Nieman DC, *et al.* A 12-week supplementation with quercetin does not affect natural killer cell activity, granulocyte oxidative burst activity or granulocyte phagocytosis in female human subjects. *Br J Nutr* 2010; 104(6): 849–857.

25 Ganio MS, Armstrong LE, Johnson EC, *et al.* Effect of quercetin supplementation on maximal oxygen uptake in men and women. *J Sports Sci* 2010; 28(2): 201–208.

26 Hertog MG, Feskens EJ, Hollman PC, *et al.* Dietary antioxidant flavonoids and risk of coronary heart disease: the Zutphen Elderly Study. *Lancet* 1993; 342(8878): 1007–1011.

27 Loke WM, Hodgson JM, Proudfoot JM, *et al.* Pure dietary flavonoids quercetin and (−)-epicatechin augment nitric oxide products and reduce endothelin-1 acutely in healthy men. *Am J Clin Nutr* 2008; 88(4): 1018–1025.

28 Di Santo A, Mezzetti A, Napoleone E, *et al.* Resveratrol and quercetin down-regulate tissue factor expression by human stimulated vascular cells. *J Thromb Haemost* 2003; 1(5): 1089–1095.

29 Janssen K, Mensink RP, Cox FJ, *et al.* Effects of the flavonoids quercetin and apigenin on hemostasis in healthy volunteers: results from an in vitro and a dietary supplement study. *Am J Clin Nutr* 1998; 67(2): 255–262.

30 Conquer JA, Maiani G, Azzini E, *et al.* Supplementation with quercetin markedly increases plasma quercetin concentration without effect on selected risk factors for heart disease in healthy subjects. *J Nutr* 1998; 128(3): 593–597.

31 Edwards RL, Lyon T, Litwin SE, *et al.* Quercetin reduces blood pressure in hypertensive subjects. *J Nutr* 2007; 137(11): 2405–2411.

32 Egert S, Bosy-Westphal A, Seiberl J, *et al.* Quercetin reduces systolic blood pressure and plasma oxidised low-density lipoprotein concentrations in overweight subjects with a high-cardiovascular disease risk phenotype: a double-blinded, placebo-controlled cross-over study. *Br J Nutr* 2009; 102(7): 1065–1074.

33 Egert S, Boesch-Saadatmandi C, Wolffram S, *et al.* Serum lipid and blood pressure responses to quercetin vary in overweight patients by apolipoprotein E genotype. *J Nutr* 2009; 140(2): 278–284.

34 Lamson DW, Brignall MS. Antioxidants and cancer, part 3: quercetin. *Altern Med Rev* 2000; 5(3): 196–208.

35 Richter M, Ebermann R, Marian B. Quercetin-induced apoptosis in colorectal tumor cells: possible role of EGF receptor signaling. *Nutr Cancer* 1999; 34(1): 88–99.

36 Murtaza I, Marra G, Schlapbach R, *et al.* A preliminary investigation demonstrating the effect of quercetin on the expression of genes related to cell-cycle arrest, apoptosis and xenobiotic metabolism in human CO115 colon-adenocarcinoma cells using DNA microarray. *Biotechnol Appl Biochem* 2006; 45(Pt1): 29–36.

37 Xing N, Chen Y, Mitchell SH, *et al.* Quercetin inhibits the expression and function of the androgen receptor in LNCaP prostate cancer cells. *Carcinogenesis* 2001; 22(3): 409–414.

38 Huynh H, Nguyen TT, Chan E, *et al.* Inhibition of ErbB-2 and ErbB-3 expression by quercetin prevents transforming growth factor alpha (TGF-alpha)- and epidermal growth factor (EGF)-induced human PC-3 prostate cancer cell proliferation. *Int J Oncol* 2003; 23(3): 821–829.

39 Lee LT, Huang YT, Hwang JJ, *et al.* Blockade of the epidermal growth factor receptor tyrosine kinase activity by quercetin and luteolin leads to growth inhibition and apoptosis of pancreatic tumor cells. *Anticancer Res* 2002; 22(3): 1615–1627.

40 El Attar TM, Virji AS. Modulating effect of resveratrol and quercetin on oral cancer cell growth and proliferation. *Anticancer Drugs* 1999; 10(2): 187–193.

41 Cureton KJ, Tomporowski PD, Singhal A, *et al.* Dietary quercetin supplementation is not ergogenic in untrained men. *J Appl Physiol* 2009; 107(4): 1095–1104.

42 Nieman DC, Henson DA, Davis JM, *et al.* Quercetin's influence on exercise-induced changes in plasma cytokines and muscle and leukocyte cytokine mRNA. *J Appl Physiol* 2007; 103(5): 1728–1735.

43 Nieman DC, Henson DA, Gross SJ, *et al.* Quercetin reduces illness but not immune perturbations after intensive exercise. *Med Sci Sports Exerc* 2007; 39 (9): 1561–1569.

44 Dumke CL, Nieman DC, Utter AC, *et al.* Quercetin's effect on cycling efficiency and substrate utilization. *Appl Physiol Nutr Metab* 2009; 34(6): 993–1000.

45 Bigelman KA, Fan EH, Chapman DP, *et al.* Effects of six weeks of quercetin supplementation on physical performance in ROTC cadets. *Mil Med* 2010; 175(10): 791–798.

46 Nieman DC, Henson DA, Davis JM, *et al.* Quercetin ingestion does not alter cytokine changes in athletes competing in the Western States Endurance Run. *J Interferon Cytokine Res* 2007; 27(12): 1003–1011.

47 Quindry JC, McAnulty SR, Hudson MB, *et al.* Oral quercetin supplementation and blood oxidative capacity in response to ultramarathon competition. *Int J Sport Nutr Exerc Metab* 2008; 18(6): 601–616.

48 Henson D, Nieman D, Davis JM, *et al.* Post-160-km race illness rates and decreases in granulocyte respiratory burst and salivary IgA output are not countered by quercetin ingestion. *Int J Sports Med* 2008; 29(10): 856–863.

49 McAnulty SR, McAnulty LS, Nieman DC, *et al.* Chronic quercetin ingestion and exercise-induced oxidative damage and inflammation. *Appl Physiol Nutr Metab* 2008; 33(2): 254–262.

50 Utter AC, Nieman DC, Kang J, *et al.* Quercetin does not affect rating of perceived exertion in athletes during the Western States endurance run. *Res Sports Med* 2009; 17(2): 71–83.

51 Nieman DC, Williams AS, Shanely RA, *et al.* Quercetin's influence on exercise performance and muscle mitochondrial biogenesis. *Med Sci Sports Exerc* 2010; 42(2): 338–345.

52 Davis JM, Carlstedt CJ, Chen S, *et al.* The dietary flavonoid quercetin increases VO(2max) and endurance capacity. *Int J Sport Nutr Exerc Metab* 2010; 20(1): 56–62.

53 Cornish KM, Williamson G, Sanderson J. Quercetin metabolism in the lens: role in inhibition of hydrogen peroxide induced cataract. *Free Radic Biol Med* 2002; 33(1): 63–70.

54 Muthian G, Bright JJ. Quercetin, a flavonoid phytoestrogen, ameliorates experimental allergic encephalomyelitis by blocking IL-12 signaling through JAK-STAT pathway in T lymphocyte. *J Clin Immunol* 2004; 24(5): 542–552.

55 Rachkauskas GS. [The efficacy of enterosorption and a combination of antioxidants in schizophrenics]. *Lik Sprava* 1998; 4: 122–124.

56 DiCenzo R, Frerichs V, Larppanichpoonphol P, *et al.* Effect of quercetin on the plasma and intracellular concentrations of saquinavir in healthy adults. *Pharmacotherapy* 2006; 26(9): 1255–1261.

57 Kim KA, Park PW, Park JY. Short-term effect of quercetin on the pharmacokinetics of fexofenadine, a substrate of P-glycoprotein, in healthy volunteers. *Eur J Clin Pharmacol* 2009; 65(6): 609–614.

58 Jin F, Nieman DC, Shanely RA, *et al.* The variable plasma quercetin response to 12-week quercetin supplementation in humans. *Eur J Clin Nutr* 2010; 64(7): 692–697.

Red yeast rice

Description

Red yeast rice has been used traditionally in China for centuries. Food supplements of red yeast rice are prepared by culturing *Monascus purpureus* (a type of yeast) at a carefully controlled temperature and growth conditions over red rice; supplements are different from red yeast rice sold in Chinese grocery stores.

Constituents

Red yeast rice contains 14 mevinic acids (known as monacolins), of which the one in highest concentration is monacolin K (mevinolin or lovastatin).[1] Supplements may contain from 0 to 5 mg statin-like substances (particularly lovastatin) in each capsule or tablet.[2] Other constituents include sterols (beta-sitosterol, campesterol, stigmasterol, and sapogenin), isoflavones, isoflavone glycosides and monounsaturated fatty acids.[3]

Action

Mevinic acids (particularly lovastatin) competitively inhibit 3-hydroxy-3-methyl-glutaryl-coenzyme A (HMG-CoA) reductase, blocking cholesterol biosynthesis, so reducing blood cholesterol.[4,5,6] Lovastatin is likely to make the greatest contribution to this cholesterol lowering effect, but all the mevinic acids and other compounds in red yeast rice supplements may have an additive effect on cholesterol lowering.[7]

Possible uses

Red yeast rice is used in Chinese medicine to reduce blood cholesterol, promote blood circulation and aid digestive problems. Western consumers have purchased this preparation mainly for cholesterol lowering. Other uses include indigestion and promotion of circulation.

Red yeast rice has been shown to lower cholesterol in several studies involving both healthy subjects and patients with dyslipidaemia. In a 12-week randomised controlled trial involving 83 healthy adults, red yeast rice 2.4 g daily in conjunction with a diet providing 30% energy from fat, significantly reduced total cholesterol, LDL cholesterol and triacylglcerol concentration compared with placebo.[4]

In a placebo-controlled 8-week trial in 79 patients with hypercholesterolaemia, red yeast rice 600 mg daily was associated with a significantly greater reduction than placebo in total cholesterol, triacylglycerols and apolipoprotein B in one paper,[8] and in another paper with significantly lower LDL cholesterol levels, and total cholesterol/HDL cholesterol, LDL/HDL cholesterol and apolipoprotein B/apolipoprotein A–I ratios.[9] In a trial evaluating red yeast rice over 6 months and fluvastatin over 12 months in 72 patients with nephrotic dyslipidaemia, both significantly reduced cholesterol.[10]

A meta-analysis of 93 randomised controlled trials (9625 participants) found that studies were generally of poor methodological quality. The combined results showed significant reduction of serum total cholesterol levels (weighted mean difference -0.91 mmol/L; 95% confidence interval (CI) -1.12 to -0.71), triglycerides levels (-0.41 mmol/L; CI -0.6 to -0.22), and LDL-cholesterol levels (-0.73 mmol/L; CI -1.02 to -0.043), and increase of HDL- cholesterol levels (0.15 mmol/L; CI 0.09 to 0.22) by red yeast rice treatment compared with placebo. The lipid modification effects appeared to be similar to pravastatin, simvastatin, lovastatin, atorvastatin, or fluvastatin. Compared with non-statin lipid-lowering agents, red yeast preparations appeared superior to nicotinate and fish oils, but equal to or less effective than fenofibrate and gemfibrozil.[5]

> **Conclusion**
> Red yeast rice should be avoided. Supplements contain varying amount of statin-like substances and are associated with the same adverse effects and interactions as statin medications. Supplements may reduce plasma cholesterol but should not be used as a substitute for licensed statin medications.

Precautions/contraindications

Red yeast rice should be avoided. It is not generally available in UK retail outlets, but is available on the Internet. In the USA, the Food and Drug Administration (FDA) considers red yeast rice supplements that contain statins to be unapproved drugs.

Pregnancy and breastfeeding

Avoid in pregnancy and breastfeeding.

Adverse effects

Because red yeast rice supplements may contain significant amounts of statin-like substances, they should be considered to have the potential for the same adverse effects as statins (e.g. myopathy, raised liver enzymes). Reports have linked red yeast rice supplements to rhabdomyolysis,[11,12] myopathy[13–15] and hepatotoxicity.[16] Red yeast rice supplements may also cause gastrointestinal side-effects (heartburn, flatulence) and dizziness.[5] Some red yeast rice products many contain citrinin, a contaminant resulting from inappropriate ferementation of red yeast.[17,18] Citrinin is nephrotoxic. Red yeast rice has also been associated with allergy and anaphylaxis.[19]

Interactions

Because red yeast rice supplements may contain statin-like substances, they could be subject to the same interactions as statins (e.g. grapefruit juice, cyclosporin, St John's wort). Red yeast rice supplements may act additively with licensed statin and other lipid-lowering medication.

Dose

Doses used in clinical trials have been 600–2400 mg.[4,5]

References

1 Li YG, Zhang F, Wang ZT, Hu ZB. Identification and chemical profiling of monacolins in red yeast rice using high-performance liquid chromatography with photodiode array detector and mass spectrometry. *J Pharm Biomed Anal* 2004; 35(5): 1101–1112.

2 Heber D, Lembertas A, Lu QY, *et al.* An analysis of nine proprietary Chinese red yeast rice dietary supplements: implications of variability in chemical profile and contents. *J Altern Complement Med* 2001; 7(2-): 133–139.

3 Ma J, Li Y, Ye Q, *et al.* Constituents of red yeast rice, a traditional Chinese food and medicine. *J Agric Food Chem* 2000; 48(11): 5220–5225.

4 Heber D, Yip I, Ashley JM, *et al.* Cholesterol-lowering effects of a proprietary Chinese red-yeast-rice dietary supplement. *Am J Clin Nutr* 1999; 69(2): 231–236.

5 Liu J, Zhang J, Shi Y, *et al.* Chinese red yeast rice (*Monascus purpureus*) for primary hyperlipidemia: a meta-analysis of randomized controlled trials. *Chin Med* 2006; 1: 4.

6 Bliznakov EG. More on the Chinese red-yeast-rice supplement and its cholesterol-lowering effect. *Am J Clin Nutr* 2000; 71(1): 152–154.

7 Li Z, Seeram NP, Lee R, *et al.* Plasma clearance of lovastatin versus chinese red yeast rice in healthy volunteers. *J Altern Complement Med* 2005; 11 (6): 1031–1038.

8 Lin CC, Li TC, Lai MM. Efficacy and safety of *Monascus purpureus* Went rice in subjects with hyperlipidemia. *Eur J Endocrinol* 2005; 153(5): 679–686.

9 Huang CF, Li TC, Lin CC, *et al.* Efficacy of *Monascus purpureus* Went rice on lowering lipid ratios in hypercholesterolemic patients. *Eur J Cardiovasc Prev Rehabil* 2007; 14(3): 438–440.

10 Gheith O, Sheashaa H, Abdelsalam M, *et al.* Efficacy and safety of *Monascus purpureus* Went rice in subjects with secondary hyperlipidemia. *Clin Exp Nephrol* 2008; 12(3): 189–194.

11 Rhabdomyolysis linked to Chinese red yeast rice. *Prescrire Int* 2008; 17(94): 64.

12 Prasad GV, Wong T, Meliton G, Bhaloo S. Rhabdomyolysis due to red yeast rice (*Monascus purpureus*) in a renal transplant recipient. *Transplantation* 2002; 74(8): 1200–1201.

13 Mueller PS. Symptomatic myopathy due to red yeast rice. *Ann Intern Med* 2006; 145(6): 474–475.

14 Smith DJ, Olive KE. Chinese red rice-induced myopathy. *South Med J* 2003; 96(12): 1265–1267.

15 Vercelli L, Mongini T, Olivero N, *et al.* Chinese red rice depletes muscle coenzyme Q10 and maintains muscle damage after discontinuation of statin treatment. *J Am Geriatr Soc* 2006; 54(4): 718–720.

16 Roselle H, Ekatan A, Tzeng J, *et al.* Symptomatic hepatitis associated with the use of herbal red yeast rice. *Ann Intern Med* 2008; 149(7): 516–517.

17 Chen F, Hu X. Study on red fermented rice with high concentration of monacolin K and low concentration of citrinin. *Int J Food Microbiol* 2005; 103 (3): 331–337.

18 Tsukahara M, Shinzato N, Tamaki Y, *et al*. Red yeast rice fermentation by selected *Monascus* sp. with deep-red color, lovastatin production but no

citrinin, and effect of temperature-shift cultivation on lovastatin production. *Appl Biochem Biotechnol* 2009; 158(2): 476–482.

19 Wigger-Alberti W, Bauer A, Hipler UC, Elsner P. Anaphylaxis due to *Monascus purpureus*-fermented rice (red yeast rice). *Allergy* 1999; 54: 1330–1331.

Resveratrol

Description

Resveratrol is a polyphenol, more specifically a phytoalexin (3,5,4′-trihydroxy-*trans*-stilbene), which exists as *cis*- and *trans*-stereoisomers.[1] It is produced by plants as a defence against infection by pathogenic micro-organisms such as fungi.

Dietary sources

The most abundant sources of resveratrol are the wine-making grapes *Vitis vinifera*, Labrusca and Muscatine. It occurs in the vines, roots, seeds and stalks, but the skin of the grape contains the highest concentration (50–100 µg/g). The resveratrol content of red wine is much higher than that of white wine. This is largely because, apart from the type of grapes used, in red wine production the skins and seeds are used, while white wine is prepared mainly from the juice, the skins being removed earlier in the process. The skins and seeds of grapes contain, in addition to resveratrol, a variety of other polyphenols including proanthocyanidins, quercetin, catechins and gallocatechins.

The resveratrol content of red wine varies considerably depending on the grapes and length of time the skins are present during the fermentation process. Red wines with the highest resveratrol content are pinot noir and cabernet sauvignon, produced in cold, humid climates (e.g. Bordeaux and Canada) rather than hot, dry climates. This is because fungal infections are more common in cooler climates, and resveratrol is produced in response to fungal infections in plants. Unfermented grape juice does not contain significant quantities of resveratrol.

Smaller amounts of resveratrol are found in mulberries and peanuts, and in other plants such as eucalyptus, lily and spruce. Resveratrol is also found in significant amounts in the dried roots and stems of the plant *Polygonium cuspidatum*, also known as Japanese knotweed. The dried root and stem of this plant are used in traditional Chinese and Japanese remedies (known as Hu Zhang, Hu Chang, tiger cane, kojo-kon and hadori-kon) for circulatory problems.[2]

Action

Knowledge of the potential benefits of resveratrol has developed partly from an appreciation of the beneficial effects of red wine on cardiovascular health.

Mechanisms for protection of the cardiovascular system that have been identified include:[3,4]

- antioxidant[5–7]
- inhibition of cholesterol synthesis
- inhibition of atherosclerosis
- inhibition of LDL oxidation
- protection and maintenance of endothelial tissue
- suppression of platelet aggregation[8–14]
- reduction of inflammatory markers (e.g. tumour necrosis factor-alpha-induced NF-κB and inflammatory gene expression)[15]
- promotion of vasodilatation
- defence against ischaemic reperfusion injury
- increasing nitric oxide through activation of endothelial nitric oxide synthase[16]
- inhibition of insulin secretion from the pancreas[17]
- oestrogenic activity.

Resveratrol has also been shown to have anticancer properties,[18] inhibiting activation of carcinogenic compounds and suppressing tumour progression.[19–21] *In vitro* studies have shown a number of protective mechanisms in relation to cancer, including inhibition of carcinogen activation, suppression of tumour initiation by inhibition of cellular-signalling cascades and influence on apoptosis,[22–24] and inhibiting cyclo-oxygenase 1 and 2.[22,25,26]

Resveratrol has also been shown to reduce cell proliferation in a human retinal epithelium cell line and may, therefore, have the ability to protect against age-related macular degeneration.[27] A study in animals indicated that resveratrol could protect cartilage in experimentally induced arthritis.[28]

Possible uses

In vitro studies have clearly demonstrated potential mechanisms for benefit of resveratrol in the prevention of cardiovascular disease (CVD) and cancer. However, these studies have been short-term and there have been very few studies in humans. Two small studies (both from the same research group in China) found that resveratrol inhibited platelet aggregation in rabbits and humans.[10,11] However, it would be premature to recommend resveratrol as a food supplement, despite the industry's claims that resveratrol is the component in red wine responsible for the beneficial effects on CVD.

Conclusion

Resveratrol is the subject of much interest as a food supplement, mainly because it is claimed to be the component in red wine responsible for its beneficial effects in CVD. *In vitro* studies have demonstrated mechanisms by which resveratrol could reduce the risk of CVD and cancer, but there have been no intervention trials in humans. The main dietary source is red wine, and care should be taken not to encourage high intake of any alcoholic drink.

Precautions/contraindications

The main dietary source of resveratrol is red wine. Recommending increased consumption of red wine to increase resveratrol intake is not necessarily responsible given the health risks, including liver damage, physical addiction and social implications of any alcoholic beverage if consumed in more than moderate amounts.

Pregnancy and breast-feeding

No problems reported, but resveratrol may be oestrogenic. Alcohol should not be consumed during pregnancy.

Adverse effects

Resveratrol is similar in structure to diethylstilbestrol (a synthetic oestrogen) and it could have the potential to stimulate breast cancer.[29] A study in rats has suggested that resveratrol could have pro-inflammatory activity in circumstances of vascular inflammation.[30] Diarrhoea has been observed with doses in humans of 2 g twice daily.[31] More studies are needed.

Interactions

None reported. However, in a study involving 42 volunteers, a dose of resveratrol 1 g daily for 4 weeks alters the activity of some cytochrome P450 enzymes.[32] Pharmacological doses of resveratrol could, therefore, lead to adverse drug effects or reduced drug activity through an influence of resveratrol on the cytochrome P450 system.

Dose

The dose is not established.

A phase I study of oral resveratrol (single doses of 0.5, 1, 2.5 or 5 g) in 10 healthy volunteers suggested that high-dose resveratrol might be insufficient to elicit systemic levels commensurate with cancer chemopreventive efficacy demonstrated in animals.[33] A study in 10 subjects found that *trans*-resveratrol 25, 50, 100 or 150 mg, six times a day similarly produced relative low plasma levels of plasma *trans*-resveratrol.[34] However, a dosing study in 40 subjects with resveratrol 0.5, 1,0, 2.5 or 5.0 g daily for 29 days demonstrated a reduction in concentrations of insulin-like growth factor-1 sufficient to contribute to a chemoprotective effect.[35] A further trial in 20 patients with colorectal cancer showed that resveratrol 0.5 or 1 g daily produced levels in the human gastrointestinal tract of an order of magnitude sufficient to elicit anticarcinogenic effects.[36]

A study in 24 healthy subjects found that the rate of absorption of *trans*-resveratrol following an oral 400 mg single dose was significantly delayed by the presence of food, but the extent of absorption was not affected in a relevant way.[37] A further trial suggested that resveratrol should be taken with a standard breakfast rather than a high-fat meal.[31]

References

1 Fremont L. Biological effects of resveratrol. *Life Sci* 2000; 66(8): 663–673.
2 Soleas GJ, Diamandis EP, Goldberg DM. Resveratrol: a molecule whose time has come? And gone? *Clin Biochem* 1997; 30(2): 91–113.
3 Hao HD, He LR. Mechanisms of cardiovascular protection by resveratrol. *J Med Food* 2004; 7(3): 290–298.
4 Wu JM, Wang ZR, Hsieh TC, *et al.* Mechanism of cardioprotection by resveratrol, a phenolic antioxidant present in red wine (Review). *Int J Mol Med* 2001; 8(1): 3–17.
5 O'Brien NM, Carpenter R, O'Callaghan YC, *et al.* Modulatory effects of resveratrol, citroflavan-3-ol, and plant-derived extracts on oxidative stress in U937 cells. *J Med Food* 2006; 9(2): 187–195.
6 Mokni M, Limam F, Elkahoui S, Amri M, Aouani E. Strong cardioprotective effect of resveratrol, a red wine polyphenol, on isolated rat hearts after ischemia/reperfusion injury. *Arch Biochem Biophys* 2007; 457(1): 1–6.
7 Ghanim H, Sia CL, Abuaysheh S, *et al.* An anti-inflammatory and reactive oxygen species suppressive effects of an extract of *Polygonum cuspidatum* containing resveratrol. *J Clin Endocrinol Metab* 2010; 95(9): E1–E8.
8 Pace-Asciak CR, Hahn S, Diamandis EP, *et al.* The red wine phenolics *trans*-resveratrol and quercetin block human platelet aggregation and eicosanoid synthesis: implications for protection against coronary heart disease. *Clin Chim Acta* 1995; 235(2): 207–219.
9 Bertelli AA, Giovannini L, Giannessi D, *et al.* Antiplatelet activity of synthetic and natural resveratrol in red wine. *Int J Tissue React* 1995; 17(1): 1–3.
10 Wang Z, Huang Y, Zou J, *et al.* Effects of red wine and wine polyphenol resveratrol on platelet aggregation in vivo and in vitro. *Int J Mol Med* 2002; 9(1): 77–79.
11 Wang Z, Zou J, Huang Y, *et al.* Effect of resveratrol on platelet aggregation in vivo and in vitro. *Chin Med J (Engl)* 2002; 115(3): 378–380.
12 Olas B, Wachowicz B. Resveratrol, a phenolic antioxidant with effects on blood platelet functions. *Platelets* 2005; 16(5): 251–260.
13 Pace-Asciak CR, Rounova O, Hahn SE, *et al.* Wines and grape juices as modulators of platelet aggregation in healthy human subjects. *Clin Chim Acta* 1996; 246(1-2): 163–182.
14 Stef G, Csiszar A, Lerea K, *et al.* Resveratrol inhibits aggregation of platelets from high-risk cardiac patients with aspirin resistance. *J Cardiovasc Pharmacol* 2006; 48(2): 1–5.
15 Csiszar A, Smith K, Labinskyy N, *et al.* Resveratrol attenuates TNF-α-induced activation of coronary arterial endothelial cells: role of NF-κB inhibition. *Am J Physiol Heart Circ Physiol* 2006; 291(4): H1694–H1699.
16 Gresele P, Pignatelli P, Guglielmini G, *et al.* Resveratrol, at concentrations attainable with moderate wine consumption, stimulates human platelet nitric oxide production. *J Nutr* 2008; 138(9): 1602–1608.
17 Szkudelski T. Resveratrol inhibits insulin secretion from rat pancreatic islets. *Eur J Pharmacol* 2006; 552(13): 176–181.
18 Soleas GJ, Grass L, Josephy PD, *et al.* A comparison of the anticarcinogenic properties of four red wine polyphenols. *Clin Biochem* 2006; 39(5): 492–497.
19 Gusman J, Malonne H, Atassi G. A reappraisal of the potential chemopreventive and chemotherapeutic properties of resveratrol. *Carcinogenesis* 2001; 22(8): 1111–1117.
20 Trincheri NF, Nicotra G, Follo C, *et al.* Resveratrol induces cell death in colorectal cancer cells by a novel pathway involving lysosomal cathepsin D. *Carcinogenesis* 2006; 28(5): 922–931.
21 Golkar L, Ding XZ, Ujiki MB, *et al.* Resveratrol inhibits pancreatic cancer cell proliferation through transcriptional induction of macrophage inhibitory cytokine-1. *J Surg Res* 2007; 138(2): 163–169.
22 Gescher AJ, Steward WP. Relationship between mechanisms, bioavailability, and preclinical chemopreventive efficacy of resveratrol: a conundrum. *Cancer Epidemiol Biomarkers Prev* 2003; 12(10): 953–957.
23 Zhang W, Fei Z, Zhen HN, *et al.* Resveratrol inhibits cell growth and induces apoptosis of rat C6 glioma cells. *J Neurooncol* 2006; 81(3): 231–240.
24 Faber AC, Chiles TC. Resveratrol induces apoptosis in transformed follicular lymphoma OCI-LY8 cells: evidence for a novel mechanism involving inhibition of BCL6 signaling. *Int J Oncol* 2006; 29(6): 1561–1566.
25 Kundu JK, Shin YK, Kim SH, *et al.* Resveratrol inhibits phorbol ester-induced expression of COX-2 and activation of NF-kappaB in mouse skin by blocking IkappaB kinase activity. *Carcinogenesis* 2006; 27(7): 1465–1474.
26 Kundu JK, Shin YK, Surh YJ. Resveratrol modulates phorbol ester-induced pro-inflammatory signal transduction pathways in mouse skin in vivo: NF-κB and AP-1 as prime targets. *Biochem Pharmacol* 2006; 72(11): 1506–1515.
27 King RE, Kent KD, Bomser JA. Resveratrol reduces oxidation and proliferation of human retinal pigment epithelial cells via extracellular signal-regulated kinase inhibition. *Chem Biol Interact* 2005; 151(2): 143–149.

28 Elmali N, Baysal O, Harma A, *et al.* Effects of resveratrol in inflammatory arthritis. *Inflammation* 2007; 30(1-2): 1–6.

29 Gehm H. Resveratrol, a polyphenolic compound found in grapes and wine, is an agonist for the estrogen receptor. *Proc Natl Acad Sci USA* 1997; 94: 557–562.

30 Cignarella A, Minici C, Bolego C, *et al.* Potential pro-inflammatory action of resveratrol in vascular smooth muscle cells from normal and diabetic rats. *Nutr Metab Cardiovasc Dis* 2006; 16(5): 322–329.

31 la Porte C, Voduc N, Zhang G, *et al.* Steady-state pharmacokinetics and tolerability of *trans*-resveratrol 2000 mg twice daily with food, quercetin and alcohol (ethanol) in healthy human subjects. *Clin Pharmacokinet* 2010; 49(7): 449–454.

32 Chow HH, Garland LL, Hsu CH, *et al.* Resveratrol modulates drug- and carcinogen-metabolizing enzymes in a healthy volunteer study. *Cancer Prev Res (Phila)* 2010; 3(9): 1168–1175.

33 Boocock DJ, Faust GE, Patel KR, *et al.* Phase I dose escalation pharmacokinetic study in healthy volunteers of resveratrol, a potential cancer chemo-preventive agent. *Cancer Epidemiol Biomarkers Prev* 2007; 16(6): 1246–1252.

34 Almeida L, Vaz-da-Silva M, Falcao A, *et al.* Pharmacokinetic and safety profile of *trans*-resveratrol in a rising multiple-dose study in healthy volunteers. *Mol Nutr Food Res* 2009; 53 (Suppl11): S7–S15.

35 Brown VA, Patel KR, Viskaduraki M, *et al.* Repeat dose study of the cancer chemopreventive agent resveratrol in healthy volunteers: safety, pharmacokinetics, and effect on the insulin-like growth factor axis. *Cancer Res* 2010; 70(22): 9003–9011.

36 Patel KR, Brown VA, Jones DJ, *et al.* Clinical pharmacology of resveratrol and its metabolites in colorectal cancer patients. *Cancer Res* 2010; 70(19): 7392–7399.

37 Vaz-da-Silva M, Loureiro AI, Falcao A, *et al.* Effect of food on the pharmacokinetic profile of *trans*-resveratrol. *Int J Clin Pharmacol Ther* 2008; 46 (11): 564–570.

Riboflavin

Description

Riboflavin is a water-soluble vitamin of the vitamin B complex.

Nomenclature

Riboflavin is the British Approved Name for use on pharmaceutical labels. It is known also as vitamin B_2.

Human requirements

See Table 1 for Dietary Reference Values for riboflavin.

Dietary intake

In the UK, the average adult diet provides: for men, 2.11 mg daily; for women, 1.60 mg.

Action

Riboflavin functions as a component of two flavin coenzymes – flavin mononucleotide (FMN) and flavin adenine dinucleotide (FAD). It participates in oxidation–reduction reactions in numerous metabolic pathways and in energy production. Examples include the oxidation of glucose, certain amino acids and fatty acids; reactions with several intermediaries of the Krebs cycle; conversion of pyridoxine to its active coenzyme; and conversion of tryptophan to niacin.

Riboflavin has a role as an antioxidant. It may be involved in maintaining the integrity of erythrocytes.

Dietary sources

See Table 2 for dietary sources of riboflavin.

Metabolism

Absorption
Riboflavin is readily absorbed by a saturable active transport system (principally in the duodenum).

Distribution
Some circulating riboflavin is loosely associated with plasma albumin, but significant amounts complex with other proteins. Conversion of riboflavin to its coenzymes occurs in most tissues (particularly in the liver, heart and kidney).

Table 1 Dietary Reference Values for riboflavin (mg/day)

Age	UK				USA		FAO/WHO RNI
						EU RDA = 1.6 mg	
	LRNI	EAR	RNI	EVM	RDA	TUL	
0–6 months	0.2	0.3	0.4		0.3	–	0.3
7–12 months	0.2	0.3	0.4		0.4	–	0.4
1–3 years	0.3	0.5	0.6		0.5	–	0.5
4–6 years	0.4	0.6	0.8		–	–	0.6
4–8 years	–	–	–		0.6	–	–
7–10 years	0.5	0.8	1.0		1.2	–	0.9[1]
9–13 years	–	–	–		0.9	–	–
Males							
11–14 years	0.8	1.0	1.2		–	–	1.2[2]
15–18 years	0.8	1.0	1.3		–	–	1.2
19–50+ years	0.8	1.0	1.3		–	–	1.3
14–70+ years				100	1.3	–	–
Females							
11–14 years	0.8	0.9	1.1		–	–	1.0[2]
14–18 years					1.0	–	1.0
15–50+ years	0.8	0.9	1.1		–	–	1.1
19–70+ years	–	–	–	100	1.1	–	–
Pregnancy	*	*	+0.3		1.4	–	1.4
Lactation	–	–	+0.5		1.6	–	1.6

* No increment.
[1]7–9 years; [2]10–14 years.
EVM = Likely safe daily intake from supplements alone.
LRNI = Lowest Reference Nutrient Intake.
RNI = Reference Nutrient Intake.
TUL = Tolerable Upper Intake Level (not determined for riboflavin).

Elimination

Riboflavin is excreted primarily in the urine (mostly as metabolites); excess amounts are excreted unchanged. Riboflavin crosses the placenta and is excreted in breast milk.

Bioavailability

Riboflavin is remarkably stable during processing that involves heat, such as canning, dehydration, evaporation and pasteurisation. Boiling in water results in leaching of the vitamin into the water, which should then be used for soups and sauces. Considerable losses occur if food is exposed to light; exposure of milk in glass bottles will result in loss of riboflavin. Animal sources of riboflavin are better absorbed and hence more available than vegetable sources.

Deficiency

Deficiency of riboflavin isolated from other B vitamin deficiencies is rare. Early symptoms

Table 2 Dietary sources of riboflavin

Food portion	Riboflavin content (mg)
Breakfast cereals	
1 bowl *All-Bran* (45 g)	0.5
1 bowl *Bran Flakes* (45 g)	0.6
1 bowl *Corn Flakes* (30 g)	0.4
1 bowl *muesli* (95 g)	0.6
1 bowl **Shreddies** (50 g)	1.1
1 bowl **Start** (40 g)	0.8
2 *Weetabix*	0.6
Milk and dairy products	
Milk, whole, semi-skimmed or skimmed (284 ml; ¹/₂ pint)	0.5
Soya milk (284 ml; ¹/₂ pint)	0.7
1 pot *yoghurt* (150 g)	0.4
Cheese (50 g)	0.2
1 *egg*, size 2 (60 g)	0.3
Meat and fish	
Beef, roast (85 g)	0.2
Lamb, roast (85 g)	0.3
Pork, roast (85 g)	0.2
1 *chicken leg* portion	0.2
Liver, lambs, cooked (90 g)	3.0
Kidney, lambs, cooked (75 g)	1.6
Fish, cooked (150 g)	0.2
Yeast	
Brewer's yeast (10 g)	0.4
Marmite, spread on 1 slice bread	0.5

Excellent sources (**bold**); good sources (*italics*).

include soreness of the mouth and throat, burning and itching of the eyes, and personality deterioration. Advanced deficiency may lead to cheilosis, angular stomatitis, glossitis (red, beefy tongue), corneal vascularisation, seborrhoeic dermatitis (of the face, trunk and extremities), normochromic normocytic anaemia, leucopenia and thrombocytopenia.

Possible uses

Supplements may be required by vegans (strict vegetarians who consume no milk or dairy produce).

Migraine

Riboflavin has been investigated for a possible role in migraine. In an open pilot study in 49 migraine patients, 26 patients were given oral riboflavin 400 mg daily or the same plus aspirin 75 mg daily for 3–5 months. The number of migraine days reduced from 8.7 ± 1.5 to 2.9 ± 1.2. There were no significant differences between the two groups.[1]

In a randomised, double-blind, placebo-controlled trial, 55 patients with a history of migraine for at least 1 year (with two to eight attacks monthly) were randomised to receive riboflavin 400 mg or placebo daily. Migraine attack frequency and duration was significantly reduced in the riboflavin group compared with placebo.[2]

A further randomised, double-blind, placebo-controlled trial evaluated the effect of a supplement providing a daily dose of riboflavin 400 mg, magnesium 300 mg and feverfew 100 mg. The placebo contained 25 mg riboflavin. Forty-nine patients completed the 3-month trial. For the primary outcome measure, a 50% or greater reduction in migraines, there was no difference between the treatment and placebo groups, achieved by 10 (42%) and 11 (44%) individuals, respectively. There were no differences in the mean number of migraines, migraine days, migraine index or triptan doses. Compared with baseline, both groups showed a significant reduction in number of migraines, migraine days and migraine index. This effect exceeds that reported for placebo agents in previous migraine trials, suggesting that riboflavin 25 mg may be an active comparator.[3]

Only one trial to date involving the use of riboflavin for migraine in children has been conducted. This was a randomised, double-blind study of riboflavin (200 mg daily) versus placebo in 48 children. The primary efficacy measure was the number of patients achieving a 50% or greater reduction in the number of migraine attacks over a 4-week period. Other outcome measures were the mean severity of migraine per day, mean duration of migraine, days with nausea or vomiting, analgesic use and adverse effects. A 50% or greater reduction in headaches was seen in 14/21 patients in the placebo group and 12/27 patients in the riboflavin group (not significant, $P = 0.125$). There were no differences between riboflavin and placebo for primary or secondary outcome variables. These results suggest that riboflavin is not an effective therapy for preventing migraine in children.[4]

Miscellaneous

A case report demonstrated successful therapy with riboflavin 50 mg daily in a patient with documented riboflavin deficiency and carpal tunnel syndrome.[5] Riboflavin has also been used successfully in the treatment of lactic acidosis induced by antiretroviral therapy in patients with AIDS.[6,7] Homocysteine metabolism is dependent on riboflavin and riboflavin has been investigated for a role in homocysteine lowering, but most studies to date have not demonstrated any clear benefit of riboflavin in lowering homocysteine.[8,9] However, a randomised, double-blind trial among 88 elderly people in seven Portugese day centres showed that 10 mg riboflavin daily lowered plasma homocysteine, but only in those elderly people with a low riboflavin status.[10] A study in 96 patients with ischaemic stroke found that a high proportion were biochemically deficient of riboflavin immediately post-infarct. Supplementation with 5 mg riboflavin for 2 weeks significantly improved riboflavin status; however, the clinical significance of these findings is not yet known.[11] Riboflavin is of unproven value for acne, mouth ulcers or muscle cramps. At present, there is no convincing scientific data to support its use in human cancer.

Conclusion

At normal doses there is no good evidence for the use of riboflavin for any indication other than riboflavin deficiency. Preliminary evidence exists that higher doses may be useful in migraine and in lactic acidosis induced by antiretroviral therapy.

Precautions/contraindications

None reported.

Pregnancy and breast-feeding

No problems reported.

Adverse effects

Riboflavin toxicity is unknown in humans. Large doses may cause yellow discoloration of the urine.

Interactions

Drugs

Alcohol: excessive alcohol intake induces riboflavin deficiency.
Barbiturates: prolonged use may induce riboflavin deficiency.
Oral contraceptives: prolonged use may induce riboflavin deficiency.
Phenothiazines: may increase the requirement for riboflavin.
Probenecid: reduces gastrointestinal absorption and urinary excretion of riboflavin.
Tricyclic antidepressants: may increase the requirement for riboflavin.

Nutrients

Adequate amounts of all B vitamins are required for optimal functioning; deficiency or excess of one B vitamin may lead to abnormalities in the metabolism of another.
Iron: deficiency of riboflavin may impair iron metabolism and produce anaemia[8].

Dose

Riboflavin is available in the form of tablets and capsules, but is mainly found as a constituent of multivitamin and mineral preparations.

Dietary supplements provide 1–3 mg daily.

References

1 Schoenen J, Lenaerts M, Bastings E. High-dose riboflavin as a prophylactic treatment of migraine: results of an open pilot study. *Cephalgia* 1994; 14: 328–329.

2 Schoenen J, Jacquy J, Lenaerts M. Effectiveness of high-dose riboflavin in migraine prophylaxis: a randomized controlled trial. *Neurology* 1998; 50: 466–470.

3 Maizels M, Blumenfeld A, Burchette R. A combination of riboflavin, magnesium and feverfew for migraine prophylaxis: a randomized trial. *Headache* 2004; 44: 885–890.

4　MacLennan SC, Wade FM, Forrest KM, *et al*. High-dose riboflavin for migraine prophylaxis in children: a double-blind, randomized, placebo-controlled trial. *J Child Neurol* 2008; 23(11): 1300–1304.

5　Folkers K, Wolaniuk A, Vadhanavikit S. Enzymology of the response of the carpal tunnel syndrome to riboflavin and to combined riboflavin and pyridoxine. *Proc Natl Acad Sci* 1984; 81: 7076–7078.

6　Fouty B, Frerman F, Reves R. Riboflavin to treat nucleoside analogue-induced lactic acidosis. *Lancet* 1998; 352: 291–292.

7　Luzzati R, Del Bravo P, Di Perri G, *et al*. Riboflavine and severe lactic acidosis. *Lancet* 1999; 353: 901–902.

8　Powers HJ. Riboflavin (vitamin B-2) and health. *Am J Clin Nutr* 2003; 77(6): 1352–1360.

9　Araki R, Maruyama C, Igarashi S, *et al*. Effects of short-term folic acid and/or riboflavin supplementation on serum folate and plasma total homocysteine concentrations in young Japanese male subjects. *Eur J Clin Nutr* 2006; 60(5): 573–579.

10　Tavares NR, Moreira PA, Amaral TF. Riboflavin supplementation and biomarkers of cardiovascular disease in the elderly. *J Nutr Health Aging* 2009; 13 (5): 441–446.

11　Gariballa S, Ullegaddi R. Riboflavin status in acute ischaemic stroke. *Eur J Clin Nutr* 2007; 61(10): 1237–1240.

Royal jelly

Description

Royal jelly is a yellow-white liquid secreted by the hypopharyngeal glands of 'nurse' worker bees from the 6th to the 12th day of their adult lives. It is an essential food for the queen bee.

Constituents

See Table 1 for the claimed nutrient composition of royal jelly.

Action

Royal jelly may have some pharmacological effects, but the only available evidence comes from *in vitro* studies and animal studies. It appears to have anti-tumour effects;[1] antioxidant effects;[2] improve the efficiency of insulin;[3] have vasodilator activity,[4] blood pressure-lowering activity[5] and wound healing activity;[6] and exhibit antimicrobial activity.[7] An ingredient, 10-hydroxy-2-decenoic acid, isolated from royal jelly has recently been found to inhibit joint destruction in rheumatoid arthritis.[8]

Possible uses

Published papers on the effects of royal jelly in humans are relatively few, and many of these are single case histories and not clinical trials.

Royal jelly has been claimed to be beneficial in anorexia, fatigue and headaches,[9] and in hypercholesterolaemia.[10,11]

Table 1　Claimed nutrient composition in a typical daily dose (500 mg) of royal jelly

Nutrient	Amount	% RNI[1]
Water (mg)	350	–
Carbohydrate (mg)	60	–
Protein (mg)	60	–
Lipids (mg)	25	–
Thiamine (µg)	2	0.2
Riboflavin (µg)	7	0.6
Niacin (µg)	20	0.1
Vitamin B$_6$ (µg)	3	0.2
Folic acid (ng)	15	0.08
Biotin (µg)	1	–
Pantothenic acid (µg)	3	–
Calcium (µg)	130	0.02
Magnesium (µg)	150	0.07
Potassium (mg)	2.5	0.07
Iron (µg)	25	0.2
Zinc (µg)	15	0.2

[1]Reference Nutrient Intake for men aged 19–50 years.

A systematic review and meta-analysis[11] examined the effect of royal jelly in 17 animal studies and nine human studies. In the animal studies, royal jelly significantly reduced serum cholesterol and total lipid levels in rats and rabbits, and slowed the progress of atheromas in rabbits fed a high-fat diet. Meta-analysis of the controlled human trials showed that royal jelly (30–100 mg daily for 3–6 weeks) resulted in a significant reduction in total serum lipids and cholesterol and normalisation of LDL and HDL cholesterol in subjects with hyperlipidaemia.

Royal jelly has been investigated in hay fever. A placebo-controlled, double-blind RCT in 80 children (aged 5–16 years) evaluated the effect of royal jelly administered 3–6 months before and throughout the pollen season. Sixty-four children completed the study. All of the patients in both groups developed hay fever symptoms during the pollen season. The severity of symptoms and need for additional hay fever treatment was similar in both groups, suggesting that royal jelly has no benefit on hay fever symptoms during the pollen season.[12]

The effects of royal jelly on serum lipids have also been evaluated. Fifteen volunteers were given either royal jelly (6 g daily) or control for 4 weeks. Total serum cholesterol and LDL decreased significantly compared with those of the control group ($P < 0.05$). There were no significant differences in serum HDL or triglyceride concentrations. Among the lipoprotein fractions, VLDL was decreased ($P < 0.05$) after royal jelly intake. These findings suggest that royal jelly decreases cholesterol and LDL cholesterol by lowering small VLDL levels.[13] A further small trail suggested that royal jelly might increase HDL cholesterol but in older people only,[14] while another trial found that royal jelly reduced serum glucose levels following a glucose tolerance test compared with placebo.[15]

Claims for the value of royal jelly in arthritis, depression, diabetes mellitus, dysmenorrhoea, eczema, morning sickness, multiple sclerosis, muscular dystrophy, myalgic encephalomyelitis and premenstrual syndrome are purely anecdotal and there is no evidence for any of these claims.

Conclusion

Anecdotally, royal jelly is thought to be beneficial in a wide range of conditions. However, there is no sound evidence to support its use.

Precautions/contraindications

Royal jelly should be avoided in asthma (adverse effects reported).

Pregnancy and breast-feeding

No problems reported, but there have not been sufficient studies to guarantee the safety of royal jelly in pregnancy and breast-feeding. Royal jelly is probably best avoided.

Adverse effects

Allergic reactions, which can be severe. Life-threatening bronchospasm has occurred in patients with asthma after ingestion of royal jelly.[16–19] Royal jelly has been responsible for IgE-mediated anaphylaxis,[20–22] leading to death in at least one individual.[23] One report of haemorrhagic colitis occurred in a 53-year-old woman after taking royal jelly for 25 days.[24]

Interactions

Evidence from a single case study indicated that an interaction between warfarin and royal jelly resulted in an increased International Normalized Ratio (INR).[25]

Dose

Royal jelly is available in the form of tablets and capsules.

The dose is not established. Dietary supplements provide 250–500 mg daily.

References

1 Tamura T, Fujii A, Kuboyama N. Antitumour effects of royal jelly. *Nippon Yakurigaku Zasshi* 1987; 89: 73–80.

2 Nagai T, Inoue R, Suzuki N, *et al.* Antioxidant properties of enzymatic hydrolysates from royal jelly. *J Med Food* 2006; 9(3): 363–367.

3 Kramer KJ, Tager HS, Childs CN, Spiers RD. Insulin-like hypoglycaemic and immunological activities in honey bee royal jelly. *J Insect Physiol* 1977; 23: 293–296.

4 Shinoda M, Nakajin S, Oikawa T, *et al.* Biochemical studies on vasodilator factor of royal jelly. *Yakugaku Zasshi* 1978; 98: 139–145.

5 Sultana A, Nabi AH, Nasir UM, *et al.* A dipeptide YY derived from royal jelly proteins inhibits renin activity. *Int J Mol Med* 2008; 21(6): 677–681.

6 Majtan J, Kumar P, Majtan T, *et al.* Effect of honey and its major royal jelly protein 1 on cytokine and MMP-9 mRNA transcripts in human keratinocytes. *Exp Dermatol* 2010; 19(8): e73–e79.

7 Fujiwara S, Imaj J, Fujiwara M, *et al.* A potent antibacterial protein in royal jelly. Purification and determination of the primary structure of royalisin. *J Biol Chem* 1990; 265: 11333–11337.

8 Yang XY, Yang DS, Wei Z, *et al.* 10-Hydroxy-2-decenoic acid from royal jelly: a potential medicine for RA. *J Ethnopharmacol* 2010; 128(2): 314–321.

9 Tamura T. Royal jelly from the standpoint of clinical pharmacology. *Honeybee Sci* 1985; 6: 117–124.

10 Cho YT. Studies on royal jelly and abnormal cholesterol and triglycerides. *Am Bee J* 1977; 117: 36–38.

11 Vittek J. Effect of royal jelly on serum lipids in experimental animals and humans with atherosclerosis. *Experientia* 1995; 51: 927–935.

12 Andersen AH, Mortensen S, Agertoft L, Pedersen S. Double-blind randomized trial of the effect of Bidro on hay fever in children. *Ugeskr Laeger* 2005; 167: 3591–3594.

13 Guo H, Saiga A, Sato M, *et al.* Royal jelly supplementation improves lipoprotein metabolism in humans. *J Nutr Sci Vitaminol (Tokyo)* 2007; 53 (4): 345–348.

14 Munstedt K, Henschel M, Hauenschild A, *et al.* Royal jelly increases high density lipoprotein levels but in older patients only. *J Altern Complement Med* 2009; 15(4): 329–330.

15 Munstedt K, Bargello M, Hauenschild A. Royal jelly reduces the serum glucose levels in healthy subjects. *J Med Food* 2009; 12(5): 1170–1172.

16 Leung R, Thien FCK, Baldo BA, *et al.* Royal jelly induced asthma and anaphylaxis: clinical characteristics and immunologic correlations. *J Allergy Clin Immunol* 1995; 96: 1004–1007.

17 Peacock S, Murray V, Turton C. Respiratory distress and royal jelly. *BMJ* 1995; 311: 1472.

18 Larporte JR, Ibaanez L, Vendrell L, *et al.* Bronchospasm induced by royal jelly. *Allergy* 1996; 51: 440.

19 Harwood M, Harding S, Beasley R, *et al.* Asthma following royal jelly. *NZ Med J* 1996; 109: 325.

20 Thien FC, Leung R, Baldo BA, *et al.* Asthma and anaphylaxis induced by royal jelly. *Clin Exp Allergy* 1996; 26: 216–222.

21 Takahama H, Shimazu T. Food-induced anaphylaxis caused by ingestion of royal jelly. *J Dermatol* 2006; 33(6): 424–426.

22 Katayama M, Aoki M, Kawana S. Case of anaphylaxis caused by ingestion of royal jelly. *J Dermatol* 2008; 35(4): 222–224.

23 Bullock RJ, Rohan A, Straatmans JA. Fatal royal jelly induced asthma. *Med J Aust* 1994; 160: 44.

24 Yonei Y, Shibagaki K, Tsukada N, *et al.* Case report: hemorrhagic colitis associated with royal jelly intake. *J Gastroenterol Hepatol* 1997; 12: 495–499.

25 Lee NJ, Fermo JD. Warfarin and royal jelly interaction. *Pharmacotherapy* 2006; 26(4): 583–586.

S-Adenosyl methionine

Description

S-Adenosyl methionine (SAMe) is synthesised in the body from the essential amino acid methionine.

Action

SAMe is involved in several biochemical pathways. It functions mainly as a methyl donor in synthetic pathways that lead to the production of DNA and RNA, neurotransmitters and phospholipids. Its involvement in phospholipid synthesis may mean that it has a role in membrane fluidity. SAMe is also involved in transulphuration reactions, regulating the formation of sulphur-containing amino acids, cysteine, glutathione (GSH) and taurine. GSH is an antioxidant, so SAMe is proposed to have antioxidant activity.

Possible uses

SAMe is being investigated for its effects on a number of conditions, such as depression, osteoarthritis, fibromyalgia and cardiovascular disease (CVD).

Depression

SAMe may be of potential use as an antidepressant. Its mechanism of action for this indication is still a matter of speculation, although there is some evidence that it may raise dopamine levels.[1] Initially it was used for this purpose by parenteral administration. However, in an uncontrolled study[2] in 20 outpatients with major depression, the group as a whole improved with oral SAMe.

In a randomised, double-blind, placebo-controlled trial involving 15 inpatients with major depression, oral SAMe was found to improve symptoms of depression. However, it induced mania in one patient with no history of the condition.[3]

The efficacy of oral SAMe was assessed in the treatment of 80 depressed postmenopausal women (aged 45–59 years). The 30-day, double-blind, placebo-controlled randomised trial found a significantly greater improvement in depressive symptoms in the group treated with 1600 mg daily of SAMe from day 10 of the study.[4]

A meta-analysis of the effect of SAMe on depression compared with placebo or tricyclic antidepressants showed a greater response rate with SAMe than placebo and an antidepressant effect comparable with tricyclic antidepressants.[5]

An in-depth literature review, which included RCTs, controlled clinical trials, meta-analyses and systematic reviews, evaluated evidence on the use of SAMe for the treatment of depression (and also osteoarthritis and liver disease). Compared with placebo, SAMe was associated with a clinically significant improvement of depression. Compared with conventional antidepressant therapy, SAMe was not associated with a statistically significant difference in outcomes.[6]

A multicentre trial found that the efficacy of 1600 mg SAMe daily taken orally[7] and 400 mg SAMe daily intramuscularly[7,8] is comparable with that of imipramine 150 mg daily, but SAMe is better tolerated.

A 6-week double-blind randomised trial in 73 patients with major depressive disorder and no response to serotonin reuptake inhibitors employed oral SAMe (target dose, 800 mg/twice daily). Patients continued to receive their SRI treatment at a stable dose throughout the 6-week trial. The primary outcome measure for the study was the response rates according to the 17-item Hamilton Depression Rating Scale (HAM-D). The HAM-D response and remission rates were higher for patients treated with adjunctive SAMe (36.1% and 25.8%, respectively) than adjunctive placebo (17.6% versus 11.7%, respectively). The number needed to treat for response and remission was approximately one in six and one in seven, respectively. There was no statistically significant difference in the proportion of SAMe- versus placebo-treated patients who discontinued the trial for any reason (20.6% versus 29.5%, respectively), because of adverse events (5.1% versus 8.8%, respectively), or because of inefficacy (5.1% versus 11.7%, respectively). The authors concluded that these preliminary results suggest that SAMe can be an effective, well-tolerated, and safe adjunctive treatment strategy for SRI non-responders with major depressive disorder and warrant replication.[9]

Osteoarthritis

SAMe appears to possess analgesic activity, and in joints there is some evidence that it stimulates the synthesis of proteoglycans by the articular chondrocytes.[10]

In a range of double-blind randomised trials, all reported in one issue of one journal, oral SAMe was found to exert the same analgesic activity as a range of NSAIDs. In one study with 734 subjects, SAMe 1200 mg daily was as effective as naproxen 750 mg daily.[11] Another study in 45 patients showed that SAMe 1200 mg daily was as effective as piroxicam (20 mg daily) in osteoarthritis of the knee.[12] Two further studies in each of 36 patients over 4 weeks, showed that SAMe 1200 mg daily was as effective as indometacin (150 mg daily)[13] or ibuprofen (1200 mg daily).[14] A 16-week study in 56 patients diagnosed with osteoarthritis of the knee found that SAMe (1200 mg daily) has a slower onset of action, but is as effective as celecoxib (200 mg daily) in the management of symptoms of knee osteoarthritis.[15]

In an uncontrolled study lasting 24 months, 108 patients received 600 mg SAMe daily for 2 weeks, then 400 mg daily thereafter. Clinical symptoms, such as morning stiffness, pain at rest and pain on movement, improved during the period of SAMe administration.[16]

Fibromyalgia

Intravenous SAMe has been shown to reduce pain in patients with fibromyalgia.[17] In a double-blind, placebo-controlled trial lasting 6 weeks and involving 44 patients, oral SAMe (800 mg) produced significant improvement in clinical disease activity, pain suffered during the last week, and fatigue. SAMe was associated with an improvement in mood on the Face Scale but not on the Beck Depression Inventory.[18]

Cardiovascular disease

Elevation of homocysteine is an independent risk factor for CVD, and SAMe controls enzymes in homocysteine metabolism. Whole-blood SAMe has been found to be lower in patients with coronary heart disease (CHD) than in controls, suggesting that low levels of SAMe might be a risk factor for the development of CHD.[19] A study with oral SAMe (400 mg in a single dose) in healthy subjects showed that SAMe did not inhibit the enzyme 5,10-methylene tetrahydrofolate reductase, which catalyses the formation of 5-methyltetrahydrofolate, the active form of folate involved in the remethylation of homocysteine to methionine. However, there were no changes in plasma homocysteine levels.[20] A more recent trial in 52 subjects found that SAMe 800 mg daily for 4 weeks did not significantly affect plasma homocysteine levels.[21]

> **Conclusion**
> Research suggests there is some evidence that SAMe has value in depression and osteoarthritis, and that it may have an influence in the metabolism of homocysteine.

Precautions/contraindications

SAMe should be used with caution in individuals with a history of bleeding or haemostatic disorders. SAMe has been reported to block platelet aggregation *in vitro*.[22]

Pregnancy and breast-feeding

No problems reported, but there have not been sufficient studies to guarantee the safety of SAMe in pregnancy and breast-feeding. SAMe is best avoided.

Adverse effects

Minor side-effects, including nausea, dry mouth and restlessness, have been occasionally reported.

Interactions

None reported, but in theory SAMe could potentiate the activity of antidepressants, anticoagulants and anti-platelet drugs.

Dose

SAMe is available in the form of tablets and capsules. A review of 13 US products found that six failed testing for content. Among those failing, the amount of SAMe was, on average, less than half of that declared on the labels.

The dose is not established. Studies have used doses of 400–1600 mg daily.

References

1 Fava M, Rosenbaum JF, MacLaughlin JR, *et al*. Neuroendocrine effects of *S*-adenosyl-L-methionine, a novel putative antidepressant. *J Psychiatr Res* 1990; 24: 177–184.

2 Rosenbaum JF, Fava M, Falk WE, *et al*. The antidepressant potential of oral *S*-adenosylmethionine. *Acta Psychiatr Scand* 1990; 81: 432–436.

3 Kagan BL, Sultzer DL, Rosenlicht N, *et al*. Oral *S*-adenosyl methionine in depression: a randomised, double-blind, placebo-controlled trial. *Am J Psychiatry* 1990; 147: 591–595.

4 Salmaggi P, Bressa GM, Nicchia G, *et al*. Double-blind, placebo-controlled study of *S*-adenosyl-L-methionine in depressed postmenopausal women. *Psychother Psychosom* 1993; 59: 34–40.

5 Bressa GM. *S*-Adenosyl-L-methionine (SAMe) as antidepressant: meta-analysis of clinical studies. *Acta Neurol Scand Suppl* 1994; 154: 7–14.

6 Agency for Healthcare Research and Evaluation. S-*Adenosyl-l-methionine for Treatment of Depression, Osteoarthritis and Liver Disease*. [Evidence Report/Technology Assessment 64; AHRQ Publication 02-E033.] Rockville, MD: Agency for Healthcare Research and Evaluation, 2002, http://www.ncbi.nlm.nih.gov/books/NBK36942/ (accessed 20April 2011).

7 Delle Chiaie R, Pancheri P, Scapicchio P. Efficacy and tolerability of oral and intramuscular *S*-adenosyl-L-methionine 1,4-butanedisulfonate (SAMe) in the treatment of major depression: comparison with imipramine in 2 multicenter studies. *Am J Clin Nutr* 2002; 76: S1172–S1176.

8 Pancheri P, Scapicchio P, Chiaie RD. A double-blind, randomized parallel-group, efficacy and safety study of intramuscular *S*-adenosyl-L-methionine 1,4-butanedisulphonate (SAMe) versus imipramine in patients with major depressive disorder. *Int J Neuropsychopharmacol* 2002; 5: 287–294.

9 Papakostas GI, Mischoulon D, Shyu I, *et al*. *S*-Adenosyl methionine (SAMe) augmentation of serotonin reuptake inhibitors for antidepressant non-responders with major depressive disorder: a double-blind, randomized clinical trial. *Am J Psychiatry* 2010; 167(8): 942–948.

10 di Padova C. *S*-Adenosylmethionine in the treatment of osteoarthritis. Review of clinical studies. *Honeybee Sci* 1987; 83(5A): 60–65.

11 Caruso I, Pietrogrande V. Italian double-blind multicenter study comparing *S*-adenosylmethionine, naproxen, and placebo in the treatment of degenerative joint disease. *Am J Med* 1987; 83 (5A): 66–71.

12 Maccagno A, Di Giorgio EE, Caston OL, *et al*. Double-blind controlled clinical trial of oral *S*-adenosylmethionine versus piroxicam in knee osteoarthritis. *Am J Med* 1987; 83(5A): 72–77.

13 Vetter G. Double-blind comparative clinical trial with *S*-adenosylmethionine and indomethacin in the treatment of osteoarthritis. *Am J Med* 1987; 83(5A): 78–80.

14 Muller-Fassbender H. Double-blind clinical trial of *S*-adenosylmethionine versus ibuprofen in the treatment of osteoarthitis. *Am J Med* 1987; 83(5A): 81–83.

15 Najm WI, Reinsch S, Hoehler F, *et al*. *S*-Adenosyl methionine (SAMe) versus celecoxib for the treatment of osteoarthritis symptoms: a double-blind crossover trial [ISRCTN362334950]. *BMC Musculoskelet Disord* 2004; 26: 5–6.

16 Konig B. A long-term (two years) clinical trial with *S*-adenosylmethionine for the treatmemt of osteoarthritis. *Am J Med* 1987; 83(5A): 89–94.

17 Volkmann H, Norregaard J, Jacobsen S, *et al*. Double-blind, placebo-controlled cross-over study of intravenous *S*-adenosyl-L-methionine in patients with fibromyalgia. *Scand J Rheumatol* 1997; 26: 206–211.

18 Jacobsen S, Danneskiold-Samsoe B, Andersen RB. Oral *S*-adenosylmethionine in primary fibromyalgia. Double-blind clinical evaluation. *Scand J Rheumatol* 1991; 20: 294–302.

19 Loehrer FM, Angst CP, Haefeli WE, *et al*. Low whole-blood *S*-adenosylmethionine and correlation between 5-methyltetrahydrofolate and homocysteine in coronary artery disease. *Arterioscler Thromb Vasc Biol* 1996; 16: 727–733.

20 Loehrer FM, Schwab R, Angst CP, *et al*. Influence of oral *S*-adenosylmethionine on plasma 5-methyltetrahydrofolate, *S*-adenosylhomocysteine, homocysteine and methionine in healthy humans. *J Pharmacol Exp Ther* 1997; 282: 845–850.

21 Thompson MA, Bauer BA, Loehrer LL, *et al*. Dietary supplement *S*-adenosyl-L-methionine (AdoMet) effects on plasma homocysteine levels in healthy human subjects: a double-blind, placebo-controlled, randomized clinical trial. *J Altern Complement Med* 2009; 15(5): 523–529.

22 De La Cruz JP, Merida M, Gonzalez-Correa JA, *et al*. Effects of *S*-adenosyl-L-methionine on platelet thromboxane and vascular prostacyclin. *Biochem Pharmacol* 1997; 53: 1761–1763.

Selenium

Description

Selenium is an essential trace element.

Human requirements

See Table 1 for Dietary Reference Values for selenium.

Dietary intake

In the UK, the average adult diet provides 39 µg daily.[1] Selenium enters the food chain through plants, which take it up from the soil. Selenium intake is low in parts of the world where soil selenium content is low, and human dietary intakes therefore vary from high to low according to geography. Selenium intakes in most parts of Europe (including the UK) are considerably lower than in the USA, European soils being a poorer source of selenium. Current UK intakes are about half the Reference Nutrient Intake, having declined considerably over the past 25 years, and this may have implications for disease risk.

Action

Selenium functions as an integral part of the enzyme glutathione peroxidase and other seleno-proteins. Glutathione peroxidase prevents the generation of oxygen free radicals that cause the destruction of polyunsaturated fatty acids in cell membranes. Selenium spares the requirement for vitamin E and vice versa. Selenium has additional effects, particularly in relation to the immune response and cancer prevention, which are not entirely due to these enzymic functions.

Thyroid function depends on selenium, which is at the active centre of the iodothyronine deiodinase enzymes that catalyse the conversion of the prohormone thyroxine to the active form of thyroid hormone, triiodothyronine.

Dietary sources

See Table 2 for dietary sources of selenium.

Metabolism

Absorption
Little is known about the intestinal absorption of selenium, but it appears to be easily absorbed.

Distribution
Selenium is stored in red cells, liver, spleen, heart, nails, tooth enamel, testes and sperm. It is incorporated into the enzyme glutathione peroxidase, the metabolically active form of selenium.

Elimination
Selenium is excreted mainly in the urine.

Deficiency

Deficiency has been associated with muscle pain and tenderness; some cases of cardiomyopathy have occurred in patients on total parenteral nutrition with low selenium status. Keshan disease (seen mainly in China) is a syndrome of endemic cardiomyopathy that is alleviated by selenium supplementation.

There is evidence that less overt selenium deficiency can have adverse consequences for health. Low selenium status has been linked to loss of immunocompetence,[2] the development of virulence and progression of some viral infections,[3] miscarriage,[4] male infertility,[5] depressed mood,[6] cognitive decline in the elderly,[7] senility and Alzheimer's disease.[6]

Low selenium status has also been associated with poor thyroid function,[8] but there was no evidence of change in thyroid hormone status with selenium in an elderly UK population,[9] an elderly New Zealand population,[10] or in North American men.[11] There appears to be no immunological benefit of selenium

Table 1 Dietary Reference Values for selenium (μg/day)

Age	UK			USA			EU RDA = none FAO/WHO
	LRNI	RNI	EVM	RDA	AI	TUL	RNI
0–3 months	4	10		–	15	45	6
4–6 months	5	13		–	15	45	6
7–9 months	5	10		–	20	45	10
10–12 months	6	10		–	20	45	10
1–3 years	7	15		20		90	17
4–6 years	10	20			–	–	22
4–8 years	–	–	–	30		150	–
7–10 years	16	30		–		–	21[1]
Males							
11–14 years	25	45		40		400	32[2]
15–18 years	40	70		50		400	32
19–50+ years	40	75	200	70		400	34[3]
Females							
11–14 years	25	45		45		400	26[2]
15–18 years	40	60		50		400	26
19–50+ years	40	60	200	55		400	26[4]
Pregnancy	*	*		65		400	28–30
Lactation	+15	+15		75		400	35–42

* No increment.
[1] 7–9 years;   [2] 10–14 years;   [3] > 65 years, 33 μg;   [4] 51–65 years, 26 μg > 65 years, 25 μg.
EVM = Safe Upper Level from supplements alone.
LRNI = Lowest Reference Nutrient Intake.
RNI = Reference Nutrient Intake.
TUL = Tolerable Upper Intake Level from diet and supplements.

supplementation among patients with autoimmune thyroiditis,[12,13] but in pregnant women who are positive for thyroid peroxidase antibodies and, therefore, prone to develop postpartum thyroid dysfunction, selenium supplementation during pregnancy and in the postpartum period reduced thyroid inflammatory activity and the incidence of hypothyroidism.[14]

Selenium deficiency has also been associated with cardiovascular disease (CVD), although results from epidemiological studies have been mixed. Thus, a two- to three-fold increase in cardiovascular mortality was found in individuals with serum selenium concentrations below 45 μg/L compared with individuals above that concentration at baseline.[15] A Danish study[16] showed that middle-aged and elderly men with serum selenium below 70 μg/L had a significantly increased risk of ischaemic heart disease. The 10-centre EURAMIC study[17] found an inverse relationship between toenail selenium levels and risk of myocardial infarction, but only in the centre with the lowest selenium (Germany). However, other studies have shown no such links.

Low selenium intake has been linked to cancer mortality. In one study,[18] dietary intake of selenium in 27 countries was found to correlate inversely with total age-adjusted cancer

Table 2 Dietary sources of selenium

Food portion	Selenium content (µg)
Cereals[1]	
2 slices **bread**	30
Milk and dairy products	
Milk (284 ml; $^1/_2$ pint)	3–30
1 egg	3–25
Meat and fish	
Beef, cooked (100 g)	3
Lamb, cooked (100 g)	1
Pork, cooked (100 g)	15
Chicken, cooked (100 g)	8
Liver (90 g)	20
Fish, cooked (150 g)	30–50
Vegetables	
1 small can baked beans (200 g)	4
Lentils, red kidney beans or other pulses, cooked (105 g)	5
Green vegetables, average, boiled (100 g)	1–3
Fruit	
1 banana	2
1 orange	2
Nuts	
20 almonds	1
10 **Brazil nuts**	200
30 peanuts	1

[1]Cereals are important sources of selenium, but the content reflects the selenium content of the soils on which they are grown and is, therefore, highly variable.
Excellent sources (**bold**); good sources (*italics*).

mortality, and low selenium status has been linked with an increased risk of cancer incidence and mortality.[19,20] A nested case-control study within a cohort of 9000 Finnish individuals showed the adjusted relative risk of lung cancer between the highest and lowest tertiles of serum selenium to be 0.41.[21] In a study looking at the association between selenium intake and prostate cancer involving 34 000 men, those in the lowest quintile of selenium status were found to have three times the likelihood of developing advanced prostate cancer as those in the highest quintile.[22]

Possible uses

Cancer (prevention)

Studies have shown that selenium supplementation may reduce the risk of certain cancers (e.g. colon, gastric, lung and prostate), but not others (breast, oesophageal and skin).

The US Nutritional Prevention of Cancer (NPC) trial[23] was the first double-blind, placebo-controlled trial in a Western population designed to test the hypothesis that selenium supplementation could reduce the risk of cancer. A total of 1312 individuals with a history of non-melanoma skin cancer were randomised to placebo or 200 µg selenium a day (as selenium yeast) for an average treatment period of 4.5 years with a total follow-up of 6.4 years. There were no statistically significant differences in incidence of basal cell carcinoma or squamous cell carcinoma. However, total cancer incidence was 37% lower in the selenium group, with 63% fewer cancers of the prostate, 58% fewer cancers of the colon and 46% fewer cancers of the lung. There were more cases of breast cancer and leukaemia-lymphoma in the selenium group, but these differences were not statistically significant. Further analysis of the trial data across the entire treatment period, which ended 3 years after the first analysis was conducted, continued to demonstrate that selenium supplementation was ineffective at preventing basal cell carcinoma, but that it increases the risk of squamous cell carcinoma and total non-melanoma skin cancer.[24] Yet further analysis of the entire treatment period of this trial continued to show a significant protective effect of selenium on the overall incidence of prostate cancer, although the effect was restricted to those with lower baseline prostate-specific antigen (PSA) levels and plasma selenium concentrations.[25]

A systematic review and meta-analysis of 16 studies concluded that selenium may reduce the risk of prostate cancer.[26] A more recent nested case–control study found that serum selenium was not associated with prostate cancer risk. However, higher serum selenium was associated with lower risks in men reporting a high vitamin E intake and in multivitamin users. Furthermore, among smokers high serum selenium was related to reduced prostate cancer risk.[27] The Selenium and Vitamin E Cancer Prevention Trial (SELECT), which was a randomised controlled trial in 35 533 healthy men aged 50 years or older, found that neither oral selenium (200 μg daily) nor vitamin E 400 IU daily, or their combination, reduced the risk of prostate cancer in this group of men.[28] A phase 2 RCT in 140 men with localised non-metastatic prostate cancer who had elected not to have active treatment showed that selenium (200 or 800 μg daily) did not show a protective effect on the progression of prostate cancer, and supplementation with the higher dose of selenium increased the risk of cancer progression among men with higher plasma selenium levels.[29] Further large randomised trials, which are ongoing, will help to throw more light on this issue.

Supplements of dietary antioxidants (including selenium) reduced the incidence of oesophageal and gastric cancer and total cancer in a study in 30 000 adults in Linxian, China,[30] an area where the incidence of oesophageal and stomach cancer is high, and the intake of certain nutrients is low. There is also some evidence that selenium may protect against colorectal cancer[31] and lung cancer.[32] A meta-analysis of small preliminary studies suggests a protective effect of selenium for bladder cancer risk[33] but additional large studies are warranted to support these findings.

Selenium has been studied for a link with breast cancer. A number of case–control studies have explored this link, but no significant associations have been found. The evidence has been summarised by Attract.[34] Low selenium status seems not to be an important factor in the development of breast cancer.

Cardiovascular disease

Selenium may have a role in the prevention of CVD, but evidence for the benefit of supplementation is limited. In a double-blind, placebo-controlled study,[35] 81 patients received either selenium-rich yeast (100 μg daily) or placebo for a 6-month period. During the study period there were four cardiac deaths in the placebo

group but none in the selenium group. There were two non-fatal reinfarctions in the placebo group, and one in the selenium group.

In a further trial, 504 participants (free of CVD) were randomised to selenium 200 μg daily and 500 participants (free of CVD) to placebo. Selenium supplementation was not significantly associated with any of the CVD end points or all CVD mortality during 7.6 years of follow-up. The authors concluded that there was no overall effect of selenium supplementation on the primary prevention of CVD in this population.[36]

In a trial involving 14 healthy subjects, selenium supplementation (110 μg daily) prevented meal-induced increase in atherogenic electro-negative LDL (LDL minus) and LDL susceptibility to oxidation. The authors concluded that the study demonstrated the efficacy of selenium in preventing post-meal oxidative stress and provide a rationale for the epidemiological evidence of the inverse correlation between selenium intake and the incidence of coronary heart disease (CHD) and other chronic conditions.[37]

A meta-analysis of 25 observational studies (14 cohort and 11 case–control studies) and six randomised trials that evaluated supplements found that selenium concentrations were inversely associated with CHD risk in the observational studies; a 50% increase in selenium concentrations was associated with a 24% reduction in CHD risk. Pooled relative risk in selenium supplementation trials compared with placebo was 0.89 (95% confidence interval (CI), 0.68 to 1.17) and findings were therefore inconclusive.[38] Evidence of benefit of selenium on endothelial function is conflicting.[39,40] Selenium has also been evaluated for an influence on homocysteine but there was no effect of selenium yeast in a preliminary study.[41] The outcomes for people with CHD require further examination.

Infertility

Selenium supplementation (selenomethionine 100 μg daily) increased sperm motility in a study involving 64 subfertile men.[42] Sperm count was unchanged after supplementation for 3 months, but sperm motility increased in 56% of the men. By the time of publication, 11% of the selenium-supplemented men had confirmed paternity, but none of the placebo group had. A further study found beneficial effects of selenium (with vitamin E) on semen quality.[43] However, another trial found a decrease in sperm motility with selenium, suggesting caution and the need for further studies to assess this potential effect.[44]

Rheumatoid arthritis

Selenium may be useful as an adjunct in the treatment of recent-onset rheumatoid arthritis. In a study, 15 women with rheumatoid arthritis of less than 5 years' duration who had been treated with NSAIDs and/or with other anti-rheumatic drugs received selenium (200 µg daily from selenium-rich yeast) supplementation for 3 months.[45] This led to improvement in subjective pain and clinical assessment of joint involvement in six out of eight of the treated subjects but none of the controls, and improvements disappeared 3 months after therapy was withdrawn, even though indicators of selenium status remained elevated. However, selenium (256 µg daily from selenium-rich yeast) was not effective in a trial of 40 men and women with an average arthritis duration of 13.5 years.[46] A further trial in 55 patients with moderate rheumatoid arthritis did not show any clinical benefit with selenium (selenium-rich yeast 200 µg daily).[47]

Diabetes mellitus

Selenium has also been evaluated for an effect on the incidence of diabetes mellitus. Secondary analysis of a randomised trial which involved administration of selenium 200 µg daily or placebo to 1202 subjects found that selenium did not appear to reduce the risk of type 2 diabetes and may increase risk. The overall hazard ratio was 1.55 (95% CI, 1.02 to 2.33). Risk was significantly increased in the highest tertile of baseline plasma selenium concentration: the hazard ratio was 2.7 (95% CI, 1.30 to 5.61).[48] In a further trial in men with prostate cancer, selenium 200 µg, 800 µg and placebo did not produce significantly different blood glucose levels.[49] More definitive studies are required to clarify the relationship between selenium and diabetes mellitus.

Miscellaneous

Selenium has been found to improve mood in some studies[50] but not others. There is some evidence that selenium may be of benefit for immune function,[51] oxidative stress and risk of pre-eclampsia and premature labour of pregnancy[52–54] and the management of HIV infection.[55,56] Evidence of benefit in asthma is conflicting;[57–59] in an observational study, selenium intake was associated with reduced incidence of arsenic-related premalignant skin lesions among populations exposed to arsenic from drinking water.[60]

> ### Conclusion
> Epidemiological research and evidence from a large controlled intervention trial suggest that selenium may reduce cancer risk. Evidence in relation to risk of cancers at specific sites is unclear. The role of selenium in heart disease is unclear and controlled clinical trials are required to identify any benefits of supplementation. Results from studies of selenium in rheumatoid arthritis are conflicting.

Precautions/contraindications

Yeast-containing selenium products should be avoided by patients taking monoamine oxidase inhibitors.

Pregnancy and breast-feeding

No problems with normal intakes.

Adverse effects

There is a narrow margin of safety for selenium. Adverse effects include hair loss, nail changes, skin lesions, nausea, diarrhoea, irritability, metallic taste, garlic-smelling breath, fatigue and peripheral neuropathy.

Interactions

There is some evidence that clozapine may reduce selenium levels and that this could be important in the pathogenesis of cardiac side-effects with clozapine.[61]

Dose

Selenium is available mainly in 'antioxidant' supplements with vitamin E and vitamin A, and is also an ingredient in multivitamin supplements.

The dose is not established; 50–100 µg daily is considered to be safe.

References

1 Ministry of Agriculture Food and Fisheries. *Total Diet Study: Aluminium, Arsenic, Cadmium, Chromium, Copper, Lead, Mercury, Nickel, Selenium, Tin and Zinc.* London: Ministry of Agriculture Food and Fisheries, 1999.

2 Spallholz JE, Boylan LM, Larsen HS. Advances in understanding selenium's role in the immune system. *Ann N Y Acad Sci* 1990; 587: 123–139.

3 Taylor EW, Nadimpalli RG, Ramanathan CS. Genomic structures of viral agents in relation to the biosynthesis of selenoproteins. *Biol Trace Elem Res* 1997; 56(1): 63–91.

4 Barrington JW, Taylor M, Smith S, *et al.* Selenium and recurrent miscarriage. *J Obstet Gynaecol* 1997; 17(2): 199–200.

5 Oldereid NB, Thomassen Y, Purvis K. Selenium in human male reproductive organs. *Hum Reprod* 1998; 13(8): 2172–2176.

6 Hawkes WC, Hornbostel L. Effects of dietary selenium on mood in healthy men living in a metabolic research unit. *Biol Psychiatry* 1996; 39(2): 121–128.

7 Akbaraly NT, Hininger-Favier I, Carriere I, *et al.* Plasma selenium over time and cognitive decline in the elderly. *Epidemiology* 2007; 18(1): 52–58.

8 Olivieri O, Girelli D, Azzini M, *et al.* Low selenium status in the elderly influences thyroid hormones. *Clin Sci (Lond)* 1995; 89(6): 637–642.

9 Rayman MP, Thompson AJ, Bekaert B, *et al.* Randomized controlled trial of the effect of selenium supplementation on thyroid function in the elderly in the United Kingdom. *Am J Clin Nutr* 2008; 87(2): 370–378.

10 Thomson CD, Campbell JM, Miller J, *et al.* Selenium and iodine supplementation: effect on thyroid function of older New Zealanders. *Am J Clin Nutr* 2009; 90(4): 1038–1046.

11 Hawkes WC, Keim NL, Diane Richter B, *et al.* High-selenium yeast supplementation in free-living North American men: no effect on thyroid hormone metabolism or body composition. *J Trace Elem Med Biol* 2008; 22(2): 131–142.

12 Karanikas G, Schuetz M, Kontur S, *et al.* No immunological benefit of selenium in consecutive patients with autoimmune thyroiditis. *Thyroid* 2008; 18(1): 7–12.

13 Bonfig W, Gartner R, Schmidt H. Selenium supplementation does not decrease thyroid peroxidase antibody concentration in children and adolescents with autoimmune thyroiditis. *Sci World J* 2010; 10: 990–996.

14 Negro R, Greco G, Mangieri T, *et al.* The influence of selenium supplementation on postpartum thyroid status in pregnant women with thyroid peroxidase autoantibodies. *J Clin Endocrinol Metab* 2007; 92(4): 1263–1268.

15 Salonen JT, Alfthan G, Huttunen JK, *et al.* Association between cardiovascular death and myocardial infarction and serum selenium in a matched-pair longitudinal study. *Lancet* 1982; 2 (8291): 175–179.

16 Virtamo J, Valkeila E, Alfthan G, *et al.* Serum selenium and the risk of coronary heart disease and stroke. *Am J Epidemiol* 1985; 122(2): 276–282.

17 Kardinaal AF, Kok FJ, Kohlmeier L, *et al.* Association between toenail selenium and risk of acute myocardial infarction in European men. The EURAMIC Study. European Antioxidant Myocardial Infarction and Breast Cancer. *Am J Epidemiol* 1997; 145(4): 373–379.

18 Schrauzer GN, White DA, Schneider CJ. Cancer mortality correlation studies IV: associations with dietary intakes and blood levels of certain trace elements, notably Se-antagonists. *Bioinorg Chem* 1977; 7(1): 35–56.

19 Combs GF,Jr Gray WP. Chemopreventive agents: selenium. *Pharmacol Ther* 1998; 79(3): 179–192.

20 Kok FJ, de Bruijn AM, Hofman A, *et al.* Is serum selenium a risk factor for cancer in men only? *Am J Epidemiol* 1987; 125(1): 12–16.

21 Knekt P, Marniemi J, Teppo L, *et al.* Is low selenium status a risk factor for lung cancer? *Am J Epidemiol* 1998; 148(10): 975–982.

22 Yoshizawa K, Willett WC, Morris SJ, *et al.* Study of prediagnostic selenium level in toenails and the risk of advanced prostate cancer. *J Natl Cancer Inst* 1998; 90(16): 1219–1224.

23 Clark LC, Combs GF,Jr Turnbull BW, *et al.* Effects of selenium supplementation for cancer prevention in patients with carcinoma of the skin. A randomized controlled trial. Nutritional Prevention of Cancer Study Group. *JAMA* 1996; 276(24): 1957–1963.

24 Duffield-Lillico AJ, Slate EH, Reid ME, *et al.* Selenium supplementation and secondary prevention of nonmelanoma skin cancer in a randomized trial. *J Natl Cancer Inst* 2003; 95(19): 1477–1481.

25 Duffield-Lillico AJ, Dalkin BL, Reid ME, *et al.* Selenium supplementation, baseline plasma selenium status and incidence of prostate cancer: an analysis of the complete treatment period of the Nutritional Prevention of Cancer Trial. *Br J Urol Int* 2003; 91(7): 608–612.

26 Etminan M, FitzGerald JM, Gleave M, *et al.* Intake of selenium in the prevention of prostate cancer: a systematic review and meta-analysis. *Cancer Causes Control* 2005; 16(9): 1125–1131.

27 Peters U, Foster CB, Chatterjee N, *et al.* Serum selenium and risk of prostate cancer: a nested case–control study. *Am J Clin Nutr* 2007; 85(1): 209–217.

28 Lippman SM, Klein EA, Goodman PJ, *et al.* Effect of selenium and vitamin E on risk of prostate cancer and other cancers: the Selenium and Vitamin E Cancer Prevention Trial (SELECT). *JAMA* 2009; 301(1): 39–51.

29 Stratton MS, Algotar AM, Ranger-Moore J, *et al.* Oral selenium supplementation has no effect on prostate-specific antigen velocity in men undergoing active surveillance for localized prostate cancer. *Cancer Prev Res (Phila)* 2010; 3(8): 1035–1043.

30 Blot WJ, Li JY, Taylor PR, *et al.* Nutrition intervention trials in Linxian, China: supplementation with specific vitamin/mineral combinations, cancer incidence, and disease-specific mortality in the general population. *J Natl Cancer Inst* 1993; 85(18): 1483–1492.

31 Jacobs ET, Jiang R, Alberts DS, *et al.* Selenium and colorectal adenoma: results of a pooled analysis. *J Natl Cancer Inst* 2004; 96(22): 1669–1675.

32 Zhuo H, Smith AH, Steinmaus C. Selenium and lung cancer: a quantitative analysis of heterogeneity in the current epidemiological literature. *Cancer Epidemiol Biomarkers Prev* 2004; 13(5): 771–778.

33 Amaral AF, Cantor KP, Silverman DT, *et al.* Selenium and bladder cancer risk: a meta-analysis. *Cancer Epidemiol Biomarkers Prev* 2010; 19(9): 2407–2415.

34 NHS Wales. Is there any evidence to suggest selenium supplementation is effective in the prevention of breast cancer? http://www.attract.wales.nhs.uk/answer.aspx?criteria=selenium&tagtrail=%2f&qid=2416&src=1 (accessed 28 April 2011).

35 Korpela H, Kumpulainen J, Jussila E, *et al.* Effect of selenium supplementation after acute myocardial infarction. *Res Commun Chem Pathol Pharmacol* 1989; 65(2): 249–2452.

36 Stranges S, Marshall JR, Trevisan M, *et al.* Effects of selenium supplementation on cardiovascular disease incidence and mortality: secondary analyses in a randomized clinical trial. *Am J Epidemiol* 2006; 163(8): 694–699.

37 Natella F, Fidale M, Tubaro F, *et al.* Selenium supplementation prevents the increase in atherogenic electronegative LDL (LDL minus) in the postprandial phase. *Nutr Metab Cardiovasc Dis* 2007; 17(9): 649–656.

38 Flores-Mateo G, Navas-Acien A, Pastor-Barriuso R, *et al.* Selenium and coronary heart disease: a meta-analysis. *Am J Clin Nutr* 2006; 84(4): 762–773.

39 Schnabel R, Lubos E, Messow CM, *et al.* Selenium supplementation improves antioxidant capacity in vitro and in vivo in patients with coronary artery disease. The Selenium Therapy in Coronary Artery Disease Patients (SETCAP) study. *Am Heart J* 2008; 156(6): 1201(6): e1–e11.

40 Hawkes WC, Laslett LJ. Selenium supplementation does not improve vascular responsiveness in healthy North American men. *Am J Physiol Heart Circ Physiol* 2009; 296(2): H256–H262.

41 Bekaert B, Cooper ML, Green FR, *et al.* Effect of selenium status and supplementation with high-selenium yeast on plasma homocysteine and B vitamin concentrations in the UK elderly. *Mol Nutr Food Res* 2008; 52(11): 1324–1333.

42 Scott R, MacPherson A, Yates RW, *et al.* The effect of oral selenium supplementation on human sperm motility. *Br J Urol* 1998; 82(1): 76–80.

43 Keskes-Ammar L, Feki-Chakroun N, Rebai T, *et al.* Sperm oxidative stress and the effect of an oral vitamin E and selenium supplement on semen quality in infertile men. *Arch Androl* 2003; 49(2): 83–94.

44 Hawkes WC, Turek PJ. Effects of dietary selenium on sperm motility in healthy men. *J Androl* 2001; 22(5): 764–772.

45 Peretz A, Neve J, Duchateau J, *et al.* Adjuvant treatment of recent onset rheumatoid arthritis by selenium supplementation: preliminary observations. *Br J Rheumatol* 1992; 31(4): 281–282.

46 Tarp U, Overvad K, Thorling EB, *et al.* Selenium treatment in rheumatoid arthritis. *Scand J Rheumatol* 1985; 14(4): 364–368.

47 Peretz A, Siderova V, Neve J. Selenium supplementation in rheumatoid arthritis investigated in a double blind, placebo-controlled trial. *Scand J Rheumatol* 2001; 30(4): 208–212.

48 Stranges S, Marshall JR, Natarajan R, *et al.* Effects of long-term selenium supplementation on the incidence of type 2 diabetes: a randomized trial. *Ann Intern Med* 20072007; 147(4): 217–223.

49 Algotar AM, Stratton MS, Stratton SP, *et al.* No effect of selenium supplementation on serum glucose levels in men with prostate cancer. *Am J Med* 2010; 123(8): 765–768.

50 Rayman M, Thompson A, Warren-Perry M, *et al.* Impact of selenium on mood and quality of life: a randomized, controlled trial. *Biol Psychiatry* 2006; 59(2): 147–154.

51 Broome CS, McArdle F, Kyle JA, *et al.* An increase in selenium intake improves immune function and poliovirus handling in adults with marginal selenium status. *Am J Clin Nutr* 2004; 80(1): 154–162.

52 Tara F, Maamouri G, Rayman MP, *et al.* Selenium supplementation and the incidence of preeclampsia in pregnant Iranian women: a randomized, double-blind, placebo-controlled pilot trial. *Taiwan J Obstet Gynecol* 2010; 49(2): 181–187.

53 Tara F, Rayman MP, Boskabadi H, *et al.* Prooxidant-antioxidant balance in pregnancy: a randomized double-blind placebo-controlled trial of selenium supplementation. *J Perinat Med* 2010; 38(5): 473–478.

54 Tara F, Rayman MP, Boskabadi H, *et al.* Selenium supplementation and premature (pre-labour) rupture of membranes: a randomised double-blind placebo-controlled trial. *J Obstet Gynaecol* 2010; 30(1): 30–34.

55 Burbano X, Miguez-Burbano MJ, McCollister K, *et al.* Impact of a selenium chemoprevention clinical trial on hospital admissions of HIV-infected participants. *HIV Clin Trials* 2002; 3(6): 483–491.

56 Hurwitz BE, Klaus JR, Llabre MM, *et al.* Suppression of human immunodeficiency virus type 1 viral load with selenium supplementation: a randomized controlled trial. *Arch Intern Med* 2007; 167(2): 148–154.

57 Allam MF, Lucane RA. Selenium supplementation for asthma. *Cochrane Database Syst Rev* 2004; (2): CD003538.

58 Shaheen SO, Newson RB, Rayman MP, *et al.* Randomised, double blind, placebo-controlled trial

of selenium supplementation in adult asthma. *Thorax* 2007; 62(6): 483–490.

59 Burney P, Potts J, Makowska J, *et al.* A case–control study of the relation between plasma selenium and asthma in European populations: a GAL2EN project. *Allergy* 2008; 63(7): 865–871.

60 Chen Y, Hall M, Graziano JH, *et al.* A prospective study of blood selenium levels and the risk of arsenic-related premalignant skin lesions. *Cancer Epidemiol Biomarkers Prev* 2007; 16(2): 207–213.

61 Vaddadi KS, Soosai E, Vaddadi G. Low blood selenium concentrations in schizophrenic patients on clozapine. *Br J Clin Pharmacol* 2003; 55(3): 307–309.

Shark cartilage

Description

Cartilage obtained from various types of shark.

Constituents

Cartilage tissue contains a mixture of glycosaminoglycans, one of which is chondroitin sulphate. Shark cartilage is also thought to contain compounds known as anti-angiogenesis factors, including sphyrnastatin 1 and 2.[1] These are factors that inhibit the growth of new blood vessels, typically seen in malignant tumours, and this mechanism could, in theory, be helpful in human cancer.

Action

It has been suggested that shark cartilage may prevent tumour growth. The proposed mechanism is that the anti-angiogenesis factors prevent tumours from developing the network of blood vessels they need to supply them with nutrients. This supposedly starves tumours and causes them to shrink. The popularity of this anti-cancer theory increased as a result of a popular book, *Sharks Don't Get Cancer*.[2]

Possible uses

Shark cartilage has been proposed as a supplement for the treatment of cancer and (because of its chondroitin content) for the treatment of osteoarthritis.

Cancer

Various *in vitro*,[2–4] animal[5] and human[6] studies have shown that shark cartilage has anti-angiogenic properties. However, there is no evidence from controlled trials that shark cartilage cures cancer in humans.

In a study of cancer patients taking shark cartilage either rectally or orally, 10 of the 20 patients reported an improved quality of life, including increased appetite and reduced pain, after 8 weeks. In addition, four of the 20 patients showed partial or complete response (50–100% reduction in tumour mass). However, information on patient selection criteria, cartilage dose and concomitant cytotoxic therapy was not provided.[7]

A 12-week open clinical trial on 60 patients with advanced cancer assessed the efficacy and safety of shark cartilage at a dose of 1 g/kg daily. No complete or partial positive responses were found, and the authors concluded that shark cartilage had no anti-cancer activity and no effect on quality of life.[8]

> **Conclusion**
> There is currently no evidence from clinical trials that shark cartilage helps to cure cancer in humans.

Precautions/contraindications

Avoid in patients with hepatic disease. There has been a single case report of hepatitis attributed to shark cartilage.[9]

Pregnancy and breast-feeding

There are no available data. Shark cartilage should be avoided.

Adverse effects

Hepatitis and various gastrointestinal effects (e.g. nausea, vomiting, constipation) have been reported. A case study has found that shark cartilage dust can be a cause of asthma. A 38-year-old man reported chest symptoms at work in association with exposure to shark cartilage dust and was diagnosed with asthma. Six months later he complained of shortness of breath and died from autopsy-confirmed asthma.[10]

Interactions

None reported.

Dose

Shark cartilage is available in the form of tablets, capsules and powder.

The dose is not established. There is no proven value of shark cartilage supplements.

References

1 McGuire TR, Kazakoff PW, Hoie EB, *et al.* Antiproliferative activity of shark cartilage with and without tumor necrosis factor-alpha in human umbilical vein endothelium. *Pharmacotherapy* 1996; 16: 237–244.

2 Lane IW. *Sharks Don't Get Cancer*, Garden City Park, New York: Avery Publishing Group; 1992: 107–118.

3 Sheu JR, Fu CC, Tsai ML, *et al.* Effect of U-995, a potent shark cartilage-derived angiogenesis inhibitor, on anti-angiogenesis and anti-tumour activities. *Anticancer Res* 1998; 18: 4435–4441.

4 Dupont E, Savard PE, Jourdain C, *et al.* Antiangiogenic properties of a novel shark cartilage extract: potential role in the treatment of psoriasis. *J Cutan Med Surg* 1998; 2: 146–152.

5 Horsman MR, Alsner J, Overgaard J. The effect of shark cartilage extracts on the growth and metastatic spread of the SCCVII carcinoma. *Acta Oncol* 1998; 37: 441–445.

6 Berbari P, Thibodeau A, Germain L, *et al.* Antiangiogenic effect of the oral administration of liquid cartilage extract in humans. *J Surg Res* 1999; 87: 108–113.

7 Mathews J. Media feeds frenzy over shark cartilage as cancer treatment. *J Natl Cancer Inst* 1993; 85: 1190–1191.

8 Miller DR, Anderson GT, Stark JJ, *et al.* Phase I/II trial of the safety and efficacy of shark cartilage in the treatment of advanced cancer. *J Clin Oncol* 1998; 16: 3649–3655.

9 Ahsar B, Vargo E. Shark-cartilage induced hepatitis. *Ann Intern Med* 1996; 125: 780–781.

10 Ortega HG, Kreiss K, Schill DP, Weissman DN. Fatal asthma from powdering shark cartilage and review of fatal occupational asthma literature. *Am J Ind Med* 2002; 42: 50–54.

Silicon

Description

Silicon is a non-metallic element found in plants, animals and most living organisms. The term silica is used to refer to naturally-occurring materials composed principally of silicon dioxide (SiO_2). It is thought to be essential for human beings.

Human requirements

Although silicon is thought to be essential, human requirements for silicon have not been established. There are no Dietary Reference Values.

Intake

The intake of dietary silicon in the UK is unknown. Intakes in the USA range from 20 to 50 mg daily.[1]

Action

Silicon is involved in the formation of bone and connective tissues. The precise mechanism is uncertain. However, it has been suggested that silicon could facilitate the formation of glycosaminoglycan and collagen components of the bone matrix through its role as a constituent of the enzyme prolyl hydrolase.

Alternatively, it may have a structural role in glycosaminoglycans and linking different polysaccharides in the bone matrix.[2] Silicon also appears to have a role in reducing the absorption of aluminium.[3]

Dietary sources

Silicon is found principally in foods derived from plants, particularly grains such as oats, barley and rice. Animal foods contain lower concentrations. Beer is also a rich source of silicon.[4] Silicon is also found in drinking water as orthosilicic acid. Consumption of 2 L a day of drinking water could result in consumption of 10 mg silicon.[2]

Metabolism

Absorption
Silicon in the form of silicic acid is readily absorbed by human beings, and absorption is increased by dietary fibre.

Distribution
Silica is freely transported in the blood and is freely diffusible into tissues from the plasma. High levels are present in bone, nails, tendons and the walls of the aorta. Lower levels are present in red blood cells and serum. Silicon has also been found in the liver, kidneys, lungs and spleen.

Elimination
Silicon is readily excreted in the urine, with smaller amounts being excreted in the faeces. Silicon excretion increases as dietary intake is increased.

Bioavailability

Silicon bioavailability depends on the solubility of the silicon compounds in question. It is thought that silicic acid is the form absorbed in the gastro-intestinal tract. Absorption of silicic acid from the gut has been reported to be 20–75%.

Deficiency

Silicon deficiency has not been observed in humans. In rats and chickens, silicon deficiency produces deformities of the skull and peripheral bones.[1] In silicon-deficient animals, glycosaminoglycan and collagen concentrations in bone are reduced. The concentration of other minerals in bone such as calcium, magnesium, zinc, sodium, iron, potassium and manganese may also be decreased in silicon-deficient animals.

Possible uses

Silicon has been claimed to have various benefits such as reducing the risk of osteoporosis and osteoarthritis, and preventing coronary heart disease and hypertension. Silicon has been shown to have an inhibitory effect on bone mass loss and stimulation of bone formation in rats.[5,6] It may have a role in reducing the risk of Alzheimer's disease, because it may reduce the absorption of aluminium.[3] It is also claimed to improve hair growth and have benefits for the skin. However, no clinical trials in humans have been identified.

Precautions/contraindications

No at-risk groups or situations have been documented.

Pregnancy and breast-feeding

No problems have been reported, but there have not been sufficient studies to guarantee the safety of silicon in pregnancy and breast-feeding.

Adverse effects

There are few data on the oral toxicity of silicon in humans. In humans, adverse effects are primarily limited to silicosis, a lung disease resulting from the inhalation of silica particles.

Interactions

Nutrients
Silicon has been reported to interact with a number of minerals, including aluminium, copper and zinc.

Drugs
None reported.

Dose

The dose is not established. Dietary supplements in the UK provide doses of up to 500 mg daily.

Upper safety levels

The Food Standards Agency Expert Vitamins and Minerals (EVM) group set a safe upper level for adults for total silicon intake (from foods and supplements) of 760 mg daily.[1]

References

1 Eckert C. Other trace elements. In: Shils ME, Shike M, Ross AC, Caballero B, Cousins RJ, eds. *Modern Nutrition in Health and Disease*, 10th edn. London: Lippincott, Williams and Wilkins, 2006: 338–350.
2 Food Standards Agency. Risk assessment. Silicon. http://www.eatwell.gov.uk/healthydiet/nutritionessentials/vitaminsandminerals/silicon (accessed 8 July 2006).
3 Edwardson JA, Moore PB, Ferrier IN, *et al.* Effect of silicon on gastrointestinal absorption of aluminium. *Lancet* 1993; 342: 211–212.
4 Bellia JP, Birchall JD, Roberts NB. Beer: a dietary source of silicon. *Lancet* 1994; 343: 235.
5 Rico H, Gallego-Lago JL, Hernandez ER, *et al.* Effect of silicon supplement on osteopenia induced by ovariectomy in rats. *Calcif Tissue Int* 2000; 66: 53–55.
6 Calomme M, Geusens P, Demeester N, *et al.* Partial prevention of long-term femoral bone loss in aged ovariectomized rats supplemented with choline-stabilized orthosilicic acid. *Calcif Tissue Int* 2006; 78: 227–232.

Spirulina

Description

Spirulina is a blue-green microscopic alga; it grows in freshwater ponds and lakes, thriving in warm and alkaline environments.

Constituents

See Table 1 for the claimed nutrient content of spirulina.

Action

Spirulina consists of approximately 65–70% crude protein, high concentration of B vitamins, phenylalanine, iron and other minerals. However all the B vitamins (including B_{12}) are thought to be in the form of analogues and nutritionally insignificant. The iron is believed to be highly bioavailable with 1.5–2 mg being absorbed from a 10-g dose of spirulina.

Possible uses

Lipid lowering

Various pilot studies have shown that spirulina may have a lipid-lowering and hypoglycaemic effect in patients with non-insulin-dependent diabetes mellitus (NIDDM). One study[1] looked at the long-term effect of spirulina supplementation (2 g daily) on blood sugar levels, serum lipid profile and glycated serum protein levels in 15 patients with NIDDM. Supplementation for 2 months resulted in a significant reduction in triglycerides and total cholesterol, as well as a reduction in blood sugar and glycated serum protein levels. Levels of HDL increased, while those of LDL fell. A further trial evaluated the lipid-lowering potential of spirulina 4.5 g daily for 6 weeks among 36 subjects. Spirulina reduced triglycerides and LDL cholesterol as well as systolic and diastolic blood pressure.[2] A randomised, double-blind placebo-controlled trial in 78 elderly Korean people demonstrated that spirulina supplementation resulted in a significant rise in plasma interleukin (IL)-2 concentration, and a significant reduction in IL-6 concentration (both anti-inflammatory compounds). A significant time-by-treatment intervention for total antioxidant status was observed between spirulina and placebo groups ($P < 0.05$). In female subjects, significant increases in IL-2 level and superoxide dismutase activity were observed ($P < 0.05$) after spirulina supplementation. There were significant reductions in total cholesterol in female subjects.[3] Further results from this study suggested that

Table 1 Claimed[1] nutrient content of spirulina

Nutrient	per 100 g	per typical dose (10 g)	% RNI[2]
Protein (g)	70	7	–
Fat (g)	7	0.7	–
Carbohydrate (g)	15	1.5	–
Beta-carotene (mg)	170	17	–
Thiamine (mg)	5.5	0.5	55
Riboflavin (mg)	4.0	0.4	33
Niacin (mg)	11.8	1.2	8
Pyridoxine (mg)	0.3	0.03	2.5
Vitamin B_{12} (µg)	200	20	1333
Folic acid (µg)	50	5	2.5
Pantothenic acid (mg)	1.1	0.1	–
Biotin (µg)	40	4	–
Vitamin E (mg)	19	0.2	–
Inositol (mg)	35	3.5	–
Calcium (mg)	132	13	2
Magnesium (mg)	192	19	6
Potassium (mg)	1540	154	4
Phosphorus (mg)	894	89	16
Iron (mg)	58	5.8	48
Zinc (mg)	4	0.4	6
Manganese (mg)	2.5	0.2	–
Selenium (µg)	40	4	2

[1]Reported on a product label;
[2]Reference Nutrient Intake for males aged 19–50 years.

spirulina may also reduce total and LDL cholesterol, particularly in those people with dyslipidaemia.[4]

Ergogenic effects
The effects of spirulina supplementation on athletic performance have been evaluated. In one open-label trial, 16 untrained students volunteered to take *Spirulina platensis* in addition to their normal diet for 3 weeks or soya protein plus their normal diet. After a treadmill exercise, plasma concentrations of malondialdehyde were significantly decreased after supplementation with spirulina ($P < 0.05$). The activity of blood superoxide dismutase was significantly raised after supplementation with spirulina or soya protein ($P < 0.05$). Both blood glutathione peroxidase and lactate dehydrogenase were significantly different between the groups with spirulina or soya protein supplementation. Blood lactate concentration was higher and the time to exhaustion was significantly extended in the spirulina group ($P < 0.05$). These results suggest that spirulina has the potential to reduce skeletal muscle damage and postpone the time of exhaustion during exercise.[5]

In a double-blind, placebo-controlled, counterbalanced crossover study, nine moderately trained men received either spirulina (6 g daily) or placebo for 4 weeks. Each subject ran on a treadmill at an intensity corresponding to 70–75% of their maximum oxygen uptake for 2 h and then at 95% of the maximum to exhaustion. Exercise performance and respiratory quotient during exercise were measured after both placebo and spirulina supplementation. Time to fatigue after the 2-h run was significantly longer after spirulina supplementation (2.05 ± 0.68 vs 2.70 ± 0.79 min). Ingestion of spirulina significantly decreased carbohydrate oxidation rate by 10.3% and increased fat oxidation rate by 10.9% during the 2-h run compared with the placebo. Reduced glutathione levels were higher after the spirulina supplementation compared with placebo at rest and 24 h after exercise. Levels of thiobarbituric acid-reactive substances increased after exercise after placebo but not after spirulina supplementation. Protein carbonyls, catalase, and total antioxidant capacity levels increased similarly immediately after and 1 h after exercise in both groups. The study conclusion was that spirulina supplementation induced a significant increase in exercise performance, fat oxidation, and reduced glutathione concentration and attenuated the exercise-induced increase in lipid peroxidation.[6]

Allergic rhinitis
Spirulina may modulate inflammatory compounds in allergic conditions. A recent double-blind crossover study investigated the effect of spirulina 1000 mg or 2000 mg daily for 12 weeks in individuals with allergic rhinitis. A dose of 2000 mg daily inhibited the production of IL-4, a type of cytokine that may be protective against allergic rhinitis.[7] In a further double-blind trial, spirulina consumption significantly improved the symptoms of allergic rhinitis compared with placebo ($P < 0.001$), including nasal discharge, sneezing, nasal congestion and itching.[8]

Miscellaneous

Spirulina has been shown *in vitro* to have anti-viral activity.[9,10]

Spirulina is claimed to act as a tonic and be beneficial in Alzheimer's disease, peptic ulcer, increasing stamina in athletes and retarding ageing. There is no evidence for any of these claims. A small trial among four physicians found no evidence that spirulina was capable of improving the symptoms of chronic fatigue.[11] When spirulina was introduced into the USA in 1979 as a slimming aid, the Food and Drug Administration could find no evidence to support these claimed benefits.

> ### Conclusion
> There is preliminary evidence that spirulina could lower lipids and have an anti-viral and anti-allergic effect. However, better controlled trials are required to confirm these effects. Evidence is emerging that spirulina can improve exercise performance.

Precautions/contraindications

Spirulina may be contaminated with mercury.

Pregnancy and breast-feeding

Avoid (contaminants – see Precautions).

Adverse effects

Effects not known (contaminants – see Precautions).

Interactions

None known.

Dose

Spirulina is available in the form of tablets, capsules and powders.

The dose is not established. There is no proven benefit of spirulina. Dietary supplements provide 6–10 g per daily dose.

References

1 Mani UV, Desai S, Iyer U. Studies on the long term effect of spirulina supplementation on serum lipid profile and glycated proteins in NIDDM patients. *J Nutraceut Funct Med Foods* 2000; 2: 25–32.

2 Torres-Duran PV, Ferreira-Hermosillo A, Juarez-Oropeza MA. Antihyperlipemic and antihypertensive effects of *Spirulina maxima* in an open sample of Mexican population: a preliminary report. *Lipids Health Dis* 2007; 6(33): 33.

3 Park HJ, Lee YJ, Ryu HK, *et al.* A randomized double-blind, placebo-controlled study to establish the effects of spirulina in elderly Koreans. *Ann Nutr Metab* 2008; 52(4): 322–328.

4 Lee EH, Park JE, Choi YJ, *et al.* A randomized study to establish the effects of spirulina in type 2 diabetes mellitus patients. *Nutr Res Pract* 2008; 2(4): 295–300.

5 Lu HK, Hsieh CC, Hsu JJ, *et al.* Preventive effects of *Spirulina platensis* on skeletal muscle damage under exercise-induced oxidative stress. *Eur J Appl Physiol* 2006; 98(2): 220–226.

6 Kalafati M, Jamurtas AZ, Nikolaidis MG, *et al.* Ergogenic and antioxidant effects of spirulina supplementation in humans. *Med Sci Sports Exerc* 2010; 42(1): 142–151.

7 Mao TK, Van de Water J, Gershwin ME. Effects of a spirulina-based dietary supplement on cytokine production from allergic rhinitis patients. *J Med Food* 2005; 8: 27–30.

8 Cingi C, Conk-Dalay M, Cakli H, *et al.* The effects of spirulina on allergic rhinitis. *Eur Arch Otorhinolaryngol* 2008; 265(10): 1219–1223.

9 Hayashi K, Hayashi T, Kojima I. A natural sulfated polysaccharide, calcium spirulan, isolated from *Spirulina platensis*: in vitro and ex vivo evaluation of anti-herpes simplex virus and anti-human immunodeficiency virus activities. *AIDS Res Hum Retroviruses* 1996; 12: 1463–1471.

10 Hayashi T, Hayashi K, Maeda M, *et al.* Calcium spirulan, an inhibitor of enveloped virus replication, from blue-green algae *Spirulina platensis*. *J Nat Prod* 1996; 59: 83–87.

11 Baicus C, Baicus A. Spirulina did not ameliorate idiopathic chronic fatigue in four N-of-1 randomized controlled trials. *Phytother Res* 2007; 21(6): 570–573.

Superoxide dismutase

Description

Superoxide dismutase (SOD) is a group of enzymes that is widely distributed in the body; several different forms exist with varying metal content. Copper-containing SOD is extracellular and present in high concentrations in the lungs, thyroid and uterus and in small amounts in plasma. SOD containing copper and zinc is present within the cells and found in high concentrations in brain, erythrocytes, kidney, liver, pituitary and thyroid.

Action

SOD enzymes act as scavengers of superoxide radicals, and protect against oxidative damage (by catalysing conversion of superoxide radicals to peroxide).

Possible uses

SOD is claimed to be useful for prevention of CVD, cancer and retardation of ageing. Such claims are partly based on studies that have used SOD by injection in clinical management. SOD is not absorbed from an oral dose and dietary supplements are therefore likely to be ineffective.

Precautions/contraindications

None reported.

Pregnancy and breast-feeding

No problems reported, but there have been insufficient studies to guarantee the safety of SOD in pregnancy and breast-feeding.

Adverse effects

None reported from oral doses.

Interactions

None reported.

Dose

SOD is available in the form of tablets and capsules. However, products may not have any of the stated activity because they are acid-labile and break down before absorption.

The dose is not established. Not recommended as a dietary supplement (probably ineffective).

Thiamine

Description

Thiamine is a water-soluble vitamin of the vitamin B complex.

Nomenclature

Thiamine is the British Approved Name for use on pharmaceutical labels. Thiamin is used to describe the vitamin present in food. It is known also as vitamin B_1 and aneurine.

Human requirements

Thiamine requirements depend on energy intake; values are, therefore, often given as milligrams per 1000 kcal and also as total values based on estimated average energy requirements for the majority of people in the UK (Table 1).

Dietary intake

In the UK, the average adult diet provides: for men, 2.0 mg daily; for women, 1.54 mg.

Action

Thiamine functions as a coenzyme in the oxidative decarboxylation of alpha-ketoacids (involved in energy production) and in the transketolase reaction of the pentose phosphate pathway (involved in carbohydrate metabolism). Thiamine is also important in nerve transmission (independently of coenzyme function).

Dietary sources

See Table 2 for dietary sources of thiamine.

Metabolism

Absorption

Absorption occurs mainly in the jejunum and ileum by both active transport and passive diffusion.

Distribution

Thiamine is transported in the plasma bound to albumin, and stored in the heart, liver, muscle, kidneys and brain. Only small amounts are stored and turnover is relatively high, so continuous intake is necessary. Thiamine is rapidly converted to its biologically active form, thiamine pyrophosphate.

Elimination

Thiamine is eliminated mainly in the urine (as metabolites). Excess beyond requirements is excreted as free thiamine. Thiamine crosses the placenta and is excreted in breast milk.

Bioavailability

Bioavailability may be reduced by alcohol. Requirements are increased by increasing carbohydrate intake. Thiamine is unstable above pH 7, and the addition of sodium bicarbonate to peas or green beans (to retain the green colour) can lead to large losses of thiamine. It is also destroyed by heat and by processing foods at alkaline pH values, high temperature and in the presence of oxygen or other oxidants. Freezing does not affect thiamine.

Thiamine antagonists (thiaminases) in coffee, tea, raw fish, betel nuts and some vegetables can lead to thiamine destruction in foods during food processing or in the gut after ingestion.

Deficiency

Thiamine deficiency may lead to beri-beri (rare in the UK). Deficiency is associated with abnormalities of carbohydrate metabolism. Early signs of deficiency (including subclinical deficiency) are anorexia, irritability and weight loss; later features include headache, weakness, tachycardia and peripheral neuropathy.

Advanced deficiency is characterised by involvement of two major organ systems: the

Table 1 Dietary Reference Values for thiamine (mg/day)

| Age | UK | | | | | USA | | FAO/WHO RNI² |
	LRNI¹	EAR¹	RNI¹	RNI²	EVM	RDA²	TUL	EU RDA = 1.6 mg
0–6 months	0.2	0.23	0.3	0.2		0.2	–	0.2
7–12 months	0.2	0.23	0.3	0.3		0.3	–	0.3
1–3 years	0.23	0.3	0.4	0.5		0.5	–	0.5
4–6 years	0.23	0.3	0.4	0.7		0.7	–	0.6
4–8 years						0.6		
7–10 years	0.23	0.3	0.4	0.7		–	0.9³	
9–13 years				0.9	–	–		
Males								
11–14 years	0.23	0.3	0.4	0.9			–	1.2⁴
15–50 years	0.23	0.3	0.4	0.9	100²		–	1.2
14–70+ years					1.2			
Females								
11–14 years	0.23	0.3	0.4	0.7			–	1.1⁴
14–18 years						1.0	–	–
15–50+ years	0.23	0.3	0.4	0.8	100²		–	1.1
19–70+ years						1.1	–	–
Pregnancy	0.23	0.3	0.4	+0.1⁵		1.4	–	+0.1
Lactation	0.23	0.3	0.4	+0.2		1.5–	–	+0.2

¹ mg/1000 kcal;
² mg/day;
³ 7–9 years;   ⁴ 10–14 years;
⁵ last trimester only.
EAR = Estimated Average Requirement.
EVM = Likely safe daily intake from supplements alone.
LRNI = Lowest Reference Nutrient Intake.
RNI = Reference Nutrient Intake.
TUL = Tolerable Upper Intake Level (not determined for thiamine).

cardiovascular system (wet beri-beri) and the nervous system (dry beri-beri, Wernicke's encephalopathy and Korsakoff's psychosis). The Wernicke–Korsakoff syndrome may be associated with a genetic variant of transketolase, which requires a higher than normal concentration of thiamine diphosphate for activity.[1] This would suggest that there may be a group of the population who have a higher than average requirement for thiamine, but the evidence is not convincing. Signs of wet beri-beri include enlarged heart with normal sinus rhythm (usually tachycardia), and peripheral oedema. Signs of dry beri-beri include mental confusion, anorexia, muscle weakness and wasting, ataxia and ophthalmoplegia.

Thiamine deficiency has been observed in HIV-positive patients,[2] those with chronic fatigue syndrome,[3] hospitalised elderly patients,[4] patients on emergency admission to hospital[5]

Thiamine deficiency also occurs in patients with both type 1 and type 2 diabetes.[6] High-dose thiamine therapy has been shown in a pilot study to produce regression in urinary albumin excretion in patients with type 2

Table 2 Dietary sources of thiamine

Food portion	Thiamine content (mg)
Breakfast cereals	
1 bowl **All-Bran** (45 g)	0.4
1 bowl **Bran Flakes** (45 g)	0.5
1 bowl **Corn Flakes** (30 g)	0.3
1 bowl **muesli** (95 g)	0.4
1 bowl **porridge** (160 g)	0.1
2 pieces *Shredded Wheat*	0.15
1 bowl **Shreddies** (50 g)	0.6
1 bowl **Start** (40 g)	0.6
2 **Weetabix**	0.4
Cereal products	
Bread, brown, 2 slices	0.2
white, 2 slices	0.15
wholemeal, 2 slices	0.2
1 chapati	0.15
1 **naan bread**	0.3
1 *white pitta bread*	0.15
Pasta, brown, boiled (150 g)	0.3
white, boiled (150 g)	0.01
Rice, brown, boiled (160 g)	0.2
white, boiled (160 g)	0.01
2 heaped tablespoons **wheatgerm**	0.3
Milk and dairy products	
Milk, whole, semi-skimmed, or skimmed (284 ml; $^1/_2$ pint)	0.1
Soya milk (284 ml; $^1/_2$ pint)	0.15
Cheese (50 g)	0.15
Meat and fish	
3 rashers **bacon, back, grilled**	0.3
Beef, roast (85 g)	0.07
Lamb, roast (85 g)	0.12
Pork, roast (85 g)	0.55
1 **pork chop, grilled** (135 g)	0.7
2 slices **ham**	0.3
1 **gammon rasher, grilled** (120 g)	1.1
1 chicken leg portion	0.1
Liver, lambs, cooked (90 g)	0.2
Kidney, lambs, cooked (75 g)	0.4
Fish, cooked (150 g)	0.15
Vegetables	
Peas, boiled (100 g)	0.3
Potatoes, boiled (150 g)	0.3
1 small can *baked beans* (200 g)	0.2
Chickpeas, cooked (105 g)	0.1
Red kidney beans (105 g)	0.2
Dahl, lentil (150 g)	0.1
Fruit	
1 apple, banana, or pear	0.04
1 *orange*	0.2
Nuts	
10 **Brazil nuts**	0.3
30 hazelnuts	0.1
30 **peanuts**	0.3
1 tablespoon sunflower seeds	0.1
Yeast	
Brewer's yeast (10 g)	1.6
Marmite, spread on 1 slice bread	0.15

[6] Excellent sources (**bold**); good sources (*italics*).

diabetes and microalbinuria, so it could improve therapy in patients with early-stage diabetic nephropathy.[7] Routine administration of thiamine could also improve endothelial function and slow development of atherosclerosis in patients with diabetes or impaired glucose tolerance.[8,9]

Long-term furosemide use may be associated with thiamine deficiency through urinary loss, contributing to cardiac insufficiency in patients with congestive heart failure (CHF).[10] It has been suggested that thiamine supplementation could improve left ventricular function, but the role of thiamine in heart failure is debatable.[11] One review suggested that, pending further studies, thiamine administration could be considered in patients receiving very large doses of diuretics and others at risk for thiamine deficiency (elderly, malnourished, alcoholic).[12] The use of spironolactone in patients taking furosemide has also been associated with improved thiamine concentrations.[13] Thiamine deficiency may play an important causative role in the deterioration of cardiac function in some patients, and this may be reversed by thiamine administration.[14]

There is also a form of diabetes that is dependent on thiamine (thiamine-responsive megaloblastic anaemia syndrome), which is the association of diabetes mellitus, anaemia and deafness, caused by mutations in a gene encoding a thiamine transporter protein. This syndrome responds to thiamine initially, but most patients become fully insulin dependent after puberty.[15]

Possible uses

Supplementary thiamine may be beneficial in older people (> 65 years), people who consume quantities of alcohol in excess of two units daily, smokers and in HIV-positive patients. However, deficiency of one B vitamin is often associated with deficiencies in other B vitamins and a multivitamin supplement is often more appropriate.

A double-blind, placebo-controlled trial in 76 elderly people found that thiamine 10 mg daily for 3 months significantly improved quality of life, and reduced blood pressure and weight in comparison with placebo, but only in subjects with low thiamine status.

There was also a non-significant trend to improvements in sleep and energy levels with supplementary thiamine, and the authors concluded that older people could benefit from increasing thiamine intake from supplements or diet.[16]

Thiamine has been considered of value in various conditions such as Alzheimer's disease and mouth ulcers.

Alzheimer's disease

Preclinical and laboratory studies show an effect of thiamine on the release and breakdown of acetylcholine. Some intellectual functions, including attention and memory, are influenced by neurons that release acetylcholine. Cholinergic function is impaired in Alzheimer's disease. It has, therefore, been hypothesised that thiamine many be beneficial in Alzheimer's disease. Biochemical abnormalities have been found in the brains of patients with Alzheimer's disease. One double-blind, placebo-controlled trial found that 3000 mg thiamine daily improved global cognitive scores compared with a niacinamide placebo, but had no effect on behavioural ratings or clinician's subjective judgement of symptoms.[17] Another small, double-blind, placebo-controlled trial using 3000 mg thiamine found no benefits of thiamine over placebo in slowing the development of Alzheimer's disease.[18] A more complex placebo-controlled trial in patients with Alzheimer's disease, designed with two phases, used doses of 3000 mg thiamine in the first phase, which lasted 1 month, and then doses of 4000–8000 mg daily over 5–13 months. In the second phase, high-dose thiamine improved scores on various neuropsychological tests, but the authors advised caution in interpretation of the results, to prevent hopes being unrealistically raised.[19] A Cochrane review[20] of three RCTs concluded that the detail in the results was insufficient to combine the results. The review therefore found no evidence of the efficacy of thiamine in people with Alzheimer's disease.

Mouth ulcers

Low erythrocyte thiamine has been found in people with recurrent mouth ulcers,[21] and replacement of B vitamins (thiamine, riboflavin and pyridoxine) led to improvement in clinical symptoms in individuals who were deficient in one or more of these vitamins.[22]

Insect repellent

Anecdotally, thiamine has been found to be of value as an insect repellent, but studies have shown it to be ineffective.[23,24] Thiamine should not be relied upon as an insect repellent in areas where malaria is endemic.

Miscellaneous

Higher doses of thiamine (25–50 mg daily) have been found to be beneficial in diabetic neuropathy,[25] HIV,[26] erectile dysfunction,[27] burns[28] and periodontal wound healing,[29] but usually only in those with poor thiamine status. Studies have sometimes used other B vitamins as well, so it is difficult to attribute any benefits to thiamine supplementation alone. One RCT has shown that thiamine (100 mg daily) could be an effective treatment for dysmenorrhoea.[30] Another RCT in male athletes has shown that thiamine (1 mg/kg body weight) causes serum lactate and heart rate to be lower than placebo and maximum oxygen consumption to be higher.[31]

> **Conclusion**
> There is some evidence that the elderly could benefit from increased thiamine intake, but evidence for a benefit of thiamine supplementation in Alzheimer's disease is equivocal, and studies have used very high doses (3000–7000 mg daily). Preliminary evidence suggests that thiamine deficiency could be associated with mouth ulcers, but further research is required to find out whether supplements can improve the condition.

Precautions/contraindications

Known hypersensitivity to thiamine.

Pregnancy and breast-feeding

No problems reported.

Adverse effects

There appear to be no toxic effects (except possibly gastric upset) with high oral doses. Large parenteral doses are generally well tolerated, but there have been rare reports of anaphylactic reactions (coughing, difficulty in breathing and swallowing, flushing, skin rash, swelling of face, lips and eyelids).

Interactions

Drugs

Alcohol: excessive alcohol intake induces thiamine deficiency.

Furosemide: may increase urinary loss of thiamine;[32] prolonged furosemide therapy may induce thiamine deficiency;[33,34] thiamine supplementation (200 mg daily) has been shown to improve left ventricular function in patients with CHF receiving furosemide therapy.[35]

Nutrients

Adequate amounts of all B vitamins are required for optimal functioning; deficiency or excess of one B vitamin may lead to abnormalities in the metabolism of another.

Dose

Thiamine is available in the form of tablets and capsules. It is also found in multivitamins and in brewer's yeast supplements.

No benefit of a dose beyond the RDA (as a food supplement) has been established.

Doses for mild and severe deficiency can be found in the *British National Formulary*. The dose for prophylaxis or treatment of Wernicke–Korsakoff syndrome caused by alcohol abuse, and the length of time that thiamine should be given after drinking has ceased, has not been clarified.[36]

Upper safety levels

The UK Expert Group on Vitamins and Minerals (EVM) has identified a likely safe total intake of thiamine for adults from supplements alone of 100 mg daily.

References

1 Bender DA. Optimum nutrition: thiamin, biotin and pantothenate. *Proc Nutr Soc* 1999; 58: 427–433.

2 Muri RM, Von Overbeck J, Furrer J, Ballmer PE. Thiamin deficiency in HIV-positive patients: evaluation by erythrocyte transketolase activity and thiamin pyrophosphate effect. *Clin Nutr* 1999; 18: 375–378.

3 Heap LC, Peters TJ, Wessely S. Vitamin B status in patients with chronic fatigue syndrome. *J R Soc Med* 1999; 92: 183–185.

4 Pepersack T, Garbusinski J, Robberecht J, *et al.* Clinical relevance of thiamine status amongst hospitalized elderly patients. *Gerontology* 1999; 45: 96–101.

5 Jamieson CP, Obeid OA, Powell Tuck J. The thiamin, riboflavin and pyridoxine status of patients on emergency admission to hospital. *Clin Nutr* 1999; 18: 87–91.

6 Thornalley P, Babaei-Jadidi R, Al Ali H, *et al.* High prevalence of low plasma thiamine concentration in diabetes linked to a marker of vascular disease. *Diabetologia* 2007; 50(10): 2164–2170.

7 Rabbani N, Alam SS, Riaz S, *et al.* High-dose thiamine therapy for patients with type 2 diabetes and microalbuminuria: a randomised, double-blind placebo-controlled pilot study. *Diabetologia* 2009; 52 (2): 208–212.

8 Arora S, Lidor A, Abularrage CJ, *et al.* Thiamine (vitamin B$_1$) improves endothelium-dependent vasodilatation in the presence of hyperglycemia. *Ann Vasc Surg* 2006; 20(5): 653–658.

9 Wong CY, Qiuwaxi J, Chen H, *et al.* Daily intake of thiamine correlates with the circulating level of endothelial progenitor cells and the endothelial function in patients with type II diabetes. *Mol Nutr Food Res* 2008; 52(12): 1421–1427.

10 Zenuk C, Healey J, Donnelly J, *et al.* Thiamine deficiency in congestive heart failure patients receiving long term furosemide therapy. *Can J Clin Pharmacol* 2003; 10(4): 184–188.

11 Sica DA. Loop diuretic therapy, thiamine balance, and heart failure. *Congest Heart Fail* 2007; 13(4): 244–247.

12 Blanc P, Boussuges A. Is thiamine supplementation necessary in patients with cardiac insufficiency? *Ann Cardiol Angeiol (Paris)* 2001; 50: 160–168.

13 Rocha RM, Silva GV, de Albuquerque DC, *et al.* Influence of spironolactone therapy on thiamine blood levels in patients with heart failure. *Arq Bras Cardiol* 2008; 90(5): 324–328.

14 Mendoza CE, Rodriguez F, Rosenberg DG. Reversal of refractory congestive heart failure after thiamine supplementation: report of a case and review of literature. *J Cardiovasc Pharmacol Ther* 2003; 8(4): 313–316.

15 Ricketts CJ, Minton JA, Samuel J, *et al.* Thiamine-responsive megaloblastic anaemia syndrome: long-term follow-up and mutation analysis of seven families. *Acta Paediatr* 2006; 95: 99–104.

16 Wilkinson TJ, Hanger HC, Elmslie J, *et al.* The response to treatment of subclinical thiamine deficiency in the elderly. *Am J Clin Nutr* 1997; 66: 925–928.

17 Blass JP, Gleason P, Brush D, *et al.* Thiamine and Alzheimer's disease. *A pilot study. Arch Neurol* 1988; 45: 833–835.

18 Nolan KA, Black RS, Sheu KF, *et al.* A trial of thiamine in Alzheimer's disease. *Arch Neurol* 1991; 48: 81–83.

19 Meador K, Loring D, Nichols M, *et al.* Preliminary findings of high-dose thiamine in dementia of Alzheimer's type. *J Geriatr Psychiatry Neurol* 1993; 6: 222–229.

20 Rodriguez JL, Qizilbash N, Lopez-Arrieta JM. Thiamine for Alzheimer's disease. *Cochrane Database. Syst Rev* 2001; (2): CD001498.

21 Haisreili-Shalish M, Livneh A, Katz J, *et al.* Recurrent aphthous stomatitis and thiamine deficiency. *Oral Surg Oral Med Oral Pathol Oral Radiol Endod* 1996; 82: 634–636.

22 Nolan A, McIntosh WB, Allam BF, *et al.* Recurrent aphthous ulceration: vitamin B1, B2 and B6 status and response to replacement therapy. *J Oral Pathol Med* 1991; 20: 389–391.

23 Holzer RB. Malaria prevention without drugs. *Schweiz Rundsch Med Prax* 1993; 82: 139–143.

24 Holzer RB. Protection against biting mosquitoes. *Ther Umsch* 2001; 58: 341–346.

25 Abbas ZG, Swai ABM. Evaluation of the efficacy of thiamine and pyridoxine in the treatment of diabetic peripheral neuropathy. *East Afr Med J* 1997; 74: 803–808.

26 Tang AM, Graham NMH, Saah AJ. Effects of multinutrient intake on survival in human immuno-deficiency type 1 infection. *Am J Epidemiol* 1996; 143: 1244–1256.

27 Tjandra BS, Jangknegt RA. Neurogenic impotence and lower urinary tract symptoms due to vitamin B1 deficiency in chronic alcoholism. *J Urol* 1997; 157: 954–955.

28 Falder S, Silla R, Phillips M, *et al.* Thiamine supplementation increases serum thiamine and reduces pyruvate and lactate levels in burn patients. *Burns* 2009; 36(2): 261–269.

29 Neiva RF, Al-Shammari K, Nociti FH, *et al.* Effects of vitamin-B complex supplementation on periodontal wound healing. *J Periodontol* 2005; 76: 1084–1091.

30 Proctor ML, Murphy PA. Herbal and dietary therapies for primary and secondary dysmenorrhoea. *Cochrane Database Syst Rev* 2001; (2): CD002124.

31 Bautista-Hernandez VM, Lopez-Ascencio R, Del Toro-Equihua M, *et al.* Effect of thiamine pyrophosphate on levels of serum lactate, maximum oxygen consumption and heart rate in athletes performing aerobic activity. *J Int Med Res* 2008; 36(6): 1220–1226.

32 Rieck J, Halkin H, Almog S, *et al.* Urinary loss of thiamine is increased by low doses of furosemide in healthy volunteers. *J Lab Clin Med* 1999; 134: 238–243.

33 Brady JA, Rock CL, Horneffer MR. Thiamin status, diuretic medications, and the management of congestive heart failure. *J Am Dietet Ass* 1995; 95: 541–544.

34 Seligmann H, Halkin H, Rauchfleish S, *et al.* Thiamin deficiency in patients with congestive heart failure receiving long-term furosemide therapy: a pilot study. *Am J Med* 1991; 91: 151–155.

35 Shimon I, Almog S, Vered Z, *et al.* Improved ventricular function after thiamine supplementation in patients with congestive heart failure receiving long-term furosemide therapy. *Am J Med* 1995; 98: 485–490.

36 Day E, Bentham P, Callaghan R, *et al.* Thiamine for Wernicke–Korsakoff Syndrome in people at risk from over-consumption of alcohol. *Cochrane Database Syst Rev* 2004; 1(1): CD004033.

Tin

Description

Tin is a metallic element usually found in the form of the dioxide (SnO_2). It has oxidation states of II and IV. Tin has not been shown to be essential in humans, but it is present in a few multivitamin/ multimineral supplements in the UK.

Human requirements

Human requirements for tin have not been established. There are no Dietary Reference Values. The Food Standards Agency Expert Vitamins and Minerals (EVM) group stated that intake of tin of up to 0.22 mg/kg body weight per day (equivalent to 13 mg tin daily in a 60-kg adult) would not be expected to have any harmful effects but did not set a safe upper level or guidance level for adults for supplemental tin intake.[1]

Intake

Mean intake of dietary tin in the UK is 1.8 mg daily, with an estimated maximum intake of 6.3 mg daily.[1]

Action

The actions of dietary tin are not known. However, it is thought that it may function as part of metalloenzymes.

Dietary sources

Tin intake is essentially dependent on food stored in tin cans. The main dietary sources of tin are canned vegetables and fruit products. The presence of tin in fresh food is highly dependent on the soil concentration of tin. Stannous chloride is a permitted food additive (E512).

Metabolism

Absorption
Tin is poorly absorbed from the gastrointestinal tract.

Distribution
Tin is concentrated principally in bone, lymph nodes, liver, kidney, lung, ovary and testis.

Elimination
The majority of ingested tin is eliminated in the faeces, with the remainder in the urine.

Bioavailability

Bioavailability varies and depends on the oxidation state of the tin salt.

Deficiency

Tin deficiency has not been observed in humans or animals.

Possible uses

No beneficial human health effects from consuming dietary tin are known. Tin has been claimed to have immune-enhancing properties in animals, but there is no evidence that tin has these effects in humans.

Precautions/contraindications

None reported.

Pregnancy and breast-feeding

No problems have been reported, but there have not been sufficient studies to guarantee the safety of tin in pregnancy and breast-feeding.

Adverse effects

Acute tin poisoning (from food or drinks) is associated with gastrointestinal effects (cramps, vomiting, nausea and diarrhoea), headaches and chills.

Interactions

None reported.

Dose

The dose is not established. Supplements in the UK contain up to 10 μg in a daily dose.

References

1 Food Standards Agency. Risk assessment. Tin. http://www.eatwell.gov.uk/healthydiet/nutritionessentials/vitaminsandminerals/tin (accessed 8 July 2006).

Vanadium

Description

Vanadium is a trace element. It is debatable whether or not it is an essential element in the diet of human beings. It exists in at least six different oxidation states. The tetravalent and pentavalent forms are the most important in higher animals.

Human requirements

Human requirements for vanadium have not been established. There are no Dietary Reference Values. It is thought that 10 μg daily is adequate. The US Food and Nutrition Board set a Tolerable Upper Intake level of 1.8 mg daily in adult men and women from the age of 19 years.

Dietary intake

The intake of dietary vanadium in the UK averages 13 μg daily.[1] Intakes in the USA range from 10 to 60 μg daily.[2]

Action

Vanadium does not have a defined function in human beings. Vanadate ions inhibit the sodium/potassium-ATPase pump and phosphate-dependent enzymes (e.g. glucose-6-phosphatase, alkaline phosphatase).

Dietary sources

Grains and grain products are significant sources of dietary vanadium. Marine organisms, brown algae, lichen, parsley, oysters, spinach and mushrooms are rich sources of vanadium.[1,3]

Metabolism

Absorption

Vanadium is poorly absorbed. Absorption occurs in the duodenum and upper gastrointestinal tract. The vanadate ion enters cells through non-specific anion channels and is reduced by glutathione.

Distribution

Vanadium is rapidly cleared from plasma and accumulates in kidney, liver, testes, bone and spleen. The vanadate ion binds to the iron-binding proteins lactoferrin, transferrin and ferritin. Tissues with the highest concentrations include lung, thyroid, teeth and bone. The quadrivalent form of vanadium is most common intracellularly, while the pentavalent form is the most common extracellularly.[2]

Elimination

Vanadium is excreted primarily through the kidney, with a small amount through the bile.

Bioavailability

Only about 5% of ingested vanadium is absorbed.

Deficiency

No cases of human vanadium deficiency have been reported, but deficiency has been suggested to be associated with cardiovascular disease.[1] Vanadium deficiency in goats leads to an increase in abortion, convulsions, bone malformations and early death. In rats, vanadium deficiency increases thyroid weight and decreases growth.

Possible uses

Diabetes mellitus

Vanadium appears to potentiate the effects of insulin and may have benefits in diabetes. *In vitro* and animal studies indicate that vanadium and other vanadium compounds increase glucose transport activity and improve glucose metabolism.

A few small human studies have investigated the effects of vanadium in diabetes. The earliest human trial involved five patients with type 1 diabetes and five patients with type 2 diabetes who were studied before and after 2 weeks of oral sodium metavanadate (125 mg daily). Glucose metabolism was not improved by vanadate therapy. There was a significant decrease in insulin requirements in the patients with type 1 diabetes, cholesterol levels decreased in both groups and there was an increase in mitogen-activated protein and S6 kinase activities in mononuclear cells from patients in both groups that mimicked the effects of insulin stimulation in controls.[4]

A further trial in six subjects with type 2 diabetes found that 3-week treatment with oral vanadyl sulphate improved hepatic and peripheral insulin sensitivity in insulin-resistant type 2 diabetics.[5] Another part of the same trial conducted by the same research group found that oral vanadyl sulphate improved hepatic and skeletal muscle insulin sensitivity in type 2 diabetics in part by enhancing insulin's inhibitory effect on lipolysis.[6]

Another trial in eight patients with type 2 diabetes found that oral vanadyl sulphate (50 mg twice daily for 4 weeks) was associated with a 20% decrease in fasting plasma glucose and a decrease in hepatic glucose output during hyperinsulinaemia (a reduction in hepatic insulin resistance).[7]

A later study investigated the effect of vanadyl sulphate at three doses in 16 patients with type 2 diabetes. Fasting glucose and haemoglobin A1c decreased significantly in the 150- and 300-mg vanadyl sulphate groups, but the mechanism on insulin action was not clear from this study.[8]

A more recent study in 11 type 2 diabetic subjects found that vanadyl sulphate 150 mg daily for 6 weeks significantly improved hepatic and muscle insulin sensitivity and improved glycaemic control, reducing fasting plasma glucose and haemoglobin A1c, while decreasing total and LDL cholesterol.[9]

A systematic review that evaluated the effect of oral vanadium supplementation for glycaemic control in type 2 diabetes identified no trials that met the inclusion criteria (placebo-controlled trial and minimum of 2 months in duration and at least 10 subjects per arm). When less restrictive criteria were used, five trials were included. These demonstrated significant treatment effects, but because of the poor study quality, findings must be interpreted with caution.[10]

Ergogenics

Vanadium has been promoted as an ergogenic aid in sports. However, a 12-week, double-blind, placebo-controlled trial of vanadyl sulphate (0.5 mg/kg body weight daily) in 31 weight-training subjects found no benefit of vanadium in improving performance.[11]

Conclusion

Vanadium is a trace element for which there is no evidence of dietary essentiality in humans. However, pharmacological doses appear to have a role in insulin and glucose metabolism. Human trials in diabetic subjects have shown beneficial effects in glycaemic control and insulin sensitivity, but they have involved small numbers of subjects and have been of poor quality. Results must therefore be treated with caution. There is no evidence that vanadium supplements have a role in sports performance.

Precautions/contraindications

See Adverse effects.

Pregnancy and breast-feeding

No problems reported, but safety studies have not been conducted.

Adverse effects

Vanadium causes abdominal cramps, diarrhoea,[10] haemolysis, increased blood pressure and fatigue. The primary toxic effect in humans occurs from inhaling vanadium dust in industrial settings. This is characterised by rhinitis, wheezing, conjunctivitis, cough, sore throat and chest pain.[2]

Interactions

None reported.

Dose

The dose is not established. Food supplements in the UK provide up to 25 µg in a daily dose.

References

1 Food Standards Agency. Risk assessment. Vanadium. http://www.food.gov.uk/multimedia/pdfs/evm_vanadium.pdf (accessed 28 April 2011).

2 Barceloux DG. Vanadium. *J Toxicol Clin Toxicol* 1999; 37: 265–278.

3 Eckert C. Other trace elements. In: Shils ME, Shike M, Ross AC, Caballero B, Cousins RJ, eds. *Modern Nutrition in Health and Disease*, 10th edn. London: Lippincott, Williams & Wilkins, 2006: 338–350.

4 Goldfine AB, Simonson DC, Folli F, *et al.* Metabolic effects of sodium metavanadate in humans with insulin-dependent and noninsulin-dependent diabetes mellitus in vivo and in vitro studies. *J Clin Endocrinol Metab* 1995; 80: 3311–3320.

5 Cohen N, Halberstam M, Shlimovich P, *et al.* Oral vanadyl sulfate improves hepatic and peripheral insulin sensitivity in patients with non-insulin-dependent diabetes mellitus. *J Clin Invest* 1995; 95: 2501–2509.

6 Halberstam M, Cohen N, Shlimovich P, *et al.* Oral vanadyl sulfate improves insulin sensitivity in

7 Boden G, Chen X, Ruiz J, *et al.* Effects of vanadyl sulfate on carbohydrate and lipid metabolism in patients with non-insulin-dependent diabetes mellitus. *Metabolism* 1996; 45: 1130–1135.

NIDDM but not in obese nondiabetic subjects. *Diabetes* 1996; 45: 659–666.

8 Goldfine AB, Patti ME, Zuberi L, *et al.* Metabolic effects of vanadyl sulfate in humans with non-insulin-dependent diabetes mellitus: in vivo and in vitro studies. *Metabolism* 2000; 49: 400–410.

9 Cusi K, Cukier S, DeFronzo RA, *et al.* Vanadyl sulfate improves hepatic and muscle insulin sensitivity in type 2 diabetes. *J Clin Endocrinol Metab* 2001; 86: 1410–1417.

10 Smith DM, Pickering RM, Lewith GT. A systematic review of vanadium oral supplements for glycaemic control in type 2 diabetes mellitus. *Q J Med* 2008; 101(5): 351–358.

11 Fawcett JP, Farquhar SJ, Walker RJ, *et al.* The effect of oral vanadyl sulfate on body composition and performance in weight-training athletes. *Int J Sport Nutr* 1996; 6: 382–390.

Vitamin A

Description

Vitamin A is a fat-soluble vitamin.

Nomenclature

Vitamin A is a generic term used to describe compounds that exhibit the biological activity of retinol. The two main components of vitamin A in foods are retinol and the carotenoids (see Carotenoids).

The term 'retinoid' refers to the chemical entity retinol or other closely related naturally-occurring derivatives. These include:

- retinal (retinaldehyde)
- retinoic acid
- retinyl esters (e.g. retinyl acetate, retinyl palmitate, retinyl propionate).

Retinoids also include structurally related synthetic analogues that may or may not have retinol-like (vitamin A) activity.

Units

The UK Dietary Reference Values express the requirement for vitamin A in terms of retinol equivalents:

$$\text{Retinol equivalents (µg)} = \text{retinol (µg)} + \frac{\text{beta-carotene equivalents (µg)}}{6}$$

The system of International Units for vitamin A was discontinued in 1954, but continues to be widely used (particularly on dietary supplement labels):

$$1 \text{ retinol equivalent (µg)} = 3.3 \text{ units}$$

One unit is equal to:
- 0.3 retinol equivalents (µg)
- 0.3 µg retinol
- 0.3 µg retinol acetate
- 0.5 µg retinol palmitate
- 0.4 µg retinol propionate.

Table 1   Dietary Reference Values for vitamin A (μg retinol equivalent/day)

Age	UK				USA		FAO/WHO
						EU RDA = 800 μg	
	LRNI	EAR	RNI	EVM	RDA	TUL	RNI
0–6 months	150	250	350		400[1]	600	375
7–12 months	150	250	350		500[1]	600	400
1–3 years	200	300	400		300	600	400
4–6 years	200	300	400		–	–	450
4–8 years	–	–	–		400	900	–
7–10 years	250	350	500		–	–	500[a]
9–13 years	–	–	–		600	1700	–
Males							
11–14 years	250	400	600		–	–	600[b]
14–18 years	–	–	–		900	2800	600
15–50+ years	300	500	700	1500	–	–	600
19–70+ years	–	–	–		900	3000	–
Females							
11–14 years	250	400	600	1500	–	–	600[b]
14–18 years	–	–	–		700	2800	600
15–50+ years	250	400	250		700	3000	500
19–70+ years	–	–	–		700		–
Pregnancy			+100		770[2]	3000[3]	800
Lactation			+350		1300[4]	3000[4]	850
Elderly 65+							600

* No increment.
[a]7–9 years.   [b]10–14 years.   [1]Adequate Intakes (AIs);   [2]aged <18 years, 750 μg;   [3]aged >18 years, 2800 μg;
[4]aged <18 years, 1200 μg.
EAR = Estimated Average Requirement.
EVM = Likely safe daily intake from supplements alone.
LRNI = Lowest Reference Nutrient Intake.
RNI = Reference Nutrient Intake.
TUL = Tolerable Upper Intake Level from foods and supplements.

Human requirements

See Table 1 for Dietary Reference Values for vitamin A.

Dietary intake

In the UK, the average adult diet provides (retinol equivalents): for men, 911 μg daily; for women, 671 μg.

Action

Vitamin A (in the form of retinal) is essential for normal function of the retina, particularly for visual adaptation to darkness. Other forms (retinol, retinoic acid) are necessary to maintain the structural and functional integrity of epithelial tissue and the immune system, cellular differentiation and proliferation, bone growth, testicular and ovarian function and embryonic development. Vitamin A may act as a cofactor in biochemical reactions.

Dietary sources

See Table 2 for dietary sources of vitamin A.

Metabolism

Absorption

Vitamin A is readily absorbed from the upper gastrointestinal tract (duodenum and jejunum) by a

Table 2 Dietary sources of vitamin A

Food portion	Retinol (µg)
Cereals	
Breads, grains, cereals	0
Milk and dairy products	
Whole milk (284 ml; ¹/₂ pint)	*150*
Semi-skimmed milk (284 ml; ¹/₂ pint)	55
Skimmed milk (284 ml; ¹/₂ pint)	2
Skimmed milk, fortified (284 ml; ¹/₂ pint)	100–150 (various brands)
2 tablespoons dried skimmed milk, fortified (30 g)	120
Single cream (35 g)	100
Whipping cream (35 g)	*190*
Double cream (35 g)	*200*
Hard cheese, e.g. cheddary (50 g)	*160*
Hard cheese, reduced fat (50 g)	80
Brie cheese (50 g)	*140*
Cream cheese (30 g)	*130*
1 carton yoghurt, low fat (150 g)	10
1 carton yoghurt, whole milk (150 g)	45
Ice cream, dairy (75 g)	90
Ice cream, non-dairy (75 g)	1
1 egg, size 2 (60 g)	*110*
Fats and oils	
Butter, on 1 slice bread (10 g)	80
Margarine, on 1 slice bread (10 g)	80
Low-fat spread, on 1 slice bread (10 g)	92
2 tablespoons ghee (30 g)	*210*
2 teaspoons cod liver oil (10 ml)	1800
Meat and fish	
Bacon, beef, lamb, pork, poultry	Trace
Kidney, lambs, cooked (75 g)	80
Liver, lambs, cooked (90 g)	**20 000**
Liver, calf, cooked (90 g)	**36 000**
Liver, ox, cooked (90 g)	**18 000**
Liver, pigs, cooked (90 g)	**21 000**
Liver paté (60 g)	**4400**
4 slices liver sausage (35 g)	**870**
White fish	Trace
2 fillets herring, cooked (110 g)	60
2 fillets kipper, cooked (130 g)	40
2 fillets mackerel, cooked (110 g)	55

Note: For dietary sources of beta-carotene, see Carotenoids monograph.
Excellent sources (**bold**); good sources (*italics*).

carrier-mediated process. Absorption requires the presence of gastric juice, bile salts, pancreatic and intestinal lipase, protein and dietary fat.

Distribution

The liver contains at least 90% of body stores (approximately 2 years' adult requirements). Small amounts are stored in the kidney and lungs. Vitamin A is transported in the blood in association with a carrier, retinol binding protein (RBP).

Elimination

Vitamin A is eliminated in the bile or urine (as metabolites). It appears in the breast milk.

Bioavailability

Absorption of vitamin A is markedly reduced if the intake of dietary fat is <5 g daily (extremely rare) and by the presence of peroxidised fat and other oxidising agents in food. Deficiencies of protein (extremely rare in the UK), vitamin E and zinc, and excessive amounts of alcohol, adversely affect vitamin A transport, storage and utilisation.

Deficiency

Vitamin A deficiency is widespread in young children in developing countries and is associated with general malnutrition in these countries. In the UK, deficiency is relatively rare (especially in adults), but marginal intakes may occur in children.

Symptoms of deficiency include night blindness (due to decreased sensitivity of rod receptors in the retina); xerophthalmia (can be irreversible) characterised by conjunctival and corneal xerosis, ulceration and liquefaction; ultimately severe visual impairment and blindness; dryness of the skin and papular eruptions (not a unique indicator of vitamin A deficiency because other nutrient deficiencies cause similar disorders); metaplasia and keratinisation of the cells of the respiratory tract and other organs; increased susceptibility to respiratory and urinary tract infections; occasionally diarrhoea and loss of appetite.

Possible uses

Children

The Department of Health advises that most children from the age of 6 months to 5 years should receive supplements of vitamins A and D, unless the adequacy of their diet can be assured.[1]

Cancer

A large number of studies have assessed the association between vitamin A and cancer, but not all of them distinguish between retinol (pre-formed vitamin A) and carotenoids. Some case–control studies reporting on the association between preformed vitamin A and breast cancer have found modest decreases in risk with higher intake,[2–4] but others[5,6] have found no association. Prospective data are compatible with a modest protective effect of preformed vitamin A.[7–9]

There is some preliminary evidence that pre-formed vitamin A may be modestly protective against colon cancer in both men[10] and women.[11] In a nested case-control study,[12] sub-jects in the highest quintile of serum retinol were at reduced risk of colon cancer for up to 9 years of follow-up. However, another study[13] failed to find any association between colon cancer and vitamin A intake.

Most data suggest that preformed vitamin A does not protect against prostate cancer, and an initial study[14] suggesting an adverse effect has not been confirmed. However, the possibility that higher intakes of vitamin A increase the risk of prostate cancer requires further investigation.

The risk of lung cancer may be related to dietary carotene intake rather than retinol, and studies have shown no benefit of vitamin A in prevention of lung cancer.[15–17]

There is some evidence that people taking vitamin A-containing supplements have a lower risk of gastric cancer than non-users.[18]

Miscellaneous

There is no evidence of any value of vitamin A in eye problems, or prevention and treatment of infections unrelated to vitamin A deficiency. Vitamin A supplements in normal safe doses have no proven benefits in skin problems (e.g. acne), but synthetic retinoids may be prescribed for this purpose.

Single case studies have appeared period-ically in the literature indicating that vitamin A may be beneficial in premenstrual syndrome, but these effects have not been confirmed in randomised trials.

Conclusion

The Department of Health recommends a sup-plement containing vitamin A (and vitamin D) in children aged 6 months to 5 years, unless a good diet can be assured. There is very little evidence for any benefit of vitamin A supple-ments except for cases of deficiency. Evidence for a role of preformed vitamin A in cancer is limited. Such evidence as exists relates more to carotenoids.

Pregnancy and breast-feeding

Excessive doses of vitamin A have been shown to be teratogenic,[19,20] although the level at which this occurs has not been firmly estab-lished. No teratogenic effects were observed in 1203 women receiving 6000 units daily at least from 1 month prior to conception until the 12th week of pregnancy,[21] and an apparent threshold of 10 000 units daily has been identified.[22] Other studies[23,24] suggest low risk with intakes up to 30 000 units daily.

The Department of Health has recommended that women who are (or may become) pregnant should not take dietary supplements that con-tain vitamin A (including fish liver oil), except on the advice of a doctor or antenatal clinic, and should also avoid liver and products containing liver (e.g. liver pate and liver sausage).

Adverse effects

Acute toxicity

Acute toxicity may be induced by single doses of 300 mg retinol (1 million units) in adults, 60 mg retinol (200 000 units) in children or 30 mg ret-inol (100 000 units) in infants.

Signs and symptoms are usually transient (usu-ally occurring about 6 h after ingestion of acute dose and disappearing after 36 h) and include severe headache (due to raised intracranial pres-sure), sore mouth, bleeding gums, dizziness, vomiting, blurred vision, hepatomegaly, irritabil-ity and (in infants) bulging of the fontanelle.

Chronic toxicity

Signs of chronic toxicity may appear when daily intake is >15 mg retinol (50 000 units) in adults and 6 mg (20 000 units) in infants and young children.

Signs may include dryness of the skin, pruritis, dermatitis, skin desquamation, skin erythema, skin rash, skin scaliness, papilloedema, disturbed hair growth, fissure of the lips, bone and joint pain, hyperostosis, headache, fatigue, irritability, insomnia, anorexia, nausea, vomiting, diarrhoea, weight loss, hepatomegaly, hepatotoxicity, raised intracranial pressure, bulging fontanelle (in infants), and hypercalcaemia (due to increase in alkaline phosphatase activity).

Not all signs appear in all patients, and relative severity varies widely among different individuals. Most signs and symptoms disappear within a week, but skin and bone changes may remain evident for several months.

Osteoporosis

Excessive vitamin A intake is thought to have a detrimental effect on bone and increase the risk of osteoporosis and fracture. Two Swedish studies, a cross-sectional study involving 175 women aged 28–74 years and a nested case–control study in 247 women aged 40–76 years, found that retinol intake was negatively associated with bone mineral density.[25] A prospective analysis begun in 1980 with 18 years' follow-up within the Nurses' Health Study, and involving 72 337 postmenopausal women aged 34–77 years, found that women in the highest quintile of vitamin A intake ($\geq$3000 μg daily of retinol equivalents) had a significantly elevated risk of hip fracture compared with women in the lowest quintile of intake ($<$ 1250 μg daily). This increased risk was attributable to retinol, not to beta-carotene, and was attenuated among women using postmenopausal oestrogens.[26] A longitudinal study in 2322 men aged 49–51 years found that the highest risk of fracture was found in men with the highest levels of serum retinol.[27] However, other studies in men,[28] perimenopausal women,[29] postmenopausal women,[30] and elderly women[31] have not found detrimental effects on bone. A review concluded that patients should be made aware of the potential risks of consuming vitamin A in amounts exceeding the RDA.[32]

Interactions

Drugs

Anticoagulants: large doses of vitamin A ($>$750 μg; 2500 units) may induce a hypoprothrombinaemic response.

Colestyramine and colestipol: may reduce intestinal absorption of vitamin A.
Colchicine: may reduce intestinal absorption of vitamin A.
Liquid paraffin: may reduce intestinal absorption of vitamin A.
Neomycin: may reduce intestinal absorption of vitamin A.
Retinoids (acitrecin, etreninate, isotretinoin, tretinoin): concurrent administration of vitamin A may result in additive toxic effects.
Statins: prolonged therapy with statins may increase serum vitamin A levels.
Sucralfate: may reduce intestinal absorption of vitamin A.

Nutrients

Iron: in vitamin A deficiency, plasma iron levels fall.
Vitamin C: under conditions of hypervitaminosis A, tissue levels of vitamin C may be reduced and urinary excretion of vitamin C increased; vitamin C may ameliorate the toxic effects of vitamin A.
Vitamin E: large doses of vitamin A increase the need for vitamin E; vitamin E protects against the oxidative destruction of vitamin A.
Vitamin K: under conditions of hypervitaminosis A, hypothrombinaemia may occur; it can be corrected by administration of vitamin K.

Dose

Vitamin A supplementation is not normally required in the UK.

Therapeutic doses may be given but only under medical supervision. For example, in cystic fibrosis, doses of 1200–3300 μg (4000–10 000 units) daily may be given.

Upper safety levels

The UK Expert Group on Vitamins and Minerals (EVM) has identified a likely safe total intake of vitamin A (retinol equivalents) for adults from supplements alone of 1500 μg daily.

References

1   Department of Health. Weaning and the weaning diet: Report of the Working Group on the Weaning Diet of the Committee on Medical Aspects of Food Policy. *Report on Health and Social Subjects No 45.* London: HMSO, 1994.

2   London SJ, Stein EA, Henderson IC. Carotenoids, retinol and vitamin E and risk of proliferative benign breast disease and breast cancer. *Cancer Causes Control* 1992; 3: 503–512.

3   Longnecker M, Newcomb P, Mittendorf PR, *et al.* Intake of carrots, spinach and supplements containing vitamin A in relation to the risk of breast cancer. *Cancer Epidemiol Biomarkers Prev* 1997; 6: 887–892.

4   Zaridze D, Lifanova Y, Maximovitch D, *et al.* Diet, alcohol consumption and reproductive factors in a case-control study of breast cancer in Moscow. *Int J Cancer* 1991; 48: 493–501.

5   Ingram DM, Nottage E, Roberts T. The role of diet in the development of breast cancer: a case-control study of patients with breast cancer, benign epithelial hyperplasia and fibrocystic disease of the breast. *Br J Cancer* 1991; 64: 187–191.

6   La Vecchia C, Decarli A, Franceschi S, *et al.* Dietary factors and the risk of breast cancer. *Nutr Cancer* 1987; 10: 205–214.

7   Graham S, Zielezny M, Marshall J. Diet in the epidemiology of breast cancer in the New York state cohort. *Am J Epidemiol* 1992; 136: 1327–1337.

8   Hunter DJ, Mason JE, Colditz GA. A prospective study of the intake of vitamins C, E and A and risk of breast cancer. *N Engl J Med* 1993; 329: 324–340.

9   Rohan TE, Howe GR, Friedenreich CM, *et al.* Dietary fiber, vitamins A, C and E, and risk of breast cancer: a cohort study. *Cancer Causes Control* 1993; 4: 29–37.

10   Graham S, Marshall B, Haughey B. Dietary epidemiology of cancer of colon in western New York. *Am J Epidemiol* 1988; 128: 490–503.

11   Heilbrun LK, Nomura A, Hankin JH, Stemmerman GN. Diet and colorectal cancer with special reference to fiber intake. *Int J Cancer* 1989; 44: 1–6.

12   Comstock GW, Helzlsouer KJ, Bush TL. Prediagnostic serum levels of carotenoids and vitamin E as related to subsequent cancer in Washington County, Maryland. *Am J Clin Nutr* 1991; 53: S260–264.

13   Potter JD, McMichael AJ. Diet and cancer of the colon and rectum: a case-control study. *J Natl Cancer Inst* 1986; 76: 557–569.

14   Graham S, Haughey B, Marshall J. Diet in the epidemiology of carcinoma of the prostate gland. *J Natl Cancer Inst* 1983; 70: 687–692.

15   Omenn GS, Goodman GE, Thornquist MD, *et al.* Effects of a combination of betacarotene and vitamin A on lung cancer and cardiovascular disease. *N Engl J Med* 1996; 334: 1150–1155.

16   De Klerk N, Musk W, Ambrosini G, *et al.* Vitamin A and cancer prevention II: comparison of the effects of vitamin A and betacarotene. *Int J Cancer* 1998; 75: 362–367.

17   Musk W, De Klerk N, Ambrosini G, *et al.* Vitamin A and cancer prevention I: observations in workers previously exposed to asbestos at Wittnoom, Western Australia. *Int J Cancer* 1998; 75: 355–361.

18   Botterweck AA, van Den Brandt PA, Goldbohm RA. Vitamins, carotenoids, dietary fiber, and the risk of gastric carcinoma: results from a prospective study after 6.3 years of follow-up. *Cancer* 2000; 88: 737–748.

19   Pinnock CB, Alderman CP. The potential for teratogenicity of vitamin A and its congeners. *Med J Aust* 1992; 157: 804–809.

20   Underwood BA. Teratogenicity of vitamin A. *Int J Vit Nutr Res Suppl* 1989; 30: (Suppl) 42–55.

21   Dudas I, Czeizel AE. Use of 6,000 IU vitamin A during early pregnancy without teratogenic effect (letter). *Teratology* 1992; 45: 335–336.

22   Rothman KJ, Moore LL, Singer MR, *et al.* Teratogenicity of high vitamin A intake. *N Engl J Med* 1995; 333: 1369–1373.

23   Mastroiacovo P, Mazzone T, Addis A, *et al.* High vitamin A intake in early pregnancy and major malformations: a multicenter prospective controlled study. *Teratology* 1999; 59: 7–11.

24   Miller RK, Hendrickx AG, Mils JL, *et al.* Periconceptual vitamin A use: how much is teratogenic? *Reprod Toxicol* 1998; 12: 75–88.

25   Melhus H, Michaelsson K, Kindmark A, *et al.* Excessive dietary intake of vitamin A is associated with reduced bone mineral density and increased risk for hip fracture. *Ann Intern Med* 1998; 129: 770–778.

26   Feskanich D, Singh V, Willet WC, Colditz GA. Vitamin A intake and hip fractures among postmenopausal women. *JAMA* 2002; 287: 47–54.

27   Michaelsson K, Lithell H, Vessby B, Melhus H. Serum retinol levels and the risk of fracture. *N Engl J Med* 2003; 348: 287–294.

28   Kawahara TN, Krieger DC, Engelke JA, *et al.* Short-term vitamin A supplementation does not affect bone turnover in men. *J Nutr* 2002; 132: 1169–1172.

29   Lim LS, Harnack LJ, Lazovich D, Folsom AR. Vitamin A intake and the risk of hip fracture in postmenopausal women: the Iowa Women's Health Study. *Osteoporosis Int* 2004; 15: 552–559.

30   Rejnmark L, Vestergaard P, Charles P, *et al.* No effect of vitamin A intake on bone mineral density and fracture risk in perimenopausal women. *Osteoporosis Int* 2004; 15: 872–880.

31   Barker ME, McCloskey E, Saha S, *et al.* Serum retinoids and beta-carotene as predictors of hip and other fractures in elderly women. *J Bone Miner Res* 2005; 20: 913–920.

32   Jackson HA, Sheehan HA. Effect of vitamin A on fracture risk. *Ann Pharmacother* 2005; 39: 2086–2090.

Vitamin B₆

Description

Vitamin B$_6$ is a water-soluble member of the vitamin B complex.

Nomenclature

Vitamin B$_6$ is a generic term used to describe compounds that exhibit the biological activity of pyridoxine. It occurs in food as pyridoxine, pyridoxal and pyridoxamine. Thus the term 'pyridoxine' is not synonymous with the generic term 'vitamin B$_6$'.

Human requirements

Vitamin B$_6$ requirements depend on protein intake; values are, therefore, given as micrograms per gram protein and also as total values (Table 1).

Dietary intake

In the UK, the average adult daily diet provides: for men, 2.9 mg; for women, 2.0 mg.

Action

Vitamin B$_6$ is converted in erythrocytes to pyridoxal phosphate and, to a lesser extent, pyridoxamine phosphate. It acts as a cofactor for enzymes that are involved in more than 100 reactions affecting protein, lipid and carbohydrate metabolism. Pyridoxal phosphate is also involved in the synthesis of several neurotransmitters; the metabolism of several vitamins (e.g. the conversion of tryptophan to niacin); and haemoglobin and sphingosine formation.

Dietary sources

See Table 2 for dietary sources of vitamin B$_6$.

Metabolism

Absorption

Absorption occurs mainly by a non-saturable process (absorption is greatest in the jejunum).

Distribution

Vitamin B$_6$ is stored in the liver, muscle and brain. Pyridoxal phosphate is transported in the plasma (bound to albumin) and in erythrocytes (in association with haemoglobin).

Elimination

Primarily in the urine (mainly as metabolites), but excess amounts are excreted largely unchanged. It also appears in breast milk.

Bioavailability

Bioavailability of vitamin B$_6$ is affected by food processing and storage. The vitamin is sensitive to light, especially in acid or neutral solutions.

Deficiency

Deficiency of vitamin B$_6$ does not produce a characteristic syndrome, but as with deficiency of the other B vitamins, symptoms such as dermatitis, cheilosis, glossitis and angular stomatitis may occur. Advanced deficiency may produce weakness, irritability, depression, dizziness, peripheral neuropathy and seizures; diarrhoea, anaemia and seizures are particular characteristics of deficiency in infants and children. Chronic deficiency may lead to secondary hyperoxaluria (increased risk of kidney stone formation) and to hypochromic, microcytic anaemia.

Possible uses

Vitamin B$_6$ has been investigated for a range of conditions, including carpal tunnel syndrome, premenstrual syndrome (PMS), asthma, diabetic neuropathy, cardiovascular disease (CVD) and autism.

Table 1   Dietary Reference Values for vitamin B$_6$ (mg/day)

Age	UK					USA		FAO/
	LRNI[1]	EAR	RNI[1]	RNI[2]	EVM	RDA[2]	TUL[2]	WHO RNI[2]
				EU RDA = 2 mg				
0–6 months	3.5	6	8	0.2		0.1[3]	–	0.1
7–9 months	6	8	10	0.3		0.3[3]	–	0.3
10–12 months	8	10	13	0.4		0.3	–	0.3
1–3 years	8	10	13	0.7		0.5	30	0.5
4–6 years	8	10	13	0.9		–	–	0.6
4–8 years	–	–	–	–		0.6	40	–
7–10 years	8	10	13	1.0		–	–	1.0[4]
9–13 years						1.0	60	–
Males								
11–14 years	11	13	15	1.2		–	–	1.3[5]
14–18 years						1.3	80	1.3
15–18 years	11	13	15	1.4				–
19–50+ years	11	13	15	1.4	10	1.3	100	1.3
51–70+ years	–	–	–	–	10	1.7	100	1.7
Females								
11–14 years	11	13	15	1.0		–	–	1.2[5]
14–18 years	–	–	–	–		1.2	80	1.2
15–18 years	11	13	15	1.2		–	–	–
19–50+ years	11	13	15	1.2	10	1.3	100	1.3
51–70+ years	–	–	–	–	10	1.5	100	1.5
Pregnancy	*	*	*	*		1.9	100[6]	1.9
Lactation	*	*	*	*		2.0	100[6]	2.0

* No increment.

[1] µg/g protein;   [2] mg/day;   [3] Adequate Intakes: [4] 7–9 years;   [5] 10–14 years;   [6] ≤ 18 years = 80 mg.

EAR = Estimated Average Requirement.
EVM = Likely safe daily intake from supplements alone.
LRNI = Lowest Reference Nutrient Intake.
RNI = Reference Nutrient Intake.
TUL = Tolerable Upper Intake Level from food and supplements.

Carpal tunnel syndrome

Idiopathic carpal tunnel syndrome, with swelling of the synovia and compression of the median nerve by the transverse carpal ligament, has been attributed to pyridoxine deficiency.[1,2] Several uncontrolled studies in the 1980s demonstrated the efficacy of vitamin B$_6$ treatment.[3–5] However, another study showed no consistent improvement in patients with carpal tunnel syndrome and normal vitamin B$_6$ status.[6] These findings led to the suggestion[7] that clinical improvement in some patients with carpal tunnel syndrome may be due to correction of unrecognised peripheral neuropathy, which could compound symptoms of the syndrome. A review article concluded that studies have not provided sufficient evidence for the use of vitamin B$_6$ as the sole treatment for carpal tunnel syndrome, but that it could be of some benefit as adjunct therapy because of its potential benefit on pain perception and increasing pain threshold.[8]

Table 2 Dietary sources of vitamin B$_6$

Food portion	Vitamin B$_6$ content (mg)
Breakfast cereals	
1 bowl **All-Bran** (45 g)	0.6
1 bowl **Bran Flakes** (45 g)	0.8
1 bowl **Corn Flakes** (30 g)	0.6
1 bowl **muesli** (95 g)	1.5
1 bowl **Start** (40 g)	1.1
2 **Weetabix**	0.4
Milk and dairy products	
Milk, whole, semi-skimmed or skimmed (284 ml, $^1/_2$ pint)	0.15
Soya milk (284 ml, $^1/_2$ pint)	0.15
Meat and fish	
Beef, roast (85 g)	0.3
Lamb, roast (85 g)	0.2
Pork, roast (85 g)	0.3
2 slices *ham*	0.3
1 *chicken leg portion*	0.3
Liver, lambs, cooked (90 g)	0.4
Kidney, lambs, cooked (75 g)	0.2
Fish, cooked (150 g)	0.5
Vegetables	
Potatoes, boiled (150 g)	0.5
1 small can *baked beans* (200 g)	0.3
Fruit	
$^1/_2$ **avocado pear**	0.4
1 *banana*	0.3
Nuts	
30 *peanuts*	0.2
Yeast	
Brewer's yeast (10 g)	0.2

Excellent sources (**bold**); good sources (*italics*).

Premenstrual syndrome

Pyridoxine has been reported to be of benefit in PMS,[9–11] but some researchers have found no significant benefit.[12–14] Doses of pyridoxine that have shown beneficial effects have been relatively high (500 mg daily) and these high doses should not be recommended because of the risk of toxicity. However, a good response has been reported with a dose of 50 mg daily.[15] Studies are complicated by the subjective nature of symptoms in PMS, and conclusions are limited by the low quality of many of the trials. Nevertheless, a systematic review[16] of nine

published trials representing 940 patients with PMS suggests that doses of vitamin B$_6$ up to 100 mg daily are likely to be of benefit in treating premenstrual symptoms and premenstrual depression.

Asthma

Low vitamin B$_6$ status has been reported in adults with asthma,[17,18] and in asthmatic children.[19] This may in part be due to use of theophylline (which was more commonly used in the USA at the time of the studies), which reduces vitamin B status.[20,21] A supplement of 15 mg of pyridoxine per day reduced side-effects of theophylline related to nervous system function.[22]

Vitamin B$_6$ supplementation (50 mg daily) reduced the severity and frequency of asthma attacks,[18] and pyridoxine (200 mg daily) reduced the need for asthma medication in children.[23] However, a dose of 300 mg daily failed to improve asthma in patients requiring steroids.[24]

Diabetic neuropathy

Peripheral neuropathy in patients with diabetes has been suggested to be associated with pyridoxine deficiency. Diabetic patients with symptoms of neuropathy and low vitamin B$_6$ status were given 150 mg of vitamin B$_6$ daily for 6 weeks.[25] Neuropathic symptoms were eliminated in all subjects. The same dose of pyridoxine gradually improved pain in patients with painful neuropathy.[26] In diabetic patients whose vitamin B$_6$ status was normal, pyridoxine supplementation resulted in no improvement in neuropathic symptoms.[27] Further studies are required to investigate the possible benefits of vitamin B$_6$ in diabetic neuropathy.

Coronary heart disease

A raised level of plasma homocysteine is associated with an increased risk of coronary heart disease (CHD). This in turn has been linked with low intake and low level of folic acid and other B vitamins, including vitamin B$_6$. However, whether vitamin B$_6$ has an influence independent of folic acid is uncertain. In the Framingham Heart Study,[28] folic acid, vitamin B$_6$ and vitamin B$_{12}$ were determinants of homocysteine levels, with folic acid showing the strongest association. In the Nurses' Health

Study,[29] those with the highest vitamin B$_6$ intake had a 33% lower risk of heart disease than those with the lowest intake, while in those with the highest intake of both vitamin B$_6$ and folate, the risk of heart disease was reduced by 45%. In a prospective, case-cohort study, heart disease was negatively associated with plasma vitamin B$_6$ in both men and women, and after correcting for a large number of risk factors, the association with pyridoxine still held, pointing to the possibility that vitamin B$_6$ offers independent protection.[30] However, two meta-analyses[31,32] concluded that although folic acid reduced plasma homocysteine, vitamin B$_6$ had no additional effect. A pharmacological dose of vitamin B$_6$ (1200 mg daily) has been found to reduce plasma homocysteine in patients with schizophrenia.[33] Several recent trials[34–36] and meta-analyses[37–39] (see Folic acid mongraph) have not provided evidence of benefit for intervention with vitamin B$_6$ combined with folic acid and B$_{12}$ for secondary prevention of CVD, although a few have indicated limited benefit in stroke prevention.[40]

Miscellaneous

Pyridoxine has also been reported to be effective in treating pregnancy sickness.[41,42] A Cochrane analysis reviewed five trials involving the use of vitamin B$_6$ in pregnancy and concluded that there was not enough evidence to detect clinical benefits of vitamin B$_6$ supplementation in pregnancy other than one trial suggesting protection against dental decay.[43] Evidence from one open trial suggested benefit in hypertension.[44] One controlled trial suggested benefit of vitamin B$_6$ supplementation in increasing immune response in critically ill patients,[45] Some studies have shown it to be effective for depression,[46,47] but a systematic review concluded that meaningful benefit was not apparent.[48]

Autism has also been shown to respond to vitamin therapy, including vitamin B$_6$, but a review of 12 studies using vitamin B$_6$ and magnesium concluded that although results were favourable, studies suffered from methodological problems of poor design, small numbers of subjects and lack of long-term follow-up.[49] A Cochrane review investigated the effect of vitamin B$_6$ and magnesium in autism but due to the small number of studies, the methodological quality and small sample sizes, the review concluded that no recommendation could be made regarding the use of vitamin B$_6$ and magnesium for autism.[50]

Vitamin B$_6$ has also been investigated for a possible role in cognitive function, on the basis of its possible homocysteine lowering effect. Homocysteine is a risk factor for cerebrovascular disease. However, a Cochrane review found no evidence from vitamin B$_6$ in improving cognitive function or mood.[51] This finding has been suggested by the results of a further trial.[52] However, vitamin B$_6$ (with other B vitamins) has been shown to reduce the risk of post-stroke depression,[53] but not of depression in older men.[54]

There is some evidence to suggest that vitamin B$_6$ may reduce the risk of colorectal cancer. A meta-analysis of 13 prospective studies (nine on vitamin B$_6$ intake and four on blood levels of pyridoxal 5'-phosphate (PLP) found that the pooled relative risk (RR) of colorectal cancer for the highest vs lowest category of vitamin B$_6$ intake and blood levels of PLP was 0.90 (95% confidence interval (CI), 0.75 to 1.07) and 0.52 (95% CI, 0.38 to 0.71), respectively. There was heterogeneity among studies of vitamin B$_6$ intake ($P = 0.01$) but not among studies of blood PLP levels ($P < 0.95$). Omitting one study that contributed substantially to the heterogeneity among studies of vitamin B$_6$ intake yielded a pooled RR of 0.80 (95% CI, 0.69 to 0.92). The risk of colorectal cancer decreased by 49% for every 100 nmol/L increase in blood PLP levels (RR, 0.51; 95% CI, 0.38 to 0.69). Overall, vitamin B$_6$ intake and blood PLP levels were inversely associated with the risk of colorectal cancer in this meta-analysis.[55]

Conclusion

The role of vitamin B$_6$ supplements in carpal tunnel syndrome, PMS and asthma is controversial, although supplements may help some individuals. Low vitamin B$_6$ status has been linked with high plasma homocysteine levels and increased risk of CHD, but whether vitamin B$_6$ has an effect independent of folic acid and vitamin B$_{12}$ is not yet clear. Further properly controlled clinical trials are needed to assess the benefit of vitamin B$_6$ supplements for all these purposes, as well as for autism, depression and pregnancy sickness.

Precautions/contraindications

Hypersensitivity to pyridoxine.

Pregnancy and breast-feeding

No problems reported with normal intakes. Large doses may result in pyridoxine dependency in infants. There has been one report of amelia of the leg at the knee in an infant whose mother had taken 50 mg pyridoxine daily during pregnancy.

Adverse effects

Peripheral neuropathy; unsteady gait; numbness and tingling in feet and hands; loss of limb reflexes; impaired or absent tendon reflexes; photosensitivity on exposure to sun; dizziness; nausea; breast tenderness; exacerbation of acne.

Adverse effects usually occur with large doses only. Doses of 100–150 mg daily over 5–10 years have not generally been associated with toxicity. However, doses averaging 117 mg daily have been associated with neurological symptoms (e.g. numbness, tingling, bone pain) in 60% of women taking supplements for 3 years, but this study has been severely criticised. Moreover, symptoms were reversed 6 months after patients stopped taking the supplement.[56] Another paper reported that women taking 500–5000 mg daily for PMS developed peripheral neuropathy over a 1- to 3-year period.[57]

Interactions

Drugs

Alcohol: increases turnover of pyridoxine.
Cycloserine: may cause anaemia or peripheral neuritis by acting as pyridoxine antagonist.
Hydralazine: may cause anaemia or peripheral neuritis by acting as pyridoxine antagonist.
Isoniazid: may cause anaemia or peripheral neuritis by acting as pyridoxine antagonist.
Levetiracetam: preliminary results from a mailed questionnaire study suggest that pyridoxine supplementation could improve behavioural side-effects observed with levetiracetam. Controlled trials are needed to characterise these findings.[58]
Levodopa: effects of levodopa are reversed by pyridoxine (even doses as low as 5 mg daily);

vitamin B$_6$ supplements should be avoided; interaction does not occur with co-beneldopa or co-careldopa.
Oestrogens: (including oral contraceptives) may increase requirement for vitamin B$_6$.
Penicillamine: may cause anaemia or peripheral neuritis by acting as pyridoxine antagonist.
Theophylline: may increase requirement for vitamin B$_6$.

Nutrients

Adequate amounts of all B vitamins are required for optimal functioning; deficiency or excess of one B vitamin may lead to abnormalities in the metabolism of another.
Vitamin C: deficiency of vitamin B$_6$ may lead to vitamin C deficiency.

Dose

As a dietary supplement, 2–5 mg daily.

References

1 Ellis JM, Azuma J, Watanabe T, *et al*. Survey and new data on treatment with pyridoxine of patients having a clinical syndrome including the carpal tunnel and other defects. *Res Commun Chem Pathol Pharmacol* 1977; 17(1): 165–177.
2 Fuhr J, Farrow A, Nelson HS Jr. Vitamin B6 levels in patients with carpal tunnel syndrome. *Arch Surg* 1989; 124: 1329–1330.
3 Driskell J, Wesley RL, Hess IE. Effectiveness of pyridoxine hydrochloride treatment on carpal tunnel syndrome patients. *Nutr Rep Int* 1986; 34: 1031–1040.
4 Ellis J, Folkers K, Levy M. Therapy with vitamin B$_6$ with and without surgery for treatment of patients having the idiopathic carpal tunnel syndrome. *Res Commun Chem Pathol Pharmacol* 1981; 33: 331–344.
5 Ellis J, Folkers K, T W. Clinical results of a cross-over treatment with pyridoxine and placebo of the carpal tunnel syndrome. *Am J Clin Nutr* 1979; 32: 2040–2046.
6 Smith G, Rudge PJ, TJ P. Biochemical studies of pyridoxal and pyridoxal phosphate status and therapeutic trial of pyridoxine in patients with carpal tunnel syndrome. *Ann Neurol* 1984; 15: 104–107.
7 Byers C, DeLisa JA, Frankel DL, *et al*. Pyridoxine metabolism in carpal tunnel syndrome with and without peripheral neuropathy. *Arch Phys Med Rehabil* 1984; 65: 712–716.

8   Jacobson MD, Plancher KD, Kleinman WB. Vitamin B$_6$ (pyridoxine) therapy for carpal tunnel syndrome. *Hand Clin* 1996; 12(2): 253–257.

9   Barr W. Pyridoxine supplements in the premenstrual syndrome. *Practitioner* 1984; 228: 425–427.

10 Day J. Clinical trials in premenstrual syndrome. *Curr Med Res Opin* 1979; 6: 40–45.

11 Kerr G. The management of premenstrual syndrome. *Curr Med Res Opin* 1977; 4: 29–34.

12 Hagen I, Neshmein BI, Tuntlund T. No effect of vitamin B$_6$ against premenstrual tension. *Acta Obstet Gynecol Scand* 1985; 64: 667–670.

13 Malmgren R, Collins A, Nilsson CG. Platelet serotonin uptake and effects of vitamin B$_6$ treatment in premenstrual tension. *Neurophysiology* 1987; 18: 83–88.

14 Smallwood J, Ah-Kye D, Taylor I. Vitamin B$_6$ in the treatment of pre-menstrual mastalgia. *Br J Clin Pract* 1986; 40: 532–533.

15 Mattes J, Martin D. Pyridoxine in premenstrual depression. *Hum Nutr Appl Nutr* 1982; 36A: 131–133.

16 Wyatt KM, Dimmock PW, Jones PW, *et al*. Efficacy of vitamin B-6 in the treatment of premenstrual syndrome: systematic review. *BMJ* 1999; 318 (7195): 1375–1381.

17 Delport R, Ubbink JB, Serfontein WJ, *et al*. Vitamin B$_6$ nutritional status in asthma: the effect of theophylline therapy on plasma pyridoxal-5′-phosphate and pyridoxal levels. *Int J Vitam Nutr Res* 1988; 58(1): 67–72.

18 Reynolds R, Natta CL. Depressed plasma pyridoxal phosphate concentrations in adult asthmatics. *Am J Clin Nutr* 1985; 41: 684–688.

19 Hall M, Thom H, Russell G. Erythrocyte aspartate aminotransferase activity in asthmatic and non-asthmatic children and its enhancement by vitamin B$_6$. *Ann Allergy* 1985; 47: 464–466.

20 Ubbink J, Vermaak WJH, R D. The relationship between vitamin B6 metabolism, asthma and theophylline therapy. *Ann NY Acad Sci* 1990; 585: 285–294.

21 Shimizu T, Maesda S, H A. Relation between theophylline and circulating levels in children with asthma. *Pharmacology* 1996; 53: 384–389.

22 Bartel PR, Ubbink JB, Delport R, *et al*. Vitamin B-6 supplementation and theophylline-related effects in humans. *Am J Clin Nutr* 1994; 60(1): 93–99.

23 Collipp P, Goldzier S, N W. Pyridoxine treatment in childhood bronchial asthma. *Ann Allergy* 1977; 35: 93–97.

24 Sur S, Camara M, Buchmeier A, *et al*. Double-blind trial of pyridoxine (vitamin B$_6$) in the treatment of steroid-dependent asthma. *Ann Allergy* 1993; 70 (2): 147–152.

25 Jones C, Gonzalez V. Pyridoxine deficiency: a new factor in diabetic neuropathy. *J Am Podiatr Ass* 1978; 68: 646–653.

26 Bernstein A, Lobitz CZ. A clinical and electrophysiologic study of the treatment of painful diabetic neuropathies with pyridoxine. In: Leklem JE &

Reynolds RD, eds. *Clinical and Physiological Applications of Vitamin B6* New York: Alan R Liss, 1988: 415–423.

27 Levin ER, Hanscom TA, Fisher M, *et al*. The influence of pyridoxine in diabetic peripheral neuropathy. *Diabetes Care* 1981; 4(6): 606–609.

28 Selhub J, Jacques PF, Wilson PW, *et al*. Vitamin status and intake as primary determinants of homocysteinemia in an elderly population. *JAMA* 1993; 270(22): 2693–2698.

29 Rimm EB, Willett WC, Hu FB, *et al*. Folate and vitamin B$_6$ from diet and supplements in relation to risk of coronary heart disease among women. *JAMA* 1998; 279(5): 359–364.

30 Folsom AR, Nieto FJ, McGovern PG, *et al*. Prospective study of coronary heart disease incidence in relation to fasting total homocysteine, related genetic polymorphisms, and B vitamins: the Atherosclerosis Risk in Communities (ARIC) study. *Circulation* 1998; 98(3): 204–210.

31 Homocysteine Lowering Trialists' Collaboration. Lowering blood homocysteine with folic acid based supplements: meta-analysis of randomised trials. *BMJ* 1998; 316(7135): 894–898.

32 Homocysteine Lowering Trialists' Collaboration. Dose-dependent effects of folic acid on blood concentrations of homocysteine: a meta-analysis of the randomized trials. *Am J Clin Nutr* 2005; 82: 806–812.

33 Miodownik C, Lerner V, Vishne T, *et al*. High-dose vitamin B$_6$ decreases homocysteine serum levels in patients with schizophrenia and schizoaffective disorders: a preliminary study. *Clin Neuropharmacol* 2007; 30(1): 13–17.

34 Potter K, Hankey GJ, Green DJ, *et al*. The effect of long-term homocysteine-lowering on carotid intima-media thickness and flow-mediated vasodilation in stroke patients: a randomized controlled trial and meta-analysis. *BMC Cardiovasc Disord* 2008; 8: 24.

35 Ebbing M, Bleie O, Ueland PM, *et al*. Mortality and cardiovascular events in patients treated with homocysteine-lowering B vitamins after coronary angiography: a randomized controlled trial. *JAMA* 2008; 300(7): 795–804.

36 Albert CM, Cook NR, Gaziano JM, *et al*. Effect of folic acid and B vitamins on risk of cardiovascular events and total mortality among women at high risk for cardiovascular disease: a randomized trial. *JAMA* 2008; 299(17): 2027–2036.

37 Marti-Carvajal AJ, Sola I, Lathyris D, *et al*. Homocysteine lowering interventions for preventing cardiovascular events. *Cochrane Database Syst Rev* 2009; 7(4): CD006612.

38 Ebbing M, Bonaa KH, Arnesen E, *et al*. Combined analyses and extended follow-up of two randomized controlled homocysteine-lowering B-vitamin trials. *J Intern Med* 2010; 268(4): 367–382.

39 VITATOPS Trial Study Group. B vitamins in patients with recent transient ischaemic attack or stroke in the VITAmins TO Prevent Stroke (VITATOPS) trial: a randomised, double-blind,

parallel, placebo-controlled trial. *Lancet Neurol* 2010; 9(9): 855–865.

40 Cui R, Iso H, Date C, *et al*. Dietary folate and vitamin B$_6$ and B$_{12}$ intake in relation to mortality from cardiovascular diseases: Japan collaborative cohort study. *Stroke* 2010; 41(6): 1285–1289.

41 Vutyavanich T, Wongtra-ngan S, Ruangsri R. Pyridoxine for nausea and vomiting of pregnancy: a randomised, double-blind, placebo-controlled trial. *Am J Obstet Gynecol* 1995; 173: 881–884.

42 Sahakian V, Rouse D, Sipes S. Vitamin B$_6$ is effective therapy for nausea and vomiting of pregnancy: a randomised, double-blind, placebo controlled study. *Obstet Gynecol* 1991; 78: 33–36.

43 Thaver D, Saeed MA, Bhutta ZA. Pyridoxine (vitamin B$_6$) supplementation in pregnancy. *Cochrane Database Syst Rev* 2006; (2): CD000179.

44 Ayback M, Sermet A, Ayyildiz MO. Effect of oral pyridoxine hydrochloride supplementation on arterial blood pressure in patients with essential hypertension. *Arzneimittelforschung* 1995; 45: 1271–1273.

45 Cheng CH, Chang SJ, Lee BJ, *et al*. Vitamin B(6) supplementation increases immune responses in critically ill patients. *Eur J Clin Nutr* 2006; 60 (10): 1207–1213.

46 Bell I, Edman JS, Marrow FD. B complex vitamin patterns in geriatric and young adult inpatients with major depression. *J Am Geriatr Soc* 1991; 39: 252–257.

47 Russ C, Hendricks TA, Chrisley BM. Vitamin B$_6$ status of depressed and obsessive-compulsive patients. *Nutr Rep Int* 1983; 27: 867–873.

48 Williams AL, Cotter A, Sabina A, *et al*. The role for vitamin B-6 as treatment for depression: a systematic review. *Fam Pract* 2005; 22(5): 532–537.

49 Pfeiffer SI, Norton J, Nelson L, *et al*. Efficacy of vitamin B$_6$ and magnesium in the treatment of autism: a methodology review and summary of outcomes. *J Autism Dev Disord* 1995; 25(5): 481–493.

50 Nye C, Brice A. Combined vitamin B$_6$-magnesium treatment in autism spectrum disorder. *Cochrane Database Syst Rev* 2005; (4): CD003497.

51 Malouf R, Grimley Evans J. The effect of vitamin B$_6$ on cognition. *Cochrane Database Syst Rev* 2003; (4): CD004393.

52 Aisen PS, Schneider LS, Sano M, *et al*. High-dose B vitamin supplementation and cognitive decline in Alzheimer disease: a randomized controlled trial. *JAMA* 2008; 300(15): 1774–1783.

53 Almeida OP, Marsh K, Alfonso H, *et al*. B-vitamins reduce the long-term risk of depression after stroke: the VITATOPS-DEP trial. *Ann Neurol* 2010; 68(4): 503–510.

54 Ford AH, Flicker L, Thomas J, *et al*. Vitamins B$_{12}$, B$_6$, and folic acid for onset of depressive symptoms in older men: results from a 2-year placebo-controlled randomized trial. *J Clin Psychiatry* 2008; 69(8): 1203–1209.

55 Larsson SC, Orsini N, Wolk A. Vitamin B$_6$ and risk of colorectal cancer: a meta-analysis of prospective studies. *JAMA* 2010; 303(11): 1077–1083.

56 Dalton K, Dalton MJ. Characteristics of pyridoxine overdose neuropathy syndrome. *Acta Neurol Scand* 1987; 76: 8–11.

57 Bernstein A. Vitamin B$_6$ in clinical neurology. *Ann NY Acad Sci* 1990; 585: 250–260.

58 Major P, Greenberg E, Khan A, *et al*. Pyridoxine supplementation for the treatment of levetiracetam-induced behavior side effects in children: preliminary results. *Epilepsy Behav* 2008; 13(3): 557–559.

Vitamin B$_{12}$

Description

Vitamin B$_{12}$ is a water-soluble member of the vitamin B complex.

Nomenclature

Vitamin B$_{12}$ is the generic term used to describe compounds that exhibit the biological activity of cyanocobalamin. It includes a range of cobalt-containing compounds, known as cobalamins. Cyanocobalamin and hydroxocobalamin are the two principal forms in clinical use.

Human requirements

See Table 1 for Dietary Reference Values for vitamin B$_{12}$.

Dietary intake

In the UK, the average adult daily diet provides: for men, 6.5 µg; for women, 4.8 µg.

Action

Vitamin B$_{12}$ is involved in the recycling of folate coenzymes and the degradation of

Table 1 Dietary Reference Values for vitamin B$_{12}$ (µg/day)

| Age | UK | | | | USA | | FAO/WHO |
	LRNI	EAR	RNI	EVM	RDA	TUL	**EU RDA** = 1 µg RNI
0–6 months	0.1	0.25	0.3		0.4	–	0.4
7–12 months	0.25	0.35	0.4		0.5	–	0.5
1–3 years	0.3	0.4	0.5		0.9	–	0.9
4–6 years	0.5	0.7	0.8			–	1.2
4–8 years					1.2	–	–
7–10 years	0.6	0.8	1.0		–	–	1.8[1]
9–13 years					1.8	–	–
Males							
11–14 years	0.8	1.0	1.2		–	–	2.4[2]
15–50+ years	1.0	1.25	1.5	1000	–	–	2.4
14–70+ years					2.4	–	–
Females							
11–14 years	0.8	1.0	1.2		–	–	2.4[2]
15–50+ years	1.0	1.25	1.5	1000	–	–	2.4
14–70+ years					2.4	–	–
Pregnancy		*			2.6	–	2.6
Lactation		+0.5			2.8	–	2.8

* No increment.
[1] 7–9 years; [2] 10–14 years.
EAR = Estimated Average Requirement.
EVM = Likely safe daily intake from supplements alone.
LRNI = Lowest Reference Nutrient Intake.
RDA = Recommended Daily Allowance.
RNI = Reference Nutrient Intake.
TUL = Tolerable Upper Intake Level from food and supplements.

valine. It is also required for nerve myelination, cell replication, haematopoiesis and nucleoprotein synthesis.

Dietary sources

See Table 2 for dietary sources of vitamin B$_{12}$.

Metabolism

Absorption

Absorption occurs almost exclusively in the terminal ileum by an active saturable process, but large amounts (>30 µg) may also be absorbed by passive diffusion (a maximum of 1.5 µg may be absorbed from oral doses of 5–50 µg). For normal absorption, the vitamin must bind to salivary haptocorrin and then to 'intrinsic factor', a highly specific glycoprotein secreted by the parietal cells of the stomach.

Distribution

Vitamin B$_{12}$ is stored mainly in the liver. In the blood, it is bound to specific plasma proteins (transcobalamins).

Elimination

Elimination is via the urinary, biliary and faecal routes. Enterohepatic recycling serves to conserve B$_{12}$. Vitamin B$_{12}$ appears in breast milk.

Table 2 Dietary sources of vitamin B$_{12}$

Food portion	Vitamin B$_{12}$ content (µg)
Breakfast cereals	
1 bowl *All-Bran* (45 g)	*0.5*
1 bowl **Bran Flakes** (45 g)	**0.8**
1 bowl *Corn Flakes* (30 g)	*0.5*
1 bowl **Start** (40 g)	**1.0**
Milk and dairy products	
Milk, whole, semi-skimmed or skimmed (284 ml; $^1/_2$ pint)	1.0
Soya milk	
Gold (284 ml; $^1/_2$ pint)	**1.5**
Plamil, diluted (284 ml; $^1/_2$ pint)	**3.2**
1 pot *yoghurt* (150 g)	*0.3*
Cheese, 50 g	**1.0**
1 *egg*, size 2 (60 g)	*0.4*
Fats and oils	
Butter, margarine, spreads, oils	Trace
Fortified margarine (vegetarian) (10 g)	**0.5**
Meat and fish	
Meat, roast (85 g)	**1.6**
Liver, lambs, cooked (90 g)	**70.0**
Kidney, lambs, cooked (75 g)	**55.0**
White fish, cooked (150 g)	**1.5–4.0**
2 fillets **herring, cooked** (110 g)	**9.0**
2 fillets **kipper, cooked** (130 g)	**8.0**
2 fillets **mackerel, cooked** (110 g)	**15.0**
Pilchards, canned (100 g)	**12.0**
Sardines, canned (70 g)	**10.0**
Tuna, canned (95 g)	**4.0**
Vegetable protein mixes	
Protoveg Burgamix (100 g)	**3.6**
Protoveg Sosmix (100 g)	**1.8**
Yeast extracts	
Marmite, spread on 1 slice bread	*0.4*
Natex, spread on 1 slice bread	*0.4*
Vecon, spread on 1 slice bread	*0.6*

Note: Plant foods (unless fortified commercially) are devoid of vitamin B$_{12}$, except for the adventitious inclusion of microbiologically formed B$_{12}$ from water or soil.
Excellent sources (**bold**); good sources (*italics*).

Deficiency

Deficiency of vitamin B$_{12}$ leads to macrocytic, megaloblastic anaemia. Symptoms include neurological manifestations (due to demyelination of the spinal cord, brain, and optic and peripheral nerves), and less specific symptoms such as weakness, sore tongue, constipation and postural hypotension. Neuropsychiatric manifestations of deficiency may occur in the absence of anaemia (particularly in the elderly).

Pernicious anaemia is a specific form of anaemia caused by lack of intrinsic factor (not lack of vitamin B$_{12}$ in the diet).

Individuals with a reduced ability to absorb vitamin B$_{12}$ develop deficiency within 2–3 years. Strict vegetarians (at risk of dietary deficiency, but with normal absorptive efficiency) may not show signs and symptoms for 20–30 years.

Possible uses

Vegans

Vitamin B$_{12}$ is found only in animal products and certain foods fortified with the vitamin (see Table 2). If vegans do not regularly consume a source of vitamin B$_{12}$, they will require a supplement. This applies particularly to vegan women during pregnancy, as the infant may suffer deficiency. Breast-fed infants whose mothers do not take a source of B$_{12}$ should be supplemented.

The elderly

Prevalence of vitamin B$_{12}$ deficiency increases with age,[1,2] especially over the age of 65 years, and elderly people should be advised to take a supplement or obtain their requirements from fortified foods (e.g. breakfast cereals, yeast spreads). Poor vitamin B$_{12}$ (and folate) status may be associated with age-related hearing dysfunction[3] and tinnitus.[4]

Cognition

Supplementation has been used with some success in reversing impaired mental function due to low vitamin B$_{12}$ status. Several studies have shown that the best responders are those with impaired memory of < 6 months' duration. In one study in 18 subjects, only those with symptoms of < 12 months' duration showed improvement with supplementation.[5]

In addition, vitamin B$_{12}$ deficiency appears to be common in patients with Alzheimer's disease.[6,7] Two Cochrane analyses[8,9] have found no evidence for vitamin B$_{12}$ for cognition and dementia.

In an RCT of 24 weeks' duration, 195 people ≥ 70 years with mild vitamin B$_{12}$ deficiency were given oral vitamin B$_{12}$ 1 mg, vitamin B$_{12}$ 1 mg plus folic acid 400 µg or placebo. Oral vitamin B$_{12}$ corrected mild B$_{12}$ deficiency, while B$_{12}$ plus folic acid also increased cell folate concentration and reduced plasma homocysteine. However, improvement in memory function was greater in the placebo group than in the group who received B$_{12}$ alone. Supplementation with neither vitamin B$_{12}$ alone nor in combination with folic acid was accompanied by any improvement in other cognitive functions.[10]

In an open trial with each subject acting as their own control, 30 subjects with mild to moderate dementia were given B$_{12}$ supplementation for 40 weeks. Various neuropsychiatric rating scales were used at baseline, and after 6, 16 and 40 weeks. Cognitive function did not significantly change over 10 months, but there was a reduction in delirium associated with dementia.[11]

A study in 56 nursing home residents (28 with low serum B$_{12}$ and 28 with normal serum B$_{12}$) evaluated the influence on cognitive function of intramuscular B$_{12}$ injection over 16 weeks in those with low serum B$_{12}$ while those with normal B$_{12}$ acted as a control group and did not receive vitamin B$_{12}$. Although B$_{12}$ replacement produced significant improvement in blood variables, it had no significant impact on cognitive or psychiatric variables.[12]

Neural tube defects

Studies have suggested that deficiency of vitamin B$_{12}$ may be a risk factor for neural tube defects (NTDs). One study[13] showed that in affected pregnancies both plasma B$_{12}$ and folate influenced the maternal red cell folate concentration and were independent risk factors for neural defects. A systematic review of 17 case–control studies concluded that there is a moderate association between low maternal vitamin B$_{12}$ status and the risk of foetal NTDs, but that study design limited the conclusions.[14] More evidence is required before a definite recommendation can be made.

Multiple sclerosis

Vitamin B$_{12}$ has been used to treat multiple sclerosis because it was thought that it might have a role in the formation of myelin, the fatty substance that coats nerve cell axons. However, results of early studies in the 1950s and 1960s were inconclusive and interest in vitamin B$_{12}$ as a treatment for multiple sclerosis declined. Case reports[15,16] have described an association between vitamin B$_{12}$ and multiple sclerosis or clinical syndromes resembling multiple sclerosis, and it is possible that vitamin B$_{12}$ deficiency may exacerbate the disease.[17] However, other researchers have concluded that serum B$_{12}$ deficiency is uncommon in multiple sclerosis.[18] Further studies into the metabolism of vitamin B$_{12}$ in multiple sclerosis are warranted.

Sleep disorders

Results from studies investigating vitamin B$_{12}$ for sleep disorders have been equivocal. One study[19] showed that 3 mg vitamin B$_{12}$ was associated with a reduction in daytime melatonin production, improved sleep quality, and improved concentration and feelings of being refreshed the next day. Another study using the same dose of vitamin B$_{12}$ found no change in mood or daytime drowsiness or night sleep compared with placebo.[20]

Cardiovascular disease

Vitamin B$_{12}$, together with folic acid, has been found to reduce plasma homocysteine levels,[21–25] and is, therefore, thought to have the potential to reduce the risk of cardiovascular disease (CVD). However, low B$_{12}$ and low folate were not found to increase the risk of fatal CVD in an Australian cohort study.[26] Two large RCTs (the Heart Outcomes Prevention Evaluation[27] and the NORVIT Trial[28]) found that B$_{12}$, folic acid and B$_6$ in combination reduced plasma homocysteine, but did not reduce the risk of major cardiovascular events in patients with CVD,[27] and did not lower the risk of recurrent CVD after acute myocardial infarction.[28] Several recent trials[29–31] and meta-analyses[32–34] (see Folic acid monograph) have not provided evidence of benefit for intervention with vitamin B$_{12}$ combined with folic acid and B$_6$ for secondary prevention of CVD, although a few have indicated limited benefit in stroke prevention.[35] A recent randomised controlled trial in 300 individuals in India showed that daily oral supplementation with vitamin B$_{12}$ (2 or 10 µg daily) significantly lowered plasma homocysteine and additional folic acid 200 µg daily has no additional effect.[36] Another Indian trial showed that higher dose vitamin B$_{12}$ reduced plasma

Vitamin B$_{12}$ **481**

homocysteine in those with high homocysteine and low vitamin B$_{12}$ levels.[37]

Miscellaneous

Vitamin B$_{12}$ has been used with some success in patients with diabetic neuropathy[38,39] and mouth ulcers.[40] A double-blind 6-month RCT in 58 primary care patients with recurrent mouth ulcers found that a sublingual dose of vitamin B$_{12}$ 1 mg produced a significant reduction in duration of mouth ulcer outbreaks, number of mouth ulcers and level of pain at 5 and 6 months regardless of the baseline plasma concentration of B$_{12}$. During the last month of the study, a number of participants in the B$_{12}$ group reached a status of 'no mouth ulcers'.[41] Low serum levels of vitamin B$_{12}$ have been found in patients with HIV,[42] and have also been associated with a faster progress towards AIDS.[43] A Japanese study in patients with stroke found that vitamin B$_{12}$ may also reduce the risk of hip fractures.[44]

> ### Conclusion
> Vitamin B$_{12}$ deficiency is a risk in elderly people and can progress to produce symptoms of dementia. The role of supplements in dementia caused by B$_{12}$ deficiency seems to depend on the duration of the symptoms, and there is no good evidence that supplements help to delay the progress of Alzheimer's disease unrelated to vitamin B$_{12}$ deficiency. Vitamin B$_{12}$ (with folic acid) reduces plasma homocysteine, but studies investigating its effects in CVD have produced conflicting results. There is some evidence that supplementation can improve symptoms of diabetic neuropathy, but the role of vitamin B$_{12}$ in multiple sclerosis is unclear. Further research is needed to confirm the benefits of vitamin B$_{12}$ for any indication other than deficiency or marginal deficiency.

Precautions/contraindications

Vitamin B$_{12}$ should not be given for treatment of deficiency until the diagnosis is fully established (administration of $> 10\,\mu g$ daily may produce a haematological response in patients with folate deficiency).

Pregnancy and breast-feeding

No problems reported with normal intakes.

Adverse effects

Vitamin B$_{12}$ may occasionally cause diarrhoea and itching skin. Signs of polycythaemia vera may be unmasked. Megadoses may exacerbate acne.

Interactions

Drugs
Alcohol: excessive intake may reduce the absorption of vitamin B$_{12}$.
Aminoglycosides: may reduce the absorption of vitamin B$_{12}$.
Aminosalicylates: may reduce the absorption of vitamin B$_{12}$.
Antibiotics: may interfere with microbiological assay for serum and erythrocyte vitamin B$_{12}$ (false low results).
Chloramphenicol: may reduce the absorption of vitamin B$_{12}$.
Colestyramine: may reduce the absorption of vitamin B$_{12}$.
Colchicine: may reduce the absorption of vitamin B$_{12}$.
Histamine H$_2$-receptor antagonists: may reduce the absorption of vitamin B$_{12}$.
Metformin: may reduce the absorption of vitamin B$_{12}$.
Methyldopa: may reduce the absorption of vitamin B$_{12}$.
Nitrous oxide: prolonged nitrous oxide anaesthesia inactivates vitamin B$_{12}$.
Oral contraceptives: may reduce blood levels of vitamin B$_{12}$.
Potassium chloride (modified release): prolonged administration may reduce the absorption of vitamin B$_{12}$.
Proton-pump inhibitors: long-term therapy may reduce serum vitamin B$_{12}$ levels.

Nutrients
Folic acid: large doses given continuously may reduce vitamin B$_{12}$ in blood.
Vitamin C: may destroy vitamin B$_{12}$ (avoid large doses of vitamin C within 1 h of oral vitamin B$_{12}$).

Dose

Vitamin B_{12} is available in the form of tablets and capsules, and is also found in many multi-vitamin supplements. In the UK, medically diagnosed deficiency of dietary origin is treated with 50–150 µg oral cyanocobalamin, while those with deficiency of non-dietary origin generally receive 1 mg hydroxocobalamin intramuscularly every 3 months. Some limited evidence (reviewed in the *Drug and Therapeutics Bulletin*[45]) suggests that most people with non-dietary deficiency could also respond to daily doses of 1 mg oral cyanocobalamin.

References

1   Baik H, Russell RM. Vitamin B_{12} deficiency in the elderly. *Ann Rev Nutr* 1999; 19: 357–377.

2   Stabler SP, Lindenbaum J, Allen RH. Vitamin B-12 deficiency in the elderly: current dilemmas. *Am J Clin Nutr* 1997; 66(4): 741–749.

3   Houston DK, Johnson MA, Nozza RJ, *et al.* Age-related hearing loss, vitamin B-12, and folate in elderly women. *Am J Clin Nutr* 1999; 69(3): 564–571.

4   Shemesh Z, Attias J, Ornan M, *et al.* Vitamin B_{12} deficiency in patients with chronic-tinnitus and noise-induced hearing loss. *Am J Otolaryngol* 1993; 14(2): 94–99.

5   Martin DC, Francis J, Protetch J, *et al.* Time dependency of cognitive recovery with cobalamin replacement: report of a pilot study. *J Am Geriatr Soc* 1992; 40(2): 168–172.

6   Abalan F, Delile JM. B_{12} deficiency in presenile dementia. *Biol Psychiatr* 1985; 20: 1251.

7   Levitt A, Karlinsky H. Folate, vitamin B_{12} and cognitive impairment in patients with Alzheimer's disease. *Acta Psychiatr Scand* 1992; 86: 301–305.

8   Malouf R, Areosa Sastre A. Vitamin B_{12} for cognition. *Cochrane Database Syst Rev* 2003; (3): CD004326.

9   Malouf M, Grimley EJ, Areosa SA. Folic acid with or without vitamin B_{12} for cognition and dementia. *Cochrane Database Syst Rev* 2003; (3): CD004514.

10   Eussen SJ, de Groot LC, Joosten LW, *et al.* Effect of oral vitamin B-12 with or without folic acid on cognitive function in older people with mild vitamin B-12 deficiency: a randomized, placebo-controlled trial. *Am J Clin Nutr* 2006; 84(2): 361–370.

11   Lam LC, Lee JS, Chung JC, *et al.* A randomized controlled trial to examine the effectiveness of case management model for community dwelling older persons with mild dementia in Hong Kong. *Int J Geriatr Psychiatry* 2010; 25(4): 395–402.

12   van Dyck CH, Lyness JM, Rohrbaugh RM, *et al.* Cognitive and psychiatric effects of vitamin B_{12} replacement in dementia with low serum B_{12} levels: a nursing home study. *Int Psychogeriatr* 2009; 21 (1): 138–147.

13   Kirke PN, Molloy AM, Daly LE, *et al.* Maternal plasma folate and vitamin B_{12} are independent risk factors for neural tube defects. *Q J Med* 1993; 86 (11): 703–708.

14   Ray J, Blom HJ. Vitamin B_{12} insufficiency and the risk of fetal neural tube defects. *Q J Med* 2003; 96: 289–295.

15   Ransohoff R, Jacobsen DW, Green R. Vitamin B_{12} deficiency and multiple sclerosis. *Lancet* 1990; 1: 1285–1286.

16   Reynolds E, Linnell JC. Vitamin B_{12} deficiency, demyelination and multiple sclerosis. *Lancet* 1987; 2: 920.

17   Reynolds E. Multiple sclerosis and vitamin B_{12} metabolism. *J Neuroimmunol* 1992; 40: 225–230.

18   Sandyk R, Awerbuch G. Vitamin B_{12} and its relationship to age of onset to multiple sclerosis. *Int J Neurosc* 1993; 71: 93–99.

19   Mayer G, Kroger M, Meier-Ewert K. Effects of vitamin B_{12} on performance and circadian rhythm in normal subjects. *Neuropsychopharmacology* 1996; 15(5): 456–464.

20   Okawa M, Takahashi K, Egashira K, *et al.* Vitamin B_{12} treatment for delayed sleep phase syndrome: a multi-center double-blind study. *Psychiatry Clin Neurosci* 1997; 51(5): 275–279.

21   Schnyder G, Roffi M, Flammer Y, *et al.* Effect of homocysteine-lowering therapy with folic acid, vitamin B_{12}, and vitamin B_6 on clinical outcome after percutaneous coronary intervention: the Swiss Heart study – a randomized controlled trial. *JAMA* 2002; 288(8): 973–979.

22   Lee BJ, Huang MC, Chung LJ, *et al.* Folic acid and vitamin B_{12} are more effective than vitamin B_6 in lowering fasting plasma homocysteine concentration in patients with coronary artery disease. *Eur J Clin Nutr* 2004; 58(3): 481–487.

23   Homocysteine Lowering Trialists' Collaboration. Dose-dependent effects of folic acid on blood concentrations of homocysteine: a meta-analysis of the randomized trials. *Am J Clin Nutr* 2005; 82: 806–812.

24   Spence J, Bang H, Chambless LE, *et al.* Vitamin Intervention for Stroke Prevention Trial: an efficacy analysis. *Stroke* 2005; 36: 2404–2409.

25   Flicker L, Vasikaran SD, Thomas J, *et al.* Efficacy of B vitamins in lowering homocysteine in older men: maximal effects for those with B_{12} deficiency and hyperhomocysteinemia. *Stroke* 2006; 37(2): 547–549.

26   Hung J, Beilby JP, Knuimaqn MW, *et al.* Folate and vitamin B_{12} and risk of fatal cardiovascular disease: cohort study from Busselton, Western Australia. *Br Med J* 2003; 326: 131.

27   Lonn E, Yusuf S, Arnold MJ, *et al.* Homocysteine lowering with folic acid and B vitamins in vascular disease. *N Engl J Med* 2006; 354(15): 1567–1577.

28   Bonaa KH, Njolstad I, Ueland PM, *et al.* Homocysteine lowering and cardiovascular events after acute myocardial infarction. *N Engl J Med* 2006; 354(15): 1578–1588.

29 Potter K, Hankey GJ, Green DJ, *et al.* The effect of long-term homocysteine-lowering on carotid intima-media thickness and flow-mediated vasodilation in stroke patients: a randomized controlled trial and meta-analysis. *BMC Cardiovasc Disord* 2008; 8: 24.

30 Ebbing M, Bleie O, Ueland PM, *et al.* Mortality and cardiovascular events in patients treated with homocysteine-lowering B vitamins after coronary angiography: a randomized controlled trial. *JAMA* 2008; 300(7): 795–804.

31 Albert CM, Cook NR, Gaziano JM, *et al.* Effect of folic acid and B vitamins on risk of cardiovascular events and total mortality among women at high risk for cardiovascular disease: a randomized trial. *JAMA* 2008; 299(17): 2027–2036.

32 Marti-Carvajal AJ, Sola I, Lathyris D, *et al.* Homocysteine lowering interventions for preventing cardiovascular events. *Cochrane Database Syst Rev* 2009; 7(4): CD006612.

33 Ebbing M, Bonaa KH, Arnesen E, *et al.* Combined analyses and extended follow-up of two randomized controlled homocysteine-lowering B-vitamin trials. *J Intern Med* 2010; 268(4): 367–382.

34 VITATOPS Trial Study Group. B vitamins in patients with recent transient ischaemic attack or stroke in the VITAmins TO Prevent Stroke (VITATOPS) trial: a randomised, double-blind, parallel, placebo-controlled trial. *Lancet Neurol* 2010; 9(9): 855–865.

35 Cui R, Iso H, Date C, *et al.* Dietary folate and vitamin B_6 and B_{12} intake in relation to mortality from cardiovascular diseases: Japan collaborative cohort study. *Stroke* 2010; 41(6): 1285–1289.

36 Deshmukh US, Joglekar CV, Lubree HG, *et al.* Effect of physiological doses of oral vitamin B_{12} on plasma homocysteine: a randomized, placebo-controlled, double-blind trial in India. *Eur J Clin Nutr* 2010; 64(5): 495–502.

37 Yajnik CS, Lubree HG, Thuse NV, *et al.* Oral vitamin B_{12} supplementation reduces plasma total homocysteine concentration in women in India. *Asia Pac J Clin Nutr* 2007; 16(1): 103–109.

38 Yaqub BA, Siddique A, Sulimani R. Effects of methylcobalamin on diabetic neuropathy. *Clin Neurol Neurosurg* 1992; 94(2): 105–111.

39 Sun Y, Lai MS, Lu CJ. Effectiveness of vitamin B_{12} on diabetic neuropathy: systematic review of clinical controlled trials. *Neurol Acta Taiwan* 2005; 14: 48–54.

40 Weusten B, van de Wile A. Aphthous ulcers and vitamin B_{12} deficiency. *Neth J Med* 1998; 53: 172–175.

41 Volkov I, Rudoy I, Freud T, *et al.* Effectiveness of vitamin B_{12} in treating recurrent aphthous stomatitis: a randomized, double-blind, placebo-controlled trial. *J Am Board Fam Med* 2009; 22(1): 9–16.

42 Paltiel O, Falutz J, Veilleux M, *et al.* Clinical correlates of subnormal vitamin B_{12} levels in patients infected with the human immunodeficiency virus. *Am J Hematol* 1995; 49(4): 318–322.

43 Tang AM, Graham NM, Chandra RK, *et al.* Low serum vitamin B-12 concentrations are associated with faster human immunodeficiency virus type 1 (HIV-1) disease progression. *J Nutr* 1997; 127(2): 345–351.

44 Sato Y, Honda Y, Iwamoto J, *et al.* Effect of folate and mecobalamin on hip fractures in patients with stroke: a randomized controlled trial. *JAMA* 2005; 293(9): 1082–1088.

45 [No authors listed]. Oral or intramuscular vitamin B12? *Drug Ther Bull* 2009; 47(2): 19–21.

Vitamin C

Description

Vitamin C is a water-soluble vitamin.

Nomenclature

Vitamin C is a generic term used to describe compounds that exhibit the biological activity of ascorbic acid. These include L-ascorbic acid (ascorbic acid) and L-dehydroascorbic acid (dehydroascorbic acid).

Human requirements

See Table 1 for Dietary Reference Values for Vitamin C.

Dietary intake

In the UK, the average adult daily diet provides: for men, 83.4 mg; for women, 81.0 mg.

Action

The functions of vitamin C are based mainly on its properties as a reducing agent. It is required for:

- the formation of collagen and other organic constituents of the intercellular matrix in bone, teeth and capillaries; and
- the optimal activity of several enzymes – it activates certain liver-detoxifying enzyme systems (including drug-metabolising enzymes)

Table 1 Dietary Reference Values for vitamin C (mg/day)

Age	UK				USA				FAO/WHO RNI
								EU RDA (for labelling purposes) = 60 mg	
	LRNI	EAR	RNI	EVM	EAR	RDA	AI	TUL	RNI
0–6 months	6	15	25		–	–	40	–	25
7–12 months	6	15	25		–	–	50	–	30
1–3 years	8	20	30		13	–	–	400	30
4–6 years	8	20	30		–	–	–	–	30
4–8 years	–	–	–		22	25	–	–	650
7–10 years	8	20	30		–	–	–	–	35[1]
9–13 years	–	–	–		39	45	–	1200	40
Males									
11–14 years	9	22	35		–	–	–	–	40[2]
14–18 years	–	–	–		63	75	–	1800	40
15–50+ years	10	25	40	1000	–	–	–	–	–
19–70+ years	–	–	–		75	90	–	2000	45
Females									
11–14 years	9	22	35		–	–	–	–	40[2]
14–18 years	–	–	–		56	65	–	1800	40
15–50+ years	10	25	40	1000	–	–	–	–	–
19–70+ years	–	–	–		60	75	–	2000	45
Pregnancy	–	–	+10		66/70[3]	80/85[3]		1800/2000[3]	55
Lactation	–	–	+30		96/100[3]	115/120[3]	1800/2000[3]	70	

[1]7–9 years;   [2]10–14 years;   [3]Up to the age of 18 years/19–50 years.
AI = Adequate Intake.
EAR = Estimated Average Requirement.
EVM = Likely safe daily intake from supplements alone.
LRNI = Lowest Reference Nutrient Intake.
RNI = Reference Nutrient Intake.
TUL = Tolerable Upper Intake Level from food and supplements.

and is involved in the synthesis of carnitine and noradrenaline and the metabolism of folic acid, histamine, phenylalanine, tryptophan and tyrosine.

Vitamin C also acts:

- as an antioxidant (reacting directly with aqueous free radicals), which is important in the protection of cellular function
- to enhance the intestinal absorption of non-haem iron.

Dietary sources

See Table 2 for dietary sources of vitamin C.

Metabolism

Absorption

Vitamin C is absorbed by passive and active transport mechanisms, predominantly in the distal portion of the small intestine (jejunum) and to a lesser extent in the mouth, stomach and proximal intestine. Some 70–90% of the dietary intake is absorbed, but absorption falls to 50% with a dose of 1.5 g.

Distribution

It is transported in the free form (higher concentrations in leukocytes and platelets than red

Table 2 Dietary sources of vitamin C

Food portion	Vitamin C (mg)	Food portion	Vitamin C (mg)
Bread and cereals[1]	0	Blackberries, stewed (100 g)	10
Milk and dairy products	0	**Blackcurrants, stewed** (100 g)	115
Meat and fish[2]	0	12 cherries	10
Vegetables		Fruit salad	
Broccoli, boiled (100 g)	44	canned (130 g)	4
Brussels sprouts, boiled (100 g)	60	fresh (130 g)	20
Cabbage, raw (100 g)	49	**¹/₂ grapefruit**	54
Cabbage, boiled (100 g)	20	Grapes (100 g)	3
Carrots, boiled (100 g)	2	**Guava** (100 g)	230
Cauliflower, boiled (100 g)	43	**1 kiwi fruit**	60
Courgette, stir-fried (100 g)	15	**Lychees** (100 g)	45
Cucumber, raw (30 g)	2	**1 mango**	50
Kale, boiled (100 g)	71	**¹/₂ melon, cantaloupe**	60
Lettuce (30 g)	2	1 slice melon, honeydew	18
Mangetout peas, boiled (50 g)	14	1 slice watermelon	20
stir-fried (50 g)	26	1 orange	90
Peas, boiled (100 g)	16	4 passion fruits	20
Peppers, green, raw (50 g)	120	1 slice pawpaw	90
Peppers, red, raw (50 g)	140	1 peach	30
Potatoes		1 pear	9
chips (250 g)	27	1 slice pineapple	15
new, boiled (150 g)	15	3 plums	6
old, boiled (150 g)	9	**Raspberries** (100 g)	32
sweet, boiled (150 g)	23	**Strawberries** (100 g)	77
Spinach, boiled (100 g)	8	1 tangerine	22
Tomatoes, raw, two (150 g)	25	**Beverages**	
Watercress (20 g)	12	1 large glass apple juice	28
Fruit		1 large glass grapefruit juice	60
1 apple	15	1 large glass orange juice	80
1 banana	16	1 large glass tomato juice	16
		1 large glass Ribena (diluted)	120

[1]A few breakfast cereals have added vitamin C (average 10 mg/portion); Excellent sources (**bold**); good sources (*italics*).   [2]liver contains approx. 15 mg/100 g.

blood cells and plasma), and is readily taken up by body tissues (highest concentration in glandular tissue, e.g. adrenals and pituitary); body stores are generally about 1.5 g.

Elimination
The urine is the main route of elimination, but very little is excreted unchanged (unless plasma concentration is >1.4 mg/100 ml).

Vitamin C crosses the placenta and is excreted in breast milk.

Bioavailability
Storage and cooking lead to loss of vitamin C through oxidation, and boiling results in leaching of the vitamin into the cooking water (cooking water should be consumed in gravies and

soups). Microwaving and stir-frying are the best cooking methods for preserving vitamin C.

Deficiency

Vitamin C deficiency may lead to scurvy. Subclinical deficiency has been associated with poor wound healing and ulceration. Early signs of deficiency may be non-specific and include general weakness, lethargy, fatigue, shortness of breath and aching of the limbs. As the disease progresses, petechiae are often prominent and may appear over the arms after application of a sphygmomanometer.

Signs of advanced deficiency include perifollicular haemorrhages (particularly about the hair follicles); swollen, bleeding gums; pallor and anaemia (the result of prolonged bleeding or associated folic acid deficiency); joints, muscles and subcutaneous tissue may become sites of haemorrhage. In children, disturbances of growth occur and bones, teeth and blood vessels develop abnormally; gum signs are only found in the presence of erupted teeth.

Groups at risk of low vitamin C status include smokers, the elderly, patients in hospitals and other institutions, and patients with diabetes.

Possible uses

Many health claims have been made for mega-dose intakes of vitamin C (i.e. 250–10 000 mg daily), including the prevention and treatment of colds, infections, stress, cancer, hypercholesterolaemia and atherosclerosis.

Respiratory conditions

Since Linus Pauling's claims about the beneficial effects of vitamin C on preventing colds and reducing their symptoms, many studies have investigated the effects of vitamin C on the common cold. A summary of 27 trials conducted between 1970 and 1986[1] concluded that vitamin C did not prevent colds, but could have a small therapeutic effect. Of these 27 trials, five were intervention trials of vitamin C or placebo given at the start of cold symptoms and for a few days, all of which found no benefit. The other 22 were double-blind controlled trials giving daily vitamin C or placebo before and during colds. Of these, 12 showed no preventive effect and no reduction in duration or severity of symptoms, five showed no prevention and only slight non-significant lessening of severity, and the other five reported no prevention and a small but significant reduction in the duration of colds.

One review of several studies indicated that vitamin C alleviates common cold symptoms,[2] although the magnitude of benefit appears to vary depending on the population group studied and the dose. A Cochrane review of 30 trials concluded that long-term daily supplementation with large doses of vitamin C does not appear to prevent colds, but there appears to be a modest benefit in terms of reducing duration of cold symptoms from ingestion of high doses. The review also found that vitamin C might be justified in people exposed to brief periods of severe physical exercise and/or cold environments, and there was also a small benefit on duration and severity of colds for those using regular vitamin C prophylaxis. The trials in which vitamin C was introduced at the onset of colds as therapy did not show any benefit in doses up to 4 g daily, but one large trial reported equivocal benefit from an 8-g therapeutic dose at the onset of symptoms.[3]

Vitamin C has also been evaluated in asthma. A Cochrane review[4] concluded that evidence to date from RCTs is insufficient to recommend a specific role for vitamin C in the treatment of asthma, and that further methodologically strong and large-scale trials are needed.

Cancer

It has been suggested that vitamin C may be useful in the prevention of cancer.[5] Possible mechanisms for this protective effect may be that vitamin C acts as an antioxidant, blocks formation of nitrosamines and faecal mutagens, enhances immune system response and accelerates detoxifying liver enzymes.

Many epidemiological studies have shown an inverse correlation between vitamin C intake and cancer incidence, but the evidence is largely indirect because it is based on the consumption of fruits and vegetables known to contain vitamin C and other nutrients such as beta-carotene and folate. The strongest evidence for a protective effect seems to be for stomach cancer.[6–9] The evidence for oesophageal cancer is not as strong. Findings are contradictory for cancers of the lung, breast, colon and rectum.

There is some evidence that vitamin C supplements may help to prevent stomach cancer,[8] reduce pre-cancerous changes in colon cancer,[10] and help to manage prostate cancer.[11] However, subjects with advanced colorectal cancer responded no better than placebo to vitamin C supplementation.[12] Vitamin C may also benefit cancer patients undergoing radiation treatment, by enabling them to withstand larger doses of radiation with fewer side-effects.[13]

Cardiovascular disease

Epidemiological studies have shown associations between low vitamin C intakes and CVD risk,[14] including stroke.[15] However, two other epidemiological studies of about 87 000 female nurses and 4000 male health professionals found no effect of vitamin C intakes from diets or supplements on cardiovascular risk.[16,17]

An association between vitamin C and atherosclerosis has been suggested in studies investigating the relationship between vitamin C and cholesterol. When 1 g of vitamin C was given to healthy young people, cholesterol levels tended to fall,[18] but in older people no significant pattern of serum cholesterol change was found. A trial of 84 patients with type 2 diabetes showed that 1000 mg vitamin C daily compared with placebo produced a significant decrease in LDL cholesterol and triglycerides as well as in blood glucose, haemoglobin A1c and serum insulin.[19] However, neither 500 mg nor 1 g vitamin C daily were sufficient to reduce LDL oxidation in elderly people with diabetes.[20] Leukocyte levels were found to be lower in patients with coronary heart disease than in patients without disease.[21] Vitamin C may also have beneficial effects on blood pressure,[22] stroke[23] and endothelial function.[24] Increased intake of vitamin C-containing foods has been linked with reduced progression of carotid atherosclerosis in elderly men.[25]

Vitamin C has been shown to reduce blood pressure in mildly hypertensive patients when given for short periods of time,[26] but not when given in the long term.[27] When given in combination with polyphenols, vitamin C has been found to be associated with raised blood pressure in hypertensive people.[28] The link between vitamin C and other cardiovascular risk factors has

also been evaluated. Vitamin C has been found to protect against lipid-induced endothelial damage,[29–32] reduce early recurrence of atrial fibrillation and associated inflammation after atrial electrical remodelling,[33] and potentially reduce triglycerides[34,35] and apo B lipoprotein.[34]

Positive effects on cardiovascular risk factors have also been shown in people with diabetes. One study found that vitamin C 500 mg daily for 1 month reduced arterial blood pressure and improved arterial stiffness.[36] A further study found that vitamin C improved thrombotic markers.[37] However, another study found no effect of vitamin C on microvascular reactivity, inflammatory cytokines and oxidised LDL cholesterol.[38] Yet another study found no significant effect of vitamin C (1.5 g daily) for 3 weeks on oxidative stress, blood pressure or endothelial function in patients with type 2 diabetes.[39]

Cataracts

Patients with cataracts have been found to have lower levels of vitamin C in the lens than patients with no cataracts,[40] and as cataracts develop, the vitamin C content of the lens declines. There is some evidence that long-term supplementation of vitamin C (>10 years) may reduce the development of age-related opacities.[41,42] Oral administration of vitamin C 2 g has been found in one study to saturate the aqueous humour, while a 1 g dose did not and higher doses did not increase aqueous humour concentration.[43]

Wound healing

Reductions in blood ascorbic acid levels have been reported in post-operative patients.[44,45] Some researchers suggest that this reduction represents increased need, while others suggest that ascorbic acid is redistributed to the tissues. Tissue ascorbic acid concentration at the site of a wound has been found to increase.[46] Studies have shown accelerated wound healing with vitamin C supplements.[46,47]

Periodontal disease

There is evidence that vitamin C status is related to periodontal disease. Vitamin C depletion in humans has been associated with significantly increased gum bleeding even though no clinical symptoms of scurvy were observed in any subject.[48] The degree of gingival inflammation was directly related to ascorbic acid status, and a reduction in bleeding was observed with vitamin C supplementation.

Smoking

Vitamin C requirements are higher in smokers than non-smokers,[49] and supplemental vitamin C may help to restore plasma vitamin C concentration in smokers. Beneficial effects of vitamin C on atherosclerotic plaque,[50] platelet aggregation,[51] oxidative stress[52] and endothelial dysfunction[53] have been found in smokers. However, one study found no such effects in smokers.[54]

Sports

Vitamin C supplementation has been investigated in sports people. One study showed that vitamin C supplementation did not counter oxidative changes during or after a marathon.[55] Two further studies concluded that vitamin C supplements could attenuate antioxidant defence.[56–58] A paper describing two studies, one in 14 men (27–36 years) training for 8 weeks, the other in 24 rats, found that the administration of vitamin C (1 g daily in the human study) reduced endurance capacity and, therefore, training efficiency through the prevention of some cellular adaptations to exercise (e.g. antioxidant enzymes, cytochrome c).[59] In a trial among 12 participants given 1500 mg vitamin C or placebo each day for 12 days, post-exercise cortisol was significantly reduced in the vitamin C group, but there was no change in immune cell function or upper respiratory tract infection.[60] A trial in 16 untrained healthy men undergoing 30 min of exercise found that vitamin C supplementation (1 g daily) prevented endurance exercise-induced lipid peroxidation and muscle damage but had no effect on inflammatory markers.[61]

Pre-eclampsia

Vitamin C has been thought to reduce the risk of pregnancy complications such as pre-eclampsia, intrauterine growth restriction and maternal anaemia. A Cochrane analysis concluded that the data are too few to say if vitamin C supplementation (alone or combined with other supplements) is beneficial during pregnancy, and it may result in increased risk of pre-term birth.[62] A trial involving 1877 women (935 women assigned to daily supplementation with 1000 mg of vitamin C and 400 IU vitamin E and 942 women to placebo) found that there was no difference between the two groups in the risk of pre-eclampsia, intrauterine growth restriction or the risk of death or serious outcomes in the infants.[63]

A further trial involving women who were considered as at increased risk of pre-eclampsia; 1199 women were randomised to 1000 mg vitamin C and 400 U vitamin E ($n = 1199$) and 1205 to matched placebo daily from the second trimester of pregnancy until delivery. Incidence of pre-eclampsia was similar in treatment and placebo groups (181 (15%) vs 187 (16%); relative risk (RR), 0.97; 95% confidence interval (CI), 0.80 to 1.17). More babies of low birthweight were born to women who took antioxidants than to controls (387 (28%) vs 335 (24%); RR, 1.15; 95% CI, 1.02 to 1.30), but small size for gestational age did not differ between groups (294 (21%) vs 259 (19%); RR, 1.12; 95% CI, 0.96 to 1.31). The authors concluded that concomitant supplementation with vitamin C and vitamin E did not prevent pre-eclampsia in women at risk but did increase the rate of babies born with a low birthweight. As such, use of these high-dose antioxidants is not justified in pregnancy.[64]

Complex regional pain syndrome

Vitamin C supplementation has been investigated for complex regional pain syndrome (CRPS), a chronic progressive disease characterised by severe pain, swelling and changes in the skin. The International Association for the Study of Pain has divided CRPS into two types based on the presence of nerve lesion following the injury: type I (reflex sympathetic dystrophy) where there are no demonstrable nerve lesions and type II (causalgia) where there is nerve damage. A prospective double-blind trial in 123 adults with 127 conservatively treated wrist fractures were randomly allocated to vitamin C 500 mg daily or placebo for 50 days. Reflex sympathetic dystrophy occurred in seven of the vitamin C-treated group and 14 of the control group.[65] In a further, but larger, trial by the same research group, 317 patients with 328 fractures were randomised to receive vitamin C (200, 500 or 1500 mg daily over 50 days) and 99 patients with 99 fractures were randomised to receive placebo. The prevalence of CRPS was 2.4% (8 of 328) in the vitamin C group and 10.1% (10 of 99) in the placebo group ($P = 0.002$); all of the affected patients were elderly women. Analysis of the different doses of vitamin C showed that the prevalence of CRPS was 4.2% (4 of 96) in the 200 mg group (RR, 0.41; 95% CI, 0.13 to 1.27), 1.8% (2 of 114) in the 500 mg group (RR, 0.17; 95% CI, 0.04 to 0.77) and 1.7% (2 of 118) in the 1500 mg group (RR, 0.17; 95% CI, 0.04 to 0.75). Early cast-related complaints predicted the development of CRPS (RR, 5.35; 95% CI, 2.13 to 13.42). The authors conclude that a daily dose of 500 mg vitamin C can reduce the prevalence of CRPS after wrist fracture.[66]

Miscellaneous

Vitamin C (500 mg daily) has been found to reduce serum uric acid, suggesting that vitamin C might be beneficial in the prevention and management of gout.[67] The vitamin may protect against gastric mucosal atrophy[68] and reduce oxidative stress[69] in patients with chronic gastritis. It has also been found to palliate response to acute stress, lowering blood pressure and cortisol;[70] to reduce oxidative stress in patients with schizophrenia on atypical antipsychotics; and to reduce C-reactive protein (an inflammatory biomarker).[71] In a trial of 312 patients with *Helicobacter pylori* infection, addition of vitamin C to the treatment regimen of amoxicillin, metronidazole and bismuth significantly increased *H. pylori* eradication rate.[72]

Conclusion

Various groups of the population are at risk of vitamin C deficiency, particularly the elderly and smokers. Vitamin C may reduce the duration of the common cold and also the severity of symptoms such as sneezing and coughing, particularly if it is taken immediately the symptoms start. Preventive effects of vitamin C supplementation appear to be limited mainly to people with low dietary intake, while therapeutic effects may occur in wider population groups. Epidemiological studies have shown a link between low blood vitamin C concentrations and CVD, cancer and cataracts. However, further controlled clinical trials are needed to confirm the value of vitamin C supplements for these conditions.

Precautions/contraindications

Vitamin C supplements should be used with caution in diabetes mellitus (because of possible interference with glucose determinations); glucose-6-phosphate dehydrogenase deficiency (risk of haemolytic anaemia); haemochromatosis; sickle cell anaemia (risk of precipitating a crisis); sideroblastic anaemia; and thalassaemia. Prolonged administration of large doses (> 1 g daily) of vitamin C in pregnancy may result in increased requirements and scurvy in the neonate.

Because ascorbic acid is a strong reducing agent it interferes with all diagnostic tests based on oxidation–reduction reactions. Vitamin C administration (megadoses only: > 1 g daily) may interfere with tests for:

- blood glucose (false negative);
- urinary glucose (false positive with analyses using cupric sulphate, e.g. Clinitest; false negative with analyses using glucose oxidase, e.g. Clinistix).

Adverse effects

Vitamin C is considered to be one of the safest of all the vitamins. There appear to be no serious health risks with doses up to 10 g daily, but doses of > 1 g daily are associated with osmotic diarrhoea (owing to the large amounts of unabsorbed ascorbic acid in the intestine), gastric discomfort and mild increase in urination.

Oxalic acid is a major metabolite of vitamin C, and there has been concern about an increased risk of renal oxalate stones with high doses. Doses of 2 g and above are associated with an increased risk of oxalate stones.[73,74]

There have been occasional reports that vitamin C destroys vitamin B_{12} in the tissues and of rebound scurvy after administration of vitamin C is stopped, but such reports remain unsubstantiated.

Prolonged use of chewable vitamin C products may cause dental erosion and increased incidence of caries.

Interactions

Drugs

Vitamin C is important for the optimal activity of some of the drug-metabolising enzymes, including the hepatic cytochrome P450 mixed-function oxidase system. Large doses (>1 g daily) of ascorbic acid (but not ascorbates) may lower urinary pH, leading to increased renal tubular re-absorption of acidic drugs and increased excretion of alkaline drugs.

Aspirin: prolonged administration may reduce blood levels of ascorbic acid.

Anticoagulants: occasional reports that vitamin C reduces the activity of warfarin.

Anticonvulsants: administration of barbiturates or primidone may increase urinary excretion of ascorbic acid.

Desferrioxamine: iron excretion induced by desferrioxamine is enhanced by administration of vitamin C.

Disulfiram: prolonged administration of large doses (>1 g daily) of vitamin C may interfere with the alcohol–disulfiram reaction.

Mexiletine: large doses (>1 g daily) of ascorbic acid may accelerate excretion of mexiletine.

Oral contraceptives (containing oestrogens): may reduce blood levels of ascorbic acid; large doses (>1 g) of vitamin C may increase plasma oestrogen levels (possibly converting low-dose oral contraceptive to high-dose oral contraceptive); possibly breakthrough bleeding associated with withdrawal of high-dose vitamin C.

Tetracyclines: prolonged administration may reduce blood levels of ascorbic acid.

Nutrients

Copper: high doses of vitamin C (>1 g daily) may reduce copper retention.

Iron: vitamin C increases absorption of non-haem iron, but not haem iron. For maximal iron absorption from a non-meat meal, a source of vitamin C providing 50–100 mg should be ingested. Vitamin C supplements appear to have no deleterious effect on iron status in patients with iron overload. Iron administration reduces blood levels of ascorbic acid (ascorbic acid is oxidised).

Vitamin A: vitamin C may reduce the toxic effects of vitamin A.

Vitamin B$_6$: deficiency of vitamin C may increase urinary excretion of pyridoxine.

Vitamin B$_{12}$: excess vitamin C has been claimed to destroy vitamin B$_{12}$, but this does not appear to occur under physiological conditions.

Vitamin E: vitamin C can spare vitamin E, and vice versa.

Heavy metals

Vitamin C may reduce tissue and plasma levels of cadmium, lead, mercury, nickel and vanadium.

Dose

Vitamin C is available in the form of tablets, chewable tablets, capsules and powders. It is found in most multivitamin preparations. A review of 26 US vitamin C products found that three of the products failed to pass the tests for labelled content of vitamin C and one failed on disintegration.

Dietary supplements contain between 25 and 1500 mg per daily dose.

References

1   Truswell A. Ascorbic acid. *N Engl J Med* 1986; 315: 709.
2   Hemila H. Vitamin C supplementation and common cold symptoms: factors affecting the magnitude of benefit. *Med Hypotheses* 1999; 52: 171–178.
3   Douglas R, Hemila H, Chalker E, *et al*. Vitamin C for preventing and treating the common cold. *Cochrane Database Syst Rev* 2007; (3): CD000980.
4   Kaur B, Rowe BH, Arnold E, Vitamin C supplementation for asthma. *Cochrane Database Syst Rev* 2009; 21(1): CD000993.
5   Blocke G, Menkes M. Ascorbic acid in cancer prevention. In: Moon TE, Micozzi MS, eds. *Nutrition and Cancer Prevention. Investigating the Role of Micronutrients*. New York: Marcel Dekker, 1989: 341–348.
6   Bjelke E. Dietary factors and the epidemiology of cancer of the stomach and the large bowel. *Klin Prax Suppl* 1978; 2: 10–17.
7   Correa P, Malcom G, Schmidt B, *et al*. Review article: antioxidant micronutrients and gastric cancer. *Aliment Pharmacol Ther* 1998; 12(Suppl1): 73–82.
8   Risch HA, Jain M, Choi NW, *et al*. Dietary factors and the incidence of cancer of the stomach. *Am J Epidemiol* 1985; 122(6): 947–959.
9   You WC, Blot WJ, Chang YS, *et al*. Diet and high risk of stomach cancer in Shandong, China. *Cancer Res* 1988; 48(12): 3518–3523.
10 Waring AJ, Drake IM, Schorah CJ, *et al*. Ascorbic acid and total vitamin C concentrations in plasma, gastric juice, and gastrointestinal mucosa: effects of gastritis and oral supplementation. *Gut* 1996; 38 (2): 171–176.
11 Paganelli GM, Biasco G, Brandi G, *et al*. Effect of vitamin A, C, and E supplementation on rectal cell proliferation in patients with colorectal adenomas. *J Natl Cancer Inst* 1992; 84(1): 47–51.

12 Moertel CG, Fleming TR, Creagan ET, *et al.* High-dose vitamin C versus placebo in the treatment of patients with advanced cancer who have had no prior chemotherapy. A randomized double-blind comparison. *N Engl J Med* 1985; 312(3): 137–141.

13 Okunieff P. Interactions between ascorbic acid and the radiation of bone marrow, skin, and tumor. *Am J Clin Nutr* 1991; 54(6Suppl): 1281S–1283S.

14 Gaby S, Singh VN. Vitamin C. In: Gaby SK, Bendich A, Sing VN, Machlin LJ, eds. *Vitamin Intake and Health, A Scientific Review.* New York: Marcel Dekker, 1991: 103–161.

15 Myint PK, Luben RN, Welch AA, *et al.* Plasma vitamin C concentrations predict risk of incident stroke over 10 y in 20 649 participants of the European Prospective Investigation into Cancer Norfolk prospective population study. *Am J Clin Nutr* 2008; 87(1): 64–69.

16 Rimm EB, Stampfer MJ, Ascherio A, *et al.* Vitamin E consumption and the risk of coronary heart disease in men. *N Engl J Med* 1993; 328(20): 1450–1456.

17 Stampfer MJ, Hennekens CH, Manson JE, *et al.* Vitamin E consumption and the risk of coronary disease in women. *N Engl J Med* 1993; 328(20): 1444–1449.

18 Spittle C. Atherosclerosis and vitamin C. *Lancet* 1972; i: 798.

19 Afkhami-Ardekani M, Shojaoddiny-Ardekani A. Effect of vitamin C on blood glucose, serum lipids and serum insulin in type 2 diabetes patients. *Indian J Med Res* 2007; 126(5): 471–474.

20 Tessier DM, Khalil A, Trottier L, *et al.* Effects of vitamin C supplementation on antioxidants and lipid peroxidation markers in elderly subjects with type 2 diabetes. *Arch Gerontol Geriatr* 2009; 48(1): 67–72.

21 Ramirez J, Flowers NC. Leucocyte ascorbic acid and its relationship to coronary artery disease in man. *Am J Clin Nutr* 1980; 33: 2079–2087.

22 Ness AR, Chee D, Elliott P. Vitamin C and blood pressure: an overview. *J Hum Hypertens* 1997; 11 (6): 343–350.

23 Gale CR, Martyn CN, Winter PD, *et al.* Vitamin C and risk of death from stroke and coronary heart disease in cohort of elderly people. *BMJ* 1995; 310 (6994): 1563–1566.

24 van Guilder GP, Hoetzer GL, Greiner JJ, *et al.* Acute and chronic effects of vitamin C on endothelial fibrinolytic function in overweight and obese adult humans. *J Physiol* 2008; 586(14): 3525–3535.

25 Ellingsen I, Seljeflot I, Arnesen H, *et al.* Vitamin C consumption is associated with less progression in carotid intima media thickness in elderly men: a 3-year intervention study. *Nutr Metab Cardiovasc Dis* 2009; 19(1): 8–14.

26 Hajjar IM, George V, Sasse EA, *et al.* A randomized, double-blind, controlled trial of vitamin C in the management of hypertension and lipids. *Am J Ther* 2002; 9(4): 289–293.

27 Kim MK, Sasaki S, Sasazuki S, *et al.* Lack of long-term effect of vitamin C supplementation on blood pressure. *Hypertension* 2002; 40(6): 797–803.

28 Ward NC, Hodgson JM, Croft KD, *et al.* The combination of vitamin C and grape-seed polyphenols increases blood pressure: a randomized, double-blind, placebo-controlled trial. *J Hypertens* 2005; 23(2): 427–434.

29 Pleiner J, Schaller G, Mittermayer F, *et al.* FFA-induced endothelial dysfunction can be corrected by vitamin C. *J Clin Endocrinol Metab* 2002; 87 (6): 2913–2917.

30 Morel O, Jesel L, Hugel B, *et al.* Protective effects of vitamin C on endothelium damage and platelet activation during myocardial infarction in patients with sustained generation of circulating microparticles. *J Thromb Haemost* 2003; 1(1): 171–177.

31 Woollard KJ, Loryman CJ, Meredith E, *et al.* Effects of oral vitamin C on monocyte:endothelial cell adhesion in healthy subjects. *Biochem Biophys Res Commun* 2002; 294(5): 1161–1168.

32 Bayerle-Eder M, Pleiner J, Mittermayer F, *et al.* Effect of systemic vitamin C on free fatty acid-induced lipid peroxidation. *Diabetes Metab* 2004; 30(5): 433–439.

33 Shidfar F, Keshavarz A, Jallali M, *et al.* Comparison of the effects of simultaneous administration of vitamin C and omega-3 fatty acids on lipoproteins, apo A-I, apo B, and malondialdehyde in hyperlipidemic patients. *Int J Vitam Nutr Res* 2003; 73(3): 163–170.

34 Korantzopoulos P, Kolettis TM, Kountouris E, *et al.* Oral vitamin C administration reduces early recurrence rates after electrical cardioversion of persistent atrial fibrillation and attenuates associated inflammation. *Int J Cardiol* 2005; 102(2): 321–326.

35 Kim MK, Sasaki S, Sasazuki S, *et al.* Long-term vitamin C supplementation has no markedly favourable effect on serum lipids in middle-aged Japanese subjects. *Br J Nutr* 2004; 91(1): 81–90.

36 Mullan BA, Young IS, Fee H, *et al.* Ascorbic acid reduces blood pressure and arterial stiffness in type 2 diabetes. *Hypertension* 2002; 40(6): 804–809.

37 Tousoulis D, Antoniades C, Tountas C, *et al.* Vitamin C affects thrombosis/fibrinolysis system and reactive hyperemia in patients with type 2 diabetes and coronary artery disease. *Diabetes Care* 2003; 26(10): 2749–2753.

38 Lu Q, Bjorkhem I, Wretlind B, *et al.* Effect of ascorbic acid on microcirculation in patients with type II diabetes: a randomized placebo-controlled crossover study. *Clin Sci (Lond)* 2005; 108(6): 507–513.

39 Darko D, Dornhorst A, Kelly FJ, *et al.* Lack of effect of oral vitamin C on blood pressure, oxidative stress and endothelial function in type II diabetes. *Clin Sci (Lond)* 2002; 103(4): 339–344.

40 Chandra DB, Varma R, Ahmad S, *et al.* Vitamin C in the human aqueous humor and cataracts. *Int J Vitam Nutr Res* 1986; 56(2): 165–168.

41 Chasan-Taber L, Willett WC, Seddon JM, *et al.* A prospective study of vitamin supplement intake and cataract extraction among US women. *Epidemiology* 1999; 10(6): 679–684.

42 Jacques PF, Taylor A, Hankinson SE, *et al.* Long-term vitamin C supplement use and prevalence of early age-related lens opacities. *Am J Clin Nutr* 1997; 66(4): 911–916.

43 Iqbal Z, Midgley JM, Watson DG, *et al.* Effect of oral administration of vitamin C on human aqueous humor ascorbate concentration. *Zhongguo Yao Li Xue Bao* 1999; 20(10): 879–883.

44 Shukla S. Plasma and urinary ascorbic acid levels in the post-operative period. *Experientia* 1969; 25: 704.

45 Irvin T, Chattopadhyay DK, Smythe A. Ascorbic acid requirements in postoperative patients. *Surg Gynaecol Obstet* 1978; 147: 49–55.

46 Crandon J, Lennihan R Jr, Mikal S, *et al.* Ascorbic acid economy in surgical patients. *Ann NY Acad Sci* 1961; 92: 246–267.

47 Ringsdorf WM Jr, Cheraskin E. Vitamin C and human wound healing. *Oral Surg* 1982; 53: 231–236.

48 Leggott PJ, Robertson PB, Rothman DL, *et al.* The effect of controlled ascorbic acid depletion and supplementation on periodontal health. *J Periodontol* 1986; 57(8): 480–485.

49 Lykkesfeldt J, Christen S, Wallock LM, *et al.* Ascorbate is depleted by smoking and repleted by moderate supplementation: a study in male smokers and nonsmokers with matched dietary antioxidant intakes. *Am J Clin Nutr* 2000; 71(2): 530–536.

50 Weber C, Erl W, Weber K, *et al.* Increased adhesiveness of isolated monocytes to endothelium is prevented by vitamin C intake in smokers. *Circulation* 1996; 93: 1488–1492.

51 Schindler TH, Lewandowski E, Olschewski M, *et al.* Effect of vitamin C on platelet aggregation in smokers and nonsmokers. *Med Klin* 2002; 97 (5): 263–269.

52 Dietrich M, Block G, Benowitz NL, *et al.* Vitamin C supplementation decreases oxidative stress biomarker f2-isoprostanes in plasma of nonsmokers exposed to environmental tobacco smoke. *Nutr Cancer* 2003; 45(2): 176–184.

53 Stamatelopoulos KS, Lekakis JP, Papamichael CM, *et al.* Oral administration of ascorbic acid attenuates endothelial dysfunction after short-term cigarette smoking. *Int J Vitam Nutr Res* 2003; 73(6): 417–422.

54 Van Hoydonck PG, Schouten EG, Manuel YKB, *et al.* Does vitamin C supplementation influence the levels of circulating oxidized LDL, sICAM-1, sVCAM-1 and vWF-antigen in healthy male smokers? *Eur J Clin Nutr* 2004; 58(12): 1587–1593.

55 Nieman DC, Henson DA, McAnulty SR, *et al.* Influence of vitamin C supplementation on oxidative and immune changes after an ultramarathon. *J Appl Physiol* 2002; 92(5): 1970–1977.

56 Khassaf M, McArdle A, Esanu C, *et al.* Effect of vitamin C supplements on antioxidant defence and stress proteins in human lymphocytes and skeletal muscle. *J Physiol* 2003; 549(Pt2): 645–652.

57 Goldfarb AH, Patrick SW, Bryer S, *et al.* Vitamin C supplementation affects oxidative-stress blood markers in response to a 30-minute run at 75% VO2max. *Int J Sport Nutr Exerc Metab* 2005; 15 (3): 279–290.

58 Dakhale GN, Khanzode SD, Khanzode SS, *et al.* Supplementation of vitamin C with atypical antipsychotics reduces oxidative stress and improves the outcome of schizophrenia. *Psychopharmacology (Berl)* 2005; 182(4): 494–498.

59 Gomez-Cabrera MC, Domenech E, Romagnoli M, *et al.* Oral administration of vitamin C decreases muscle mitochondrial biogenesis and hampers training-induced adaptations in endurance performance. *Am J Clin Nutr* 2008; 87(1): 142–149.

60 Carrillo AE, Murphy RJ, Cheung SS. Vitamin C supplementation and salivary immune function following exercise-heat stress. *Int J Sports Physiol Perform* 2008; 3(4): 516–530.

61 Nakhostin-Roohi B, Babaei P, Rahmani-Nia F, *et al.* Effect of vitamin C supplementation on lipid peroxidation, muscle damage and inflammation after 30-min exercise at 75% VO2max. *J Sports Med Phys Fitness* 2008; 48(2): 217–224.

62 Rumbold A, Crowther CA. Vitamin C supplementation in pregnancy. *Cochrane Database Syst Rev* 2005; (2): CD004072.

63 Rumbold AR, Crowther CA, Haslam RR, *et al.* Vitamins C and E and the risks of preeclampsia and perinatal complications. *N Engl J Med* 2006; 354(17): 1796–1806.

64 Poston L, Briley AL, Seed PT, *et al.* Vitamin C and vitamin E in pregnant women at risk for pre-eclampsia (VIP trial): randomised placebo-controlled trial. *Lancet* 2006; 367(9517): 1145–1154.

65 Zollinger PE, Tuinebreijer WE, Kreis RW, *et al.* Effect of vitamin C on frequency of reflex sympathetic dystrophy in wrist fractures: a randomised trial. *Lancet* 1999; 354(9195): 2025–2028.

66 Zollinger PE, Tuinebreijer WE, Breederveld RS, *et al.* Can vitamin C prevent complex regional pain syndrome in patients with wrist fractures? A randomized, controlled, multicenter dose-response study *J Bone Joint Surg Am* 2007; 89(7): 1424–1431.

67 Huang HY, Appel LJ, Choi MJ, *et al.* The effects of vitamin C supplementation on serum concentrations of uric acid: results of a randomized controlled trial. *Arthritis Rheum* 2005; 52(6): 1843–1847.

68 Sasazuki S, Sasaki S, Tsubono Y, *et al.* The effect of 5-year vitamin C supplementation on serum pepsinogen level and *Helicobacter pylori* infection. *Cancer Sci* 2003; 94(4): 378–382.

69 Sasazuki S, Hayashi T, Nakachi K, *et al.* Protective effect of vitamin C on oxidative stress: a

randomized controlled trial. *Int J Vitam Nutr Res* 2008; 78(3): 121–128.

70 Brody S, Preut R, Schommer K, *et al.* A randomized controlled trial of high dose ascorbic acid for reduction of blood pressure, cortisol, and subjective responses to psychological stress. *Psychopharmacology (Berl)* 2002; 159(3): 319–324.

71 Block G, Jensen CD, Dalvi TB, *et al.* Vitamin C treatment reduces elevated C-reactive protein. *Free Radic Biol Med* 2009; 46(1): 70–77.

72 Zojaji H, Talaie R, Mirsattari D, *et al.* The efficacy of *Helicobacter pylori* eradication regimen with and without vitamin C supplementation. *Dig Liver Dis* 2009; 41(9): 644–647.

73 Massey L, Liebman M, Kynast-Gales SA. Ascorbate increases human oxaluria and kidney stone risk. *J Nutr* 2005; 135: 1673–1677.

74 Traxer O, Huet B, Poindexter J, *et al.* Effect of ascorbic acid consumption on urinary stone risk factors. *J Urol* 2003; 170(2Pt1): 397–401.

Vitamin D

Description

Vitamin D is a fat-soluble vitamin.

Nomenclature

Vitamin D is a generic term used to describe all sterols that exhibit the biological activity of cholecalciferol. These include:

- vitamin D_1 (calciferol)
- vitamin D_2 (ergocalciferol)
- vitamin D_3 (colecalciferol, cholecalciferol)
- $1(OH)D_3$ (1-hydroxycholecalciferol; alfacalcidol)
- $25(OH)D_3$ (25-hydroxycholecalciferol; calcifediol)
- $1,25(OH)_2D_3$ (1,25-dihydroxycholecalciferol; calcitriol)
- $24,25(OH)_2D_3$ (24,25-dihydroxycholecalciferol)
- dihydrotachysterol.

Vitamin D_2 is the form most commonly added to foods and dietary supplements.

Units

One international unit of vitamin D is defined as the activity of 0.025 µg of cholecalciferol. Thus: 1 µg vitamin D = 40 units vitamin D and: 1 unit vitamin D = 0.025 µg vitamin D.

Human requirements

See Table 1 for Dietary Reference Values for vitamin D.

In addition, there is growing evidence that higher levels of vitamin D are associated with prevention of various conditions.[1,2] Although there is no consensus on optimal levels of serum $25(OH)D_3$, vitamin D deficiency is defined as a $25(OH)D_3$ level of < 50 nmol/L (20 ng/mL). However, some experts suggest that a desirable $25(OH)D_3$ concentration is ≥ 75 nmol/L (30 ng/mL),[1] while others have suggested 60 ng/mL to be an appropriate level.[3] Achieving this blood level could require a daily vitamin D intake of 20–25 µg, with some experts saying that the dietary values are too low.[1]

Dietary intake

In the UK, the average adult daily diet provides: for men, 3.7 µg; for women, 2.8 µg.

Cutaneous synthesis

More than 90% of the vitamin D requirement for most people comes from casual exposure to sunlight. The skin has a large capacity to produce vitamin D. Adult men and women in bathing suits exposed to 1 minimum erythemal dose (MED) of UVB radiation on a tanning bed had increases in blood vitamin D concentrations equivalent to those observed with oral doses of 250–500 µg of vitamin D.[4,5] In another study, at least once weekly use of a tanning bed was associated with 90% higher blood vitamin D concentrations than no use of a tanning bed.[6] A British nursing home study reported that daily exposure of approximately 20% of the skin to

Table 1 Dietary Reference Values for vitamin D (μg/day)

Age	UK		USA		FAO/WHO RNI
	RNI	EVM	AI	TUL	EU RDA = 5 μg
					FAO/WHO RNI
Males and females					
0–6 months	8.5		5	25	5
7–12 months	7.0		5	25	5
1–3 years	7.0		5	50	5
4–18 years	0[1]		5	50	5
19–50 years	0[1]	25	5	50	5
51–65 years	–	–	–	–	10
65+ years	10	25	–	–	2.5
51–70+ years	–	25	10	50	–
> 65 years	–	–	–	–	15
> 70 years	–	–	15	50	–
Pregnancy and lactation	10	–	5	50	10

[1] If skin is exposed to adequate sunlight.
AI = Adequate Intake.
EVM = Likely safe daily intake from supplements alone.
RNI = Reference Nutrient Intake.
TUL = Tolerable upper intake level from diet and supplements.

UVB radiation equivalent to 15 min of summer sunshine was effective in improving vitamin D status, leading the author to suggest that the use of UVB lamps in British nursing homes was the most effective means of maintaining blood vitamin D levels.[7]

The amount of vitamin D synthesised in the skin depends on several factors, including latitude, season and time of day. Very little vitamin D is produced in the skin in regions north of 37° latitude during the winter months. Seasonal variation in $25(OH)D_3$ is well known in Northern Europe with low winter vitamin D status found in children[8] and middle-aged adults in Britain,[9] postmenopausal women in Ireland[10] and adolescents[11,12] and elderly women[11] in Finland. Even in the summer, vitamin D skin synthesis is low in the early morning and late afternoon.

Age also has an influence on skin synthesis. For an equal amount of sun exposure, a person aged 70 years produces 25% of the vitamin D made by a 20-year old.[5] In addition, people with dark skins require longer exposure to sunlight to make the same amount of vitamin D as light-skinned people. Obese people also exhibit smaller increases in blood plasma vitamin D concentrations than non-obese people following the same UVB exposure.[13] This is because vitamin D is stored in the adipose tissue and is not bioavailable. Pollution may also reduce skin synthesis. High levels of atmospheric pollution have also been associated with lower blood $25(OH)D_3$ levels.[14]

Sunscreens have a substantial influence on vitamin D synthesis, but their use is recommended because of concern about exposure to sunlight causing skin cancer and wrinkling. However, a sunscreen with a sun protection factor (SPF) of 8 reduces the capacity of the skin to produce vitamin D by > 95%, while a properly applied sunscreen with a SPF of 15 reduces the capacity by 98%.[5] On this basis, a US researcher has suggested that exposure to sunlight for 5–15 min without a sunscreen between the hours of 10 am and 3 pm during the spring, summer and autumn would be sufficient to improve vitamin D status in people with skin type II (burns easily, tans moderately) or III (burns moderately, tans gradually), with the recommendation that a sunscreen of SPF ≥ 15 should be applied following this exposure.[5] However, UK guidance on skin cancer prevention emphasises the importance of appropriate sun protection, including the use of sunscreens and spending time in the shade between 11 am and 3 pm.[15]

Action

Vitamin D is essential for promoting the absorption and utilisation of calcium and phosphorus and normal calcification of the skeleton. Along with parathyroid hormone (PTH) and calcitonin, it regulates serum calcium concentration by altering serum calcium and phosphate blood levels as needed, and mobilising calcium from bone. It maintains neuromuscular function and various other cellular processes, including the immune system and insulin production.

Dietary sources

See Table 2 for dietary sources of vitamin D.

Metabolism

Absorption (dietary source)
Vitamin D is absorbed with the aid of bile salts from the small intestine via the lymphatic system and its associated chylomicrons. The efficiency of absorption is estimated to be about 50%.

Distribution
Vitamin D is converted by hydroxylation (predominantly in the liver) to $25(OH)D_3$; this is the major circulating form of vitamin D. Further hydroxylation of $25(OH)D_3$ to form $1,25(OH)_2D_3$ (calcitriol), which is the main biologically active form of vitamin D, is now known to occur at several sites in addition to the kidney, including the breast, colon, prostate gland, heart and cells of the immune system.[1] Renal hydroxylation of $25(OH)D_3$ produces the $1,25(OH)_2D_3$ responsible for the traditionally recognised actions of vitamin D in increasing calcium and phosphorus absorption in the intestine, resulting in decreased PTH synthesis, calcium homeostasis and effects on bone. Renally produced $1,25(OH)_2D_3$ also plays a role in blood

pressure control via inhibition of renin production.[16] Extra-renal hydroxylation of $25(OH)D_3$ was discovered as a result of the identification of vitamin D receptors on non-renal cells where production of $1,25(OH)_2D_3$ results in effects different from those traditionally associated with vitamin D. These effects include regulation of immune function,[17] cellular growth, maturation, differentiation and apoptosis,[18,19] and help to explain vitamin D's emerging role in immune function and protection against cancer, heart disease and autoimmune disorders.[1,2] $25(OH)D_3$ is also converted to $24,25(OH)_2D_3$.

Synthesis is regulated mainly by circulating levels of $1,25(OH)_2D_3$. When levels of $1,25(OH)_2D_3$ are high, synthesis is low and vice versa. Synthesis is also stimulated by hypocalcaemia, hypophosphataemia and PTH, and inhibited by hypercalcaemia. A second metabolite of vitamin D, $24,25(OH)_2D_3$, is produced in the kidney. Both $1,25(OH)_2D_3$ and $24,25(OH)_2D_3$ may be required for the biological activity of vitamin D.

Vitamin D is transported in the plasma bound to a specific vitamin D-binding protein, which is its main storage form. Small amounts are stored in the liver, and also in adipose tissue, which may cause a relative deficiency in obese people. Some vitamin D derivatives are excreted in breast milk.

Deficiency

Deficiency of vitamin D results in inadequate intestinal absorption of calcium and phosphate; hypocalcaemia, hypophosphataemia and increase in serum alkaline phosphatase activity; and hyperparathyroidism. Demineralisation of bone leads to rickets in children and osteomalacia in adults. Infants may develop convulsions and tetany. Rickets was thought to be a disease of the past, but has recently re-emerged in the UK, in particular among black children, but the disease is also seen in white children, usually in areas of urban deprivation.[20] A high prevalence of hypovitaminosis D has also been found among young UK Asian women,[21,22] and also in white adolescent UK women.[21]

UK research suggests that the wider community is also at risk of poor vitamin D status, particularly during the winter and early spring.[8,9] Low concentrations of plasma $25(OH)D_3$ have been demonstrated in older people in the UK during the winter months.[23] In a large

Table 2 Dietary sources of vitamin D

Food portion	Vitamin D content (µg)
Breakfast cereals	
1 bowl All-Bran (45 g)	0.8
1 bowl Bran Flakes (45 g)	1.0
1 bowl Corn Flakes (25 g)	0.5
1 bowl Frosties (45 g)	1.0
1 bowl Rice Krispies (35 g)	0.7
1 bowl Special K (35 g)	0.9
Muesli, porridge, Shredded Wheat, Sugar Puffs, Weetabix	0
Bread	0
Milk and dairy products	
Whole milk (284 ml; $^1/_2$ pint)	0.1
Semi-skimmed milk (284 ml; $^1/_2$ pint)	0.03
Skimmed milk (284 ml; $^1/_2$ pint)	0
Skimmed milk, fortified (284 ml; $^1/_2$ pint)	0.2–0.5 (various brands)
2 tablespoons dried skimmed milk, fortified (30 g)	1.0
Hard cheese (50 g)	0.1
Feta cheese (50 g)	0.25
1 carton whole-milk yoghurt (150 g)	0.06
1 carton low-fat yoghurt (150 g)	0.01
1 egg, size 2 (60 g)	1.0
Fats and oils	
Butter, on 1 slice bread (10 g)	0.25
Margarine, on 1 slice bread (10 g)	2.5
Low-fat spread, on 1 slice bread (10 g)	2.5
2 tablespoons ghee (30 g)	0.6
2 teaspoons **cod liver oil** (10 mL)	21.0
Meat and fish	
Liver, lambs, cooked (90 g)	0.5
Liver, calf, cooked (90 g)	0.3
Liver, ox, cooked (90 g)	1.0
Liver, pig, cooked (90 g)	1.0
White fish	Trace
Sardines (70 g)	5.6
Tinned salmon (100 g)	12.5
Tinned pilchards (100 g)	8.0
Tinned tuna (100 g)	5.0
2 fillets **herring, cooked** (110 g)	20.0
2 fillets **kipper, cooked** (130 g)	20.0
2 fillets **mackerel, cooked** (110 g)	21.0
Beverages	
1 mug Ovaltine[1] (300 mL)	0.7
1 mug Horlicks[1] (300 mL)	0.7
1 mug Build-Up[1] (300 mL)	3.0
1 mug *Complan*[2] (300 mL)	1.5

[1] Made with milk (whole or skimmed). [2] Made with water.
Excellent sources (> 5 µg/portion) (**bold**); good sources (> 1.5 µg/portion) (*italics*).

multinational study involving 18 countries, more than 60% of women taking medication for osteoporosis had levels of $25(OH)D_3 < 75$ nmol/L.[24] Evidence suggests that some people have low vitamin D status despite abundant UV exposure.[3]

Possible uses

Requirements may be increased and/or supplements necessary in:

- Infants who are breast-fed without supplemental vitamin D or who have minimal exposure to sunlight: the UK Department of Health[14] advises that all children from the age of 1–5 years should receive supplements of vitamins A and D. These can be obtained free, for those entitled, through the Healthy Start scheme.
- Pregnancy, as women who have low intake of vitamin D during pregnancy have been shown to produce low birthweight infants.[25] Maternal vitamin D insufficiency during pregnancy has been associated with reduced bone-mineral accrual in the offspring during childhood.[26]
- Breast-feeding (particularly with babies born in the autumn).
- The elderly, whose exposure to sunlight may be reduced because of poor mobility.
- Individuals with dark skins.
- Strict vegetarians and vegans.
- Those who do not get much exposure to sunlight.
- Patients with malabsorption conditions (e.g. coeliac disease, cystic fibrosis, Crohn's disease, short bowel syndrome).

Lack of vitamin D has been associated with a range of different conditions, such as osteoporosis, cancer, cardiovascular disease, multiple sclerosis, diabetes mellitus and poor immune function.[1] In addition, a recent meta-analysis of 18 RCTs, including 57 311 participants found that intake of ordinary doses of vitamin D supplements (mean daily dose 528 IU) was associated with a 7% reduction in death from all causes.[27] Outcomes from randomized controlled trials (RCTs), systematic reviews and further meta-analyses are shown in Table 3.

Osteoporosis

Vitamin D (independently of calcium) may be useful in the prevention of osteoporosis. Some

Table 3 Clinical trials and systematic reviews evaluating vitamin D

Reference	Duration and type of trial	Dose of vitamin D	Study group	Outcome measures	Observed effects
Dawson-Hughes et al. (1991)[28]	1-year double-blind placebo-controlled trial	400 IU	249 postmenopausal women with vitamin D intake of 100 IU (all taking Ca 377 mg/day)	Bone loss in the winter and BMD	Reduction in late wintertime bone loss and improved net BMD of the spine with vitamin D 400 IU
Ooms et al. (1995)[29]	2-year randomised controlled trial	400 IU	348 women (≥ 70 years)	BMD of both hips (femoral neck and trochanter) and the distal radius; biochemical markers of bone turnover	Increased BMD at the femoral neck; no change in markers of bone turnover
Dawson-Hughes et al. (1995)[30]	2-year double-blind placebo-controlled trial	2.5 μg (100 IU) or 17.5 μg (700 IU)	247 postmenopausal women with vitamin D intake of 100 IU (all taking Ca 500 mg/day)	Bone loss in the winter and BMD	5.0 μg (200 IU) vitamin D/day limited bone loss from the spine and whole body but was not adequate to minimise bone loss from the femoral neck
Lips et al. (1996)[31]	3.5 year randomised controlled trial	400 IU vitamin D₃	2578 (1916 women, 662 men) ≥ 70 years of age (mean age 80 years; SD 6) living independently in apartments or homes for elderly persons	Incidence of hip and peripheral fractures	No change in incidence of hip or peripheral fractures
Meier et al. (2004)[32]	1 year prospective study followed by an intervention in parts of year 2	Vitamin D₃ (500 IU/day) and Ca (500 mg/day) during the winter months of year 2	55 healthy subjects	Bone turnover and bone loss	Prevented wintertime bone loss and change in bone turnover
Bischoff-Ferrari et al. (2004)[33]	Meta-analysis of 5 randomised controlled trials	Various	1237 elderly participants (mean age, 60 years)	Falls	Vitamin D supplementation reduced risk of falls by >20%
Avenell et al. (2005)[34]	Systematic review of 17 trials	Various	18 668 elderly people	Fractures	No significant of vitamin D alone on hip fracture, vertebral fracture or any new fracture; vitamin D with Ca (in patients in institutions) marginally reduced hip fracture and non-vertebral fracture, but had no effect on vertebral fracture
Bischoff-Ferrari et al. (2005)[35]	Meta-analysis of 5 randomised controlled trials for hip fracture and 7 randomised controlled trials for non-vertebral fracture	Oral vitamin D ± Ca	Elderly patients: 9924 (hip fracture); 9820 (non-vertebral fracture)	Fracture	700–800 IU vitamin D reduced hip and non-vertebral fracture; 400 IU was insufficient to impact fracture

(Continued)

Table 3 *(Continued)*

Reference	Duration and type of trial	Dose of vitamin D	Study group	Outcome measures	Observed effects
Viljakainen et al. (2006)[36]	1-year randomised controlled trial	Oral vitamin D (5 and 10 μg/day)	228 girls (mean age, 11.4 years; SD 0.4)	BMC augmentation	BMC augmentation in the femur was 14.3% and 17.2% higher in the groups receiving 5 and 10 μg vitamin D, respectively, compared with the placebo group; only 10 μg increased lumbar spine BMC augmentation significantly
Schleitoff et al. (2006)[37]	9 month randomised controlled trial	50 μg vitamin D_3/day plus 500 mg Ca/day or placebo plus 500 mg Ca/day	123 patients	Survival rate and different biochemical variables in congestive heart failure	No difference in survival rates; compared with baseline, PTH and interleukin-10 were significantly higher in vitamin D group
Hsia et al. (2007)[38]	7-year randomised controlled trial	Calcium carbonate 500 mg with vitamin D 200 IU twice daily or placebo	36 282 postmenopausal women (50–79 years)	Cardiovascular risk	Ca/vitamin D supplementation neither increased nor decreased coronary or cerebrovascular risk
Broe et al. (2007)[39]	Secondary data analysis of a previous randomised controlled trial (5 months duration)	200, 400, 600, 800 IU	124 nursing home residents (mean age, 89 years)	Risk of falls	Highest vitamin D (800 IU) resulted in lower risk of falls than lower doses or placebo
Izaks et al. (2007)[40]	Meta-analysis of 11 trials	Various (400–800 IU)	Various	Fracture risk	Low-dose vitamin D (400 IU) was not effective in reducing fracture; high dose (800 IU) was effective in reducing risk of fracture (hip and non-vertebral) in institutionalised elderly only
Jackson et al. (2007)[41]	Meta-analysis	Various	9 studies in postmenopausal women	Risk of fall and fracture	Trend towards reduction in fall with vitamin D_3
Boonen et al. (2007)[42]	Meta-analysis	Oral vitamin D with or without Ca supplementation vs. placebo/no treatment	Postmenopausal women or older men reporting risk of hip fracture; 4 randomised controlled trials in 9083 patients involving vitamin D alone; 6 randomised controlled trials (45 509 patients) involving Ca and vitamin D	Risk of hip fracture	Oral vitamin D reduced risk of hip fracture only when Ca added

Reference	Study type	Intervention/dose	Participants	Outcome	Findings
Pittas et al. (2007)[43]	Systematic review and meta-analysis	Oral vitamin D and Ca (intervention); blood levels of vitamin D and Ca (observational)	Observational and intervention trials	Glycaemic control	Vitamin D and Ca insufficiency may negatively influence glycaemia, whereas combined supplementation with both nutrients may be beneficial in optimising glucose metabolism
Lappe et al. (2007)[44]	A 4-year, population-based, double-blind, randomised placebo-controlled trial	Supplemental 1400–1500 mg Ca/day alone or plus 1100 IU vitamin D$_3$/day; or placebo	1179 community-dwelling women randomly selected from the population of healthy postmenopausal women (age > 55 years)	Cancer	Ca + vitamin D reduced all cancer risk
Autier et al. (2007)[27]	Meta-analysis of 18 randomised controlled trials	300–2000 IU	57 311 participants	Mortality	Intake of vitamin D was associated with reduced mortality
Tang et al. (2007)[45]	Meta-analysis of 29 randomised controlled trials	Ca (1200 mg) alone or + vitamin D (800 IU)	63 897 participants (> 50 years)	Fracture and BMD	Ca + vitamin D associated with best outcomes in reduced risk of fracture and bone loss
Cranney et al. (2007)[46]	Meta-analysis of observational and randomised controlled trials	Vitamin D (> 700 IU/day) ± Ca, or placebo	112 randomised controlled trials, 19 prospective cohorts, 30 case-controls and six before–after studies	Fracture and BMD	Compared with placebo, vitamin D$_3$ with Ca supplementation had a small beneficial effect on BMD and reduced the risk of fractures and falls, although benefit may be confined to specific subgroups
Prince et al. (2008)[47]	1-year double-blind randomised controlled trial	Vitamin D 1000 IU day or placebo (both groups received calcium citrate 1000 mg/day)	302 participants (70–90 years) in a sunny climate with a history of falling and vitamin D insufficiency	Falls	Vitamin D reduced risk of falling by 19%
Wei et al. (2008)[48]	Meta-analysis of epidemiological studies	7 studies involved people taking vitamin D, others evaluated dietary intake and/or blood levels	17 studies	Colorectal adenoma	Both circulating 25(OH)D$_3$ and vitamin D intake were inversely associated with colorectal adenoma incidence and recurrent adenomas
Jorde et al. (2008)[49]	1-year cross-sectional study followed by double-blind randomised controlled trial	20 000 or 40 000 IU vitamin D per week	441 subjects (21–70 years)	Depression	Serum 25(OH)D$_3$ of > 40nmol/L was associated with less depression than serum levels of < 40nmol/L
Gissel et al. (2008)[50]	Meta-analysis	100–400 IU vitamin D daily in most studies	6 studies	Breast cancer	No association with breast cancer overall; trend to reduced breast cancer with intakes > 400 IU/day
Parker et al. (2009)[51]	Meta-analysis	Various	28 studies in 99 745 participants	Vitamin D levels and cardiometabolic disorders	Highest levels of vitamin D were associated with a 43% reduced risk of cardiometabolic disorders
Yin et al. (2009)[52]	Meta-analysis	Various	11 longitudinal studies	Prostate cancer	Serum 25(OH)D$_3$ not associated with prostate cancer risk

(Continued)

Table 3 (Continued)

Reference	Duration and type of trial	Dose of vitamin D	Study group	Outcome measures	Observed effects
Chen et al. (2009)[53]	Meta-analysis	Various	36 studies (involving vitamin D intake and/or serum 25(OH)D$_3$ Ca intake	Breast cancer	Highest levels of 25(OH)D$_3$ and/or Ca associated with reduced risk of breast cancer
Bischoff-Ferrari et al. (2009)[54]	Meta-analysis of 8 randomised controlled trials	Various (200–1000 IU/day) supplemental vitamin D	2426 subjects aged 65 years or older	Falls	Doses of 700–1000 IU reduced falls by 19%; lower doses did not reduce falls
Bischoff-Ferrari et al. (2009)[54]	Meta-analysis of 12 randomised controlled trials	Various	Various	Fracture	Vitamin D > 400 IU associated with 20% reduced risk of non-vertebral fracture in elderly people
Molgaard et al. (2009)[55]	12 month randomised controlled trial	5 or 10 μg vitamin D	221 girls (11–12 years)	Bone mass and bone turnover according to genotype	No overall effect of vitamin D on bone health; benefit of vitamin D on BMD in a subgroup with a specific genotype
Moreira-Pfrimer et al. (2009)[56]	6-month randomised controlled trial	Supplementation with Ca and vitamin D$_3$ (December to May): daily Ca plus monthly placebo or daily Ca plus oral vitamin D$_3$ (150 000 IU once a month during the first 2 months, followed by 90 000 IU once a month for the last 4 months)	Institutionalised elderly	Biochemical parameters and muscle strength	Vitamin D enhanced serum 25(OH)D$_3$ and improved lower limb muscle strength
Glendenning et al. (2009)[57]	Randomised controlled trial	Vitamin D$_2$ or D$_3$ (both 1000 IU/day)	90 inpatients with hip fracture and vitamin D insufficiency	Change in serum 25(OH)D$_3$ and PTH	Vitamin D$_3$ increased serum 25(OH)D$_3$ compared with vitamin D$_2$ but no change in PTH
Witham et al. (2009)[58]	Meta-analysis of randomised controlled trials	Various	11 randomised controlled trials	Blood pressure	Weak evidence of a small fall in blood pressure with vitamin D in people with hypertension; no fall in blood pressure in normotensive patients
Aljabri et al. (2010)[59]	Non-blinded, non-'randomised controlled trial	4000 IU vitamin D$_3$ plus Ca to ensure Ca intake of 1200 mg/day	80 patients with type 1 diabetes mellitus and serum 25(OH)D$_3$ < 50 nmol/L	Glycaemic control	Improved glycaemic control in those who achieved vitamin D repletion

Reference	Study type	Intervention	Subjects	Outcome	Results
Zhu et al.[60] (2010)	Randomised controlled trial	Vitamin D_2 (1000 IU/day) or placebo (calcium citrate 1000 mg/day in both groups)	322 women (70–90 years) with serum $25(OH)D_3 < 24 ng/mL$	Muscle strength and function	Improved muscle function with vitamin D in those who were weakest and slowest at baseline
Winzenberg et al.[61] (2010)	Meta-analysis of 6 randomised controlled trials	Various	541 subjects receiving vitamin D for at least 3 months (age 1 month to < 20 years)	BMC, BMD	Vitamin D may improve BMD in vitamin D-deficient children but not in those with adequate vitamin D status
Patel et al.[62] (2010)	4-month randomised controlled trial	400 or 1200 IU vitamin D_3	Subjects with type 2 diabetes and serum $25(OH)D_3 < 25 ng/mL$	Glucose control and insulin sensitivity	Improved (but not optimal) vitamin D levels did not improve glycaemia or insulin sensitivity of lipid levels
Ward et al.[63] (2010)	Randomised controlled trial	4 doses of 150 000 IU vitamin D_2 over 1 year	73 females (12–14 years)	BMD, bone strength, muscle power	No effect on bone or muscle measures
Wu et al.[64] (2010)	Meta-analysis of 4 randomised controlled trials	Various	429 participants	Blood pressure	Vitamin D reduced systolic but not diastolic blood pressure
Grandi et al.[65] (2010)	Meta-analysis	Serum $25(OH)D_3$ levels	9 prospective studies	Cardiovascular risk	Inverse association between $25(OH)D_3$ and cardiovascular risk
Kalyani et al.[66] (2010)	Meta-analysis of 10 trials	Various	Elderly people > 60 years	Falls	200–1000 IU vitamin D resulted in 14% lower risk of falls than Ca alone or placebo
Sanders et al.[67] (2010)	Double-blind randomised controlled trial	50 000 IU vitamin D_3 or placebo each winter for 3–5 years	2256 community dwelling women (> 70 years)	Falls and fractures	High-dose vitamin D resulted in reduced falls and fractures
Yin et al.[68] (2010)	Meta-analysis	Various	10 case–control studies	Breast cancer	$25(OH)D_3$ measured after diagnosis (but not before diagnosis) inversely associated with breast cancer
Parekh et al.[69] (2010)	4-week double-blind randomised controlled trial	Not stated	28 Asian patients with type 2 diabetes	Glucose tolerance	No improvement in glucose tolerance, insulin sensitivity or insulin secretion
Urashima et al.[70] (2010)	3-month double-blind randomised controlled trial	1200 IU (in winter months)	Schoolchildren	Influenza A	Reduction influenza A with vitamin D
Salovaara et al.[71] (2010)	3 year randomised controlled trial	800 IU vitamin D_3 + 1000 mg Ca	3432 women (65–71 years)	Fracture	No significant effect of Ca and vitamin D on fracture
Wang et al.[72] (2010)	Systematic review	Various	17 prospective studies and randomised controlled trials in adults	Cardiovascular events	Vitamin D at moderate to high doses may reduce cardiovascular risk; Ca had minimal effects
Pittas et al.[73] (2010)	Meta-analysis	Various	13 observational studies and 14 trials	Cardiometabolic outcomes	No clinical significant effects of vitamin D in doses given

(Continued)

Table 3 (Continued)

Reference	Duration and type of trial	Dose of vitamin D	Study group	Outcome measures	Observed effects
Witham et al. (2010)[74]	Double-blind parallel group randomised controlled trial	100 000 IU vitamin D_2 or placebo at baseline and after 6 weeks	Patients (> 70 years) with systolic heart failure and 25(OH)D_3 < 20 ng/mL	Functional capacity, quality of life	No significant effect on measured variables
Karkkainen et al. (2010)[75]	3-year randomised population-based open trial	800 IU vitamin D_3 + Ca 1000 mg daily	1566 people	Falls	No association between Ca and vitamin D and risk of falls; post hoc analysis suggested reduced risk of multiple falls
Jagannath et al. (2010)[76]	Meta-analysis	Not stated	1 trial	Multiple sclerosis	Some evidence of benefit, but a low-powered trial
Winzenberg et al. (2011)[77]	Meta-analysis of 6 trials	Various	541 children and adolescents receiving vitamin D	BMD	Lumbar spine BMD and total BMC may improve in vitamin D deficient children and adolescents

BMC, bone mineral content; BMD, bone mineral density; Ca, calcium; PTH, parathyroid hormone.

research has shown that women with hip fractures have lower levels of plasma vitamin D.[78] People with a certain type of vitamin D receptor may be more susceptible to osteoporosis, and women with different types of vitamin D receptor seem to respond differently to vitamin D supplements.[79]

There is some evidence that vitamin D supplementation helps to reduce bone loss, fracture risk and improve functional outcome after hip fracture. Evidence suggests that vitamin D in combination with calcium may enhance the effect of hormone replacement therapy.[80] However, other studies have not shown any reduction in rates of fracture with vitamin D supplementation (see Table 3). Furthermore the Oxford arm of the European Prospective Investigation into Cancer and Nutrition found no evidence of an association between plasma $25(OH)D_3$ and fracture risk for men or women.[81]

Several meta-analyses have addressed the issue of vitamin D supplementation and fracture. One meta-analysis of four RCTs, each of which used a dose of 20 µg (800 IU) vitamin D daily, found that this dose prevents approximately 30% of hip or non-vertebral fractures compared with placebo in adults over the age of 65 years, and concluded that lower intakes are not effective.[82] Another meta-analysis, which included five RCTs for hip fracture and seven RCTs for non-vertebral fracture risk, concluded that oral vitamin D supplementation between 700 and 800 IU daily appears to reduce the risk of hip and any non-vertebral fractures in ambulatory or institutionalised elderly persons, but that an oral vitamin D dose of 400 IU daily is not effective.[35] An extension of this meta-analysis selected RCTs of oral vitamin D with or without calcium supplementation vs placebo/ no treatment in postmenopausal women and/ or older men (≥ 50 years) specifically reporting a risk of hip fracture. The pooled relative risk for vitamin D alone was 1.10 (95% confidence interval (CI) 0.89 to 1.36) and for vitamin D with calcium was 0.82 (95% CI, 0.71 to 0.94). The authors concluded that these findings suggest that oral vitamin D appears to reduce the risk of hip fractures only when calcium supplementation is added.[42] A more recent meta-analysis of 12 RCTs added more weight to the earlier findings that higher doses of vitamin D (> 400 IU daily) are needed to produce a significant reduction in risk of fracture.[54]

Whether vitamin D or vitamin D analogues have a different effect on fracture incidence is unclear. With regard to postmenopausal osteoporosis, there is evidence that vitamin D analogues (rather than plain vitamin D) may have bone-sparing actions. This may be because the type of vitamin D deficiency is a reflection of $1,25(OH)_2D_3$ deficiency or resistance and plain vitamin D will have no effect. Thus, a vitamin D analogue (e.g. $1,25(OH)_2D_3$) could reduce bone loss as a result of a pharmacological action rather than replenishing a deficiency.

A meta-analysis found that the vitamin D analogues, $1(OH)D_3$ and $1,25(OH)_2D_3$, were superior to plain vitamin D in preventing spinal fractures.[83] A Cochrane review found no evidence for this and also concluded that vitamin D alone had no significant effect on hip fracture, vertebral fracture or any new fracture, while vitamin D given with calcium was associated with fewer hip and other non-vertebral fractures.[34] The anti-fracture effect of vitamin D and calcium is likely to be due to their effect on bone mineral density, although again the results of controlled trials are inconsistent.

Falls

Vitamin D may also improve neuromuscular coordination, preserve muscle function[56,60] and as a consequence decrease the risk of falling and falling-related fractures (see Table 3).[84–86] A meta-analysis of five RCTs involving 1237 participants found that vitamin D reduced the risk of falls among both ambulatory and institutionalised older people by 2%.[33] A trial published more recently found that supplementation with both colecalciferol (700 IU daily) and calcium (500 mg daily) over a 3-year period reduced the risk of falling in ambulatory older women by 46% and in less active women by 65%, but supplements had no effect in men.[87] A further trial in 124 nursing home residents (average age 89) who received 200, 400, 600 or 800 IU or placebo daily for 5 months found that the proportion of participants with falls was 44% in the placebo group, 58% in the 200 IU group, 60% in the 400 IU group and 20% in the 800 IU group. Participants in the 800 IU group had a 72% lower adjusted-incidence rate ratio of falls than those taking placebo over the 5 months. No significant differences were observed for the adjusted fall rates compared with placebo in any of the other supplement groups.[39] More recent RCTs have continued to show benefit of vitamin D supplementation (in doses of 700–1000 IU) in reducing the risk of falls by approximately 20%.[47,88] A 2010 meta-analysis concluded that vitamin D in a dose range 200–1000 IU resulted in a 14% lower risk of falls than calcium alone or placebo.[66]

Cancer

Evidence from epidemiological studies suggests that enhanced sunlight exposure is associated with reduced death rates from certain common cancers, including cancer of the colon, breast, pancreas, prostate and ovary.[89–91] Vitamin D intake and low vitamin D levels have also been associated with overall cancer risk. A prospective study in men found an inverse association between low vitamin D levels and risk of total cancer and mortality, particularly for cancers of the digestive system.[92] A 4-year RCT in 1179 women (aged > 55 years) living in the community compared calcium (1400–1500 mg daily) alone or with vitamin D (1100 IU daily) or placebo on cancer incidence. Calcium plus vitamin D reduced all-cause cancer risk by 58% (relative risk (RR), 0.42; $P = 0.01$). In the calcium alone group RR was 0.532 ($P = 0.06$). Calcium plus vitamin D significantly reduced all-cancer risk.[44] Reductions in cancer mortality from intake of 1000 IU (25 µg) daily of vitamin D have been estimated to be 7% for men and 9% for women in the USA and 14% for men and 20% for women in Western European countries below 50° latitude.[93]

Vitamin D intake > 800 IU daily has been associated with a small decrease in risk of breast cancer,[94] although no relationship between serum 25(OH)D$_3$ and breast cancer was found in another prospective study.[95] Conclusions from three recent meta-analyses have also been inconsistent. One showed no relationship between vitamin D intake and breast cancer overall, but there was a trend to reduced breast cancer incidence with vitamin D intakes > 400 IU daily[60] while another showed that the highest levels of 25(OH)D$_3$ were linked with reduced breast cancer.[53] A meta-analysis of 10 case–control studies found that 25(OH)D$_3$ measured after (but not before) diagnosis was inversely associated with breast cancer.[68]

Prospective studies show relative risks for colon cancer of 0.33 to 0.74 with higher vitamin D intake or concentrations of 25(OH)D$_3$ > 65

nmol/L.[2,96,97] Supplemental vitamin D and calcium has been associated with reduced recurrence of colorectal adenomas, although the association was weak.[96] However, an RCT involving 36 282 postmenopausal women found that daily supplementation for 7 years with calcium 1000 mg daily and vitamin D 400 units daily had no effect on the incidence of colorectal cancer.[98] A quantitative meta-analysis found a 50% lower risk of colorectal cancer with a serum 25(OH)D$_3$ level $\geq$ 33 ng/mL compared with < 12 ng/mL and concluded that a daily intake of 1000–2000 IU (25–50 µg) vitamin D$_3$ could reduce the incidence of colorectal cancer with minimal risk.[99] A pooled analysis by the same research group found a 50% lower risk of breast cancer with a serum 25(OH)D$_3$ level of 52 ng/mL compared with < 13 ng/mL, which would correspond to an intake of 4000 IU (100 µg daily) vitamin D. However, the US safe upper level is 2000 units (50 µg) daily. The authors suggest that a 25(OH)D$_3$ level of 52 ng/mL could be maintained by an intake of 2000 units (50 µg) of vitamin D with, when possible, very moderate exposure to sunlight.[100] A recent meta-analysis of 17 epidemiological studies (seven of which involved people taking vitamin D) found that both circulating 25(OH)D$_3$ and vitamin D intake were inversely associated with colorectal adenoma and recurrent adenomas.[48]

Prostate cancer risk has been found to be higher in men with low serum 25(OH)D$_3$ concentrations, but this protective role seems to be strongest in younger men when serum androgen levels are higher[101] and may be affected by genotype.[102] A meta-analysis of longitudinal studies evaluating serum 25(OH)D$_3$ and prostate cancer found no indication that serum 25(OH)D$_3$ is associated with prostate cancer incidence.[103]

Cardiovascular disease and diabetes

Epidemiological studies have demonstrated a weak inverse relationship between serum 25(OH)D$_3$ levels and cardiovascular risk[65,104] and blood pressure.[58,105] There is also evidence that poor vitamin D status is associated with high concentrations of various inflammatory markers (e.g. tumour necrosis factor and interleukin-6) that contribute to the development of atherosclerosis, and that vitamin D supplementation can improve the profile of these markers.[106]

Reduced vitamin D status is also associated with a higher incidence of both type 1 and type 2 diabetes mellitus, insulin resistance, low insulin concentrations and glycaemic control in some studies,[4,59,107] but not others.[62,73] Insufficiency of both vitamin D and calcium may predispose to type 2 diabetes while combined supplementation with both nutrients may be beneficial in optimising glucose metabolism.[43,106]

Miscellaneous

Vitamin D has an important role in the immune system. There is growing evidence for an involvement of vitamin D in infections,[108–110] particularly in tuberculosis,[111] and also in various autoimmune and inflammatory conditions such as rheumatoid arthritis, multiple sclerosis and inflammatory bowel diseases, including ulcerative colitis and Crohn's disease.[1] Vitamin D supplementation has been shown to improve symptoms of rheumatoid arthritis and multiple sclerosis.[106] Vitamin D may also protect against age-related macular degeneration[112] and maternal pre-eclampsia.[113] Low levels of vitamin D have also been associated with cognitive decline in elderly people[114] and depression.[49]

> ### Conclusion
> Vitamin D is important for bone health, and some research has shown that supplementation with vitamin D may reduce the risk of osteoporosis and fracture. It is unclear whether most benefit is achieved from vitamin D alone or from vitamin D with calcium, and what the appropriate doses are. Epidemiological studies have found a link between colon cancer and low vitamin D, but whether supplements can reduce the risk of cancer is unknown.

Precautions/contraindications

Vitamin D should be avoided in hypercalcaemia; and renal osteodystrophy with hyperphosphataemia (risk of metastatic calcification).

Vegetarians

Supplements containing vitamin D_3 (cholecalciferol) are obtained from animal sources (usually as a by-product of wool fat) and are not suitable for strict vegetarians (vegans). Vitamin D_2 (ergocalciferol) is obtained from plant sources and can be recommended.

Pregnancy and breast-feeding

No problems reported with normal intakes. There is a risk of hypercalcaemic tetany in breast fed infants whose mothers take excessive doses of vitamin D.

Adverse effects

Vitamin D is the most likely of all the vitamins to cause toxicity; the margin of safety is very narrow. There is a wide variation in tolerance to vitamin D, but doses of 250 µg (10 000 IU) daily for 6 months may result in toxicity. Infants and children are generally more susceptible than adults; prolonged administration of 45 µg (1800 units) daily may arrest growth in children. Some infants seem to be hyper-reactive to small doses. There is no risk of vitamin D toxicity from prolonged exposure to sunlight.

Excessive intake leads to hypercalcaemia and its associated effects. These include apathy, anorexia, constipation, diarrhoea, dry mouth, fatigue, headache, nausea and vomiting, thirst and weakness.

Later symptoms are often associated with calcification of soft tissues and include bone pain, cardiac arrhythmias, hypertension, renal damage (increased urinary frequency, decreased urinary concentrating ability; nocturia, proteinuria), psychosis (rare) and weight loss.

Interactions

Drugs

Anticonvulsants (phenytoin, barbiturates or primidone): may reduce effect of vitamin D by accelerating its metabolism; patients on long-term anticonvulsant therapy may require vitamin D supplementation to prevent osteomalacia. High dose vitamin D therapy (4000 IU (100 µg) daily) in adults substantially increased bone mineral density at several skeletal sites compared with low dose vitamin D (400 IU (10 µg) daily). In children and adolescents, both high dose (2000 IU (50 µg) daily) and low dose (400 IU (10 µg) daily) vitamin D resulted in comparable increases in bone mass.[115]

Calcitonin: effect of calcitonin may be antagonised by vitamin D.

Colestyramine, colestipol: may reduce intestinal absorption of vitamin D.

Digoxin: caution because hypercalcaemia caused by vitamin D may potentiate effects of digoxin, resulting in cardiac arrhythmias.

Liquid paraffin: may reduce intestinal absorption of vitamin D (avoid long-term administration of liquid paraffin).

Sucralfate: may reduce intestinal absorption of vitamin D.

Thiazide diuretics: may increase risk of hypercalcaemia.

Vitamin D analogues (alfacalcidol, calcitriol, dihydrotachysterol): increased risk of toxicity with vitamin D supplements.

Nutrients

Calcium: may increase risk of hypercalcaemia.

Dose

Vitamin D is available in the form of tablets and capsules, as well as in multivitamin preparations and fish oils. Available supplements (both prescription and OTC) contain either ergocalciferol (vitamin D_2) or cholecalciferol (vitamin D_3). Comparisons have been made between the ability of these two forms to increase blood vitamin D levels. The majority of studies to date have found a significantly greater increase in serum $25(OH)D_3$ levels in response to cholecalciferol compared with ergocalciferol,[116–119] while one study found both equally effective.[120]

A suitable dose of vitamin D in most cases is 10 μg (400 IU) daily.

For prevention of fracture in older people, there is evidence that a higher dose of 20 μg (800 IU)[39,54] with calcium 1200 mg daily is required.

Higher doses, higher RDAs and higher upper safety levels are being discussed worldwide.[1,121] One review suggests an intake for all adults of 1000 IU (40 μg) vitamin D (cholecalciferol) daily is needed to bring vitamin D concentrations in no less than 50% of the population up to 75 nmol/L. A recent analysis suggests that mean serum $25(OH)D_3$ levels of about 75 to 110 nmol/l provide optimal benefits for health and disease endpoints investigated to date without increasing health risks, and that these levels can be best obtained with oral doses in the range 1800 to 4000 IU (45–100 μg) vitamin D per day.[122] RCTs in Ireland suggested that to ensure that the vitamin D requirement is met by the vast majority (> 97.5%) of adults aged > 20 years (including elderly people) during winter, between 7.2 and 42.8 μg vitamin D each is required, depending on summer sun exposure and the threshold of adequacy of $25(OH)D_3$.[123,124] The oral dose of vitamin D_2 required to rapidly achieve adequate levels of plasma $25(OH)D_3$ is seemingly much higher than the often recommended vitamin D_3 dose (20 μg daily). A 3 month trial in postmenopausal women with osteopaenia or osteoporosis showed that 250 μg/day of vitamin D_2 most effectively raised plasma $25(OH)D_3$ levels to 85 nmol/l in 75% of the treated women.[119] However, further work is still needed to better define the doses that will achieve optimal blood levels in the large majority of the population.

Upper safety levels

The UK Expert Group on Vitamins and Minerals (EVM) has identified a likely safe total intake of vitamin D for adults from supplements alone of 25 μg daily.

The US upper level for vitamin D established by the Food and Nutrition Board (FNB) is 50 μg (2000 units). However, recent research[93] has suggested that the absence of toxicity in trials conducted in healthy adults using vitamin D doses of up to 250 μg daily (10 000 IU vitamin D_3) supports the confident selection of this value as the Tolerable Upper Intake Level.[121]

References

1 Holick MF. Vitamin D deficiency. *N Engl J Med* 2007; 357(3): 266–281.

2 Zitterman A. Vitamin D in preventive medicine: are we ignoring the evidence? *Br J Nutr* 2003; 89: 552–572.

3 Binkley N, Novotny R, Krueger D, *et al.* Low vitamin D status despite abundant sun exposure. *J Clin Endocrinol Metab* 2007; 92(6): 2130–2135.

4 Holick M. Vitamin D: importance in the prevention of cancers, type 1 diabetes, heart disease, and osteoporosis. *Am J Clin Nutr* 2004; 79(3): 362–371.

5 Holick M. Sunlight and vitamin D for bone health and prevention of autoimmune diseases, cancers, and cardiovascular disease. *Am J Clin Nutr* 2004; 80(6): 1678S–1688S.

6 Tangpricha V, Turner A, Spina C, *et al.* Tanning is associated with optimal vitamin D status (serum 25-hydroxyvitamin D concentration) and higher bone mineral density. *Am J Clin Nutr* 2004; 80(6): 1645–1649.

7   Chuck A, Todd J, Diffey B. Subliminal ultraviolet-B irradiation for the prevention of vitamin D deficiency in the elderly: a feasibility study. *Photodermatol Photoimmunol Photomed* 2001; 17(4): 168–171.

8   Davies PS, Bates CJ, Cole TJ, *et al.* Vitamin D: seasonal and regional differences in preschool children in Great Britain. *Eur J Clin Nutr* 1999; 53(3): 195–198.

9   Hypponen E, Power C. Hypovitaminosis D in British adults at age 45 y: nationwide cohort study of dietary and lifestyle predictors. *Am J Clin Nutr* 2007; 85(3): 860–868.

10 Hill TR, O'Brien MM, Lamberg-Allardt C, *et al.* Vitamin D status of 51–75-year-old Irish women: its determinants and impact on biochemical indices of bone turnover. *Public Health Nutr* 2006; 9 (2): 225–233.

11 Andersen R, Molgaard C, Skovgaard LT, *et al.* Teenage girls and elderly women living in northern Europe have low winter vitamin D status. *Eur J Clin Nutr* 2005; 59(4): 533–541.

12 Outila TA, Karkkainen MU, Lamberg-Allardt CJ. Vitamin D status affects serum parathyroid hormone concentrations during winter in female adolescents: associations with forearm bone mineral density. *Am J Clin Nutr* 2001; 74(2): 206–210.

13 Wortsman J, Matsuoka LY, Chen TC, *et al.* Decreased bioavailability of vitamin D in obesity. *Am J Clin Nutr* 2000; 72(3): 690–693.

14 Agarwal KS, Mughal MZ, Upadhyay P, *et al.* The impact of atmospheric pollution on vitamin D status of infants and toddlers in Delhi, India. *Arch Dis Child* 2002; 87(2): 111–113.

15 Cancer Research UK. SunSmart. The UK's national skin cancer prevention campaign. http://www.sunsmart.org.uk/ (accessed 25 April 2011).

16 Dusso AS, Brown AJ, Slatopolsky E. Vitamin D. *Am J Physiol Renal Physiol* 2005; 289(1): F8–F28.

17 Adams JS, Liu P, Chun R, *et al.* Vitamin D in defense of the human immune response. *Ann N Y Acad Sci* 2007; 1117: 94–105.

18 Billiet L, Furman C, Larigauderie G, *et al.* Enhanced VDUP-1 gene expression by PPARgamma agonist induces apoptosis in human macrophage. *J Cell Physiol* 2008; 214(1): 183–191.

19 Chen S, Sims GP, Chen XX, *et al.* Modulatory effects of 1,25-dihydroxyvitamin D_3 on human B cell differentiation. *J Immunol* 2007; 179(3): 1634–1647.

20 Wharton B, Bishop N. Rickets. *Lancet* 2003; 362: 1389–1400.

21 Das G, Crocombe S, McGrath M, *et al.* Hypovitaminosis D among healthy adolescent girls attending an inner city school. *Arch Dis Child* 2006; 91(7): 569–572.

22 Roy DK, Berry JL, Pye SR, *et al.* Vitamin D status and bone mass in UK South Asian women. *Bone* 2007; 40(1): 200–204.

23 Hegarty V, Woodhouse P, Khaw K. Seasonal variation in 25-hydroxyvitamin D and parathyroid hormone concentrations in healthy elderly people. *Age and Ageing* 1994; 23: 478–482.

24 Lips P, Hosking D, Lippuner K, *et al.* The prevalence of vitamin D inadequacy amongst women with osteoporosis: an international epidemiological investigation. *J Intern Med* 2006; 260(3): 245–254.

25 Mannion CA, Gray-Donald K, Koski KG. Association of low intake of milk and vitamin D during pregnancy with decreased birthweight. *CMAJ* 2006; 174(9): 1273–1277.

26 Javaid M, Crozier S, Harvey N, *et al.* Maternal vitamin D status during pregnancy and childhood bone mass at age 9 years: a longitudinal study. *Lancet* 2006; 367: 36–43.

27 Autier P, Gandini S. Vitamin D supplementation and total mortality: a meta-analysis of randomized controlled trials. *Arch Intern Med* 2007; 167(16): 1730–1737.

28 Dawson-Hughes B, Dallal GE, Krall EA, *et al.* Effect of vitamin D supplementation on wintertime and overall bone loss in healthy postmenopausal women. *Ann Intern Med* 1991; 115(7): 505–512.

29 Ooms ME, Roos JC, Bezemer PD, *et al.* Prevention of bone loss by vitamin D supplementation in elderly women: a randomized double-blind trial. *J Clin Endocrinol Metab* 1995; 80(4): 1052–1058.

30 Dawson-Hughes B, Harris SS, Krall EA, *et al.* Rates of bone loss in postmenopausal women randomly assigned to one of two dosages of vitamin D. *Am J Clin Nutr* 1995; 61(5): 1140–1145.

31 Lips P, Graafmans WC, Ooms ME, *et al.* Vitamin D supplementation and fracture incidence in elderly persons. A randomized, placebo-controlled clinical trial. *Ann Intern Med* 1996; 124: 400–406.

32 Meier C, Woitge HW, Witte K, *et al.* Supplementation with oral vitamin D_3 and calcium during winter prevents seasonal bone loss: a randomized controlled open-label prospective trial. *J Bone Miner Res* 2004; 19(8): 1221–1230.

33 Bischoff-Ferrari H, Dawson-Hughes B, Willett W, *et al.* Effect of vitamin D on falls: a meta-analysis. *JAMA* 2004; 291(16): 1999–2006.

34 Avenell A, Gillespie WJ, Gillespie LD, *et al.* Vitamin D and vitamin D analogues for preventing fractures associated with involutional and postmenopausal osteoporosis. *Cochrane Database Syst Rev* 2005; 20(3): CD000227.

35 Bischoff-Ferrari HA, Willett WC, Wong JB, *et al.* Fracture prevention with vitamin D supplementation: a meta-analysis of randomized controlled trials. *JAMA* 2005; 293(18): 2257–2264.

36 Viljakainen HT, Natri AM, Karkkainen M, *et al.* A positive dose-response effect of vitamin D supplementation on site-specific bone mineral augmentation in adolescent girls: a double-blinded randomized placebo-controlled 1-year intervention. *J Bone Miner Res* 2006; 21(6): 836–844.

37 Schleithoff SS, Zittermann A, Tenderich G, *et al.* Vitamin D supplementation improves cytokine profiles in patients with congestive heart failure: a double-blind, randomized, placebo-controlled trial. *Am J Clin Nutr* 2006; 83(4): 754–759.

38 Hsia J, Heiss G, Ren H, *et al.* Calcium/vitamin D supplementation and cardiovascular events. *Circulation* 2007; 115(7): 846–854.

39 Broe KE, Chen TC, Weinberg J, *et al.* A higher dose of vitamin d reduces the risk of falls in nursing home residents: a randomized, multiple-dose study. *J Am Geriatr Soc* 2007; 55(2): 234–239.

40 Izaks GJ. Fracture prevention with vitamin D supplementation: considering the inconsistent results. *BMC Musculoskelet Disord* 2007; 8: 26.

41 Jackson C, Gaugris S, Sen SS, *et al.* The effect of cholecalciferol (vitamin D$_3$) on the risk of fall and fracture: a meta-analysis. *Q J Med* 2007; 100(4): 185–192.

42 Boonen S, Lips P, Bouillon R, *et al.* Need for additional calcium to reduce the risk of hip fracture with vitamin D supplementation: evidence from a comparative metaanalysis of randomized controlled trials. *J Clin Endocrinol Metab* 2007; 92(4): 1415–1423.

43 Pittas AG, Lau J, Hu FB, *et al.* The role of vitamin D and calcium in type 2 diabetes. a systematic review and meta-analysis. *J Clin Endocrinol Metab* 2007; 92(6): 2017–2029.

44 Lappe JM, Travers-Gustafson D, Davies KM, *et al.* Vitamin D and calcium supplementation reduces cancer risk: results of a randomized trial. *Am J Clin Nutr* 2007; 85(6): 1586–1591.

45 Tang BM, Eslick GD, Nowson C, *et al.* Use of calcium or calcium in combination with vitamin D supplementation to prevent fractures and bone loss in people aged 50 years and older: a meta-analysis. *Lancet* 2007; 370(9588): 657–666.

46 Cranney A, Horsley T, O'Donnell S, *et al. Effectiveness and Safety of Vitamin D in Relation to Bone Health.* [Evidence Report/Technology Assessment No. 158.] Rockville, MD: Agency for Healthcare Research, 2007.

47 Prince RL, Austin N, Devine A, *et al.* Effects of ergocalciferol added to calcium on the risk of falls in elderly high-risk women. *Arch Intern Med* 2008; 168(1): 103–108.

48 Wei MY, Garland CF, Gorham ED, *et al.* Vitamin D and prevention of colorectal adenoma: a meta-analysis. *Cancer Epidemiol Biomarkers Prev* 2008; 17(11): 2958–2969.

49 Jorde R, Sneve M, Figenschau Y, *et al.* Effects of vitamin D supplementation on symptoms of depression in overweight and obese subjects: randomized double blind trial. *J Intern Med* 2008; 264(6): 599–609.

50 Gissel T, Rejnmark L, Mosekilde L, *et al.* Intake of vitamin D and risk of breast cancer: a meta-analysis. *J Steroid Biochem Mol Biol* 2008; 111(35): 195–199.

51 Parker J, Hashmi O, Dutton D, *et al.* Levels of vitamin D and cardiometabolic disorders: systematic review and meta-analysis. *Maturitas* 2009; 65 (3): 225–236.

52 Yin L, Grandi N, Raum E, *et al.* Meta-analysis: longitudinal studies of serum vitamin D and colorectal cancer risk. *Aliment Pharmacol Ther* 2009; 30(2): 113–125.

53 Chen P, Hu P, Xie D, *et al.* Meta-analysis of vitamin D, calcium and the prevention of breast cancer. *Breast Cancer Res Treat* 2009; 121(2): 469–477.

54 Bischoff-Ferrari HA, Willett WC, Wong JB, *et al.* Prevention of nonvertebral fractures with oral vitamin D and dose dependency: a meta-analysis of randomized controlled trials. *Arch Intern Med* 2009; 169(6): 551–561.

55 Molgaard C, Larnkjaer A, Cashman KD, *et al.* Does vitamin D supplementation of healthy Danish Caucasian girls affect bone turnover and bone mineralization? *Bone* 2009; 46(2): 432–439.

56 Moreira-Pfrimer LD, Pedrosa MA, Teixeira L, *et al.* Treatment of vitamin D deficiency increases lower limb muscle strength in institutionalized older people independently of regular physical activity: a randomized double-blind controlled trial. *Ann Nutr Metab* 2009; 54(4): 291–300.

57 Glendenning P, Chew GT, Seymour HM, *et al.* Serum 25-hydroxyvitamin D levels in vitamin D-insufficient hip fracture patients after supplementation with ergocalciferol and cholecalciferol. *Bone* 2009; 45(5): 870–875.

58 Witham MD, Nadir MA, Struthers AD. Effect of vitamin D on blood pressure: a systematic review and meta-analysis. *J Hypertens* 2009; 27(10): 1948–1954.

59 Aljabri KS, Bokhari SA, Khan MJ. Glycemic changes after vitamin D supplementation in patients with type 1 diabetes mellitus and vitamin D deficiency. *Ann Saudi Med* 2010; 30(6): 454–458.

60 Zhu K, Austin N, Devine A, *et al.* A randomized controlled trial of the effects of vitamin D on muscle strength and mobility in older women with vitamin D insufficiency. *J Am Geriatr Soc* 2010; 58(11): 2063–2068.

61 Winzenberg TM, Powell S, Shaw KA, *et al.* Vitamin D supplementation for improving bone mineral density in children. *Cochrane Database Syst Rev* 2010; 6(10): CD006944.

62 Patel P, Poretsky L, Liao E. Lack of effect of subtherapeutic vitamin D treatment on glycemic and lipid parameters in type 2 diabetes: a pilot prospective randomized trial. *J Diabetes* 2010; 2(1): 36–40.

63 Ward KA, Das G, Roberts SA, *et al.* A randomized, controlled trial of vitamin D supplementation upon musculoskeletal health in postmenarchal females. *J Clin Endocrinol Metab* 2010; 95(10): 4643–4651.

64 Wu SH, Ho SC, Zhong L. Effects of vitamin D supplementation on blood pressure. *South Med J* 2010; 103(8): 729–737.

65 Grandi NC, Breitling LP, Brenner H. Vitamin D and cardiovascular disease: systematic review and meta-analysis of prospective studies. *Prev Med* 2010; 51(34): 228–233.

66 Kalyani RR, Stein B, Valiyil R, *et al*. Vitamin D treatment for the prevention of falls in older adults: systematic review and meta-analysis. *J Am Geriatr Soc* 2010; 58(7): 1299–1310.

67 Sanders KM, Stuart AL, Williamson EJ, *et al*. Annual high-dose oral vitamin D and falls and fractures in older women: a randomized controlled trial. *JAMA* 2010; 303(18): 1815–1822.

68 Yin L, Grandi N, Raum E, *et al*. Meta-analysis: serum vitamin D and breast cancer risk. *Eur J Cancer* 2010; 46(12): 2196–2205.

69 Parekh D, Sarathi V, Shivane VK, *et al*. Pilot study to evaluate the effect of short-term improvement in vitamin D status on glucose tolerance in patients with type 2 diabetes mellitus. *Endocr Pract* 2010; 16(4): 600–608.

70 Urashima M, Segawa T, Okazaki M, *et al*. Randomized trial of vitamin D supplementation to prevent seasonal influenza A in schoolchildren. *Am J Clin Nutr* 2010; 91(5): 1255–1260.

71 Salovaara K, Tuppurainen M, Karkkainen M, *et al*. Effect of vitamin D(3) and calcium on fracture risk in 65- to 71-year-old women: a population-based 3-year randomized, controlled trial: the OSTPRE-FPS. *J Bone Miner Res* 2010; 25(7): 1487–1495.

72 Wang L, Manson JE, Song Y, *et al*. Systematic review: vitamin D and calcium supplementation in prevention of cardiovascular events. *Ann Intern Med* 2010; 152(5): 315–323.

73 Pittas AG, Chung M, Trikalinos T, *et al*. Systematic review: vitamin D and cardiometabolic outcomes. *Ann Intern Med* 2010; 152(5): 307–314.

74 Witham MD, Crighton LJ, Gillespie ND, *et al*. The effects of vitamin D supplementation on physical function and quality of life in older patients with heart failure: a randomized controlled trial. *Circ Heart Fail* 2010; 3(2): 195–201.

75 Karkkainen MK, Tuppurainen M, Salovaara K, *et al*. Does daily vitamin D 800 IU and calcium 1000 mg supplementation decrease the risk of falling in ambulatory women aged 65–71 years? A 3-year randomized population-based trial (OSTPRE-FPS) *Maturitas* 2010; 65(4): 359–365.

76 Jagannath VA, Fedorowicz Z, Asokan GV, *et al*. Vitamin D for the management of multiple sclerosis. *Cochrane Database Syst Rev* 2010; 8(12): CD008422.

77 Winzenberg T, Powell S, Shaw KA, *et al*. Effects of vitamin D supplementation on bone density in healthy children: systematic review and meta-analysis. *BMJ* 2011; 342(25): c7254.

78 LeBoff MS, Kohlmeier L, Hurwitz S, *et al*. Occult vitamin D deficiency in postmenopausal US women with acute hip fracture. *JAMA* 1999; 281: 1505–1511.

79 Graafmans WC, Lips P, Ooms ME, *et al*. The effect of vitamin D supplementation on the bone mineral density of the femoral neck is associated with vitamin D receptor genotype. *J Bone Miner Res* 1997; 12: 1241–1245.

80 Recker RR, Davies KM, Dowd RM, *et al*. The effect of low-dose continuous estrogen and progesterone therapy with calcium and vitamin D on bone in elderly women. A randomized, controlled trial. *Ann Intern Med* 1999; 130: 897–904.

81 Roddam AW, Neale R, Appleby P, *et al*. Association between plasma 25-hydroxyvitamin D levels and fracture risk: the EPIC–Oxford Study. *Am J Epidemiol* 2007; 166(11): 1327–1336.

82 Vieth R. The role of vitamin D in the prevention of osteoprosis. *Annals of Medicine* 2005; 37(4): 278–285.

83 Richy F, Schacht E, Bruyere O, *et al*. Vitamin D analogs versus native vitamin D in preventing bone loss and osteoporosis-related fractures: a comparative meta-analysis. *Calcif Tissue Int* 2005; 76(3): 176–186.

84 Janssen HC, Samson MM, Verhaar HJ. Vitamin D deficiency, muscle function, and falls in elderly people. *Am J Clin Nutr* 2002; 75(4): 611–615.

85 Bischoff-Ferrari H, Dietrich T, Orav E, *et al*. Higher 25-hydroxyvitamin D concentrations are associated with better lower extremity function in both active and inactive persons aged 60 years or more. *Am J Clin Nutr* 2004; 80: 752–758.

86 Snijder MB, van Schoor NM, Pluijm SM, *et al*. Vitamin D status in relation to one-year risk of recurrent falling in older men and women. *J Clin Endocrinol Metab* 2006; 91(8): 2980–2985.

87 Bischoff-Ferrari H, Orav EJ, Dawson-Hughes B. Effect of cholecalciferol plus calcium on falling in ambulatory older men and women. *Arch Intern Med* 2006; 166: 424–430.

88 Bischoff-Ferrari HA, Dawson-Hughes B, Staehelin HB, *et al*. Fall prevention with supplemental and active forms of vitamin D: a meta-analysis of randomised controlled trials. *BMJ* 2009; 339(339): b3692.

89 Guyton K, Kensler T, Posner G. Cancer chemoprevention using natural vitamin D and synthetic analogs. *Annu Rev Pharmacol Toxicol* 2001; 41: 421–442.

90 Garland C, Garland F, Gorham E, *et al*. The role of vitamin D in cancer prevention. *Am J Public Health* 2006; 96(2): 252–261.

91 Skinner HG, Michaud DS, Giovannucci E, *et al*. Vitamin D intake and the risk for pancreatic cancer in two cohort studies. *Cancer Epidemiol Biomarkers Prev* 2006; 15(9): 1688–1695.

92 Giovannucci E, Liu Y, Rimm E, *et al*. Prospective study of predictors of vitamin D status and cancer incidence and mortality in men. *J Natl Cancer Inst* 2006; 98(7): 451–459.

93 Grant WB, Garland CF, Gorham ED. An estimate of cancer mortality rate reductions in Europe and

the US with 1,000 IU of oral vitamin D per day. *Recent Results Cancer Res* 2007; 174: 225–234.

94   Robien K, Cutler GJ, Lazovich D. Vitamin D intake and breast cancer risk in postmenopausal women: the Iowa Women's Health Study. *Cancer Causes Control* 2007; 18(7): 775–782.

95   Jacobs ET, Thomson CA, Flatt SW, *et al*. Vitamin D and breast cancer recurrence in the Women's Healthy Eating and Living (WHEL) Study. *Am J Clin Nutr* 2011; 93(1): 108–117.

96   Hartman T, Albert P, Snyder K, *et al*. The association of calcium and vitamin D with risk of colorectal adenomas. *J Nutr* 2005; 135(2): 252–259.

97   Freedman DM, Looker AC, Chang S-C, *et al*. Prospective study of serum vitamin D and cancer mortality in the United States. *J Natl Cancer Inst* 2007; 99(21): 1594–1602.

98   Wactawski-Wende J, Kotchen J, Anderson J, *et al*. Calcium plus vitamin D supplementation and the risk of colorectal cancer. *N Engl J Med* 2006; 354 (7): 684–696.

99   Gorham ED, Garland CF, Garland FC, *et al*. Optimal vitamin D status for colorectal cancer prevention: a quantitative meta analysis. *Am J Prev Med* 2007; 32(3): 210–216.

100   Garland CF, Gorham ED, Mohr SB, *et al*. Vitamin D and prevention of breast cancer: pooled analysis. *J Steroid Biochem Mol Biol* 2007; 103(3): 708–711.

101   Tuohimaa P, Lyakhovich A, Aksenov N, *et al*. Vitamin D and prostate cancer. *J Steroid Biochem Mol Biol* 2001; 76: 125–134.

102   Li H, Stampfer MJ, Hollis JB, *et al*. A prospective study of plasma vitamin D metabolites, vitamin D receptor polymorphisms, and prostate cancer. *PLoS Med* 2007; 4(3): e103.

103   Yin L, Raum E, Haug U, *et al*. Meta-analysis of longitudinal studies: serum vitamin D and prostate cancer risk. *Cancer Epidemiol* 2009; 33(6): 435–445.

104   Grandi NC, Breitling LP, Vossen CY, *et al*. Serum vitamin D and risk of secondary cardiovascular disease events in patients with stable coronary heart disease. *Am Heart J* 2010; 159(6): 1044–1051.

105   Forman JP, Giovannucci E, Holmes MD, *et al*. Plasma 25-hydroxyvitamin D levels and risk of incident hypertension. *Hypertension* 2007; 49 (5): 1063–1069.

106   Zittermann A. Vitamin D and disease prevention with special reference to cardiovascular disease. *Prog Biophys Mol Biol* 2006; 92(1): 39–48.

107   Pittas AG, Dawson-Hughes B, Li T, *et al*. Vitamin D and calcium intake in relation to type 2 diabetes in women. *Diabetes Care* 2006; 29 (3): 650–656.

108   Liu PT, Stenger S, Li H, *et al*. Toll-like receptor triggering of a vitamin D-mediated human antimicrobial response. *Science* 2006; 311(5768): 1770–1773.

109   Schauber J, Dorschner RA, Coda AB, *et al*. Injury enhances TLR2 function and antimicrobial peptide expression through a vitamin D-dependent mechanism. *J Clin Invest* 2007; 117(3): 803–811.

110   Gombart AF, Borregaard N, Koeffler HP. Human cathelicidin antimicrobial peptide (CAMP) gene is a direct target of the vitamin D receptor and is strongly up-regulated in myeloid cells by 1,25-dihydroxyvitamin D₃. *FASEB J* 2005; 19(9): 1067–1077.

111   Martineau AR, Wilkinson RJ, Wilkinson KA, *et al*. A single dose of vitamin D enhances immunity to mycobacteria. *Am J Respir Crit Care Med* 2007; 176(2): 208–213.

112   Parekh N, Chappell RJ, Millen AE, *et al*. Association between vitamin D and age-related macular degeneration in the Third National Health and Nutrition Examination Survey, 1988 through 1994. *Arch Ophthalmol* 2007; 125(5): 661–669.

113   Bodnar LM, Catov JM, Simhan HN, *et al*. Maternal vitamin D deficiency increases the risk of preeclampsia. *J Clin Endocrinol Metab* 2007; 92(9): 3517–3522.

114   Llewellyn DJ, Lang IA, Langa KM, *et al*. Vitamin D and risk of cognitive decline in elderly persons. *Arch Intern Med* 2010; 170(13): 1135–1141.

115   Mikati MA, Dib L, Yamout B, *et al*. Two randomized vitamin D trials in ambulatory patients on anticonvulsants: impact on bone. *Neurology* 2006; 67(11): 2005–2014.

116   Armas LA, Hollis BW, Heaney RP. Vitamin D₂ is much less effective than vitamin D₃ in humans. *J Clin Endocrinol Metab* 2004; 89(11): 5387–5391.

117   Houghton LA, Vieth R. The case against ergocalciferol (vitamin D₂) as a vitamin supplement. *Am J Clin Nutr* 2006; 84(4): 694–697.

118   Trang H, Cole D, Rubin L, *et al*. Evidence that vitamin D₃ increases serum 25-hydroxy-vitamin D more efficiently than does vitamin D₂. *Am J Clin Nutr* 1998; 68: 854–858.

119   Mastaglia SR, Mautalen CA, Parisi MS, *et al*. Vitamin D₂ dose required to rapidly increase 25OHD levels in osteoporotic women. *Eur J Clin Nutr* 2006; 60(5): 681–687.

120   Rapuri PB, Gallagher JC, Haynatzki G. Effect of vitamins D₂ and D₃ supplement use on serum 25 (OH)D concentration in elderly women in summer and winter. *Calcif Tissue Int* 2004; 74(2): 150–156.

121   Hathcock JN, Shao A, Vieth R, *et al*. Risk assessment for vitamin D. *Am J Clin Nutr* 2007; 85(1): 6–18.

122   Bischoff-Ferrari HA, Shao A, Dawson-Hughes B, *et al*. Benefit-risk assessment of vitamin D supplementation. *Osteoporos Int* 2010; 21(7): 1121–1132.

123   Cashman KD, Wallace JM, Horigan G, *et al*. Estimation of the dietary requirement for vitamin D in free-living adults ≥ 64 y of age. *Am J Clin Nutr* 2009; 89(5): 1366–1374.

124   Cashman KD, Hill TR, Lucey AJ, *et al*. Estimation of the dietary requirement for vitamin D in healthy adults. *Am J Clin Nutr* 2008; 88(6): 1535–1542.

Vitamin E

Description

Vitamin E is a fat-soluble vitamin.

Nomenclature

Vitamin E is a generic term used to describe all tocopherol and tocotrienol derivatives that exhibit the biological activity of alpha-tocopherol.

Units

To determine the number of milligrams of alpha-tocopherol in a supplement expressed in International Units, use the following conversion factors. If the form of vitamin E in the supplement is natural, i.e. *d*-alpha-tocopherol or (*R,R,R*)-alpha-tocopherol, multiply international units by 0.67. Thus, 100 IU of natural vitamin E is 66.7 mg alpha-tocopherol (100 × 0.67). If the form of vitamin E in the supplement is synthetic (i.e. *d,l*-alpha-tocopherol or *all-rac*-alpha-tocopherol), multiply the international units by 0.45. Thus, 100 IU of synthetic vitamin E is 45 mg alpha-tocopherol (30 × 0.45).

Human requirements

See Table 1 for Dietary Reference Values for vitamin E.

There is an increased requirement for vitamin E in diets high in polyunsaturated fatty acids (PUFAs), but many items high in PUFA (e.g. vegetable oils and fish oils) are also high in vitamin E (see Table 2). In general, the requirement for vitamin E appears to be 0.4 mg/g linoleic acid; 3–4 mg/g eicosapentaenoic and docosahexaenoic acid combined.

Dietary intake

In the UK, the average adult daily diet provides 8.3 mg.

Action

Vitamin E is an antioxidant, protecting PUFAs in membranes and other critical cellular structures from free radicals and products of oxidation. It works in conjunction with dietary selenium (a cofactor for glutathione peroxidase), and also with vitamin C and other enzymes, including superoxide dismutase and catalase.

Dietary sources

See Table 2 for dietary sources of vitamin E.

Metabolism

Absorption

Absorption of vitamin E is relatively inefficient (20–80%); the efficiency of absorption falls as the dose increases. Normal bile and pancreatic secretion are essential for maximal absorption. Absorption is maximal in the median part of the intestine; it is not absorbed in the large intestine to any great extent.

Distribution

Vitamin E is taken up principally via the lymphatic system and is transported in the blood bound to lipoproteins. More than 90% is carried by the LDL fraction. There is some evidence that a greater proportion is transported by the HDL fraction in females than in males. Vitamin E is stored in all fatty tissues, in particular adipose tissue, liver and muscle.

Elimination

The major route of elimination is the faeces; usually < 1% of orally administered vitamin E is excreted in the urine. Vitamin E appears in breast milk.

Bioavailability

Absorption is enhanced by dietary fat; medium-chain triglycerides enhance absorption whereas polyunsaturated fats are inhibitory.

Table 1 Dietary Reference Values for vitamin E (mg/day)

						EU RDA = 10 mg
Age	UK Safe Intake	EVM	USA			FAO/WHO RNI
			EAR	RDA	TUL	
0–6 months	0.4 mg/g PUFA[1]	–	–	4[2]	–	2.7
7–12 months	0.4 mg/g PUFA[1]	–	–	6[2]	–	2.7
1–3 years	0.4 mg/g PUFA[1]	–	5	6	200	5.0
4–8 years	–	–	6	7	300	5.0[3]
9–13 years	–	–	9	11	600	–
10–65+ years	–	–			–	7.5[4]/10.0[5]
14–70+ years	–	–	12	15	1000[6]	
Males						
11–50+ years	>4	–	–	727	–	–
Females						
11–50+ years	>3	–	–	–	–	–
Pregnancy	–	–	16	19	800/1000[7]	
Lactation	–	–	16	19	800/1000[7]	

[1]PUFA = polyunsaturated fatty acid;   [2]Adequate Intakes (AI);   [3]7–9 years, 7.0 mg;   [4]women;   [5]men;
[6]14–18 years, 800 mg;   [7]up to 18 years/19–50 years.
EAR = Estimated Average Requirement.
EVM = Likely safe daily intake from supplements alone.
RDA = Recommended Daily Allowance.
TUL = Tolerable Upper Intake Level from diet and supplements.

Vitamin E is not very stable; significant losses from food may occur during storage and cooking. Losses also occur during food processing, particularly if there is significant exposure to heat and oxygen. There can be appreciable losses of vitamin E from vegetable oils during cooking.

Water-miscible preparations are superior to fat-soluble preparations in oral treatment of patients with fat malabsorption syndromes. The bioavailability of natural vitamin E is greater than that of synthetic vitamin E. However, several studies indicate that these differences may be even greater than originally thought.[1–4]

Deficiency

Deficiency of vitamin E is not generally recognised as a clearly definable syndrome. In premature infants, deficiency is associated with haemolytic anaemia, thrombocytosis, increased platelet aggregation, intraventricular haemorrhage and increased risk of retinopathy (but prophylaxis is controversial – see Precautions/contraindications).

The only children and adults who show clinical signs of vitamin E deficiency are those with severe malabsorption (i.e. in abetalipoproteinaemia, chronic cholestasis, biliary atresia and cystic fibrosis), or those with familial isolated vitamin E deficiency (rare inborn error of vitamin E metabolism). Clinical signs of deficiency include axonal dystrophy, reduced red blood cell half-life and neuromuscular disturbances.

Possible uses

A large number of claims for vitamin E have been made, but they are generally difficult to evaluate because they are often anecdotal or deduced from poorly designed trials.

Table 2 Dietary sources of vitamin E

Food portion	Vitamin E content (mg)	Food portion	Vitamin E content (mg)
Breakfast cereals		Kidney (75 g)	0.3
1 bowl All-Bran (45 g)	1.0	Sardines (70 g)	0.3
1 bowl **muesli** (95 g)	3.0	*Tinned salmon* (100 g)	1.5
2 pieces Shredded Wheat	0.5	Tinned pilchards (100 g)	0.7
1 bowl **Start** (35 g)	6.2	Tinned tuna (100 g)	0.5
2 Weetabix	0.5	2 fillets herring, cooked (110 g)	0.3
Cereal products		2 fillets kipper, cooked (130 g)	0.4
Brown rice, boiled (160 g)	0.5	*Vegetables*	
Brown pasta	0	Broccoli, boiled (100 g)	1.3
Wholemeal bread, 2 slices	1.5	Brussels sprouts, boiled (100 g)	0.9
2 heaped tablespoons **wheatgerm**	3.6	**Sweet potatoes, boiled** (150 g)	6.5
Milk and dairy products		*2 tomatoes*	1.8
Whole milk (284 ml; $^1/_2$ pint)	0.08	1 small can baked beans (200 g)	0.75
Soya milk (284 ml; $^1/_2$ pint)	1.7	*Chickpeas, cooked* (105 g)	1.6
Hard cheese, 50 g	0.25	Red kidney beans, cooked (105 g)	0.2
1 egg, size 2 (60 g)	0.6		
Fats and oils		*Fruit*	
Butter, on 1 slice bread (10 g)	0.2	1 apple	0.4
Margarine, on 1 slice bread (10 g)	0.8	$^1/_2$ **avocado pear**	3.0
Low-fat spread, on 1 slice bread (10 g)	0.6	1 banana	0.3
2 tablespoons ghee (30 g)	1.0	*Blackberries, stewed* (100 g)	2.0
1 tablespoon olive oil	1.0	1 orange	0.3
1 tablespoon **sunflower seed oil**	10	3 plums	0.6
1 tablespoon **wheatgerm oil**	27	*Nuts*	
2 teaspoons *cod liver oil*	2.0	20 **almonds**	4.8
Meat and fish		10 *Brazil nuts*	2.5
Liver, lambs, cooked (90 g)	0.3	30 **hazelnuts**	6.2
Liver, calves, cooked (90 g)	0.4	30 **peanuts**	3.3
Liver, ox, cooked (90 g)	0.3	1 tablespoon **sunflower seeds**	7.5
		Peanut butter, on 1 slice bread (10 g)	0.5

Excellent sources (> 3.0 mg/portion) (**bold**); good sources (> 1.5 mg/portion) (*italics*).

Cancer

Vitamin E has been suggested to be protective against cancer, and several epidemiological studies have found either low dietary intakes of vitamin E and/or lower serum levels of vitamin E in patients who have cancer than in people without cancer. However, not all studies have shown protective effects.

The prospective Iowa Women's Health Study[5] showed that a reduced risk of colon cancer was associated with high intakes of supplemental vitamin E in women under 65 years of age. Further data from this study showed that higher intakes of vitamin E are linked to lower risk of gastric, oesophageal, oral and pharyngeal cancers.[6] High

dietary intake of vitamin E has been associated with reduced risk of breast cancer,[7] but another study showed no protective effect.[8] There is some evidence that high plasma vitamin E levels protect against cervical cancer,[9] lung cancer,[10] and prostate cancer.[11] A 5-year US prospective study among 295 344 men found that dietary intake of gamma-tocopherol (the most commonly consumed form of vitamin E in the USA) was significantly inversely related to the risk of advanced prostate cancer, but use of vitamin E supplements was not related to prostate cancer risk.[12]

A large Finnish study involving 29 133 male smokers showed that vitamin E supplementation (50 mg daily) reduced the incidence of prostate cancer by 32% and the risk of prostate cancer deaths by 41% compared with those who took no vitamin E.[13] The study also detected a somewhat lower incidence of colorectal cancer in the vitamin E arm compared with the no vitamin E arm, but this was not statistically significant.[14] Further data from this study showed that neither of the treatments used (vitamin E or beta-carotene) had a statistically significant effect on the incidence and mortality rate of pancreatic cancer and incidence of lung and urinary tract cancers.[15]

More recent trials have shown no significant benefit of vitamin E supplementation in cancer. A randomised, double-blind, placebo-controlled international trial (the initial Heart Outcomes Prevention Evaluation (HOPE) trial and the ongoing HOPE trial) investigated the effect of vitamin E (400 IU daily) on cardiovascular events and primary prevention of cancer with a median follow-up of 7 years. There were no significant differences for cancer incidence and cancer deaths.[16] In the Women's Health Study, which tested the effect of vitamin E 600 IU on alternate days on cardiovascular events and cancer, there were no significant effects on total cancer, breast cancer, lung cancer, colon cancer or cancer deaths.[17]

A 2003 systematic review concluded that there is insufficient evidence to recommend for or against the use of routine vitamin E supplementation for the prevention of cancers other than lung cancer (i.e. oesophageal, stomach, colorectal, urological and prostate) in the general population. The reviewers also concluded that there is good evidence to recommend against the use of routine vitamin E supplementation for the prevention of lung cancer.[18]

A systematic review of four placebo-controlled trials on vitamin E role for primary prevention of colorectal cancer which included 94 069 participants aged 40 years or above found no sufficient evidence of vitamin E role for decreasing risk of colorectal cancer incidence (relative risk (RR), 0.89; 95% confidence interval (CI), 0.76 to 1.05; $P = 0.18$). The authors recommended further studies, but on diverse populations, to determine the role vitamin E for the primary prevention of colorectal cancer.[19]

Cardiovascular disease

Epidemiological studies have shown that low dietary intakes of vitamin E are associated with an increased risk of cardiovascular disease (CVD) in both men[20] and women.[21] Plasma vitamin E levels have also been found to be low in patients with variant angina.[22]

Several randomised, placebo-controlled trials have looked at the effects of vitamin E supplementation in CVD. The Cambridge Heart Antioxidant Study (CHAOS),[23] which involved a total of 2002 subjects with angiographically proven CVD, showed that those who received vitamin E (400 or 800 IU daily) had a 47% reduction in death from cardiovascular death and non-fatal myocardial infarction. This effect was due to a significant reduction (77%) in the risk of non-fatal myocardial infarction.

However, there was no effect on death from CVD alone. A non-significant increase in death from CVD was found in the supplemented group. However, a subsequent analysis of the deaths[24] showed that, of the 59 deaths from ischaemic heart disease, six were in the group of patients that complied with vitamin E supplementation, 21 were in the non-compliant group and 32 in the placebo group. This subsequent analysis has reduced concern about the possible adverse effects of vitamin E in this group of patients with established CVD.

An Italian trial, the Gruppo Italiano per lo Studio Della Sopravvivenza nell'Infarto Miocardio (GISSI),[25] involved 11 324 patients who had survived a myocardial infarction within the 3-month period before enrolment. The four arms of the study included vitamin E, n-3 PUFA, a mixture of the two, or placebo, and the primary end points were death, non-fatal myocardial infarction and stroke. Vitamin E reduced the risk for the primary end points by 11%, and the n-3 PUFA by 15%, with only the latter reaching statistical significance. Possible explanations for the differences in the results between CHAOS and GISSI have been suggested, and include the fact that 50% of the GISSI subjects were on lipid-lowering drugs and that they presumably ate a Mediterranean diet with a high intake of fruit and vegetables.

The Alpha-Tocopherol, Beta-Carotene Cancer Prevention (ATBC) Study, involving 27 271 men, was designed to investigate the influence of antioxidant supplements on cancer in Finnish smokers. However, an analysis of heart disease[26] in this trial showed that vitamin E

(50 mg) reduced the risk of primary major coronary events by 4% and the incidence of fatal CHD by 8%. Neither of these benefits was found to be statistically significant, but the trial used a small dose of a synthetic vitamin E supplement. A further analysis of the prevention of recurrence of angina for subjects in the ATBC trial[27] showed no significant protective effect of vitamin E.

The Heart Outcomes Prevention Evaluation (HOPE) study[28] enrolled a total of 2545 women and 6996 men aged 55 years or older who were at high risk of cardiovascular events, either because they had CVD or diabetes in addition to one other risk factor. They were assigned to natural vitamin E (400 IU daily), an ACE inhibitor or placebo for a mean of 4.5 years. In comparison with placebo, there were no significant differences in the number of deaths from cardiovascular causes, myocardial infarction and stroke with vitamin E. Further analysis of the HOPE study in people with mild-to-moderate renal insufficiency found that vitamin E supplementation had no apparent effect on cardiovascular outcomes.[29] Extension of the HOPE trial by a further 4 years (HOPE-TOO) indicated that there were no differences in cardiovascular events but higher rates of heart failure and hospitalisations for heart failure.[16] The Women's Health Study[17] also concluded that 600 IU vitamin E every other day over an average of 10.1 years provided no overall benefit for major cardiovascular events, but it reduced cardiovascular mortality in healthy women.

A double-blind RCT compared vitamin E (1200 IU daily) for 2 years with placebo in 90 patients with coronary artery disease. This high-dose vitamin E supplement significantly reduced plasma biomarkers of oxidative stress and inflammation (C-reactive protein, urinary F_2-isoprostanes, monocyte superoxide anion, tumour necrosis factor), but had no significant effect on carotid intimal medial thickness over 2 years.[30] Another trial evaluated the influence of vitamin E dosage on inflammatory markers and plasma lipoproteins in 12 healthy subjects and 12 patients with coronary heart disease (CHD). In this study, the patients appeared to require lower doses of vitamin E supplements than healthy subjects to exert effects on lipoproteins and inflammatory markers.[31] Another controlled supplementation trial (400 IU daily alpha-tocopherol for 6 weeks) in healthy men found that vitamin E supplementation had little effect on cardiovascular risk factors in this group of healthy men.[32]

Systematic reviews[18,33,34] and meta-analyses[35] have concluded that there is no benefit of vitamin E in the prevention of cardiovascular events. A further meta-analysis found that high-dose vitamin E supplements (400 IU daily) may increase all-cause mortality and should be avoided.[36] In a recent epidemiological study, use of vitamin E supplements was unrelated to overall mortality, but the authors concluded that this represented a combination of increased mortality in those with severe cardiovascular disease and a possible protective effect for those without.[37]

Supplementation may have benefits in particular patient subgroups. In a controlled trial in 39 876 women, vitamin E 600 IU daily reduced the risk of venous thromboembolism, particularly those with a prior history or genetic predisposition.[38]

Cataract

Epidemiological evidence suggests an association between cataract incidence and antioxidant status. Subjects with a low to moderate intake of vitamin E from foods had a higher risk of cataract relative to subjects with higher intakes,[39] and low serum levels of vitamin E and beta-carotene were related to increased risk of cataract in a Finnish study,[40] a French study,[41] and a US study.[42] However, an analysis of the ATBC Study showed that vitamin E (50 mg daily) had no effect on cataract prevalence in middle-aged smoking men.[43] Another study in 750 elderly people with cataracts[44] showed that those who took vitamin E supplements halved the risk of their cataracts progressing over a period of 4.5 years. A further trial in 1193 people with early or no cataract found that vitamin E 500 IU daily given for 4 years did not reduce the incidence or progression of nuclear, cortical or posterior subcapsular cataracts.[45] A recent analysis from the US Health Professionals' Study among 39 876 female health professionals with 9.7 years of treatment and follow-up indicated that 600 IU natural-source vitamin E taken every other day provided no benefit for age-related cataract or subtypes.[46]

Diabetes

Vitamin E has been evaluated for possible benefit in diabetes, in both prevention and management.

In a large US randomised placebo-controlled trial involving 38 716 apparently healthy women, the intervention group received 600 IU of vitamin E on alternate days. However, there was no evidence of an effect on development of diabetes with vitamin E supplementation.[47]

In a double-blind, placebo-controlled crossover study, 25 elderly patients with type 2 diabetes were randomised to receive 900 mg vitamin E or placebo daily for 3 months. Vitamin E supplementation was associated with a significant reduction in plasma glucose, haemoglobin A1c, triglycerides, free fatty acids, total and LDL cholesterol and apoprotein B levels. The authors concluded that daily vitamin E supplementation produces a small but significant improvement in metabolic control in type 2 diabetes, but that more studies are needed to draw conclusions about the safety of long-term supplementation.[48]

Vitamin E could help to decrease the development of vascular disease in diabetes. Vitamin E supplementation (1200 IU for 3 months) in 75 subjects who were diabetic or diabetic with vascular disease reduced the oxidation of LDL cholesterol, and reduced free radical levels and other markers of inflammation.[49] However in this study, the diabetics with or without vascular disease were not distinguishable by any of the markers of inflammation. Much larger, longer-term studies are needed to show that vitamin E has an anti-inflammatory effect in patients with vascular disease.

In another trial, 1434 middle aged individuals with type 2 diabetes and haptoglobin (a major antioxidant protein and determinant of cardiovascular events in patients with type 2 diabetes) were randomised to vitamin E 400 IU daily or placebo. The primary composite outcome was myocardial infarction, stroke and cardiovascular death. Eighteen months after starting the study, the primary outcome was reduced in individuals receiving vitamin E (2.2%) compared with placebo (4.7%) and led to termination of the study. The authors concluded that vitamin E appears to reduce cardiovascular events in individuals with diabetes mellitus and the haptoglobin (*Hp*) gene.[50]

Increased cardiovascular risk in people with type 2 diabetes is associated with decreased fibrinolysis, mainly linked to high plasminogen activator inhibitor type 1 production, together with a reduced bioavailability of nitric oxide and an impairment in sodium/potassium-ATPase. A study among 37 type 2 diabetics found that vitamin E 500 IU/day for 10 weeks produced beneficial differences in these markers of endothelial function compared with placebo, suggesting that that vitamin E counteracts endothelial activation in type 2 diabetes.[51] A further study among Chinese women with diabetes showed that vitamin E, 100, 200 and 300 IU reduced oxidative stress levels and improved lipid profile.[52]

Neuropsychiatric disorders

Vitamin E supplementation has been associated with some success in tardive dyskinesia.[53,54]

In a double-blind, placebo-controlled study, 341 patients with Alzheimer's disease were randomised to receive 2000 IU alpha-tocopherol, 10 mg selegiline, selegiline plus alpha-tocopherol or placebo. There was no significant difference in outcomes between the groups, but after adjustment for confounding factors, there were significant improvements in outcome with all three treatment groups compared with placebo. Vitamin E led to the greatest improvement, followed by selegiline, followed by the combination.[55]

Cognitive impairment

Vitamin E has been studied for a role in cognitive impairment and Alzheimer's disease. In a recent RCT, long-term use of vitamin E supplements was not associated with cognitive benefits in healthy older women.[56] A further trial in 57 patients with Alzheimer's disease (33 finished the study) treated with 800 IU vitamin E or placebo found that some people responded to vitamin E while others did not. In the vitamin E responders, blood oxidized glutathione (a marker of oxidation) fell and scores on measured cognitive tests were maintained. Subjects who did not respond to vitamin E in relation to reduced oxidative stress experienced decreased cognition. These results suggest that vitamin E lowers oxidative stress in some patients with Alzheimer's disease and maintains cognitive status; however, it appears to be detrimental in terms of cognition in those for whom vitamin E does not prevent oxidative stress. The authors recommend that supplementation with vitamin E for patients with Alzheimer's disease cannot be recommended without determination of its antioxidant effect in each patient.[57]

A Cochrane review in which only two studies matched the selection criteria found no overall evidence of efficacy of vitamin E in the prevention or treatment of people with Alzheimer's disease or mild cognitive impairment.[58]

Infection

Vitamin E supplementation (50 mg daily) was associated with a 28% reduction in cold incidence in the ATBC study. However, further analysis of the ATBC study found that in subjects of 72 years or older at the follow-up, the effect of vitamin E on common cold incidence varied. Among those smoking 5–14 cigarettes a day at baseline and living in cities, vitamin E reduced common cold risk, whereas among those smoking more and living away from cities, vitamin E increased common cold risk.[59]

Further analysis of the ATBC study found that vitamin E supplementation seems to increase transiently the risk of tuberculosis in heavy smokers with a high vitamin C intake. Vitamin E had no overall effect on the incidence of tuberculosis.[60]

Miscellaneous

Some studies have shown that vitamin E reduces oxidative damage in exercise,[61,62] reduces DNA damage in older adults,[63] improves lung function,[64] and improves immune function in the elderly.[65] Low serum vitamin E has been associated with subsequent decline in physical function among community-living older adults,[66,67] but vitamin E supplementation did not improve physical performance beyond that of aerobic exercise alone in older sedentary adults.[68] Low maternal vitamin E intake has been associated with asthma in 5-year-old children.

Vitamin E has been suggested to be of benefit in a vast range of conditions including arthritis, asthma, infertility and Parkinson's disease. Preliminary trials have shown some positive benefits, but larger trials are required to confirm these findings.

A recent trial among 72 women with menstrual migraine suggested that, compared with placebo, vitamin E 400 IU for 5 days in each of two cycles was effective in relieving symptoms of migraine, including pain severity, photophobia and nausea.[69]

Evidence from the US Women's Health Study, a RCT involving 39 876 female health professionals, suggests that alternate day supplementation with 600 IU vitamin E is not associated with a significant reduction in the development of rheumatoid arthritis.[70]

There is some evidence that vitamin E (together with vitamin C) may raise the tolerance to UV and, therefore, reduce the risk of sunburn.

A trial in 21 adults undergoing acute exercise suggested that vitamin E supplementation represents an important factor in the defence against oxidative stress and muscle damage but not against the inflammatory response in humans.[71] A double-blind clinical trial among 75 women with cyclical mastalgia found that vitamin E for 2 months had beneficial therapeutic effects.[72]

Conclusion

Several epidemiological studies have shown a link between low vitamin E intakes and CHD. There is some evidence that supplements (>100 IU daily) reduce the risk of CHD, but some studies do not demonstrate a benefit. Evidence therefore remains promising but inconclusive. There is little evidence of benefit with vitamin E supplements in cancer prevention. There is preliminary evidence that vitamin E supplements improve immune function and lung function, and reduce oxidative damage in exercise. They may also improve glucose utilisation and lipid profile in diabetes, reduce the risk of cataract, and improve symptomology in tardive dyskinesia. However, further research is required before vitamin E can be recommended as a supplement for these purposes. There is insufficient evidence from trials to date to suggest that vitamin E supplementation has a role in Alzheimer's disease. A recent commentary on vitamin E research argues that studies to date may be meaningless because the levels of vitamin E to reduce oxidative stress are far higher (i.e. 1600–3200 IU daily, as measured by markers of lipid peroxidation) than those commonly used in clinical trials and this could help to explain the inconsistencies in results of vitamin E trials evaluating its effects in cardiovascular disease and other chronic conditions.[73]

Precautions/contraindications

Vitamin E supplements should be avoided: by patients taking oral anticoagulants (increased bleeding tendency); in iron-deficiency anaemia (vitamin E may impair haematological response to iron) and hyperthyroidism.

In a case control study of 276 mothers of a child with CHD and 324 adults with their children, high maternal vitamin E by diet and supplements was associated with an increased risk of offspring with CHD. In this study, periconception use of vitamin E supplements in addition to a high dietary vitamin E intake above 14.9 mg daily generated up to a nine-fold increased CHD risk.[74]

Vitamin E supplements (IN DOSES HIGHER THAN RECOMMENDED DOSES) should be avoided.

Pregnancy and breast-feeding

No problems reported at normal intakes.

Adverse effects

Vitamin E is relatively non-toxic (fractional absorption declines rapidly with increasing intake, thereby preventing the accumulation of toxic concentrations of vitamin E in the tissues). Most adults can tolerate 100–800 mg daily and even doses of 3200 mg daily do not appear to lead to consistent adverse effects.

Large doses (> 1000 mg daily for prolonged periods) have occasionally been associated with the following side-effects: increased bleeding tendency in vitamin K-deficient patients; altered endocrine function (thyroid, adrenal and pituitary); rarely, blurred vision, diarrhoea, dizziness, fatigue and weakness, gynaecomastia, headache and nausea.

However, a recent meta-analysis found that high-dose vitamin E supplements (≥ 400 IU daily) may increase all-cause mortality and concluded that they should be avoided.[32]

Interactions

Drugs

Anticoagulants: large doses of vitamin E may increase the anticoagulant effect.

Anticonvulsants (phenobarbitone, phenytoin, carbamazepine): may reduce plasma levels of vitamin E.

Colestyramine or colestipol: may reduce intestinal absorption of vitamin E.

Digoxin: requirement for digoxin may be reduced with vitamin E (monitoring recommended).

Insulin: requirement for insulin may be reduced by vitamin E (monitoring recommended).

Liquid paraffin: may reduce intestinal absorption of vitamin E (avoid long-term use of liquid paraffin).

Oral contraceptives: may reduce plasma vitamin E levels.

Sucralfate: may reduce intestinal absorption of vitamin E.

Tamoxifen: supplemental vitamin E may reduce the inhibitory effect of tamoxifen on the proliferation of oestrogen receptor-positive breast cancer cells and eliminate the rapid rise in intracellular calcium that leads to apoptosis stimulated by tamoxifen.[75]

Nutrients

Copper: large doses of copper may increase requirement for vitamin E.

Iron: large doses of iron may increase requirements for vitamin E; vitamin E may impair the haematological response in iron-deficiency anaemia.

Polyunsaturated fatty acids: the dietary requirement for vitamin E increases when the intake of PUFA increases.

Vitamin A: vitamin E spares vitamin A and protects against some signs of vitamin A toxicity; very high levels of vitamin A may increase requirement of vitamin E; excessive doses of vitamin E may deplete vitamin A.

Vitamin C: vitamin C can spare vitamin E; vitamin E can spare vitamin C.

Vitamin K: large doses of vitamin E (1200 mg daily) increase the vitamin K requirement in patients taking anticoagulants.

Zinc: zinc deficiency may result in reduced plasma vitamin E levels.

Dose

Vitamin E is available in the form of tablets and capsules and is an ingredient of multivitamin preparations. Dietary supplements provide 10–1000 mg per daily dose.

Doses for use as an over-the-counter supplement above the RDA have not been established to be of value. There is no evidence to recommend doses higher than 400 IU daily.

References

1 Ferslew KE, Acuff RV, Daigneault EA, *et al.* Pharmacokinetics and bioavailability of the *RRR* and all racemic stereoisomers of alpha-tocopherol in humans after single oral administration. *J Clin Pharmacol* 1993; 33(1): 84–88.

2 Acuff RV, Thedford SS, Hidiroglou NN, *et al.* Relative bioavailability of *RRR*- and *all-rac*-alpha-tocopheryl acetate in humans: studies using deuterated compounds. *Am J Clin Nutr* 1994; 60(3): 397–402.

3 Kiyose C, Muramatsu R, Kameyama Y, *et al.* Biodiscrimination of alpha-tocopherol stereoisomers in humans after oral administration. *Am J Clin Nutr* 1997; 65(3): 785–789.

4 Burton GW, Traber MG, Acuff RV, *et al.* Human plasma and tissue alpha-tocopherol concentrations in response to supplementation with deuterated natural and synthetic vitamin E. *Am J Clin Nutr* 1998; 67(4): 669–684.

5 Bostick RM, Potter JD, McKenzie DR, *et al.* Reduced risk of colon cancer with high intake of vitamin E: the Iowa Women's Health Study. *Cancer Res* 1993; 53(18): 4230–4237.

6 Zheng W, Sellers TA, Doyle TJ, *et al.* Retinol, antioxidant vitamins, and cancers of the upper digestive tract in a prospective cohort study of postmenopausal women. *Am J Epidemiol* 1995; 142(9): 955–960.

7 London SJ, Stein EA, Henderson IC, *et al.* Carotenoids, retinol, and vitamin E and risk of proliferative benign breast disease and breast cancer. *Cancer Causes Control* 1992; 3(6): 503–512.

8 Hunter DJ, Manson JE, Colditz GA, *et al.* A prospective study of the intake of vitamins C, E, and A and the risk of breast cancer. *N Engl J Med* 1993; 329(4): 234–240.

9 Palan PR, Mikhail MS, Basu J, *et al.* Plasma levels of antioxidant beta-carotene and alpha-tocopherol in uterine cervix dysplasias and cancer. *Nutr Cancer* 1991; 15(1): 13–20.

10 Comstock GW, Helzlsouer KJ, Bush TL. Prediagnostic serum levels of carotenoids and vitamin E as related to subsequent cancer in Washington County, Maryland. *Am J Clin Nutr* 1991; 53(1Suppl): 260S–264S.

11 Eichholzer M, Stahelin HB, Ludin E, *et al.* Smoking, plasma vitamins C, E, retinol, and carotene, and fatal prostate cancer: seventeen-year follow-up of the prospective basel study. *Prostate* 1999; 38(3): 189–198.

12 Wright ME, Weinstein SJ, Lawson KA, *et al.* Supplemental and dietary vitamin E intakes and risk of prostate cancer in a large prospective study. *Cancer Epidemiol Biomarkers Prev* 2007; 16(6): 1128–1135.

13 Heinonen OP, Albanes D, Virtamo J, *et al.* Prostate cancer and supplementation with alpha-tocopherol and beta-carotene: incidence and mortality in a controlled trial. *J Natl Cancer Inst* 1998; 90(6): 440–446.

14 Rautalahti MT, Virtamo JR, Taylor PR, *et al.* The effects of supplementation with alpha-tocopherol and beta-carotene on the incidence and mortality of carcinoma of the pancreas in a randomized, controlled trial. *Cancer* 1999; 86(1): 37–42.

15 Virtamo J, Edwards BK, Virtanen M, *et al.* Effects of supplemental alpha-tocopherol and beta-carotene on urinary tract cancer: incidence and mortality in a controlled trial (Finland). *Cancer Causes Control* 2000; 11(10): 933–939.

16 Lonn E, Bosch J, Yusuf S, *et al.* Effects of long-term vitamin E supplementation on cardiovascular events and cancer: a randomized controlled trial. *JAMA* 2005; 293(11): 1338–1347.

17 Lee IM, Cook NR, Gaziano JM, *et al.* Vitamin E in the primary prevention of cardiovascular disease and cancer: the Women's Health Study: a randomized controlled trial. *JAMA* 2005; 294(1): 56–65.

18 Alkhenizan A, Palda VA and the Canadian Task Force on Preventive Health Care. *The Role of Vitamin E Supplements in the Prevention of Cardiovascular Disease and Cancer: Systematic Review and Recommendations.* London, Ontario: Canadian Task Force on Preventive Health Care, 2003.

19 Arain MA, Abdul Qadeer A. Systematic review on 'vitamin E and prevention of colorectal cancer'. *Pak J Pharm Sci* 2010; 23(2): 125–130.

20 Rimm EB, Stampfer MJ, Ascherio A, *et al.* Vitamin E consumption and the risk of coronary heart disease in men. *N Engl J Med* 1993; 328(20): 1450–1456.

21 Kushi LH, Fee RM, Sellers TA, *et al.* Intake of vitamins A, C, and E and postmenopausal breast cancer. The Iowa Women's Health Study. *Am J Epidemiol* 1996; 144(2): 165–174.

22 Miwa K, Miyagi Y, Igawa A, *et al.* Vitamin E deficiency in variant angina. *Circulation* 1996; 94(1): 14–18.

23 Stephens NG, Parsons A, Schofield PM, *et al.* Randomised controlled trial of vitamin E in patients with coronary disease: Cambridge Heart Antioxidant Study (CHAOS). *Lancet* 1996; 347 (9004): 781–786.

24 Mitchinson MJ, Stephens NG, Parsons A, *et al.* Mortality in the CHAOS trial. *Lancet* 1999; 353 (9150): 381–382.

25 Gruppo Italiano per lo Studio della Sopravvivenza nell'Infarto miocardico. Dietary supplementation with n-3 polyunsaturated fatty acids and vitamin E after myocardial infarction: results of the GISSI-Prevenzione trial. *Lancet* 1999; 354(9177): 447–455.

26 Virtamo J, Rapola JM, Ripatti S, *et al.* Effect of vitamin E and beta carotene on the incidence of primary nonfatal myocardial infarction and fatal coronary heart disease. *Arch Intern Med* 1998; 158(6): 668–675.

27 Rapola JM, Virtamo J, Ripatti S, *et al.* Effects of alpha tocopherol and beta carotene supplements on symptoms, progression, and prognosis of angina pectoris. *Heart* 1998; 79(5): 454–458.

28 Yusuf S, Dagenais G, Pogue J, *et al.* Vitamin E supplementation and cardiovascular events in high-risk patients. The Heart Outcomes Prevention Evaluation Study Investigators. *N Engl J Med* 2000; 342(3): 154–160.

29 Mann JF, Lonn EM, Yi Q, *et al.* Effects of vitamin E on cardiovascular outcomes in people with mild-to-moderate renal insufficiency: results of the HOPE study. *Kidney Int* 2004; 65(4): 1375–1380.

30 Devaraj S, Tang R, Adams-Huet B, *et al.* Effect of high-dose α-tocopherol supplementation on biomarkers of oxidative stress and inflammation and carotid atherosclerosis in patients with coronary artery disease. *Am J Clin Nutr* 2007; 86(5): 1392–1398.

31 Leichtle A, Teupser D, Thiery J. Alpha-tocopherol distribution in lipoproteins and anti-inflammatory effects differ between CHD-patients and healthy subjects. *J Am Coll Nutr* 2006; 25(5): 420–428.

32 Woollard KJ, Rayment SJ, Bevan R, *et al.* Alpha-tocopherol supplementation does not affect monocyte endothelial adhesion or C-reactive protein levels but reduces soluble vascular adhesion molecule-1 in the plasma of healthy subjects. *Redox Rep* 2006; 11(5): 214–222.

33 Shekelle PG, Morton SC, Jungvig LK, *et al.* Effect of supplemental vitamin E for the prevention and treatment of cardiovascular disease. *J Gen Intern Med* 2004; 19 , 4, 380–389.

34 Eidelman RS, Hollar D, Hebert PR, *et al.* Randomized trials of vitamin E in the treatment and prevention of cardiovascular disease. *Arch Intern Med* 2004; 164(14): 1552–1556.

35 Vivekananthan DP, Penn MS, Sapp SK, *et al.* Use of antioxidant vitamins for the prevention of cardiovascular disease: meta-analysis of randomised trials. *Lancet* 2003; 361(9374): 2017–2023.

36 Miller ER 3rd, Pastor-Barriuso R, Dalal D, *et al.* Meta-analysis: high-dosage vitamin E supplementation may increase all-cause mortality. *Ann Intern Med* 2005; 142(1): 37–46.

37 Hayden KM, Welsh-Bohmer KA, Wengreen HJ, *et al.* Risk of mortality with vitamin E supplements: the Cache County study. *Am J Med* 2007; 120(2): 180–184.

38 Glynn RJ, Ridker PM, Goldhaber SZ, *et al.* Effects of random allocation to vitamin E supplementation on the occurrence of venous thromboembolism. report from the Women's Health Study. *Circulation* 2007; 116(13): 1497–1503.

39 Jacques PF, Chylack LT Jr. Epidemiologic evidence of a role for the antioxidant vitamins and carotenoids in cataract prevention. *Am J Clin Nutr* 1991; 53(1Suppl): 352S–355S.

40 Knekt P, Heliovaara M, Rissanen A, *et al.* Serum antioxidant vitamins and risk of cataract. *BMJ* 1992; 305(6866): 1392–1394.

41 Delcourt C, Cristol JP, Tessier F, *et al.* Age-related macular degeneration and antioxidant status in the POLA study. POLA Study Group. Pathologies Oculaires Liees a l'Age. *Arch Ophthalmol* 1999; 117(10): 1384–1390.

42 Lyle BJ, Mares-Perlman JA, Klein BE, *et al.* Serum carotenoids and tocopherols and incidence of age-related nuclear cataract. *Am J Clin Nutr* 1999; 69 (2): 272–277.

43 Teikari JM, Virtamo J, Rautalahti M, *et al.* Long-term supplementation with alpha-tocopherol and beta-carotene and age-related cataract. *Acta Ophthalmol Scand* 1997; 75(6): 634–640.

44 Leske MC, Chylack LT,Jr He Q, *et al.* Antioxidant vitamins and nuclear opacities: the longitudinal study of cataract. *Ophthalmology* 1998; 105(5): 831–836.

45 McNeil JJ, Robman L, Tikellis G, *et al.* Vitamin E supplementation and cataract: randomized controlled trial. *Ophthalmology* 2004; 111(1): 75–84.

46 Christen WG, Glynn RJ, Chew EY, *et al.* Vitamin E and age-related cataract in a randomized trial of women. *Ophthalmology* 2008; 115(5): 822–829.

47 Liu S, Lee IM, Song Y, *et al.* Vitamin E and risk of type 2 diabetes in the Women's Health Study randomized controlled trial. *Diabetes* 2006; 55(10): 2856–2862.

48 Paolisso G, D'Amore A, Galzerano D, *et al.* Daily vitamin E supplements improve metabolic control but not insulin secretion in elderly type II diabetic patients. *Diabetes Care* 1993; 16(11): 1433–1437.

49 Devaraj S, Jialal I. Low-density lipoprotein postsecretory modification, monocyte function, and circulating adhesion molecules in type 2 diabetic patients with and without macrovascular complications: the effect of alpha-tocopherol supplementation. *Circulation* 2000; 102(2): 191–196.

50 Milman U, Blum S, Shapira C, *et al.* Vitamin E supplementation reduces cardiovascular events in a subgroup of middle-aged individuals with both type 2 diabetes mellitus and the haptoglobin 2-2 genotype: a prospective double-blinded clinical trial. *Arterioscler Thromb Vasc Biol* 2008; 28(2): 341–347.

51 Vignini A, Nanetti L, Moroni C, *et al.* A study on the action of vitamin E supplementation on plasminogen activator inhibitor type 1 and platelet nitric oxide production in type 2 diabetic patients. *Nutr Metab Cardiovasc Dis* 2008; 18(1): 15–22.

52 Wang Q, Sun Y, Ma A, *et al.* Effects of vitamin E on plasma lipid status and oxidative stress in Chinese women with metabolic syndrome. *Int J Vitam Nutr Res* 2010; 80(3): 178–187.

53 Lohr JB, Caligiuri MP. A double-blind placebo-controlled study of vitamin E treatment of tardive dyskinesia. *J Clin Psychiatry* 1996; 57(4): 167–173.

54   Adler LA, Edson R, Lavori P, *et al*. Long-term treatment effects of vitamin E for tardive dyskinesia. *Biol Psychiatry* 1998; 43(12): 868–872.

55   Sano M, Ernesto C, Thomas RG, *et al*. A controlled trial of selegiline, alpha-tocopherol, or both as treatment for Alzheimer's disease. The Alzheimer's Disease Cooperative Study. *N Engl J Med* 1997; 336(17): 1216–1222.

56   Kang JH, Cook N, Manson J, *et al*. A randomized trial of vitamin E supplementation and cognitive function in women. *Arch Intern Med* 2006; 166 (22): 2462–2468.

57   Lloret A, Badia MC, Mora NJ, *et al*. Vitamin E paradox in Alzheimer's disease: it does not prevent loss of cognition and may even be detrimental. *J Alzheimers Dis* 2009; 17(1): 143–149.

58   Isaac MG, Quinn R, Tabet N. Vitamin E for Alzheimer's disease and mild cognitive impairment. *Cochrane Database Syst Rev* 2008; 16(3): CD002854.

59   Hemila H, Virtamo J, Albanes D, *et al*. The effect of vitamin E on common cold incidence is modified by age, smoking and residential neighborhood. *J Am Coll Nutr* 2006; 25(4): 332–339.

60   Hemila H, Kaprio J. Vitamin E supplementation may transiently increase tuberculosis risk in males who smoke heavily and have high dietary vitamin C intake. *Br J Nutr* 2008: 1–7.

61   Meydani M, Evans WJ, Handelman G, *et al*. Protective effect of vitamin E on exercise-induced oxidative damage in young and older adults. *Am J Physiol* 1993; 264(5): R992–R998.

62   Tsakiris S, Karikas GA, Parthimos T, *et al*. Alpha-tocopherol supplementation prevents the exercise-induced reduction of serum paraoxonase 1/aryl-esterase activities in healthy individuals. *Eur J Clin Nutr* 2009; 63(2): 215–221.

63   Chin SF, Hamid NA, Latiff AA, *et al*. Reduction of DNA damage in older healthy adults by Tri E tocotrienol supplementation. *Nutrition* 2007; 24(1): 1–10.

64   Dow L, Tracey M, Villar A, *et al*. Does dietary intake of vitamins C and E influence lung function in older people? *Am J Respir Crit Care Med* 154(5): 1401–1404.

65   Meydani SN, Han SN, Wu D. Vitamin E and immune response in the aged: molecular mechanisms and clinical implications. *Immunol Rev* 2005; 205: 269–284.

66   Bartali B, Frongillo EA, Guralnik JM, *et al*. Serum micronutrient concentrations and decline in physical function among older persons. *JAMA* 2008; 299 (3): 308–315.

67   Devereux G, Turner SW, Craig LC, *et al*. Low maternal vitamin E intake during pregnancy is associated with asthma in 5-year-old children. *Am J Respir Crit Care Med* 2006; 174(5): 499–507.

68   Nalbant O, Toktas N, Toraman NF, *et al*. Vitamin E and aerobic exercise: effects on physical performance in older adults. *Aging Clin Exp Res* 2009; 21 (2): 111–121.

69   Ziaei S, Kazemnejad A, Sedighi A. The effect of vitamin E on the treatment of menstrual migraine. *Med Sci Monit* 2009; 15(1): CR16–CR19.

70   Karlson EW, Shadick NA, Cook NR, *et al*. Vitamin E in the primary prevention of rheumatoid arthritis: the Women's Health Study. *Arthritis Rheum* 2008; 59(11): 1589–1595.

71   Silva LA, Pinho CA, Silveira PC, *et al*. Vitamin E supplementation decreases muscular and oxidative damage but not inflammatory response induced by eccentric contraction. *J Physiol Sci* 2009; 60(1): 51–57.

72   Parsay S, Olfati F, Nahidi S. Therapeutic effects of vitamin E on cyclic mastalgia. *Breast J* 2009; 15(5): 510–514.

73   Blumberg JB, Frei B. Why clinical trials of vitamin E and cardiovascular diseases may be fatally flawed. Commentary on 'The relationship between dose of vitamin E and suppression of oxidative stress in humans'. *Free Radic Biol Med* 2007; 43(10): 1374–1376.

74   Smedts HP, de Vries JH, Rakhshandehroo M, *et al*. High maternal vitamin E intake by diet or supplements is associated with congenital heart defects in the offspring. *BJOG* 2009; 116(3): 416–423.

75   Peralta EA, Viegas ML, Louis S, *et al*. Effect of vitamin E on tamoxifen-treated breast cancer cells. *Surgery* 2006; 140(4): 607–614 discussion 614–615.

Vitamin K

Description

Vitamin K is a fat-soluble vitamin.

Nomenclature

Vitamin K is a generic term for 2-methyl-1,4-naphthaquinone and all derivatives that exhibit qualitatively the biological activity of phytomenadione. The form of vitamin K present in foods is phytomenadione (vitamin K_1). The substances synthesised by bacteria are known as menaquinones (vitamin K_2). The parent compound of the vitamin K series is known as menadione (vitamin K_3); it is not a natural substance

Table 1 Dietary Reference Values for vitamin K (µg/day)

Age	UK Safe Intake	EVM	US RDA	FAO/WHO RNI
0–6 months	10		2.0[1]	5
7–12 months	10		2.5[1]	10
1–3 years	–		30[1]	15
4–6 years	–		–	20
4–8 years	–		55[1]	–
7–9 years	–		–	25
9–13 years	–		60	–
10–18 years	–		–	35–55
14–18 years	–		75	–
Males				
19–70+ years	1 µg/kg body weight	1000	120	65
Females				
19–70+ years	1 µg/kg/body weight	1000	90	55
Pregnancy	1 µg/kg/body weight		90	–
Lactation	1 µg/kg/body weight		90	–

Some of the requirement for vitamin K is met by synthesis in the intestine.
[1] Adequate Intakes (AI).
EVM = Likely safe daily intake from supplements alone.
RDA = Recommended Daily Allowance.
RNI = Reference Nutrient Intake.

and is not used in humans. Menadiol sodium phosphate is a water-soluble derivative of menadione.

Human requirements

See Table 1 for Dietary Reference Values for vitamin K.

Action

Vitamin K is an essential cofactor for the hepatic synthesis of proteins involved in the regulation of blood clotting. These are prothrombin (factor II), factors VII, IX, X and proteins C, S and Z. Vitamin K is responsible for the carboxylation of the bone protein, osteocalcin, to its active form. Osteocalcin regulates the function of calcium in bone turnover and mineralisation. Vitamin K is also required for the biosynthesis of some other proteins found in plasma and the kidney.

Dietary sources

See Table 2 for dietary sources of vitamin K.

Table 2 Dietary sources of vitamin K

Food portion	Vitamin K content (µg)
Broccoli, boiled (100 g)	175
Brussels sprouts, boiled (100 g)	100
Cabbage, boiled (100 g)	125
Cauliflower, boiled (100 g)	150
Kale, boiled (100 g)	700
Lettuce (30 g)	45
Spinach, boiled (100 g)	400
Soya beans, cooked (100 g)	190
Meat, average, cooked (100 g)	50
Cheese (100 g)	50
Bread and cereals (100 g)	< 10
Fruit (100 g)	< 10

Excellent sources (> 100 µg/portion) (**bold**).

Metabolism

Absorption

Vitamin K is absorbed into the lymphatic system, predominantly in the upper part of the small intestine (jejunum and ileum), by a process that requires bile salts and pancreatic juice. The absorption of the different forms of vitamin K differs. Vitamin K_1 (phytomenadione) is absorbed by an active energy-dependent process from the proximal portion of the small intestine; menadione is absorbed by a passive non-carrier-mediated process from both the small and large intestines.

There is evidence that bacterially synthesised vitamin K can be a source of the vitamin for humans, although the availability of a sufficient concentration of bile salts for absorption is questionable (plasma levels of menaquinones suggest that some absorption occurs).

Distribution

Vitamin K is transported in the plasma and metabolised in the liver. Vitamin K_1 is concentrated and retained in the liver. Menadione is poorly retained by the liver but widely distributed in all other tissues.

Elimination

Vitamin K is eliminated partly in the bile (30–40%) and partly in the urine (15%).

Bioavailability

The effect of cooking and food processing on vitamin K has not been carefully studied, but it appears to be relatively stable.

Deficiency

Vitamin K deficiency is rare and usually only occurs in people who have malabsorption problems or liver disease. However, it can occur in newborn babies, and all newborns should be given vitamin K. Deficiency leads to a prolonged prothrombin time, which can be corrected by vitamin K supplementation.

Possible uses

Bone strength and osteoporosis

Vitamin K is not in common use as a dietary supplement, and few products contain it.

However, there is increasing evidence that vitamin K deficiency may contribute to osteoporosis by reducing the carboxylation of osteocalcin in bone. Low serum levels of vitamin K and high levels of under-carboxylated osteocalcin have been reported in both postmenopausal women and individuals who have sustained hip fractures,[1–3] and low intakes of vitamin K may increase the risk of low bone mineral density[4] and hip fracture.[5,6] In addition, some studies have shown that patients taking oral anticoagulants (which are vitamin K antagonists) are at increased risk of osteoporosis. High dietary phylloquinone intake has been shown to modestly reduce bone resorption in postmenopausal women.[7]

Intervention trials have shown mixed effects on bone and risk of fracture, and the different preparations and doses used in the trials will likely have contributed to these inconsistencies. A study in which vitamin K_2 45 mg daily was given by mouth to 120 subjects with osteoporosis was found to reduce the risk of fractures and to sustain lumbar bone mineral density (BMD).[8] Six months of 600 µg daily vitamin K_1 supplementation did not improve regional BMD in a group of pre- and perimenopausal women.[9] Daily supplementation with vitamin K_1 (5 mg) for 2 to 4 years did not protect against age-related decline in BMD, but it may protect against fractures and cancers in postmenopausal women with osteopaenia.[10] Phylloquinone supplementation in a dose attainable in the diet did not confer any additional benefit for bone health at the spine or hip in a 3-year RCT among 452 men and women (aged 60–80 years) when taken with recommended amounts of calcium and vitamin D.[11]

Combined administration of vitamin K_2 (45 mg daily) and vitamin D_3 (1-alpha-hydroxy-vitamin D_3 0.75 µg daily) increased the BMD of the lumbar spine in postmenopausal women with osteoporosis compared with treatment with calcium.[12] Combined therapy with vitamin K_2 and vitamin D_3 has been found to increase BMD more than vitamin K_2 alone.[13] Vitamin K_1 1 mg daily (co-administered with calcium, magnesium, zinc and vitamin D) reduced bone loss at the femoral neck in postmenopausal women between 50 and 60 years of age to a greater extent than vitamin D and the minerals alone.[14]

In a Dutch study in postmenopausal women, 80 µg of vitamin K_1 daily for 1 year increased carboxylated osteocalcin to pre-menopausal levels.[15] In another study, vitamin K_2 (45 mg daily) in elderly women with osteoporosis reduced serum under-carboxylated osteocalcin levels within 2 weeks, without any significant change in intact osteocalcin, suggesting that under-carboxylated osteocalcin is changed to carboxylated osteocalcin with potentially beneficial effects on bone metabolism.[16]

In a further Dutch study, 325 postmenopausal women received 45 mg daily of vitamin K_2 or placebo for a period of 3 years. Measurements were made of bone mineral content (BMC), hip geometry and BMD. Vitamin K_2 did not affect BMD, but BMC and the femoral neck width increased relative to placebo. In the vitamin K_2-treated group, hip bone strength remained unchanged during the 3-year intervention period while in the placebo group, bone strength decreased significantly.[17]

A trial in 31 postmenopausal women in which volunteers were supplemented with 200 and 500 µg phylloquinone daily or placebo plus 10 µg of vitamin D daily found that supplementation increased vitamin K status but had no effect on bone turnover.[18]

In a 12-month RCT among 381 postmenopausal women who received phylloquinone (1 mg daily), menaquinone (45 mg daily) or placebo (with all three groups taking calcium and vitamin D), no effect of either vitamin K supplement was seen on BMD at the lumbar spine or proximal femur.[19]

A meta-analysis investigated the role of vitamin K supplementation in bone turnover and fracture. Thirteen trials were identified with data on bone loss, and seven reported fracture data. All studies but one showed an advantage of phytonadione and menaquinone in reducing bone loss. All seven trials that reported fracture effects were Japanese and used menaquinone. Pooling the seven trials with fracture data in a meta-analysis, the researchers found an odds ratio (OR) favouring menaquinone of 0.40 (95% confidence interval (CI), 0.25 to 0.65) for vertebral fractures, an OR of 0.23 (95% CI, 0.12 to 0.47) for hip fractures, and an OR of 0.19 (95% CI, 0.11 to 0.35) for all non-vertebral fractures. The conclusion drawn from this systematic review was that supplementation with phytonadione and menaquinone-4 reduced bone loss. In the case of the latter, there was a strong effect on incident fractures among Japanese patients.[20]

A further meta-analysis of seven RCTs (with criteria of approximately 50 or more subjects per group and study period of 2 years or longer) showed that vitamin K_1 and vitamin K_2 supplementation reduced serum under-carboxylated osteocalcin levels regardless of dose but that it had inconsistent effects on serum total osteocalcin levels and no effect on bone resorption. Despite the lack of a significant change or the occurrence of only a modest increase in BMD, high-dose vitamin K_1 and vitamin K_2 supplementation improved indices of bone strength in the femoral neck and reduced the incidence of clinical fractures.[21]

There is some evidence of synergy between vitamin K, vitamin D and calcium to enhance BMC. A 2-year RCT randomised 244 healthy Scottish women ≥ 60 years to either placebo, vitamin K_1 (200 µg daily) or vitamin D (10 µg daily) plus calcium (1000 mg daily) or combined vitamin D, vitamin K and calcium. Significant bone loss was seen only at the mid-distal radius with no differences between groups. However, women who took combined vitamin K and vitamin D plus calcium showed a significant sustained increase in both BMD and BMC at the site of the ultradistal radius. Over 2 years, serum vitamin K increased by 157% and the percentage of undercarboxylated osteocalcin decreased by 51% ($P < 0.001$). These effects, if replicated in other studies, may have long-term benefits and the vitamin K intakes in the study are potentially achievable by diet.[22]

Vitamin K_2 has also been found to be protective in glucocorticoid-induced bone loss. In one study involving 60 patients, vitamin K_2 alone (45 mg daily), vitamin K_2 plus vitamin D_3 (alfacalcidol 0.5 µg daily) and vitamin D_3 alone prevented BMD loss at the lumbar spine caused by prednisolone.[23] Results from a further study suggested that vitamin K_2 (15 mg daily) could help to prevent glucocorticoid-induced bone loss.[24]

Osteoarthritis

Low vitamin K status has been associated with risk of osteoarthritis. In an observational study among 672 subjects (mean age 65.6 years), low plasma vitamin K plasma levels were associated with increased prevalence of osteo-arthritis manifestations in the hand and knee.[25] In an ancillary study designed to look at vita-min K and bone loss, 378 participants (193 in vitamin K arm, 185 in placebo arm) were evaluated for arthritis. There were no effects of randomisation to vitamin K for radiographic osteoarthritis outcomes. However, those with insufficient vitamin K at baseline who attained sufficient concentrations at follow-up had trends towards 47% less joint space narrowing ($P < 0.02$).[26]

Cardiovascular disease

In another observational study involving 40 087 men who participated in the Health Professionals' Follow-up Study, there was a trend ($P = 0.05$) for the relative risk of total cor-onary heart disease (CHD) events to fall with increased vitamin K intake. However, the risk for CHD events and strokes did not remain sig-nificantly associated with vitamin K intake after adjustment for lifestyle and other lifestyle fac-tors, suggesting that high vitamin K intake may be a marker of dietary patterns associated with CHD risk.[27] A high intake of vitamin K_2 (espe-cially menaquinones 8, 9 and 10) has been linked with a reduced risk of CHD in a prospect-ive study (hazard ratio, 0.91 (95% CI, 0.85 to 1.00) per 10 μg vitamin K_2 daily intake.[28] In a rat study, high vitamin K intake was shown to reverse arterial calcification (an independent risk factor for cardiovascular morbidity and mortality) and the resulting arterial distensibility.[29]

A systematic review of five studies (one trial, four cohort studies) found no associations between vitamin K_1 intake and CHD (four cohorts) or stroke (two cohorts) in multivariate analyses. Two cohorts examined the effects of vitamin K_2 intake on the incidence of CHD; both found significant associations where higher vitamin K_2 intake was associated with fewer CHD events.[30]

In a controlled trial in 388 healthy men and postmenopausal women, 200 received a multi-vitamin with 500 μg phylloquinone daily (treat-ment), and 188 received a multivitamin alone (control). In an intention-to-treat analysis, there was no difference in coronary artery calcifica-tion progression between the phylloquinone group and the control group. In a subgroup analysis of 367 participants who were > 85% adherent to supplementation, there was less pro-gression of calcification in the phylloquinone group than in the control group ($P = 0.03$). Of those with pre-existing calcification, those who received phylloquinone supplements had 6% less progression than did those who received the multivitamin alone ($P = 0.04$).[31]

Glucose metabolism

Vitamin K has a potentially beneficial effect on glucose and insulin metabolism. In an ancillary study of a 36-month, randomised, double-blind, controlled trial designed to assess the impact on bone loss of supplementation with 500 μg phyl-loquinone daily, older non-diabetic subjects (213 women, 142 men; aged 60–80 years) were evaluated for insulin resistance. Compared with placebo, insulin resistance was significantly lower in the men supplemented with vitamin K but not in the women.[32] A 12 month RCT in 21 postmenopausal women receiving phylloquin-one (1 mg daily) found no change in insulin secretion in this group of women.[33]

Precautions/contraindications

None reported (except Interactions; see below).

Pregnancy and breast-feeding

No problems reported.

Adverse effects

Oral ingestion of natural forms of vitamin K is not associated with toxicity. A rare hypersensi-tivity reaction (occasionally results in death) has been reported after intravenous administration of phytomenadione (especially if rapid).

Interactions

Drugs

Antibiotics: may increase requirement for vita-min K.

Anticoagulants: Evidence suggests that altera-tions in the dietary intake of vitamin K can affect anticoagulant response to warfarin. Several recent trials have attempted to evaluate this potential interaction. A systematic dose–response study in healthy volunteers who have been stably anticoagulated and maintained on their individual doses for 13 weeks evaluated the response to weekly incremental doses (50–100 µg) of vitamin K_1 taken daily for 7 days. The threshold K_1 dose causing a statistically significant lowering of the International Normalised Ratio (INR) was 150 µg daily. The response to vitamin K-rich food items (spinach and broccoli) was short lived. The authors concluded that short-term variability in intake of K_1 is less important to INR than has been assumed, and that supplements providing 100 µg of vitamin K_1 daily do not significantly interfere with oral anticoagulant therapy.[34]

A further study found that for each increase of 100 µg in the daily dietary intake of vitamin K, the INR was reduced by 0.2. Analysis showed that dietary vitamin K had no effect on warfarin dose requirements. However, a certain phenotype (CYP2C9) and also age significantly contributed to interpatient variability in warfarin dose requirements. The authors concluded that, overall, a consistent vitamin K intake could reduce intrapatient variability in anticoagulation response and improve the safety of warfarin therapy.[35]

In another study, patients with unstable control of anticoagulation had lower dietary intakes of vitamin K than those with stable control. During the 2 weeks of the study, changes in vitamin K intake were negatively correlated with changes in INR among the unstable patients. The authors suggested that daily supplementation with oral vitamin K in unstable patients could lead to a more stable anticoagulation response to warfarin.[36] The same research group conducted an RCT in 70 warfarin-treated patients with unstable anticoagulant control, randomising them to 150 µg oral vitamin K or placebo for 6 months. Vitamin K supplementation resulted in a significantly greater decrease in standard deviation of INR and a significantly greater increase in percentage time within target INR range. Anticoagulation control improved in 33/35 patients receiving vitamin K and 19 patients achieved good anticoagulant control. However, only 24/33 patients receiving placebo showed some degree of improvement with only seven patients achieving good anticoagulant control.[37]

In a small study involving eight patients (45–79 years), supplementation with low-dose oral vitamin K significantly increased the number of INR values in range and decreased INR fluctuation.[38]

A retrospective study among 43 patients requiring interruption of warfarin for surgery showed that 1 mg oral vitamin K on the day before surgery can normalize the INR by the day of surgery and may not confer resistance to warfarin re-anticoagulation after surgery.[39] Improved stability of anticoagulant therapy was also observed in a RCT among 200 patients who took 100 µg vitamin K with their anticoagulant therapy.[40] Concomitant supplementation with vitamin K has also been shown to improve anticoagulant control in patients with unexplained instability in response to warfarin.[41] A dose-finding study which evaluated the effect of vitamin K_1 (100, 150 or 200 mg daily) in patients taking anticoagulant therapy found that time spent within the therapeutic range for anticoagulant was improved with all doses of vitamin K_1, but there was no difference between the doses.[42]

A prospective dietary assessment study in 60 outpatients (43 completed the study) receiving warfarin indicated that a weekly change of 714 µg of dietary vitamin K significantly altered INR by 1 unit, suggesting that patients who markedly change their vitamin K intake are at risk of unstable anticoagulant outcomes.[43] Case studies have indicated that low doses of vitamin K (i.e. 25 µg) found in multivitamin supplements can alter anticoagulant control. This is most likely to occur in patients who are vitamin K depleted.[44,45] A singe case study has shown that vitamin K supplementation removal can increase INR.[46]

Colestyramine or colestipol: may reduce intestinal absorption of vitamin K.

Liquid paraffin: may reduce intestinal absorption of vitamin K (avoid long-term use of liquid paraffin).

Sucralfate: may reduce intestinal absorption of vitamin K.

Nutrients

Vitamin A: under conditions of hypervitaminosis A, hypothrombinaemia may occur; it can be corrected by administering vitamin K.

Vitamin E: large doses of vitamin E (1200 mg daily) increase the vitamin K requirement in patients taking anticoagulants, but there is no confirmed effect in individuals not taking anticoagulants.

Conclusion

Vitamin K deficiency may contribute to osteoporosis by reducing the carboxylation of osteocalcin in bone. Low intakes of vitamin K have been associated with low BMD and fracture. RCTs employing vitamin K have shown variable results in influencing BMD but a variety of different doses and preparations have been used, which make comparison difficult. Further research is warranted. Vitamin K (both dietary and supplemented) can influence anticoagulant control and it is important not to make changes in intakes of vitamin K while an anticoagulant is being taken. However, there is emerging evidence that low-dose vitamin K can help to improve anticoagulant control particularly in patients whose control is poor. Evidence is emerging that vitamin K may be protective against CVD and metabolic syndrome but further work is needed.

Dose

Vitamin K is not generally available in isolation as a supplement. It is an ingredient in some multivitamin preparations. No dose has been established.

Two forms of vitamin K are available for inclusion in food supplements. The synthetic vitamin K_1 is the most commonly used type, but the natural longer chain menaquinone-7 (MK-7) has also become available. Both types are absorbed well, with peak serum concentrations four hours after intake. However, MK-7 has a much longer half life, resulting in more stable serum levels and accumulation to higher levels during prolonged intake. MK-7 has also been shown to induce more complete carboxylation of osteocalcin, and preparations supplying $\geq 50\,\mu g$ daily of MK-7 may interfere with oral anticoagulant treatment.[47]

Upper safety levels

The UK Expert Group on Vitamins and Minerals (EVM) has identified a safe upper level of vitamin K for adults from supplements alone of $1000\,\mu g$ daily.

References

1 Binkle NC, Suttie JW. Vitamin K nutrition and osteoporosis. *J Nutr* 1995; 125: 1812–1821.

2 Kanai T, Takagi T, Masuhiro K, *et al.* Serum vitamin K level and bone mineral density in post-menopausal women. *Int J Gynaecol Obstet* 1997; 56: 25–30.

3 Vermeer C, Gijsbers BL, Cracium AM, *et al.* Effects of vitamin K on bone mass and bone metabolism. *J Nutr* 1996;, suppl4, 1187S–1191S.

4 Booth SL, Broe KE, Gagnon DR, *et al.* Vitamin K intake and bone mineral density in women and men. *Am J Clin Nutr* 2003; 77(2): 512–516.

5 Feskanich D, Weber P, Willett WC, *et al.* Vitamin K intake and hip fractures in women: a prospective study. *Am J Clin Nutr* 1999; 69: 74–79.

6 Booth SL, Tucker KL, Chen H, *et al.* Dietary vitamin K intakes are associated with hip fracture but not with bone mineral density in elderly men and women. *Am J Clin Nutr* 2000; 71(5): 1201–1208.

7 Martini LA, Booth SL, Saltzman E, *et al.* Dietary phylloquinone depletion and repletion in postmenopausal women: effects on bone and mineral metabolism. *Osteoporos Int* 2006; 17(6): 929–935.

8 Shikari M, Shikari Y, Aoki C, Miura M. Vitamin K_2 (menatetranone) effectively prevents fractures and sustains lumbar bone mineral density in osteoporosis. *J Bone Miner Res* 2000; 15: 515–521.

9 Volpe SL, Leung MM, Giordano H. Vitamin K supplementation does not significantly impact bone mineral density and biochemical markers of bone in pre- and perimenopausal women. *Nutr Res* 2008; 28(9): 577–582.

10 Cheung AM, Tile L, Lee Y, *et al.* Vitamin K supplementation in postmenopausal women with osteopenia (ECKO trial): a randomized controlled trial. *PLoS Med* 2008; 5(10): e196.

11 Booth SL, Dallal G, Shea MK, *et al.* Effect of vitamin K supplementation on bone loss in elderly men and women. *J Clin Endocrinol Metab* 2008; 93(4): 1217–1223.

12 Iwamoto J, Takeda T, Ichimura S. Effect of combined administration of vitamin D_3 and vitamin K_2 on bone mineral density of the lumbar spine in postmenopausal women with osteoporosis. *J Orthop Sci* 2000; 5: 546–551.

13 Braam LA, Knapen MH, Geusens P, *et al.* Vitamin K_1 supplementation retards bone loss in postmenopausal women between 50 and 60 years of age. *Calcif Tissue Int* 2003; 73: 21–26.

14 Schaafsma A, Muskiet FA, Storm H, *et al.* Vitamin D_3 and vitamin K_1 supplementation of Dutch postmenopausal women with normal and low bone mineral densities: effects of serum 25-hydroxyvitamin D and carboxylated osteocalcin. *Eur J Clin Nutr* 2000; 54: 626–631.

15 Miki T, Nakatsuka K, Naha H, *et al.* Vitamin K_2 (menaquinone 4) reduces serum undercarboxylated osteocalcin level as early as 2 weeks in elderly

women with established osteoporosis. *J Bone Miner Metab* 2003; 21: 161–165.

16 Ushiroyama T, Ikeda A, Ueki M. Effect of continuous combined therapy with vitamin K_2 and vitamin D_3 on bone mineral density and coagulofibrinolysis function in postmenopausal women. *Maturitas* 2002; 41: 211–221.

17 Knapen MH, Schurgers LJ, Vermeer C. Vitamin K_2 supplementation improves hip bone geometry and bone strength indices in postmenopausal women. *Osteoporos Int* 2007; 18(7): 963–972.

18 Bugel S, Sorensen AD, Hels O, *et al.* Effect of phylloquinone supplementation on biochemical markers of vitamin K status and bone turnover in postmenopausal women. *Br J Nutr* 2007; 97(2): 373–380.

19 Binkley N, Harke J, Krueger D, *et al.* Vitamin K treatment reduces undercarboxylated osteocalcin but does not alter bone turnover, density, or geometry in healthy postmenopausal North American women. *J Bone Miner Res* 2009; 24(6): 983–991.

20 Cockayne S, Adamson J, Lanham-New S, *et al.* Vitamin K and the prevention of fractures: systematic review and meta-analysis of randomized controlled trials. *Arch Intern Med* 2006; 166(12): 1256–1261.

21 Iwamoto J, Sato Y, Takeda T, Matsumoto H. High-dose vitamin K supplementation reduces fracture incidence in postmenopausal women: a review of the literature. *Nutr Res* 2009; 29(4): 221–228.

22 Bolton-Smith C, McMurdo ME, Paterson CR, *et al.* Two-year randomized controlled trial of vitamin K_1 (phylloquinone) and vitamin D_3 plus calcium on the bone health of older women. *J Bone Miner Res* 2007; 22(4): 509–519.

23 Yonemura K, Fukasawa H, Fujigaki Y, Hishida A. Protective effect of vitamin K2 and D_3 on prednisolone-induced loss of bone mineral density in the lumbar spine. *Am J Kidney Dis* 2004; 43: 63–60.

24 Sasaki N, Kusano E, Takahashi H, *et al.* Vitamin K_2 inhibits glucorticoid-induced bone loss partly by preventing the reduction of osteoprotegerin (OPG). *J Bone Miner Metab* 2005; 23: 41–47.

25 Neogi T, Booth SL, Zhang YQ, *et al.* Low vitamin K status is associated with osteoarthritis in the hand and knee. *Arthritis Rheum* 2006; 54(4): 1255–1261.

26 Neogi T, Felson DT, Sarno R, Booth SL. Vitamin K in hand osteoarthritis: results from a randomised clinical trial. *Ann Rheum Dis* 2008; 67(11): 1570–1573.

27 Erkkila AT, Booth SL, Hu FB, Jacques PF, Lichtenstein AH. Phylloquinone intake and risk of cardiovascular diseases in men. *Nutr Metab Cardiovasc Dis* 2007; 17(1): 58–62.

28 Gast GC, de Roos NM, Sluijs I, *et al.* A high menaquinone intake reduces the incidence of coronary heart disease. *Nutr Metab Cardiovasc Dis* 2009; 19 (7): 504–510.

29 Schurgers LJ, Spronk HMH, Soute BAM, *et al.* Regression of warfarin-induced medial elastocalcinosis by high intake of vitamin K in rats. *Blood* 2007; 109(7): 2823–2831.

30 Rees K, Guraewal S, Wong YL, *et al.* Is vitamin K consumption associated with cardio-metabolic disorders? A systematic review. *Maturitas* 2010; 67(2): 121–128.

31 Shea MK, O'Donnell CJ, Hoffmann U, *et al.* Vitamin K supplementation and progression of coronary artery calcium in older men and women. *Am J Clin Nutr* 2009; 89(6): 1799–1807.

32 Yoshida M, Jacques PF, Meigs JB, *et al.* Effect of vitamin K supplementation on insulin resistance in older men and women. *Diabetes Care* 2008; 31(11): 2092–2096.

33 Kumar R, Binkley N, Vella A. Effect of phylloquinone supplementation on glucose homeostasis in humans. *Am J Clin Nutr* 2010; 92(6): 1528–1532.

34 Schurgers LJ, Shearer MJ, Hamulyak K, Stocklin E, Vermeer C. Effect of vitamin K intake on the stability of oral anticoagulant treatment: dose-response relationships in healthy subjects. *Blood* 2004; 104 (9): 2682–2689.

35 Khan T, Wynne H, Wood P, *et al.* Dietary vitamin K influences intra-individual variability in anticoagulant response to warfarin. *Br J Haematol* 2004; 124(3): 348–354.

36 Sconce E, Khan T, Mason J, *et al.* Patients with unstable control have a poorer dietary intake of vitamin K compared to patients with stable control of anticoagulation. *Thromb Haemost* 2005; 93(5): 872–875.

37 Sconce E, Avery P, Wynne H, Kamali F. Vitamin K supplementation can improve stability of anticoagulation for patients with unexplained variability in response to warfarin. *Blood* 2007; 109(6): 2419–2423.

38 Reese AM, Farnett LE, Lyons RM, *et al.* Low-dose vitamin K to augment anticoagulation control. *Pharmacotherapy* 2005; 25(12): 1746–1751.

39 Woods K, Douketis JD, Kathirgamanathan K, Yi Q, Crowther MA. Low-dose oral vitamin K to normalize the international normalized ratio prior to surgery in patients who require temporary interruption of warfarin. *J Thromb Thrombol* 2007; 24(2): 93–97.

40 Rombouts EK, Rosendaal FR, van der Meer FJ. Daily vitamin K supplementation improves anticoagulant stability. *J Thromb Haemost* 2007; 5 (10): 2043–2048.

41 Sconce E, Avery P, Wynne H, Kamali F. Vitamin K supplementation can improve stability of anticoagulation for patients with unexplained variability in response to warfarin. *Blood* 2007; 109(6): 2419–2423.

42 Gebuis EP, Rosendaal FR, van Meegen E, van der Meer FJ. Vitamin K_1 supplementation to improve stability of anticoagulation therapy with vitamin K antagonists: a dose-finding study. *Haematologica* 2011; 96(4): 583–589.

43 Couris R, Tataronis G, McCloskey W, *et al*. Dietary vitamin K variability affects international normalized ratio (INR) coagulation indices. *Int J Vitam Nutr Res* 2006; 76(2): 65–74.

44 Kurnik D, Lubetsky A, Loebstein R, Almog S, Halkin H. Multivitamin supplements may affect warfarin anticoagulation in susceptible patients. *Ann Pharmacother* 2003; 37(11): 1603–1606.

45 Kurnik D, Loebstein R, Rabinovitz H, *et al*. Over-the-counter vitamin K1-containing multivitamin supplements disrupt warfarin anticoagulation in vitamin K_1-depleted patients. A prospective, controlled trial. *Thromb Haemost* 2004; 92(5): 1018–1024.

46 Miesner AR, Sullivan TS. Elevated international normalized ratio from vitamin K supplement discontinuation. *Ann Pharmacother* 2010; 45(1): e2.

47 Schurgers LJ, Teunissen KJF, Hamulyak K, *et al*. Vitamin K-containing dietary supplements: comparison of synthetic vitamin K_1 and natto-derived menaquinone-7. *Blood* 2007; 109(8): 3279–3283.

Wheat germ oil

Description

Wheat germ oil is extracted from the germ of the wheat kernel.

Constituents

Wheat germ oil is high in vitamin E and contains the essential fatty acids, linoleic acid and linolenic acid, and also oleic acid and palmitic acid (see Table 1). It is particularly high in octacosanol. Octacosanol (see Octacosanol) is a 28-carbon long-chain saturated primary alcohol found in a number of different vegetable waxes. Octacosanol

Table 1 Average nutrient composition of wheat germ oil

Nutrient	Per teaspoon (4 g)	% DRV (approx.)
Energy	119 kcal (498 kJ)	6%
Total fat	13.5 g	21%
Saturated fat	2.5 g	13%
Monounsaturated fat	2.0 g	–
Polyunsaturated fat	8.3 g	–
Total omega-3 fatty acids	932 mg	–
Total omega-6 fatty acids	7398 mg	–
Phytosterols	74.7 mg	–
Vitamin E	20.2 mg	200% of EU RDA
Vitamin K	3.3 µg	–
Choline	2.7 mg	–

DRV = Dietary Reference Value.

has been studied in CVD and as an exercise and physical performance enhancing agent.

Possible uses

Wheat germ oil is a useful source of vitamin E and of essential fatty acids. A small study in 32 subjects with hypercholesterolaemia found that wheat germ oil rich in alpha-linolenic acid (1 tablespoon/day) reduced oxidative stress and CD40 ligand (a marker of inflammation and thrombosis).[1]

Precautions/contraindications

Not reported.

Pregnancy and breast-feeding

No problems reported.

Adverse effects

No problems reported.

Interactions

Not reported.

Dose

Wheat germ oil is available in the form of an oil (administered by dropper) and capsules.

References

1 Alessandri C, Pignatelli P, Loffredo L, *et al*. Alpha-linolenic acid-rich wheat germ oil decreases oxidative stress and CD40 ligand in patients with mild hypercholesterolemia. *Arterioscler Thromb Vasc Biol* 2006; 26: 2577–2578.

Zinc

Description

Zinc is an essential trace mineral.

Human requirements

See Table 1 for Dietary Reference Values for zinc.

Dietary intake

In the UK, the average adult daily diet provides: for men, 10.2 mg; for women, 7.4 mg.

Action

The human body contains approximately 2 g of zinc, making this trace element the most abundant in the body after iron. Zinc is an essential component of over 200 enzymes.[1] It plays an important role in the metabolism of proteins, carbohydrates, lipids and nucleic acids. It is a cofactor in a range of biochemical processes, including the synthesis of DNA, RNA and protein.[2] Zinc is also required for the hepatic synthesis of retinol-binding protein, the protein involved in transporting vitamin A. Without adequate zinc, symptoms of vitamin A deficiency can appear even if supplements of vitamin A are taken.[3]

Zinc is also crucial for maintaining the structure and integrity of cell membranes. Reduction in the concentration of zinc in biomembranes results in increased susceptibility to oxidative damage and alteration in specific transport systems and receptor sites, and may underlie some of the disorders associated with zinc deficiency.[4] Accumulation of zinc in cell membranes can block receptor sites for histamine release, leading to reduction in release of histamine from mast cells.[5]

Another important structural role for zinc is the so-called zinc-finger motif in proteins.[6] Zinc fingers enable polypeptides that are too small to fold by themselves to fold stably when stabilised by bound zinc. Zinc finger proteins regulate gene expression[7] by acting as transcription factors (binding to DNA and influencing the transcription of specific genes). These proteins are involved in the metabolism of reproductive hormones (e.g. androgens, oestrogens and progesterone). Prostaglandins and nuclear receptors for steroids are also zinc finger proteins. Zinc has regulatory roles in cell signalling and influences nerve impulse transmission. It also has a role in apoptosis (gene-directed cell death), a critical cellular regulatory process with implications for growth and development, as well as a number of chronic diseases.[8]

Zinc plays a role in immune function, which explains why it has been investigated for possible benefit in infections, such as colds. It is involved in the function of cells contributing to non-specific immunity, such as neutrophils and natural killer cells. Zinc also plays a role in T-lymphocyte function and the development of acquired immunity.[9] Normal serum zinc concentrations in nursing home elderly people are associated with a decreased incidence and duration of pneumonia, a decreased number of new antibiotic prescriptions and a decrease in the days of antibiotic use.[10] Zinc supplementation has been associated with reduced incidence of infections in the elderly[11] and in patients with sickle cell disease,[12] and also with a reduction in the number of days of oral antibiotics used to treat respiratory tract infections in children with cystic fibrosis.[13]

Zinc is essential for reproduction. It is necessary for the metabolism of reproductive hormones, ovulation, testicular function, the formation and maturation of sperm, fertilisation and the health of the mother and foetus during pregnancy.[14] Deficiency of zinc during early development can be teratogenic. In men, the prostate gland has the highest concentration of zinc of any organ in the body.

Other roles for zinc include wound healing, behaviour and learning, taste and smell, blood clotting, thyroid hormone function and insulin

Table 1　Dietary Reference Values for zinc (mg/day)

							EU RDA = 15 mg
Age	UK				USA		FAO/WHO RNI[1]
	LRNI	EAR	RNI	EVM	RDA	TUL	
0–3 months	2.6	3.3	4.0		2.0[2]	0	1.1–6.6
4–6 months	2.6	3.3	4.0		2.0[2]	0	1.1–6.6
7–12 months	3.0	3.8	5.0		3.0	5.0	2.5–8.4
1–3 years	3.0	3.8	5.0		3.0	7.0	2.4–8.3
4–6 years	4.0	5.0	6.5		–	–	2.9–9.6
4–8 years	–	–	–		5.0	12.0	–
7–10 years	4.0	5.4	7.0		–	–	3.3–11.2[3]
Males							
11–14 years	5.3	7.0	9.0		–	–	5.1–17.1[4]
14–18 years	–	–	–		11.0	34.0	5.1–17.1
15–18 years	5.5	7.3	9.5		–	–	–
19–50 + years	5.5	7.3	9.5	25	11.0	40.0	–
19–65 + years	–	–	–		–	–	4.2–14.0
Females							
11–14 years	5.3	7.0	9.0		–	–	4.3–14.4[4]
14–18 years	–	–	–		9.0	34.0	4.3–14.4
15–18 years	4.0	5.5	7.0		–	–	–
19–50 + years	4.0	5.5	7.0	25	8.0	40.0	–
19–65 + years	–	–	–		–	–	3.0–9.8
Pregnancy	*	*	*		11.0[5]	40.0[6]	–
Lactation	–	–	–		12.0[7]	40.0[6]	–
0–4 months			+6.0		–	–	–
4 + months			+2.5		–	–	–

* No increment.
[1] Recommended intake varies from diet of high to low zinc bioavailability;　[2] Adequate Intakes (AIs);　[3] 7–9 years;
[4] 10–14 years;　[5] aged < 18 years, 13 mg daily;　[6] aged < 18 years, 34 mg daily;　[7] aged < 18 years, 14 mg daily.
EAR = Estimated Average Requirement.
EVM = Likely safe daily intake from supplements alone.
LRNI = Lowest Reference Nutrient Intake.
RNI = Reference Nutrient Intake.
TUL = Tolerable Upper Intake Level from diet and supplements.

action. Present in high concentrations in the eye, particularly in the retina and choroid, zinc plays a role in the maintenance of vision.[15]

Zinc also acts as an antioxidant, restricting endogenous free radical production and acting as a structural component of the extracellular antioxidant enzyme, superoxide dismutase. It also helps to protect against depletion of vitamin E and maintains tissue concentrations of metallothionein – a possible scavenger of free radicals.[15] Zinc supplementation may have favourable effects on antioxidant–oxidant balance in patients with chronic obstructive pulmonary disease (COPD).[16] In healthy adolescent athletes, zinc supplementation benefits antioxidant capacity but impairs copper and iron nutritional status.[17] However, in a population of apparently healthy, free-living elderly people, zinc supplementation did not alter oxidative stress markers and antioxidant defences (except an increase in copper/zinc superoxide dismutase),[18] and had no effect on copper-induced low-density lipoprotein (LDL) oxidation.[19] Zinc also influences folate and vitamin B_{12} metabolism, but zinc supplementation in older people has been shown to have no effect on folate, B_{12} or homcysteine.[20]

Dietary sources

See Table 2 for dietary sources of zinc.

Metabolism

Absorption

Absorption occurs throughout the length of the small intestine, mostly in the jejunum, both by a carrier-mediated process and by diffusion.

Distribution

Zinc is transported in association with albumin, amino acids and a 2-macroglobulin. Zinc is principally an intracellular ion and approximately 95% is found within the cells. Approximately 57% of the body pool is stored in skeletal muscle, 29% in bone and 6% in the skin, but zinc is found in all body tissues and fluids, including the liver, kidneys, pancreas, prostate gland and retina.[2]

Elimination

Elimination of zinc is mainly in the faeces; smaller amounts are excreted in the urine and via the skin.

Bioavailability

Absorption of zinc is enhanced by certain amino acids such as cysteine and histidine: meat, dairy produce and fish contain these amino acids and therefore their zinc is efficiently absorbed. Humans absorb zinc more efficiently from low-zinc diets.[21] Current dietary zinc intake seems to have a greater effect on fractional zinc absorption than does longer-term zinc intake,[22] but there is evidence from a study in postmenopausal women that there may be adaptation to absorb a uniform amount of zinc despite wide variation in dietary intake.[23] Zinc from wholegrain cereals, including bran products, and also soya protein, is less available, partly because of the presence of phytate. The effect of non-starch polysaccharides (dietary fibre), tannic acid and caffeine is equivocal. High calcium intake may reduce absorption, but this is likely only at higher than recommended intakes of calcium. One study in 10 healthy women found that dietary calcium intakes of 700 mg daily and 1800 mg daily did not impair zinc absorption.[24]

Zinc supplementation (15 or 30 mg daily for 6 months) significantly increased the size of the exchangeable zinc pool[25] and serum zinc levels and urinary zinc excretion[26,27] but did not significantly modify erythrocyte zinc levels or erythrocyte copper/zinc superoxide dismutase activity.[26,27] A trial in healthy adult men showed that zinc supplementation raised plasma zinc levels above those of placebo within 5 days, while zinc plasma levels following discontinuation of zinc fell to those of placebo within 14 days.[28]

Bioavailability of zinc from supplements varies and depends on the form of the zinc. There is evidence that absorption of zinc from zinc gluconate is higher than from zinc oxide,[29] and that organic yeast salts[30] and zinc bisglycinate[31] are more biologically available than zinc gluconate.

Deficiency

Clinical manifestations of severe zinc deficiency include alopecia, diarrhoea, dermatitis, psychiatric disorders, weight loss, intercurrent infection (due to impaired immune function), hypogonadism in males, and poor ulcer healing. Signs of mild to moderate deficiency include growth retardation, male hypogonadism, poor appetite, rough skin, mental lethargy, delayed wound healing and impaired taste acuity.

Maternal zinc deficiency before and during pregnancy may lead to intrauterine growth retardation and congenital abnormalities in the foetus.

Table 2 Dietary sources of zinc

Food portion	Zinc content (mg)	Food portion	Zinc content (mg)
Breakfast cereals		**1 beef steak** (155 g)	7.0
1 bowl **All-Bran** (45 g)	3.0	**Minced beef, lean, stewed** (100 g)	6.0
1 bowl *Bran Flakes* (45 g)	1.5	1 *chicken leg* (190 g)	2.0
1 bowl Corn Flakes (30 g)	0.1	**Liver, lambs, cooked** (90 g)	4.0
1 bowl *muesli* (95 g)	2.0	**Kidney, lambs, cooked** (75 g)	3.0
2 pieces Shredded Wheat	1.0	***Fish***	
2 Weetabix	1.0	*Pilchards, canned* (105 g)	1.5
		Sardines, canned (70 g)	2.0
Cereal products		**Crab** (100 g)	5.5
Bread, brown, 2 slices	0.7	1 dozen **oysters**	78.7
white, 2 slices	0.4	***Vegetables***	
wholemeal, 2 slices	1.3	Green vegetables, average, boiled (100 g)	0.4
1 chapati	0.7	Potatoes, boiled (150 g)	0.5
Pasta, brown, boiled (150 g)	1.5	1 small can baked beans (200 g)	1.0
white, boiled (150 g)	0.7	Lentils, kidney beans or other pulses (105 g)	1.0
Rice, brown, boiled (165 g)	1.0	*Dahl, chickpea* (155 g)	1.5
white, boiled (165 g)	1.0	*lentil* (155 g)	1.5
Milk and dairy products		Soya beans, cooked (100 g)	1.0
Milk, whole, semi-skimmed or skimmed (284 ml; $^1/_2$ pint)	1.0		
1 pot yoghurt (150 g)	1.0	***Fruit***	
Cheese, Brie (50 g)	1.0	8 dried apricots	0.2
Camembert (50 g)	1.3	4 figs	0.3
Cheddar (50 g)	1.1	Half an avocado pear	0.3
Cheddar, reduced fat (50 g)	1.4	1 banana	0.2
Cottage cheese (100 g)	0.5	Blackberries (100 g)	0.2
Cream cheese (30 g)	0.2	Blackcurrants (100 g)	0.3
Edam (50 g)	1.1	***Nuts***	
Feta (50 g)	0.4	20 almonds	0.6
Fromage frais (100 g)	0.3	10 Brazil nuts	1.0
White cheese (50 g)	1.5	30 hazelnuts	0.7
1 egg, size 2 (60 g)	0.8	1 small bag peanuts (25 g)	1.0
Meat and fish			
Red meat, roast (85 g)	4.0		

Excellent sources (**bold**); good sources (*italics*).

Possible uses

Anorexia nervosa

It has been suggested that zinc deficiency is involved in the aetiology of anorexia nervosa. Teenage girls who are restricting their food intake during the period of rapid growth may develop a state of zinc deficiency and anorexia nervosa. A daily supplement of 45 mg zinc, as zinc sulphate, has been reported to result in weight gain in 17 young female patients with long-standing anorexia nervosa.[32] The weight gain continued over a 4-year follow-up period. Compared with placebo, a daily dose of 100 mg of zinc gluconate doubled the rate of increase in body mass index in 35 female patients with anorexia.[33]

Wound healing

Zinc is essential in wound healing and zinc supplementation is valuable in cases of wounds where there is zinc deficiency or malnutrition. According to one review, zinc administered orally or topically to wounds can promote healing and reduce infection.[34] In patients with low serum zinc levels, topical zinc oxide has been shown to promote cleansing and re-epithelialisation of leg ulcers, reducing deterioration of ulcers and the risk of infection.[35] A Cochrane review assessed six placebo-controlled trials of zinc supplementation in arterial and venous leg ulcers and found no overall benefit on the number of ulcers healed.[36] However, in people with low serum zinc levels, there is some evidence that oral zinc might improve healing of leg ulcers.

Common cold

The use of zinc lozenges within 24 h of the onset of cold symptoms and continued every 2–3 h while awake has been advocated for reducing the duration of the common cold. One proposed mechanism is that zinc may bind with proteins of critical nerve endings in the respiratory tract and surface proteins of the rhinovirus, thereby interrupting virus infection.[37] However, results from RCTs in humans are conflicting. A meta-analysis of six RCTs reported no statistical benefit of using zinc lozenges to reduce cold duration.[38] Two additional analyses of RCTs of zinc for the common cold found that evidence is inconclusive.[39,40] A more recent US trial in 50 volunteers recruited within 24 h of developing common cold symptoms found that taking zinc lozenges (containing 13.3 mg zinc as zinc acetate) one every 2–3 h was associated with reduced duration of cold (4.0 vs 7.1 days, $P < 0.0001$) and shorter duration of cough (2.1 vs 5.0 days, $P < .0001$) and nasal discharge (3.0 vs 4.5 days, $P < 0.02$) compared with placebo. Symptom severity also decreased significantly in the zinc group. These improvements were related to changes in antioxidant and anti-inflammatory markers (plasma interleukin-1 receptor antagonist, soluble tumor necrosis factor receptor 1 and adhesion molecules).[41]

Researchers have suggested that discrepancies may be caused by inadequate placebo control and differences in lozenge formulation (including formulations with relatively low concentrations of ionic zinc[42]), administration and dosage. The amount of available ionised zinc may influence the effectiveness of zinc and this varies with different lozenge formulations. The addition of flavouring agents such as citric acid, mannitol or sorbitol to zinc gluconate lozenge preparations decreases the effect of zinc ionisation, and hence its release, while the addition of glycine to zinc gluconate lozenges does not.[43] Positive results in the common cold are generally associated with zinc gluconate or zinc acetate, while other forms are less effective.

Some researchers question the clinical relevance of oral zinc levels because the rhinovirus replicates in the nasal mucosa. Zinc nasal preparations have also been investigated for the common cold. One study showed that a nasal gel formulation reduced cold duration compared with placebo when used within 24 h of onset of symptoms,[44] while others showed no effect of a nasal spray on duration of cold symptoms.[45,46] A recent meta-analysis of three studies has evaluated the effect of intranasal zinc used to treat the common cold. In two studies, high doses of intranasal zinc preparation (2.1 mg zinc daily) were reported to shorten the duration and reduce the symptom severity of common cold in healthy adults, when started within 24 to 48 h of onset of illness. A lower dose study (0.044 mg zinc daily) found no benefit in resolution but did report a significant improvement in symptoms at day 1 and day 3. Combining the three studies, the relative risk for benefit at day 3 was 0.62 (95% confidence interval, 0.18 to 2.19) (random effects), i.e. the benefit was non-significant.[47]

Taking lozenges every 2–3 h while awake may result in daily zinc intakes above the safe upper level of 25 mg daily. Short-term use of zinc lozenges (up to 5 days) has not resulted in serious side-effects, although some individuals experience gastrointestinal irritation. Use of zinc at above the upper limit for prolonged periods (e.g. 6–8 weeks) is not recommended and may lead to copper deficiency.

Two randomised, controlled trials from Turkey have addressed the influence of zinc intervention in the common cold in children. In the first study, a total of 200 healthy children were randomly assigned to receive oral zinc sulphate or placebo. Zinc sulphate (15 mg zinc) or placebo syrup were administered for prophylaxis once daily during a 7-month study period. The dose was increased to twice a day (30 mg zinc) at the onset of a cold, until symptoms resolved. The mean number of colds in the zinc group was significantly less than in the placebo group (1.2 vs 1.7 colds per child; $P = 0.003$). The mean cold-related school absence was 0.9 days per child in the zinc group versus 1.3 days in the placebo group ($P = 0.04$). Compared with the placebo group, the zinc group had shorter mean duration of cold symptoms and decreased total severity scores for cold symptoms ($P < 0.0001$). Adverse effects were mild and similar in both groups.[48] In the second study, children presenting with at least two of 10 symptoms of common cold within the 24–48 h of the onset of illness were randomised to receive either oral zinc containing zinc sulphate or placebo. A diary was completed to record symptoms and adverse effects. Symptoms were scored as absent (0), mild (1), moderate (2), or severe (3). A total of 150 children participated in the study, and 120 children were included in the final analysis. The median duration of all cold symptoms was 6 days ($P = 0.20$), and the median duration of nasal symptoms was 5 days in both groups ($P = 0.09$). However, total symptom severity scores were significantly lower in the zinc group, starting from the second day of the study. The lower scores in the zinc group were largely due to improvement of nasal symptom scores. Adverse effects were similar in both groups.[49] In the first of these trials zinc reduced the duration of cold symptoms while in the second study it did not. Both trials showed that zinc supplementation appeared to be effective in reducing the severity of the cold symptoms in healthy children.

Diabetes mellitus

Zinc is important for insulin function. The pancreas contains a high concentration of zinc and levels are decreased in diabetes. Zinc is involved in the pathology of diabetes, mainly as a result of its antioxidant function (e.g. as a part of the superoxide dismutase enzyme and the Zn–metallothionein complex[50,51]) and its contribution to insulin resistance.[52] Zinc interaction with hormones such as leptin and melatonin may be of significance in the metabolism of obese patients

with diabetes.[53–56] Low serum zinc concentrations in patients with diabetes are associated with increased the risk for myocardial infarction and death from coronary heart disease.[57] In the large prospective Nurses Health Study, there was a mild trend for higher zinc intake to be associated with lower risk of developing type 2 diabetes.[58]

A Cochrane review has evaluated the effects of zinc supplementation in the prevention of type 2 diabetes. Only one study met the inclusion criteria for the review. There were 56 normal glucose-tolerant, obese women (aged 25 to 45 years, body mass index 36.2 2.3 kg/m^2). Follow-up was 4 weeks. The outcomes measured were decrease of insulin resistance, anthropometric and diet parameters, leptin and insulin concentration, zinc concentration in the plasma and urine, lipid metabolism and fasting plasma glucose. There were no statistically significant differences favouring participants receiving zinc supplementation compared with placebo concerning any outcome measured by the study. The reviewers' conclusions were that there is currently no evidence to suggest the use of zinc supplementation in the prevention of type 2 diabetes mellitus. Future trials will have to standardise outcome measures such as incidence of type 2 diabetes mellitus, decrease of the insulin resistance, quality of life, diabetic complications, all-cause mortality and costs.[59]

A more recent clinical trial from Iran has tested the effect of zinc supplements for diabetics on renal function. This was a randomised, controlled trial of crossover design on 50 patients with type 2 diabetes with microalbuminuria, given zinc (30 mg daily for 30 days) or placebo with a 4-week wash out. Zinc supplementation resulted in a 9.5% reduction in urine albumin excretion ($P < 0.01$).[60] A further Iranian trial in 60 obese, prepubertal children found that zinc supplementation 20 mg daily for 8 weeks reduced fasting plasmal glucose, insulin and insulin resistance with no change in body mass index, waist circumference, LDL cholesterol and triglycerides.[61]

Male fertility

Zinc is necessary for growth, sexual maturation and reproduction. Infertile men have been reported to have reduced seminal and serum zinc levels compared with fertile men.[62–64] However, other research has shown no statistically significant relationship between zinc in serum or seminal plasma and semen quality or IgA or IgG antisperm antibody. In the same study, zinc levels had no influence on sperm capacity to penetrate cervical mucus *in vitro* or *in vivo* and had no effect on subsequent fertility.[65,66] A randomised, controlled trial involving 45 Kuwait men with > 40% immobile sperm found that zinc therapy alone, in combination with vitamin E or with vitamin E plus vitamin C, was associated with improved sperm parameters, less oxidative stress, sperm apoptosis and sperm DNA fragmentation compared with placebo, suggesting the mechanisms by which zinc could improve sperm mobility in this group of men.[67]

Age-related macular degeneration

Several studies have investigated the effects of zinc and antioxidant vitamins on the progression of age-related macular degeneration (ARMD). The highest profile study is the Age-Related Eye Disease Study (AREDS) in which high-dose zinc supplements (80 mg daily, which is about 10 times the Reference Nutrient Intake; RNI), together with antioxidants, were shown to reduce the risk of progression to advanced ARMD among patients who already had extensive drusen.[66] An ancillary study of AREDS found that zinc supplementation reduced one marker of oxidative stress (plasma cystine) compared with placebo.[68] A Cochrane review looked at the overall evidence to date, including AREDS, and concluded that current data are insufficient to state that antioxidant vitamin and mineral supplementation should be taken during early signs of the disease and that more research is needed.[69]

A 2008 study assessed the effect of a novel zinc-monocysteine compound in ARMD. Both zinc and placebo groups enrolled 40 participants, with best corrected visual acuity 20/25 to 20/70, macular drusen and pigment changes. Eligible, consenting patients were randomised to either zinc monocysteine 25 mg or placebo twice daily for 6 months. By 6 months, the zinc monocysteine group showed improved visual acuity ($P < 0.0001$) and contrast sensitivity ($P < 0.0001$). Macular light flash recovery time shortened in the zinc monocysteine group at 3 months by 2.1 s (left eye, $P = 0.0001$) to 3.6 s (right eye, $P < 0.0001$), and at 6 months by 7.2 s (left eye, $P < 0.0001$) to 7.4 s (right eye, $P < 0.0001$). There was no improvement in this variable in the placebo group. Gastrointestinal irritation rate in the zinc monocysteine group was below 2%. The study concluded that zinc monocysteine 25 mg twice daily was well tolerated and was associated with improved macular function in comparison to a placebo in persons with dry ARMD.[70]

Taste acuity

Adequate intake of zinc may be important in determining the sensory experience of food, appetite, and hence dietary quality. In the European multi-centre ZENITH study in older people, higher erythrocyte zinc status was associated with better taste acuity for salt and taste in the whole surveyed sample ($n = 385$). Higher serum zinc levels were associated with greater sensitivity to sour taste in older groups (aged 79–90 years). There was no apparent link between serum or erythrocyte zinc status and acuity for bitter or sweet tastes, irrespective of age.[71] In healthy young adults (aged 25–40 years), higher dietary zinc intake has been associated with better taste acuity for salt in women but not men. Acuity for bitter taste appeared to be related to zinc intake in women but not men. Among those whose average intake was below the RNI, men were less sensitive than women to sour and bitter taste. A randomised, controlled trial among 91 healthy older European adults (aged 70–87 years) recruited to the same ZENITH study determined taste acuity in response to zinc supplementation (15 or 30 mg) or placebo. Results differed depending on geographical region. Salt taste acuity was greater in response to zinc (30 mg) than placebo post-intervention among those recruited in Grenoble. There was no apparent change in acuity for sweet, sour or bitter taste in response to zinc.[72] These preliminary findings suggest that zinc does play a role in taste acuity and that age, gender and geographical region should be taken into account when studying links between zinc and taste acuity.

Cognitive function

A link has been suggested between zinc and cognitive function. A randomised, double-blind, placebo-controlled trial investigated the effects of zinc supplementation on cognitive function in 387 healthy adults aged 55–87 years. Several measures of visual memory, working memory, attention and reaction time were obtained at baseline and then after taking zinc 15 or 30 mg daily or placebo for 3 and 6 months. Younger adults (< 70 years) performed significantly better on all tests than older adults (> 70 years), and performance improved with practice on some measures. For two out of eight dependent variables, there were significant interactions indicating a beneficial effect (at 3 months only) of both 15 and 30 mg daily on one measure of spatial working memory and a detrimental effect of 15 mg daily on one measure of attention. Whether these findings generalise to older adults in poorer mental and physical health and with less adequate zinc intake and status than the present sample is unclear and must await the findings of further research.[73]

Miscellaneous

There is limited evidence that zinc may play a role in the treatment of benign prostatic hyperplasia and exercise performance.[74] In AIDS patients receiving zidovudine supplemented with zinc for 30 days, body weight was stabilised and the frequency of opportunistic infections reduced in the following 2 years.[75] Long-term (18-month) zinc supplementation at nutritional levels was shown to delay immunological failure and decreased diarrhoea over time in HIV-infected adults.[76] However, further controlled trials are needed.

The role of zinc supplements in acne, white spots on the finger nails and treatment of brittle nails is controversial. One recent trial indicated that zinc sulphate 100 mg daily improved symptoms of rosacea.[77]

Small studies in animals and humans have suggested that zinc may affect lipoprotein metabolism. However, in a meta-analysis of 33 studies, no effect zinc supplementation on plasma lipoproteins was detected in the overall analysis although zinc supplementation was associated with a decrease in HDL cholesterol concentrations in individuals classified as healthy, which could contribute to an increased risk of coronary heart disease.[78] A small study in Japan suggested that zinc supplementation may be effective in reducing anger and depression.[79]

Conclusion
Results from studies investigating the effect of zinc supplements on the common cold are conflicting. There is limited evidence for a benefit of zinc in male infertility and immune function. Further controlled trials are needed.

Adverse effects

Signs of acute toxicity (doses > 200 mg daily) include gastrointestinal pain, nausea, vomiting and diarrhoea. Prolonged exposure to doses > 50 mg daily may induce copper deficiency (marked by low serum copper and caeruloplasmin levels, microcytic anaemia and neutropenia), and iron deficiency. Doses > 150 mg daily may reduce serum HDL levels, depress immune function and cause gastric erosion. Data from the AREDS, a randomised, controlled trial which involved 3640 patients with ARMD, found that zinc supplementation 80 mg daily increased hospitalization for urinary complications compared with placebo, and suggested that high-dose zinc supplementation may have a negative effect on urinary system physiology.[80]

Interactions

Drugs
Ciprofloxacin: reduced absorption of ciprofloxacin.
Oral contraceptives: may reduce plasma zinc levels.
Penicillamine: reduced absorption of penicillamine.
Tetracyclines: reduced absorption of zinc and vice versa.
Imipramine: Zinc supplementation may augment the efficacy and speed of onset of therapeutic response to imipramine treatment, particularly in patients previously non-responsive to antidepressant pharmacotherapies. These findings suggest the participation of disturbed zinc/glutamatergic transmission in the pathophysiology of drug resistance.[81]

Nutrients
Copper: large doses of zinc may reduce absorption of copper.

Folic acid: may reduce zinc absorption (raises concern about pregnant women who are advised to take folic acid to reduce the risk of birth defects).

Iron: reduces absorption of oral iron and vice versa (raises concern about pregnant women who are often given iron; this may reduce zinc status and increase the risk of intrauterine growth retardation and congenital abnormalities in the foetus).

Dose

Zinc is available in the form of tablets and capsules and as an ingredient in multivitamin preparations.

The dose beyond the RDA is not established. Dietary supplements contain 5–50 mg (elemental zinc) per daily dose.

The zinc content of some commonly used zinc salts is as follows: zinc amino acid chelate (100 mg/g); zinc gluconate (130 mg/g); zinc orotate (170 mg/g); zinc sulphate (227 mg/g).

Upper safety limits

The UK Expert Groups on Vitamins and Minerals has identified a safe upper limit of zinc for adults from supplements alone of 25 mg daily.

References

1 Grahn B, Paterson PG, Gottschall-Pass KT, *et al.* Zinc and the eye. *J Am Coll Nutr* 2001; 20: 106–118.

2 King J, Keen CL. Zinc. In: Shils ME, Olson JA, Shike M, Ross AC, eds. *Modern Nutrition in Health and Disease*, 9th edn. Philadelphia, PA: Lippincott Williams & Wilkins, 1998: 223–239.

3 Christian P, Khatry SK, Yamini S, *et al.* Zinc supplementation might potentiate the effect of vitamin A in restoring night vision in pregnant Nepalese women. *Am J Clin Nutr* 2001; 73(6): 1045–1051.

4 Bettger W, Fish TJ, O'Dell BL. Effects of copper and zinc status of rats on erythrocyte stability and superoxide dismutase activity. *Proc Soc Exp Biol Med* 1978; 158: 279–282.

5 Kazimierczak W, Adamas B, Maslinski C. The action of the complexes of lidocaine with zinc on histamine release from isolated rat mast cells. *Biochem Pharmacol* 1978; 27: 243–249.

6 Klug ADR. 'Zinc fingers': a novel protein motif for nucleic acid recognition. *Trend Biochem Sci* 1987; 12: 464–469.

7 Cousins RJ, Blanchard RK, Moore JB, *et al.* Regulation of zinc metabolism and genomic outcomes. *J Nutr* 2003; 133(5Suppl1): 1521S–1526S.

8 Thompson C. Apoptosis in the pathogenesis and treatment of disease. *Science* 1995; 267: 1456–1462.

9 Shankar A, Prasad AS. Zinc and immune function: the biological basis of altered resistance to infection. *Am J Clin Nutr* 1998; 68: 447S–463S.

10 Meydani SN, Barnett JB, Dallal GE, *et al.* Serum zinc and pneumonia in nursing home elderly. *Am J Clin Nutr* 2007; 86(4): 1167–1173.

11 Prasad AS, Beck FW, Bao B, *et al.* Zinc supplementation decreases incidence of infections in the elderly: effect of zinc on generation of cytokines and oxidative stress. *Am J Clin Nutr* 2007; 85(3): 837–844.

12 Bao B, Prasad AS, Beck FW, *et al.* Zinc supplementation decreases oxidative stress, incidence of infection, and generation of inflammatory cytokines in sickle cell disease patients. *Transl Res* 2008; 152(2): 67–80.

13 Abdulhamid I, Beck FW, Millard S, *et al.* Effect of zinc supplementation on respiratory tract infections in children with cystic fibrosis. *Pediatr Pulmonol* 2008; 43(3): 281–287.

14 Barceloux D. Zinc. *J Toxicol Clin Toxicol* 1999; 37: 279–292.

15 Powell S. The antioxidant properties of zinc. *J Nutr* 2000; 130: 1447S–1454S.

16 Kirkil G, Hamdi Muz M, Seckin D, *et al.* Antioxidant effect of zinc picolinate in patients with chronic obstructive pulmonary disease. *Respir Med* 2008; 102(6): 840–844.

17 de Oliveira K de J, Donangelo CM, de Oliveira AV Jr, *et al.* Effect of zinc supplementation on the antioxidant, copper, and iron status of physically active adolescents. *Cell Biochem Funct* 2009; 27(3): 162–166.

18 Andriollo-Sanchez M, Hininger-Favier I, Meunier N, *et al.* No antioxidant beneficial effect of zinc supplementation on oxidative stress markers and antioxidant defenses in middle-aged and elderly subjects: the Zenith study. *J Am Coll Nutr* 2008; 27(4): 463–469.

19 Feillet-Coudray C, Meunier N, Bayle D, *et al.* Effect of zinc supplementation on in vitro copper-induced oxidation of low-density lipoproteins in healthy French subjects aged 55–70 years: the Zenith Study. *Br J Nutr* 2006; 95(6): 1134–1142.

20 Ducros V, Andriollo-Sanchez M, Arnaud J, *et al.* Zinc supplementation does not alter plasma homocysteine, vitamin B$_{12}$ and red blood cell folate concentrations in French elderly subjects. *J Trace Elem Med Biol* 2009; 23(1): 15–20.

21 Hunt JR, Beiseigel JM, Johnson LK. Adaptation in human zinc absorption as influenced by dietary zinc and bioavailability. *Am J Clin Nutr* 2008; 87(5): 1336–1345.

22 Chung CS, Stookey J, Dare D, *et al.* Current dietary zinc intake has a greater effect on fractional zinc absorption than does longer term zinc consumption in healthy adult men. *Am J Clin Nutr* 2008; 87(5): 1224–1229.

23 Beiseigel JM, Klevay LM, Johnson LK, *et al.* Zinc absorption adapts to zinc supplementation in post-menopausal women. *J Am Coll Nutr* 2009; 28(2): 177–183.

24 Hunt JR, Beiseigel JM. Dietary calcium does not exacerbate phytate inhibition of zinc absorption by women from conventional diets. *Am J Clin Nutr* 2009; 89(3): 839–843.

25 Feillet-Coudray C, Meunier N, Rambeau M, *et al.* Long-term moderate zinc supplementation increases exchangeable zinc pool masses in late-middle-aged men: the Zenith Study. *Am J Clin Nutr* 2005; 82(1): 103–110.

26 Hininger-Favier I, Andriollo-Sanchez M, Arnaud J, *et al.* Age- and sex-dependent effects of long-term zinc supplementation on essential trace element status and lipid metabolism in European subjects: the Zenith Study. *Br J Nutr* 2007; 97(3): 569–578.

27 Intorre F, Polito A, Andriollo-Sanchez M, *et al.* Effect of zinc supplementation on vitamin status of middle-aged and older European adults: the ZENITH Study. *Eur J Clin Nutr* 2008; 62(10): 1215–1223.

28 Wessells KR, Jorgensen JM, Hess SY, *et al.* Plasma zinc concentration responds rapidly to the initiation and discontinuation of short-term zinc supplementation in healthy men. *J Nutr* 2010; 140(12): 2128–2133.

29 Siepmann M, Spank S, Kluge A, *et al.* The pharmacokinetics of zinc from zinc gluconate: a comparison with zinc oxide in healthy men. *Int J Clin Pharmacol Ther* 2005; 43(12): 562–565.

30 Tompkins TA, Renard NE, Kiuchi A. Clinical evaluation of the bioavailability of zinc-enriched yeast and zinc gluconate in healthy volunteers. *Biol Trace Elem Res* 2007; 120(13): 28–35.

31 Gandia P, Bour D, Maurette JM, *et al.* A bioavailability study comparing two oral formulations containing zinc (Zn bis-glycinate vs. Zn gluconate) after a single administration to twelve healthy female volunteers. *Int J Vitam Nutr Res* 2007; 77(4): 243–248.

32 Safai-Kutti S. Oral zinc supplementation in anorexia nervosa. *Acta Psychiatr Scand Suppl* 1990; 361(82): 14–17.

33 Birmingham C, Goldner EM, Bakan R. Controlled trial of zinc supplementation in anorexia nervosa. *Int J Eat Disord* 1994; 15: 251–255.

34 Landsdown A. Zinc in the healing wound. *Lancet* 1996; 346: 706–707.

35 Agren M. Studies in zinc wound healing. *Acta Derm Venereol* 1990; 154(Suppl): 1–36.

36 Wilkinson E, Hawke CI. Oral zinc for arterial and venous leg ulcers. *Cochrane Database Syst Rev* 1998; (4): CD001273.

37 Novick S, Godfrey JC, Pollack RL, *et al.* Zinc-induced suppression of inflammation in the respiratory tract, caused by infection with human rhinovirus and other irritants. *Med Hypotheses* 1997; 49: 347–357.

38 Jackson J, Peterson C, Lesho E. A meta-analysis of zinc salts lozenges and the common cold. *Arch Intern Med* 1997; 157: 2373–2376.

39 Jackson J, Lesho E, Peterson C. Zinc and common cold: a meta-analysis revisited. *J Nutr* 2000; 130: 1512S–1515S.

40 Marshall I. Zinc and the common cold. *Cochrane Database Syst Review* 2000; (4): CD001364.

41 Prasad AS, Beck FW, Bao B, *et al.* Duration and severity of symptoms and levels of plasma interleukin-1 receptor antagonist, soluble tumor necrosis factor receptor, and adhesion molecules in patients with common cold treated with zinc acetate. *J Infect Dis* 2008; 197(6): 795–802.

42 Eby GA, 3rd. Zinc lozenges as cure for the common cold: a review and hypothesis. *Med Hypotheses* 2009; 74(3): 482–492.

43 Eby G. Zinc ion availability: the determinant of efficacy in zinc lozenge treatment of common colds. *J Antimicrob Chemother* 1997; 40: 483–493.

44 Hirt M, Nobel S, Barron E. Zinc nasal gel for the treatment of common cold symptoms: a double-blind, placebo-controlled trial. *Ear Nose Throat J* 2000; 79(77880): 782.

45 Belongia E, Berg R, Liu K. A randomized trial of zinc nasal spray for the treatment of upper respiratory illness in adults. *Am J Med* 2001; 111: 103–108.

46 Turner R. Ineffectiveness of intranasal zinc gluconate for prevention of experimental rhinovirus colds. *Clin Infect Dis* 2001; 33: 1865–1870.

47 D'Cruze H, Arroll B, Kenealy T. Is intranasal zinc effective and safe for the common cold? A systematic review and meta-analysis *J Prim Health Care* 2009; 1(2): 134–139.

48 Kurugol Z, Akilli M, Bayram N, *et al.* The prophylactic and therapeutic effectiveness of zinc sulphate on common cold in children. *Acta Paediatr* 2006; 95(10): 1175–1181.

49 Kurugol Z, Bayram N, Atik T. Effect of zinc sulfate on common cold in children: randomized, double blind study. *Pediatr Int* 2007; 49(6): 842–847.

50 Chausmer AB. Zinc, insulin and diabetes. *J Am Coll Nutr* 1998; 17(2): 109–115.

51 Maret W. A role for metallothionein in the pathogenesis of diabetes and its cardiovascular complications. *Mol Genet Metab* 2008; 94(1): 1–3.

52 Salgueiro MJ, Krebs N, Zubillaga MB, *et al.* Zinc and diabetes mellitus: is there a need of zinc supplementation in diabetes mellitus patients? *Biol Trace Elem Res* 2001; 81(3): 215–228.

53 Marreiro DN, Geloneze B, Tambascia MA, *et al.* Effect of zinc supplementation on serum leptin levels and insulin resistance of obese women. *Biol Trace Elem Res* 2006; 112(2): 109–118.

54   Gomez-Garcia A, Hernandez-Salazar E, Gonzalez-Ortiz M, et al. [Effect of oral zinc administration on insulin sensitivity, leptin and androgens in obese males]. Rev Med Chil 2006; 134(3): 279–284.

55   Hussain SA, Khadim HM, Khalaf BH, et al. Effects of melatonin and zinc on glycemic control in type 2 diabetic patients poorly controlled with metformin. Saudi Med J 2006; 27(10): 1483–1488.

56   Islam MS, Loots du T. Diabetes, metallothionein, and zinc interactions: a review. Biofactors 2007; 29 (4): 203–212.

57   Soinio M, Marniemi J, Laakso M, et al. Serum zinc level and coronary heart disease events in patients with type 2 diabetes. Diabetes Care 2007; 30(3): 523–528.

58   Sun Q, vanDam RM, Willett WC, et al. Prospective study of zinc intake and risk of type 2 diabetes in women. Diabetes Care 2009; 32(4): 629–634.

59   Beletate V, ElDib RP, Atallah AN. Zinc supplementation for the prevention of type 2 diabetes mellitus. Cochrane Database Syst Rev 2007; (4): CD005525.

60   Parham M, Amini M, Aminorroaya A, et al. Effect of zinc supplementation on microalbuminuria in patients with type 2 diabetes: a double blind, randomized, placebo-controlled, cross-over trial. Rev Diabet Stud 2008; 5(2): 102–109.

61   Hashemipour M, Kelishadi R, Shapouri J, et al. Effect of zinc supplementation on insulin resistance and components of the metabolic syndrome in pre-pubertal obese children. Hormones (Athens) 2009; 8(4): 279–285.

62   Mohan H, Verma J, Singh I. Inter-relationship of zinc levels in serum and semen in oligospermic infertile patients and fertile males. Indian J Pathol Microbiol 1997; 40: 451–455.

63   Kvist U, Bjornadahl L, Kjellberg S. Sperm nuclear zinc, chromatin stability and male fertility. Scanning Microsc 1987; 1: 1241–1247.

64   Chia S, Ong CN, Chua LH, et al. Comparisons of zinc concentrations in blood and seminal plasma and the various sperm parameters between fertile and infertile men. J Androl 2000; 21: 53–57.

65   Eggert-Kruse W, Zwick EM, Batschulat K, et al. Are zinc levels in seminal plasma associated with seminal leukocytes and other determinants of semen quality? Fertil Steril 2002; 77(2): 260–269.

66   Age Related Eye Disease Study Research Group. A randomized, placebo-controlled, clinical trial of high-dose supplementation with vitamins C and E, beta carotene, and zinc for age-related macular degeneration and vision loss: AREDS Report No. 8. Arch Ophthalmol 2001; 119: 1417–1436.

67   Omu AE, Al-Azemi MK, Kehinde EO, et al. Indications of the mechanisms involved in improved sperm parameters by zinc therapy. Med Princ Pract 2008; 17(2): 108–116.

68   Moriarty-Craige SE, Ha KN, Sternberg P Jr, et al. Effects of long-term zinc supplementation on plasma thiol metabolites and redox status in patients with age-related macular degeneration. Am J Ophthalmol 2007; 143(2): 206–211.

69   Evans J. Antioxidant vitamin and mineral supplements for age-related macular degeneration. Cochrane Database Syst Rev 2006; (4): CD000254.

70   Newsome DA. A randomized prospective, placebo-controlled clinical trial of a novel zinc-monocys-teine compound in age-related macular degeneration. Curr Eye Res 2008; 33(7): 591–598.

71   Stewart-Knox BJ, Simpson EE, Parr H, et al. Zinc status and taste acuity in older Europeans: the ZENITH study. Eur J Clin Nutr 2005; 59 (Suppl2): S31–S36.

72   Stewart-Knox BJ, Simpson EE, Parr H, et al. Taste acuity in response to zinc supplementation in older Europeans. Br J Nutr 2008; 99(1): 129–136.

73   Maylor EA, Simpson EE, Secker DL, et al. Effects of zinc supplementation on cognitive function in healthy middle-aged and older adults: the ZENITH Study. Br J Nutr 2006; 96(4): 752–760.

74   Krotkiewski M, Gudmundsson M, Backstrom P, et al. Zinc and muscle strength and endurance. Acta Physiol Scand 1982; 116(3): 309–311.

75   Mocchegiani E. Benefit of oral zinc supplementation as an adjunct to zidovudine (AZT) therapy against opportunistic infections in AIDS. Int J Immunopharmacol 1995; 17: 719–727.

76   Baum MK, Lai S, Sales S, et al. Randomized, controlled clinical trial of zinc supplementation to prevent immunological failure in HIV-infected adults. Clin Infect Dis 2010; 50(12): 1653–1660.

77   Sharquie KE, Najim RA, Al-Salman HN. Oral zinc sulfate in the treatment of rosacea: a double-blind, placebo-controlled study. Int J Dermatol 2006; 45 (7): 857–861.

78   Foster M, Petocz P, Samman S. Effects of zinc on plasma lipoprotein cholesterol concentrations in humans: a meta-analysis of randomised controlled trials. Atherosclerosis 2009; 210(2): 344–352.

79   Sawada T, Yokoi K. Effect of zinc supplementation on mood states in young women: a pilot study. Eur J Clin Nutr 2010; 64(3): 331–333.

80   Johnson AR, Munoz A, Gottlieb JL, et al. High dose zinc increases hospital admissions due to genitourinary complications. J Urol 2007; 177(2): 639–643.

81   Siwek M, Dudek D, Paul IA, et al. Zinc supplementation augments efficacy of imipramine in treatment resistant patients: a double blind, placebo-controlled study. J Affect Disord 2009; 118(13): 187–1895.

Appendix 1

Guidance on safe upper levels of vitamins and minerals

Vitamin/mineral	EU RDA	EVM UK	TUL USA	SCF EU
Vitamin A (retinol equivalent µg)	800	1500[1]	3000	3600
Vitamin B$_1$ (thiamine) mg	1.1	100[1]	–	
Vitamin B$_2$ (riboflavin) mg	1.4	100[1]	–	–
Vitamin B$_6$ (pyridoxine) mg	1.4	10[2]	100	25
Vitamin B$_{12}$ (cobalamin) µg	2.5	1000[1]	–	–
Vitamin C (ascorbic acid) mg	80	1000[1]	2000	–
Vitamin D (cholecalciferol) µg	5	25[1]	100	50
Vitamin E (tocopherol) mg	12	727[2]	1000	300
Niacin mg	16		30	
Nicotinamide mg	–	500[1]		900
Nicotinic acid mg	–	17[1]		10
Biotin µg	50	970[1]	–	–
Folic acid µg	200	1000[1]	1000	1000
Pantothenic acid mg	6	200[1]	–	–
Calcium mg	800	1500[1]	2500	2500
Iodine µg	150	500[1]	1100	600
Iron mg	14	17[1]	45	
Magnesium mg	375	400[1]	350	250
Phosphorus mg	700	250[1]	4000	
Zinc mg	10	25[2]	40	25
Vitamin K mg	–	1[1]	–	–
Beta-carotene mg		7[2]	–	20
Chromium µg	40	–	–	
Copper mg	1[2]	10	5	
Manganese mg	2	4[1]	11	–
Molybdenum µg	50	–	2000	600
Selenium µg	55	200[2]	400	300
Boron mg	–	5.9[2]	20	
Nickel mg	–		1	
Vanadium mg	–		1.8	–

EU RDA: the Recommended Daily Allowance considered sufficient to prevent deficiency in most individuals in the population.
EVM: draft figures (2002) produced by the Food Standards Agency (FSA) Expert Vitamin and Mineral (EVM) group.
TUL: Tolerable Upper Intake Levels defined by the Food and Nutrition Board of the US National Academy of Sciences as the highest total level of a nutrient (diet plus supplements) that could be consumed safely on a daily basis, which is unlikely to cause adverse health effects to almost all individuals in the general population. As intakes rise above the TUL, the risk of adverse effects increases. The TUL describes long-term intakes, so an isolated dose above the TUL need not necessarily cause adverse effects. The TUL defines safety limits and is not a recommended intake for most people most of the time.
SCF: Tolerable Upper Intake Levels defined by the European Commission's Scientific Committee on Food (SCF) as the maximum level of chronic daily intake of a nutrient (from all sources) judged to be unlikely to pose a risk of adverse effects to humans. http://ec.europa.eu/comm./food/fs/sc/scf/out80_en.html.
[1] Likely safe total daily intake from supplements alone.
[2] Safe upper level from supplements alone.
Note: dashes (–) indicate that the nutrient has been considered but no level set. Where the column is blank, the nutrient has not been considered.

Appendix 2

Drug and supplement interactions

Drug	Food/ nutrient	Effect	Intervention
Drugs acting on the gastrointestinal system			
Antacids	Iron	Aluminium-, magnesium- and calcium-containing antacids and sodium bicarbonate reduce absorption of iron	Separate administration of antacids and iron by at least 2 h
Sulfasalazine	Folic acid	Sulfasalazine can reduce absorption of folic acid	Monitor and give a supplement if necessary
Stimulant laxatives	Potassium	Prolonged use of stimulant laxatives can precipitate hypokalaemia	Avoid prolonged use of laxatives
Liquid paraffin	Fat-soluble vitamins	Liquid paraffin reduces absorption of vitamins A, D, E and K	Avoid prolonged use of liquid paraffin
Drugs acting in the treatment of diseases of the cardiovascular system			
Thiazide diuretics	Calcium/ vitamin D	Excessive serum calcium levels can develop in patients given thiazides with supplements of calcium and/or vitamin D	Concurrent use of thiazides with calcium and/or vitamin D need not be avoided but serum calcium levels should be monitored
ACE inhibitors	Potassium	Concurrent use of ACE inhibitors with potassium may induce severe hyperkalaemia	Avoid
Potassium-sparing diuretics	Potassium	Concurrent use of potassium-sparing diuretics and either potassium supplements or potassium-containing salt substitutes may induce severe hyperkalaemia	Avoid concurrent use of potassium-sparing diuretics and potassium supplements unless potassium levels are monitored; warn patients about risks of salt substitutes
Calcium-channel blockers	Calcium	Therapeutic effects of verapamil can be antagonised by calcium	Calcium supplements should be used with caution in patients taking verapamil
Hydralazine	Vitamin B_6	Long-term administration of hydralazine may lead to pyridoxine deficiency	Vitamin B_6 supplement may be needed if symptoms of peripheral neuritis develop

Drug	Food/ nutrient	Effect	Intervention
Anticoagulants	Vitamin E	Effects of warfarin may be increased by large doses of vitamin E (>100 IU daily)	Avoid high-dose vitamin E supplements
	Vitamin K	Effects of anticoagulants can be reduced or abolished by large intakes of vitamin K	Avoid excessive intake of vitamin K (e.g. check labels of enteral feeds)
	Bromelain	Effects of anticoagulants may be increased by these supplements	Care with these supplements in people taking anticoagulants, aspirin and antiplatelet drugs. Avoid if possible, otherwise monitor carefully
	Chondroitin		
	Fish oils		
	Garlic		
	Ginkgo biloba		
	Ginseng Glucosamine		
	Grape seed extract		
	Green tea		
	S-adenosyl-methionine		
Colestyramine	Fat-soluble vitamins	Prolonged use of these drugs may result in deficiency of fat-soluble vitamins	Supplements of vitamins A, D, E and K may be needed if these drugs are administered for prolonged periods
Colestipol			

Drugs acting on the central nervous system

Drug	Food/ nutrient	Effect	Intervention
Phenothiazines	Evening primrose oil	Evening primrose oil supplements may increase the risk of epileptic side-effects	Avoid evening primrose oil supplements
Monoamine oxidase inhibitors	Brewer's yeast	Brewer's yeast may provoke a hypertensive crisis	Avoid brewer's yeast supplements
Anti-epileptics[1]	Folic acid	Anti-epileptics may cause folate deficiency, but use of folic acid supplements may lead to a fall in serum anticonvulsant levels and reduced seizure control	Folic acid supplements should be given only to those folate-deficient patients on anti-epileptics who can be monitored
	Vitamin B_6	Large doses of vitamin B_6 may reduce serum levels of phenytoin and phenobarbital	Avoid large doses of vitamin B_6 from supplements (>10 mg daily)

Drug	Food/ nutrient	Effect	Intervention
	Vitamin D	Anti-epileptics may disturb metabolism of vitamin D leading to osteomalacia	Susceptible individuals should take 10 µg vitamin D daily
	Vitamin K	Anti-epileptics have been associated with foetal haemorrhage. This is because the drug crosses the placenta and decreases vitamin K status, resulting in bleeding in the infant	Vitamin K should be provided to the newborn infant
Levodopa	Iron	Iron reduces the absorption of levodopa	Separate doses of iron and levodopa by at least 2 h
	Vitamin B_6	Effects of levodopa are reduced or abolished by vitamin B_6 supplements (> 5 mg daily), but dietary vitamin B_6 has no effect	Avoid all supplements containing any vitamin B_6. Suggest co-careldopa or co-beneldopa as an alternative to levodopa

Drugs used in the treatment of infections

Drug	Food/ nutrient	Effect	Intervention
Tetracyclines	Iron	Absorption of tetracyclines is reduced by iron and vice versa	Separate doses of iron and tetracyclines by at least 2 h
	Calcium/ magnesium/ zinc	Absorption of tetracyclines may be reduced by mineral supplements and vice versa	Separate doses of mineral supplements and tetracyclines by at least 2 h
Trimethoprim	Folic acid	Folate deficiency in susceptible individuals	Folic acid supplement may be needed if drug used for prolonged periods
4-Quinolones	Iron/zinc	Absorption of 4-quinolones may be reduced by mineral supplements and vice versa	Separate doses of mineral supplements and 4-quinolones by at least 2 h
Cycloserine	Folic acid	Folate deficiency in susceptible individuals	Monitor folate status and give supplement if necessary
Isoniazid	Vitamin B_6	Long-term administration of isoniazid may lead to pyridoxine deficiency	Vitamin B_6 supplement may be needed if symptoms of peripheral neuritis develop
Rifampicin	Vitamin D	Rifampicin may disturb metabolism of vitamin D leading to osteomalacia in susceptible individuals	Monitor serum vitamin D levels

Drug	Food/ nutrient	Effect	Intervention
Drugs used in the treatment of disorders of the endocrine system			
Oral hypoglycaemics and insulin	Aloe vera	These supplements could theoretically potentiate the effects of oral hypoglycaemics and insulin	Care in people on medication for diabetes
	Alpha-lipoic acid		
	Chromium		
	Glucosamine	Glucosamine might reduce the effects of oral hypoglycaemics and insulin	Care in people on medication for diabetes
Oestrogens (including HRT and oral contraceptives)	Vitamin C	Concurrent administration of oestrogens and large doses of vitamin C (1 g daily) increases serum levels of oestrogens	Avoid high-dose vitamin C supplements
	DHEA	May potentiate hormonal effects	Care in people using HRT
	Isoflavones	May potentiate hormonal effects	Care in people using HRT
Bisphosphonates	Calcium	May lead to reduced absorption of bisphosphonate	Take 2 h apart
Thyroid medication	Kelp/iodine	May lead to poor control of thyroid condition	Avoid without a doctor's advice
Drugs used in the treatment of musculo-skeletal and joint diseases			
Penicillamine	Iron/zinc	Absorption of penicillamine reduced by mineral supplements and vice versa	Separate doses of mineral supplements and penicillamine by at least 2 h

[1]This interaction applies to the older anti-epileptic drugs (e.g. phenytoin, primidine, phenobarbitone, valproate and carbamazepine). There is little information on newer anti-epileptic drugs except with the possibility of lamotrigine, which may have anti-epileptic properties. (Gilman JT. Lamotrigine: an antiepileptic agent for the treatment of partial seizures. *Ann Pharmacother* 1995; 29: 144–151.)

Appendix 3

Additional resources

Government web sites related to dietary supplements

United Kingdom

UK Food Standards Agency has published UK National Diet and Nutrition Surveys across various population groups and more recently a rolling programme including all age groups. Resposibility for these surveys will pass to the Department of Health (http://www.dh.gov.uk). Archived material is available at: http://tna.europarchive.org/20110116113217/http://www.food.gov.uk/science/dietarysurveys/

UK Food Standards Agency Expert Group on Vitamins and Minerals (EVM)
A group of independent experts established to consider the safety of vitamins and minerals sold under food law. Produced a report, *Safe Upper Levels for Vitamins and Minerals*, in May 2003. http://www.food.gov.uk/multimedia/pdfs/vitmin2003.pdf

Medicines and Healthcare products Regulatory Agency (MHRA)
The UK body that licenses medicines. Provides information on legislation relating to herbals and supplements.
http://www.mhra.gov.uk

Europe

European Union Food Safety web site
Gives details of all EU regulation on food supplements.
http://www.efsa.europa.eu/

European Food Safety Authority (EFSA)
Nutrition and health claims: gives details of legislation and EFSA opinions on health claims.
http://www.efsa.europa.eu/en/topics/topic/nutrition.htm

USA

US Food and Drug Administration (FDA)
Dietary Supplements: provides information on dietary supplements legislation and FDA remit.
http://www.fda.gov/Food/DietarySupplements/default.htm
FDA alerts and safety information on dietary supplements
http://www.fda.gov/Food/DietarySupplements/Alerts/default.htm

National Institutes of Health Office of Dietary Supplements
http://dietary-supplements.info.nih.gov

Associations representing industry

Association of the European Self-Medication Industry (AESGP)

European trade association representing the over-the-counter healthcare products industry
http://www.aesgp.be

Council for Responsible Nutrition (CRN)
Provides member companies with legislative guidance, regulatory interpretation, scientific information on supplement benefits and safety issues and communications expertise.
UK web site: http://www.crnuk.org/
US web site: http://www.crnusa.org

Health Food Manufacturers' Association (HFMA)
A trade association that acts as a voice for the industry; covers food supplements, health foods, herbal remedies, etc.
http://www.hfma.co.uk

International Alliance of Dietary/Food Supplement Associations (IADSA)
Aims to facilitate a sound legislative and political environment to build growth in the

international market for dietary supplements based on scientific principles.
http://www.iadsa.org

Proprietary Association of Great Britain (PAGB)
UK trade association representing the consumer healthcare industry.
http://www.pagb.co.uk

Health Supplement Information Service (HSIS)
Developed by the Proprietary Association of Great Britain (PAGB) to present the facts about health supplements in a straightforward way. Aims to eliminate confusion and provide reliable data about individual nutrients and supplements.
http://www.hsis.org

Journals and newsletters

American Journal of Clinical Nutrition
Official journal of the American Society for Clinical Nutrition. Published monthly.
http://www.ajcn.org

Focus on Alternative and Complementary Therapies (FACT)
Provides summaries and commentaries on various aspects of complementary medicine, including vitamins, minerals and supplements. Published quarterly.
http://www.pharmpress.com

Journal of Dietary Supplements
A peer-reviewed academic publication, providing the latest information on food supplements. Published quarterly.
http://informahealthcare.com/jds

On-line research information and comment

Arbor Nutrition Guide
Provides regular updates on nutritional issues, including those with relevance to supplements.
http://arborcom.com (for subscriptions, see http://www.nutritionupdates.org/sub/sub01.php?item=3)

Medline
The US National Library of Medicine's bibliographic database providing extensive coverage of medicine and healthcare from approximately 3900 current biomedical journals, published in about 70 countries.
http://www.ncbi.nlm.nih.gov/pubmed

Medline Dietary Supplements
http://ods.od.nih.gov/Research/PubMed_Dietary_Supplement_Subset.aspx

Medline Plus Vitamins
http://www.nlm.nih.gov/medlineplus/vitamins.html

Medline Plus Herbs and Supplements
http://www.nlm.nih.gov/medlineplus/druginfo/herb_All.html

Other information

Consumer Lab
Tests the content of diet supplements in the USA and provides reports on its work (subscription required).
http://consumerlab.com

Food portion	Zinc content (mg)	Food portion	Zinc content (mg)
Breakfast cereals		**1 beef steak** (155 g)	7.0
1 bowl **All-Bran** (45 g)	3.0	**Minced beef, lean, stewed** (100 g)	6.0
1 bowl *Bran Flakes* (45 g)	1.5	1 *chicken leg* (190 g)	2.0
1 bowl Corn Flakes (30 g)	0.1	**Liver, lambs, cooked** (90 g)	4.0
1 bowl *muesli* (95 g)	2.0	**Kidney, lambs, cooked** (75 g)	3.0
2 pieces Shredded Wheat	1.0	***Fish***	
2 Weetabix	1.0	*Pilchards, canned* (105 g)	1.5
		Sardines, canned (70 g)	2.0
Cereal products		**Crab** (100 g)	5.5
Bread, brown, 2 slices	0.7	**1 dozen oysters**	78.7
white, 2 slices	0.4	***Vegetables***	
wholemeal, 2 slices	1.3	Green vegetables, average, boiled (100 g)	0.4
1 chapati	0.7	Potatoes, boiled (150 g)	0.5
Pasta, brown, boiled (150 g)	1.5	1 small can baked beans (200 g)	1.0
white, boiled (150 g)	0.7	Lentils, kidney beans or other pulses (105 g)	1.0
Rice, brown, boiled (165 g)	1.0	*Dahl, chickpea* (155 g)	1.5
white, boiled (165 g)	1.0	*lentil* (155 g)	1.5
Milk and dairy products		Soya beans, cooked (100 g)	1.0
Milk, whole, semi-skimmed or	1.0		
skimmed (284 ml; ¹/₂ pint)		***Fruit***	
1 pot yoghurt (150 g)	1.0	8 dried apricots	0.2
Cheese, Brie (50 g)	1.0	4 figs	0.3
Camembert (50 g)	1.3	Half an avocado pear	0.3
Cheddar (50 g)	1.1	1 banana	0.2
Cheddar, reduced fat (50 g)	1.4	Blackberries (100 g)	0.2
Cottage cheese (100 g)	0.5	Blackcurrants (100 g)	0.3
Cream cheese (30 g)	0.2	***Nuts***	
Edam (50 g)	1.1	20 almonds	0.6
Feta (50 g)	0.4	10 Brazil nuts	1.0
Fromage frais (100 g)	0.3	30 hazelnuts	0.7
White cheese (50 g)	1.5	1 small bag peanuts (25 g)	1.0
1 egg, size 2 (60 g)	0.8		
Meat and fish			
Red meat, roast (85 g)	4.0		